RNA
TUMOR
VIRUSES

MOLECULAR BIOLOGY OF TUMOR VIRUSES

SECOND EDITION

CONTRIBUTORS

A. Bernstein *Ontario Cancer Institute, Toronto*
J.M. Bishop *University of California, San Francisco*
D. Blair *National Cancer Institute*
J. Coffin *Tufts University School of Medicine*
C. Dickson *Imperial Cancer Research Fund*
R. Eisenman *Fred Hutchinson Cancer Research Center*
H. Fan *University of California, Irvine*
W. Hardy *Memorial Sloan-Kettering Cancer Center*
S. Hughes *Cold Spring Harbor Laboratory*
E. Hunter *University of Alabama Medical School*
M. Linial *Fred Hutchinson Cancer Research Center*
T. Mak *Ontario Cancer Institute, Toronto*
R. Swanstrom *University of California, San Francisco*
N. Teich *Imperial Cancer Research Fund*
H. Varmus *University of California, San Francisco*
R. Weiss *Institute of Cancer Research*
J. Wyke *Imperial Cancer Research Fund*

RNA TUMOR VIRUSES

Edited by

Robin Weiss
Institute of Cancer Research

Natalie Teich
Imperial Cancer Research Fund

Harold Varmus
University of California, San Francisco

John Coffin
Tufts University School of Medicine

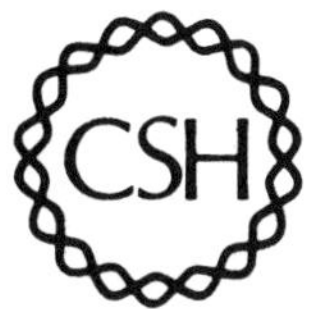

Cold Spring Harbor Laboratory
1982

COLD SPRING HARBOR MONOGRAPH SERIES

The Lactose Operon
The Bacteriophage Lambda
The Molecular Biology of Tumour Viruses
Ribosomes
RNA Phages
RNA Polymerase
The Operon
The Single-Stranded DNA Phages
Transfer RNA:
  Structure, Properties, and Recognition
  Biological Aspects
Molecular Biology of Tumor Viruses, Second Edition:
  DNA Tumor Viruses
  RNA Tumor Viruses
The Molecular Biology of the Yeast Saccharomyces:
  Life Cycle and Inheritance
  Metabolism and Gene Expression
Mitochondrial Genes
Lambda II

RNA TUMOR VIRUSES
Molecular Biology of Tumor Viruses, Second Edition

Printed in the United States of America

Cover and book design by Emily Harste

Library of Congress Cataloging in Publication Data
Main entry under title:

RNA tumor viruses.

(Molecular biology of tumor viruses ;)
(Cold Spring Harbor monograph series ; 10C)
Includes index.
1. Viruses, RNA. 2. Oncogenic viruses.
I. Weiss, Robin. II. Bernstein, A. (Alan)
III. Title: R.N.A. tumor viruses. IV. Series:
Molecular biology of tumor viruses (2nd ed.) ;
V. Series: Cold Spring Harbor monograph
series ; 10C.
QR372.O6M64 1979 616.99'20194s 81-69062
[QR395] [616.99'20194] AACR2
ISBN 0-87969-132-8

All Cold Spring Harbor Laboratory publications are available through booksellers or may be ordered directly from Cold Spring Harbor Laboratory, Box 100, Cold Spring Harbor, New York 11724.

SAN 203-6185

Contents

Preface

Almost a decade has passed since the publication of the first edition of *The Molecular Biology of Tumor Viruses.* In the interim, so much has happened in the field of tumor virology that the current volume can only dimly be viewed as a revision of the first. In the first edition, RNA tumor viruses commanded about 200 pages of the 700 or so in the entire volume; now RNA tumor viruses (or, more properly, retroviruses) require a massive volume of their own, with almost 1400 pages of text and appendixes. This profusion of information has required an editorial consortium, a large collection of authors and critics, and a major effort by the Cold Spring Harbor Publications staff to assemble a monograph that is almost entirely new, but one, we hope, that preserves the qualities that made the first edition so useful for both new and old members of the tumor virus community. Of the material appearing in the first edition, only a little remains—some historical perspectives to be found in Chapter 1 and a scattering of figures and tables throughout the remainder of the book.

The enthusiasm required to assemble this large book has been fired by remarkable progress during the past several years in efforts to describe the major biochemical and genetic features of the curious viruses we study: the organization of viral RNA and proviral DNA; the strategies for viral replication and gene expression; the nature and origin of viral transforming genes; and the structure and function of endogenous viral genomes. Although retroviruses are dauntingly numerous and some isolates disconcertingly idiosyncratic, the gratifying theme that has pervaded the work of the past decade is one of unity of design. It is that theme that we have exploited in the construction of this book. Thus, we have emphasized conceptual rather than taxonomic categories in the choice of chapter topics, in the belief that the occasional exceptions to the general rules are more usefully discussed in the context of accounts of how most retroviruses work. The rapid expansion of our information about retroviruses, particularly since the introduction of recombinant DNA and DNA sequencing methods, has been sufficiently great to forbid a graceful blending of all the pertinent facts within the text. To remedy this situation, we have appended compilations of restriction endonuclease maps of viral genomes and of nucleotide and amino acid sequences.

A word should be said about the manner in which we expect this book to be used. We have attempted to create a text that will meet the needs of students learning about retroviruses for the first time and of working scientists—both those who are new to the field and those who have grown up with it. To achieve such general utility, we have had to sacrifice the virtue of brevity. Thus, for the uninitiated, we have provided the historical and experimental perspectives that nurtured the theoretical conclusions and factual detail now available; and, for the expert, we have provided the inclusive descriptions, bibliographies, and information relevant to current experimentation as appropriate for a standard reference work. To diminish the dangers of making this book all things to all people, we have copiously subdivided the chapters and listed the subdivisions at the start of each chapter, abstracted much of the detailed material into tables within chapters and placed the rest in the appendices, and provided a detailed index that should facilitate, in particular, the retrieval of information about individual viruses from chapters organized around conceptual principles. What emerges is not a text to be read from cover to cover, but one that can be readily dissected into components germane to readers with different backgrounds and different demands. For example, each chapter begins with an overview that should serve as an introduction to its central ideas and as a guide to further reading within the chapter or elsewhere. To minimize overlaps, we have made abundant use of cross-references between chapters. Several figures and tables, in addition to the Appendixes, should be helpful throughout the book. These include Tables 2.3 (a list of retroviruses), 4.1 (viral genes), 6.1 (viral proteins), and 9.1 (*onc* genes); Figures 4.1 (genome structures), 5.1 (the replication cycle), and 6.1 (proteins and virion structure); and the tables following Chapter 7 (a catalog of viral mutants).

We have considered it appropriate to designate by name the individuals chiefly responsible for the composition of each of the chapters (other than Chapter 1, which was derived mainly from Chapter 1 of the first edition). However, we have also attempted to make this book one that reflects the consensus of the community of retrovirologists; to this end, we have relied heavily upon short contributions to, and critical readings of, most of these chapters by many of our colleagues. We hope to have obtained from this wide participation the balanced viewpoints that should characterize the standard reference text in a field as diverse as our own.

Compensation for working on a production such as this is never equal to the task; all we can offer is our sincere gratitude to those who contributed to it in one way or another. Many of the named authors made significant, unattributed contributions to other chapters, and several other colleagues helped with drafts that become obsolete with the passage of time or wrote (or rewrote) short portions of the various chapters that now appear. Among these otherwise unsung contributors are David Baltimore, Karen Beemon, Henry Bose, June East, Ray Erikson, Ashley Haase, Nancy Hogg, Wally Mangel, Jim Neil, Roel Nusse, Gordon Peters, Naomi Rosenberg, David Steffen, George Vande Woude, and Lu-Hai Wang. Detailed editorial assistance was provided by too many colleagues to list, but the special efforts of several (Bob Weinberg, John Wyke, Chuck Sherr, Harriet Robinson, and Craig Cohen) deserve special mention. Even the extraordinary persistence of Steve Hughes in compiling the appendixes would have been insufficient without the cooperation of many colleagues, especially Dennis Schwartz, Chuck Van Beveren, Tom Shinnick, Steve Oroszlan, and others, who provided unpublished and annotated maps and sequences. We are also indebted to Betsy Matthews for assembling the index, to Audrey Simson for typing a large portion of the text, and to Audrey Simons, Gerry Leach, Mike Ockler, and Fran Cefalu for producing the excellent graphics. Last, but far from least, we are grateful to Nancy Ford and members of her staff (Dorothy Brown, Judy Cuddihy, Joan Ebert, Gail Anderson) for their patience and extraordinary editorial skills, displayed throughout this long and arduous undertaking. Without their conviction that there would one day be a complete product, this volume would probably not exist.

The Editors

RNA
TUMOR
VIRUSES

1

Origins of Contemporary RNA Tumor Virus Research

INTRODUCTION

Most, if not all, complex eukaryotic organisms are subject to disorders of cell growth and differentiation that result in the appearance of localized or disseminated tumors. Although a large number of physical, chemical, and biological agents have been implicated in the etiology of neoplastic growth (Hiatt et al. 1977), it is generally agreed that some stage of tumorigenesis usually involves specific genetic alterations in individual cells whose progeny constitute the tumor mass (Cairns 1975, 1980). Those genetic alterations may be multiple (Armitage and Doll 1957), they may be inherited (Ponder 1980), or they may be induced or contributed by some of the agents implicated in tumorigenesis. Such a statement implies that the etiology of cancer is complex, a view that is reinforced by the study of the pathology and clinical behavior of tumors arising in the many cell lineages in higher organisms.

The great attraction of oncogenic viruses for experimentalists interested in cancer depends in large part on the apparent simplicity of many of these agents and on the correlative hope that a detailed understanding of the genetic contribution such viruses make to a cell will enlarge our understanding of neoplastic conversion in general. In the happiest of all experimental situations, a virus introduces into a normal cell a single gene whose product is capable of initiating and maintaining the oncogenic state. This state of affairs appears to apply to some viral agents, prompting a number of immediate questions to which at least partial answers are now available: Where do tumor genes come from? How is the gene introduced, reproduced, and expressed? What kind of protein does such a gene make?

What does the protein do, directly or indirectly, to the metabolism of host cells? As knowledge accrues from such simple systems, more complex viruses, as well as nonviral agents that effect genetic change by more elusive means, are becoming accessible targets for experimental work.

Tumor viruses, like other viruses, are conventionally categorized according to the chemical composition, organization, and size of their genomes. In a companion volume in this series (Tooze 1980), the pertinent properties of tumor viruses carrying DNA genomes have been reviewed. Virtually all classes of DNA viruses include members that manifest some property sufficient to implicate them as tumor viruses: induction of tumors in certain hosts, alteration of the morphological and growth properties of cultured cells (transformation), or epidemiological associations with tumors of uncertain etiology. Thus, the field of DNA tumor virology is, in fact, a conglomeration of several virological subspecialties dealing with papovaviruses, adenoviruses, herpesviruses, and even hepatitis viruses.

The RNA tumor viruses, in contrast, include members of only a single taxonomic group of RNA viruses. Although RNA tumor viruses have been isolated from an extraordinarily diverse group of animals (Chapter 2) and can produce a vast array of pathological consequences (Chapter 8) through a variety of mechanisms (Chapter 9), they are unified by the nature of their genomes (Chapter 4), their means of entering cells (Chapter 3), their composition and structure (Chapter 6), and their mode of replication via a DNA-intermediate (Chapter 5). The last property, more than any other, distinguishes this class of viruses from other RNA viruses. As a result, viruses that use virus-coded, RNA-directed DNA polymerases to replicate their RNA genomes are grouped together as "retroviruses" regardless of whether they are capable of producing the biological effects expected of true tumor viruses. Some nontumorigenic retroviruses are mutants, or closely related natural variants of tumor viruses, and some are related to the tumorigenic retroviruses only by the fundamental principles guiding virus replication and morphology. In either case, it is instructive to consider all members of the retrovirus group within a volume that concentrates principally on its oncogenic members.

Retrovirology has now progressed to a point where it is possible to confront the central themes of genetic organization, replication, and oncogenesis as they apply to the entire class of viruses, rather than to describe what is known about each of the isolated members of the class in turn. This perspective promotes economy and stimulates consideration of design and mechanism, but it does not necessarily provide the uninitiated student with an adequate sense of the slow and ungainly pace at which the threads were drawn together to form the conceptual fabric upon which disciples of this field now rely. The study of RNA tumor viruses, like most other scientific enterprises, has its roots in a number of serendipitous observations, some refractory to study at the time and some promptly and profitably exploited. Some candidate tumor viruses have been ignored out of prejudice or set aside for want of suitable techniques. Others have been much more productive of informative research because of certain inherent biological properties or because they were delivered into the right hands at the right time. Much of the intriguing history of tumor virology has been admirably summarized by Gross (1970), but the ensuing pages recapitulate some of the major moments in the experimental approach to the most useful of RNA tumor viruses.

ROUS SARCOMA VIRUS

Discovery

The first tumor virus to be studied seriously proved ultimately to be the most useful of the RNA tumor viruses and was found in 1911 by Peyton Rous, working in New York at the Rockefeller Institute. For several years he had been studying a spontaneous chicken sarcoma (tumor of connective tissue) that he had been passaging through closely related Plymouth Rock chickens (Rous 1910). With each passage, the tumor acquired heightened transplantability and showed a greater tendency to spread from the original graft site. Rous then tested to see whether cell-free filtrates could also induce a tumor to grow at the inoculation site. Although previous experiments with extracts of transplantable tumors of rats, mice, and dogs failed, Rous immediately succeeded, first using material that passed through ordinary filter paper and then using filters known to hold back bacteria, thereby establishing a virus as the etiological cause of the tumor (Rous 1911). Now the name Rous sarcoma virus (RSV) is given not only to the original virus isolated by Rous, but also to a number of independently isolated chicken viruses that induce sarcomas by a similar genetic mechanism (Chapters 2 and 9).

Immunological Responses to RSV

In Rous's original experiments, very large numbers of viral particles were injected for every visible tumor produced. Tumors arose most frequently when young chickens were inoculated, and especially large numbers of viral particles had to be injected in order to induce tumors in adult chickens. Moreover, when adult chickens were used as recipients, the tumors frequently regressed; as we now realize, the high frequency of takes in young chickens probably reflected their lesser ability to mount an immunological response. Most likely, for every visible tumor produced, even in very young chickens, thousands of cells were transformed into cancer cells and only a small fraction somehow overcame immunological attack. Already in 1913, Rous could distinguish antibodies against the infectious viral particles from those against the tumor cells, but the immature state of immunology at that time prevented a real understanding of what was happening (Rous 1913; Rous and Murphy 1914).

Host Range of RSVs

The first isolated strains of RSV had restricted host ranges; they would induce tumors in only a few strains of chickens. Continued passage of such RSV, however, led to a much wider host range, and tumors were induced in young turkeys, ducks, guinea fowl, and pigeons. It had been thought that RSV would not induce tumors in mammals, but in 1957 Zilber and Svet-Moldavsky in Moscow showed that infection by the Carr-Zilber RSV strain induced a fatal hemorrhagic disease in adult rats (Svet-Moldavsky 1957; Zilber and Kriukova 1957). The following year, Svet-Moldavsky (1958) observed the formation of sarcomas after inoculating newborn rats with the same RSV strain, although RSV will not establish a productive infection in mammalian cells.

Growth of RSV in Embryonated Eggs

As early as 1911, Rous and Murphy realized that RSV would grow in embryonated chicken eggs. Both the embryo itself and its surrounding membranes contain cells that can be transformed by the virus. Most important, at this stage, no immunological response exists and tumor regression does not complicate studies of cell transformation. But it was not until 1938 that Keogh in England employed growth of RSV on the chorioallantoic membrane as a quantitative assay for RSV (Keogh 1938). Following direct inoculation on the membrane, small tumors developed, and their number was directly proportional to the concentration of the virus suspension. This result established the very important principle that infection by a single RSV particle can transform a normal cell into a cancer cell.

Transformation of Cultured Cells

Over the past two decades, most work with RSV and retroviruses generally has involved the use of cultured cells. In cultures of chicken fibroblasts, RSV grows to high titers and morphologically altered transformed cells become visible several days after infection (Manaker and Groupe 1956). When chick fibroblasts growing as monolayers on petri dishes are infected with RSV, the transformed sarcoma cells stand out as easily countable foci, the number of foci being directly proportional to the concentration of virus added (Temin and Rubin 1958) (see Chapters 3 and 8).

Host Susceptibility and Virus Interference

Occasionally, fibroblasts prepared from a chicken embryo prove totally resistant to RSV. Such resistant cells frequently contain closely related leukemia viruses that multiply in chicken fibroblasts without causing obvious morphological changes (Rubin 1960, 1961). A number of different strains of such avian leukemia viruses (ALVs) exist, each conferring a distinctive pattern of resistance to infection by RSV (Vogt and Ishizaki 1966). The resistance or sensitivity of chick cells to infection by particular strains of RSV is also controlled by chromosomal genes that are inherited in a simple Mendelian fashion. Sensitivity is dominant and usually reflects the presence at the cell surface of specific sites that allow particular strains of RSV to bind to and penetrate the cells. Both of these mechanisms are considered in Chapter 3.

Morphology and Biochemical Properties of RSV Particles

Although Claude et al. (1947) first observed RSV in the electron microscope, the morphology of the viral particle was not learned until methods for examining thin sections of cells were developed (Gaylord 1955; Bernhard et al. 1956). Sections of cells infected with RSV often reveal the presence on the cell-surface membranes of large numbers of spherical particles, about 70–80 nm in diameter. Each such particle is surrounded by an external lipid-containing membrane within which is a centrally located body called the nucleoid. Subsequent biochemical characterization showed that the genetic material located in the nucleoid is RNA (Crawford and Crawford 1961); each RSV particle contains perhaps as much as 10^7 daltons of RNA.

The RSV particles seen on the outer surfaces of infected cells are progeny viral particles just ready to be released. Prior to this stage of the virus life cycle, the nascent RNA-containing nucleoids move into contact with the cell membrane to begin an enveloping process, at the conclusion of which mature RSV particles bud off from the cell membrane. Budding somehow occurs such that the integrity of the outer membrane is maintained even though many new particles are released every hour (Chapter 6).

Defectiveness and Helper Viruses

In the 1950s and early 1960s, many investigators concentrated their work on an RSV strain, obtainable in very high titers, that was isolated by W. R. Bryan of the National Institutes of Health. High yields of virus were obtained when each cell was infected with large numbers of viral particles. But when the cells were infected instead with only single viral particles, they did not seem to yield any progeny particles even though they became morphologically transformed and could initiate tumors (Prince 1959). Several years later, this phenomenon was shown by Temin (1962) at Madison, Wisconsin, and Vogt and Rubin (1962) at Berkeley to involve the simultaneous presence of related leukemia virus (see below). Only cells simultaneously infected with both the Bryan RSV strain and the leukemia virus were found to produce infectious progeny particles containing an RSV genome. The Bryan strain of RSV was thus a defective virus, genetically unable to manufacture its outer membrane proteins, and therefore dependent on a "helper" leukemia virus to provide envelope components necessary for infection (Chapters 3 and 7). This component, as we now know, can be supplied either by a coinfecting ALV or by an endogenous ALV genome inherited by chicks as a cellular gene. It is important to remember, however, that the Bryan RSV strain can transform cells once it has entered them; its defectiveness has nothing to do with the ability to transform cells per se. Although other strains of RSV are nondefective for replication as well as transformation, most RNA tumor viruses capable of transforming cells in culture are also defective for replication.

Evidence for a DNA Provirus

As soon as cultured cells were available, it became possible to study the effects of a variety of metabolic inhibitors on the various stages of RSV multiplication. These experiments did not give the answer expected for a virus with an RNA genome. Infection by RNA viruses should not be directly influenced by compounds that inhibit DNA synthesis. Yet, if the DNA inhibitor bromodeoxyuridine is present during the first 12 hours of infection, it blocks both transformation by and multiplication of RSV (Bader 1964, 1965). Likewise, addition of actinomycin D, a drug that specifically inhibits DNA-dependent RNA polymerase, immediately blocks formation of new progeny particles by transformed cells (Temin 1963). To explain these results, Temin (1964) proposed that the infecting RNA genomes were used as templates to make DNA genomes, which in turn were then integrated as proviruses into one or more chicken chromosomes. Almost no one else espoused this idea until, in the spring of 1970, Temin and Mizutani and, independently, Baltimore of MIT located RNA-dependent DNA polymerase activity within mature particles of RSV and other RNA tumor viruses (Baltimore 1970; Temin and Mizutani 1970). As discussed in great detail in Chapter 5, the study of proviruses dominates much of the current work on RNA tumor viruses.

Evidence for a Transforming Gene of RSV

Observations that RSV could induce fibrosarcomas in animals and initiate transformation of cultured fibroblasts fired speculation that the virus carried a gene (or genes) directly responsible for these pathogenic effects. Not until the past decade, however, was there genetic or biochemical support for these speculations (Chapters 4, 7, and 9). Because many strains of RSV are replication-competent, it is not difficult to clone transforming viruses. In addition, RSV strains often segregate deletion mutants lacking most or all of the transforming gene (Chapter 7). These features have been indispensable for the use of RSV as a prototype virus for investigations leading to identification of transforming genes, their products, and the progenitors of transforming genes in normal cellular genomes (Chapter 9).

AVIAN LEUKEMIA VIRUSES

Pathology

Leukemia and other related diseases of the blood-forming tissues in chickens are sometimes caused by viruses. This was first realized by Ellermann and Bang (1908, 1909) who, working in Denmark, transmitted chicken leukemia by injecting an extract of leukemia cells that had been filtered to remove bacteria. Because leukemia was not then clearly designated as a form of cancer, their discovery did not create the major impact that followed Rous's proof that a virus could cause a solid tumor (Rous 1911). However, in subsequent years, a large number of avian viruses capable of inducing a variety of hematological neoplasms have been identified. Pathological events initiated by these agents in vivo and, more recently, in vitro are described in detail in Chapters 8 and 9, and additional attributes are considered in Chapters 4, 5, and 7.

Study of avian leukosis viruses (ALVs) has been complicated in the past by varied manifestations of disease, by the lack of appropriate cell-culture systems for studying transformation, and by the frequent presence of more than one type of leukemia virus in virus stocks. Despite such difficulties, one type of ALV, the avian myeloblastosis virus (AMV), has been particularly useful as a source of biological and biochemical reagents. AMV has been intensively studied since 1952 by Beard and his colleagues at Duke University (Beard et al. 1952). For over 150 passages through chickens, it has maintained the property of inducing the proliferation of very large numbers of myeloblasts. Cell counts as high as 2×10^6/ml are found in diseased blood, and attendant virus titers frequently are on the order of 10^{11} particles/ml (Sharp and Beard 1952). AMV-diseased chickens have provided the most convenient source of material for biochemical study of avian RNA tumor viruses, yielding much greater amounts of virus than are obtained from RSV-induced tumors.

It has recently been recognized that certain ALVs, like AMV, can induce leukemia rapidly, will transform certain hematopoietic cells in culture, carry specific transforming genes, and are defective for virus replication (Chapters 4, 8, and 9). Thus, like the Bryan strain of RSV, these so-called acute, defective leukemia viruses must be propagated in the presence of a helper virus. The helper virus is usually an avian lymphoid leukosis virus (LLV) which itself produces tumors, albeit inefficiently, lacks a transforming gene, and is competent to replicate (Chapter 8). These viruses are also referred to frequently as Rous associated viruses (RAVs), since helper ALVs were first recognized in association with the Bryan high-titer strain of RSV (see above).

Inapparent Infections

ALV particles are not only found in diseased animals; in fact, many embryos and chickens carry these viruses as apparently harmless passengers without any evidence of disease (Rubin 1960; Vogt and Rubin 1962). The viruses apparently multiply in a variety of normal cells without regularly transforming them into their cancerous counterparts; conceivably, the rare normal cell is transformed but then quickly destroyed by an immunological response. Within a few months of hatching, however, the birds develop leukemia and eventually die of the disease.

When cells from carrier embryos are used for experiments, the viruses they harbor may interfere with infections by closely related RSV. Indeed, one strain of ALV was first noticed by Rubin because of its ability to inhibit multiplication of RSV, and the virus was therefore named RIF (Rous interfering factor; Rubin 1960).

Vertical Transmission

Much past work on ALV has been generated by a desire to find a way to decrease the incidence of the various chicken leukemias. Lymphoblastosis, in particular, is of great economic importance. The densely crowded conditions in contemporary poultry farms clearly favor spread of the virus from one chicken to another, and so the disease may reach epidemic proportions. Infection (horizontal transmission) is not, however, the only way in which chickens become infected by ALV. Some birds inherit the viral genome through eggs and sperms of their parents, a phenomenon known as vertical transmission. Embryos that inherit ALV vertically often contain multiplying viral particles (Cottral et al. 1954). When the immune system comes into existence, the ALV particles are recognized as "normal" cell components, and so antibodies against ALV are never made throughout the life of the bird (Rubin et al. 1961, 1962). During the past decade, it has been shown that ALV-related genomes can also be inherited as proviruses present in the germ line of chickens; similar findings have been made with several other hosts and viruses, as summarized in Chapter 10. In the case of chickens and several mammalian species, however, the viruses transmitted as endogenous proviruses do not appear to be pathogenic.

MURINE LEUKEMIA VIRUSES

Development of Mouse Strains with High and Low Incidences of Leukemia

The possibility that leukemia in mice, as well as in birds, had a viral origin was seriously considered long before 1951, when Ludwik Gross of the Bronx Veterans Hospital did the first definitive experiments. During the early 1930s, several inbred mouse strains were noticed to have high frequencies of spontaneous leukemia. Particularly useful in subsequent work have been the C58 strain developed by MacDowell at Cold Spring Harbor Laboratory and the various Ak strains bred by Jacob Furth, then of the Cornell University Medical College (Richter and MacDowell 1929; Furth et al. 1933). Leukemia in these strains tends to develop between 6 and 18 months of age, with as many as 85% of the mice developing detectable disease before the time of natural death. During the same period, a number of mouse strains, developed for other reasons, were found to have relatively low (1–2%) leukemia incidences during their normal life spans. One of these strains, C3H, was initially bred at the Jackson Laboratory for its high incidence (90%) of mammary cancer (Strong 1935). Thus, an increased tendency to develop one type of cancer need not be correlated with an increased tendency to develop a different cancer.

Tumor Transplantation

The existence of these strains led to experiments in which leukemic cells were injected into individuals of both the same strain and unrelated strains (Korteweg 1929; Richter and MacDowell 1929; Furth and Strumia 1931). In general, leukemia developed in the recipient animals only when they were of the same strain as the donor, although occasional takes between unrelated strains did occur. If, however, newborn mice are inoculated, then strain barriers break down with, for example, newborn C3H mice readily accepting Ak leukemic cells (Gross 1950). The Ak cells that grow in newborn C3H mice retain their own specificity, however, because they remain unable to grow after subsequent transfer to adult C3H mice while retaining their transplantability to Ak mice (Gross 1943).

When leukemia cells are serially passaged through mice, they frequently become progressively more virulent so that leukemia develops more quickly in recipients. These "transplantable leukemias" also tend to lose some of their immunological specificity, occasionally becoming able to multiply in unrelated adult mice. In most experiments with transplantable leukemia, the number of leukemic cells that must be injected into a single animal in order to ensure a high probability of take is very large. Probably very large cell numbers are usually needed to overcome the cell-mediated immunological response that must be generated following appearance of the "foreign" leukemia cells.

Throughout the decade when transplantable leukemia strains were being developed, there were frequent attempts to pass the disease by means of extracts of leukemia cells and, thereby, implicate viruses as the ultimate cause of murine leukemia. In such experiments, extracts made from leukemic cells arising in a high-leukemia strain were injected into adult mice from strains that normally have very low incidence. All the well-done experiments, however, consistently gave negative results (Furth et al. 1933; MacDowell et al. 1939; Engelbreth-Holm 1948). As we now realize, this was inevitable for two reasons. First and foremost, the use of adult recipients guaranteed that any newly infected cells would stimulate cellular immune responses. Second, the murine leukemia viruses (MLVs) have different host ranges; some mice resist infection by some strains of virus but are susceptible to infection by other strains.

Discovery by Gross of MLV

Gross's search for leukemia viruses also was done without foreknowledge of the discovery of immunological tolerance. Fortunately, he started his experiments in 1945 with young mice, guessing that previous failures might have resulted from the use of adult mice as recipients. Because Andervont and Bryan (1944) and Bittner (1944) had caused mammary tumors to develop by injecting the Bittner strain of mouse mammary tumor virus (MMTV; see below) into 7- to 21-day-old mice, Gross began using mice of this age. He failed, however, to transmit leukemia to 7- to 21-day-old mice with cell-free extracts of leukemia cells. Success did not come until 1950, when he switched to even younger mice and inoculated 1-day-old suckling C3H mice with cell-free material from Ak leukemia cells (Gross 1951). Then, over 50% of the inoculated mice developed leukemia in comparison to a control frequency of less than 1%. As proof that his extracts were actually cell-free, he showed that the newly developed leukemia cells had the immunological specificity of the recipient C3H mice, not that of the donor Ak cells used to make the cell-free extracts.

Not all of Gross's subsequent experiments, however, gave the same high incidence of induced leukemia. Apparently, the leukemia virus he first studied was easily inactivated as he prepared the filtered extracts. Continued passage of this virus through many generations of suckling mice gradually produced a much more stable virus that regularly induced leukemia 2.5 to 3.5 months after inoculation (Gross 1957). In contrast, the virus preparations used in his first successful experiments did not produce leukemia until some 6 to 12 months after inoculation.

Isolation of Other MLVs

The isolation of the Gross leukemia virus quickly led to attempts to find viruses responsible for other forms of cancer in mice. But when extracts made from a variety of different transplantable sarcomas and carcinomas (cancers of epithelial tissue) were injected into newborn mice, the cancers that occasionally arose were usually leukemias, not the form of cancer used to prepare the cell-free extracts. In contrast to the Gross virus, several of these more recently isolated MLVs usually cause disseminating myeloid leukemias, but they may also lead to the lymphatic form. Probably, like their avian counterparts, each isolate of MLV has the capacity to transform more than one type of normal cell and may indeed be a mixture of different viruses. Frequently, however, stocks of MLV preferentially transform one particular cell type.

In the absence of any rational taxonomic nomenclature, the various isolates of MLV are named after the persons who first isolated them. The Graffi virus (Graffi et al. 1955), the Moloney virus (Moloney 1960), the Friend virus (Friend 1957), and the Rauscher virus (Rauscher 1962) have been studied in some detail. At first there was a temptation to believe that each of these viruses was the causative agent of the sarcoma or carcinoma from which it was isolated. But very similar viruses have now been isolated from normal cells as well as from transplantable tumor cells, and so it may well be that these various strains of MLV were passengers and perhaps not the causative agents of the tumors from which they were obtained (Chapters 2 and 8).

MLV and Induced Leukemias

When mice of a low-leukemia strain are exposed to large sublethal X-ray doses, they frequently develop leukemia (Krebs et al. 1930; Kaplan 1947; Kaplan and Brown 1952). For example, 400 rads of whole-body radiation to several-week-old C3H mice leads to leukemia in up to 60% of the exposed mice (Gross et al. 1959). From many of these X-ray-induced leukemias, infectious MLV particles have been isolated (Gross 1959; Gross et al. 1959). In contrast, extracts of tissue from nonirradiated animals fail to yield any infectious material. Thus, somehow, the radiation treatment seems to bring about the appearance of MLV particles.

Most important, within several days of the radiation treatment, viruses are seen in thin sections in the electron microscope, and after several months, appreciable numbers of leukemia cells appear (Gross and Feldman 1968). This implies that the first step in some forms of

X-ray oncogenesis is the conversion of a latent leukemia virus to a form that multiplies within normal cells. Then, some time later, some of these newly produced MLV particles presumably transform the appropriate blood precursors into leukemic cells.

Injection of several chemical carcinogens also increases the incidence of leukemia in low-leukemia strains. Extracts made from such leukemia cells generally yield infectious MLV particles, leading to the suggestion that chemical carcinogens also can activate latent leukemia viruses. Among the carcinogens that produce infectious extracts are methylcholanthrene (Irino et al. 1963), dimethylbenzanthracene (Zilber and Postnikova 1966), and urethan (Ribacchi and Giraldo 1966). All these agents also induce other forms of cancer; it is not known whether or not they act indirectly by activating RNA tumor viruses.

Inheritance of MLV through Germ Cells

For laboratory mice, MLV is normally acquired vertically through the germ cells, not horizontally by infection from other mice (Gross and Dreyfuss 1967). Crosses of high-leukemia and low-leukemia mouse strains yield F_1 progeny that behave largely like the high-leukemia parent and develop leukemia independently of whether the male or female parent was of the high-leukemia line (MacDowell and Richter 1935; Cole and Furth 1941). Thus, MLV is transmitted through both the egg and the sperm, presumably as endogenous proviruses (Chapter 10).

Adaptation of MLV to Cross Species Barriers: Xenotropic MLV

With time, the number of species in whose cells MLV and murine sarcoma virus (MSV) can grow has steadily widened. Graffi and Gimmy (1957) first showed that MLV induced leukemia in newborn rats, and subsequent work has shown that after only several rat-to-rat passages, it grows in rats as well as, if not better than, in mice. After such passages, it can induce leukemia in greater than 95% of the rats tested within several months after inoculation (Gross 1963). Rat-adapted MLV does not lose its ability to grow in mice; its capacity to cause leukemia remains unaltered after many rat passages.

MSV and MLV have been found to grow, albeit poorly, in human fibroblasts. Continued passage of the resulting viruses in human cells, however, leads to strains that grow best in human cells, losing at the same time the capacity to grow in mice (Aaronson 1971). These adapted strains are antigenically distinct from the original mouse virus and have been found to contain mouse viruses with a marked preference for growth in foreign, rather than murine, cells (Chapter 3). These so-called xenotropic viruses (Levy 1973) are transmitted as endogenous proviruses in many mouse strains but have yet to be shown to have pathological potential (Chapters 2 and 8).

Isolation of MSVs

The first MSV to be found was isolated in London by Jennifer Harvey (1964). After passaging the Moloney strain of MLV in rats, she obtained a virus preparation that produced pleomorphic sarcomas as well as leukemias. Subsequently, Moloney (1966) reported the induction of multiple rhabdomyosarcomas by injecting high doses of the Moloney MLV into newborn BALB/c mice, and Kirsten and Mayer (1967) isolated MSV in stocks of the Kirsten MLV strain that had been passaged in rats. Naturally occurring strains of MSV have also been isolated (Chapter 2).

Attempts to separate the sarcoma-inducing capacity from the ability to induce leukemia consistently failed, leading to the recognition by Hartley and Rowe (1966) that MSV is a defective virus that multiplies only in the presence of a related leukemia virus. Pure MSV preparations, therefore, cannot be obtained, and all MSV preparations also contain morphologically identical MLV particles. In other words, strains of MSV resemble the Bryan strain of RSV (see above); they can transform cells in the absence of a leukemia helper virus, but they cannot multiply to produce infectious progeny in the absence of a helper virus.

Morphology of Retroviral Particles

The MLVs and MSVs and their avian counterparts have very similar morphologies and gross chemical compositions. Frequently, mature RNA sarcoma and leukemia viruses are collectively described as C-type particles; this term and two others, A-type particles and B-type particles, were coined by Bernhard in 1960 to distinguish the different sorts of particles he had observed in thin sections of infected cells in the electron microscope. A complete description of these types of particles, as well as the more recently identified D-type particle, is provided in Chapters 2 and 6.

MOUSE MAMMARY TUMOR VIRUS

Origins

The discovery that a virus is the cause of the mammary tumors that "spontaneously" develop in female mice had its origin in studies of the formal genetics of the mouse that began in the early 1900s at W.B. Castle's laboratory in the Bussey Institute of Harvard University. There C.C. Little, a student of Castle, began developing various inbred strains of mice by brother-sister matings. Several strains were selectively inbred for high incidence of mammary cancers (for review, see Little 1947). Particularly important were the C3H and A strains selected by Strong (1935, 1936, 1942), a mouse geneticist who first joined Little at Ann Arbor, going with him to Bar Harbor, Maine, where in 1929 Little created the Jackson Laboratory for the study of fundamental cancer biology.

Transmission through a Milk Factor

By 1933 sufficient crosses had been done between the high-incidence (C3H) and the low-incidence (C57) strains to show that the pattern of inheritance of susceptibility to mammary tumors depended on whether the male or female parent carried the high-incidence trait. When the females were from the C3H strain, greater than 90% of the female progeny developed mammary cancers, whereas when the C3H parent was the male, less than 10% of the female progeny developed mammary tumors (Staff of the Roscoe B. Jackson Memorial Laboratory 1933). These results led the Bar Harbor group to conclude that a nonchromosomal factor was transmitted from parent to offspring through the female parent. Soon afterward, Korteweg (1934, 1936) in Holland, using mice from Bar Harbor, arrived at the same conclusion.

One conceivable explanation for such maternal inheritance was transmission of a factor through the cytoplasm of the egg, while another possibility was intrauterine infection. A third possibility, the one quickly shown to be correct, was transmission through the milk of the mother. In experiments done at Bar Harbor between 1934 and 1936 by John Bittner, newborn mice were removed from their high-incidence A mothers and subsequently nursed by mothers of the low-incidence CBA strain. The resulting incidence of cancer would be much lower than expected if their natural mothers had been the nurse (Bittner 1936). Correspondingly, when newborn mice of a low-incidence strain were nursed by a high-incidence strain, most of the female offspring developed mammary tumors. Subsequent experiments showed that a few drops of milk were sufficient to transmit the high-incidence trait. Newborn mice, therefore, must be transferred immediately to foster parents if they are to remain free of the milk factor.

Hormonal-dependent Tumor Growth

Mammary cancer normally develops only in female mice of susceptible strains. Injection of female hormones (estrogens) into male mice of the same strain causes the disease (Lacassagne 1932). In contrast, similar treatment to males of low-incidence strains never results in mammary tumors (Bittner 1942). Thus, estrogens are carcinogenic only when the milk factor is present. How they act still remains a puzzle, although work with tissue cultures shows that mammary cells often multiply only in the presence of suitable estrogens (Furth 1953), and also that virus replication itself is often strongly regulated by steroid hormones (Parks et al. 1974).

B-type Particles in Mice with Milk Factor

In 1942 Bittner found that the milk factor was a virus when he passed infectious material through Seitz filter pads that trap bacteria (Bittner 1942; Andervont and Bryan 1944). Today Bittner's virus and other closely related viruses discovered subsequently are called MMTVs. The first convincing electron micrographs of these MMTVs were taken by Dmochowski (1954) and Bernhard and Bauer (1955). They saw large numbers of 75-nm-diameter bodies in the cytoplasm of mammary tumor cells, while budding off from the cell surfaces were very distinctive 105-nm-diameter bodies (B-type particles) with eccentrically placed nucleoids. The intracytoplasmic particles seem to be precursors that eventually move to surface sites where they acquire lipid-containing membranes and become the mature B-type particles.

However, the eccentric location of nucleoids in B-type particles does not appear to reflect a fundamental difference between MMTV and the more symmetrical C-type viruses (see Chapters 4, 5, 6, and 8).

Several Forms of MMTV

The simple idea that MMTV is transmitted only through the milk was quickly complicated by the observation that when males of the high-incidence C3H strain are mated to females of certain low-incidence strains (e.g., BALB/c), the female progeny frequently develop mammary tumors (Andervont 1945; Muhlbock 1950, 1952; Bittner 1952). At first, the possibility was considered that the female parents become infected by MMTV during mating. This hypothesis, however, could not account for the fact that supposedly MMTV-free C3H males nursed on MMTV-free milk also pass the disease to their progeny (Andervont and Dunn 1948). Thus, for many years the significance of the Bittner agent remained controversial.

Recently, the MMTV story was clarified when it was realized that more than one strain of MMTV exists and that virus can be transmitted as endogenous proviruses as well as infectious agents in milk (Muhlbock and Bentvelzen 1968) (Chapter 10). Thus, C3H mice also carry a less-virulent strain of MMTV in the germ line. When C3H progeny are foster-nursed on an MMTV-free strain, they lose the milk-borne strain but retain the endogenous strain (Pitelka et al. 1964). The latter virus went unnoticed for a long time because of its low oncogenic potential; the tumor it induces usually takes over a year to become visible and only seldom becomes malignant (Chapter 8).

A third strain of MMTV was first isolated from the European mouse strain GR (Muhlbock 1965) and is as virulent as the milk-borne strain in C3H mice. It induces pregnancy-dependent neoplastic lesions, which start as plaquelike growths that become noticeable within the first 100 days of life. The virus is easily transmitted both through the milk and through the germ line of the GR strain (Bentvelzen 1968; Muhlbock and Bentvelzen 1968) as a recently well-defined proviral element (Chapter 10).

FELINE LEUKEMIA AND SARCOMA VIRUSES

Leukemia is one of the most frequent cancers of cats. It usually takes the form of a generalized lymphosarcoma, although late in the disease, circulating cancerous blood cells are sometimes seen. From these leukemias, it has proved relatively easy to isolate infectious virus that transmits leukemia to other cats. Jarrett and his colleagues isolated the first feline leukemia virus (FeLV) in 1964. In the following years, several new isolations of FeLV were reported, and it seems likely that all cat leukemia may be of viral origin (Kawakami et al. 1967; Rickard et al. 1969). Interestingly, it has proved impossible to isolate infectious FeLV from a large proportion of tumors, which, on epidemiological grounds, are almost certainly due to FeLV infection (Hardy et al. 1980).

More recently, infectious agents have also been isolated from several feline fibrosarcomas that cause new fibrosarcomas when inoculated into newborn cats (Snyder and Theilen 1969; Gardner et al. 1970; McDonough et al. 1971). Stocks of feline sarcoma virus (FeSV) contain an excess of FeLV and in this respect resemble MLVs (Sarma et al. 1971). Interestingly, stocks of FeSV not only infect newborn cats, but also induce solid tumors when injected into adult cats. Such tumors, however, generally regress, most likely because of cell-mediated immunological responses.

FeLV and FeSV induce leukemias and sarcomas when injected into neonatal dogs (Rickard et al. 1969; Theilen et al. 1970). FeSV also induces solid tumors in young rabbits, marmosets, and monkeys. In the rabbit and monkey, the tumors regress (Theilen et al. 1970), but in the marmoset they can grow until they kill their host (Deinhardt 1970).

These experiments with various species of animals clearly indicate that FeSV and FeLV are no respecters of species barriers; both viruses will grow in human cells. Sarma et al. (1970), for example, reported that FeSV morphologically transforms human embryo cells in culture, and in the previous year Jarrett et al. (1969) had reported that FeLV grows to high titers in human cells without prior adaptation. This finding raised the possibility that some cases of human leukemia might originate by infection with FeLV. Epidemiological studies (Dorn et al. 1970) suggest that there is no connection between the occurrence of leukemia and the presence of cats in the affected households, but the possibility deserves further investigation.

RETROVIRUSES FROM OTHER SPECIES

Many of the lessons derived from the pioneering studies of virus-induced diseases of birds, mice, and cats have been applied to searches for candidate tumor viruses in a large number of species. Animals as varied as vipers, pike, mink, deer, cows, and several subhuman primates have been found to harbor retroviruses; several of these viruses are oncogenic in the laboratory and some are economically significant agents of natural disease. An account of the discoveries and fundamental properties of these diverse agents is the topic of the ensuing chapter. A summary of efforts to identify similar viruses in man is presented in the concluding chapter.

REFERENCES

Aaronson, S.A. 1971. Common genetic alterations of RNA tumour viruses grown in human cells. *Nature* **230:**445–447.

Andervont, H.B. 1945. Fate of the C3H milk influence in mice of strains C and C57 Black. *J. Natl. Cancer Inst.* **5:**383–390.

Andervont, H.B. and W.R. Bryan. 1944. Properties of the mouse mammary-tumor agent. *J. Natl. Cancer Inst.* **5:**143–149.

Andervont, H.B. and T.B. Dunn. 1948. Mammary tumors in mice presumably free of the mammary tumor agent. *J. Natl. Cancer Inst.* **8:**227–233.

Armitage, P. and R.A. Doll. 1957. A two-stage theory of carcinogenesis in relation to the age distribution of human cancer. *Br. J. Cancer* **11:**161–169.

Bader, J.P. 1964. The role of deoxyribonucleic acid in synthesis of Rous sarcoma virus. *Virology* **22:**462–468.

———. 1965. The requirement for DNA synthesis in the growth of Rous sarcoma and Rous-associated viruses. *Virology* **26:**253–261.

Baltimore, D. 1970. RNA-dependent DNA polymerase in virions of RNA tumour viruses. *Nature* **226:**1209–1211.

Beard, J.W., D.G. Sharp, E.A. Eckert, D. Beard, and E.B. Mommaerts. 1952. Properties of the virus of the fowl erythromyeloblastic disease. *Natl. Cancer Conf. Proc.* **2:**1396–1411.

Bentvelzen, P. 1968. *Genetical control of the vertical transmission of the Mühlbock mammary tumour virus in the GR mouse strain.* Hollandia, Amsterdam.

Bernhard, W. 1960. The detection and study of tumor viruses with the electron microscope. *Cancer Res.* **20:**712–727.

Bernhard, W. and A. Bauer. 1955. Mise en evidence de corpuscules d'aspect virusal dans des tumeurs mammaires de la souris. Etude au microscope électronique. *C. R. Acad. Sci.* **240:**1380–1382.

Bernhard, W., C. Oberling, and P. Vigier. 1956. Ultrastructure de virus dans le sarcome de Rous, leur rapport avec le cytoplasme des cellules tumorales. *Bull. Cancer* **43:**407–422.

Bittner, J.J. 1936. Some possible effects of nursing on the mammary gland tumor incidence in mice. *Science* **84:**162.

———. 1942. The milk-influence of breast tumors in mice. *Science* **95:**462–463.

———. 1944. Inciting influences in the etiology of mammary cancer in mice. *Res. Conf. Cancer. Am. Assoc. Adv. Sci. Publ.*, pp. 63–96.

———. 1952. Transfer of the agent for mammary cancer in mice by the male. *Cancer Res.* **12:**387–398.

Cairns, J. 1975. Mutation selection and the natural history of cancer. *Nature* **255:**197–200.

———. 1980. The origins of human cancers. *Nature* **289:**353–357.

Claude, A., K.R. Porter, and E.G. Pickels. 1947. Electron microscope study of chicken tumor cells. *Cancer Res.* **7:**421–430.

Cole, R.K. and J. Furth. 1941. Experimental studies on the genetics of spontaneous leukemia in mice. *Cancer Res.* **1:**957–965.

Cottral, G.E., B.R. Burmester, and N.F. Waters. 1954. Egg transmission of avian lymphomatosis. *Poultry Sci.* **33:**1174–1184.

Crawford, L.V. and E.M. Crawford. 1961. The properties of Rous sarcoma virus purified by density gradient centrifugation. *Virology* **13:**227–232.

Deinhardt, F. 1970. Induction of tumors in marmoset monkeys with ST-feline fibrosarcoma virus. In *Comparative leukemia research 1969* (ed. R.M. Dutcher), pp. 401–402. Karger, Basel.

Dmochowski, L. 1954. Discussion in: Proceedings, symposium on 25 years of progress in mammalian genetics and cancer. *J. Natl. Cancer Inst.* **15:**785–787.

Dorn, C.R., D.O.N. Taylor, and R. Schneider. 1970. Epidemiology of canine leukemia and lymphoma. In *Comparative leukemia research 1969* (ed. R.M. Dutcher), pp. 403–407, Karger, Basel.

Ellermann, V. and O. Bang. 1908. Experimentelle Leukämie bei Hühnern. *Zentralbl. Bakteriol.* **46:**595–609.

———. 1909. Experimentelle Leukämie bei Hühnern. *Z. Hyg. Infektionskr.* **63:**231–272.

Engelbreth-Holm, J. 1948. Is is possible to transmit or accelerate the development of mouse leukemia by tissue extracts? *Blood* **3:**862–866.

Friend, C. 1957. Cell-free transmission in adult Swiss mice of a disease having the character of a leukemia. *J. Exp. Med.* **105:**307–319.

Furth, J. 1953. Conditioned and autonomous neoplasms: A review. *Cancer Res.* **13:**477–492.

Furth, J. and M. Strumia. 1931. Studies on transmissible lymphoid leukemia of mice. *J. Exp. Med.* **53:**715–731.

Furth, J., H.R. Seibold, and R.R. Rathbone. 1933. Experimental studies on lymphomatosis of mice. *Amer. J. Cancer* **19:**521–604.

Gardner, M.B., R.W. Rongey, P. Arnstein, J.D. Estes, P. Sarma, R.J. Huebner, and C.G. Rickard. 1970. Experimental transmission of feline fibrosarcoma to cats and dogs. *Nature* **226:**807–809.

Gaylord, W.H., Jr. 1955. Virus-like particles associated with the Rous sarcoma as seen in sections of the tumor. *Cancer Res.* **15:**80–83.

Graffi, A. and J. Gimmy. 1957. Erzeugung von Leukosen bei der Ratte durch ein leukämogenes Agens der Maus. *Naturwissenschaften* **44:**518–519.

Graffi, A., H. Bielka, F. Fey, F. Scharsach, and R. Weiss. 1955. Gehauftes Auftreten von Leukämien nach Injektion von Sarkom-Filtraten. *Wien. Klin. Wochenschr.* **105:**61–64.

Gross, L. 1943. Intradermal immunization of C3H mice against a sarcoma that originated in an animal of the same line. *Cancer Res.* **3:**326–333.

———. 1950. Susceptibility of suckling-infant and resistance of adult mice of the C3H and the C57 lines to inoculation with Ak leukemia. *Cancer* **3:**1073–1087.

———. 1951. "Spontaneous" leukemia developing in C3H mice following inoculation, in infancy, with Ak-leukemic extracts, or Ak-embryos. *Proc. Soc. Exp. Biol. Med.* **76:**27–32.

———. 1957. Development and serial cell-free passage of a highly potent strain of mouse leukemia virus. *Proc. Soc. Exp. Biol. Med.* **94:**767–771.

———. 1959. Serial cell-free passage of a radiation-activated mouse leukemia agent. *Proc. Soc. Exp. Biol. Med.* **100:**102–105.

———. 1963. Serial cell-free passage in rats of the mouse leukemia virus. Effect of thymectomy. *Proc. Soc. Exp. Biol. Med.* **112:**939–945.

———. 1970. *Oncogenic viruses*, 2nd edition. Pergamon Press, New York.

Gross, L. and Y. Dreyfuss. 1967. How is the mouse leukemia virus transmitted from host to host under natural life conditions? In *Carcinogenesis: A broad critique. 20th Annual*

Symposium on Fundamental Cancer Research, pp. 9–21. Williams and Wilkins, Baltimore.

Gross, L. and D.G. Feldman. 1968. Electron microscopic studies of radiation-induced leukemia in mice: Virus release following total-body X-ray irradiation. *Cancer Res.* **28:** 1677–1685.

Gross, L., B. Roswit, E.R. Mada, Y. Dreyfuss, and L.A. Moore. 1959. Studies on radiation-induced leukemia in mice. *Cancer Res.* **19:** 316–320.

Hardy, W.D., Jr., A.J. McClelland, E.E. Zuckerman, H.W. Snyder, Jr., E.G. MacEwen, D.P. Francis, and M. Essex. 1980. Immunology and epidemology of feline leukemia virus nonproducer lymphosarcomas. *Cold Spring Harbor Conf. Cell Proliferation* **7:** 677–697.

Hartley, J.W. and W.P. Rowe. 1966. Production of altered cell foci in tissue culture by defective Moloney sarcoma virus particles. *Proc. Natl. Acad. Sci.* **55:** 780–786.

Harvey, J.J. 1964. An unidentified virus which causes the rapid production of tumours in mice. *Nature* **204:** 1104–1105.

Hiatt, H.H., J.D. Watson, and J.A. Winsten, eds. 1977. Origins of human cancer. *Cold Spring Harbor Conf. Cell Proliferation* **4.**

Irino, S., Z. Ota, T. Sezaki, M. Suzaki, and K. Hiraki. 1963. Cell-free transmission of 20-methylcholanthrene-induced RF mouse leukemia and electron microscopic demonstration of virus particles in its leukemia tissue. *Gann* **54:** 225–238.

Jarrett, O., H.M. Laird, and D. Hay. 1969. Growth of feline leukaemia virus in human cells. *Nature* **224:** 1208–1209.

Jarrett, W.F.M., E.M. Crawford, W.B. Martin, and F. Davey. 1964. Leukaemia in the cat. A virus-like particle associated with leukaemia (lymphosarcoma). *Nature* **202:** 567–568.

Kaplan, H.S. 1947. Observations on radiation-induced lymphoid tumors of mice. *Cancer Res* **7:** 141–147.

Kaplan, H.S. and M.B. Brown. 1952. Protection against radiation-induced lymphoma development by shielding and partial-body irradiation of mice. *Cancer Res.* **12:** 441–444.

Kawakami, T.G., G.H. Theilen, D.L. Dungworth, R.J. Munn, and S.G. Beall. 1967. "C"-type viral particles in plasma of cats with feline leukemia. *Science* **158:** 1049–1050.

Keogh, E.V. 1938. Ectodermal lesions produced by the virus of Rous sarcoma. *Br. J. Exp. Pathol.* **19:** 1–9.

Kirsten, W.H. and L.A. Mayer. 1967. Morphologic responses to a murine erythroblastosis virus. *J. Natl. Cancer Inst.* **39:** 311–355.

Korteweg, R. 1929. Eine überimpfbare Leukosarkomatose bei der Maus. *Z. Krebsforsch.* **29:** 455–476.

———. 1934. Proefondervindelijke onderzoekingen aangaande erfelijheid van kanker. *Ned. Tijdschr. Geneeskde.* **78:** 240–245.

———. 1936. On the manner in which the disposition to carcinoma of the mammary gland is inherited in mice. *Genetics* **18:** 350–371.

Krebs, C., H.C. Rask-Nielsen, and A. Wagner. 1930. The origin of lymphosarcomatosis and its relation to other forms of leucosis in white mice. *Acta Radiol.* (Suppl.) **10:** 1–53.

Lacassagne, A. 1932. Apparition de cancers de la mammelle chez la souris mâle, soumise à des injections de folliculine. *C. R. Acad. Sci.* **195:** 630–632.

Levy, J.A. 1973. Xenotropic viruses: Murine leukemia viruses associated with NIH Swiss, NZB, and other mouse strains. *Science* **182:** 1151–1153.

Little, C.C. 1947. The genetics of cancer in mice. *Biol. Rev.* **22:** 315–343.

MacDowell, E.C. and M.N. Richter. 1935. Mouse leukemia. IX. The role of heredity in spontaneous cases. *Arch. Pathol.* **20:** 709–724.

MacDowell, E.C., J.S. Potter, M. Bovarnick, M.N. Richter, M.J. Taylor, E.N. Ward, T. Laanes, and M.P. Wintersteiner. 1939. Experimental leukemia. *Carnegie Inst. Wash. Yearbook* **38:** 191–195.

Manaker, R.A. and V. Groupe. 1956. Discrete foci of altered chicken embryo cells associated with Rous sarcoma virus in tissue culture. *Virology* **2:** 838–840.

McDonough, S.K., S. Larsen, R.S. Brodey, N.D. Stock, and W.D. Hardy, Jr. 1971. A transmissible feline fibrosarcoma of viral origin. *Cancer Res* **31:**953–956.

Moloney, J.B. 1960. Biological studies on a lymphoid-leukemia virus extracted from Sarcoma 37. I. Origin and introductory investigations. *J. Natl. Cancer Inst.* **24:**933–951.

———. 1966. A virus-induced rhabdomyosarcoma of mice. *Natl. Cancer Inst. Monogr.* **22:**139–142.

Muhlbock, O. 1950. Mammary tumor-agent in the sperm of high-cancer-strain male mice. *J. Natl. Cancer Inst.* **10:**861–864.

———. 1952. Studies on the transmission of the mouse mammary tumor agent by the male parent. *J. Natl. Cancer Inst.* **12:**819–837.

———. 1965. Note on a new inbred mouse strain GR/A. *Eur. J. Cancer* **1:**123–124.

Muhlbock, O. and P. Bentvelzen. 1968. The transmission of the mammary tumor viruses. *Perspect. Virol.* **6:**75–87.

Parks, W.P., E.M. Scolnick, and E.H. Kozikowski. 1974. Dexamethasone stimulation of murine mammary tumor virus expression: A tissue culture source of virus. *Science* **184:**158–160.

Pitelka, D.R., H.A. Bern, S. Nandi, and K.B. DeOme. 1964. On the significance of virus-like particles in mammary tissues of C3Hf mice. *J. Natl. Cancer Inst.* **33:**867–885.

Ponder, B.A.J. 1980. Genetics and cancer. *Biochim. Biophys. Acta* **605:**369–410.

Prince, A.M. 1959. Quantitative studies on Rous sarcoma virus. IV. An investigation of the nature of "noninfective" tumors induced by low doses of virus. *J. Natl. Cancer Inst.* **23:**1361–1381.

Rauscher, F.J. 1962. A virus-induced disease of mice characterized by erythrocytopoiesis and lymphoid leukemia. *J. Natl. Cancer Inst.* **29:**515–543.

Ribacchi, R. and G. Giraldo. 1966. Leukemia virus release in chemically or physically induced lymphomas in BALB/c mice. *Natl. Cancer Inst. Monogr.* **22:**701–711.

Richter, M.N. and E.C. MacDowell. 1929. The experimental transmission of leukemia in mice. *Proc. Soc. Exp. Biol. Med.* **26:**362–364.

Rickard, C.G., J.E. Post, F. Noronha, and L.M. Barr. 1969. A transmissible virus-induced lymphatic leukemia of the cat. *J. Natl. Cancer Inst.* **42:**987–1014.

Rous, P. 1910. A transmissible avian neoplasm: Sarcoma of the common fowl. *J. Exp. Med.* **12:**696–705.

———. 1911. A sarcoma of the fowl transmissible by an agent separable from the tumor cells. *J. Exp. Med.* **13:**397–411.

———. 1913. Resistance to a tumor-producing agent as distinct from resistance to the implanted tumor cells. Observations with a sarcoma of the fowl. *J. Exp. Med.* **18:** 416–427.

Rous, P. and J.B. Murphy. 1911. Tumor implantations in the developing embryo. Experiments with a transmissible sarcoma of the fowl. *J. Am. Med. Assoc.* **56:**741–742.

———. 1914. On immunity to transplantable chicken tumors. *J. Exp. Med.* **20:**419–432.

Rubin, H. 1960. A virus in chick embryos which induces resistance in vitro to infection with Rous sarcoma virus. *Proc. Natl. Acad. Sci.* **46:**1105–1119.

———. 1961. The nature of a virus-induced cellular resistance to Rous sarcoma virus. *Virology* **13:**200–206.

Rubin, H., A. Cornelius, and L. Fanshier. 1961. The pattern of congenital transmission of an avian leukosis virus. *Proc. Natl. Acad. Sci.* **47:**1058–1069.

Rubin, H., L. Fanshier, A. Cornelius, and W.F. Hughes. 1962. Tolerance and immunity in chickens after congenital and contact infection with an avian leukosis virus. *Virology* **17:**143–156.

Sarma, P.S., R.V. Gilden, and R.J. Huebner. 1971. Complement-fixation test for feline leukemia and sarcoma viruses (the COCAL test). *Virology* **44:**137–145.

Sarma, P.S., R.J. Huebner, J.F. Basker, L. Vernon, and R.V. Gilden. 1970. Feline leukemia and sarcoma viruses: Susceptibility of human cells to infection. *Science* **168:**1098–1100.

Sharp, D.G. and J.W. Beard. 1952. Counts of virus particles by sedimentation on agar and electron micrography. *Proc. Soc. Exp. Biol. Med.* **81:**75–79.

Snyder, S.P. and G.H. Theilen. 1969. Transmissible feline fibrosarcoma. *Nature* **221:**1074–1075.

Staff of Roscoe B. Jackson Memorial Laboratory. 1933. The existence of non-chromosomal influence in the incidence of mammary tumors in mice. *Science* **78:**465–466.

Strong, L.C. 1935. The establishment of the C3H inbred strain of mice for the study of spontaneous carcinoma of the mammary gland. *Genetics* **20:**586–591.

———. 1936. The establishment of the "A" strain of inbred mice. *J. Hered.* **27:**21–24.

———. 1942. The origin of some inbred mice. *Cancer Res.* **2:**531–539.

Svet-Moldavsky, G.J. 1957. Development of multiple cysts and of haemorrhagic affections of internal organs in albino rats treated during the embryonic or new-born period with Rous sarcoma virus. *Nature* **180:**1299–1300.

———. 1958. Sarcoma in albino rats treated during the embryonic stage with Rous virus. *Nature* **182:**1452–1453.

Temin, H. 1962. Separation of morphological conversion and virus production in Rous sarcoma virus infection. *Cold Spring Harbor Symp. Quant. Biol.* **27:**407–414.

———. 1963. The effects of actinomycin D on growth of Rous sarcoma virus *in vitro*. *Virology* **20:**577–582.

———. 1964. Nature of the provirus of Rous sarcoma. *Natl. Cancer Inst. Monogr.* **17:**557–570.

Temin, H.M. and S. Mizutani. 1970. RNA-directed DNA polymerase in virions of Rous sarcoma virus. *Nature* **226:**1211–1213.

Temin, H.M. and H. Rubin. 1958. Characteristics of an assay for Rous sarcoma virus and Rous sarcoma cells in tissue culture. *Virology* **6:**669–688.

Theilen, G.H., S.P. Snyder, L.G. Wolfe, and J.C. Landon. 1970. Biological studies with viral induced fibrosarcomas in cats, dogs, rabbits and non-human primates. In *Comparative leukemia research 1969* (ed. R.M. Dutcher), pp. 393–400. Karger, Basel.

Tooze, J., ed. 1980. *The molecular biology of tumor viruses, Part 2. DNA tumor viruses,* 2nd edition. Cold Spring Harbor Laboratory, Cold Spring Harbor, New York.

Vogt, P.K. and R. Ishizaki. 1966. Patterns of viral interference in the avian leukosis and sarcoma complex. *Virology* **30:**368–374.

Vogt, P.K. and H. Rubin. 1962. The cytology of Rous sarcoma virus infection. *Cold Spring Harbor Symp. Quant. Biol.* **27:**395–405.

Zilber, L.A. and I.N. Kriukova. 1957. Haemorrhagic disease of rats caused by Rous sarcoma virus. *Vopr. Virusol.* **2:**239–243.

Zilber, L.A. and Z.A. Postnikova. 1966. Induction of a leukemogenic agent by a chemical carcinogen in inbred mice. *Natl. Cancer Inst. Monogr.* **22:**397–403.

2

Taxonomy of Retroviruses

I. INTRODUCTION

Although the bulk of this text is concerned with the biology and molecular biology of the RNA tumor viruses, we consider here and, to some extent, in Chapters 6 and 8 the entire Retroviridae virus family. The family encompasses all viruses containing an RNA genome and an RNA-dependent DNA polymerase (reverse transcriptase) enzymic activity (Fenner 1975). The family is divided into three subfamilies: (1) Oncovirinae, including all the oncogenic members and many closely related nononcogenic viruses; (2) Lentivirinae, the "slow" viruses, such as visna virus; and (3) Spumavirinae, the "foamy" viruses that induce persistent infections without any clinical disease. The latter two subfamilies are generally given summary treatment in discussions on retroviruses and, therefore, we propose to present at least some of their salient features. The spumaviruses provide an excellent model system for chronic viral disease, whereas the lentiviruses are in the mystical realm of slow neurological diseases.

To some extent, a taxonomical description is, of necessity, a tedious job and relatively unimaginative, since the essence of the matter is covered in the chapters to follow. What we propose to do here is to cover the viruses isolated (or particles seen but without infectious transmission) in the different invertebrate and vertebrate genera. Obviously, much of the focus in later chapters is devoted to the viruses from the best-characterized systems: chickens, mice, cats, cattle, and monkeys. Therefore, the coverage here of the more familiar isolates may seem disproportionately small with respect to the plethora of available data; needless to say, such data are presented in the subsequent chapters where appropriate. However, studies on the less-familiar virus isolates often illuminate by contrasts or similarities the functional significance of features common to the broad retrovirus family.

A. Criteria for Retrovirus Classification

All retroviruses have common morphological, biochemical, and physical properties that justify their inclusion into a single virus family; these parameters are summarized in Table 2.1. The next few chapters cover the RNA genome, the replication cycle, and the structural proteins (Chapters 4–6), with the emphasis on the well-defined retrovirus groups. Therefore, general properties only are described here.

The genomic RNA is a 60S–70S dimer complex composed of two identical subunits, which resemble mRNA molecules in that there is a methylated cap structure at one end (the 5′ end) and a polyadenylate tract at the other end (the 3′ end). The genome is positive-sense in that it can be used to direct protein synthesis in experimental translation systems in vitro. The genomes of all replication-competent retroviruses contain three genes encoding the structural proteins: *gag* codes for the internal structural proteins, *pol* codes for the reverse transcriptase, and *env* encodes the envelope proteins. The order of these three genes is so far invariable in all retroviruses: 5′-*gag-pol-env*-3′. By convention (August et al. 1974), the gene products are annotated by prefixing p, pp, or gp (for protein, phosphoprotein, or glycoprotein, respectively) to the molecular weight ($\times 10^{-3}$). Polyprotein precursors are designated by the prefix Pr. For clarification, when necessary, the protein may be ascribed as a particular gene product by using the gene name as a superscript. Thus, $pp12^{gag}$ would be a phosphorylated internal structural *gag*-gene product with a molecular weight of 12,000 daltons. Additionally, a number of the oncogenic retroviruses contain sequences essential for their oncogenicity in vivo

Table 2.1 Taxonomic features of Retroviridae

Nucleic acid	linear positive-sense single-stranded RNA (60S–70S) composed of identical subunits (30S–35S); 5′ structure ($m^7G^5ppp^{5\prime}NmpNp$); polyadenylated 3′ end; repeated sequences at 3′ and 5′ ends; tRNA base-paired to genome complex
Protein	about 60% by weight; *gag,* internal structural proteins (4–5); *pol,* reverse transcriptase (1–2); *env,* envelope proteins (1–2)
Lipid	about 35% by weight; derived from cell membrane
Carbohydrate	about 4% by weight; associated with *env* proteins
Physicochemical properties	density 1.16–1.18 g/ml in sucrose, 1.16–1.21 g/ml in cesium chloride; sensitive to lipid solvents, detergents, and heat inactivation (56°C, 30 min); highly resistant to UV- and X-irradiation
Morphology	spherical enveloped virions (80–120-nm diameter), variable surface projections (8-nm diameter), icosahedral capsid containing a ribonucleoprotein complex with a core shell (nucleoid)

and, when applicable, for their ability to elicit morphological transformation of cells in vitro. These sequences have been called *onc* (for oncogene) sequences or *onc* genes for which there are generally homologous counterparts in normal cells (see Chapter 9).

The fact that retroviruses code for and package the enzyme, reverse transcriptase, which has both RNA-dependent and DNA-dependent DNA polymerase activities, conforms to their mode of replication involving double-stranded DNA intermediates. These intermediates may exist as unintegrated forms (linear molecules or covalently closed circles) or as integrated (proviral) forms within the cellular DNA of the infected host. From this integrated state, they are transcribed (or not transcribed) in a manner similar to cellular genes (see Chapter 5). A schematic representation of a retroviral RNA genome and its integrated provirus is shown in Figure 2.1.

All retroviruses have very similar overall chemical compositions. They comprise about 60–70% protein, 30–40% lipid, 2–4% carbohydrate, and about 1% RNA (for review, see Beard 1963). The envelope of retroviral particles is derived from the cell-surface membrane, and most, if not all, of the lipids in viral particles are located in the unit-membrane envelope of the virion. Bonar and Beard (1959) and Rao et al. (1966) have reported that avian and murine retroviruses contain phospholipids. Quigley et al. (1971) analyzed the phospholipid content of chick embryo fibroblasts and their plasma membranes, before and after infection with the Schmidt-Ruppin strain of the avian Rous sarcoma virus (RSV), and the phospholipid composition of the progeny virions. Infection with RSV did not significantly change the overall phospholipid content of the cells.

The phospholipid composition of the RSV virions, however,

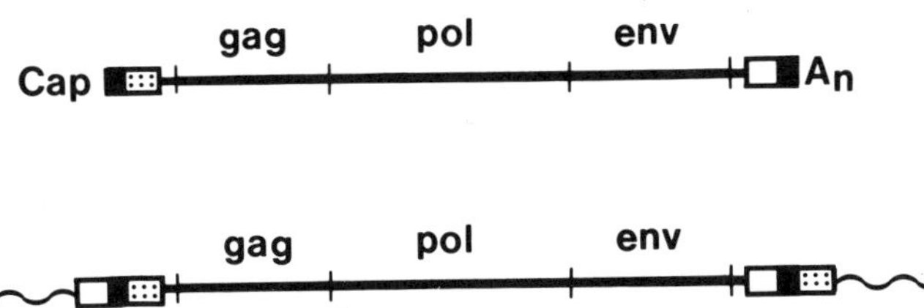

Figure 2.1 Schematic representation of one subunit of a retroviral genome (*top*) and of an exogenously infected integrated provirus (*bottom*).

differs significantly from that of the plasma membrane of infected cells. Apparently, RSVs are budded from areas of the plasma membrane exceptionally rich in sphingomyelin and poor in phosphatidylcholine. Studies of antigens on the surfaces of infected cells also indicate that the retroviruses are budded from particular areas of the cell surface. For example, the virus-specific Gross cell-surface antigen (GCSA) and the cell-specific H-2 antigen are localized in patches on the surfaces of murine cells infected with murine leukemia virus (MLV) of the Gross subgroup (Aoki et al. 1970). Progeny viruses are budded from areas of the surface that do not contain either of these antigens, which, as a result, are not present in the envelopes of the virions.

B. Morphological Classification of Retroviruses

The original formulation of one family of animal viruses containing several members now recognized as retroviruses was based upon similarities in physical structure in electron micrographs. Because early studies were mainly concerned with the oncogenic viruses, the family has been called by various names through the years, including RNA tumor viruses, oncornaviruses (an acronym for oncogenic RNA viruses), leukoviruses, C-type viruses, and retraviruses. The standard nomenclature now is generally satisfactory, but several problems remain. Where does one place a virus that (1) does not elicit the foamy type of cytopathic effects in cultured cells (as do the spumaviruses), (2) does not cause slow disease (as do the lentiviruses), and (3) does not cause any neoplasia (as do the oncoviruses)? For the most part, if they do not share any detectable antigenic relationship with spumaviruses or lentiviruses, these orphans have been classified among the oncoviruses. The same procedure has been adopted for particles observed by electron microscopy that show at least some criteria of a retrovirus, although they may never occur as extracellular infectious entities. Such particles are best described by morphological criteria. However, morphology has also served a very useful function in delineating the infectious viruses as well.

The structure of retroviruses has been repeatedly investigated by electron microscopists during the past two decades (for review, see Gross 1970; Vigier 1970); these investigators have used successively thin-sectioning techniques, negative staining of intact particles, and, most recently, negative staining followed by freeze-drying and freeze-etching (Nermut et al. 1972).

The earliest electron microscopy studies established that most retroviruses are roughly spherical structures about 100 nm in diameter (Sharp et al. 1952; Bernhard et al. 1958). They comprise a core or nucleoid enclosed in an outer envelope made of a unit membrane, with spikes projecting from the outer surfaces (Eckert et al. 1963; de Thé et al. 1964). The projecting spikes are particularly prominent in some retrovirus groups, whereas they are seen much less frequently on the surfaces of sectioned or negatively stained viruses of other groups. We now know (Rifkin and Compans 1971) that these spikes are made of the glycoproteins (see below). By virtue of their morphology, as revealed in the electron microscope, retroviruses can be classified into four categories, so-called A-type, B-type, C-type, and D-type particles (Fig. 2.2) (for review, see Bernhard 1958, 1960; Sarkar et al. 1972; Fine and Schochetman 1978).

1. A-type Particles

A-type particles occur as intracellular forms only and do not have any infectivity, even when isolated in large amounts from cells containing them. The particles are generally 60–90 nm in diameter, with an electron-lucent center surrounded by a double shell. The location of these particles has led to a further subdivision: intracisternal and intracytoplasmic forms. The role of the intracisternal A-type particles is totally unknown, although they have often been observed, particularly in cells producing C-type or D-type particles. On the other hand, intracytoplasmic A-type particles are apparently precursor forms to B-type mouse mammary tumor virus (MMTV) virions (discussed in Chapter 6).

2. B-type Particles

The prototype member of the B-type particle group is MMTV. There are two distinguishing features in the morphology of this group. First, budding particles at the plasma membrane show toroidal (doughnut-shaped) cores about 75 nm in diameter, and long spikes are seen at the cell surface. Second, after budding, the mature forms contain electron-dense nucleoids that are eccentri-

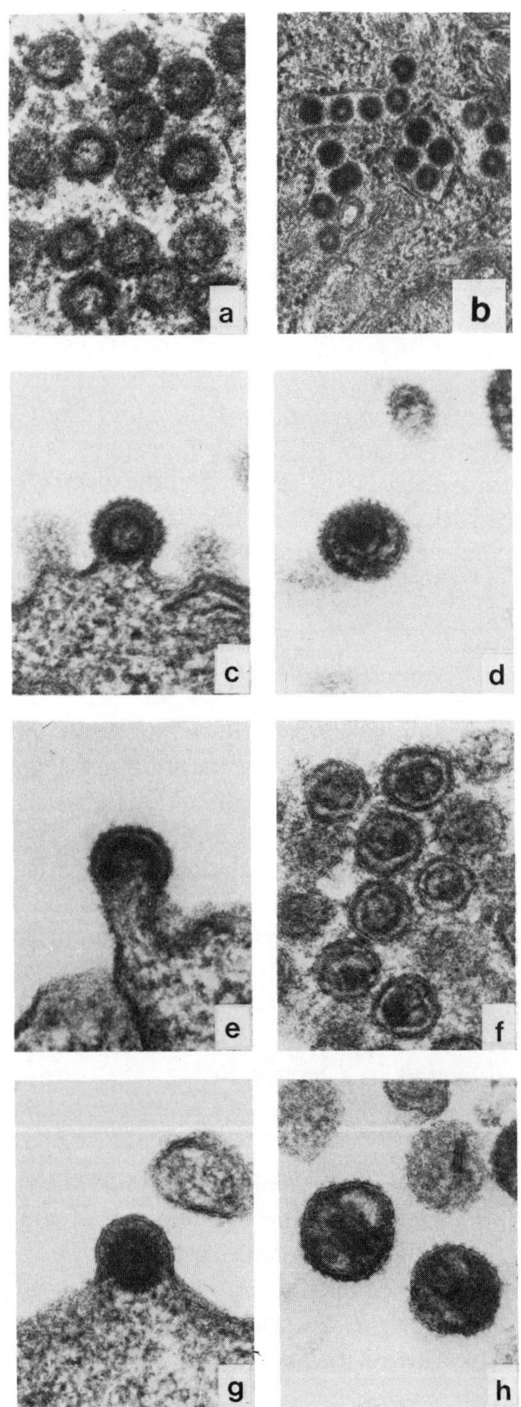

Figure 2.2 *(See facing page for legend.)*

cally located within the enveloped particle (125–130-nm diameter) (see Fig. 2.2).

3. C-type Particles

By far, the majority of retroviruses isolated to date are of the C-type morphology. One of the key features of this class is that, in general, no intracytoplasmic viral structures are observed until budding has commenced at the plasma membrane. In a few cases, particles apparently bud into cytoplasmic vacuoles; it is not known whether these vacuoles are destined to be extruded into the extracellular space.

At the plasma membrane, the first distinct viral structure is an electron-dense crescent-shaped form that is to become the core of the particle. Sometimes the spikes of the virion envelope can be seen protruding from the surface of the cell in areas where core formation is noted; however, such spikes are generally not as well defined or as long as those seen on B-type particles. As virus maturation proceeds, the core is eventually seen as a sphere with an electron-lucent center, and the cell plasma membrane begins to pinch off as it surrounds this structure. Finally, extracellular forms (80–110-nm diameter) with centrally located electron-lucent cores (immature C-type particles) or centrally located electron-dense cores (mature C-type particles) are observed (Fig. 2.2). Some members of this group have easily discernible spikes, whereas others do not; thus, the presence or absence of spikes is not a very useful criterion. The cardinal features of C-type particles are the lack of identifiable intracytoplasmic precursor forms, other than the crescent-shaped core at the cell membrane, and the centrally located core in extracellular particles.

4. D-type Particles

The definition of D-type particles has arisen since the last edition of this book (Tooze 1973), devolving from detailed electron microscopy studies on the Mason-Pfizer monkey virus (MPMV).

Figure 2.2 Electron micrographs of intracellular and extracellular viral particles. (*a*) Intracytoplasmic A-type particles; (*b*) intracisternal A-type particles; (*c*) budding B-type particle; (*d*) extracellular B-type particle; (*e*) budding C-type particle; (*f*) extracellular C-type particle; (*g*) budding D-type particle; (*h*) extracellular D-type particle. Micrographs were provided by D.L. Fine and M. Gonda (Fine and Schochetman 1978).

Because this virus was clearly a member of the Retroviridae family, as judged by biochemical criteria, and yet could not be easily classified among B-type or C-type particles, a new morphological subdivision was created. There are now several more retrovirus isolates within this subdivision; all of these isolates have been made from primate species.

D-type particles are associated with both intracellular and extracellular forms. The intracellular particles are ring-shaped, 60–95 nm in diameter, and are generally most abundant near the plasma membrane; these are called immature D-type particles. The extracellular or mature D-type particles measure 100–120 nm in diameter, contain an electron-dense nucleoid that is eccentrically located, and bear shorter surface spikes than those on B-type MMTV (Fig. 2.2).

C. Definitions

1. Origin

A unique feature of retroviruses is that they may occur in nature not as infectious elements but as stably integrated proviruses within cellular DNA of the host. Such endogenous viruses are thus genetically transmitted as inherited genes from one generation to the next. These viruses may remain latent, they may be partially transcribed to produce viral mRNA and translated to produce virus-specific proteins, or they may become activated to undergo a complete replication cycle with subsequent virus production, viremia, and perhaps neoplasia. On the other hand, the exogenous viruses are those which are not represented as integrated viral DNA copies until after infection of the animal at a cellular level; after this "infection from without," a new DNA provirus may be synthesized and then incorporated into the cellular genome. If this occurs in cells of the germ line, then the exogenous virus may become an endogenous virus and thus become a stable heritable trait.

2. Host-range Variants

A second important concept is that of cell-tropism, i.e., defining properties of the virus and of those cells in which the virus will undergo a complete replication cycle. The ecotropic viruses are those that will grow in cells of the species from which they were isolated, e.g., a mouse virus that propagates best in mouse cells and to a limited or undetectable level in cells of other species. Most ecotropic mouse retroviruses undergo a low level of replication in cells from other rodents, like rats or hamsters, but are generally incapable of replication in cells of higher mammalian species. This phenomenon is attributable to the absence of appropriate receptors for the virus on the surface of the resistant cell (see Chapter 3).

In contrast to the ecotropic viruses are the xenotropic viruses. These are viruses that are endogenous to one species but cannot replicate well in that species, generally because of a receptor block (see below). On the other hand, they tend to have a wide range for replication in cells of heterologous species. A great number of animal species contain endogenous viruses (or parts thereof), which, in addition to being called proviruses, are sometimes called virogenes (see Chapter 10). The majority of endogenous viruses, once activated, display a xenotropic host range. None of the xenotropic viruses has yet been shown to be pathogenic in any animal. On the other hand, both endogenous ecotropic and exogenous ecotropic viruses may be pathogenic. Moreover, a retrovirus need not undergo a complete cycle of replication in order to produce disease. For example, nonproductive infection of heterologous hosts can lead to tumor formation (e.g., avian Rous sarcoma virus [RSV] in rats or murine sarcoma virus [MSV] in hamsters). Further host-range restrictions that pertain to retroviruses are discussed in the appropriate sections and in Chapter 3.

3. Transmission

The etiological agents of infectious diseases are usually transmitted from host to host within a population by contact, aerosols, insect vectors, or other methods. Retroviruses, like other viruses, may be transmitted from one host animal to another by contact, but a frequent mode of transmission is from parent to offspring. Gross (1944, 1970) distinguished these two routes of transmission from one organism to another as horizontal transmission and vertical transmission, respectively. We now recognize two modes of vertical transmission, congenital infection and genetic transmission, which are quite different at the molecular level and are consequently affected by different biological controls.

Congenital infection occurs when infectious viral particles released by the mother infect the offspring. The virus may infect the egg of a bird or be transmitted via the placenta or milk of a mammal, but in each case the virus is transmitted as an infectious particle bearing an RNA genome. It must be released from a maternal cell and then enter a cell of the offspring, where viral DNA is synthesized and integrated into the cell genome. Thus, similar host-range restrictions will apply to congenital infection and to horizontal transmission.

During genetic transmission, on the other hand, the viral genome is vertically transmitted from one generation to the next as a DNA provirus and is maintained as part of the genetic complement of the gametes. Bentvelzen (1972) called this viral genome a germinal provirus to distinguish it from somatic proviruses acquired by infection. Although congenital infection usually occurs through the mother, genetic transmission may be either maternal or paternal, and, because the viral genome is not transmitted as a viral particle, genetic transmission bypasses host-range restrictions.

The three modes of transmission, horizontal infection, congenital infection, and genetic transmission of provirus, are exemplified in Figure 2.3 for avian leukosis viruses in the chicken. In this host species, all three modes of transmission occur naturally and with different consequences, although genetic transmission is restricted to the apathogenic viral genomes encoding subgroup-E envelope specificity (see Chapters 3 and 10). If chicks become horizontally infected when they are more than a few days old posthatching, they are very unlikely to develop leukemia, but after a transient viremia, they become immune to further infection and virus replication, largely through the development of neutralizing antibodies (Rubin et al. 1962). If, on the other hand, the virus is transmitted congenitally (Burmester et al. 1955), the chick typically becomes viremic during embryogenesis and remains immunologically tolerant to viral antigens throughout life (Rubin et al. 1961, 1962). The bird grows normally but frequently develops leukemia when adult. Such birds are a major source of horizontal infection, as well as further congenital infection, because they are continually shedding virus (Zeigel et al. 1964).

In a morphological study, Di Stefano and Dougherty (1966) observed very large concentrations of viral particles in the female reproductive organs, including the ovarian follicles and the oviducts; thus, the gametes and zygote must be exposed to high con-

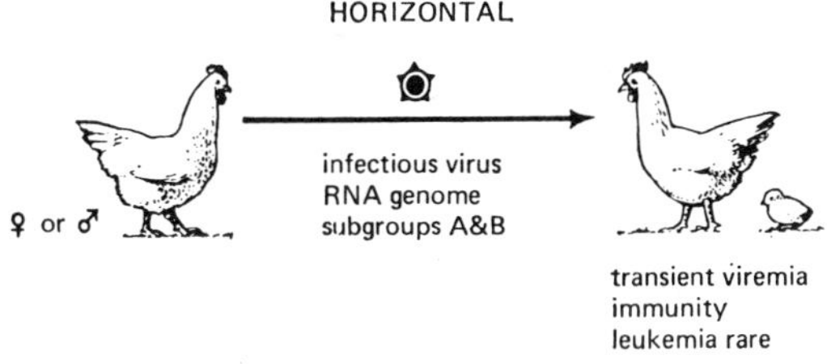

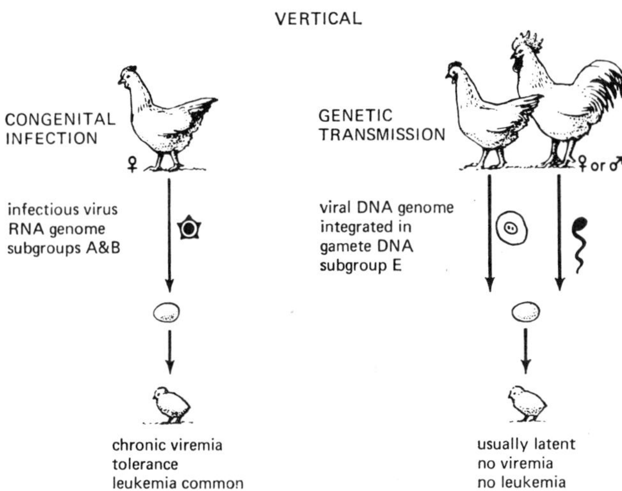

Figure 2.3 Modes of transmission of avian leukosis virus.

centrations of virus. Budding particles, however, were not observed on the germ cells themselves, which may be resistant to infection by subgroup-A or subgroup-B viruses. But much virus is shed from the oviducts into the ovalbumin and subsequently infects the developing embryo.

Cats are also susceptible both to horizontal infection and to congenital, transplacental infection by feline leukemia virus (FeLV). In contrast to the situation in chickens, however, horizontal infection can cause leukemia or anemia, whereas congenital infection usually leads to abortion or fatal runting of newborn kittens before hematopoietic neoplasms can develop (W. Jarrett 1971).

The best-known example of congenital infection is that of mammary carcinoma induced by MMTV in C3H mice (Bittner 1942a,b). Viral particles secreted in the milk are transmitted to newborn mice, and the females subsequently develop mammary tumors and perpetuate the cycle of infection. Such milk-borne transmission can be eliminated by foster nursing the neonates on surrogate mothers lacking infectious MMTV in the milk.

Germ-line transmission is not a very important mode of viral oncogenesis except in special cases of particular inbred strains of mice. These include AKR mice, which have a high incidence of leukemia due to their endogenous viruses, and GR mice, which have a high incidence of mammary carcinoma due to endogenous MMTV. Other strains have had new endogenous viruses experimentally introduced into the germ line via exogenous infection of pre- or postimplantation embryos (see Chapter 10).

D. In Vitro Assay Systems

A number of the methods used to detect, analyze, or titrate retroviruses are presented in Chapter 3. However, because the taxonomic description of a retrovirus includes some of the parameters defined by such assays, a brief account of some of their features is given here.

First, electron microscopy can be used to determine the presence of viruslike particles and, as mentioned in Section I.B., has led to the categories of A-, B-, C-, and D-type viral particles. However, on its own, this technique does not permit the classification of a particle as a virus, although it may often provide the first glimmer of the presence of particles. On the other hand, using immunological reagents (immunoelectron microscopy), one can determine whether a particle shares antigenic determinants with specific viruses or virion components.

Second, well-established or more recently developed immunological techniques have been applied to the identification of viruses and to the analysis of cross-reacting antigenic determinants. For example, complement fixation, immunodiffusion, and immunofluorescence assays have been used in determining whether cells, cell extracts, viral particles, or virus extracts contain antigens capable of binding antibodies that have been raised to specific antigens. In general, these are qualitative, rather than quantitative, assays. But much of the older literature describes the use of such techniques in retrovirus research for detecting "gs-1" cross-reactivity (most likely related to group-specific antigens) or "gs-3" cross-reactivity (related to interspecies-specific antigens). For example, all MLV isolates share common (gs-1) antigens that are nonreactive with FeLV or gibbon ape leukemia virus (GALV) antigenic determinants; however, all three virus groups show relatedness using antisera detecting the broadly reactive gs-3 determinants. Because the antisera employed were generally not well defined and were rarely monospecific, it is difficult to assess whether the reactivities, in the case of antisera to virion components, were directed to *gag* or *env* antigens or to both.

Third, more recently developed immunological assays involve the use of better-defined reagents (antigens and/or antibodies) coupled with radiological or fractionation techniques to define more precisely and to titrate the formation of antigen-antibody complexes. For example, radioimmunoassays (RIAs) involve the use of one radiolabeled reagent (antigen or antibody) and assess the radioactivity present in the antigen-antibody complex; this technique allows quantitative measurements. Such RIAs might be used to determine the level of a particular antigen in a tissue or in cells. By further modification, the competition RIA was developed in which known amounts of antigen and an antibody specific to it (one of which is radiolabeled) are tested in a system to which an unknown material is added; in such a system, one is looking for "displacement" or a decrease in binding between the components of the specific complex. Dilution of the unknown material allows the titration of the level of its cross-reactivity in terms of absolute amounts and in terms of specificity. This type of reaction is known as the homologous competition RIA and is generally useful for type-specific or group-specific antigens. However, one can also look at less closely related antigenic determinants (e.g., interspecies antigens) in the heterologous competition RIA. For example, if two antigens cross-react, but are known to be nonidentical, one antigen and the antibody specifically directed to the second antigen (i.e., a heterologous antibody) are used as the standard reagents in the mixture to which the test material is added. As in the homologous RIA, one titrates the level at which the unknown material competes with the standard reactants.

Structural and nonstructural viral products can be assessed by a number of chromatographic or fractionation procedures (see Chapter 6). The degree of definition is extended when such methods are conjoined with specific immunological reagents. One of the most widely used techniques for separating and identifying viral products or their precursors is SDS-polyacrylamide gel electrophoresis, in which the migration of proteins is governed, for the most part, by their molecular weights. Thus, by using standardized markers whose molecular weights are known, the molecular weights of other proteins can be approximated, while recognizing that modifications, such as glycosylation and phosphorylation, may cause aberrant migration patterns.

Nucleic acid hybridization reactions that have been used to assess the relatedness of viral nucleic acids are compared among various virus isolates or the presence of virus-related information in cellular DNA or cellular RNA. There are numerous variations in the manner in which such reactions can be performed, including (1) solution reactions versus solid-phase reactions, (2) metabolically labeled materials versus reactants labeled in vitro, (3) DNA-DNA analysis or DNA-RNA analysis, and (4) the use of viral genomic RNA versus a complementary DNA (cDNA) synthesized in vitro. Depending on a number of reaction conditions, particular specificity of reagents employed, and the temperature at which the reactions are performed, the level of hybridization can be increased, often accompanied, however, by the loss of specificity. All of these situations affect the stringency (highly specific reactivity) of the final analysis. The nucleic acid hybridization studies described in this chapter are based on these types of reactions. However, in the past few years, recombinant DNA technology and improved methods for nucleic acid sequencing have been developed and provide more sophisticated and more precise measurements of nucleic acid homologies. These newer techniques will be used in the ensuing years to repeat some of the previous experiments and will, in the end, resolve some of the anomalies and catalog the homologies at the levels of distinct nucleotide sequences. In the meantime, the data provided in this chapter still pertain, given the caveat that the levels of relatedness or lack thereof will be further defined in the future.

Infectivity measurements are a further step in the classification of a virus as an infectious entity. The most widely used technique in animal virology is the analysis of distinctive patterns of cytopathic effects (CPE) or cytocidal plaques in tissue-culture cells. For the most part, however, retroviruses rarely induce CPE; the exceptions to this rule are indicated in the appropriate sections of this chapter. A second major technique is the analysis of foci of morphologically transformed cells in infected-cell cultures (some parameters of transformation in vitro are discussed in Chapter 3). This technique is generally limited to a minority of the retroviruses, the transforming viruses, that generally contain genetic information (called *onc*-gene sequences) whose gene products in some way mediate this response in infected host cells. Most of the viruses that are called sarcoma viruses can elicit this type of response. In cells that are neither transformed nor lytically infected, analysis of retrovirus infection must be monitored by other methods. In some cases, assays specific to one or to a few virus groups have been developed. For example, there is the XC syncytial plaque assay in which a focus of syncytia (multinucleated giant cells) appears in response to contact with cells producing many of the ecotropic MLV or simian sarcoma-associated virus (SSAV)/GALV (see Chapter 3, Fig. 3.4). A similar assay, using the KC cell line, has been used for the endogenous cat virus RD114 and for some primate viruses, including baboon endogenous virus (BaEV) and MPMV. One obtains not only a linear dose response as a quantitative measurement of virus titers, but also a further criterion for virus subclassification (e.g., XC^+ vs. XC^- ecotropic MLV). Furthermore, the replication of a retrovirus for which there is no convenient assay may be monitored by the production of reverse transcriptase activity in extracellular particles (except for mutants or variants lacking polymerase activity), providing a semiquantitative measurement.

In many cases, the isolation of retroviruses, particularly the endogenous retroviruses, has not been achieved by direct-infectivity studies on tissues explanted from the host animal. However, activation of the expression and possibly production of endogenous virus elements has often been established by treatment of the cultured cells with a variety of agents, which have been called inducers. A more detailed description of the induction procedure and its significance is presented in Chapter 10; however, for the purposes of this chapter, it suffices to mention that the most efficacious agents in the past decade have been the halogenated pyrimidines, 5-bromo-2′-deoxyuridine (BrdU) and 5-iodo-2′-deoxyuridine (IdU). Another important method for activating viral gene expression and for isolating infectious virus has been the use of cocultivation techniques, which involve mixing test cells, purported to contain an endogenous provirus, with a variety of test cells in which an induced virus might actively replicate. This technique has been particularly useful in the isolation of a variety of endogenous retroviruses that have a xenotropic host range and hence do not replicate in cells derived from the animal in which they are maintained as proviruses. As described above and in Chapter 3, the xenotropic nature of a retrovirus is generally caused by its envelope proteins and their interaction with glycoprotein receptors on cell surfaces, both of which are genetically determined. In addition, intracellular restrictions sometimes apply. The use of the cocultivation procedure has, often serendipitously, provided the means to overcome these receptor and intracellular restrictions.

A further situation that applies to retroviruses is the replication defectiveness of a number of virus isolates that occur both in nature and in experimental situations. The virus may express particular proteins or antigens in infected cells or noninfectious particles may be produced. In most cases, however, these viruses can still be assayed by means of genetic complementation of the defects by coinfection of cells with related replication-competent viruses. In some cases, defective particles may require the provision of a biochemical function, e.g., polymerase activity, to complete a replicative cycle. The most general case, however, is when the replication-defective virus requires structural virion proteins in which to assemble and encapsidate its genome. These two situations are examples of infectious rescue mediated by complementation at the phenotypic level and result in the formation of progeny infectious for one replicative cycle only. Recombination between viruses, leading to the generation of a fully competent virus, is a less frequent occurrence (see Chapter 7). The complementation of structural proteins or phenotypic mixing leads to the formation of mosaic particles containing the genome of one virus and some or all of the structural components of another virus. All of the mammalian sarcoma viruses and many of the avian viruses are replication-defective and, when isolated, they exist as "pseudotypes" (see Chapter 3) with proteins provided by the helper virus. These phenotypic interactions between retroviruses are discussed in detail in Chapters 3 and 7. However, for this chapter, it is necessary to present the accepted nomenclature for describing such particles. A particle whose envelope proteins are provided by a helper virus is indicated by first citing the viral genome and then showing, within parentheses, the helper virus providing the *env* components. For example, the replication-defective Moloney strain of MSV (Mo-MSV), when found as a pseudotype with its natural helper, the Moloney strain of MLV (Mo-MLV), is denoted as Mo-MSV(Mo-MLV); however, when the Mo-MSV genome is rescued from a nonproducer cell, for example, by the endogenous feline virus, RD114, then the pseudotype formed is denoted Mo-MSV (RD114). In many cases, this specification is not required for the discussion and, therefore, will be omitted. However, it must be remembered that a pseudotype particle shows the host-range, interference, and neutralization properties of the particle supplying the virion envelope (see Chapters 3 and 7). There are several advantages of the pseudotype system; e.g., the defective genome can be introduced into a host cell that is normally nonpermissive to that virus (and hence eliminate complications of related nucleic acid sequences in the cellular genome that cross-react with the viral genome) or the defective viral genome can be studied separately from its natural helper (from which it may have been derived and with which it may share a large proportion of nucleic acid sequences).

E. Distribution of Retroviruses

The retroviruses are fairly widely distributed throughout vertebrates and perhaps invertebrates as well. A summary of the phylogenetic classes in which retroviruslike particles have been observed by electron microscopy or from which infectious retroviruses have been isolated is presented in Table 2.2. All of the noninfectious particles and those nononcogenic viruses lacking antigenic or nucleic acid homology to spumaviruses and lentiviruses have been listed among the oncoviruses. A number of isolates from human materials, normal or pathological sources, have been made. The ones resembling spumaviruses are discussed in this chapter, whereas the remainder are discussed in Chapter 11. This chapter is subdivided in a fashion similar to the Retroviridae family (i.e., by subfamilies) and the isolates are discussed below in phylogenetic order. In addition, viruses are listed in Table 2.3 along with the abbreviations used throughout this volume.

Table 2.2 Retroviridae distribution

Class	Order	Animal host	Infectious virus	Particles
		(a) Subfamily I: Oncovirinae		
Cestoda	Pseudophyllidea	tapeworm		(+)
Insecta	Diptera	fruit fly		+
Osteichthyes	Teleostei	northern pike	+	
Reptilia	Squamata	snakes	+	
Aves	Galliformes	chickens	+	
	Galliformes	pheasants	+	
	Galliformes	turkeys	+	
	Anseriformes	ducks	+	
Mammalia	Marsupialia	dunnart		(+)
	Rodentia	mice	+	
	Rodentia	rats	+	
	Rodentia	hamsters	+	
	Rodentia	guinea pigs	+	
	Lagomorpha	rabbits		+
	Carnivora	cats	+	
	Carnivora	mink	+	
	Artiodactyla	pig	+	
	Artiodactyla	deer	+	
	Artiodactyla	cattle	+	
	Perissodactyla	horse	+	
	Primates	prosimians	+	
	Primates	monkeys and apes	+	
	Primates	humans	(+)	(+)
		(b) Subfamily II: Lentivirinae		
Mammalia	Artiodactyla	sheep	+	
	Artiodactyla	goats	+	
		(c) Subfamily III: Spumavirinae		
Mammalia	Carnivora	cats	+	
	Artiodactyla	cattle	+	
	Primates	prosimians	+	
	Primates	monkeys and apes	+	
	Primates	humans	+	

The parentheses indicate a degree of uncertainty; in the column for particles, the parentheses denote that the particles have been identified by electron microscopy only and that other parameters of retroviruses have not yet been detected or sought. With regard to human oncoviruses, the complications and controversies are discussed in Chapter 11.

II. TAXONOMY OF ONCOVIRUSES

As mentioned above, the ensuing sections cover the oncogenic and related nononcogenic retroviruses, the isolates that are difficult to classify in a retrovirus subfamily, and the noninfectious retrovirus-like particles. The discussion thus ranges from the C-type particles observed in cestodes to the C-type and D-type viruses isolated from nonhuman primates, touching on many of the taxonomic classes between the two. Whenever possible, the original reports on detection and/or isolation are cited; additionally, many of the earliest papers describing the criteria fulfilled for classifying the isolate as a retrovirus are provided. Such an approach is an exhaustive task for the much studied viruses and therefore only the most vital sources are noted for these virus groups; however, several review articles are referenced to counteract this abridgment.

A. Tapeworm C-Type Particles

Whether or not these parasites are hosts to retroviruses is a moot question. However, as shown in Figure 2.4, electron micrographs taken cross-sectionally through the excretory ducts of the spargana form of the tapeworm *Spirometra mansonoides* show particles closely resembling C-type retroviruses, both as budding and extracellular forms, and with the classical crescent-shaped immature core (Dougherty et al. 1975). Similar particles have also been noted in other tapeworms (*Diphyllobothrium ditremum* and *Ligula intestinalis*). The hypothesis that these particles represent viruses has been put forward by a number of investigators (Mueller and Strano 1974a,b; Daly et al. 1975), but the one attempt to identify RNA within these particles was unsuccessful (Dougherty et al. 1975). Although the nature of these particles remains to be resolved, these results emphasize that more than morphological evidence is required to establish the existence of a virus.

B. *Drosophila* A-type Particles

One cultured cell line from the fruit fly, *Drosophila melanogaster,* has been reported to contain particles with morphological properties similar to retroviral A-type particles (Heine et al. 1980). The

Table 2.3 Retroviruses

Virus	Species of isolation	Type[a]	Disease[b]	Section
AEV (avian erythroblastosis virus	chicken	C,X,T	E,S	II.E.1
ALV (avian leukosis virus)	chicken	C,N or X,N	L, others	II.E.1
AMV (avian myeloblastosis virus)	chicken	C,X,T	L	II.E.1
ASV (avian sarcoma virus)	chicken	C,X,T	S	II.E.1
BEV (baboon endogenous virus)	baboon (*Papio spp.*)	C,N,N	none	II.T.3
B1LN	*P. hamadryas*			
M7	*P. cynocephalus*			
M28	*P. cynocephalus*			
PP-1-Lu	*P. papio*			
TG-1-K	gelada			
BLV (bovine leukemia virus)	cow	C,X,N	L	II.R
BSV (bovine syncytial virus)	cow	S,X,N	none	IV
CAEV (caprine arthritis-encephalitis virus)	goat	L,X,N	Ar,N,P	III
CERV-CI, CERV C-II	*Mus cervicolor*	C,N,N	none	II.G.2
CCC	cat	C,N,N	none	II.M.2
CPC-1	colobus monkey	C,N,N	?	II.T.6
CSRV (corn snake retrovirus)	corn snake	C,?,?	?	II.D
CSV (chick syncytial virus)	chicken	C,X,N	various	II.E.3
DIAV (duck infectious anemia virus)	duck	C,X,N	various	II.E.3
DKV (deer kidney virus)	black-tailed deer	C,N,N	?	II.P
DPC-1	agouti	C,N,N	?	II.K.2

EIAV (equine infectious anemia virus)	horse	C,X,N	A	II.Q
ESV (Esh sarcoma virus)	chicken	C,X,T	S	II.E.1
FeLV (feline leukemia virus)	cat	C,N or X,N	L	II.M.1
FeSV (feline sarcoma virus)	cat	C,X,T	S	II.M.1
GA (Gardner-Arnstein)				
SM (McDonough)				
ST (Snyder-Theilen)				
FS-1	*Felis sylvestris* (wildcat)	C,N,N	none	II.M.2
FSFV (feline syncytium-forming virus)	cat	S,X,N	none	IV
FuSV (Fujinami sarcoma virus)	chicken	C,X,T	S	II.E.1
GALV (gibbon ape leukemia virus)	gibbon	C,X,N	L	II.T.2
GLV (goat leukoencephalitis virus)	see CAEV			
GPV (golden pheasant virus)	golden pheasant	C,N,N	?	II.E.2
HaLV (hamster leukemia virus)	hamster	D,N,N	?	II.J
ILV (induced leukemia virus)	chicken	C,N,N	none	II.E.1
LLV (lymphoid leukosis virus)	see ALV			
LPDV (lymphoproliferative disease of turkeys)	turkey	C,X,T		II.E.3
M432	*Mus cervicolor*	B,N,N	none	II.G.4
M832	*Mus caroli*	B,N,N	none	II.G.4
MAC-1	stumptail monkey	C,N,N	none	II.T.4
Maedi	sheep	L,X,N	P,N	III
MAV (myeloblastosis-associated virus)	chicken	C,X,N	L,O	II.E.1

Table 2.3 (Continued)

Virus	Species of isolation	Type[a]	Disease[b]	Section
MC29 (myelocytomatosis virus)		C,X,T,	S,C,L	II.E.1
MCF (mink cell focus-inducing virus)	mouse	C,NR,N	L	II.G.1
MH2 (myelocytomatosis virus)	chicken	C,X,T	S,C,L?	II.E.1
MiLV (mink leukemia virus)	mink	C,N,N	?	II.N
MLV (murine leukemia virus)	mouse	C,X or N,N or T	L,N	II.G.1
Ab (Abelson)		C,X,T,	L	
Fr (Friend)		C,X,N	A,E	
Graffi		C,X,N	A,E,L	
Gross		C,N,N	L	
Ki (Kirsten)		C,X,N	L	
Mo (Moloney)		C,X,N	L	
Ra (Rauscher)		C,X,N	L,E	
MMC-1	rhesus monkey	C,N,N	none	II.T.4
MMTV (mouse mammary tumor virus)	mouse	B,X or N,N	M	II.G.3
MPMV (Mason-Pfizer monkey virus)	rhesus monkey	D,X,N	none	II.T.7
MSV (murine sarcoma virus)	mouse	C,X,T	S	II.G.1
BALB				
FBJ (Finkel-Biskis-Jinkins)				
FBR				
Gz (Gazdar)				
Ha (Harvey)				
Ki (Kirsten)				

Mo (Moloney)				
MPV (myeloproliferative)				
OS2 (osteosarcoma)				
MyLV (myeloid leukemia)	mouse	C,X,N	L	II.G.1
OK10 (myelocytomatosis virus)	chicken	C,X,T	C	II.E.1
OMC-1	owl monkey	C,N,N	none	II.T.5
PK-15	pig	C,N,N	?	II.O
PO-1-Lu	langur	D,N,N	none	II.T.9
PPV (progressive pneumonia virus)	sheep	L,X,N	P	III
PRCII, PRCIV (Poultry Research Centre)	chicken	C,X,T	S	II.E.1
R-35	rat	C,X?,T	?	II.H
RaLV (rat leukemia virus)	rat	C,X,N	none	II.H
RaSV (rat sarcoma virus)	rat	C,X,T	S	II.H
RAV-*n* (Rous-associated virus)	see ALV			
RAV-0 (Rous-associated virus 0)	chicken	C,N,N	none	II.E.1
RAV-60 (Rous-associated virus 60)	chicken	C,R,N,	L, others	II.E.1
RAV-61 (Rous-associated virus 61)	ring-necked pheasant	C,R,N	?	II.E.1
RD114	cat	C,N,N	none	II.M.2
REAV (reticuloendotheliosis-associated virus)	turkey	C,X,N	various	II.E.3
REV (reticuloendotheliosis virus)	birds	C,X,N	various	II.E.3
REV-T (reticuloendotheliosis virus-transforming)	turkey	C,X,T		II.E.3
RIF (Rous interference factor)	see ALV			

Table 2.3 (Continued)

Virus	Species of isolation	Type[a]	Disease[b]	Section
RPL-*n* (Regional Poultry Laboratory)	see ALV			
RPV (ring-necked pheasant virus)	ring-necked pheasant	C,R,N	L	II.E.2
RSV (Rous sarcoma virus)	chicken	C,X,T	S	II.E.1
B77 (Bratislava)				
BH (Bryan high titer)				
BS (Bryan standard)				
CZ (Carr-Zilber)				
EH (Engelbreth-Holm)				
HA (Harris)				
PR (Prague)				
SR (Schmidt-Ruppin)				
SFV-*n* (simian foamy virus)	monkey	S,X,N	none	IV
SFFV (spleen focus-forming virus)	mouse	C,X, or R N or T	E,A	II.G.1
Friend				
MPV				
Rauscher				
SiSV (simian sarcoma virus)	see SSV			
SLV (simian lymphoma virus)	see GALV			
SMRV (squirrel monkey retrovirus)	squirrel monkey	D,N,N	none	II.T.9
SMV (simian myelogenous leukemia virus)	see GALV			
SSAV (simian sarcoma-associated virus)	woolly monkey	C,X,N	L	II.T.2
SSV (simian sarcoma virus)	woolly monkey	C,X,T	S	II.T.2

TRV-1	tree shrew	C,N,N	?	II.T.1
UR-*n* (University of Rochester)	chicken	C,X,T	S	II.E.1
Vand C-I	tree mouse	C,N,N	none	II.I
Visna	sheep	L,X,N	N,P	III
VRV (viper retrovirus)	Russell's viper	C,N,?	?	II.D
WMV (woolly monkey virus)	see SSV			
WoLV (woolly monkey leukemia virus)	see SSAV			
Y73 (Yamaguchi 73)	chicken	C,X,T	S	II.E.1

[a]The first letter denotes classification: (B) oncovirus, B-type; (C) oncovirus, C-type; (D) oncovirus, D-type; (L) lentivirus; (S) spumavirus. The second letter denotes: (N) endogenous; (X) exogenous; (R) recombinant. The third letter denotes: (T) transforming (i.e., containing an *onc* sequence); (N) nontransforming; (?) unknown.

[b](L) Leukemia (of various sorts); (S) sarcoma; (E) erythroleukemia; (O) osteopetrosis; (C) carcinoma; (N) neurological disorders; (P) progressive pneumonia; (A) anemia; (Ar) arthritis; (M) mammary carcinoma. n.d. indicates not done.

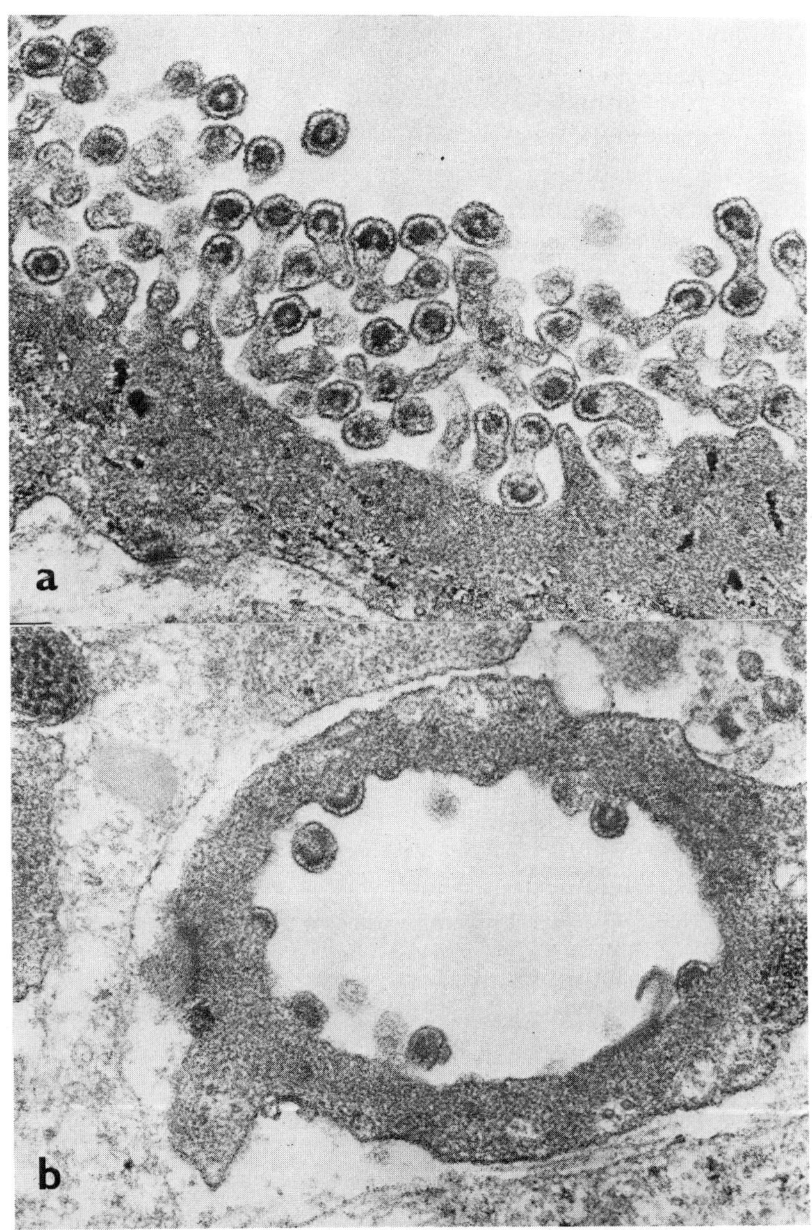

Figure 2.4 Electron micrographs of particles resembling retroviruses in the excretory ducts of the spargana of two pseudophyllidean cestodes. (*a*) *Spirometra mansonoides;* (*b*) *Spirometra mansoni.* Micrographs were provided by R.M. Dougherty (Dougherty et al. 1975).

toroidal (doughnut-shaped) particles are smaller in diameter (40 nm) than intracisternal A-type particles (70–100 nm) or intracytoplasmic A-type particles (60–70 nm). However, particles sedimenting at 1.22 g/ml in sucrose possess the following characteristics associated with retroviruses: polyadenylated 70S RNA, which dissociates after heating into 35S subunits; reverse transcriptase activity (preferentially stimulated by Mn^{++}); and RNase-H activity. Extracellular fluids contain little reverse transcriptase activity, suggesting that the particles are not readily released; however, the activity can be enhanced following treatment of the cells with IdU. Furthermore, it is interesting that *Drosophila* cells contain transposable elements, known as *copia,* which can exist both as integrated forms and as extrachromasomal covalently closed circles, and that these elements possess structural similarities to forms of retroviral DNA proviruses (Flavell and Ish-Horowicz 1981). No infectivity of the A-type particles has yet been demonstrated, but the above findings open the possibility that invertebrates may also harbor retroviral particles or related nucleic acid sequences.

C. Fish C-type Retroviruses

The most primitive class of vertebrates in which C-type viruses have been observed is the bony fish. Up to 21% of northern pike (*Esox lucius*) in Old World waters (Mulcahy 1963; Ljungberg and Lange 1968) and in North American waters (Sonstegard 1976) bear lymphosarcomas characterized by multiple cutaneous lesions. This tumor has a higher relative incidence than any other known neoplasm in wild populations of vertebrates. In North America, horizontal transmission is believed to occur during sexual contact, because the tumor occurs only in sexually mature adults and is usually restricted to the posterior half of the body, although in the Old World, the primary site of tumor development is the jaw (M. Mulcahy, pers. comm.). In a high proportion of northern pike, the tumor spontaneously regresses, but in a related species, the muskellunge of Ontario (*Esox masquinongy*) (Sonstegard 1975), the tumor is also prevalent and seldom, if ever, regresses.

The first evidence suggesting a viral etiology came from transmission experiments with cell-free extracts of tumor material; tumors arose in the jaw or as diffuse lymphomas (Mulcahy and

O'Leary 1970). Although many cell-free transmission experiments have not been successful, one study (Brown et al. 1975) reports an 89% incidence of lymphosarcoma 7 weeks after young fish are inoculated. C-type particles have not been seen in sections of the lymphosarcoma cells, but intracytoplasmic viruslike particles have been observed in cells derived from epidermal hyperplasia, which occurs as an epizootic disease in the watersheds endemic with lymphosarcoma (Winqvist et al. 1968, 1973). More recently, post-mitochondrial fractions of lymphosarcoma tissue have been found to exhibit reverse transcriptase activity (pI = 5.5) and to contain C-type particles with a buoyant density of 1.16 g/ml (Papas et al. 1976, 1977). Comparable fractions from normal tissues have neither reverse transcriptase activity nor C-type particles. The reverse transcriptase activity in the tumor-cell extracts has a temperature optimum of 20°C and retains 82% maximal activity at 5°C; the enzymes present in retroviruses of higher vertebrates have an optimum temperature of about 37°C. The etiological significance of these biochemical observations is not yet known, but it is interesting that the appearance of the tumors in pike shows seasonal periodicity; the tumors develop during the colder months (at water temperatures of 4–12°C). Moreover, Brown et al. (1976) found that the transplantability of tumor cells was greatest in fish kept at 4–7°C. The high activity of the reverse transcriptase at low temperatures (Papas et al. 1976) may be related to this periodicity, and the parallels between the seasonal periodicities of the lymphosarcoma of pike and the herpesvirus-induced Lucké renal adenocarcinomas of the leopard frog (Tooze 1980) are striking. Perhaps both reflect the temperature sensitivity of a viral nucleic acid polymerase.

The evidence that C-type viruses have a predominant role in the etiology of pike lymphosarcoma is only circumstantial; proof will depend on transmission experiments with purified virus. It is clear from the work of Brown et al. (1973, 1976) that, in nature, other environmental factors, particularly organic pollution of the water, directly affect the frequency, growth rate, and severity of the tumors.

There are two other fish genera in which retroviruslike particles have been observed in neoplastic tissue. One is the walleye pike perch (*Stizostedion vitreum*), where intracytoplasmic and budding viruslike forms have been detected in electron micrographs of dermal sarcomas, which occur at an incidence of about 5% (Walker 1969; Yamamoto et al. 1976). Maturation of particles occurs at the membrane where dense crescent-shaped cores are seen. After budding from the cell membrane, particles of about 100 nm are seen. Another disease of this fish, epidermal hyperplasia, is also associated with particles of similar morphology, but smaller size (80 nm); however, both diseases can occur simultaneously in an individual fish. The second fish involved is the Atlantic salmon (*Salmo salar*), in which particles have been observed in swim-bladder fibrosarcomas (Duncan 1978). Relatively little detail is discerned in the intracytoplasmic particles, often found in aggregates near the membrane; however, budding particles (120 nm) look much like typical C-type particles with a crescent-shaped nucleoid, and extracellular particles have centrally located cores and spiked surface projections. The viruses mentioned here have not yet been propagated in vitro, nor have cell-free transmission experiments been attempted.

D. Reptilian C-type Retroviruses

As one moves up the phylogenetic tree, it is noted that no amphibian C-type viruses have yet been observed. However, retroviruses have been isolated from snakes. In 1969 a large precardial swelling in an Asian viper (*Vipera russelli*) was diagnosed as an adenomatous myxofibroma. Viral particles were not detected in the tumor cells (Zeigel and Clark 1969, 1971), but a permanent cell line derived from the spleen of the same animal contained intracytoplasmic A-type particles (65-nm diameter) with radiating spikelike projections (Lunger and Clark 1977) and spontaneously liberated C-type viral particles resembling those isolated from warm-blooded vertebrates. These particles have distinct antigens that show no cross-reactions with the *gag* antigens of characterized murine and avian viruses (Gilden et al. 1970).

As viper retrovirus (VRV) can be obtained in relatively large amounts, its structure and composition have been investigated. The molecular weight of the reverse transcriptase from viper viruses, as determined by glycerol gradient centrifugation, is estimated to be 109,000 daltons, significantly less than the $\alpha\beta$ complex of avian enzyme (160,000 m.w.) but greater than the mature murine enzyme (70,000 m.w.). VRV reverse transcriptase, like the avian enzyme, has a preferential requirement for Mg^{++}, rather than for Mn^{++} (Twardzik et al. 1974). In addition, the viral enzyme shows maximal activity at 40° C, whereas virus production in reptilian cells shows a 30° C optimum and is undetectable at 37° C (Twardzik et al. 1974; Menko et al. 1976).

SDS-polyacrylamide gel electrophoresis of the virion proteins revealed 16 polypeptides with molecular weights ranging from 11,000 to 97,000 daltons. Three of these polypeptides accounted for 75% of the total protein, and some of the minor species are presumably of host origin. The three chief polypeptides have been designated p24 (47% of total protein), p18 (18%), and p13 (10%) (Menko et al. 1976). Clark et al. (1979) also detected a p12 component. Whether any of the virion polypeptides are glycosylated remains to be tested.

In other respects, VRV resembles other C-type viruses. It contains 70S RNA, is labile to ether, has a buoyant density of 1.76 g/ml in sucrose, and its replication is inhibited by actinomycin D (Gilden et al. 1970). All these data indicate that VRV is a typical C-type retrovirus but also that it is not at all closely related to either avian or mammalian C-type viruses.

Regarding the second reptilian retrovirus isolate, Lunger et al. (1974) reported numerous viral particles at various stages of morphogenesis in electron micrographs through sections of the multiple subcutaneous rhabdomyosarcomas of a corn snake (*Elaphe guttata*). Although early attempts to transmit this virus to cultivated reptilian cells failed, a variety of timber rattlesnake cell lines support the replication of the corn snake retrovirus (CSRV), whereas piscine, mammalian, and a variety of other reptilian cell lines do not (Clark et al. 1979). In all infected cell lines, virus replication induces syncytia formation, which may eventually lead to the destruction of the monolayer.

CSRV can be observed budding from plasma and vacuolar membranes with a crescent-shaped nucleoid. The fully mature particle is 105–115 nm in diameter but has a very small core (45–55 nm); in this respect, it resembles avian C-type viruses more than mammalian C-type viruses. The virus bands at 1.16 g/ml in sucrose, and the viral reverse transcriptase shows a divalent cation preference for Mg^{++}, as does VRV.

Analysis of disrupted CSRV by polyacrylamide gel electrophoresis reveals the presence of four major polypeptides; gp72, p24, p16, and p13, and one minor polypeptide, p12. Using antisera raised in rabbits to either CSRV or VRV, the major antigenic specificities (presumably p24) do not cross-react in immunodiffusion tests (Clark et al. 1979). However, immunoprecipitates of viral proteins have not yet been assayed by gel electrophoresis; therefore, it is not yet possible to determine whether or not there are some immunological cross-reactions between these two viruses. Of interest, but still unexplained, is the detectable antigenic cross-reactivity between VRV and the major *gag* polypeptide of the primate D-type viruses, MPMV and the endogenous langur virus (Andersen et al. 1979).

Andersen et al. (1979) showed that sequences related to VRV are endogenous to vipers, occurring at about 15–20 copies per haploid genome. Homologous sequences are not found in the rattlesnake, and, despite the antigenic cross-reaction to the primate D-type viruses, no nucleic acid homology is detected between VRV and MPMV. It is not yet known whether CSRV is endogenous to the corn snake or whether either of the two reptilian viruses are tumorigenic.

Thus, on the basis of immunological criteria, the two retroviruses obtained from reptiles are apparently unique isolates; this finding fits well with the taxonomic classification of the host species, i.e., the corn snake is a New World colubrid, whereas the pit viper is of Old World origin.

E. Avian Retroviruses

Retroviruses have been isolated from gallinaceous birds, such as the domestic fowl (henceforth called the chicken), turkey, and quail, and from the domestic duck. In all probability, retroviruses parasitize other avian orders, but their presence has not been studied.

The avian retroviruses are C-type viruses and fall into four groups: (1) avian sarcoma and leukosis viruses of chickens (ASLVs), (2) endogenous viruses of certain pheasant and quail species, (3) reticuloendotheliosis virus of turkeys and related viruses of ducks and chickens, and (4) lymphoproliferative disease virus of turkeys.

1. Avian Sarcoma and Leukosis Viruses

The ASLVs constitute a large group with close genomic and antigenic homologies to an endogenous C-type virus of chickens. The endogenous virus, called RAV-0 (Vogt and Friis 1971), appears to be apathogenic, or at least its oncogenicity is very low (see Chapters 8 and 10). The exogenous leukosis viruses typically cause lymphoid neoplasms originating in the bursa of Fabricius, the avian lymphopoietic organ that gives rise to B lymphocytes. Leukosis viruses are infectiously transmitted, either horizontally or vertically, through the egg. Acutely oncogenic viruses, such as the sarcoma viruses and the defective leukemia viruses, have been isolated on rare occasions and have then been subjected to intense laboratory study. They carry specific transforming genes acquired by recombination with host genes (see Chapter 9). Lymphoid leukosis is endemic in many domestic flocks, whereas sarcoma and acute leukemia occur only sporadically, although rare epizootics have been noted (Purchase and Burmester 1978). Thus, we do not know whether the acutely transforming viruses are naturally transmitted or whether each case represents the generation of a new recombinant.

The study of a viral etiology to avian neoplasms dates from the observations by Ellermann and Bang (1908) in Denmark that leukemia in chickens was infectious and from the demonstration by Rous (1911) that a fibrosarcoma in the chicken was transmissible by a cell-free filtrate of the tumor. Rous observed no lymphoma or leukemia in the chickens in New York between 1910 and 1915, although he collected some 60 solid tumors, mostly sarcomas, of which 3 tumors yielded sarcoma virus. Since that time, leukosis viruses have become very widespread. It is possible that viral leukosis did not become endemic in the United States until the introduction from Europe of new stocks of white leghorns in the 1920s, just as bovine leukosis has spread in more recent times, from northwestern Europe throughout the world via exportation of cattle. However, lymphoma was recognized in chickens more than 100 years ago, and three cases in the United States were described in 1905 (see Purchase and Burmester 1978).

The classification of avian tumor viruses is based on their pathogenicities and the biological properties of the envelope glycoproteins (see Chapters 3 and 8). Because retroviruses often occur as mixtures and because there is a high frequency of recombination between closely related retroviral genomes (Vogt 1971a), it is not sensible to regard isolates as pure strains. The defective leukemia and sarcoma viruses can only be passaged in the presence of helper leukosis viruses that provide the missing viral proteins (see Chapter 7), but recombination between helper virus and defective transforming virus can occur (Hanafusa and Hanafusa 1971). Furthermore, up to 10% of the progeny of exogenous viruses passaged through chicken cells can be recombinants with endogenous virus elements for the *env* gene alone (Weiss et al. 1973). Thus, there is frequent recombination of viral structural genes, and strains should only be regarded as "pure" with respect to transforming genes of viruses that have been biologically or molecularly cloned.

The envelope classification of ASLVs is based on the properties of host range, interference, and neutralization by antibodies, which are discussed in detail in Chapter 3. The chicken viruses are divided by these criteria into five subgroups, A, B, C, D, and E. Subgroups A and B represent the commonly occurring field strains of leukosis (Calnek 1968); subgroups C and D have not been isolated from the field except in Scandinavia (Sandolin and Estola 1974). Subgroup-D viruses and B77 virus (subgroup C) are able to infect mammalian cells. Subgroup E is the envelope specificity determined by the endogenous virus, RAV-0 and its related genetic elements. Table 2.4 summarizes some of the better-known strains of ASLVs.

a. Avian Sarcoma Viruses. Rous isolated three separate sarcoma-inducing viruses, but all the current strains of RSV are probably derivatives of his "number-1 agent" (Gross 1970). The earliest extant stock, RSV-29, dates from material lyophilized in 1929 and recovered in 1963 (Simons and Dougherty 1963). Most RSV strains are named after the scientists who used them, e.g., Bryan standard (BS-RSV) and Bryan high-titer (BH-RSV) strains (Bryan 1955), Schmidt-Ruppin (SR-RSV) (Schmidt-Ruppin 1964), and Harris strain (HA-RSV) (Harris and Chesterman 1964), or after the locations where the work was carried out, e.g., Prague (PR-RSV) and Bratislava (B77-RSV). The BS-RSV and BH-RSV strains, which were routinely used by American virologists in the 1950s and 1960s, are defective in the *env* gene (Hanafusa et al.

Table 2.4 Laboratory strains of chicken leukosis and sarcoma viruses

Virus	Envelope subgroup					Defective
	A	B	C	D	E	
Sarcoma	SR-RSV-A PR-RSV-A EH-RSV RSV-29	SR-RSV-B PR-RSV-B HA-RSV	B77 PR-RSV-C	SR-RSV-D CZ-RSV	SR-RSV-E PR-RSV-E	BH-RSV BS-RSV FuSV PRCII PRCIV
Myeloblastosis						AMV-BAI/A AMV-E26
Myelocytoma						MC29 MH2 CMII OK10
Erythroblastosis						AEV-ES4 AEV-R
Lymphoid leukosis	RAV-1 RAV-3 RAV-5 MAV-1 RPL12 HPRS42 RIF-1	RAV-2 RAV-6 MAV-2 *td* PR-RSV-B	RAV-7 RAV-49 NT B77 *td* B77	RAV-50 CZAV	RAV-60	
Endogenous					RAV-0 ILV	

1963) (see Chapter 7). In contrast, the Engelbreth-Holm (EH-RSV), SR-RSV, Carr-Zilber (CZ-RSV) (Zilber 1961), PR-RSV (Svoboda and Grozdanovic 1959), and B77-RSV (Thurzo et al. 1963) strains, which were all developed in European laboratories, are nondefective. It would be interesting, therefore, to investigate the defectiveness of RSV-29. B77 was thought to be an independent isolate of sarcoma virus, but its molecular structure is almost indistinguishable from PR-RSV of subgroup C (PR-RSV-C), which casts doubt on its separate provenance.

The *src* gene of RSV (see Chapter 9) determines the malignant property of the virus, as well as the transformation of fibroblasts in culture. The different strains of RSV transform fibroblasts (and also epithelial cells) to characteristic cell morphologies. The most obvious difference is between the rounded (morph-r) and fusiform (morph-f) substrains of BH-RSV, first defined by Temin (1960).

Not long after Rous first isolated his agent, Fujinami and Inamoto (1914) in Japan also isolated a virus that became known as Fujinami sarcoma virus (FuSV). During subsequent decades, further sarcoma viruses were described, such as PRCII and PRCIV from the Poultry Research Centre (Edinburgh) by Carr and Campbell (1958) and Esh sarcoma virus (ESV) (Wallbank et al. 1966) and, more recently, Y73 (Kawai et al. 1980) and UR1 and UR2 (Balduzzi et al. 1981). These viruses, which are all replication-defective, carry transforming genes quite distinct from the *src* gene of RSV (see Chapters 4 and 9). Furthermore, among the defective leukemia viruses, avian erythroblastosis virus (AEV) and myelocytoma viruses (MC29 and MH2) cause sarcomas or carcinomas when injected subcutaneously or intramuscularly, and these viruses also transform fibroblasts in vitro (see Chapter 8). The myeloblastosis viruses, however, are not sarcomagenic.

b. Avian Defective Leukemia Viruses. The genetics and pathogenesis of these viruses are described in Chapters 7 and 8. Like the sarcoma viruses, the defective leukemia viruses (DLVs) have acquired host transforming genes that confer transforming properties to these viruses for specific cell types in vitro and in vivo (see Chapter 9). They are all defective and rely on helper lymphoid leukosis viruses (LLVs) for their propagation. Two strains of avian myeloblastosis virus (AMV), E26 and BAI/A (Graf and Beug 1978), transform myeloblasts or monocytes and bear similar transforming genes. Four independent isolates of myelocytoma viruses, MC29, MH2, CMII, and OK10, belong to a second group of DLVs, and two substrains of AEV (Engelbreth-Holm and Rothe Meyer 1932), AEV-ES4 and AEV-R, constitute a third group.

The BAI/A strain of AMV (Eckert et al. 1951) has been used for many years to induce acute myeloblastic leukemia in chickens. During the short leukemic phase of the disease, very high titers of virus are shed into the plasma, which has been a source of virus for biochemical studies.

c. Lymphoid Leukosis Viruses. These are the common field strains of virus that typically cause B-cell lymphomas and leukemias. Erythroid or myeloid leukemia, hemangiomias (endotheliomas), nephroblastomas, fibrosarcomas, and osteopetrosis are also associated with these viruses (Frederickson et al. 1964); but substrains can be selected for the prevalence of one kind of disease, e.g., osteopetrosis (Smith and Moscovici 1969). The viruses are not defective, and specific transforming genes have not so far been associated with these viruses. Proposed mechanisms for their oncogenic potential are presented in Chapters 8 and 9.

Numerous field isolates of LLVs have been made (Biggs and Payne 1964; Frederickson et al. 1964; Purchase and Burmester 1978). The best known and most widely used is the RPL12 virus from the Regional Poultry Laboratory (East Lansing, Michigan). The virus is derived from a transmissible lymphoid tumor of the chicken first studied by Olson (1941). Cell-free transmission was demonstrated by Burmester et al. (1946), and after further in vivo passages, the virus strain eventually became known as RPL12 (Gross et al. 1959).

Many LLVs are called RIF or RAV. RIF stands for resistance-inducing factor and stems from the discovery (Rubin 1960) of the presence of an LLV in chick embryo cells that conferred resistance to infection by RSV. The resistance proved to be an interference phenomenon whereby cell-surface receptors were blocked to challenge by RSV possessing envelope glycoproteins of the same subgroup. The RIF, like other LLVs, does not transform fibroblasts, but preinfection interferes with RSV infection. RAV stands for Rous-associated virus and stems from the discovery (Rubin and Vogt 1962) that stocks of BH-RSV contained an excess of RIFs.

Upon the discovery of the defectiveness of BH-RSV (Temin 1963; Hanafusa et al. 1963), it was realized that the "contaminating" RAV was, in fact, essential as a helper virus for the continued propagation of the RSV. RAV-1 and RAV-2 belong to envelope subgroups A and B, respectively, and were isolated from BH-RSV; RAV-3 and RAV-6 were similarly isolated from BS-RSV. Further RAV isolates were made from other RSV strains, and indeed RAV came to denote fibroblast nontransforming viruses in general, e.g., the endogenous virus RAV-0 that had not been associated with RSV but could act as a helper virus. More "associated" helper or nontransforming viruses were isolated from stocks of acutely transforming viruses; thus, MAV-1 and MAV-2 are the subgroup-A and subgroup-B helper viruses, respectively, associated with AMV, and FAV-1 is associated with FuSV. CZAV is the RAV associated with Carr-Zilber sarcoma virus and belongs to envelope subgroup D.

Nondefective strains of RSV readily generate nontransforming deletion mutants that have lost all or a portion of the *src* gene (see Chapter 7). These viruses were originally referred to as nontransforming (*nt*) viruses (Vogt 1971b) and were subsequently called transformation-defective (*td*) viruses (Vogt et al. 1974). Nontransforming viruses associated with nondefective strains of RSV, such as CZAV, probably reflect the presence of transformation-defective mutants within such a stock.

All the RIF, RAV, MAV, nontransforming, and transformation-defective viruses that have been tested in vivo behave as LLVs, with the possible exception of RAV-0. Therefore, although the profusion of names must remain for defining strain isolates, they are best referred to collectively as LLV, ALV, or transformation-defective viruses.

2. *Retroviruses of Pheasant, Quail, and Partridge*

Endemic diseases caused by retroviruses have not been described in gallinaceous birds other than chickens and turkeys. Several species, however, carry endogenous genetic elements partially related to avian leukosis viruses, which have been revealed using RAV-0 or LLV probes in nucleic acid hybridization studies (Neiman 1973a; Kang and Temin 1974; Varmus et al. 1974; Tereba et al. 1975; Fujita et al. 1978; Frisby et al. 1979, 1980). The presence of LLV-related sequences in avian host DNA does not fit any discernible pattern either of phylogeny or of geographical distribution (Frisby et al. 1979, 1980). Red jungle fowl (*Gallus gallus*), from which domestic chickens have descended, carry RAV-0-related genomes (Weiss et al. 1971; Weiss and Biggs 1972), whereas other closely related species of jungle fowl (*G. sonnerati, G. lafayetti,* and *G. varius*) have no RAV-0-related sequences at all (Frisby et al. 1979). Other species carrying endogenous genes related to RAV-0 include the ring-necked pheasant (*Phasianus colchicus*), gray partridge (*Perdix perdix*), red-legged partridge (*Alectoris rufa*), and red grouse (*Lagopus lagopus*) (Frisby et al. 1980).

C-type viruses have been induced or "rescued" both from birds carrying RAV-0-related sequences and from species with no related sequences. In almost all cases where an experimentally usable titer was obtained, the virus was obtained after passage of RSV or RAV through the cells carrying the endogenous genome, and many of the rescued viruses are recombinants (Hanafusa and Hanafusa 1973; Fujita et al. 1974; Hanafusa et al. 1976; Chen and Vogt 1977). The rescued viruses were identified by novel host-range and interference patterns, and molecular hybridization studies indicate that at least their *env* genes are unrelated to LLV and RAV-0 (Hanafusa et al. 1976; Fujita et al. 1978).

The recombinant viruses bearing novel *env* genes have been assigned to additional envelope subgroups in the classification of avian retroviruses. The virus rescued from ring-necked pheasant (*P. colchicus*) is called RAV-61 and is assigned to subgroup F (Hanafusa and Hanafusa 1973; Fujita et al. 1974). Although this host species contains several endogenous genetic elements that show partial homology with LLV (Kang and Temin 1974; Frisby et al. 1979), the *env* gene of the rescued virus is not homologous to that of LLV (Fujita et al. 1978). Viruses rescued from golden pheasant and Lady Amherst pheasant (*Chrysolophus* spp.) are assigned to subgroup G (Fujita et al. 1974; Hanafusa et al. 1976). A retrovirus that infects mammalian cells was obtained from the Chinese quail (*Excalfactoria chinensis*) by Chen and Vogt (1977), and cells of two genera of partridge (*Alectoris* and *Perdix*) complement *env*-defective BH-RSV to produce pseudotypes, again with a novel host range (Hanafusa et al. 1976; Chen and Vogt 1977; H. Murphy et al., pers. comm.).

3. Reticuloendotheliosis Viruses

Reticuloendotheliosis viruses (REVs) constitute a group of pathogenic avian retroviruses that are antigenically distinct from, and genetically unrelated to, ASLVs (Theilen et al. 1966; Kang and Temin 1973; Maldonado and Bose 1973). There are five members of this group: reticuloendotheliosis virus strain T (REV-T) (Robinson and Twiehaus 1974), reticuloendotheliosis-associated virus (REAV) (Hoelzer et al. 1979), duck infectious anemia virus (DIAV) (Ludford et al. 1972), Trager duck spleen necrosis virus (SNV) (Trager 1959), and chick syncytial virus (CSV) (Cook 1969). These viruses have similar morphologies (Kang et al. 1975), a common group-reactive antigen (Maldonado and Bose 1976), and an extensive RNA sequence homology (Kang and Temin 1973) and will be called collectively REV. With the exception of REV-T, which is a replication-defective virus, the members of the REV group can be distinguished from one another only on the basis of pathogenicity and cross-neutralization tests; both criteria probably reflect differences in virion surface glycoproteins (Purchase and Witter 1975).

REV-T, the prototype member, was isolated from the tissue of an adult turkey that died with visceral reticuloendotheliosis and infiltrative nerve lesions (Campbell et al. 1971; Robinson and Twiehaus 1974). The other members of the REV group cause a wide variety of syndromes, including visceral reticuloendotheliosis, splenic enlargement and necrosis, lymphoproliferative nerve lesions, and B-cell lymphomas (Purchase et al. 1973; Witter and Crittenden 1979). Further details on pathogenicity are presented in Chapter 8.

Nondefective REVs contain a single-stranded RNA genomic component of approximately 60S (Kang and Temin 1973; Maldonado and Bose 1973), which dissociates into 35S subunits, suggesting a dimeric genomic structure composed of similarly sized subunits (Halpern et al. 1973). Beemon et al. (1976) have shown by oligonucleotide mapping that the REAV genome has a complexity of about 3.9×10^6 daltons. DNA-transfection studies have shown that unintegrated double-stranded DNA from REV-infected cells has a functional size of 6×10^6 daltons, corresponding to 3×10^6 daltons of RNA (Fritsch and Temin 1977). The dimeric structure of REAV RNA has been confirmed by electron microscopy, with linkage at the 5′ ends in a fashion similar to that in the genomes of mammalian retroviruses (Bender et al. 1978; Gonda et al. 1980) (see Chapter 4). The nucleotide sequences of the four nondefective REVs show greater than 90% homology, although their sequences are not identical (Kang and Temin 1973) and they are not related to other avian or mammalian retroviruses (Simek and Rice 1980). Some homology has recently been detected with the MAC-1 group of primate viruses (G. Lovinger and G. Schochetman, pers. comm.). Furthermore, the RNA primer for the reverse transcriptase of REV is $tRNA^{Pro}$ (Peters and Glover 1980), the same primer used by MLV (Waters 1975). REV-T RNA subunits are smaller (30S) than those of the nondefective REVs and contain an extensive deletion in the *gag-pol* region (Hu et al. 1981) and a unique region, the putative *rel* oncogene sequence, toward the 3′ end (Wong and Lai 1981). Further details of the REV genome are presented in Chapter 4.

The structural proteins of REV are described in Chapter 6. Briefly, the *gag*-gene peptides are p29, p15, and p13 and those of *env* are gp73 and gp22, whereas *pol* is a molecule of either 68,000 or 84,000 daltons (see Chapter 6). Several biological properties indicate a lack of relationship of REV to RSV and ALV. First, there is no cross interference in host range (Bose and Levine 1967; Halpern et al. 1973). Second, REAV fails to complement RSV mutants that are temperature-sensitive in the *pol* and/or *gag* genes (Halpern et al. 1973). REV group members are, however, able to form infectious pseudotypes with BH-RSV, indicating that the glycoprotein-defective BH-RSV(−) can utilize REV glycoprotein (Sawyer and Hanafusa 1977; Vogt et al. 1977). Notably, however, the efficiency of phenotypic mixing between REAV and BH-RSV(−) is considerably lower than that obtained between BH-RSV(−) and ALV. In contrast, REV-T phenotypically mixes efficiently with the nondefective members of the REV group (Hoelzer et al. 1980).

Extensive cytopathic effects are observed in avian fibroblast cultures infected by the nondefective REV; these changes led to the development of a plaque assay (Temin and Kassner 1974; Moscovici et al. 1976). Cells surviving the acute phase of infection divide and form persistently infected cultures that are morphologically similar to uninfected fibroblasts (Temin and Kassner 1975). In addition, REAV establishes persistent infection of canine thymus cells (Allen et al. 1979; Simek and Rice 1980). Although the non-transforming REVs do not morphologically transform fibroblasts or hematopoietic cells in vitro, they do induce lymphatic leukemia in chickens after a very protracted latent period (Witter and Crittenden 1979), and cell lines have been isolated from bursal cells of chickens infected with CSV and REAV (Nazerian et al. 1980).

Initially, it was reported that REV-T did not transform cultured cells (Witter et al. 1970; Temin and Kassner 1974). However, this simply reflected the loss of the transforming virus from the stock following serial propagation in vitro (Witter et al. 1970; Halpern et al. 1973; Breitman et al. 1980). REV-T-transformed fibroblasts display disoriented morphology, increased cell density, and decreased serum requirement, and the cells proliferate in soft agar (Franklin et al. 1974; Hoelzer et al. 1979). Although the life span of REV-T-transformed fibroblasts increases in comparison with that of uninfected avian fibroblasts, cellular senescence occurs after 20–30 passages. A quantitative transformation assay has been developed for REV-T using quail embryo fibroblasts (Hoelzer et al. 1979) or hematopoietic cells (Hoelzer et al. 1980).

REV-T-transformed nonproducer cells do not make detectable levels of any of the viral polypeptides synthesized in productively infected cells (Hoelzer et al. 1980). Efforts to precipitate a putative transformation-specific protein encoded by REV-T from nonproducer cells, using antiserum to REAV or p29, have failed. It is possible that the transformation-specific protein encoded by REV-T could be synthesized in low concentration, or it could be very unstable. Another possibility is that the REV-T transformation-specific protein does not contain helper-virus-related peptides. Recent data indicate that in vitro translation of REV-T-specific RNA produces a 58,000-dalton protein (T. Wong and M. Lai, pers. comm.) (see Chapter 9); however, the significance of this protein to the transforming phenotype is as yet unknown.

The origin of nondefective REVs is unclear; homologous sequences are not found in avian or mammalian cellular DNA and, therefore, presumably they are exogenous viruses. On the other hand, the REV-T-specific sequences, *rel*, are detected in avian cells (with the highest level of hybridization to turkey), although, interestingly, no homology with mammalian cells has been observed (Wong and Lai 1981).

4. Lymphoproliferative Disease Virus of Turkeys

Lymphoproliferative disease virus (LPDV) has been identified in turkeys with a lymphoproliferative disease distinct from the lymphomas induced by REV (Biggs et al. 1974, 1978; McDougall et al. 1978). LPDV is a retrovirus that is not related to REV or ALV and is not endogenous in turkeys (Gazit et al. 1979; Yaniv et al. 1979). The virus spreads horizontally in turkey flocks, and, in contrast to other oncogenic retroviruses, experimental infection of 4-week-old turkeys results in a higher incidence of disease than infection of hatchlings (McDougall et al. 1978). No culture system has yet been found to support LPDV replication.

F. Marsupial A-type Particles

There has been one recent report (Hamilton et al. 1979) based on electron microscopic observations of particles resembling enveloped ("mature") A-type particles in two cell lines derived from the fat-tailed dunnart (*Sminthopsis crassicaudata*), a mouse-size marsupial carnivore of southern Australia. The first observable sign of particle formation is a small electron-dense core (about 75 nm) in the Golgi region, which eventually progresses through horseshoe-shaped and doughnut-shaped stages. This last form is usually considered a typical A-type particle. Next, these particles are found budding at the cell membrane, generally into cytoplasmic vacuoles. No mature particles were observed; extracellular particles about 85 nm in diameter (now enveloped) did not show any later condensation of the core. As yet, no biological or biochemical tests have been used to determine whether these particles manifest the cardinal characteristics of a retrovirus, nor have attempts to propagate the particles been reported. However, since neither foamy degeneration nor cytopathic effects are observed in the marsupial cells, the particles would not seem to belong among the spumavirus or lentivirus subfamilies. Moreover, they have been tentatively called members of the Retroviridae family on the basis of morphological appearance alone.

G. Murine Retroviruses

The most extensively studied of the mammalian retroviruses are those of murine origin. Although the historical survey of mouse leukemia, sarcoma, and carcinoma does not date as far back as that on the avian neoplasms described by Ellermann and Bang (1908) and Rous (1911), the availability of inbred strains of mice has greatly enhanced the identification and experimental manipulations of the murine retroviruses. The treatise presented by Gross (1970) gives a very detailed account of the chronological advances and pathologies of these diseases; some further details of pathogenesis are presented in Chapter 8.

The incidence of mammary adenocarcinomas was early noted to be influenced by the tumor incidence in the ancestors of the maternal parents, even in partially inbred strains (Lathrop and Loeb 1918). The development of inbred strains of mice at the Jackson Memorial Laboratory (Bar Harbor, Maine) led to more fundamental conclusions on the nature of the inheritance of this disease via an extrachromosomal element transmitted from the mother to the offspring (Staff of Roscoe B. Jackson Memorial Laboratory 1933; Korteweg 1934). Following these observations, Bittner performed his classical foster-nursing experiments, which involved the nursing of progeny of high-incidence mouse strains, C3H and A, on females of low-incidence strains, and demonstrated the presence of a milk-borne factor (Bittner 1936, 1939). The Bittner agent or milk-borne factor was, in fact, what we now call the mouse mammary tumor virus. MMTV particles became the prototype for the B-type retroviruses, as described earlier, because of their unusual morphogenic characteristics, compared with those of the majority of retroviruses. We now know that MMTV genomes are encoded within the chromosomal DNAs of most mice and that, depending on the strain of mice, the transmission of the disease can be genetic (vertical) or congenital (horizontal). The different strains of MMTV are discussed in Section II.G.3, and their pathogenic properties are presented in Chapter 8.

During the same period, it was noted that there were several inbred strains of mice in which the incidence of spontaneous leukemia was greater than 90%; perhaps the most familiar of these strains are the albino strain Ak (later derivatives became known as AKR) and the C58 strain. Numerous attempts to transmit leukemia by cell-free extracts of tumor cells from these strains failed until 1946, when Zilber reported the induction of tumors from cell-free extracts of chemically induced tumors. In 1951 Gross also successfully transmitted leukemia by inoculating neonatal C3H mice with extracts of Ak leukemia cells. The viral particles transmitted in these filtrates were the C-type MLV. (Incidentally, Gross also discovered and transmitted the DNA tumor virus polyoma in some of these inocula.)

Since the pioneering work of Gross, several strains of MLV and MSV have been isolated. Many of the oncogenic isolates from inbred mouse strains are discussed individually and in greater detail in Section II.G.1. In fact, the numbers of different retroviruses obtained from mice have proved to be quite extraordinarily large. Estimates of the proportion of chromosomal DNA occupied by viral genomes or elements have reached 0.04% of the total mouse DNA complement. The interactions of these endogenous viruses with one another, with exogenous viruses, and with nonviral cellular DNA have led to substantial diversification in their numbers, serological and biochemical relationships, nucleic acid homologies, and pathogenic properties; such properties are discussed in Chapters 4 and 6 through 10. The aim of this chapter is to present the taxonomic diversity among the more commonly described strains, i.e., to provide a description of the origin and possible interrelationships among these viruses. All replication-competent murine C-type retroviruses are collectively termed MLV, although the majority are nonleukemogenic.

At the beginning, however, it is advisable to provide some useful definitions. The concepts of ecotropic versus xenotropic host-range variants were discussed earlier (see Section I.C.2), because they can be applied to all retroviral systems. However, the original definition arose in connection with MLV. Levy (1973) coined the terms ecotropic and xenotropic, respectively, to distinguish between the host-range properties of the commonly studied MLVs and the virus isolated from the NZB strain of mice. For further discussion of MLV, these categories must be defined with greater detail, and new host-range categories must be introduced. The ecotropic MLVs propagate best in mouse cells and to a lesser extent in rat cells and generally do not replicate in cells of other mammalian species. Tropism can be further subdivided according to the particular mouse strains in which ecotropic viruses can grow. It has been found that all inbred mice have a single genetic locus, designated *Fv-1,* that controls susceptibility or resistance to different virus strains (for review, see Lilly and Pincus 1973). Two alleles have been identified at this locus, $Fv\text{-}1^{n}$ and $Fv\text{-}1^{b}$; n denotes the prototype NIH-Swiss mouse and b, the prototype BALB/c mouse (Hartley et al. 1970; Pincus et al. 1971a,b, 1975). Those mice carrying the *Fv-1*^{n} allele at both loci are designated *Fv-1*^{nn}; these mice are susceptible to a class of naturally occurring MLVs (called N-tropic viruses) and are relatively resistant to another class of MLVs (called B-tropic viruses). Mice with the genotype *Fv-1*^{bb} show the reciprocal susceptibility pattern. Both alleles are dominant for resistance, as F_1 hybrids (*Fv-1*^{nb}) between *Fv-1*^{n} and *Fv-1*^{b} mice are resistant to both N-tropic and B-tropic viruses. There is yet another type of ecotropic virus, called NB tropic, that is not regulated by the *Fv-1* gene and thus can grow in *Fv-1*^{nn}, *Fv-1*^{bb}, and *Fv-1*^{nb} cells. An example of this type of virus is Mo-MLV. A few cell lines, derived from feral (SC-1; Hartley and Rowe 1975) and random-bred (3T3 FL; Gisselbrecht et al. 1974) mice, do not exhibit any *Fv-1* restriction and have been designated *Fv-1*$^{-/-}$ (for review, see Pincus 1980).

Table 2.5 illustrates the main features of this discussion. The classical Gross passage-A-type virus (or AKR-MLV) (Gross 1951) is the prototype N-tropic virus, the Tennant strain of MLV from BALB/c mice (Tennant 1962) is a standard B-tropic virus, and

Table 2.5 Titration of ecotropic MLV on fibroblasts derived from different mouse strains

		Log_{10} XC pfu/ml		
Mouse strain	Genotype	N-tropic MLV	B-tropic MLV	NB-tropic MLV
N type	*Fv-1*^{nn}			
NIH		5.2	1.5	6.3
AKR		5.9	2.6	6.6
Restricted N type	*Fv-1*$^{nr/nr}$			
129		4.0	1.2	6.2
NZB		3.3	1.4	5.7
B type	*Fv-1*^{bb}			
BALB/c		2.8	4.8	6.2
C57BL		2.0	4.6	6.1
NB type	*Fv-1*^{nb}			
(NIH × BALB/c)		2.9	2.5	6.5
Nil type	*Fv-1*$^{-/-}$			
SC-1		6.0	4.9	6.5

Some of these data are taken from Pincus et al. (1971a). However, the data for *Fv-1*$^{-/-}$ cell lines, such as SC-1 (Hartley and Rowe 1975) and 3T3 FL (Gisselbrecht et al. 1974), have been added with titer estimates to illustrate the lack of *Fv-1* restriction in these cell lines. Also, the definition of restricted N-type cells (Fv-1^{nn}) was not made at the time of the Pincus et al. study.

Mo-MLV (Moloney 1960a,b) is an NB-tropic prototype. A few salient points can be made at this stage:

1. It is important to remember that the resistance conferred by the *Fv-1* gene is relative and not absolute and can be overcome, to a great extent, by high-multiplicity infection (Decleve et al. 1975; Pincus et al. 1975; O'Donnell et al. 1976). Further details on the mechanism of *Fv-1* restriction are discussed on Chapters 3 and 5. Viruses grown in the cells of the nonpermissive *Fv-1* type still replicate to a limited extent. This is in contrast to the absolute resistance of different chicken cells to the various subgroups of avian leukosis virus and of most mouse cells to xenotropic MLV, as determined by the presence or absence of specific cell-surface receptors (see Chapter 3).
2. Virus tropism should not be confused with the type of cells from which a virus is isolated; e.g., both B-tropic and N-tropic viruses can be isolated from $Fv\text{-}1^{bb}$ BALB/c mice (Tennant 1962; Hartley et al. 1969; Peters et al. 1973; Chang et al. 1975) or by induction from $Fv\text{-}1^{bb}$ cells cultured in vitro (Stephenson and Aaronson 1976; Gelmann et al. 1978; Moll et al. 1979). However, B-tropic viruses have never been isolated from $Fv\text{-}1^{n}$ mice, and N-tropic isolates are the most frequent isolates from young $Fv\text{-}1^{b}$ mice. Furthermore, B-tropic viruses seem to arise by recombination of endogenous N-tropic MLV with endogenous ecotropic or xenotropic viral sequences (Robbins et al. 1977; Benade et al. 1978; Gautsch et al. 1978a; Rommelaere et al. 1978; Benade and Barbacid 1980; Benade and Ihle 1980) (see Chapter 4).
3. NB-tropic viruses are considered laboratory variants as they have not been isolated as naturally occurring viruses.

Xenotropic viruses are endogenous to one species but cannot replicate well in that species (Levy 1973), due basically to a lack of specific receptors on the cells of its host (see Chapter 3). On the other hand, they tend to have a wide host range in heterologous species. It appears that all mice, inbred and feral, have endogenous, xenotropic viruses and/or viral sequences. Although the genomes and proteins of these viruses are related to components of their leukemogenic ecotropic counterparts, no known pathology, neoplastic or otherwise, has been associated with any xenotropic murine virus.

A third class of murine C-type virus is represented by the amphotropic viruses, which have a broad host range and replicate in both homologous and heterologous cells. The most important criterion defining this group is that they do not show cross interference or cross neutralization with the ecotropic and xenotropic viruses. This is due to the fact that their *env* glycoproteins are unrelated to those of ecotropic and xenotropic viruses. Thus far, the amphotropic viruses have been isolated from feral mice only (*Mus musculus*) (Hartley and Rowe 1976; Rasheed et al. 1976a). Some isolates induce lymphomas and/or paralysis (see Section II.G.2 and Chapter 8). They replicate in a variety of mammalian cells, but not in duck cells (which are permissive for xenotropic MLV replication). They show N tropism for mouse cells but do not trigger the XC-cell syncytial response. The amphotropic viruses are defined as belonging to the MLV family on the basis of serological reactivity with a group-specific serum in an immunofluorescence assay and with anti-MLV p30 serum in radioimmunoassays and by reverse transcriptase activity (Hartley and Rowe 1976).

Finally, there exist dualtropic (or now more commonly called polytropic) recombinant variants of ecotropic and xenotropic viruses that, like amphotropic viruses, replicate in both homologous and heterologous cells. Unlike amphotropic viruses, however, they are neutralized by antiserum to the major *env* glycoprotein, gp70, of both ecotropic and xenotropic MLVs and are also subject to cross interference with either of the two virus groups. These viruses were designated mink cell focus-forming (MCF) viruses because of their ability to induce focal growth or morphological alterations in monolayers of a mink lung cell line (Hartley et al. 1977); this assay is used to quantitate MCF virus infectivity. The original isolates of MCF viruses were obtained from thymus extracts of preleukemic or leukemic mice of strains that develop a high incidence of spontaneous leukemia. Several other MCF isolates have since been obtained from other sources (see Section II.G.1.d). The comparative host ranges of infectivity of these four MLV groups (ecotropic, xenotropic, amphotropic, and MCF) are summarized in Table 2.6.

Numerous retroviruses have been obtained from inbred strains of mice since Gross first started his work on the AKR leukemia system. Because many of these viruses have no biological relevance with regard to disease induction, a catalog of all of the isolates reported would be an exhausting effort with little import

Table 2.6 Host range of murine C-type retroviruses

Cells	Ecotropic MLV	Xenotropic MLV	Amphotropic MLV	MCF-MLV
Mouse[a]	+	–	+	+
Rat	+	+	+	+
Hamster	–	–	–	–
Guinea pig	–	+	+	+
Rabbit	–	+	+	+
Mink	–	+	+	+
Cat	–	+	+	+
Dog	–	+	+	?[b]
Bat	–	–	?	?
Pig	–	–	?	?
Cow	–	+	–[c]	?
Deer	–	+	+	?
Horse	–	+	?	?
Monkey	–	+	+	?
Human	–	+	+	–[d]
Chicken	–	–	–[c]	?
Duck, quail	–	+	–	?
Pheasant	–	+	?	?
Turkey	–	+	?	?

Some variations are noted, dependent on particular cell line and virus strain; consensus data are presented. (+) Replication-positive; (–) no replication; (?) no information available.

[a]Replication in mouse cells is subject to *Fv-1* restriction of particular cells used (e.g., primary cells vs. established cell lines). Xenotropic MLV replication in mouse cells is subject to receptor restriction and intracellular restriction (for further discussion, see Chapter 3).

[b]Although not tested formally, MCF-MLV should replicate in all cells permissive to xenotropic MLV.

[c]One isolate replicates in bovine and chicken cells (Rasheed et al. 1977) (see Section II.G.2).

[d]Only one cell line tested (Hartley and Rowe 1976).

to the overall picture. Thus, the following sections will focus on the viruses of historical or pathological importance. In summary, ecotropic MLVs have been isolated from nearly every mouse strain from which they have been sought; three notable exceptions include the NIH-Swiss, strain 129, and NZB mice. Xenotropic MLVs have been obtained from NIH and NZB mice (see Section II.G.1.c); however, infectious virus has never been isolated from strain-129 mice. Interestingly, strain-129 mice contain endogenous virus sequences like those of every other mouse examined (Lowy et al. 1974) and were used to define the G_{IX} antigen found on normal thymocytes of this strain and on leukemic thymocytes (Geering et al. 1966; Stockert et al. 1971), an antigen now known to be the product of an endogenous virus *env* gene (Tung et al. 1975) (see Chapters 4, 6, and 10).

The proteins of murine retroviruses are described in great detail in Chapter 6. Briefly, for the C-type isolates, the *gag* proteins are 5′-p15-pp12-p30-p10-3′, the *env* proteins are 5′-gp70-p15(E)-3′, and the *pol* product is p80. For the B-type MMTV family, the *gag* proteins are 5′-p10-pp21-p27-p14-3′, the *env* proteins are 5′-gp52-gp36-3′, and the *pol* product is p100. Only minor differences in these proteins, indicating substantial polymorphism in the genes and manifested by novel antigenic reactions, are discerned among the murine retroviruses; the few exceptions are noted where appropriate.

In the following sections, the retroviruses of inbred mice are divided into ecotropic, xenotropic, and MCF classes. The ecotropic viruses are roughly separated into leukemia- and sarcoma-inducing categories; the latter class is somewhat artificially defined here to include all of the replication-defective viruses that produce foci of morphologically altered cells in tissue. Recall that the pathogenic potential of a given virus may be greatly influenced by a number of factors, such as age and strain of mouse (or other species), hormonal conditions, and experimental manipulations (e.g., thymectomy or splenectomy). The manifestations of these factors may render an animal completely resistant, or, conversely, enhance its susceptibility, to the virus or may result in a different type of tumor (see Chapter 8).

1. C-type Retroviruses of Inbred Mouse Strains

a. Leukemia Viruses. The extensive efforts by Gross to demonstrate the viral etiology in AKR thymic leukemias set forth the paradigms for dissecting potential retrovirus involvement, whether of endogenous or exogenous source, in other tumors. Despite the complexities of multiple viruses and their interactions with host and environmental factors, the Gross passage-A virus remains one of the more interesting oncogenic isolates. It is an N-tropic, ecotropic XC^+ MLV, as are many isolates from AKR mice that are nonetheless nonleukemogenic; e.g., the readily inducible AKR viruses (Lowy et al. 1971) are not pathogenic, a situation encountered with most other endogenous viruses induced in vitro. In the analysis of the specific regions of nonhomology between different AKR virus isolates, molecular comparisons are currently providing an area of great and intensive interest (Buchhagen et al. 1980; Pedersen et al. 1981). In addition, N-tropic, ecotropic XC^{-}MLVs have been isolated from preleukemic thymus tissues (Rapp and Nowinski 1976; Hays and Vredevoe 1977; Nowinski et al. 1977), and many of these, derived from spontaneous leukemias and thus called SL viruses, are proving to be highly oncogenic per se or active in assays for acceleration of leukemia in AKR mice (see Chapter 8). Finally, there are the MCF isolates from AKR mice (see Section II.G.1.d), which can also be oncogenic or enhance the rate of tumor development. Thus, the AKR mouse seems to be unusually burdened with endogenous oncogenic viruses. Dissecting the intimate relationships among these viruses in vivo is another area of current research in many laboratories (see Chapter 10).

There is a long history to the study of radiation-induced tumors in mice (for review, see Gross 1970), which culminated in the identification of a number of presumably radiation-induced endogenous viruses capable of producing bone tumors (see Section II.G.1.b) and thymic lymphomas (thymomas or disseminated leukemias) (Gross 1959; Lieberman and Kaplan 1959). The sensitivity of the C57BL mouse strain to X-irradiation leukemogenesis was extensively analyzed by Lieberman and Kaplan and their colleagues in the ensuing years (see Chapter 8). As with AKR spontaneous leukemias, the C57BL radiation-induced tumors contain a plethora of viruses: ecotropic (N-tropic and B-tropic viruses that infect fibroblasts efficiently, as well as B-tropic isolates that infect and replicate in fibroblasts only very poorly, but show a high infectivity in the thymus and hence are called thymotropic), xenotropic, and MCF types (Decleve et al. 1976, 1977, 1978; Haas et al. 1977; Haas 1978). In addition, an RNA species smaller than genomic size has been detected in virus stocks, suggesting the possible presence of a replication-defective particle (Manteuil-Brutlag et al. 1980) (see Chapter 4). Therefore, the connotation of a radiation leukemia virus (previously called RadLV) has been modified in the last few years. Molecular discrimination between the different viral elements and analysis of their individual leukemogenic activities have been the subject of many recent studies (see Chapter 8). At this time, it is unclear which of the MCF isolates of the thymotropic viruses are the most important agents in the generation of radiation-induced leukemia in C57BL mice.

Mo-MLV was obtained from the passage of a cell-free extract of the Sarcoma-37 transplantable tumor in neonatal mice. The general pathology includes thymic leukemia, disseminated lymphosarcoma, or lymphatic leukemia and hepatosplenomegaly (Moloney 1960a,b) and resembled the pathology induced by the Gross passage-A virus. One difference from Gross virus is the NB tropism of Mo-MLV; this may have occurred by selection during the numerous passages in BALB/c mice or may have arisen during the many years that the Sarcoma-37 tumor was transplanted in rats and mice.

The derivation of Kirsten MLV (Ki-MLV) involves an extensive in vivo-passage history. Thymic lymphoma extracts from C3Hf mice inoculated with human leukemia extracts induced lymphoid leukemias or erythroblastic splenomegaly and severe anemia in recipient mice and rats (Kirsten et al. 1967). The role of the human leukemia extracts was probably nil, and one assumes that Ki-MLV arose from an endogenous C3H virus. However, its NB-tropic host range and erythroblastic properties suggest that it may have been generated by successive recombinational events.

The erythroleukemia-inducing Friend virus (FV) complex is covered in great detail elsewhere (see Chapters 4 and 8). The original isolate was obtained from a Swiss mouse that had received an injection of Ehrlich ascites mouse carcinoma cells 2 weeks previously (Friend 1957). Cell-free extracts, after further passage in Swiss mice, were highly potent in inducing the hallmarks of Friend disease: splenomegaly, hepatomegaly, and eventually erythroleukemia. Unlike the majority of MLVs, the FV complex does not induce abnormal pathology in the thymus. In her original experiments, Friend noted marked anemia in recipient mice. Later virus preparations induced polycythemia (Mirand 1967). It is now known that there are two forms of the Friend virus complex (FV-A and FV-P for anemia and polycythemia, respectively) and that each is composed of two virus components, a replication-competent helper virus (designated Fr-MLV_A and Fr-MLV_P) and a replication-defective component that induces foci of erythroid proliferation in spleens of infected mice (the SFFV strains, $SFFV_A$ and $SSFV_P$) (Axelrad and Steeves 1964; Dawson et al. 1966; Steeves et al. 1971). The various helper viruses are nearly identical and have been shown to induce splenomegaly and anemia in neonatal mice of certain strains (Troxler and Scolnick 1978; MacDonald et al. 1980a). In addition, Fr-MLV can induce erythroleukemia in adult mice after long latency periods (Dawson et al. 1979). On the other hand, distinct differences can be detected between the genomes of $SFFV_A$ and $SFFV_P$, although both are recombinant viruses between Fr-MLV and endogenous xenotropic viral sequences (Troxler et al. 1977a, 1980; MacDonald et al. 1980b). The glycoprotein, gp55 (Racevskis and Koch 1977; Dresler et al. 1979; Ruscetti et al. 1979), encoded by the recombinant *env* gene is closely linked to the oncogenic potential of the virus (see Chapter 8). The manifestations of Friend virus disease due to SFFV are observed in adult mice of most inbred strains and occur within a few weeks. Interestingly, an MCF virus component is induced in the spleens of infected mice (Troxler et al. 1978). Fr-MLV can also induce anemia in newborn mice of a few strains (e.g., NIH-Swiss and BALB/c). Further details of the biochemical and pathogenic properties of the different components are found in Chapter 8.

Since Friend's report a number of other isolates capable of inducing the same disease spectrum have been identified: (1) strain WM1-B obtained from a wild house mouse and passaged through newborn mice (Pope 1961, 1962), (2) an isolate from Swiss mice inoculated with Sarcoma-37 cells (cf. Mo-MLV) (Bather 1961), (3) virus from an erythroleukemia induced by injection of the myeloid leukemia Graffi virus (Fey and Graffi 1965), and (4) BSB virus complex, derived from Friend virus but having an expanded in vivo host range (Steeves et al. 1970) (see Chapter 8). None of these viruses have been extensively characterized. There is also a regressor strain of Friend virus, known as RFV, in which the disease is transitory (Rich et al. 1969); apparently, this property of regression is due to the helper Fr-MLV and not the SFFV component (Dietz et al. 1977). Additionally, Ki-MLV (described above) and the Rauscher virus complex, Ki-MSV, Harvey (Ha)-MSV, and myeloproliferative sarcoma virus (MPV-MSV) have effects on the erythroid hematopoietic cell compartments (see below and Section II.G.2.b). Spleen focus induction, however, is associated only with Friend virus, Rauscher, BSB, and MPV-MSV.

The origin of the Rauscher virus complex involved a great number of in vivo passages through different strains of mice of a variety of different tumor-cell materials (Rauscher 1962); hence, it is difficult to establish when or where the viruses arose. Biologically, the Rauscher virus most closely resembles the anemia strain of Friend virus: (1) It contains a Rauscher SFFV (Ra-SFFV) (Pluznik and Sachs 1964), which is replication-defective, and a replication-competent NB-tropic helper virus (Ra-MLV) (Bentvelzen et al. 1972). (2) The pathogenesis mimics FV-A in both pathological manifestations and responses to host resistance genes (Rauscher 1962; Boiron et al. 1965). (3) An MCF component is found in the spleens of infected mice (Van Griensven and Vogt 1980) (see Chapter 8). However, it is not yet known at the molecular level how closely the Rauscher virus components are related to those of FV-A.

Early serological analyses on the above-mentioned viruses by Old et al. (1964, 1965) led to the definition of two neutralization serotypes: (1) Gross-AKR type, shared by the spontaneously occurring viruses, and (2) FMR type, defined by Fr-MLV, Mo-MLV, and Ra-MLV. The development of monoclonal antibodies with which one can distinguish and localize specific antigenic epitopes has relegated these serological categories more to a historical, rather than a practical, place.

A number of tumor extracts containing viruses capable of inducing myeloid leukemias have been described in the past. However, few of these have been subjected to biochemical or molecular characterization. Because of the ubiquity of endogenous viruses and the promiscuity that occurs among retroviruses, especially during in vivo passage, it is difficult to attribute the pathological process to a single agent in any of these stocks at this time. No doubt resurrection of these isolates from long-frozen tumors or extracts will shortly give rise to molecularly cloned viruses for detailed characterization. Some of the tumorigenicity studies with these myelogenous leukemia viruses are described in Chapter 8; a brief catalog of these viruses follows.

Graffi and his colleagues studied extensively the pathological and immunological properties of cell-free extracts of a variety of transplantable mouse tumors (Ehrlich carcinoma, Sarcoma 37, Landschutz sarcomas 1 and 2, and SOV 16, a myeloid leukemia derivative of a sarcoma-1-inoculated animal), each of which induced a fairly high incidence of chloroleukemia (a form of myeloid leukemia characterized by greenish discoloration of involved lymph nodes) in particular inbred or random-bred mice (Graffi 1957; Graffi et al. 1966, 1968). Although other types of leukemias arose occasionally, the predominant affected cell was of the myeloid lineage (see Chapter 8). Studies on Graffi virus have generally involved the use of extracts derived from tumors, rather than virus propagated in tissue-culture cells; altered proportions or numbers of different retrovirus components during in vivo passage could explain the "hematological diversification" described by Graffi. Nevertheless, the pathology induced by Graffi virus is significantly distinct from those of all the mouse leukemia viruses that had been derived up till that time, and thus further studies would be welcome.

Another retrovirus, called Stansly virus or sometimes Soule virus, was isolated from BALB/c mice inoculated with Ehrlich ascites tumor cells (cf. Graffi and Friend virus derivations) or with a cell-free extract of the tumor (Stansly and Soule 1962). The tumor was diagnosed as a reticulum-cell sarcoma, accompanied by splenomegaly and lymph node enlargement. Later studies using virus produced by a tumor cell line established in vitro showed a more predominant incidence of myeloid leukemia (Soule and Arnold 1970; Nooter and Bentvelzen 1976).

The myeloid inducing virus, MyLV, isolated by McGarry et al. (1974), was derived by passaging a polycythemia Friend virus strain through C57BL and Swiss Ha/ICR mice numerous times. The eventual outcome was a virus stock that was capable of inducing chloroleukemia, with hepatosplenomegaly and occasional involvement of the thymus. It was concluded that the SFFV component of the Friend virus complex was lost along the way with a concomitant gain of an agent(s) or variant with a new oncogenic spectrum.

Myeloid leukemia is also a frequent consequence of X-irradiation of the RF mouse strain (Upton et al. 1958). Cell-free extracts of spleens from the leukemic mice contain retroviral particles and produce myeloid leukemia (and, in some cases, thymic leukemia) in recipient neonatal or adult mice with a relatively short latency (Jenkins and Upton 1963). The RF system has not been examined further; resurrection of frozen filtrates in the future might cast some light on the nature of the oncogenic agent(s).

MPV-MSV (see Section II.G.1.b) also affects myeloid-cell differentiation in vivo and, under certain circumstances, particularly neonatal thymectomy, myeloid leukemias are induced by Gross passage-A virus (Gross 1960) and Mo-MLV (Moloney 1962).

b. Sarcoma Viruses. Despite the fact that mice develop a variety of solid tumors with age, the number of isolates of MSV, whether naturally occurring or experimentally generated (by radiation or inoculation of MLV), is quite small (see Table 2.7). It is interesting that osteosarcomas are the most prevalent source of MSV, although as yet it is difficult to assess how many and to what degree the various osteosarcoma isolates are related. The pathogenic properties of these viruses are described in Chapter 8, and other characteristics of the well-studied viruses are presented in the appropriate chapters.

The first of the naturally occurring MSV isolates is the Finkel-Biskis-Jinkins (FBJ) osteogenic sarcoma virus complex obtained from a spontaneous osteosarcoma in an old CF-1 mouse (Finkel et al. 1966a). The complex consists of an N-tropic nonleukemogenic helper virus (FBJ-MLV) and a replication-defective transforming virus (FBJ-MSV), of which the latter is responsible for the induction of osteosarcomas (Finkel et al. 1966b; Kelloff et al. 1969; Yumoto et al. 1970; Levy et al. 1973, 1975, 1978).

Historically, the next naturally occurring MSV isolate is the Gazdar strain of MSV (Gz-MSV) (Gazdar et al. 1972a,b) derived from a spontaneous tumor in a 6-month-old $(NZB \times NZW)F_1$

Table 2.7 Murine sarcoma virus isolates

Isolate	Oncogene sequence	Predominant oncogenic potential
Ab-MLV	*abl*	pre-B-cell leukemia, lymphosarcoma
Mo-MSV	*mos*	rhabdomyosarcoma, pleomorphic sarcoma
Gz-MSV	*mos*	undifferentiated sarcoma
MPV-MSV	*mos*	erythroid and myeloid leukemia
Ball-MSV	*mos*	rhabdomyosarcoma
Ha-MSV	*ras*	erythroleukemia, fibrosarcoma
Ki-MSV	*ras*	erythroleukemia, lymphosarcoma
BALB-MSV	*ras*	hemangiosarcoma
FBJ-MSV	?	osteosarcoma
FBR-MSV	?	osteosarcoma
RFB-MSV	?	osteoma
OS2-MSV	?	osteosarcoma
R^+FC3-MSV	?	undifferentiated sarcoma
Carc2-MSV	?	lung adenocarcinoma
AK-T8-MSV	?	?
V793-MSV	?	?

mouse. Injection into neonatal rodents induces undifferentiated sarcomas, accompanied by angiomatous formation, inflammation, fibrosis, and splenomegaly. Interestingly, the helper virus is NB tropic. As mentioned previously, NB-tropic isolates appear to derive by alterations during experimental manipulations, rather than occurring spontaneously; thus, the presence of an NB-tropic helper in Gz-MSV stocks is unusual and raises speculation that the "rescue" of the MSV genome in vivo might have occurred because of exogenous infection by an NB-tropic helper virus. In addition, the *onc*-gene sequences of Gz-MSV are highly related, if not identical, to those (*mos*) of Mo-MSV (Pang et al. 1977; Donoghue et al. 1979), although their location within the genome is different from the arrangement in Mo-MSV, suggesting that the two viruses arose independently (see below and Chapter 4).

The derivation of the 138-MSV strain, now known as BALB-MSV, involved the cell-free transmission of blood from an 18-month-old BALB/c mouse with a spontaneous chloroleukemia (Peters et al. 1974). The original filtrate induced a variety of neoplasms following inoculation of newborn BALB/c mice, including hemangiosarcomas, lymphosarcomas, and lymphoreticular tumors. However, later passages from hemangiosarcoma tissue produced predominantly the same type of neoplasm. The initial virus preparation contained a B-tropic helper virus as well as the replication-defective MSV. Preliminary data (P. Andersen et al., pers. comm.) suggest that the *onc*-gene sequences are related to those found in Ha-MSV and Ki-MSV (i.e., *ras*), although the derivation of the BALB-MSV never involved rats, and thus the sequences probably represent acquisition of the mouse cellular *ras* counterpart.

In 1973 Finkel et al. reported the isolation of a second osteogenic sarcoma virus complex, called FBR, from a strontium-90-induced osteosarcoma in an X/Gf mouse. The helper virus is B tropic (X/Gf mice are of *Fv-1*^{b} genotype), and the complex induces osteosarcomas rapidly in X/Gf mice but is poorly oncogenic for CF-1 mice (from which the FBJ-MSV was isolated) (Finkel et al. 1975; Lee et al. 1979).

A benign bone tumor in a CF-1 mouse was the source of isolation of an osteoma-inducing virus, RFB (Finkel et al. 1976; Reilly and Finkel 1976). At the present time, little is known about this virus other than its pathogenic properties (see Chapter 8).

An osteosarcoma-inducing virus (called OS2) has also been isolated from radium-224-induced tumors in (C3H × 101)F_1 mice (Erfle et al. 1979, 1980). No information has yet appeared on the number of virus components, tropism, or relationship to other osteosarcoma viruses.

Two fibroblast-transforming viruses, with no known oncogenic capacity, have been described. First, the AK-T8 virus was isolated from an AKR thymoma cultured in vitro (Staal et al. 1977). Second, Bentvelzen et al. (1978) isolated a fibroblast-transforming virus (V793) from a spontaneous osteosarcoma in a 19-month-old BALB/c mouse. Although the original cells were nonproducers, this virus was obtained following cocultivation with BALB/3T3 cells chronically infected with Ra-MLV. Little is known regarding the relationship of these viruses to better-characterized strains.

Although the viruses mentioned above were from tumors, spontaneously arising or derived by radiation treatment, historically and by far the best-understood MSV isolates were derived following experimental procedures that involved injecting various MLV isolates into mice or rats, from which viruses with both fibroblast-transforming and sarcomagenic properties were obtained.

The first mammalian sarcoma virus was isolated by Harvey in 1964. The plasma from an outbred Chester Beatty rat with a thymoma induced by Mo-MLV inoculation caused sarcomas in newborn BALB/c mice, rats, and hamsters. In addition, the virus causes anemia, splenomegaly (due to erythroblastic proliferation) (Harvey 1964), and erythroleukemia (Scher et al. 1975) (see Chapter 8). The fibroblast-transforming virus, henceforth called Ha-MSV, is now known to have arisen by recombination of Mo-MLV with rat-cell sequences (*ras*) (Scolnick and Parks 1974) (see Chapters 4 and 9).

Biologically and biochemically related to Ha-MSV is the strain isolated by Kirsten and Mayer (1967), now known as Ki-MSV. After two passages in Wistar/Furth rats, the erythroblastic Ki-MLV strain (described above) had the capacity to induce in rats multiple sarcomas, osteolytic lesions, and petechial hemorrhages, in addition to the erythroblastic splenomegaly. Mo-MLV pseudotypes of Ki-MSV also induce the erythroid disease (Scher et al. 1975) (see Chapter 8). The replication-defective focus-forming virus also contains rat-cell-derived *ras* sequences (Scolnick et al. 1973) (see Chapters 4 and 9). Mutants of Ki-MSV have been extremely useful in defining the functions of the *ras* sequences (see Chapters 7 and 9).

Whereas Ha-MSV and Ki-MSV were isolated from rats inoculated with MLV, two fibroblast-transforming viruses arose following infection of mice with MLV: the Moloney and Abelson strains. The Moloney strain of MSV was isolated from a rhabdomyosarcoma induced in a BALB/c mouse inoculated at birth with Mo-MLV (Moloney 1966). As discussed in greater detail in Chapters 4 and 7, the original uncloned Mo-MSV stock contained a number of different replication-defective variants (including viruses later known as MSV-124, the hamster tumor isolate HT-1 MSV, and m1 MSV). Each of the variants studied contains Mo-MLV-derived sequences as well as the specific oncogene sequence *mos*. The location of *mos* within the MSV genome, the differential expression of the adjacent MLV sequences, and the positions of the deletions in the parental MLV *pol* and *env* regions suggest that Mo-MSV may have arisen from one initial recombinational event but that the variants arose later through some sort of genetic instability of the resultant genome.

Injection of MLV spontaneously produced by the JLS-V9 cell line into neonatal CFW/D, NIH-Swiss, C3H/Bi, or C57BL/6J mice led to a high incidence of rhabdomyosarcomas and granulomas (Ball et al. 1973). Plasma filtrates from tumor-bearing animals contained fibroblast-transforming sarcoma viruses; the virus obtained from CFW/D mice has been called the Ball-MSV or 1712-MSV isolate. However, the close similarity between this isolate and Mo-MSV isolates, determined by RNA oligonucleotide mapping (Deng and Wimmer 1978) and heteroduplex mapping (Donoghue et al. 1979), suggests that it might be a variant rather than an independent isolate.

MPV-MSV is a variant of Mo-MSV that arose following passage of plasma from tumor-bearing animals in BALB/c mice (Chirigos et al. 1968). This variant contains the *mos* sequences of Mo-MSV (Pragnell et al. 1981) but has an altered pathological range, including erythroid and myeloid leukemias and myelofibrosis of spleen and bone marrow, and it induces spleen foci in infected mice, a property similar to that of SFFV (Le Bousse-Kerdiles et al. 1980; Ostertag et al. 1980) (see Chapter 8). Thus, it might be called MPV-SFFV synonymously with MPV-MSV.

Abelson and Rabstein (1970a,b) noted that one BALB/c mouse,

out of many that had been inoculated with Mo-MLV at birth and subsequently had been given repeated doses of prednisolone (a steroid that leads to thymic atrophy), developed a thymic-independent lymphosarcoma. The virus complex isolated from this tumor contained Mo-MLV and a replication-defective component (known as Abelson [Ab]-MLV or Ab-MSV). Ab-MLV transforms both fibroblasts (Scher and Siegler 1975) and lymphoid cells in vitro (Sklar et al. 1974; Rosenberg et al. 1975) and is the agent responsible for the induction of pre-B-cell leukemias in vivo (Boss et al. 1979; Siden et al. 1979). The Ab-MLV genome is clearly derived from recombination between Mo-MLV and mouse-cell sequences (*abl*) (Reynolds et al. 1978; Witte et al. 1978; Baltimore et al. 1980; Goff et al. 1980) and thus is distinct from all other acutely transforming viruses. Further details on this virus and some mutants obtained from it are discussed in Chapters 4, 7, 8, and 9.

Finally, there is a group of new agents comprised of sarcoma- and carcinoma-inducing viruses that have been generated in vitro (Rapp and Todaro 1978a,b, 1980). The protocol involved using a BrdU-induced endogenous ecotropic MLV from C3H mouse cells for infection of spontaneously transformed NIH-3T3 cells or methylcholanthrene-transformed C3H cells, passage of the harvest onto untransformed cells (mouse C3H cells for leukemia and sarcoma viruses and mink cells for carcinoma viruses), and, finally, selection of morphologically altered foci of soft-agar-grown colonies. Viruses recovered from the cells produced sarcomas (e.g., R^{+}FC3-MSV), lung adenomas or adenocarcinomas (e.g., Carc2-MSV), or ovarian carcinomas; viruses extracted from the tumor cells reproduced the same disease, suggesting stability of the new genomes. The molecular analysis of these viruses is eagerly awaited.

c. Xenotropic Viruses. Initially, the virological situation in the NZB mouse strain presented an enigma in that C-type particles were detected microscopically in these mice throughout life, as well as in late-term embryos (Mellors and Huang 1966; East et al. 1967b; Yumoto and Dmochowski 1967; Prosser 1968), and in animals produced by caesarian section and fostered on germ-free mothers of another strain, indicating that the virus was endogenous and transmitted via the placenta and/or germ cells (East et al.

1967a). But biological description of virus from NZB mice showed that it replicated in rat and human cells, but not in mouse cells, and that it shared group-specific antigenic determinants with other MLV isolates, yet neither produced XC syncytia nor was effectively neutralized by anti-MLV sera. At first this was regarded as an interesting problem of host range and antigenic variation (Levy and Pincus 1970). With the advent of the data supporting the concept of endogenous viruses and the definition of xenotropism (Levy 1973), the NZB virological picture fell into its natural place as a classic example of an endogenous xenotropic virus. Since that time, it has been shown that the activation of xenotropic MLV in vitro from a repressed state is quite sensitive to a variety of inducing agents or treatments (see Chapter 10), followed by cocultivation with heterologous cells to facilitate the replication of these viruses to high titers. Hence, numerous xenotropic MLV have been isolated from nearly every inbred mouse strain studied (for review, see Levy 1978). The one known exception is the 129 strain of mice which, as mentioned previously, also does not release any ecotropic virus in vivo or from cells cultured in vitro, even following cocultivation or treatment with inducing agents (Levy et al. 1979).

Mouse cells lack receptors for xenotropic MLV (discussed in Chapter 3); therefore, activation of such viruses in vivo is not readily detected because the barrier to reinfection abrogates the establishment of a chronic virus-producing state. However, one of the most common situations of xenotropic MLV production in vivo is in mice bearing xenogeneic tumor transplants. This can be particularly confusing and annoying for investigators who use nude mice or immunologically suppressed animals to grow tumor cells that are not easily amenable to establishment in vitro, because upon reexamination of the tumors thus grown, chronic production of xenotropic virus can occur, concomitant with the expression of virus-specific antigens. The discovery of the prototype xenotropic MLV, AT-124, of NIH-Swiss mice was accomplished in this way (Todaro et al. 1973c). Many more examples involving xenotropic MLV production during heterotransplantation now abound (Suzuki et al. 1977; Crawford et al. 1979).

A number of different xenotropic MLVs have been compared using liquid hybridization techniques. Most of the xenotropic MLVs from inbred mouse strains are relatively highly related;

however, the isolates from NZB and NIH mice are apparently quite distinct from the other isolates. For example, Callahan et al. (1975) have determined that RNA from many xenotropic MLVs show virtually 100% hybridization to a probe derived from a BALB/c xenotropic MLV, whereas the NZB isolate hybridizes only 65% and the NIH isolate hybridizes 35%. The latter two mouse strains are somewhat interesting with regard to xenotropic MLV production per se, in that no ecotropic MLV has ever been isolated from either strain. Furthermore, NZB mice chronically produce high titers of xenotropic virus throughout life, and most of the embryo-derived cell lines are also spontaneous virus producers.

Polymorphism of the structural virion proteins among xenotropic MLVs can be detected serologically. For example, type-specific differences on the pp12 *gag* protein and the gp70 *env* glycoprotein, which correlated roughly with the hybridization data mentioned above, were noted (Stephenson et al. 1974a,b, 1975; Hino et al. 1976). Whether the differences in pp12 antigens are reflected in the specific binding properties of pp12 for its homologous viral RNA (see Chapter 6) has not been determined. The gp70 molecules are generally the targets for neutralizing antisera; yet the antigenic differences noted in RIAs are not expressed in neutralization tests with appropriate antisera (Levy 1973) and therefore may not be associated with functional domains of the molecule. However, tryptic peptide analyses reveal a unique pattern for the NZB-MLV compared with all other xenotropic MLVs, including NIH-MLV (Lerner et al. 1976; Elder et al. 1977a). Obviously, such differences could reflect only subtle changes in amino acid sequence and may not be immunogenic.

Despite the absence of xenotropic MLV production in most mouse strains, it is interesting that molecules related to the NZB-MLV gp70 are found in the sera of strains of laboratory mice and feral mice (Hino et al. 1976; Lerner et al. 1976; Elder et al. 1977a; Bryant et al. 1978). The other type of xenotropic gp70 has also been detected in mouse sera (McClintock et al. 1977). However, the physiological role of the serum gp70 in the life of its host is totally unknown.

Uniquely, NZB adults and embryos spontaneously produce high titers of xenotropic virus. Patterns of expression in a variety of NZB hybrid crosses suggest that one (Stephenson and Aaronson

1974; Levy et al. 1979) or two (Datta and Schwartz 1976; Chused and Morse 1978) independently segregating autosomal dominant loci may be involved. The latter two, designated *Nzv-1* and *Nzv-2,* are held responsible for high and low levels of virus expression, respectively, and are considered to be regulatory genes, rather than structural genes (Datta and Schwartz 1977). On the basis of infectivity patterns in vitro (Chused and Morse 1978) and gp70 protein analysis (Elder et al. 1980), two distinct xenotropic NZB viruses have been observed. One (NZB-X1) spontaneously produced by NZB mice is unique and has the gp70 protein that is otherwise only found free in the sera of normal strains. The second (NZB-X2), revealed by IdU induction of NZB fibroblasts, has a gp70 resembling that of complete xenotropic MLV recovered from other strains. Furthermore, X1 and X2 may correspond to the high-titer and low-titer viruses regulated by the genetic loci *Nzv-1* and *Nzv-2,* respectively (Elder et al. 1980). Although a single locus (*Bxv-1*) for the induction of xenotropic virus has been mapped to the same site on chromosome 1 in five non-NZB strains, it is not thought to be the NZB inducibility gene and may represent viral sequences, rather than a regulatory locus (Kozak and Rowe 1978). The second NZB locus has not been examined for chromosome-1 linkage.

Mouse lymphocytes express cell-surface antigens (XenCSA) that cross-react with the gp70 of xenotropic MLV, but the amount differs greatly between strains and is largely independent of the level of infectious virus produced by the cells (Morse et al. 1979a,b). Such viral *env*-related antigens expressed on thymocytes and splenocytes apparently carry the determinants of NZB-X2 (Elder et al. 1980).

Although ecotropic MLV coexists with xenotropic MLV in many mouse strains, none have been isolated from adults or embryos of five different NZB colonies, either as infectious virus or as viral antigen after induction (Levy 1975; Stephenson et al. 1975; Datta and Schwartz 1978). There is also no evidence in vivo that ecotropic MLV or viral antigen is present in the lymphoid organs of preleukemic or leukemic NZB mice that have been X-irradiated or immunologically suppressed (Harvey et al. 1979a,b). This correlates well with the finding that no MCF viruses have been reported from NZB mice (Harvey et al. 1979b).

d. MCF Viruses. The first isolations of MCF viruses were from preleukemic or leukemic thymus tissues from strains of mice with high incidences of naturally occurring leukemias, e.g., AKR and C58 mice (Hartley et al. 1977). The prototype strain for many of the biological and biochemical studies is MCF 247. Although the viruses are dualtropic or polytropic (i.e., grow in mouse and heterologous cells), they can be distinguished from the wild-mouse amphotropic viruses on the basis of their neutralization and interference patterns; treatment with sera that neutralize either ecotropic MLV or xenotropic MLV destroys the infectivity of MCF viruses (Hartley et al. 1977). This phenomenon suggested that MCF viruses represent true genetic recombinants, a theory that has been confirmed and extended by several ensuing studies: (1) The MCF *env*-gene product gp70 contains tryptic peptides characteristic of both ecotropic and xenotropic MLVs (Elder et al. 1977b; Fischinger et al. 1978). (2) The location of the MCF recombinant *env* region has been defined to the carboxyterminal half of the gp70-coding region by oligonucleotide analysis (Faller et al. 1978; Rommelaere et al. 1978; Shih et al. 1978; Green et al. 1980), by reactivity with monoclonal antibodies (Niman and Elder 1980; O'Donnell and Nowinski 1980), and by heteroduplex mapping (Chien et al. 1978; Donoghue et al. 1978; Bosselman et al. 1979) (see Chapter 4).

Since the initial report and definition of the MCF virus group were made by Hartley et al. (1977), a number of other MCF viruses have been described. First, there are the isolates from preleukemic or leukemic tissues from other strains of mice that have a high incidence of leukemia: (1) from BALB/Mo mice, which contain an artificially introduced Mo-MLV in the germ line (Vogt 1979) (see Chapter 10); (2) from splenic reticulum-cell sarcomas (Cloyd et al. 1980); (3) from tissues of preleukemic or leukemic HRS/J mice (Green et al. 1980); and (4) from C3H thymomas and C3H/Fg leukemic spleens (Cloyd et al. 1980). Second, MCF viruses appear to be activated in mice exogenously infected with other MLV: (1) from spleens of mice inoculated with Friend virus (Troxler et al. 1978) and (2) from serum of SJL/J mice infected with the Rauscher leukemia virus complex (Van Griensven and Vogt 1980). Third, MCF-MLV has been identified in a BALB/c mouse inoculated with a cell-free extract of a graft-versus-host-induced nonthymic reticulum-cell neoplasm (Armstrong et al. 1980). Fourth, MCF virus was obtained from a pristane-induced transplantable plasmacytoma of BALB/c mice (Cloyd et al. 1980). Fifth, cell lines derived from radiation-induced thymomas contain MCF, as in the thymic epithelium cell lines from C57BL mice (Decleve et al. 1977; Haas 1978; Haas and Rashef 1980). Finally, MCF viruses appear to be frequent passengers in stocks of Mo-MLV: the HIX isolate (Fischinger et al. 1975), the Mo-MLV_{83} isolate (Troxler et al. 1977b), and the SMX-1 virus (Stockert et al. 1980). As expected, the N-tropic or B-tropic host-range pattern of the isolate reflects the ecotropic virus parent; e.g., those derived from NB-tropic Mo-MLV, Friend, or Rauscher viruses are NB tropic, those from highly leukemic mouse strains (all of which are *Fv-1*^{n} mice) are N tropic, and the isolates from *Fv-1*^{b} mice (BALB/c and C57BL) are B tropic. However, in no case has the xenotropic parent of the recombinant been identified.

BALB/c myeloma (immunoglobulin-producing B-cell) tumors, passaged in vivo or in vitro, have been reported to spontaneously produce virus with MCF activity (Spriggs et al. 1980). Furthermore, an NB-tropic host-range pattern was observed in mouse cells. Also uniquely, these isolates do not cross-interfere with either ecotropic or xenotropic MLV, although virus neutralization was accomplished with normal mouse sera that had neutralizing activity for xenotropic MLV, and the gp70 molecules contained tryptic peptides analogous to ecotropic and xenotropic gp70 molecules (and analogous to that of the BALB/c plasmacytoma MCF isolate described above) (Spriggs and Krueger 1981). Additionally, these myeloma isolates appeared to contain recombinant ecotropic and xenotropic *gag*-gene proteins (Spriggs and Krueger 1980). Further comparison of these isolates with other MCF viruses for serological and nucleic acid homologies should provide information on the origins of these viruses.

Most MCF isolates, and only one ecotropic MLV, induce a unique cell-surface antigen, $G^{(AKSL2)}$, on productively infected fibroblasts; this antigen is also found on cells of the thymus and other hematopoietic organs of preleukemic animals from strains that develop a high incidence of leukemia. In addition, animals expressing this antigen also contain detectable serum antibody to it (Stockert et al. 1979). The relevance of this antigen to leukemogenesis in these animals is at present unknown.

Cloyd et al. (1979) have obtained sera that detect antigens specific to MCF isolates. Three antigenic specificities have been determined: (1) MCFA-1, common to all MCF viruses; (2) MCFA-2, shared by the naturally occurring isolates only; and (3) MCFA-3, expressed by some, but not all, MCF isolates, without any specificity regarding origin. In terms of pathogenic properties, the MCF isolates fall into four categories: (1) those that are nonpathogenic, (2) those that prevent or decrease leukemia induced by other isolates (e.g., SMX-1), (3) those that accelerate naturally occurring leukemia in high-incidence strains of mice, and (4) those that are leukemogenic per se (see Chapter 8).

2. C-type Retroviruses of Feral Mice

A number of C-type retroviruses have been obtained from different subspecies of *M. musculus* and from other species of the genus *Mus*. The isolates fall into ecotropic, xenotropic, and amphotropic classes, and some appear to be quite distinct from any of the prototype viruses obtained from inbred mouse strains.

Certain demes (small, isolated populations) of wild mice (*Mus musculus domesticus*) in the La Puente and Lake Casitas regions of California have a high prevalence of MLV infection associated with a high incidence of spontaneous lymphoma and hind-limb paralysis disease of the central nervous system (Gardner et al. 1973a,b). Three classes of C-type viruses have been isolated directly from organs of these animals or from IdU-treated cultures of embryo cells. One is an N-tropic isolate that replicates in mouse cells only and elicits an XC syncytial cell response. However, it has immunological properties distinct from those of standard ecotropic and xenotropic MLVs of laboratory mice (Bryant and Klement 1976; Hartley and Rowe 1976). Generally, these ecotropic viruses were obtained only from those mice with paralysis and are capable of inducing hind-limb paralysis and/or nonthymic lymphomas about 6 months after injection into newborn NIH-Swiss mice (for review, see Gardner 1978) (Chapter 8).

The second virus type, which has been designated amphotropic (see discussion above), shows N tropism for mouse cells but also replicates in rat, rabbit, mink, guinea pig, cat, dog, and human cells (Hartley and Rowe 1976; Rasheed et al. 1976a). At least one isolate capable of replication in chicken cells (unlike all other MLVs studied) has been obtained (Rasheed et al. 1977). Amphotropic viruses, whether grown in mouse cells or in cells of heterologous species, do not elicit the XC syncytial cell response characteristic of many ecotropic MLVs. Furthermore, these viruses show interference and neutralization patterns distinct from those of standard ecotropic and xenotropic MLVs (Bryant and Klement 1976; Hartley and Rowe 1976) and neutralizing antibodies to the prototype La Puente strain (1504-A) do not neutralize the prototype Lake Casitas strain (4070-A) (Hartley and Rowe 1976). The latter results suggest that there is some polymorphism in the *env* antigenic determinants among various amphotropic MLV.

In populations of wild mice in which amphotropic MLV is prevalent, the major mode of infection appears to be transuterine or via exogenous infection, rather than the genetic transmission observed with MLV of laboratory mice (Gardner et al. 1976).

Amphotropic MLVs contain nucleic acid sequences not found in the genomes of a variety of ecotropic, xenotropic, and MCF viruses and are found in multiple copies within mouse-cell DNA (Chattopadhyay et al. 1978, 1980a; Rands et al. 1981). Some sequence diversity is also observed between different amphotropic isolates (Chattopadhyay et al. 1978). However, there is some controversy on the issue of the endogenous origin of these viruses, since Barbacid et al. (1979) claim that only part of the viral genomic sequences can be found in cellular DNA. This issue should be resolved by using either probes that are carefully monitored to represent the entire genome or probes obtained from molecularly cloned viruses. More homology is detected between amphotropic and ecotropic MLVs from wild mice than between the wild-mouse isolates and ecotropic or xenotropic isolates from inbred mice (Bryant et al. 1978b; Chattopadhyay et al. 1978; Barbacid et al. 1979).

In addition, using RIAs, there is diversity among the gp70 molecules isolated from different amphotropic MLVs (Barbacid et al. 1979). As determined by tryptic peptide analysis, the gp70 molecules from wild-mouse ecotropic isolates resemble those of other ecotropic MLVs, and the amphotropic gp70 molecules are more closely related to those of the xenotropic MLVs of AKR and NIH mice than to those of the NZB xenotropic MLV (Bryant et al. 1978).

The third type of isolate from these California mice is xenotropic in host range (Chattopadhyay et al. 1978) and can be induced from cultured embryo cells by IdU treatment followed by cocultivation with heterologous cells. Whether these xenotropic isolates are related to xenotropic MLVs from inbred strains of mice or to xenotropic MLVs from other species of *Mus* (see below) has not been reported.

Both ecotropic and xenotropic MLVs have been isolated from the Japanese subspecies *M. m. molossinus* (Bedigian and Meier 1975; Lieber et al. 1975c; Chattopadhyay et al. 1980a,b). The ecotropic isolate is N tropic, shares p30 antigenicity with ecotropic MLV isolated from laboratory mice, and exhibits a partial cross-reactivity with reverse transcriptase of Ra-MLV. Restriction enzyme analysis reveals that the ecotropic isolate from *M. m. molossinus* is essentially identical with the endogenous ecotropic MLV of AKR mice (Chattopadhyay et al. 1980a; Rands et al. 1981). The xenotropic isolate has a broad host range, infecting cells of rat, rabbit, dog, cat, horse, monkey, and human. It too shares common antigens with the p30 and reverse transcriptase of standard MLV (Lieber et al. 1975c). In nucleic acid hybridization studies, the *M. m. molossinus* xenotropic isolate shows about 95% homology with most xenotropic MLVs of inbred mouse strains; only 75% hybridization occurs to the xenotropic NZB isolate and only 44% to that from NIH mice (Callahan et al. 1975).

Yet another subspecies that originates in eastern Asia, *M. m. castaneus,* has provided a xenotropic MLV. This isolate shares host range and immunological properties with the xenotropic viruses of laboratory mice and of *M. m. molossinus* (Lieber et al. 1975c; Chattopadhyay et al. 1980a).

A heart cell line from the Asian mouse, *M. caroli,* following treatment with BrdU and cocultivation with heterologous cells, released an endogenous virus distinct from the viruses of laboratory and feral mice mentioned above (Lieber et al. 1975d; Benveniste et al. 1977). The virus has a limited host range, replicating in normal cat cells and nonproducer mink cells transformed by MSV, but not in cells derived from any *Mus* species. There is no cross-reaction with the species-specific and interspecies-specific determinants of the p30 of standard ecotropic or xenotropic MLV. However, a limited cross-reaction is noted with the reverse transcriptase of xenotropic MLV. Interestingly, the *M. caroli* virus, as judged by these same immunological criteria, shows marked homology with the infectious primate viruses, SSAV/GALV.

However, nucleic acid hybridization studies show less than 10% homology with ecotropic MLV, xenotropic MLV, or SSAV (despite the shared antigenic determinants). Still, the unexpected serological relationship between the *M. caroli* virus and SSAV/GALV suggests that it, or an ancestor, may be a progenitor of these primate viruses, or vice versa.

Finally, we should mention *M. cervicolor,* a mouse of southeast Asia that contains at least four distinct endogenous viruses. Two of these viruses more closely resemble B-type particles and are discussed in Section II.G.4. In addition, it is possible to induce two distinct C-type viruses from *M. cervicolor* (Benveniste et al. 1977). One, called CERV-CI, has a p30 and a reverse transcriptase related antigenically to the xenotropic virus of *M. caroli* and to the infectious SSAV/GALV primate viruses. As determined by nucleic acid hybridization, CERV-CI and the *M. caroli* virus are about 55% homologous with each other, which may account, in part, for some of the antigenic determinants they both share with SSAV/GALV. Less than 10% hybridization to any other retrovirus is observed. CERV-CI is endogenous to *M. cervicolor* (about six copies per haploid-cell genome) and has a xenotropic host range, replicating in rabbit, cat, and rhesus monkey cells, but not in mouse, rat, or human cells. The second isolate, CERV-CII, multiplies in cells of *M. musculus* (both $Fv\text{-}1^n$ and $Fv\text{-}1^b$) and in cells of other *Mus* species, with the exception of *M. cervicolor.* CERV-CII shows about 50% homology with ecotropic MLV and about 25% homology with xenotropic MLV, but less than 10% homology with CERV-CI.

On the basis of immunological criteria and, in some cases, nucleic acid hybridization studies, the retroviruses from *Mus* species other than *M. musculus* fall into at least four groups. First, there is the group that shares homology with SSAV/GALV; this includes isolates from *M. caroli, M. cervicolor* (CERV-CI), *M. cookii, M. dunni,* and *M. shortridgei.* All that is known about the latter three isolates is that they are antigenically related to other members of this group (Callahan and Todaro 1978). The second group contains those isolates related to ecotropic MLV of inbred mice; this group contains isolates from *M. cervicolor* (CERV-CII) and *M. cookii* (Callahan and Todaro 1978). The third and fourth groups are described in Section II.G.4 and comprise the M432 isolate of *M. cervicolor,* the M832 virus from *M. caroli,* and the

MMTV-related isolates from *M. cervicolor* and *M. cookii,* respectively. With the exception of the viruses of Californian wild mice mentioned above, no pathological role has been attributed to any of these C-type viruses of feral mice.

3. B-type Retroviruses of Inbred Mouse Strains

In the 1930s the development of several strains of inbred mice by repeated brother × sister matings was pursued by Little and later in collaboration with Strong. A few of these mouse strains exhibited high incidences of different neoplastic diseases and were carefully maintained. Two particularly interesting strains, C3H and A, were selected because about 90% of the females developed "spontaneous" mammary adenocarcinomas within 1 year of age (for review, see Little 1947). Classic genetic breeding experiments showed that the inheritance of this disease was transmitted to the offspring by the female parent in an extrachromosomal manner (Staff of Roscoe B. Jackson Memorial Laboratory 1933; Korteweg 1934, 1936). Several conceivable modes of disease transmission were considered, including the presence of an episomal cytoplasmic factor, intrauterine infection, and the presence of a factor in the milk of lactating mothers. In 1936 Bittner showed that the last possibility was correct, and subsequently, Bittner (1942b) and Andervont and Bryan (1944) presented evidence that the factor was a virus present in the milk. The advent of electron microscopy allowed Bernhard and Bauer (1955) to visualize the virus. The virus appeared as a particle 100–120 nm in diameter bound by a discrete membrane with an eccentrically located electron-dense nucleoid of about 70–75 nm in diameter, and it could be seen budding from the tumor-cell membranes. The extracellular form of the virus was called a B-type particle and is the morphological structure of what was then called the Bittner virus, milk-borne factor, or milk agent, which we now know as MMTV.

Since these early studies, many investigators have studied the structure, replication, and virus-host interactions of MMTV (see Chapters 5, 6, 8, and 10). Many studies have been hindered by the lack of an in vitro biological assay for this virus, a problem that still exists today. For this reason, the different virus strains isolated were classified according to the mouse strain of origin and their potency as a tumor agent. More recently, the use of sophisticated molecular techniques has resulted in many of the MMTVs being further classified by their proviral structure, often in conjunction with a genetic locus and chromosomal location (see below).

The results from many of the experiments performed in the 1950s and 1960s were confusing and led to controversy over the significance of MMTV as an important feature in mammary tumorigenesis (for review, see Hilgers and Bentvelzen 1978). Interpretation of these studies became easier with the discovery that many mouse strains harbor more than one MMTV, and these additional MMTVs were transmitted as endogenous genetic elements (see Chapters 8 and 10). Also, the finding that retroviruses replicate via a chromosomally integrated DNA intermediate made the vehicle of genetic transmission easier to comprehend. As several other chapters in this volume deal in some detail with the transmission, susceptibility to infection, and pathogenesis of MMTV in general (see Chapters 8 and 10), it will suffice here to outline the major findings in order to provide a framework to describe the classification of the most common MMTV strains.

Several inbred mouse strains that demonstrate a high incidence of mammary tumors carry a milk-borne (exogenous) MMTV, demonstrating the transmission characteristics originally described by Bittner (1936). A prototype mouse strain carrying this type of virus is C3H, and the virus isolated from this strain was initially designated MMTV-S (see Table 2.8). There are several other strains carrying similar MMTVs (e.g., A, RIII, and DBA/2) that are often considered to harbor MMTV-S. However, structural analyses (Michalides and Schlom 1975; Friedrich et al. 1976; Drohan et al. 1977; Gautsch et al. 1978b) and immunological analyses (Blair 1970, 1971; Hageman et al. 1972; Daams et al. 1973; Teramoto et al. 1977; Zavada et al. 1977; Teramoto and Schlom 1978; Massey et al. 1980) revealed differences between most of these MMTVs; hence, MMTVs represent a family of related polymorphic variants. Analysis of the proviral DNA structure using restriction endonucleases also shows MMTVs to be a multigene family (see Chapters 8 and 10). This has led many investigators to adopt a different classification scheme in which the MMTV is suffixed with the mouse strain of origin in parentheses, e.g., MMTV(RIII) (see Table 2.8). However, many of the strains also contain additional MMTV proviruses that are genetically transmitted (see Hilgers and Bentvelzen 1978; Moore et al. 1979; and Chapter 10, Tables 10.5 and 10.6).

Table 2.8 Common inbred mouse strains and their associated mouse mammary tumor viruses

Common name	Classification		Host mouse strain	Transmission	Genetic locus	Chromosomal allocation	Phenotype
	previous	present					
Bittner virus	MMTV-S	MMTV(C3H)	C3H	milk	n.a.[a]	n.a.	very oncogenic
Nodule-inducing virus	MMTV-L	MMTV(C3Hf)	C3H C3Hf	genetic (milk)	*mtv*-1[b]	7	weakly oncogenic
—	MMTV-P	MMTV(GR)	GR	genetic (milk)	*mtv*-2	18	very oncogenic
—	—	MMTV(RIII)	RIII	milk	n.a.	n.a.	very oncogenic
—	—	MMTV(RIIIf)	RIII RIIIf	genetic	?	?	weakly oncogenic
—	—	MMTV(DBA)	DBA	milk	n.a.	n.a.	oncogenic
—	—	MMTV(DBAf)	DBA DBAf	genetic (milk)	*mtv*-1[b]	7	weakly oncogenic
—	—	MMTV(A)	A	milk	n.a.	n.a.	oncogenic with pregnancy

[a]n.a. indicates not applicable; integration of proviruses varies considerably due to reinfections.
[b]MMTV(C3Hf) and MMTV(DBAf) are probably the same.

Foster nursing of neonatal mice that carry the highly oncogenic exogenous (milk-borne) virus on virus-free mothers (low-incidence strains such as C57BL) result in the loss of the milk-transmitted virus in descendants of the foster-nursed mice, whereas the genetically transmitted virus is retained and often expressed in the milk of lactating mothers (Pitelka et al. 1964; Hageman et al. 1968). Virus isolated from the milk of foster-nursed strains (e.g., C3Hf, the f designating that it is fostered and no longer contains the milk-transmitted MMTV) has a low oncogenic activity when injected into other susceptible mouse strains (Hageman et al. 1972) (see Table 2.8). In the C3Hf and DBAf mouse strains, the endogenous viruses, designated MMTV(C3Hf) or MMTV (DBAf), previously MMTV-L, are responsible for the low oncogenic activity and are identified in genetic breeding experiments as the *mtv-1* locus on chromosome 7 (see Chapters 8 and 10). The presence of these weakly oncogenic virus strains (40% tumors after 1–2 years) still remaining endogenous to foster-nursed C3H animals caused a lot of the early controversy over whether MMTV, in this case MMTV(C3H), was really responsible for mammary tumorigenesis or only accelerated the disease.

The GR/A strain of mouse (Mühlbock 1965) is unusual in that it harbors a highly oncogenic MMTV that is transmitted genetically (Bentvelzen 1968). This virus induces a tumor that is initially dependent on the hormonal changes induced by pregnancy; the early tumor is called a plaque, hence the original classification of the virus as MMTV-P (see Table 2.8). This mouse strain has been extensively studied, and the biologically active endogenous provirus was identified at a single locus (*mtv-2*) (see Chapters 8 and 10).

Molecular analyses have demonstrated the presence of multiple MMTV proviral elements in many strains of inbred mice. A few, like the *mtv-1* and *mtv-2* loci, have been associated with biologically active MMTV, both in terms of virus replication and oncogenicity. Many other endogenous proviral elements of similar molecular structure have been identified in mouse strains of both high- and low-incidence mice, but these have not been associated with either expression or disease. The reason these proviruses are not expressed remains an important question for future studies. It is possible that some of these proviruses may be structurally defective, representing pseudoproviruses analogous to the recently identified pseudogenes, or they may be suppressed, as are most genes in cells in which their differentiation-specific products are not normally expressed.

One other feature concerning the distribution of MMTV proviruses should be noted: not all feral mice contain endogenous MMTV proviruses (Cohen and Varmus 1979), suggesting that the acquisition of these elements in evolutionary terms is a very recent event for *M. musculus*. On the other hand, several other mouse species do contain MMTV-like elements, as determined by DNA hybridization (Morris et al. 1977) and by immunological criteria (Hand et al. 1980; Teramoto et al. 1980). Furthermore, MMTV-related viruses have been isolated from at least two other *Mus* species (see Section II.G.4). Thus, MMTVs are a multigene family existing in both endogenous and exogenous forms that are associated with most mouse strains.

4. B-type Retroviruses of Feral Mice

M. cervicolor mice from Thailand contain at least four endogenous viruses. Two of these were morphologically C-type and have been discussed in Section II.G.2. The third isolate, called M432, was isolated by cocultivation of spleen cells with cells of heterologous species and appears to have morphological and biochemical characteristics that are intermediate between B-type and C-type viruses (Callahan et al. 1976a). For example, the virions resemble B-type particles in that (1) intracytoplasmic A-type particles are observed, (2) particles with doughnut-shaped nucleoids are seen to bud from the plasma membrane, and (3) its reverse transcriptase activity is Mg^{++}-dependent. On the other hand, the virions differ from MMTV B-type particles in that (1) the intracytoplasmic (83-nm diameter) and the extracellular (110-nm diameter) particles are smaller, (2) the nucleoids are central rather than eccentric, and (3) the particles lack surface spikes. Furthermore, no immunological relatedness to MMTV has been detected.

M432 virions contain the major structural proteins, gp65, gp32, p24, p16, pp12, and a reverse transcriptase of 70,000 daltons (Callahan et al. 1977). Antigenic cross-reactivity between p24 and the major protein (p73) of intracisternal A-type particles is detectable in RIAs, although as yet the other structural proteins, including reverse transcriptase, appear unrelated (Kuff et al. 1980). This finding is supported by the degree of homology (20–30%) observed in nucleic acid hybridization studies between the two types of particles (Kuff et al. 1978).

The host range of M432 virus is limited to *M. musculus* cells of both *Fv-1*^{n} and *Fv-1*^{b} types and, as judged by viral reverse transcriptase activity, replication is greater in the *Fv-1*^{n} cells; it fails to replicate in *M. cervicolor* cells and in xenogeneic cells (Callahan et al. 1976a). As judged from nucleic acid hybridization, the genome of M432 virus of *M. cervicolor* is not related to ecotropic MLV, xenotropic MLV of laboratory mice, xenotropic virus of *M. caroli,* the two endogenous C-type viruses of *M. cervicolor,* MMTV, MPMV, or bovine leukemia virus (BLV). The cells of *M. cervicolor* appear to contain about 25 endogenous copies of the viral genome per haploid-cell genome, and some related sequences can also be detected in *M. musculus* and *M. caroli* (Benveniste et al. 1977).

An endogenous virus immunologically and biochemically closely related to M432 has been isolated from the Japanese mouse *M. caroli* (Callahan et al. 1977; Callahan and Todaro 1978). The virus (M832) was spontaneously released from a heart cell line after more than 3 years in culture and replicates in *M. musculus,* but not in *M. caroli,* cells. M832 shares antigenic determinants with M432 on the reverse transcriptase and the major core protein p24. About 25% sequence homology is also detected between the two viruses in hybridization experiments in which no significant homology is observed with any other B-type, C-type, or D-type retroviruses. Thus, it would appear that these two viruses represent a unique class of retroviruses.

In addition to the M432 isolate, particles closely resembling B-type viruses have been observed in the milk of the subspecies *M. cervicolor popaeus* (Schlom et al. 1978). These particles, called MC-MTV, exhibit a partial cross-reactivity to antigens on the major *gag* protein p27 and the major *env* glycoprotein gp52 of MMTV. No cross-reactivity is observed with other B-type viruses (e.g., the endogenous guinea pig retrovirus) or C-type viruses. However, particles obtained from milk extracts of mammary tumor cells from another wild-mouse species, *M. cookii,* also share the antigen displayed on MMTV p27 (Hand et al. 1980). Morphologically, the *M. cervicolor popaeus* and *M. cookii* particles appear indistinguishable from MMTVs obtained from inbred strains of mice. Additionally, the reverse transcriptase reaction is enhanced preferentially by Mg^{++}, rather than by Mn^{++}.

Although high levels of expression of these wild-mouse MMTV-related isolates occur in lactating mammary glands and in mammary tumors (Hand et al. 1980), it is not yet known whether the viruses are etiological agents of the mammary carcinomas that occur in these feral populations. Interestingly, none of these Asian mice seem to lack MMTV-like proviruses, whereas a few of the wild mice (*M. musculus*) found in the Lake Casitas region of California (Cohen and Varmus 1979) and mice from certain demes of Morocco (*M. musculus brevirostris*) and Czechoslovakia (*M. musculus musculus*) (W. Drohan et al., pers. comm.) do not contain any MMTV-related cellular DNA sequences. One can argue that these findings suggest that MMTV proviruses are a recent acquisition by the germ line or, conversely, that they are slowly being eliminated during the course of evolution; this is a moot question at the moment.

On the basis of experiments reported here and in Section II.G.1, *M. cervicolor* is a species that contains four endogenous retroviruses (representing about 0.04% of the total cellular genome); this species is resistant to infection (i.e., all the recovered viruses have had xenotropic host ranges), although it supports the replication of a xenotropic virus from BALB/c mice. Moreover, the four *M. cervicolor* viruses share less than 10% homology with one another. The issue of multigene families and the origins of the various endogenous retroviruses are the subjects of further discussion in Chapter 10.

H. Rat C-type Retroviruses

During the last decade, C-type particles have been observed in, or isolated from, a number of cell lines derived from several rat tumors, including spontaneous mammary carcinomas (Engle et al. 1969; Chopra et al. 1970b), chemically induced mammary carcinomas (Bergs et al. 1970; Chopra and Taylor 1970), the transplantable Novikoff hepatoma (Karasaki 1969), chemically induced hepatomas (Weinstein et al. 1972), tumors induced by MSV (Ting 1968; Aaronson 1971a; Gilden et al. 1971), and spontaneous leukemias (Chopra et al. 1970a). C-type viruses have also been detected in normal or chemically transformed rat kidney cell lines (Rhim et al. 1972, 1973a; Freeman et al. 1973) and spontaneously transformed rat embryo fibroblasts (Gazzolo et al. 1971; Bergs et al.

1972; Rhim et al. 1972). Particles have been observed in the junctional zone between maternal and fetal cell layers of placentas obtained from normal healthy rats (Gross et al. 1975), and sporadic production of virus also occurs in cultures of morphologically normal rat cell lines (Teitz et al. 1971; Klement et al. 1973; Rasheed et al. 1976c). It is also possible to induce virus production with the halogenated pyrimidines, IdU and BrdU (Aaronson 1971b; Klement et al. 1971, 1972; Grolle et al. 1973; Verwoerd and Sarma 1973). As these observations have been made with a wide range of tissues from a variety of inbred strains of rats, it is safe to conclude that C-type particles are ubiquitous in rats.

The infectivity of rat C-type viruses (called rat leukemia virus, although none are leukemogenic) is rather low, and those that have been studied replicate only in rat cells; i.e., they are ecotropic. Furthermore, although many attempts have been made to induce neoplastic disease in neonatal rats with purified virus, none have been successful. It appears, therefore, that these viruses have no oncogenic potential despite their isolation from a variety of tumor cells (Grolle et al. 1973; Klement et al. 1973).

The viral particles have the classic C-type morphological, biochemical, and biophysical properties; they have a buoyant density in sucrose of 1.16 g/ml and they contain 70S RNA and reverse transcriptase activity with Mn^{++} preference. The major structural polypeptides are gp70, p30, p 5, p12, and p10; the latter two are phosphorylated (Pal et al. 1975) and it is thought that p10 may be a breakdown product of p12 (Parks et al. 1974). The p30 protein contains the interspecies-specific antigenicity that cross-reacts with hamster and cat C-type viruses more strongly than with the murine viruses (Oroszlan et al. 1972a; Charman et al. 1974; Scolnick et al. 1974a). Neither spontaneous nor chemically induced isolates exhibit any type-specific antigenic differences on the p30 molecule, as determined by RIAs (Charman et al. 1974, 1976b), on the gp70 protein (Bergs et al. 1972; Pearson et al. 1972) or on the p12 molecule (Scolnick et al. 1974a), as measured by immunofluorescence or neutralization kinetics. The particles induced by halogenated pyrimidines appear, however, to be more fragile than spontaneously released particles; most of the virion RNA in the former is of low molecular weight, and the particles often have little or no biological activity (Klement et al. 1973).

Although there seems to be serological identity among the different endogenous rat viruses, molecular hybridization studies can detect some differences in the RNA sequences. Approximately 70–95% homology is detected among the three rat isolates, VNRK, RT21C, and CCL38 (Benveniste and Todaro 1973; Scolnick et al. 1974a). However, essentially no cross-hybridization is detected to MLV, FeLV, RD114, or SSAV/GALV.

Nucleic acid hybridization reveals that there are endogenous proviral sequences in the cellular DNA extracted from several rat strains (Tsuchida et al. 1975). There appear to be about 100 copies of sequences homologous to approximately 85% of the viral genome and about 10 copies homologous to the remaining 15% in each haploid-cell genome. There also are multiple copies of the DNA of viruslike 30S RNA in rat cells, and the level of transcription is increased by exposing the cells to BrdU (Scolnick et al. 1974a; Tsuchida et al. 1975). Moreover, the 30S sequences are often packaged into virions produced by rat cells after exogenous infection with MLV or other mammalian C-type viruses (Scolnick et al. 1974a, 1976a); 30S RNA molecules, discussed in greater detail in Chapter 10, are associated with the generation of Ki-MSV and Ha-MSV (see Chapters 4 and 9).

R-35 is a rat-tropic virus with transforming potential in vitro (Ahmed et al. 1972). It was isolated from an adenocarcinoma that arose during the in vivo passage of a spontaneous rat mammary fibroadenoma. R-35 induces foci in cultures of mammary tissue from lactating rats that have been treated with hydrocortisone but does not transform other rat cell types; therefore, it is possible that the target cell for transformation is a glandular epithelial cell rather than stromal fibroblasts. As one of the few rat C-type viruses with transforming potential, this virus deserves greater attention.

As mentioned above, Ha-MSV and Ki-MSV were derived by passage of MLV in rats (see Section II.G.1) and represent recombinants between the endogenous 30S RNA elements of rat cells, endogenous rat oncogene sequences (called *c-ras*), and the helper MLV (see Chapters 4 and 9). The two MSVs are highly related and encode a similar *ras*-gene product (Scolnick and Parks 1974; Shih et al. 1979) (see Chapter 9). Interestingly, the rescue of related transformation-specific *ras* sequences has been accomplished in vitro and resulted in the generation of stable rat sarcoma viruses (Rasheed et al. 1978; Rasheed 1980). The procedure involved cocultivation of a Sprague-Dawley rat embryo cell culture (SD-1-T), a spontaneously transformed line that releases an endogenous C-type virus, i.e., Sprague-Dawley rat leukemia virus, with any of three chemically transformed rat tumor cell lines. Cell-free supernates from these cocultures induced focus formation with two-hit kinetics on rat cells, although no foci were detectable on mink, cat, bat, or human cells. Rat sarcoma virus can be rescued from nonproducer transformed cells by a variety of mammalian retroviruses; however, superinfection of the original rat tumor cell lines by any of these helper viruses does not result in the generation of a rat sarcoma virus, suggesting that there is a very specific interaction between Sprague-Dawley rat leukemia virus and the endogenous cellular *ras* sequences. Although cells transformed by rat sarcoma virus form transplantable tumors in rats, this is also a property of the parental SD-1-T cells; there is no direct evidence yet for tumor induction in vivo by rat sarcoma virus.

The relationship between viral DNA sequences endogenous to rat cells and carcinogenesis is unclear. There is a strong positive correlation between the expression of endogenous virus genes and the efficiency of spontaneous or chemical transformation in vitro of rat embryo cells (Freeman et al. 1973); the appearance of detectable amounts of viral antigens or virus production often precedes spontaneous transformation. Moreover, infection of rat cells with rat leukemia virus renders them more susceptible to transformation. The tumorigenicity of rat cells in vivo does not, however, correlate with the production of viral particles, but rather with the appearance of morphological changes in vitro (Rasheed et al. 1976b).

I. Tree Mouse C-type Retrovirus

The number of isolates of retrovirus from rodent species has recently been increased by the isolation of a virus from the long-tailed tree mouse *Vandeleuria oleracea* (Callahan et al. 1979) belonging to the family Muridae.

The virus was isolated from a kidney cell line derived from *V. oleracea* after 24 weeks in culture and can be propagated easily in human and cat cells. It also replicates in rabbit, bat, and mink cells, but not in chimpanzee, dog, or a variety of mouse (*M. cervic-*

olor, M. caroli, M. dunni, M. shortridgei, and *M. musculus*) cell lines. In this respect, the virus designated Vand C-I, might be considered xenotropic in host range.

Antigenically, two viral structural proteins, p30 and reverse transcriptase, show cross-reactivity with the respective proteins of the SSAV/GALV group of viruses, whereas no homology has been detected with any murine retroviral proteins. The degree of competition detected in RIAs suggests that Vand C-I is partially, but not completely, related to these primate viruses. In addition, the virus shows some cross-reactivity to porcine C-type virus. No further biochemical analysis of Vand C-I has yet been reported.

A cDNA probe made from the Vand C-I viral RNA showed that the virus is endogenous to *V. oleracea* (the only member of the *Vandeleuria* genus), with some related sequences in DNA samples from most other rodents, proportional to the evolutionary divergence. It is interesting that about 75 copies of viral genetic material are detected per haploid-cell genome in *Vandeleuria,* with T_m values indicating extensive mismatching. This suggests that there are other partially related endogenous virogenes in this genus.

As determined by nucleic acid hybridization reactions, little homology is detected between Vand C-I and any other virus tested, including several rodent isolates and SSAV/GALV isolates with which it shares some antigenic specificities.

J. Hamster C-type Retroviruses

The presence of C-type particles within a hamster tumor (Stenback et al. 1966) and the cell-free transmission of leukemia using an extract of the tumor cells suggested a viral etiology for the disease (Graffi et al. 1968). However, it was not until a number of investigators had induced tumors in newborn hamsters with MSV that the existence of an infectious hamster virus was realized (Bassin et al. 1968; Klement et al. 1969; Perk et al. 1969; Kelloff et al. 1970a–c, 1971, 1973; Sarma et al. 1970a). Hamster tumors induced by MSV were found to release an infectious focus-forming virus that had lost the ability to infect mouse cells. Although the focus-forming and sarcomagenic potentials of this hamster virus are derived from the defective MSV used to induce the hamster tumors, the helper virus, designated HaLV, which rescues the defective

MSV genome, was shown by immunological tests to be of nonmurine origin.

The hamster-tropic, focus-forming pseudotypes of MSV, designated MSV(HaLV), do not contain antigens that cross-react in complement fixation or immunodiffusion tests with the group-specific antigenic determinant of the MLVs. (This determinant, originally called gs-1, is now known to be one of the antigenic sites of the major internal virion core protein, p30.) However, as expected, these MSV pseudotypes contain an antigen that cross-reacts with the interspecies-specific determinant gs-3 of the mammalian C-type viruses (Kelloff et al. 1970b; Freeman et al. 1971; Nowinski et al. 1971a,b; Oroszlan et al. 1971). It is interesting that in all stocks of MSV(HaLV) pseudotypes tested so far, the murine internal core protein p30 could not be detected. This suggests that when propagated in hamster cells, the MSV genome either loses the p30 component of the *gag* gene or cannot properly express it, so that only the hamster internal polypeptide is available for incorporation into progeny virions.

Focus formation by MSV(HaLV) cannot be neutralized by antiserum to MSV(MLV), but antiserum to one isolate of MSV(HaLV) neutralizes any other isolate of the pseudotype. Furthermore, from endpoint titration of focus formation by a stock of MSV(HaLV), a pool of HaLV free of any MSV pseudotypes was isolated, and this HaLV specifically interfered with focus formation by other MSV-(HaLV) pseudotypes (Kelloff et al. 1970a). These findings prove that in addition to acquiring a new major core polypeptide, MSV(HaLV) pseudotypes have envelope specificities distinct from those of murine viruses.

Although Kelloff et al. (1970a) obtained a stock of HaLV by endpoint titration, it has proved difficult to obtain HaLV routinely in this way. Two factors appear to reduce the chances of success in cloning HaLV free of MSV(HaLV). First, the HaLV helper is only at about a ten-fold excess of the focus-forming MSV(HaLV). Second, HaLV proves not to be highly infectious. Why this is the case has not been established, but the reverse transcriptase of HaLV has only a low capacity to synthesize DNA in vitro using the endogenous template (Somers et al. 1973; Verma et al. 1974), and, therefore, it may be that the majority of HaLV particles are incapable of making a provirus.

The obstacles to obtaining pure HaLV have been circumvented

in three ways: (1) Chemical transformation of hamster embryo cells in vitro with 3-methylcholanthrene, 7,12-dimethylbenzanthracene, or with extracts of cigarette smoke and subsequent serial transplantation of the transformed cells has led to the "activation" of HaLV in the tumor tissues (Freeman et al. 1971). (2) Chemical induction of tumors in hamsters in vivo by these same compounds or by the papovaviruses (SV40 and polyoma virus) has given rise to infectious HaLV (Freeman et al. 1974). (3) Treatment of Chinese or Syrian hamster cell lines with IdU (Lieber et al. 1973; Todaro 1973) or with dibutyryl cAMP (Tihon and Green 1973) has been an efficient means of inducing virus. Stocks of MSV-free HaLV have been obtained from these sources, and the virus has been biochemically characterized.

Electron microscopy reveals that the morphology and morphogenesis of HaLV are typical of C-type viruses, and in sucrose the particles have the characteristic buoyant density of 1.16 g/ml. The reverse transcriptase, which requires Mn^{++} for activity (Gazdar et al. 1971), is a protein with a molecular weight of 120,000 daltons, consisting of two subunits, with molecular weights estimated from their electrophoretic mobilities in SDS-polyacrylamide gels to be 68,000 and 53,000 daltons (Verma et al. 1974). The major internal polypeptide, originally reported to have a molecular weight of 35,000–37,000 (Oroszlan et al. 1971), has a molecular weight of only 27,000 (Charman et al. 1974). RIAs fail to reveal any type-specific differences between different HaLV isolates; however, the interspecies-specific antigenic determinant of p27 is more closely related to those of feline and rat viruses than to those of murine viruses (Charman et al. 1974).

Nucleic acid hybridization experiments have led to three major conclusions: (1) All HaLV isolates show marked sequence homology with one another, but little homology with any other retroviruses. (2) Sequences homologous to a large portion of the viral RNA occur in the cellular DNA of all inbred hamster strains tested, both in embryo and adult tissues. This confirms the conclusion from induction experiments that HaLV is an endogenous ecotropic virus of this species. (3) Hybridization experiments indicate that one of the MSV(HaLV) pseudotypes, $GLOH^-$, may be a recombinant virus between the endogenous hamster virus and the tumor-inducing MSV(MLV) and, as such, is an interesting virus for further study (Okabe et al. 1974).

Although the sarcomagenic potential of stocks of MSV(HaLV) has been repeatedly demonstrated by injecting the virus into susceptible hamsters, very little indeed is known about the leukemogenic activities of pure HaLV isolates. However, nucleic acid hybridization studies have revealed that the amount of virus-specific RNA is significantly greater in tumor tissue than in normal tissue, implying that the neoplastic process or environment is correlated with the activation of expression of endogenous HaLV (Tsuchida et al. 1975).

Finally, it is worth mentioning that the spontaneous release, at a low level, of HaLV from cultured hamster cells has been reported; the spontaneously released viruses infect hamsters cells, but attempts to infect mouse, rat, cat, monkey, and human cells have failed (Lieber et al. 1973).

K. Cavian Retroviruses

The Caviomorpha suborder contains the New World rodents and diverged from the Myomorpha suborder (consisting of the Old World rodents such as mice, rats, and hamsters) about 50–55 million years ago. Two distinct retroviruses have been isolated from cavian genera: (1) the B-type virus of guinea pigs (*Cavia porcellus*) and (2) the C-type virus of the agouti (*Dasyprocta punctata*).

1. Guinea Pig B-type Retrovirus

Guinea pigs (cavies) have their own endogenous retrovirus that, in the past, has often been called a C-type virus. Morphological and biochemical studies, however, now indicate that this virus more closely resembles the B-type viruses.

The L2C strain of transplantable guinea pig leukemia arose spontaneously (Congdon and Lorenz 1954) in the strain-2 inbred line of guinea pigs. Later, intracellular and extracellular viruslike particles were observed in these cultured cells (Nadel et al. 1967; Opler 1967). The intracellular particles appear to bud from membranes of the rough endoplasmic reticulum into intracisternal spaces (Feldman and Gross 1970) and, in this way, resemble intracisternal A-type particles seen in the mouse. Similar particles have been observed in primordial germ cells (principally in gonocytes of testes and oogonia of ovaries) of fetal guinea pigs (Black 1974), in spleen germinal centers of normal guinea pigs (Ma et al. 1969), and in a chemically induced guinea pig hepatoma (Dunkel et al. 1974). Extracellular particles have been reported in the tissues of leukemic guinea pigs in the absence of any apparent budding of virions from the plasma membrane (Feldman and Gross 1970) and in the plasma of animals carrying the transplantable leukemia (Nayak et al. 1975).

Studies of the virus were greatly advanced by the discovery that treatment of guinea pig cells (normal and leukemic) with the halogenated pyrimidines BrdU and IdU induces production of viral particles from previously virus-negative cells (Hsiung 1972; Nayak and Murray 1973; Rhim et al. 1973b, 1974). The induced guinea pig virus appears to be morphologically and biochemically similar to the virus present in the plasma of leukemic guinea pigs (Michalides et al. 1976).

Several parameters of the induced virus are more closely related to those of the B-type MMTV than to those of the C-type mammalian viruses:

1. Buoyant density. Although these particles have often been reported to band at 1.16 g/ml in sucrose and 1.17 g/ml in cesium chloride gradients (Gross et al. 1973; Nayak and Murray 1973), there is one report claiming densities of 1.18 g/ml and 1.2 g/ml in sucrose and cesium chloride, respectively (Michalides et al. 1975).
2. Divalent cation preference of the virion reverse transcriptase. The reverse transcriptase of guinea pig virus preferentially uses Mg^{++}, rather than Mn^{++}, in the presence of exogenous template primer (Nayak and Murray 1973; Michalides et al. 1975).
3. Interspecies-specific (gs-3) antigen. Neither MMTV nor the guinea pig virus cross-react in numerous immunological assays with the gs-3 antigens of mouse, rat, feline, hamster, and woolly monkey C-type viruses (Rhim et al. 1973b).
4. Morphological features. The difficulty in assigning the guinea pig virus to the C-type or B-type class arises because it shares some properties with both classes and has other features that are atypical and make it unique. A survey of the reported morphological studies includes descriptions of intracisternal particles, intracytoplasmic particles, and extracellular particles. Early studies on leukemic lymphocytes cultured in vitro re-

vealed the presence of intracisternal particles that are attached to the membranes of the rough endoplasmic reticulum (Nadel et al. 1967; Opler 1967; Feldman and Gross 1970). In BrdU-treated cultures, intracytoplasmic particles and extracellular particles are observable (Gross et al. 1973; Nayak and Murray 1973; Dahlberg et al. 1974; Fong and Hsiung 1976; Michalides et al. 1976). The intracytoplasmic particles are approximately 80 nm in diameter with a central electron-lucent nucleoid. The extracellular particles are larger (100–110 nm) with either a central or eccentric electron-dense nucleoid, and some have long surface spikes. Those particles seen budding from the plasma membrane always appear to have complete nucleoids (Dahlberg et al. 1974; Fong and Hsiung 1976). Studies on normal guinea pig tissues from embryos and adults revealed predominantly intracisternal particles of 90–100 nm (Ma et al. 1969; Feldman and Gross 1970; Anderson and Jeppesen 1972; Rhim et al. 1973b; Black 1974; Hsiung et al. 1974; Fong and Hsiung 1976).

Analysis of the structural proteins of the virion by polyacrylamide gel electrophoresis revealed five major peaks: gp70, gp36, p24, p18, and p16 (Murray and Nayak 1974). The virion RNA has been shown to be a 65S–70S complex that dissociates in formamide to yield 36S subunits (Nayak and Murray 1973). Estimates of the molecular weights of the RNA are 7×10^6 to 10×10^6 for the 70S molecule and 2.6×10^6 for the subunit (Nayak 1974; Michalides et al. 1975).

Radiolabeled viral RNA has been utilized in nucleic acid hybridization reactions to clarify several points: (1) No homology has been detected between the guinea pig viral RNA and the genomic RNAs of MLV, MMTV, HaLV, or MPMV (Michalides et al. 1975). (2) Over 90% sequence homology has been detected between the induced guinea pig virus and the virus found in the plasma of leukemic guinea pigs (Michalides et al. 1976). (3) Sequences complementary to the guinea pig viral RNA has been detected in the cellular DNA isolated from normal, as well as leukemic, guinea pigs, but not from tissues derived from heterologous species. Michalides et al. (1976) estimate that there are approximately 80 copies of complementary DNA per haploid-cell genome, whereas Nayak (1974) detected about 2–3 copies of about 60% of the viral genome and 150 copies homologous to the rest of the viral genome. These estimates have now been revised to 2 copies and 12 copies, respectively (Nayak and Davis 1976). Studies with molecularly cloned virus could resolve these issues. The cardinal point, however, is that the virus is an endogenous one and therefore is transmitted by inheritance.

Attempts to propagate the virus in cultured cells from guinea pigs, mice, rats, or humans have been unsuccessful (Murray and Nayak 1974). The only productive system in vitro appears to be guinea pig cells grown in the continuous presence of BrdU. Likewise, transmission of the disease has been accomplished only by inoculation of animal with spleen cells or plasma from leukemic hosts (Hsiung et al. 1973; Murray and Nayak 1974). Preparations of purified virus have not caused disease in newborn or adult guinea pigs, although hepatosplenomegaly has been observed in animals receiving the retrovirus and a guinea pig herpesvirus simultaneously (Hsiung et al. 1973).

2. Agouti C-type Retrovirus

The isolation of a retrovirus from the agouti was accomplished by cocultivation of agouti tissue with a variety of cell lines. After 2 months, reverse transcriptase activity was detected in the cocultures with the cell line A547 from a human lung tumor (Sherwin et al. 1979). The virus, called DPC-1, was readily transmitted to human and cat cells, but not to cells of the bat, dog, mink, rabbit, mouse, or owl monkey. In contrast to the endogenous guinea pig retrovirus isolate, DPC-1 shows features characteristic of C-type viruses in morphology and Mn^{++} requirement for reverse transcriptase activity.

DPC-1 virus is not closely related by hybridization of a cDNA probe to any known endogenous retroviruses. Nevertheless, there is cross-reaction of interspecies determinants between its p30 structural protein and those of SSAV, mouse, and pig retroviruses. Furthermore, the activity of DPC-1 viral polymerase can be partially inhibited by antisera to rat, SSAV, and FeLV polymerases.

Hybridization of DPC-1 cDNA to cellular DNA derived from a variety of mammals shows that the virus is endogenous to the agouti. Very little homology can be detected with the closely related guinea pig or with other rodents and mammals. The kinetics of hybridization suggest that there are 75–100 copies of viral sequences in agouti cellular DNA. Thus, DPC-1 represents the first transmissible endogenous C-type virus from a New World rodent species.

L. Rabbit C-type Particles

Viruslike particles have recently been induced from lymphosarcoma material derived from the WH/J strain of rabbits (Bedigian et al. 1978). Electron microscopic examination of the cells revealed no viral particles until after treatment with IdU; the particles are about 95 nm in diameter and are observed to bud from the cell membrane. Further cultivation of the lymphosarcoma material led to the loss of reticulum cells and to the appearance of predominantly fibroblasts; at this stage the cells were no longer susceptible to IdU induction. No particles were induced from normal rabbit tissues.

After the IdU treatment, there is a transient appearance of RNA-directed DNA polymerase activity at 2–3 days posttreatment. Subsequently, the reverse transcriptase activity declines, although it is reinducible with IdU; both particles and enzyme activity band isopycnically at 1.17 g/ml in sucrose. The enzyme shows a preferential requirement for Mn^{++} and can be partially inhibited by antisera to the polymerases of FeLV, GALV, and RT21C (an endogenous rat virus). An antigen cross-reacting with broadly reactive p30 antisera is also detected after induction (Bedigian et al. 1976, 1978), although the concentration is low.

Unfortunately, it has not yet been possible to find a permissive host cell for the replication of this viruslike particle, making further characterization difficult. However, a cDNA probe from the particle RNA detects related sequences in normal rabbit liver as well as in the lymphosarcomatous material, but not in mouse-cell DNA, suggesting that the particle is endogenous to rabbits.

M. Feline C-type Retroviruses

Another recently burgeoning field of interest in retrovirology is that of C-type viruses among the feline species, particularly the domestic cat (*Felis catus*). The accumulated knowledge on this subject in the last 8 years has changed the mention of feline retroviruses from the status of text ancillary to that of other retroviruses (as in Tooze 1973) into an extensive coverage. The existence of C-type viruses associated with leukemias, lymphomas, and fibrosarcomas of cats is particularly significant, not only because of the infective and oncogenic nature of the viruses, but also because of the association of the viruses with naturally occurring neoplasms in an outbred mammalian population (Jarrett et al. 1964a,b; Kawakami et al. 1967; Rickard et al. 1967; Snyder and Theilen 1969; for review see, Essex 1975 and Hardy et al. 1980).

There are several distinct types of feline C-type viruses: (1) FeLVs are ecotropic viruses and are classified into several subgroups according to serological and host-range properties. They are responsible for a wide spectrum of diseases, including lymphatic leukemia, lymphosarcoma, thymoma, myeloid leukemia, monocytoid leukemia, erythroleukemia, myelosclerosis, anemia, polycythemia vera, panmyelosis, immunosuppression, glomerulonephritis, reproductive failure, and abortion (for review, see Jarrett 1975; Jarrett 1980). The diversity of these diseases suggests that specific virus isolates may be responsible for a particular pathogenic process. For example, FeLV isolates of one serotype (see below) are always obtained from anemic, rather than leukemic, cats and predominantly cause anemia (Jarrett 1980); similar limitations in pathogenic potential may soon be discerned for other isolates. Further details on pathogenicity are presented in Chapter 8. (2) FeSVs are replication-defective (similar to MSV) and are thus always isolated as pseudotypes of FeLV. Because FeSVs are derived by recombination of FeLV with cellular *onc* sequences (see Chapter 9), they are highly related to FeLV by nucleic acid homology and immunological criteria. Together, FeLV and FeSV constitute a single related group. (3) The endogenous xenotropic viruses, including the RD114 and CCC isolates, form a second virus group and can be distinguished from the prototype FeLV/ FeSV class by host-range patterns (Fischinger et al. 1973; Livingston and Todaro 1973; Sarma et al. 1973), serology (Boone et al. 1973; Oroszlan et al. 1972b, 1973; Gilden et al. 1974), and molecular and biophysical characterization (Oroszlan et al. 1972b; East et al. 1973). In addition, none of the RD114/CCC group members are oncogenic.

The most important finding of this model system, however, is the very strong evidence for a horizontal mode of transmission of feline leukemia/sarcoma (Rickard et al. 1969; Brodey et al. 1970; Essex and Snyder 1973; W. Jarrett et al. 1973), and even animals infected as adults can transmit the virus and cause viremia and tumors in other adults (see Chapter 8).

1. Feline Leukemia and Sarcoma Viruses

The conventional FeLV was first isolated from a naturally occurring lymphosarcoma, the most common hematopoietic neoplasm in the cat. Jarrett et al. (1964a,b) showed unequivocally that the etiological agent was a virus that could be experimentally transmitted to young kittens. Electron microscopy studies showed the obvious morphological relationship to the avian and murine C-type viruses (Jarrett et al. 1964b). Subsequently, FeLV was demonstrated in a number of field cases of the disease (Kawakami et al. 1967; Laird et al. 1967; Rickard et al. 1967; Hertz et al. 1970). As with many of the original avian and murine retrovirus isolates, the isolates of FeLV from tumors often contained more than one type of particle, distinguishable by host-range and neutralization properties, which led to the division of these isolates into three serologically defined subgroups: A, B, and C. All naturally occurring isolates of B or C subgroups also contain a subgroup-A virus, although this virus can be obtained independently (Sarma and Log 1971, 1973; O. Jarrett et al. 1973).

The host range of infectivity for the different FeLV subgroups often provides the means for separating components in mixed stocks (O. Jarrett et al. 1973; Sarma and Log 1973). Subgroup-B FeLV has the broadest host range, replicating in cells of cat, dog, human, monkey, bovine, pig, and hamster origins. Subgroup-A viruses show the narrowest host range, growing well in cat cells and only very poorly in dog cells, although two subgroup-A isolates do replicate in embryonic human cells. Subgroup-C FeLVs replicate equally well in cat and human cells and are the only FeLV isolates that grow in guinea pig cells (Sarma et al. 1975).

Rangan et al. (1972) developed a test for ecotropic FeLV that is essentially similar to the XC test used for some of the ecotropic MLVs (Rowe et al. 1970). The same XC rat line, derived from an RSV-induced rat tumor, undergoes syncytium formation in the presence of cells producing FeLV. The assay is quantitative and shows a one-hit dose-response curve. Although the assay was suitable for the Snyder-Theilen strain of FeLV, it was not possible to demonstrate a syncytial response with cells infected with the Rickard strain of FeLV (Rangan et al. 1973).

The protein constituents of FeLV are summarized and are compared with those of RD114/CCC in Chapter 6. The protein products of *gag* are p26, p15, pp12, and p10, those of *env* are gp70 and p15(E), and that of *pol* is a p70 molecule (Schafer et al. 1971; Oroszlan et al. 1973; Velicer and Graves 1974; Rho and Gallo 1979). All strains of FeLV are highly related, with the greatest differences discerned in the type-specific antigenic determinants on *env* products; the latter are reflected in neutralization assays (Sarma and Log 1973) and cross-interference analysis (Sarma and Log 1971) and presumably equate with host-range patterns as well. More-sensitive neutralization studies suggest that all subgroup-A isolates may be monotypic, whereas there are detectable antigenic variations between individual members of subgroups B and C (Russell and Jarrett 1978). It seems likely that isolates obtained as mixed virus stocks are envelope mosaics.

Studies of FeSV have concentrated on the three early isolates: the Snyder-Theilen (ST) strain (Snyder and Theilen 1969), the Gardner-Arnstein (GA) strain (Gardner et al. 1970), and the McDonough (SM) strain (McDonough et al. 1971). However, FeSVs can be isolated from other cats with naturally occurring fibrosarcomas (Snyder 1971; Essex and Snyder 1973), and it is possible that other distinct strains may exist. As discussed elsewhere, analyses of their genomes and gene products show that they have arisen by recombination of FeLV with cellular *onc* sequences (*fes* in the case of ST-FeSV and Ga-FeSV and *fms* in the case of SM-FeSV) (see Chapters 4 and 9).

The presence of a tumor-specific antigen on the surface of cultured feline lymphoma cells was first detected by the use of sera from FeSV(FeLV)-infected cats (Essex et al. 1971a,b) and is called feline oncornavirus-associated cell-membrane antigen (FOCMA). This antigen has prognostic significance for FeLV/FeSV-induced tumor formation in vivo and is also of possible prophylactic importance (see Chapter 8). Normal or FeLV-infected cells do not express FOCMA, whereas FeSV-transformed producer and non-producer cells of various species are FOCMA-positive (Sliski et al. 1977; Stephenson et al. 1977a; Essex et al. 1979). Many feline lymphoma cells, including those not expressing any FeLV *gag* proteins, are also FOCMA-positive (Hardy et al. 1977, 1978; Stephenson et al. 1977a; Essex et al. 1978, 1979; Snyder et al. 1978, 1980). More recently, the antigen has been analyzed at a molecular level. The term FOCMA-S was proposed for the protein detectable on FeSV-transformed nonproducer cells and in defective FeSV virions (Sherr et al. 1978b,c); this molecule contains peptides of the *gag* p15 and pp12 proteins (Stephenson et al. 1977a; Khan et al. 1978; Sherr et al. 1978b,c) and, in at least one strain, some antigenic determinants of p30 as well (Porzig et al. 1979). The molecular weight of FOCMA-S varies from 80,000 to 160,000 daltons depending on the strain of FeSV, the larger molecules being associated with SM-FeSV. These data correlate well with the genetic structures (Chapter 4) and with the size of the *gag-onc* fusion proteins generated by each FeSV strain (see Chapter 9). The term FOCMA-L was suggested to define FOCMA-reactive molecules on lymphoid cells or in freshly biopsied tissues (Sherr et al. 1978c), which have a molecular weight of 70,000 daltons and lack *gag* antigens (see Chapter 8).

Although FeLVs are transmitted horizontally in the cat population, partially related sequences can be found in the DNA of the domestic cat, as well as in some other Felidae species (Ruprecht et al. 1973; Benveniste and Todaro 1974c; Quintrell et al. 1974, Benveniste et al. 1975; Koshy et al. 1980). The kinetics of the hybridization reaction suggest that there are about 7–9 copies per haploid genome (Benveniste and Todaro 1975b). FeLV-related sequences have also been detected in cellular DNA from cats maintained free of exogenous FeLV infection and in which there was no evidence of subclinical infections (Okabe et al. 1976). Such studies, together with the detection of similar sequences in other Felidae from which no retroviruses have been isolated, rule out the possibility that the FeLV sequences were due to exogenous infections in the population. In addition, related sequences can also be found in rodents, suggesting that there was a common ancestral virus. These sequence homologies are also reflected in a low level of hybridization between FeLV and MLV isolates, for example, and in the common determinants detected in interspecies-specific antigenic analyses. Despite the presence of these endogenous FeLV-related species, however, no one has yet been able to activate an FeLV-related virus from cat cells, suggesting that the sequences do not represent the full genome of a replication-competent virus or are not present in a single contiguous unit. Recombinant DNA technology should soon resolve these issues.

2. Endogenous Retroviruses

The original isolate of this group, RD114, was discovered in a study both fortuitous and (at that time) controversial. McAllister et al. (1972) injected human rhabdomyosarcoma cells into the brain of a fetal cat and subsequently recovered a retrovirus from cultures of the transplanted tumor. This virus was clearly not related to the known FeLV/FeSV isolates with regard to serological characteristics of its *gag*-gene or *env*-gene products (Klement and McAllister 1972; McAllister et al. 1972; Fischinger et al. 1973; Sarma and Log 1973), virus-induced cell-membrane antigens (Boone et al. 1973; Oshiro et al. 1974), or nucleic acid sequences (Baluda and Roy-Burman 1973; Benveniste and Todaro 1973; East et al. 1973), and thus a transient interest in RD114 as a putative human retrovirus arose. However, this possibility was soon eliminated unequivocally by numerous nucleic acid hybridization studies showing that cat-cell DNA and RNA contained all of the RD114 genetic sequences, whereas human DNA did not (Baluda and Roy-Burman 1973; Fujinaga et al. 1973; Gillespie et al. 1973; Neiman 1973b; Okabe et al. 1973a,b; Ruprecht et al. 1973). Thus, the xenotropic nature of RD114 led first to the misinterpretation of its origin and second to an increased awareness of endogenous xenotropic viruses.

Several RD114-related viruses have since been obtained from cultured cat cells (Fischinger et al. 1973; Livingston and Todaro 1973; Sarma et al. 1973, 1974; Todaro et al. 1973b), generally following IdU treatment and cocultivation with heterologous cell lines. The CCC isolate of Livingston and Todaro (1973), as well as of others, has been shown to be highly related to RD114, and thus this group of endogenous feline viruses became known as the RD114/CCC group.

Sequences related to the RD114/CCC group are detected in other Felidae family, including the European wildcat (*F. sylvestris*) and, to a lesser extent, the sand cat (*F. margarita*) and the jungle cat (*F. chaus*) (Benveniste and Todaro 1974b,c). These data prompted the in vitro study of tissues from the wildcat. Lieber et al. (1975a) obtained two retrovirus isolates from cocultivations of spleen and kidney with a variety of indicator cell lines. One virus elicited the syncytia and CPE characteristic of foamy viruses. The second virus, designated FS-1, showed properties related to RD114: reverse transcriptase cross interference, similar p30 antigens, extensive nucleic acid homology, and a similar host range of infectivity.

The KC cell line, a human glioma cell transformed by RSV, forms syncytia by fusion in response to infection by RD114 or to cocultivation with RD114-infected cells (Rand and Long 1972, 1973). The fusion-inducing component appears to be the envelope glycoprotein (Rand et al. 1975). KB cells, of human epidermoid carcinoma origin, also form syncytia in response to infection with RD114 (Klement and McAllister 1972). One difference in this system from the XC and KC assays mentioned above is that pretreatment of the cells with DEAE-dextran decreases, rather than increases, the response. No detectable differences in the levels of sensitivity of KB and KC cells have been found (Nelson-Rees et al. 1973).

One unusual shared feature between RD114 and FeLV is the ability to induce aggregation and syncytia formation in Epstein-Barr virus (EBV) containing human lymphoid cell lines (Hampar et al. 1973). Although viral particles are produced, fusion does not continue after a second wave at around 3 weeks postinfection. However, a virus-carrier state is established; such RD114-carrier cultures are resistant to fusion by superinfection with RD114 or FeLV, but FeLV-carrier cultures are susceptible to RD114-induced fusion. Interestingly, there is a transient heightened expression of EBV early antigens in the syncytia.

Perhaps the most striking feature of RD114-related viruses is their usually high degree of relatedness to BaEV. This is reflected in the host range, antigenic determinants, protein sequences, and nucleic acid homology. To avoid reiteration, these properties are presented in Section II.T.3 in the discussion of BaEV isolates.

N. Mink C-type Retrovirus

Recently, there have been several articles dealing with the isolation and characterization of an endogenous mink C-type retrovirus from the Mv-1-Lu mink (*Mustela vison*) lung cell line (Barbacid et al. 1978; Klement et al. 1978; Sherr et al. 1978a). The method of virus isolation in each case was different: spontaneous production after long-term passage (100 generations), production after coculture with BrdU-treated mouse cells, and production after BaEV infection of a Ki-MSV-transformed nonproducer mink-cell derivative, respectively. However, the properties of each isolate are very similar, and one can now assume that a single virus type has been isolated and characterized by the different laboratories.

The virus, designated mink leukemia virus (MiLV), is apparently highly infectious for dog and donkey cells, weakly infectious for mink cells, and consistently noninfectious for mouse, rat, goat, human, and monkey cells, whereas the data for cat and rabbit cells are inconsistent. These differences may be resolved following serological, biochemical, and molecular comparisons of the different isolates.

The isolates display typical C-type morphology in both budding and extracellular particles of approximately 100 nm with a 80-nm nucleoid and show a buoyant density of 1.16 g/ml in sucrose. Protein analysis has distinguished the following components: gp70, p30, p15, pp12, and p10. Serologically, the p30 of MiLV is closely related to that of FeLV and less closely related to that of an endogenous rat leukemia virus. Some interspecies cross-reactivity is also observed with AKR-MLV, RD114, BaEV, and SSAV. Antiserum to MiLV gp70 precipitates FeLV gp70, but not the gp70 molecules of a variety of other retroviruses. On the other hand, p15 shows no cross-reactivity to FeLV p12 (Sherr et al. 1978a). The viral polymerase requires Mn^{++} as a divalent cation and can be inhibited by antiserum to rat and mouse, but not feline, viral polymerases (Sherr et al. 1978a).

The use of MiLV cDNA probes in nucleic acid hybridization experiments with a variety of cellular DNA species indicates that MiLV is an endogenous virus of mink, with about 20 virus copies per haploid-cell genome (Sherr et al. 1978a). There is considerably less homology detected in DNA from other members of the *Mustela* genus and virtually none in DNA from other carnivores and mammals. A higher degree of hybridization (13–17%) to mouse-cell DNA has been reported by Klement et al. (1978) and could possibly reflect those sequences coding for the cross-reacting antigens. Both groups of workers reported that there was a low, but detectable, level of hybridization to mink-cell RNA, suggesting that viral gene expression may be a common phenomenon in cultured mink cells.

O. Porcine C-type Retroviruses

Since the first descriptions of C-type viral particles in normal pig kidney cell cultures appeared (Breese 1970; Armstrong et al. 1971) and the finding of such viruses in lymphosarcomas obtained from minipigs fed with strontium 90 (Howard et al. 1968), it has become increasingly more obvious that these viruses are common in domestic pigs (*Sus scrofa*).

The viruses are associated with lymphosarcomas, tumors that occur at a frequency varying from 3 to 50 per 1 million animals, and account for more than 25% of neoplasms detected in the populations at the slaughterhouse (Bostock and Owen 1973). The tumors generally appear in animals less than 6 months of age, and a genetic predisposition is seen at a higher frequency in brother-sister matings in certain high-incidence herds.

Several continuous cell lines derived from pigs spontaneously produce C-type virus; these include the porcine kidney PK-15 cultures mentioned above, the 38A-1 lymph node cell line (Strandstrom et al. 1974; Moennig et al. 1974), a swine testis cell line, and a minipig kidney cell line (Lieber et al. 1975b). In fact, only two of all the porcine cell cultures, a second swine testis line (Lieber et al. 1975b) and a fallopian tube cell line (Bouillant et al. 1975), have been found to be virus-negative, although the latter of these two is inducible with BrdU treatment.

The host range of the porcine retrovirus is extremely limited. Infection of the one virus-negative porcine cell line has been accomplished, whereas a wide variety of other mammalian cell lines has proved resistant to infection with this virus (Lieber et al. 1975b). Biological studies of the virus are therefore minimal, but biochemical characterization has been extensive owing to the availability of cultures that are high virus producers. The porcine virus is similar to the other mammalian C-type viruses by morphological, biological, biochemical, and immunological criteria. The particles are most frequently observed extracellularly or budding from the cell plasma membrane, although some intracisternal particles have also been identified (Woods et al. 1973). The viruses band at the characteristic 1.16 g/ml in sucrose gradients, contain a 70S RNA, and a reverse transcriptase of 70,000 daltons (Woods et al. 1973; Moennig et al. 1974; Todaro et al. 1974a). The reverse transcriptase and the p30 internal viral protein exhibit some immunological cross-reactions with those of murine and primate (SSAV/GALV) origin, whereas there does not seem to be any cross-reaction with viruses of rat, hamster, or feline systems (Moennig et al. 1974; Todaro et al. 1974a; Sherr et al. 1975).

Nucleic acid hybridization studies using a single-stranded DNA probe complementary to the PK-15 viral RNA indicate little, if any, sequence homology of the PK-15 virus with any of the other mammalian viruses tested (Todaro et al. 1974a). A similar probe was used to examine whether the porcine retrovirus is an endogenous virus of pigs and related ungulates. Viral sequences are present in multiple copies in the cellular DNAs of domestic pigs, wild boars, bush pigs, and warthogs but are absent from the South American peccary, hippopotami, and sheep (Benveniste and Todaro 1975a). Less hybridization was detected to the cellular DNAs of rodents (mouse, rat, and hamster, in decreasing frequency), and in these cases, the thermal-denaturation profiles of the hybrids formed are considerably depressed, indicating base-pair mismatching. From studies on the evolutionary divergence of the species, it appears that an ancestral endogenous xenotropic MLV was infectiously transmitted and subsequently became integrated into the germ line of pigs. This transspecies infection must have occurred after the divergence of pigs from other related ungulates, such as the New World peccary, and before the divergence between domestic pigs and warthogs and is estimated at 5–10 million years ago (Benveniste and Todaro 1975a).

Once again, the etiological significance of the porcine C-type virus is unknown. The studies described above show that all normal pig tissues contain the information of the complete viral genome and that the majority of cell lines established from normal tissues are spontaneous and chronic virus producers. Also, pig-cell RNA does not contain sequences homologous to the C-type virus; therefore, although the information is present, it is not being transcribed in normal, nonleukemogenic tissue (Todaro et al. 1974a).

P. Deer C-type Retrovirus

Aaronson et al. (1976a) reported the isolation of a C-type virus from the Colombian black-tailed deer, *Odocoileus hemionus*. The virus (DKV), which was obtained following cocultivation of *O. hemionus* kidney cells with a variety of cell lines, shows a narrow xenotropic host range; it replicates in some human and horse cells, but not in cells of other primates or in cow, dog, cat, rat, hamster, mouse, and *O. hemionus*. As might be expected from its xenotropism, nucleic acid hybridization studies indicate that the virus is endogenous to the deer. There appear to be 30–40 copies of proviral DNA per haploid genome of *O. hemionus,* but there is only partial homology between the viral sequences and the DNAs from tissues of five separate genera of deer that evolved in the Old World (moose, elk, caribou, muntjac, and fallow deer), as well as sheep and antelope. These latter two bovid species shared a common ancestor with deer some 25–30 million years ago. No homology was detected between the viral sequences and the DNA of llama or pig species that have been genetically distinct from deer for at least 55 million years (Tronick et al. 1977). In addition, nucleic acid hybridization reactions detect no genetic homologies with C-type viruses from chicken, mouse, rat, cat, or primates; the B-type MMTV; or the D-type MPMV.

The deer virus reverse transcriptase shows a preferential divalent-cation requirement for Mn^{++} and is only partially inhibited by antisera to MLV, RD114, or SSAV enzymes. Cross-reactivity of the major structural protein, p30, is most evident with those of the endogenous cat and baboon viruses (Aaronson et al. 1976a).

Q. Horse C-type Retrovirus

Historically, equine infectious anemia is one of the first diseases to have a viral ("filterable") etiology (Vallee and Carre 1904). The disease occurs worldwide and is characterized by recurrent episodes of fever, hemolytic anemia, bone marrow depression, lymphoproliferation, immune-complex glomerulonephritis, and persistent viremia (McGuire and Henson 1973; Henson and McGuire 1974; Umphenour et al. 1974; Ishii and Ishitani 1975). However, no neoplasms are associated with the disease spectrum. Transmission generally occurs from mares to foals via insect vectors (Stein et al. 1944, 1972; Kemen and Coggins 1972). The wide range of pathogenic properties can be attributed to a single C-type retrovirus, called the equine infectious anemia virus (EIAV); this is not an unusual phenomenon (see Chapter 8).

The host range of EIAV in vitro is limited to horse peripheral blood leukocytes or bone marrow (Kobayashi 1961a,b), and this has hindered progress on the biochemical characterization of the virus. However, it is interesting to note that, although viral antigens can be detected in virtually all tissues of infected horses, the macrophages are the predominant population of infected cells. The replication of virus in this cell could account for the persistence of the virus in vivo and may also suggest a limited target cell for the virus (Kono et al. 1970a; McGuire et al. 1971). Virus infection apparently gives rise to CPE in vitro; however, it is difficult to distinguish this CPE clearly from the normal degeneration of the cell cultures. Thus, investigators have often relied on measurements of complement-fixing (CF) group-specific antigens (Kono and Kobayashi 1966; Henson et al. 1970) or on the use of infected horse serum in an immunofluorescence assay to determine virus titers (Ushimi et al. 1970, 1972; Crawford et al. 1971; Norcross and Coggins 1971; Coggins et al. 1972); the antigen detected is the major internal structural protein. There are apparently at least eight different serotypes; all share the common group-specific antigen but are distinguished by neutralizing antisera (Kono et al. 1971). This serology has been confirmed by cross-protection studies in vivo using attenuated virus stocks (Kono et al. 1970b).

The virus has generally been isolated from the blood of infected horses and then inoculated onto horse leukocytes. As determined by electron microscopy, the earliest evidence of virus production is the appearance of a crescent-shaped nucleoid under the plasma membrane, typical of C-type particles. Some aggregates of mature particles are observed in membrane-bound vesicles or vacuoles, although particles are never seen free in the cytoplasm, suggesting that such vesicles may represent invaginations of the plasma membrane. Extracellular particles are about 80–120 nm in diameter, with a pleomorphic spherical or rod-shaped electron-dense nucleoid of about 40–60 nm. Thin surface projections and an inner shell around the nucleoid are sometimes observed. On the basis of these observations, it was proposed that EIAV resembled members of the retrovirus family (Nakajima et al. 1969a,b; Tajima et al. 1969;

Ito et al. 1969; Henson et al. 1970; Kono et al. 1970a). EIAV also shares other characteristics with the retrovirus family: sensitivity to ether (Nakajima and Obara 1964), sensitivity to IdU during the early stages of replication (Kono et al. 1970a), buoyant density of 1.15 g/ml (Nakajima et al. 1969a), an RNA genome (Nakajima et al. 1970; Cheevers et al. 1977), and an RNA-dependent DNA polymerase (Archer et al. 1977).

It is only in the last few years that sufficient virus has been available for detailed biochemical analysis. The genome sediments as 60S–70S RNA and is composed of two single-strand subunits of approximately 34S. The reverse transcriptase is about 70,000 daltons and requires Mg^{++} for its divalent cation (Charman et al. 1976a; Archer et al. 1977; Cheevers et al. 1978). The enzyme is apparently quite effective in an endogenous reaction, yielding a product of approximately genomic length (8000 nucleotides) (Rice and Coggins 1979).

SDS-polyacrylamide gel electrophoresis has provided information on the virion structural proteins. The major structural core protein shows an apparent molecular weight of about 28,000 daltons (Nakajima et al. 1970). Other nonglycosylated proteins include some lower-molecular-weight species: p13, p11, and p9 (Charman et al. 1976a; Cheevers et al. 1978; Ishizaki et al. 1978; Parekh et al. 1980). The major glycoproteins are gp90 and gp45 and are not linked by disulfide bonds. Using broadly reactive antisera to *gag* structural components, EIAV does not cross-react with a variety of oncoviruses (Charman et al. 1976a) or lentiviruses (Stowring et al. 1979). Thus, EIAV has unique antigenic determinants.

No nucleic acid sequence homology is detected between EIAV and the following retroviruses: MLV, MMTV, rat leukemia virus, HaLV, AMV, BLV, FeLV, RD114, BaEV, SMRV, and MPMV. In addition, no homologous sequences could be found in normal horse tissue or in other equine species and a variety of other mammals (Rice et al. 1978). Therefore, EIAV is not an endogenous virus of the horse and remains quite distinct from other retroviruses. Whether the insect vectors are passive or whether they support active replication of the virus is unknown but merits further study.

The disease syndrome itself is quite interesting (as a model for persistent virus infections and for immune-complex disease) and a brief account is given. There are several reviews available on this subject (Ishii 1963; Hyslop 1966; Johnson 1966; Squire 1968; Henson et al. 1970), and an account of persistent retrovirus infection is given in Chapter 8 in relation to visna virus. EIAV viremia persists for the lifetime of the animal, and increases in virus titers are associated with the recurrence and exacerbation of the acute illness. In addition, EIAV-neutralizing antibodies are detected in horse sera years after the initial infection (Tanaka and Sakaki 1962; Kobayashi et al. 1969; Kono 1968; Coggins and Norcross 1970; Henson et al. 1970, 1971). Infectious virus-antibody complexes are also detected (McGuire et al. 1972) and probably account for the glomerulonephritis. Because of the chronic nature of EIAV-induced disease, EIAV is sometimes called a lentivirus; however, the absence of antigenic relatedness to visna virus described above does not substantiate this classification. Another feature of the disease is hemolytic anemia, which is due to a chronic hypoferremia because of iron retention in macrophages (the infected cell) and immunologically mediated hemolysis. In addition, antivirus antibody has been detected on the surfaces of erythrocytes (McGuire and Henson 1973). The mechanism of virus persistence in equine infectious anemia and other persistent virus infections is not known. This question represents an important challenge in infectious-disease research, and the complex interaction between host and virus in equine infectious anemia should provide valuable information.

R. Bovine C-type Retroviruses

Enzootic bovine leukosis or lymphosarcoma is an important disease of cattle (Anderson and Jarrett 1968). Herds with a high incidence of leukemia are found as clusters, and this pattern is associated with European cattle whose importation into the New World led to massive spreading of the virus-induced disease. In some regions, the high frequency of lymphosarcoma or the benign persistent lymphocytosis has made the disease an economically important problem. Early seroepidemiological studies demonstrated the phenomenon of cohort clustering of the disease and suggested that horizontal transmission is of primary importance (Piper et al. 1975). There is also evidence that transmission of the disease may occur congenitally or through the colostrum from the dam to her calf. However, a second disease spectrum, called sporadic lymphosarcoma/leukemia, occurs infrequently throughout the world and is not associated with a retrovirus. A most excellent and comprehensive review of bovine leukemia has been prepared by Burny et al. (1980).

Electron microscopic examination of lymphocytes from leukemic animals first revealed the presence of C-type viral particles (Enke et al. 1961; Dutcher et al. 1964; Enke 1964). Particles have also been observed infrequently in milk. Subsequently, C-type viruses were isolated from peripheral leukocytes from cattle with lymphosarcoma (Miller et al. 1969; Dutta et al. 1970; Olson et al. 1970) or from cattle with persistent lymphocytosis (Van der Maaten et al. 1972). The infected bovine lymphocytes are capable of inducing lymphosarcomas in neonatal calves (Mammerickx 1972; Miller et al. 1972), and inoculation of chimpanzees gives rise to an erythroleukemia (McClure et al. 1974). More recently, cell-free extracts of tumor cells have been successfully used to transmit lymphosarcoma (Van der Maaten and Miller 1976).

Biological and biochemical studies of BLVs have yielded evidence of some similarities to and some distinct differences from the major mammalian C-type viruses. Morphologically, the particle is somewhat atypical and is often seen budding from intracytoplasmic vacuolar membranes (Calafat et al. 1974; Van der Maaten et al. 1974). Some of the particles are seen to have complete cores during budding, and many of the extracellular particles have surface spikes like those of B-type particles; however, the nucleoid remains central like those of C-type particles (Weiland et al. 1974). The particles band at 1.15 g/ml in sucrose and contain a high-molecular-weight RNA of approximately 70S. Unlike other mammalian C-type viruses, the BLV reverse transcriptase has an absolute requirement for Mg^{++} (Gilden et al. 1975), which is a property associated with the B-type and D-type mammalian viruses (MMTV, MPMV, and guinea pig endogenous virus) and the avian C-type leukemia and sarcoma viruses. The major viral structural protein is p24; this molecule does not seem to have the interspecies-specific determinants cross-reactive with other retroviruses (Ferrer 1972).

SDS-polyacrylamide gel electrophoresis of virion structural proteins reveals the following peptides: gp55, gp45, p24, and p18 (Onuma et al. 1976). Size estimates on the major structural protein have varied from 23,000 to 25,000 daltons; the isoelectric point of this molecule is extremely variable: pI 8.6 (Gilden et al. 1975), pI 7.2 (Onuma et al. 1976), pI 6.4–6.6 (McDonald et al. 1976), and pI 6.6–6.8 (McDonald and Ferrer 1976). Using radioimmunoprecipitation assays, no cross-reactivity of the BLV p24 is detected to the following retroviruses: MLV, MMTV, FeLV, RD114, porcine PK-15, BaEV, SSAV, MPMV, AMV, or REV (McDonald and Ferrer 1976; McDonald et al. 1976). Detectable homology is observed only with the oncovirus isolated from sheep with lymphosarcoma (see Section II.S), and it is thought that the disease in sheep is actually caused by interspecies horizontal transmission of BLV (Paulsen et al. 1974; Pauli et al. 1977; Rohde et al. 1978). Experimental inoculation of sheep with BLV causes a high incidence of lymphosarcoma (Olson and Baumgartener 1976), although apparently there is no horizontal transmission between sheep (Hoss and Olson 1974; for review, see Burny et al. 1980).

Nucleic acid hybridization studies using radiolabeled viral RNA or in vitro-synthesized cDNA do not detect any sequence homologies with MPMV, SSAV, FeLV, or AMV. In addition, although proviral sequences have been detected in tumor-cell DNA, there are no integrated viral genomes in normal bovine tissues; therefore, the disease is acquired by infection with an exogenous virus, rather than by endogenous virogenes (Callahan et al. 1976b; Kettmann et al. 1976b, 1980).

The host range of the virus in vitro is rather broad; it infects human, bovine, simian, ovine, caprine, canine, and bat cells, but rodent cells appear to be refractory to infection. BLV induces syncytia in most of the types of cells that it infects in vitro (Diglio and Ferrer 1976; Graves and Ferrer 1976; Ogura et al. 1977), and this property can be used as a quantitative assay of virus infectivity. Apparently, the syncytia result from cell fusion of the infected cells, rather than from endomitosis. However, because bovine foamy viruses (see Section IV) are also common and also lead to syncytia formation, it is important that virus stocks be carefully cloned to eliminate the possibility of a mixed virus population.

There is a good correlation between the titer of antibodies to p24 in cattle and the leukosis status of the herd. Human contacts on the farms or in the slaughterhouses do not have any detectable antibody (Devare et al. 1976). More recently, it has been found that sera from leukemic animals contain antibodies that specifically inhibit the activity of BLV reverse transcriptase. However, sera from virus-infected nonleukemic animals that show reactivity to the major viral structural protein do not possess this anti-reverse transcriptase activity (Wuu et al. 1977). Also, infected animals produce antibodies to the *env* gp55 capable of neutralizing virus, and these antibodies can be readily detected for seroepidemiological surveys by neutralization of BLV pseudotypes of vesicular stomatitis virus (VSV) (Zavada et al. 1978, 1979). The economic importance of the disease is a strong stimulus for devising methods for preventing infection.

S. Sheep C-type Retroviruses

Lymphocyte cultures from sheep with spontaneous leukemia produce viral particles that resemble the classical C-type viruses (Paulsen et al. 1972). Biochemical and biophysical analyses have shown that the particles band at a density of 1.16 g/ml in sucrose and contain a high-molecular-weight RNA and an RNA-dependent DNA polymerase activity (Paulsen et al. 1976). Furthermore, purified viral particles can experimentally produce leukemia in inoculated sheep (Paulsen et al. 1975). The low yield of virus from the lymphocyte cultures has precluded extensive biochemical characterization of the virus; however, it appears that the major structural protein of the virus is approximately 21,000 daltons. The ovine retrovirus p21 cross-reacts immunologically with BLV p24 and with serum from leukemic animals, cattle as well as sheep (Paulsen et al. 1974).

No in vitro assay has yet been developed for this virus, so further comparisons with the bovine virus have not been made. It would be interesting to determine whether these viruses are identical, as such information would provide evidence that the virus isolated from sheep has been transmitted in nature from one species to another.

T. Primate Retroviruses

In the past decade, numerous retrovirus isolates have been made from many of the primate genera, and these can be subdivided on the basis of several criteria: (1) oncoviruses or spumaviruses; (2) species of origin, i.e., prosimian or New World monkeys or Old World monkeys or apes; (3) C-type or D-type particle morphology; and (4) exogenous or endogenous derivation. By these criteria, the primate retroviruses fall into seven distinct classes: (1) the prosimian C-type isolate; (2) the exogenous C-type viruses isolated from New World and Old World primates (woolly monkey and gibbon ape); (3) the endogenous C-type viruses of Old World monkeys, of which there are three unrelated groups (from baboons, macaques, and the colobus monkey); (4) the endogenous C-type virus of a New World monkey (owl monkey); (5) the exogenous D-type virus (MPMV) from an Old World monkey (macaque); (6) the endogenous D-type virus from an Old World monkey (langur); and (7) the endogenous D-type virus from a New World monkey (squirrel monkey). For simplicity, Figure 2.5 illustrates schematically the evolution of primates and the types of retroviruses reco-

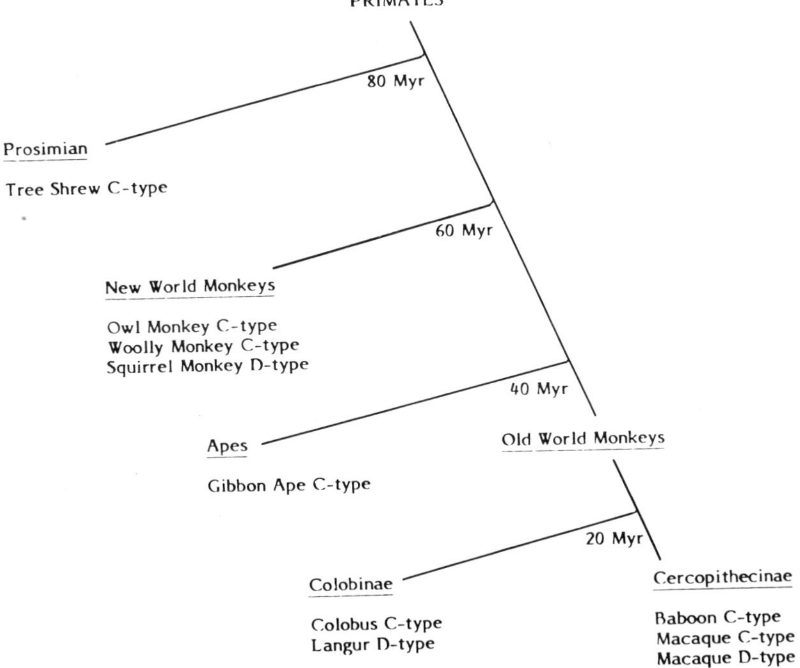

Figure 2.5 Schematic representation of the evolution of primates, showing the retrovirus isolates associated with the various suborders. The scale is given in millions of years (Myr) but is meant as a tentative estimate only.

vered from primate families and subfamilies. The spumavirus isolates from primates (discussed in Section IV) and the putative human oncovirus isolates (discussed in Chapter 11) are omitted from this figure. Of all the isolates tested so far, only SSV and GALV are oncogenic, although experimental inoculation of MPMV, for example, does cause some abnormal pathology.

Antigenic cross-reactions and nucleic acid homologies between different primate retroviruses frequently arise. This is often reflected as a high degree of conservation in the amino acid sequence of the structural virion proteins (see Chapter 6 and Appendix C).

Among the endogenous viruses, homologous cellular sequences in species related to the species from which the retrovirus was isolated appear to mirror the phylogenetic divergence, suggesting that ancestral provirus progenitors have evolved along with nonvirogenic cellular genes. In addition, unexpected homologies between primate retroviruses and isolates from lower vertebrates also occur. These findings have led to speculation about the infectious transmission of retroviruses from one species to another, the possibility of acquiring new proviruses in the germ line from the exogenous infection, and the possibility of as yet undetected retroviruses in the other primate genera.

1. Prosimian C-type Retroviruses

There has been one report on the activation of a retrovirus from the prosimian tree shrew (*Tupaia belangeri*) (Flugel et al. 1978). IdU treatment of cultured cells derived from placenta, embryo fibroblasts, or juvenile skin fibroblasts was positive for retrovirus expression, i.e., electron microscopic particles, reverse transcriptase activity, and 70S RNA detected in particles banding at 1.16 g/ml in sucrose. The virus, designated TRV-1, did not replicate in human, marmoset, or mink cells, although it did grow in dog thymus cells. Cocultivation with XC cells of the producer dog cells, but not the producer tree shrew cells, led to the formation of syncytia; this discrepancy remains to be explained. No further reports on this prosimian retrovirus have appeared.

2. Simian Sarcoma and Gibbon Ape Leukemia C-type Retroviruses

An extensive literature on this group of retroviruses has accrued since the initial description of C-type particles in a New World woolly monkey with multiple fibrosarcomas (Theilen et al. 1971). Further virus isolates from the Old World gibbon apes proved to be remarkably similar in biological and immunological assays and have promoted classification of all of these viruses into a single group.

In 1971, histological examination of tissues from a 3-year-old male woolly monkey (*Lagothrix* sp.) with multiple sarcomas, myelofibrosis, and myeloid metaplasia revealed the presence of numerous budding C-type particles, particularly in fibroblasts, histiocytic cells, bone marrow, and tumor tissue (Theilen et al. 1971). Some of these tissues were used for the isolation of infectious virus which was named simian sarcoma virus (SSV) type 1 (Wolfe et al. 1971). SSV itself is replication-defective like other mammalian sarcoma viruses; the helper virus with which it was isolated is known as simian sarcoma-associated virus (SSAV). There is some ambivalence in the literature regarding nomenclature of these viruses; other sobriquets include SiSV, WMV, and WoLV (for woolly monkey leukemia virus). It is necessary to keep in mind that there has been only this one isolate from a woolly monkey (a pet in a California household shared with several cats, dogs, and a gibbon ape). SSV(SSAV) is tumorigenic in a variety of primates; well-differentiated fibrosarcomas or fibromas arise in marmosets and squirrel monkeys inoculated as neonates (Rabin 1971; Wolfe et al. 1971; Deinhardt et al. 1972, 1973; Wolfe and Deinhardt 1972; Theilen et al. 1973), and the viruses could be readily recovered from tumor explants. Thus, SSV is truly an oncogenic virus.

C-type virus isolates from gibbon apes (*Hylobates lar*) have been more numerous. The first infectious virus described was obtained, in California, from a 3.5-year-old female gibbon with disseminated lymphosarcoma (Kawakami et al. 1972). Electron microscopy showed wide-spread occurrence of particles in tissues from this animal, and explanted lymphoid cells produced particles with the typical criteria of C-type retroviruses: high-molecular-weight RNA in particles of 1.16 g/ml buoyant density in sucrose, with associated reverse transcriptase activity. Further isolates were made from two animals with lymphosarcoma in the same gibbon colony (Kawakami et al. 1973; Snyder et al. 1973). All of these animals had received several low doses of X-ray exposure. There have also been several isolates from five animals in a colony in Thailand

(SEATO), where there was a high incidence of granulocytic leukemia among the gibbons (De Paoli et al. 1973; Kawakami and Buckley 1974); many of the animals in this colony had received injections of blood from people with malaria. These virus isolates can induce granulocytic leukemias in primate hosts (Kawakami et al. 1975, 1978, 1980). Another three isolates (GBr-1, GBr-2, and GBr-3) were obtained from the brains of nonleukemic animals from the same SEATO colony (Todaro et al. 1975); two of the three animals from which virus was isolated had been inoculated with brain extracts from patients with kuru. Finally, an isolate (GALV-H) from a leukemic animal in Bermuda has been reported (Gallo et al. 1978; Krackower et al. 1978; Reitz et al. 1979). The viruses have at times been designated SLV (simian lymphoma virus) and SMV (simian myelogenous leukemia virus), but they have now been named collectively GALV (gibbon ape leukemia-lymphoma viruses).

The host range of replication of all of the SSV/GALV isolates is extremely broad, including cells of human, monkey, cat, dog, cow, bat, mink, rabbit, rat (but not Chinese hamster or mouse), pheasant, quail, turkey, duck, and guinea fowl (but not chicken) (Kawakami et al. 1972; Wolfe et al. 1972; Rangan et al. 1973; Teich et al. 1975; Todaro et al. 1975; Weiss and Wong 1977). There do not seem to be any cell lines that can distinguish the different isolates. All the isolates belong to a single receptor-interference group (Rangan 1974). As with FeLV and some MLVs, the SSAV/GALV group of viruses elicit syncytial formation in XC cells (Wolfe and Deinhardt 1972; Rangan et al. 1972, 1973), allowing quantitative measurement of helper-virus infectivity.

One distinguishing feature of the defective SSV component is its ability to induce foci of transformed cells (Wolfe et al. 1972; Scolnick and Parks 1973; Aaronson et al. 1976b; Scolnick et al. 1976b). Rescue of the sarcoma genome from nonproducer cells by a variety of mammalian leukemia helper viruses from different species shows that there is no specificity for its own helper (Scolnick and Parks 1973).

The analyses of viral structural proteins of the SSAV/GALV are discussed in Chapter 6. There are four major *gag*-gene products (p27, p15, pp12, and p10), two *env*-gene proteins (gp70 and p15[E]), and one *pol*-gene product (p70). In general, it has been difficult to identify type-specific determinants on the gp70 molecules of SSAV and all GALV isolates. Antisera to the gp70 antigens of one virus can effectively neutralize the other isolates with similar titers (Kawakami et al. 1973; Kawakami and Buckley 1974; Rangan 1974; Todaro et al. 1975). Of interest is the marked cross interference between the SSAV/GALV group and the one endogenous virus isolated from the Asian feral mouse, *M. caroli* (Lieber et al. 1975d). However, by using stringent competition radioimmunoprecipitation assays, it is possible to distinguish between SSAV and at least two GALV isolates (the original GALV-1 and the GALV-SEATO viruses) (Hino et al. 1975). The precipitating antibodies often show little, if any, neutralizing activity and therefore are most likely reacting with different antigenic determinants.

The major structural virion protein p27 has been studied in great detail (Hoekstra and Deinhardt 1973; Gilden et al. 1974; Oroszlan et al. 1975) (see Chapter 6). The isoelectric point of the SSAV protein is approximately 6.4 (Parks et al. 1973a; Sherr and Todaro 1974; Oroszlan et al. 1975) and that of GALV is 6.2 (Oroszlan et al. 1975). In nearly every assay based on cross-reactivities of the major *gag*-gene products, the SSAV/GALV group stands alone. Comparison within this group gives estimates of almost total identity (Kawakami et al. 1972; Parks and Scolnick 1972; Parks et al. 1973a; Hoekstra and Deinhardt 1973; Gilden et al. 1974; Kawakami and Buckley 1974; Tronick et al. 1974a; Sherr et al. 1975; Todaro et al. 1975). Although the p27 molecules of SSAV/ GALV are antigenically distinct from those of other primate and mammalian retroviruses, several cross-reactive determinants have been identified. The strongest cross-reactivity, as pointed out earlier for gp70, is with the endogenous virus from *M. caroli*. The p30 of this murine virus competes efficiently and almost completely in homologous competition RIAs for the GALV p27, whereas that of Ra-MLV shows little, if any, competition (Lieber et al. 1975d). Weaker interspecies determinants also exist on SSAV/GALV p27. Antisera to SSAV and GALV p27 precipitate MLV p30 in both immunodiffusion (Gilden et al. 1974) and RIAs (Parks et al. 1973a), although only at much higher concentrations than are required for the homologous protein. In broadly cross-reactive competition RIAs designed to recognize interspecies determinants, both SSAV and GALV compete, although the extent of competition varies considerably in the hands of different investigators

(Hoekstra and Deinhardt 1973; Parks et al. 1973a; Sherr et al. 1974a; Lieber et al. 1975d; Stephenson et al. 1977b). There is also a low, but detectable, reaction with Ra-MLV and the endogenous porcine virus PK-15 (Sherr et al. 1975). The aminoterminal amino acid residues of p27 of GALV and SSAV have been sequenced and are identical for at least the first 28 residues (Oroszlan et al. 1975, 1977) (see Appendix C). This could account for the fact that the p27 molecules of SSAV/GALV have a strong group-specific determinant and a weak or negligible interspecies determinant.

The small internal pp12 *gag* phosphoprotein has the strongest type-specific antigens and has been used to detect differences among the SSAV/GALV isolates. Using RIA, one can distinguish between SSAV and GALV-1 or between GALV-1 and GALV-SEATO. These assays show a partial cross-reaction among the isolates, which suggests that the pp12 molecules contain both unique and shared determinants (Tronick et al. 1974a, 1975). With the exception of shared determinants on the *M. caroli* and pig endogenous viruses, no interspecies reactivities are present on SSAV/GALV pp12 (Tronick et al. 1974a; Stephenson et al. 1977b). The pp12 molecule binds with type-specificity to its homolgous 70S and subunit 35S virion RNA (Sen and Todaro 1976) (see Chapter 6); comparative binding studies suggest that (1) SSAV is probably more distantly related to the GALV isolates than are the GALV isolates to one another and (2) the gibbon brain isolates, although from animals in the SEATO colony, are more distantly related to the original GALV-SEATO than is the GALV-1 isolate from the California colony. Less than 15 molecules of pp12 bind to the 70S RNA: this is substantially less than the amount of pp12 found in each virion and suggests that there might be two pp12 populations (Sen et al. 1976). Sen and his colleagues have suggested that the pp12-RNA interaction may play a role in viral RNA synthesis and processing.

The reverse transcriptase provides another means of establishing the similarity or dissimilarity between various retroviruses, based on the inhibition of reverse transcriptase enzymic activity by antisera to heterologous reverse transcriptase. The data show (1) nearly complete inhibition of SSAV/GALV enzymes by antisera to any individual isolate of the group, (2) some inhibitory activity of the endogenous porcine viral enzyme and the *M. caroli* viral enzyme by antisera to SSAV/GALV enzymes, and (3) little or no cross-inhibition to other viral enzymes (Kawakami et al. 1972; Scolnick et al. 1972a,b; Kawakami and Buckley 1974; Tronick et al. 1974a; Lieber et al. 1975d; Sherr et al. 1975; Todaro et al. 1975).

It was shown very early that neither SSAV nor the GALV isolates are endogenous to woolly monkeys, gibbon apes, or a variety of other primates (Scolnick et al. 1974b; Benveniste and Todaro 1974b; Sherr et al. 1974a; Wong-Staal et al. 1975), although a low level of homologous sequences, related to a small fraction of the genome, is detected in the DNAs of mice and, to a lesser extent, in the DNAs of primates and pigs. These findings correlate with the cross-reactions between the endogenous *M. caroli* and the SSAV/GALV group described above and has led to the interpretation that Muridae, pig, and SSAV/GALV viruses had a common evolutionary ancestor (Lieber et al. 1975d).

Electron micrographic studies show that SSAV genomic RNA is somewhat shorter (8.5 kb/subunit) than that of either RD114 or BaEV. The genome does exhibit a looped structure on each subunit, which is a regular feature of the mammalian C-type viruses (Kung et al. 1976). On the basis of the RNA sequence homology, one can classify the different isolates into four subgroups: subgroup A containing SSAV, subgroup B containing the original GALV-1 (California) isolate, subgroup C containing the SEATO (Thailand) isolates, and subgroup D containing the SEATO gibbon brain (GBVr) isolates (Todaro et al. 1975). This subgroup classification correlates with the pp12 reactivities as well. Furthermore, there appear to be relatively few homologous sequences to most of the retroviruses, with the exception of MLV, again corresponding well with the viral nucleic acid hybridization with mouse-cell DNA and with the antigenic cross-reactivities observed with the *M. caroli* wild-mouse isolate.

SSV-transformed nonproducer cells have been assayed for the expression of virus-specific proteins in an attempt to elucidate the coding sequences of the SSV genome. Varying levels and numbers of *gag*-gene products may be found: two cell lines had low, but detectable, levels of p12 and p27 antigens, one had only p12, and one had neither; gp70 could not be detected in any of these clones (Tronick et al. 1974a; Aaronson et al. 1976b).

One very interesting use of nonproducer cells is the production of interspecies pseudotypes for nucleic acid hybridization studies to determine the proportion of sequences overlapping in SSAV and SSV. In one such study by Scolnick et al. (1976b), the SSV genome was rescued from a nonproducer cell line by infection with an amphotropic MLV. Velocity sedimentation showed that the RNA extracted from this SSV(MLV) and MLV population contained two major species, 70S and 45S. The 70S RNA hybridized to MLV and not to SSAV, whereas the 45S RNA hybridized exclusively to SSAV. This study provided evidence that heterodimers did not form between RNA subunits of the two parental types. Further proof of homodimers was provided when the two species were denatured; the 70S RNA gave rise to 33S–35S subunits, whereas the 45S RNA dissociated into 24S–26S subunits. Hybridization of an SSAV DNA probe to the smaller RNA indicated that approximately 50% of the SSAV genome is present in the SSV RNA molecule. A DNA probe transcribed from the SSV RNA hybridized to SSAV and SSV, with a slight increase in hybridization to SSV. This difference may be interpreted to represent the oncogene sequences of SSV (called *sis*); more direct means for assessing this gene are discussed in Chapter 9.

Neither SSAV nor GALV is an endogenous virus of primates; and their origins are still unknown. Hybridization experiments suggest that, among various primates, the *sis* sequences of SSV have most likely come from the cellular genome of the woolly monkey, but the source of the helper virus has not been identified conclusively. Yet it is evident from the epidemiological surveys that GALV is horizontally transmitted and leads to a substantial incidence of leukemia in gibbon colonies. Some serological studies have further substantiated this conclusion. Kawakami et al. (1973) analyzed sera from gibbons in five geographically distinct gibbon colonies for antibodies that reacted with virus-producing cells or that neutralized GALV. The groups that contained the highest proportion of antibody-positive animals were from those colonies where leukemia had been reported and from which virus had been isolated. These antibodies were further shown to be specific for viral envelope antigens in an immunoelectron-microscopy study (Aoki et al. 1976). Species of gibbon other than *H. lar* have not been studied, and all *H. lar* colonies may be derived from a small breeding stock from Thailand; feral colonies of gibbons have not been studied for infectious virus or antibody.

If we consider, retrospectively, the original isolate of this group, SSV(SSAV) plus SSAV, it is of interest that the woolly monkey, from whose fibrosarcoma the viruses were isolated, was maintained in a California household that included a gibbon. Although SSAV can be distinguished immunologically and biochemically from the GALV members of the group and although a transforming virus has not been isolated from gibbons, it is possible that the initial infection of the monkey was from a horizontally transmitted gibbon virus. Furthermore, all SSAV/GALV isolates are from animals that have been in close contact with humans and/or have received injections of human materials (blood from leukemia or malarial patients or brain material from kuru patients) and/or have been experimentally manipulated (e.g., exposed to X-rays). These exposures may be entirely fortuitous. On the other hand, the possibility exists that human biological materials may have played some role in the evolution of these leukemogenic viruses (see Chapter 11).

3. Baboon C-type Retroviruses

The existence of baboon C-type viruses was first predicted from early electron micrography studies of normal baboon tissues. Numerous typical C-type particles were seen to bud from the membranes of syncytiotrophoblast cells of placentas taken from all stages of pregnancy (Kalter et al. 1973), and also from preimplantation embryos (Kalter et al. 1974), follicular oocytes, and tubal ova (Kalter et al. 1975b). In addition, baboon testicular cells infected with FeSV gave rise to a transforming pseudotype population with a new host range (Melnick et al. 1973; Todaro et al. 1973a), which suggested the production of a baboon helper virus. This led to the isolation of an infectious baboon C-type virus, initially by cocultivation of a normal baboon full-term placenta with a variety of cell lines (Benveniste et al. 1974a). The technique of cocultivation has subsequently proved to be not just useful but also essential for the isolation of infectious baboon C-type viruses, which have now been obtained from at least four baboon species (*Papio papio,* the western baboon; *P. anubis,* the dogface baboon; *P. cynocephalus,* the yellow baboon; and *P. hamadryas,* the royal baboon) and from the closely related gelada (*Therapithecus gelada*). A wide spectrum of tissues has provided the isolates: placenta, amnion, chorionic fluid, umbilicus, ovary, testes, spleen, liver, kidney, skin, heart, lung, intestines, brain, lymph nodes, bone marrow, and whole embryos (Benveniste et al. 1974a; Goldberg et al. 1974; Todaro et al. 1974c, 1976; Heberling et al. 1976; Lapin 1976). Pretreatment of the baboon cells with halogenated pyrimidines has always increased the frequency of virus recovery.

In the electron microscope the baboon C-type virus appears as a 50-nm electron-lucent core, surrounded by three layers to give an overall diameter of approximately 100 nm; no conspicuous surface spikes have been observed. The BaEV particles have cross-reacting serological and biochemical properties with the endogenous feline C-type virus RD114 (Strickland et al. 1973; Hellman et al. 1974; Sherr et al. 1974b; Todaro et al. 1974b); the significance of this will be discussed later. The most frequently cited isolates are M7 and M28 (from *P. cynocephalus*), B1LN (from *P. hamadryas*), PP-1-Lu (from *P. papio*), and TG-1-K (from the gelada).

The relatedness of the BaEV and RD114/CCC and their classification as a distinct group of mammalian retroviruses are based on nucleic acid homology and antigenic relatedness. The structural proteins of BaEV are described in detail in Chapter 6, and therefore only the antigenic specificities are presented here. In homologous competition RIAs, where either BaEV p28 or RD114 p28 is precipitated with its homologous antiserum, both RD114 and BaEV compete with similar efficiency (Goldberg et al. 1974; Sherr and Todaro 1974; Sherr et al. 1974b; Todaro et al. 1974b; Stephenson et al. 1976a; Barbacid et al. 1977), although in most cases the slope of the competition curve and the final extent of competition do allow the differentiation of the two viruses. The p28 peptides from all BaEV isolates, including those from different genera, compete well (57–100%) (Goldberg et al. 1974; Todaro et al. 1974b), whereas no competition is observed with viruses of the SSAV/GALV group or with those from lower mammals (e.g., MLV and FeLV). The p28 molecules of BaEV and RD114 carry interspecies antigenic determinants that are cross-reactive with those of MLV and FeLV. This is observed most strongly when antiserum to BaEV is used to precipitate MLV p30. These determinants are not shared with the exogenous C-type primate viruses. Some cross-reactivity, however, is observed with the p26 of MAC-1 virus, an endogenous virus of rhesus monkeys (Bryant et al. 1978; Todaro et al. 1978c), a result predicted from the observation that a protein cross-reactive with RD114 and BaEV p28 is detected in normal rhesus monkey tissues (Stephenson et al. 1976a). The major core proteins of BaEV and RD114, however, are readily distinguishable by isoelectric focusing; the isoelectric point of RD114 is 8.8 and that of the BaEV is 7.1 (Sherr and Todaro 1974).

The reverse transcriptase has a molecular weight of 70,000 daltons and exhibits a Mn^{++} divalent-cation preference (Benveniste et al. 1974b). Antisera to reverse transcriptases of many mammalian C-type viruses do not inhibit the activity of the baboon viral enzyme; however, there is a partial inhibition of activity (about 50%) by serum prepared against RD114 reverse transcriptase.

The gp70 confers similar neutralization and host-range (see below) characteristics on both BaEV and RD114 (Benveniste et al. 1974a; Hellman et al. 1974; Todaro et al. 1974c). As might be expected, cells infected with either BaEV or RD114 are resistant to superinfection by MSV pseudotypes of either virus (Hellman et al. 1974). Immunological studies using highly sensitive competition RIAs have nevertheless shown the presence of highly type-specific determinants on both virus groups. In addition to the group-specific antigenic determinants that are shared by BaEV and RD114, a novel group of interspecies antigenic determinants have been identified. These do not cross-react with the analogous polypeptides of MLV, FeLV, or SSAV/GALV, but do cross-react with the glycoproteins of the D-type primate retroviruses (MPMV, SMRV, and langur virus) (Stephenson et al. 1976b; Bryant et al. 1978; Devare et al. 1978a). Also, gp70 proteins of BaEV and RD114 and those of the primate D-type viruses share functional determinants, since complete virus interference is observed between viruses from these two groups (Sacks et al. 1978; Chatterjee and Hunter 1980; Fine et al. 1980).

The genomic RNA in baboon C-type viral particles is a complex with a sedimentation coefficient of 52S, corresponding to a molecular weight of about 6×10^6, and it can be irreversibly dissociated into two equal subunits. In the 52S dimer, the subunits are joined near their 5′ ends along a region of about 400 nucleotides. Electron microscopy reveals a characteristic large loop that occurs symmetrically in each subunit. Although the size of the RNA subunit of baboon C-type virus is slightly smaller than that of RD114 (9.4 kb vs. 10.0 kb), the size and location of the loops in each molecule are remarkably similar (Kung et al. 1976) (see Chapter 4, Fig. 4.3). These data provide further evidence of a relationship between BaEV and RD114.

Cocultivation of baboon cells with, or infection of, heterogeneic cells was found to be essential for the isolation of infectious virus; this reflects the xenotropic host range. The *P. cynocephalus, P. hamadryas,* and *T. gelada* isolates replicate in human, rhesus monkey, dog, and bat cells. The *P. papio* isolate apparently replicates in rhesus monkey cells only. None of these isolates replicate in baboon, cat, mink, rat, mouse, or avian cells (Benveniste et al. 1974a; Goldberg et al. 1974; Todaro et al. 1974b,c, 1976). The pattern mirrors, for the most part, that seen with RD114, except that one cat cell line (FFc60WF) is susceptible to RD114 infection but resistant to the baboon viruses (Todaro et al. 1974c). Cells infected with either BaEV or RD114 elicit a syncytial response in human KC cells upon cocultivation (Hellman et al. 1974; Ahmed et al. 1975); however, the often high background of spontaneous syncytia with the KC cell line renders this assay unsatisfactory for quantitative measurement of virus titers.

One expects a virus with a xenotropic host range to exist as an endogenous provirus, and this is indeed the case with the baboon viruses; endogenous virus DNA sequences can readily be detected in normal baboon-cell DNA (Benveniste and Todaro 1974a; Benveniste et al. 1974a; Sherr et al. 1974a) at a concentration of about 7–10 copies of viral DNA per haploid-cell genome (Benveniste and Todaro 1974b, 1976). The search for baboon proviral sequences in cellular DNAs of other primates and mammals revealed (1) that sequences related to BaEV occur in the DNAs of other Old World monkeys, but not in the DNAs of apes or New World monkeys to any significant extent, and (2) that the DNA of the domestic cat (and European wildcat) is unique among nonprimates in exhibiting a substantial homology with baboon viral sequences. The latter finding substantiates all the other biochemical and serological data that indicate an evolutionary relationship between BaEV and RD114. There is extensive homology between the viral RNA genomes of different BaEV and gelada isolates (greater than 50%) and a notable amount of homology (10–20%) with endogenous xenotropic cat viruses, but little homology is found with other C-type viruses (Benveniste et al. 1974b; Todaro et al. 1974b).

The presence of DNA sequences related to the sequences of the endogenous baboon viruses in the cellular genome of all the Old World monkeys that have been tested suggests that these genes have been conserved during speciation, perhaps because they provide functions that confer a selective evolutionary advantage

(Todaro et al. 1975). On the other hand, the recent work by Wong-Staal and Josephs (1981) suggests that BaEV may be like other endogenous viruses in having entered the germline postspeciation, albeit ubiquitously. It is also interesting that the extent of these sequence homologies correlates closely with taxonomic relationships of the monkey species on the basis of anatomical criteria and fossil records and thus may provide another measurement of evolutionary divergence. Reservations about this type of analysis are discussed in Chapter 10. Analysis of the thermal-elution profiles of the hybrids formed between the cDNAs of the baboon viruses and the cellular DNAs of various monkeys suggests that during speciation, there has been base-pair alteration involving the entire proviral genome, rather than the preservation (without change) of only a small segment of the proviruses (Benveniste and Todaro 1974a).

The unexpected finding that baboon proviral sequences are present in the cellular DNAs of some, but not all, members of the cat family promoted the notion of interspecies transmission of retroviruses. Models for this horizontal transmission between unrelated species and the ontogeny of proviral sequences have been proposed by Benveniste and Todaro (1974c), taking into account that sequences related to the genomes of RD114 and BaEV are found in the cellular genomes of all anthropoid primates and some members of the Felidae family. The most suitable model postulates that the endogenous primate virus infected an ancestor of the domestic cat about 5–10 million years ago. Other examples of horizontal transmission of retroviruses between species that are only remotely related are described elsewhere in this chapter.

The extent to which the baboon proviral sequences are expressed in the cellular RNA of normal baboon tissues is debatable. Benveniste et al. (1974b) initially reported that approximately 40% of the sequences are transcribed in placental tissue, compared with 2% in liver tissue; which would suggest differential transcription of proviral sequences in these tissues (Benveniste et al. 1974b). Subsequently, Benveniste et al. (1974a) detected transcripts corresponding to 10% of the proviral sequences in liver, to 30–40% in testes, spleen, and lung, and to 70% in placenta. A third report from this group indicates that spleen-, lung-, testes-, and liver-cell RNAs all contain transcripts of 40% of the endogenous viral sequences (Sherr et al. 1974a). The extent to which variation between individual animals accounts for these differences remains to be seen.

Since baboon C-type viruses are endogenous to baboons and since the endogenous proviruses appear to be partially expressed in a variety of tissues, one might perhaps expect baboons to be immunologically unresponsive or tolerant to viral antigens. Antibodies of IgG and IgA classes that bind to intact viral particles, however, have been detected in radioimmunoprecipitation assays with baboon sera (Weislow et al. 1976). These antibodies do not bind to viruses disrupted with ether, which may indicate they are directed specifically against the surface glycoproteins of the viral particles. On the other hand, they fail to neutralize the virus, and so it is presently unclear precisely which antigenic determinants of the virus provoke their production.

Isolates of baboon C-type viruses have been injected into a variety of primates and other mammals but without pathological consequences (Heberling et al. 1976; Weislow et al. 1976). There are, however, several instances in which these viruses have been associated with neoplastic diseases. The one isolate that has been obtained from a royal baboon (*P. hamadryas*) came from tissues of a lymphomatous animal (Goldberg et al. 1974), but the ease with which these viruses are isolated from tissues of other baboons suggests that the neoplastic state of this particular animal may well have been fortuitous. Another example of an association of baboon virus with lymphoproliferative disease is more intriguing. Lapin (1976) described an outbreak of leukemia in *P. hamadryas* baboons that had been inoculated with, or had been in contact with animals inoculated with, human leukemic blood samples. C-type virus was regularly observed in many tissues in such animals. Sediments of virus-containing urine injected into *P. hamadryas* or *Macaca arctoides* (stumptail macaque) induced a lymphoproliferative disease. A herpesvirus, morphologically and serologically related to EBV, was consistently found, however, in the sick animals in association with the C-type virus. Whether either virus alone is oncogenic or whether they are coleukemogenic has yet to be determined. These observations call to mind the coleukemogenic effect of the guinea pig retrovirus and herpesvirus (see Section II.K.1), and they suggest that further studies of the interactions between RNA and DNA tumor viruses might prove interesting.

Finally, although all the known baboon retroviruses are typical C-type particles, Kalter et al. (1975a), using electron microscopy, observed structures resembling A-type and B-type retroviruses in baboon prostate tissue. Three years previously, these animals had received injections of dimethylbenzanthracene in this site, but no tumors had developed. Whether or not these observations foreshadow the discovery of a baboon B-type retrovirus remains to be seen.

4. Macaque C-type Retroviruses

A new class of endogenous primate C-type virus was isolated from a continuous tissue-culture cell line of the stumptail monkey *Macaca arctoides* (Todaro et al. 1978a), thus representing the second C-type virus obtained from Old World primates. The virus was obtained after long-term (150 days) cocultivation of a stumptail monkey spleen cell with the human alveolar carcinoma cell line A549. Similar cocultivations with dog, bat, rhesus, MSV-transformed mink, and other human cells were unsuccessful. The particles closely resemble C-type viruses by electron microscopy, and neither cytoplasmic A-type particles nor D-type particles were observed. The host range of the isolate, designated MAC-1, includes feline and human cells, but the virus does not replicate in the original stumptail monkey cells or in those of other Old World monkeys (rhesus and African green monkeys). The isolate is apparently distinct serologically from other C-type viruses, as indicated by the failure to detect p30 or reverse transcriptase cross-reactivity in group-specific assays (Todaro et al. 1978a).

A second isolate from a macaque, the rhesus monkey (*M. mulatta*), was reported by Rabin et al. (1979). This isolate was derived from a spontaneous esophageal carcinoma that was established in culture, treated with IdU, and then cocultivated with canine cells. This second isolate, MMC-1, is related to MAC-1, as the p30 molecules of MAC-1 and MMC-1 show a line of identity in immunodiffusion tests (Rabin et al. 1979). It is not yet clear whether type-specific determinants which could differentiate the two viruses exist on the p30 molecules. Interspecies determinants common with RD114/BaEV, MLV, and FeLV are present (Bryant et al. 1978; Rabin et al. 1979), but the most closely related virus yet found seems to be the REV group of avian viruses (Section II.E.3).

An isolate from the pig-tailed macaque (*M. nemestrina*) is apparently unrelated to MAC-1 and MMC-1 by immunological and nucleic acid criteria (E. Hefti and S. Panem, pers. comm.).

However, these distinctions will have to be assessed further to determine the degree by which the new isolate differs from the stumptail monkey and rhesus monkey isolates.

Hybridization of a MAC-1 viral cDNA probe to a variety of primate cellular DNAs showed complete hybridization to stumptail monkey DNA and lesser, although high (72–96%), hybridization to DNAs from other species of macaques and closely related Old World monkeys, whereas no homology was detected with New World species (Todaro et al. 1978a; Bonner and Todaro 1979). These data provide good evidence that MAC-1 is an endogenous virus of stumptail monkeys, present at 50–150 copies per haploid genome, and suggest that primate species closely related to stumptail macaques contain related viral gene sequences in their cellular DNAs. In addition the MAC-1 cDNA transcripts hybridize to cat-cell DNA at significant levels, compared with various other mammalian cellular DNAs. Hybridization is detected to all members of the Felidae family whether or not they contain endogenous RD114 or FeLV sequences. However, hybridization to the viral RNAs from RD114 and FeLV, as well as reciprocal hybridizations with cDNA transcripts of the feline viruses and MAC-1 viral RNA, establishes that the sequences detected in Felidae cellular DNA are not related to either of the two groups of feline C-type viruses. Therefore, the MAC-1 viral transcripts detect sequences in Felidae that may correspond to genes in viruses that have yet to be isolated. The fact that MAC-1-related sequences are present in a number of carnivores suggests that the sequences may have been present for at least 40 million years (Bonner and Todaro 1979).

MAC-1 virus was also shown to be unrelated to other previously isolated endogenous primate retroviruses. Therefore, the sequences related to MAC-1 in cellular DNA of baboons and other Old World monkey species are not of the baboon C-type viral gene class. A second set of endogenous virus sequences can therefore be detected in the genomes of various primates which also appear to diverge with the host genome. This finding raises the possibility that there exist still other retroviral gene sequences in primates in addition to the ones that have so far been identified.

5. Owl Monkey C-type Retrovirus

An established cell culture of owl monkey (*Aotus trivirgatus*) kidney cells was the source of a new virus, called OMC-1 (Todaro et al. 1978c). The virus is morphologically of C-type and its crescent-shaped nucleoid appears to condense at the plasma membrane, forming budding particles and extracellular particles 110–120 nm in diameter. This size is somewhat larger than the baboon C-type viruses (100–110 nm) and smaller than the langur D-type virus (120–130 nm). The host range is apparently limited to cells from the owl monkey, cat, and bat. Therefore, this is the only endogenous primate retrovirus (C type or D type) that reinfects cells of its own host species.

The virus contains a genomic RNA of 60S–65S, which after heat denaturation sediments as 32S. The viral reverse transcriptase shows a preferential requirement for Mg^{++}, although its reduced requirement for divalent cations (3.5 mM Mg^{++} and 0.09 mM Mn^{++}) can be used to differentiate OMC-1 from other mammalian retroviruses. The enzyme is also not inhibited by antisera to the reverse transcriptase from other primate C-type or D-type viruses.

Tryptic peptide analyses show that the p30 of OMC-1 is distinct from other primate retroviral p30 proteins, and this polypeptide is unreactive in most of the RIAs commonly used to detect interspecies antigenic determinants on various mammalian viruses (Todaro et al. 1978c; Barbacid et al. 1980). Nevertheless, a hyperimmune serum to OMC-1 p30 precipitates the analogous polypeptides from REV, SSAV, and deer kidney virus (DKV) with varying avidity. The common determinants on SSAV and DKV are also shared by other mammalian viruses and REV, but not by viruses of the BaEV/RD114 group or by members of the B-type or D-type virus groups (Barbacid et al. 1980).

In competition RIAs designated to detect interspecies determinants shared by the glycoproteins of many primate C-type and D-type viruses, the major OMC-1 *env*-gene product gp70 shows no competition (Barbacid et al. 1980). Therefore, the polypeptides of this virus appear to have diverged significantly from those of the other retroviruses.

Hybridization of OMC-1 cDNA to a variety of cellular DNAs shows that OMC-1 is endogenous to owl monkeys and that fewer, although related, sequences can be found in other New World monkeys (Todaro et al. 1978c). In contrast, the extent of hybridization to DNA from Old World monkeys and nonprimates is considerably less. The kinetics of hybrid formation suggest that there are 30–40 copies of OMC-1 viral sequences per haploid genome of owl monkey cells. No hybridization was detected with cDNA from other primate retroviruses.

6. Colobus Monkey C-type Retrovirus

A virus, CPC-1, was isolated recently from the colobus monkey (*Colobus polykomos*) and appears to be related to the macaque viruses. An early culture of normal colobus kidney cells was cocultivated with a variety of cell lines and treated with IdU. After 7 months, virus activity was detected in the coculture with the human carcinoma A549 cells, although similar experiments with bat and dog cells remained virus-negative (Sherwin and Todaro 1979).

The CPC-1 viral reverse transcriptase requires Mn^{++} and is inhibited, as are the polymerases of most mammalian C-type viruses, by a broadly reactive antiserum to RD114 polymerase. Viral cDNA transcripts, used in hybridization experiments, showed that the virus is endogenous to the colobus. The kinetics of hybridization suggest that there are about 50–70 copies of the CPC-1 genome in colobus cells. Significant levels of hybridization (about 20%) were also detected in the cellular DNA of the other Old World monkey subfamily (Cercopithecinae), which includes the macaques and baboons. Essentially no homology with New World monkey DNA was obtained.

CPC-1 and the macaque virus MAC-1 show similar host-range patterns, replicating in human and cat cells, but not in cells of bat, rhesus or African green monkey, dog, mink, or mouse. This similarity suggests that the two viruses may have related *env*-gene proteins, although this has not yet been formally demonstrated.

The macaque and colobus monkey isolates are further related in immunological assays of the major core proteins (approximately 50%). It is interesting that this endogenous C-type isolate from the Colobinae family is so highly related to the macaque (Cercopithecinae) C-type virus, whereas it is unrelated to the D-type retrovirus isolated from langurs (also Colobinae), because the two subfamilies of Old World monkeys are thought to have diverged genetically about 20 million years ago.

7. Mason-Pfizer Monkey D-Type Retrovirus

MPMV was first discovered by electron microscopy of a spontaneous mammary adenocarcinoma that arose in an 8-year-old female rhesus monkey (*M. mulatta*) (Chopra and Mason 1970; Jensen et al. 1970; Mason et al. 1972). Attempts to establish long-term cultures of the carcinoma cells were unsuccessful, but cocultivation of the tumor cells with fetal monkey cells resulted in the development of a cell line that continuously shed the virus (Jensen et al. 1970). Further studies showed that secondary monkey embryo cells, fetal monkey lung cells, a chimpanzee lung cell line, embryonic human cells, and human lymphoblastoid cell lines were susceptible to infection by MPMV. On the other hand, attempts to infect mouse bone marrow cells, baby hamster kidney cells, rhesus monkey kidney cells, African green monkey cells, and baboon or chimpanzee lymphocytes have failed. The ability of MPMV-infected human cells to form easily identifiable syncytia when overlaid in culture with KC cells (a human glioma cell transformed by RSV) led to the development of a plaque assay (Rand et al. 1974). Preexposure of the KC cells to RD114 gp70 blocked the formation of syncytia by both RD114 and MPMV (Rand et al. 1975). This study foreshadowed the detection of immunological relatedness between the envelope glycoproteins of these two viruses (see below). Although infection of permissive cells with MPMV generally has no accompanying cytopathic effects, infection of rhesus monkey and human foreskin cultures or embryonic rhesus monkey lung cultures results directly in syncytia formation (Fine et al. 1971, 1975); such syncytia are clearly distinguishable on the basis of size, extent of vacuolization, and time of appearance from those induced by primate spumaviruses.

The morphogenesis of MPMV proved to be unusual compared with that of standard B-type and C-type viruses. The virus matures by the budding of intracytoplasmic A-type particles, similar to the intracellular form of MMTV, but extracellular mature virions have a smooth envelope and a centrally located nucleoid typical of C-type viruses (Chopra and Mason 1970; Kramarsky et al. 1971; Manning and Hackett 1972). Thus, the new category of D-type viral particles was introduced (see Section I.B.).

MPMV fulfills all the criteria for retroviruses: It contains an aggregate 60S–70S RNA with an associated reverse transcriptase (Nowinski et al. 1971a; Schlom and Spiegelman 1971; Manning and Hackett 1972; Abrell and Gallo 1973). The viral RNA is a dimer structure composed of subunits, each with a complexity of about 2.8×10^6 daltons (Schochetman and Schlom 1975) and containing a polyadenylic acid tract (Gillespie et al. 1972). The reverse transcriptase has an apparent molecular weight of 80,000 daltons (Abrell and Gallo 1973) and shows preferential use of Mg^{++} (Yaniv et al. 1974).

The structural proteins of MPMV are gp68, gp20, pp14, p12, and p10 (Tronick et al. 1974b; Schochetman et al. 1975, 1976) and are discussed in detail in Chapter 6. Serological analysis allows MPMV to be distinguished from B-type and C-type viruses, including the foamy viruses (spumaviruses; see Section IV) often associated with monkey cells. Nowinski et al. (1971a) detected no cross-reactivity in immunodiffusion assays of MPMV with MLV, FeLV, MMTV, visna, or primate foamy viruses (types 1, 2, and 3). In more sensitive radioimmunoprecipitation assays, no cross-reactivity was detected between the MPMV p27 and the major internal proteins of MLV, RD114, FeLV, and SSAV/GALV isolates (Parks and Scolnick 1972; Tronick et al. 1974b). Similarly, antiserum to MPMV reverse transcriptase does not inhibit other retroviral enzymes (Yaniv et al. 1974). However, Stephenson et al. (1976b) reported some cross-reactions between the major glycoproteins of MPMV and the endogenous BaEV and RD114 viruses. MPMV transforms certain fibroblast cultures of rhesus monkey, human, and horse cells (Pienta et al. 1972; Fine et al. 1974; Ahmed et al. 1976, 1977). Transformed cells show anchorage-independent growth, loss of contact inhibition of movement, altered morphology, and decreased serum requirements.

The virus has been detected in cell cultures derived from normal breast, fetal, and placental tissues of healthy rhesus monkeys (Ahmed et al. 1974). However, neither these animals nor various primates experimentally inoculated with MPMV show evidence of tumor formation (Fine et al. 1972, 1975). However, in neonatally infected rhesus monkeys, the virus can be detected in many organs, including lymph nodes, spleen, thymus, bone marrow, and brain, in which cytopathological changes are observed (Fine et al. 1975). Infection also induces thymic involution and a consequent depletion of lymphocytes. Furthermore, many animals showed symptoms more typical of other retrovirus infections, e.g., runting and thymic atrophy, like Fr-MLV in mice (Takeichi et al. 1974); neurological abnormalities including hind-limb paralysis, like some MLV isolates from wild mice (Gardner et al. 1973b); and persistent infection with concomitant antibody production, like the lentiviruses (see Chapter 8). These pathological manifestations are described in detail elsewhere (Fine and Schochetman 1978).

Nucleic acid hybridization has shown that MPMV is not an endogenous virus of rhesus monkeys (Old World Cercopithecinae) (Parks et al. 1973b; Drohan et al. 1976; Schlom et al. 1976), since only 20% sequence homology is detected between the MPMV genome and rhesus DNA. However, a higher degree of hybridization (32–45%) is obtained with cellular DNA from the other Old World monkey subfamily Colobinae (which includes colobus and langur monkeys) (Benveniste and Todaro 1977). The kinetics of hybridization in the latter situation indicate that MPMV sequences are present at about 20–50 copies per cell. These data are also reflected in studies of nucleic acid homologies between primate retroviruses. No detectable homology is observed with any B-type or C-type viruses or with the D-type squirrel monkey isolate (Colcher et al. 1977a). However, about 30% homology is observed with the D-type retrovirus isolated from the spectacled langur (PO-1-Lu) (Todaro et al. 1978b) (see Section II.S.8). In fact, it has been suggested that MPMV was derived by infection of rhesus monkeys by an endogenous langur virus and that it persists among rhesus monkeys by horizontal transmission.

MPMV or very similar viruses have also been isolated on numerous occasions from cultures of human cells. It appears most likely, however, that these represent laboratory contamination (Parks et al. 1973b; see Chapter 11).

8. Langur D-type Retrovirus

Recently, a D-type virus was isolated from the lung tissue (treated with IdU) of a spectacled langur (*Presbytis obscurus*) following long-term cocultivation (about 6 months) with bat cells (Todaro et al. 1978b). The virus, designated PO-1-Lu, is morphologically a D-type retrovirus. Intracytoplasmic A-type particles are seen, as are budding particles with completed nucleoids at the cell membrane. The mature extracellular particles are pleomorphic in shape and generally contain a cylindrically shaped nucleoid separated from the viral envelope by an electron-dense intermediate layer, often resembling a line or bar (see Fig. 2.2). The virus has a very limited host range, growing in bat and human cells only. This distinguishes it from MPMV (which replicates in human and rhesus monkey cells) and SMRV (which has a broader host range).

The proteins of the langur virus and MPMV are very similar (see Chapter 6).

The langur virus and MPMV p27 proteins are indistinguishable in homologous competition RIAs, but no competition is observed with any B-type or C-type viruses of mammalian or avian origin (Bryant et al. 1978; Colcher et al. 1978; Todaro et al. 1978b). However, the p27 proteins of MPMV and PO-1-Lu do share common antigenic determinants with the major structural polypeptide, p35, of SMRV (Colcher et al. 1977b; Hino et al. 1977; Devare et al. 1978b). These interspecies determinants are not shared by the RD114/BaEV or SSAV/GALV groups of viruses and thus may reflect an evolutionary relatedness of the Old World and New World D-type viruses. A second rather unusual interspecies determinant on MPMV/PO-1-Lu p27 is shared by the analogous protein of the viper retrovirus (VRV) (Andersen et al. 1979) and poses interesting questions as to the origins of such cross-reactive determinants.

In homologous competition RIAs, the major glycoproteins of langur virus and SMRV do not inhibit MPMV gp70 precipitation (Devare et al. 1978a; Todaro et al. 1978b). However, antiserum to MPMV precipitates both langur and SMRV gp70 peptides and, in heterologous RIAs where antiserum to MPMV precipitates SMRV gp70, both MPMV and SMRV compete equally well. This correlates with the partial interference observed between D-type retroviruses (Chatterjee and Hunter 1980). The endogenous RD114 and BaEV also compete efficiently in this assay (Devare et al. 1978a), indicating that the interspecies determinants shared by MPMV and SMRV are common to a second "primate" virus group. Indeed, antiserum to MPMV precipitates BaEV gp70. This cross-reactivity is the basis for the interspecies RIAs (Stephenson et al. 1976b; Bryant et al. 1978; Devare et al. 1978a). This conservation of antigenic determinants might be expected in light of the cross interference observed between the D-type and RD114 virus groups (Sacks et al. 1978; Fine et al. 1980).

The viral reverse transcriptase has a molecular weight of 85,000–90,000 daltons and exhibits a preferential requirement for Mg^{++}. The reverse transcriptases of MPMV and PO-1-Lu viruses are not inhibited by antisera to the enzymes of several mammalian and primate B-type or C-type viruses (Bryant et al. 1978). Furthermore, in reciprocal experiments, antiserum to partially purified reverse transcriptase of MPMV does not inhibit the polymerases from several other viruses (MLV, FeLV, MMTV, and SSAV) (Yaniv et al. 1974; Harewood and Ahmed 1977).

Hybridization to cellular DNAs has shown that PO-1-Lu is endogenous to langurs and that related sequences are found in other Old World monkeys (Todaro et al. 1978b). The virus shows about 30% homology with the MPMV genome and none with SMRV or BaEV. Thus far, the langur virus represents the only endogenous D-type virus from an Old World monkey.

9. Squirrel Monkey D-type Retrovirus

Heberling et al. (1977) reported the isolation of a retrovirus from a variety of adult and fetal squirrel monkey (*Saimiri sciureus*) tissues that had been cocultivated with established dog or chimpanzee cell lines. Morphologically, this virus (called SMRV) resembles the prototype D-type virus (MPMV), as there are intracytoplasmic A-type (60–75-nm) particles, budding particles, and extracellular (100–140-nm) particles (Smith et al. 1977). The fully mature particles display an electron-dense centrally located nucleoid, which is generally spherical, although sometimes rod-shaped. Between the core and the envelope, there is an electron-lucent space and an electron-dense shell; no surface spikes are visible.

The virus is able to replicate in cell lines derived from dog, mink, bat, chimpanzee, rhesus monkey, and human, but not in baboon, marmoset, owl monkey, howler monkey, or squirrel monkey cells. In view of this host range, it would appear that SMRV is a xenotropic virus of squirrel monkeys.

The virus bands at 1.16–1.17 g/ml in sucrose and contains a 70S RNA. Polypeptide analysis of the virus by SDS-polyacrylamide gel electrophoresis reveals four to six major proteins: gp75, p53, p35, p16, pp12, and p9. The major core component is p35, showing an apparent molecular weight much higher than the characteristic value for most other retroviruses (Schochetman et al. 1977). SMRV p35 is distinct both structurally and immunologically from the p27 proteins of MPMV and langur viruses and from the p30 proteins of other primate C-type viruses (Bryant et al. 1978). It does, however, share common antigenic determinants with the other two D-type viruses that are not shared with other primate or mammalian C-type viruses. These assays also indicate that the major core polypeptide of langur virus is more closely related to that of SMRV than to that of MPMV (Colcher et al. 1977a; Hino et al. 1977; Schochetman et al. 1977; Bryant et al. 1978; Devare et al. 1978a). The virus is antigenically distinct from MPMV in that it is not neutralized by MPMV-neutralizing antiserum. In addition, serum that labels MPMV-producing cells in immunoelectron microscopy fails to react with SMRV-infected cells. It is interesting to note that SMRV-infected cells can induce the formation of syncytia in cocultures with the KC cell line.

In homologous RIAs, MPMV cannot compete for SMRV gp75 binding, but antiserum to MPMV can precipitate the New World viral peptide efficiently. Heterologous RIAs utilizing this cross-reactivity also detect common antigenic determinants on RD114/BaEV glycoproteins, and, in fact, antiserum to SMRV gp75 precipitates RD114/BaEV glycoprotein (Devare et al. 1978a). The presence of these common antigenic determinants on the RD114/BaEV and primate D-type viral glycoproteins has raised the possibility that, during evolution of these viruses, a recombinational event has taken place between ancestral viruses of the two groups.

The reverse transcriptase reaction shows a preferential requirement for Mg^{++}, as does that of MPMV. The viral polymerase of 80,000 daltons displays an interesting feature: In the presence of a high monovalent cation concentration (160 mM KCl), the enzyme shows a shift toward the preferential utilization of Mn^{++}, a shift not observed with other retroviruses (Colcher et al. 1977b). The polymerase of SMRV appears similar to, but distinguishable from that of MPMV, as antiserum to the latter causes only a partial (40%) inhibition of SMRV polymerase activity.

Nucleic acid hybridization experiments using a ^{3}H-labeled SMRV RNA show that the virus is probably endogenous to squirrel monkeys and that its genes occur in multiple copies in all squirrel monkey tissues. There is little hybridization of viral RNA to cellular DNA from other Old World primates, suggesting that the acquisition of the virus was relatively recent in evolutionary terms. Despite the slight antigenic relatedness of SMRV and MPMV, Colcher et al. (1977b) detected no nucleic acid homology between the two retroviruses. SMRV thus represents the first xenotropic endogenous D-type virus isolated from a New World primate.

III. TAXONOMY OF LENTIVIRUSES

Slow virus infection is a term coined by Sigurdsson (1954a) to describe the natural history of a group of diseases of Icelandic sheep distinguished by a prolonged incubation period and a protracted symptomatic disease phase. These diseases include a chronic pneumonia, *maedi* (meaning shortness of breath) and *visna* (meaning wasting due to progressive neurological impairment), with inflammation of the central nervous system. Both diseases were introduced into Iceland by the importation of 20 sheep, apparently latently infected, from Germany in 1933. In the next two decades, several hundred thousand sheep died from these illnesses, and the introduction of a mass slaughter program was eventually the means of eradication of visna and maedi.

Sigurdsson (1954b) later showed that visna and maedi could be transmitted by cell-free filtrates from affected organs. The period from inoculation to clinical manifestations spanned several months or even years, and the subsequent course of disease was very long. Further details of the pathogenesis are presented in Chapter 8 (for review, see Haase 1975; DeBoer and Houwers 1979; Petursson et al. 1979; Brahic and Haase 1981).

Several viruses related to, if not nearly identical with, visna virus have been isolated from sick sheep and goats in various locales. The isolates from sheep are called visna, maedi (Gudnadottir and Palsson 1967), zwoegerziekte (De Boer 1975), and progressive pneumonia virus (PPV) (Kennedy et al. 1968), and there has been one isolate of a related virus from goats, called caprine encephalitis-arthritis virus (CAEV) (Cork et al. 1974). These five viruses presently comprise the lentivirus subfamily. A recently isolated retrovirus that causes arthritis in sheep is antigenically related to visna virus and may prove to be a sixth member of this group (unpubl. data from O. Narayan and J. Gorham cited in Narayan et al. 1980). As discussed below, it appears likely that all of these viruses may represent strains of a single isolate which are capable of producing distinct but related pathological syndromes, perhaps dependent upon the initial site of the infection (Gudnadottir 1974).

The initial isolation of visna virus was performed by identification of an agent that caused CPE in cell cultures from sheep choroid plexus (SCP) (Sigurdsson et al. 1960). Similarly, the agents of maedi and progressive pneumonia were obtained. Taken as the prototype of lentiviruses, visna virus replicates in cells of many vertebrate species, but virus production is most efficient in ovine cells, particularly SCP cultures (Thormar and Sigurdsardottir 1962; Harter et al. 1968) The CPE in SCP cells consists of the formation of multinucleated cells and focal areas of degeneration. These effects led to the development of quantitative assays in vitro (Sigurdsson et al. 1960; Harter and Choppin 1967a,b). Plaque assays allowed the clonal isolation of visna virus (Haase and Levinson 1973), as well as small-plaque and large-plaque variants (Trowbridge 1974). Despite the slow progression of the virus-induced disease in vivo, replication of visna virus in vitro occurs with the same kinetics as other retroviruses.

Electron micrographs of cells infected with visna virus showed particles with a narrow crescent-shaped core at the cell membrane. The mature virions are 80–120 nm in diameter, with a central electron-dense core (40 nm) and prominent spikes (8–10 nm) (Thormar 1961a; Thormar and Cruickshank 1965; Chippaux-Hyppolite et al. 1972; Dubois-Dalcq et al. 1976). The close proximity of the crescent to the envelope in budding and newly budded virions is slightly different from the majority of C-type particles (see Fig. 2.6).

Other early studies demonstrating retrovirus characteristics in-

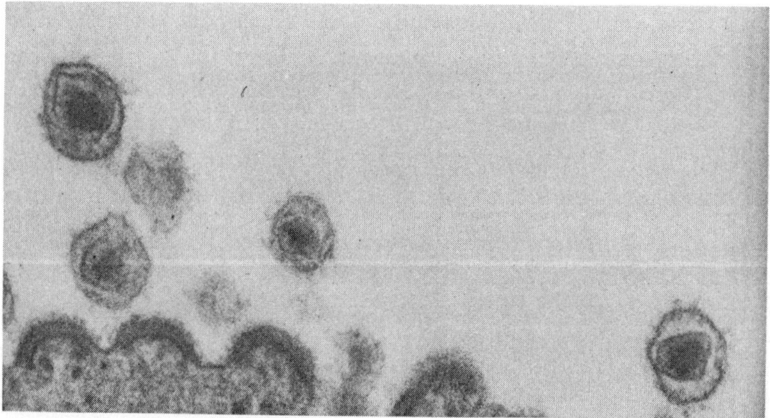

Figure 2.6 Electron micrograph of budding and extracellular particles of visna virus. Note the close proximity of the core shell to the outer membrane. (Micrograph kindly provided by A. Haase and J. Baringer.)

cluded buoyant density of 1.16 g/ml in sucrose (Stone et al. 1971b); sensitivity to lipid solvents and thermal inactivation (Thormar 1961b, 1965); 60S–70S RNA composed of 35S subunits (Brahic et al. 1971, 1973; Harter et al. 1971; Lin and Thormar 1971; Haase et al. 1974a), showing a complexity of 3×10^6 to 3.5×10^6 daltons (Beemon et al. 1976; Vigne et al. 1977); and reverse transcriptase activity (Lin and Thormar 1971, 1972; Schlom et al. 1971; Stone et al. 1971a,b). Similar properties have been confirmed for maedi virus and PPV.

The structural proteins of visna and related viruses are discussed in Chapter 6 (Mountcastle et al. 1972; Haase and Baringer 1974; Lin and Thormar 1970, 1973, 1974). The major low-molecular-weight protein of 25,000 daltons bears antigenic determinants shared by visna, maedi, PPV, and zwoegerziekte viruses (Stowring et al. 1979). There are two other peptides, p16 and p14; the p14 peptide is found in association with the viral RNA (Lin and Thormar 1974) and may be equivalent to the virion RNA-binding proteins of other retroviruses. Four glycoproteins are detected: gp135, gp90, gp51, and gp46. The largest of these constitutes 12% of the mass of the virion and thus is considered to be the major envelope glycoprotein. As discussed in Chapter 6, this molecule could represent a stable complex of several components whose interactions resist standard denaturing techniques. One phosphoprotein, pp97, is also detected. Immunoprecipitation of purified virions and of extracts from infected cells should clarify which of these proteins are virus-encoded and whether some represent uncleaved precursors. Initially the reverse transcriptase molecule of visna virus was reported to have a molecular weight of 125,000 daltons (Lin et al. 1973), but later studies indicated that it is a dimeric structure with a molecular weight of 68,000 daltons per subunit (Haase et al. 1974b; Lin and Papini 1978).

Visna and maedi viruses share common antigenic determinants, as judged by reciprocal neutralization patterns with sera from infected sheep (Thormar and Helgadottir 1965) and by immunofluorescence assays (Takemoto et al. 1971). Furthermore, no cross-reactivities to oncoviruses have been detected (Thormar 1965; Harter et al. 1971); however, type-specific determinants can be discerned on the gp135 molecule, as measured by neutralization and by differences in the peptide maps (Mountcastle et al. 1972; Bruns and Frenzel 1979; Lin and Thormar 1979; Scott et al. 1979).

The agent that causes the leukoencephalomyelitis-arthritis syndrome (Cork et al. 1974; Cork and Narayan 1980), originally called CAEV and later GLV for goat leukoencephalitis virus (Narayan et al. 1980), has been shown to be related to the prototypic lentivirus visna (Crawford et al. 1980; Narayan et al. 1980). Morphologically, the virus resembles visna virus in both its intracellular and extracellular forms. Reverse transcriptase activity, utilizing Mg^{++} as divalent cation, is detected at 1.15 g/ml in sucrose. The agent differs somewhat from visna virus in its biological properties in vivo (see Chapter 8) and in vitro. First, serological relatedness is detected to visna p30 in immunodiffusion tests, but the virus is not neutralized by highly neutralizing anti-visna serum (Crawford et al. 1980; Narayan et al. 1980); the latter property suggests that CAEV *env*-gene antigens are quite distinct from those of visna. Second, although visna virus replicates well in sheep, goat, and cow cells, CAEV replication is restricted to goat cells, most particularly cultures of synovial membrane (predominantly macrophages). Persistence of CAEV in SCP cells for at least 2 weeks without detectable virus production is suggested by cocultivation rescue experiments (Narayan et al. 1980).

Replication of visna virus occurs through proviral DNA intermediates, like that of other retroviruses (Haase and Varmus 1973; Weiss et al. 1975; Haase et al. 1976; Brahic et al. 1977). DNA synthesis occurs in a biphasic manner, corresponding to the latency and exponential phase of the replication cycle (Clements et al. 1979). Interestingly, 80–90% of the viral DNA is found in an unintegrated form in the nucleus (Haase and Varmus 1973; Haase et al. 1976; Vigne et al. 1978; Clements et al. 1979). Also in opposition to oncoviruses, nondividing cells support virus replication, suggesting that cellular DNA synthesis and/or mitosis is not required.

Takemoto and Stone (1971) reported that visna virus and PPV could transform mouse cells. These nonproducer cells contained virus rescuable by fusion to permissive sheep cells and produced tumors upon injection into irradiated mice. On the other hand, Brown and Thormar (1975) contended that mouse and hamster cells could be latently infected by visna virus but that there were no signs of morphological transformation. Macintyre et al. (1972) observed morphological alterations in visna-virus-infected human astrocytoma cells and sheep cells using a virus strain passaged through human cells. The situation is probably best explained by concluding that lentiviruses can cause cytopathic effects of morphological alterations that resemble morphological transformation and that the tumors induced in mice were probably the result of spontaneous transformation of the infected mouse cell line or the interaction between visna virus and an endogenous mouse virus or mouse cellular *onc* sequences. The latter possibility would certainly be an interesting model for further investigation.

Three species of virus-specific mRNAs are detectable, with sedimentation coefficients of 35S, 28S, and 21S (Filippi et al. 1979). By analogy to the oncoviruses, the largest and smallest species would represent the mRNAs for *gag*- and *env*-gene precursors, respectively, but the analogy does not account for the 28S RNA. Comparison of immunofluorescence and hybridization data shows that only 0.02% of cells containing viral DNA express viral mRNA or synthesize the major *gag* protein, suggesting that there is a strong block to transcription (Haase et al. 1977, 1978). Hybridization data show that there is extensive homology between visna and maedi viruses, but not between these two viruses and PPV (Weiss et al. 1975), whereas there is no detectable homology of lentiviruses with oncoviruses (Harter et al. 1973; Quintrell et al. 1974). Neither visna virus nor PPV sequences are detected in sheep-cell DNA (Haase and Varmus 1973; Weiss et al. 1975) and therefore these lentiviruses are not endogenous. This finding is not surprising considering the epidemiology of the disease described earlier in this section.

IV. TAXONOMY OF SPUMAVIRUSES

Foamy viruses, which constitute the third subfamily, Spumavirinae, of the Retroviridae, are present in a number of mammalian species and induce persistent infections without evident pathogenesis in their natural hosts. They have been isolated primarily as contaminants of primary cell cultures in which they induce a characteristic "spontaneous" foamy degeneration after a few weeks of culture.

Although induction of a foamy appearance in cell cultures is a criterion of this group, this property is shared by viruses of other families. The foamy viruses are classified within the retrovirus family because of their physical and chemical structures and the presence of reverse transcriptase. In morphology, the foamy viruses clearly resemble oncoviruses. Intracellular particles are 35–50 nm in diameter, with an inner electron-lucent core surrounded by an electron-opaque shell. Extracellular particles or those within cytoplasmic vacuoles are larger (100–140 nm) and show clearly defined radiating spikes 5–15 nm in length (Clarke et al. 1967, 1969a,b; Clarke and Attridge 1968; Malmquist et al. 1969; Clarke and McFerran 1970; Chopra et al. 1972; Hooks et al. 1972, 1973; Epstein et al. 1974).

Rustigian et al. (1955) described the isolation of the first foamy virus. This agent, from macaque cells, was designated simian foamy virus (SFV) type 1. There are now at least nine SFV serotypes (Johnston 1961, 1971; Stiles et al. 1964; Rogers et al. 1967; Gajdusek et al. 1969; Hooks et al. 1972, 1973; Rabin et al. 1976). Types 1 through 3 are associated with Old World monkeys; types 4, 8, and 9 with New World monkeys; types 6 and 7 with apes (chimpanzees); and type 5 with prosimians. No common group-specific antigen has been detected among these isolates and neutralization is apparently type-specific (Hooks and Gibbs 1975).

Bovine syncytial virus (BSV) can be isolated easily from normal cattle and from cattle with leukosis (Malmquist et al. 1969). It is worth reiterating here that some of the properties attributed to BLV, which has been studied extensively and discussed earlier (see Section II.R), could have been due to contaminating foamy virus. Several properties of BLV are clearly related to those of foamy viruses: (1) the induction of cytopathology with extensive syncytia formation, (2) a morphology described as intermediate between typical B-type and C-type particles, and (3) the lack of *gag* protein reactivity with other oncoviruses. Although BSV and BLV can be distinguished serologically (Burny et al. 1980), their widespread prevalence implies that they may often occur simultaneously in an animal or tissue, and thus it will be important to reevaluate BSV and BLV stocks with the newer availability of monospecific antisera and of biological and molecular cloning methods.

Feline syncytium-forming virus (FSFV) has been isolated from healthy cats (Hackett et al. 1970; Jarrett et al. 1974), as well as from cats with a variety of nonneoplastic diseases (Zook et al. 1968; Fabricant et al. 1969; Ward and Pederson 1969; Gaskin and Gillespie 1972) and neoplasms (Kasza et al. 1969; Riggs et al. 1969; McKissick and Lamont 1970; Hackett and Manning 1971). In addition, isolates have been obtained from fetuses and from primary embryonic cell cultures (Hackett and Manning 1971; O. Jarrett 1971), and there is one isolate from a European wildcat (Lieber et al. 1975a). No cross neutralization among foamy viruses of simian, bovine, and feline origins is observed (Hooks et al. 1972; Gillespie and Scott 1973; Epstein et al. 1974).

There have been two reports of foamy viruses from hamster cells, one of which involved induction using IdU (Fabisch et al. 1973; Rossignol et al. 1975). It is not known whether these isolates represent distinct serotypes.

Finally, there have been several reports of foamy virus isolates from human tissues. The first isolate was from a patient with nasopharyngeal carcinoma (NPC) (Achong et al. 1971; Epstein et al. 1974). On the basis of seroepidemiology, this group concluded that inhabitants of Kenya, particularly those with oropharyngeal tumors, were susceptible to virus infection, as detected by the presence of antibodies in immunofluorescence assays (Achong and Epstein 1978). However, another group reported this isolate to be closely related by complement-fixation, fluorescence, and neutralization tests to SFV type 6 (Brown et al. 1978; Nemo et al. 1978). The latter investigators also conducted a seroepidemiological survey and found no naturally occurring antibody to the human isolate or to SFV type 6 in 256 humans from diverse geographical areas, although sera obtained from chimpanzees naturally infected with SFV type 6 neutralized either virus. Thus, they concluded that the isolate was probably a variant of the chimpanzee virus. This conclusion was challenged by a further seroepidemiological survey conducted by Achong, Epstein, and their colleagues (Muller et al. 1980), showing that by immunofluorescence, 3.4% of 493 sera from healthy inhabitants of Uganda reacted positively, whereas sera from inhabitants of Kenya and Tanzania showed reaction only when obtained from patients with nasopharyngeal carcinoma (9 of 57 positive sera from NPC, none from 80 non-NPC sera). They therefore concluded that foamy virus infection of humans was a natural and not infrequent phenomenon. One recent study found that 6.9% of sera from 1717 inhabitants of nine Pacific islands also had antibodies reactive with the human isolate in fluorescence and neutralization assays (Loh et al. 1980). These authors argue that such data provide evidence for human infection, as neither chimpanzees nor other simian populations are found naturally on these islands. It is possible, then, that in the African population, a human foamy virus infects monkeys or that the reverse (i.e., a zoonosis) could be true. The final debate awaits finer serological and molecular characterizations of these viruses.

Several other foamy virus isolates from human tissues have been reported. Peripheral blood cells from a patient with leukemia yielded a virus related serologically to SFV type 1 (Young et al. 1973). Several isolates were obtained from patients with de Quervian subacute granulomatous thyroiditis (Stancek and Gressnerova 1974; Stancek et al. 1975). Although originally considered to be paramyxoviruses, these isolates showed morphological properties and induced cytopathic alterations characteristic of foamy viruses (Werner and Gelderblom 1979). The most recent identification of a human foamy virus was from the brain of a patient with dialysis encephalopathy (Cameron et al. 1978). It should perhaps be noted that in most cases the isolates were obtained directly from the human tissues or by injection of tissue homogenates into cell cultures, including human cells. Such techniques would tend to rule out the possibility that the viruses were induced from the cells used as indicators of cytopathic changes. Further analyses of these isolates have not been reported.

Foamy viruses replicate in cells cultured from numerous species, including fibroblast and epithelial cells of human, monkey, rabbit, pig, cat, dog, mink, rat, and chicken origins. In addition, SFV type 1 establishes a nonproducer state in Hep-2 and BHK-21 cells (Clarke et al. 1970), although no viral envelope antigens can be detected by membrane immunofluorescence (Gould and Hartley 1979). Cytopathic changes involve multinucleated cells that enlarge and vacuolate; it is not known whether syncytia formation is due to fusion from within (i.e., due to some aspect of virus replication) or from without (i.e., due to membrane contact with a specific protein). These effects have provided the basis of plaque assays for titrating foamy viruses in vitro, using either liquid culture or an agar-overlay system with or without antibody to foamy virus to inhibit virus spread (Parks and Todaro 1972; Chiswell and Pringle 1977; Loh et al. 1977).

As with other retroviruses, attachment and penetration apparently occur by association of the envelope spikes with the cell membrane followed by engulfment (Dermott and Samuels 1973a). During this process, the envelope of the virus and the plasma membrane appear to fuse and the virion is carried into the cell within a vacuole. By fluorescence microscopy, viral antigens are detected within the nucleus by 20 hours postinfection. This nuclear fluorescence is a distinguishing feature of the Spumavirinae subfamily (Carski 1960; Malmquist et al. 1969; Fleming and Clarke 1970; Hooks et al. 1972; Parks and Todaro 1972). Dermott and her colleagues (Dermott et al. 1971; Dermott and Samuels 1973b) have demonstrated intranuclear viruslike particles by electron microscopy in cells infected with BSV or SFV type 1. The viral particles mature within the cytoplasm in areas containing much endoplasmic reticulum and may be seen budding into intracytoplasmic vacuoles or from the plasma membrane; at this stage, envelope spikes are clearly seen.

There have been few studies on the biochemical characterization of virus-infected cells in vitro. For example, although virus has been isolated from embryo cells, no attempts have been made to determine whether the foamy viruses exist as endogenous proviruses directly. However, using transfection techniques, Chiswell and Pringle (1977, 1978, 1979b) have shown that FSFV-infected cells contain infectious DNA molecules of approximately 6×10^6 daltons. This finding demonstrates that viral DNA is synthesized and suggests, but does not prove, that the foamy virus replicative cycle progresses through an integrated proviral DNA state.

The only structural virion protein that has been investigated in any detail is the reverse transcriptase. In all isolates examined, the required divalent cation for an exogenous (template-directed) reaction is Mn^{++} (Scolnick et al. 1970; Parks et al. 1971; Hruska and Takemoto 1975; Liu et al. 1977; Chiswell and Pringle 1979a). Liu et al. (1977) estimated that the partially purified enzyme from a simian isolate had a molecular weight of about 80,000 daltons and that it was unrelated serologically to the reverse transcriptases of several oncoviruses (RD114, SSAV, Ra-MLV, and AMV). There are no reports on the molecular weights of other structural virion proteins.

With regard to viral RNA, there is one report on the biophysical properties of the genomic RNA of a hamster foamy virus (Hruska and Takemoto 1975). Viral particles contained a 62S RNA molecule; however, upon heat treatment similar to that which causes dissociation of oncoviral RNA to 30S–35S subunits, the foamy virus RNA migrated uniformly as 18S–20S molecules, with some

4S–7S RNA species. If this finding is not due to contaminating ribosomal RNA, a possibility considered but thought to be unlikely by these authors, then two explanations for this disparity with the oncovirus group can be put forward: (1) The foamy virus RNA might be more sensitive to degradation. (2) The genome might be multisegmented (i.e., trimeric or tetrameric) with identical or nonidentical subunits. Future work should resolve these issues.

One of the distinguishing features of foamy viruses is that they do not induce clinical disease in their natural hosts, and the virus persists despite the presence of high levels of circulating antibody (Johnston 1961; Hooks et al. 1972). Injection of virus into seronegative animals results in seroconversion, persistence of virus, but no signs of clinical disease (Ruckle 1958a; Johnston 1961, 1971; Stiles et al. 1964).

The mechanism of virus spread within a population is not well understood. In monkeys, virus persists in the throat, and thus horizontal spread could occur by direct contact or by aerosols (Johnston 1961). On the other hand, vertical transmission has been suggested by the isolation of foamy viruses from fetuses of cats (Hackett and Manning 1971), cattle (Scott et al. 1973; Gould et al. 1978), or monkeys (Asher and Hooks, cited in Hooks and Gibbs 1975), although it is not known whether this is due to genetic transmission or congenital infection.

Within an infected animal, virus can be detected in numerous tissues (Malmquist et al. 1969; Gaskin and Gillespie 1972; Gillespie and Scott 1973). Antibody too is widespread within natural host populations and is, for example, quite commonly detected in fetal or adult bovine sera (Gould et al. 1978). There is a high degree of correlation between the presence of antibody and the ability to recover virus from an individual (Ruckle 1958a,b; Carski 1960; Johnston 1961, 1971; Stiles 1968; Riggs et al. 1969; Hooks et al. 1972, 1973).

Simian foamy viruses can establish chronic infections following experimental inoculation of rabbits (Swack and Hsiung 1975; Hooks and Detrick-Hooks 1979). As with other persistent virus infections (see Chapter 8 for possible mechanisms of virus persistence of oncoviruses and lentiviruses), foamy viruses can suppress immune responses. Injection of SFV type 7 into rabbits causes transient depression of cell-mediated immunity, as measured by a decreased response to mitogens and an absence of immune-interferon production (Hooks and Detrick-Hooks 1979). Thus, foamy virus can adversely affect a persistently infected host. For further details about the foamy viruses, see the most recent review by Hooks and Gibbs (1975).

For the present, it would seem that the absence of pathological disease has relegated this virus subfamily to a minor place, compared with its Oncovirinae and Lentivirinae relatives. Future studies may provide more information about the basic features of this subfamily. Several aspects of their nature and their role in nature remain unanswered at present.

1. Epidemiological. Are there bona fide human isolates, considering the absence of substantive evidence for human oncoviruses (without even implying any etiological function)? Are the antibodies in human sera detecting carbohydrate moieties rather than specific protein determinants? Do foamy viruses exist as endogenous elements? Are spumavirus isolates restricted to mammals only and to so few mammalian orders?
2. Pathological. Is immunosuppression a general feature of foamy viruses? If so, does a latent infection alter the host's response and the course of the disease induced by other biological agents?
3. Biological. Is the classic retrovirus life cycle utilized by this group? What are the nature and function of the intranuclear antigen(s) detected by immunofluorescence? How is syncytium formation induced? What is the nature of cell-surface receptors for virus adsorption/penetration which confers the broad host range reported for these viruses?
4. Biochemical. Is the organization of the virion structural components comparable to other retroviruses? Is the genomic RNA a dimeric structure? Are the absence of a group-specific antigen and the presence of type-specificity for neutralization within a group such as the SFV isolates indicative of little or no RNA sequence homology? Does recombination occur between spumaviruses or with other retroviruses? Is the organization of the coding sequences and postulated signal sequences arranged as in other retroviruses?

REFERENCES

Aaronson, S.A. 1971a. Isolation of a rat-tropic helper virus from M-MSV-O stocks. *Virology* **44:** 29–36.

———. 1971b. Chemical induction of focus-forming virus from nonproducer cells transformed by murine sarcoma virus. *Proc. Natl. Acad. Sci.* **68:** 3069–3072.

Aaronson, S.A., S.R. Tronick, and J.R. Stephenson. 1976a. Endogenous type C RNA virus of *Odocoileus hemionus,* a mammalian species of New World origin. *Cell* **9:** 489–494.

Aaronson, S.A., S.R. Tronick, J.R. Stephenson, and S. Hino. 1976b. Immunological analysis of structural polypeptides of woolly monkey-gibbon ape type C viruses. In *Comparative leukemia research 1975* (ed. J. Clemmesen and D.S. Yohn), pp. 102–109. Krager, Basel.

Abelson, H.T. and L.S. Rabstein. 1970a. Influence of prednisolone on Moloney leukemogenic virus in BALB/c mice. *Cancer Res.* **30:** 2208–2212.

———. 1970b. Lymphosarcoma: Virus-induced thymic-independent disease in mice. *Cancer Res.* **30:** 2213–2222.

Abrell, J.W. and R.C. Gallo. 1973. Purification, characterization, and comparison of the DNA polymerases from two primate RNA tumor viruses. *J. Virol.* **12:** 431–439.

Achong, B.G. and M.A. Epstein. 1978. Preliminary seroepidemiological studies on the human syncytial virus. *J. Gen. Virol.* **40:** 175–181.

Achong, B.G., P.W.A. Mansell, M.A. Epstein, and P. Clifford. 1971. An unusual virus in cultures from a human nasopharyngeal carcinoma. *J. Natl. Cancer Inst.* **46:** 299–307.

Ahmed, M., W. Korol, G. Schidlovsky, and S.A. Mayyasi. 1976. Defective virus clones of Mason-Pfizer virus. *Proc. Am. Assoc. Cancer Res.* **17:** 165.

Ahmed, M., W. Korol, D.L. Larson, K.R. Harewood, and S.A. Mayyasi. 1975. Interactions between endogenous type-C virus and oncogenic viruses. I. Syncytium induction and development of infectivity assay. *Int. J. Cancer* **16:** 747–755.

Ahmed, M., W. Korol, D. Larson, H. Molnar, and G. Schidlovsky. 1972. Transformation of rat mammary cell cultures by R-35 virus isolated from spontaneous rat mammary adenocarcinoma. *J. Natl. Cancer Inst.* **48:** 1077–1083.

Ahmed, M., G. Schidlovsky, W. Korol, G. Vidrine, and J.L. Cicmanec. 1974. Occurrence of Mason-Pfizer monkey virus in healthy rhesus monkeys. *Cancer Res.* **34:** 3504–3508.

Ahmed, M., J. Yeh, H.E. Holden, W. Korol, G. Schidlovsky, and S.A. Mayyasi. 1977. Characterization of Mason-Pfizer monkey virus induced transformation *in vitro. Arch. Virol.* **55:** 93–107.

Allen, J.A., C.L. Mullins, A. Hellman, R.F. Garry, and M.R.F. Waite. 1979. Replication of reticuloendotheliosis virus in mammary cells. In *Annual Meeting of American Society for Microbiology,* p. 256 (Abstr.).

Andersen, P.R., M. Barbacid, S.R Tronick, H.F. Clark, and S.A. Aaronson. 1979. Evolutionary relatedness of viper and primate endogenous retroviruses. *Science* **204:** 318–321.

Anderson, H.K. and T. Jeppesen. 1972. Virus-like particles in guinea pig oogonium and oocytes. *J. Natl. Cancer Inst.* **49:** 1403–1410.

Anderson, L.J. and W.F.H. Jarrett. 1968. Lymphosarcoma (leukemia) in cattle, sheep and pigs in Great Britain. *Cancer* **22:** 398–405.

Andervont, H.B. and W.R. Bryan. 1944. Properties of the mouse mammary-tumor agent. *J. Natl. Cancer Inst.* **5:** 143–149.

Aoki, T., M. Liu, M.J. Walling, G.S. Bushar, P.B. Brandchaft, and T.G. Kawakami. 1976. Specificity of naturally occurring antibody in normal gibbon serum. *Science* **191:** 1180–1183.

Archer, B.G., T.B. Crawford, T.C. McGuire, and M.E. Frazier. 1977. RNA-dependent DNA polymerase associated with equine infectious anemia virus. *J. Virol.* **22:** 16–22.

Armstrong, J.S., J.S. Porterfield, and A.T. deMadrid. 1971. C-type virus particles in pig kidney cell lines. *J. Gen. Virol.* **10:** 195–198.

Armstrong, M.Y.K., R.B. Weininger, D. Binder, C.A. Himsel, and F.F. Richards. 1980. Role of endogenous leukemia virus in immunologically triggered lymphoreticular tumors. II. Isolation of B-tropic mink cell focus-inducing (MCF) murine leukemia virus. *Virology* **104:** 164–173.

August, J.T., D.P. Bolognesi, E. FLeissner, R.V. Gilden, and R.C. Nowinski. 1974. A proposed nomenclature for the virion proteins of oncogenic RNA viruses. *Virology* **60:** 595–601.

Alxerad, A.A. and R.A. Steeves. 1964. Assay for Friend leukemia virus: Rapid quantitative method based on enumeration of macroscopic spleen foci in mice. *Virology* **24:** 513–518.

Balduzzi, P.C., M.F.D. Notter, H.R. Morgan, and M. Shibuya. 1981. Some biological properties of two new avian sarcoma viruses. *J. Virol.* **40:** 268–275.

Ball, J.K., D. Harvey, and J.A. McCarter. 1973. Evidence for naturally occurring murine sarcoma virus. *Nature* **241:** 272–274.

Baltimore, D., A. Shields, G. Otto, S. Goff, P. Besmer, O. Witte, and N. Rosenberg. 1980. Structure and expression of the Abelson murine leukemia virus genome and its relationship to a normal cell gene. *Cold Spring Harbor Symp. Quant. Biol.* **44:** 849–854.

Baluda, M.A. and P. Roy-Burman. 1973. Partial characterization of RD114 virus by DNA-RNA hybridization studies. *Nat. New Biol.* **244:** 59–62.

Barbacid, M., M.D. Daniel, and S.A. Aaronson. 1980. Immunological relationships of OMC-1, an endogenous virus of owl monkeys, with mammalian and avian type C viruses. *J. Virol.* **33:** 561–566.

Barbacid, M., K.C. Robbins, and S.A. Aaronson. 1979. Wild mouse RNA tumor viruses. A nongenetically transmitted virus group closely related to exogenous leukemia viruses of laboratory mouse strains. *J. Exp. Med.* **149:** 254–266.

Barbacid, M., J.R. Stephenson, and S.A. Aaronson. 1977. Evolutionary relationships between *gag* gene-coded proteins of murine and primate endogenous type C RNA viruses. *Cell* **10:** 641–648.

Barbacid, M., S.R. Tronick, and S.A. Aaronson. 1978. Isolation and characterization of an endogenous type C RNA virus of mink (Mv1Lu) cells. *J. Virol.* **25:** 129–137.

Bassin, R.H., P.J. Simons, F.C. Chesterman, and J.J. Harvey. 1968. Murine sarcoma virus (Harvey). Characteristics of focus formation in mouse embryo cell cultures and virus production by hamster tumor cells. *Int. J. Cancer* **3:** 265–272.

Bather, R. 1961. Observations on murine monocytic leukaemia induced by a virus isolated from S37 sarcoma. *Br. J. Cancer* **15:** 114–119.

Beard, J.W. 1963. Avian virus growths and their etiologic agents. *Adv. Cancer Res.* **7:** 1–127.

Bedigian, H.G. and H. Meier. 1975. Isolation of an endogenous C-type RNA virus from *Mus musculus molossinus. J. Natl. Cancer Inst.* **55:** 1007–1010.

Bedigian, H.G., R.R. Fox, and H. Meier. 1976. Presence of a high molecular-weight RNA and RNA-directed DNA polymerase in rabbit hereditary lymphosarcoma. *Cancer Res.* **36:** 4693–4698.

———. 1978. Induction of type C RNA virus from cultured rabbit lymphosarcoma cells. *J. Virol.* **27:** 313–319.

Beemon, K.L., A.J. Faras, A.T. Haase, P.H. Duesberg, and J.E. Maisel. 1976. Genomic complexities of murine leukemia and sarcoma, reticuloendotheliosis, and visna viruses. *J. Virol.* **17:** 525–537.

Benade, L.E. and M. Barbacid. 1980. Polymorphism among the major core proteins of C57BL B-tropic murine leukemia viruses. *Virology* **106:** 387–390.

Benade, L.E. and J.N. Ihle. 1980. Different serotypes of B-tropic murine leukemia viruses and association with endogenous ecotropic viral loci. *Virology* **106:** 374–386.

Benade, L.E., J.N. Ihle, and A. Decleve. 1978. Serological characterization of B-tropic viruses of C57BL mice: Possible origin by recombination of endogenous N-tropic and xenotropic viruses. *Proc. Natl. Acad. Sci.* **75:** 4553–4557.

Bender, W., Y.-H. Chien, S. Chattopadhyay, P.K. Vogt, M.B. Gardner, and N. Davidson. 1978. High-molecular-weight RNAs of AKR, NZB, and wild mouse viruses and avian reticuloendotheliosis virus all have similar dimer structures. *J. Virol.* **25:** 888–896.

Bentvelzen, P. 1968. "Genetic control of the vertical transmission of the Mühlbock mammary tumor virus in the GR mouse strain." Ph.D thesis, Hollandia, Amsterdam.

———. 1972. Hereditary infections with mammary tumor viruses in mice. In *RNA viruses and host genome in oncogenesis* (ed. P. Emmelot and P. Bentvelzen), pp. 309–337. North-Holland, Amsterdam.

Bentvelzen, P., A.M. Aarssen, and J. Brinkhof. 1972. Defectivity of Rauscher murine erythroblastosis virus. *Nat. New. Biol.* **239:** 122–123.

Bentvelzen, P., K. Nooter, and B.F. Deys. 1978. Rescue of a transforming virus from a spontaneous nonproducing osteosarcoma in BALB/c mice. *J. Natl. Cancer Inst.* **60:** 401–403.

Benveniste, R.E. and G.J. Todaro. 1973. Homology between type-C viruses of various species as determined by molecular hybridization. *Proc. Natl. Acad. Sci.* **70:** 3316–3320.

———. 1974a. Evolution of type C viral genes: I. Nucleic acid from baboon type C virus as a measure of divergence among primate species. *Proc. Natl. Acad. Sci.* **71:** 4513–4518.

———. 1974b. Multiple divergent copies of endogenous C-type virogenes in mammalian cells. *Nature* **252:** 170–173.

———. 1974c. Evolution of C-type viral genes: Inheritance of exogenously acquired viral genes. *Nature* **252:** 456–459.

———. 1975a. Evolution of type C viral genes: Preservation of ancestral murine type C viral sequences in pig cellular DNA. *Proc. Natl. Acad. Sci.* **72:** 4090–4094.

———. 1975b. Segregation of RD-114 and FeLV-related sequences in crosses between domestic cat and leopard cat. *Nature* **257:** 506–508.

———. 1976. Evolution of type C viral genes: Evidence for an Asian origin of man. *Nature* **261:** 101–108.

———. 1977. Evolution of primate oncornaviruses: An endogenous virus from langurs (*Presbytis* spp.) with related virogene sequences in other Old World monkeys. *Proc. Natl. Acad. Sci.* **74:** 4557–4561.

Benveniste, R.E., C.J. Sherr, and G.J. Todaro. 1975. Evolution of type C viral genes: Origin of feline leukemia virus. *Science* **190:** 886–888.

Benveniste, R.E., R. Callahan, C.J. Sherr, V. Chapman, and G.J. Todaro. 1977. Two distinct endogenous type C viruses isolated from the Asian rodent *Mus cervicolor:* Conservation of virogene sequences in related rodent species. *J. Virol.* **21:** 849–862.

Benveniste, R.E., R. Heinemann, G.L. Wilson, R. Callahan, and G.J. Todaro. 1974a. Detection of baboon type C viral sequences in various primate tissues by molecular hybridization. *J. Virol.* **14:** 56–67.

Benveniste, R.E., M.M. Lieber, D.M. Livingston, C.J. Sherr, G.J. Todaro, and S.S. Kalter. 1974b. Infectious C-type virus isolated from a baboon placenta. *Nature* **248:** 17–20.

Bergs, V.V., M. Bergs, and H.C. Chopra. 1970. A virus (RMTDV) derived from chemically-induced rat mammary tumors. I. Isolation and general characteristics. *J. Natl. Cancer Inst.* **44:** 913–921.

Bergs, V.V., G. Pearson, H.C. Chopra, and W. Turner. 1972. Spontaneous appearance of cytopathology and rat C-type virus (WF-1) in a rat embryo cell line. *Int. J. Cancer* **10:** 165–173.

Bernhard, W. 1958. Electron microscopy of tumor cells and tumor viruses. A review. *Cancer Res.* **18:** 491–509.

———. 1960. The detection and study of tumor viruses with the electron microscope. *Cancer Res.* **20:** 712–727.

Bernhard, W. and A. Bauer. 1955. Mise en evidence de corpuscules d'aspect virusal dans des tumeurs mammaires de la souris. Etude au microscope electronique. *C. R. Acad. Sci.* **240:** 1380–1382.

Bernhard, W., R.A. Bonar, D. Beard, and J.W. Beard. 1958. Ultrastructure of viruses of myeloblastosis and erythroblastosis isolated from plasma of leukemic chickens. *Proc. Soc. Exp. Biol. Med.* **97:** 48–52.

Biggs, P.M.and L.N. Payne. 1964. Relationship of Marek's disease (neural lymphomatosis) to lymphoid leukosis. *Natl. Cancer Inst. Monogr.* **17:** 83–98.

Biggs, P.M., J.S. McDougall, J.A. Frazier, and B.S. Milne. 1978. Lymphoproliferative disease of turkeys. I. Clinical aspects. *Avian Pathol.* **7:** 131–139.

Biggs, P.M., B.S. Milne, J.A. Frazier, J.S. McDougall, and J.C. Stuart. 1974. Lymphoproliferative disease in turkeys. In. *Proceedings of the 15th World Poultry Congress,* pp. 55–57. World Poultry Society of America, Washington.

Bittner, J.J. 1936. Some possible effects of nursing on the mammary gland tumor incidence in mice. *Science* **84:** 162.

———. 1939. Relation of nursing to the extra-chromosomal theory of breast cancer in mice. *Am. J. Cancer* **35:** 90–97.

———. 1942a. Possible relationship of the estrogenic hormones, genetic susceptibility, and milk influence in the production of mammary cancer in mice. *Cancer Res.* **2:** 710–721.

———. 1942b. The milk-influence of breast tumors in mice. *Science* **95:** 462–463.

Black, V.H. 1974. Virus particles in primordial germ cells of fetal guinea pigs. *J. Natl. Cancer Inst.* **52:** 545–551.

Blair, P.B. 1970. Immunology of the mouse mammary tumor virus: Comparison of the antigenicity of mammary tumor virus obtained from several strains of mice. *Cancer Res.* **30:** 625–631.

———. 1971. Strain specificity in mouse mammary tumor virus virion antigens. *Cancer Res.* **31:** 1473–1477.

Boiron, M., J.-P. Levy, J. Lasneret, S. Oppenheim, and J. Bernard. 1965. Pathogenesis of Rauscher leukemia. *J. Natl. Cancer Inst.* **35:** 865–884.

Bonar, R.A. and J.W. Beard. 1959. Virus of avian myeloblastosis. XII. Chemical constitution. *J. Natl. Cancer Inst.* **23:** 183–197.

Bonner, T.I. and G.J. Todaro. 1979. Carnivores have sequences in their cellular DNA distantly related to the primate endogenous virus, MAC-1. *Virology* **94:** 224–227.

Boone, C.W., E.C. Church, and R.M. McAllister. 1973. Testing by the "paired-label" antibody binding technique for feline leukemia virus-induced cell surface antigens (FeLV-CSA) on the surface of human rhabdomyosarcoma cells releasing RD-114 virus. *Virology* **55:** 157–162.

Bose, H.R., Jr. and A.S. Levine. 1967. Replication of the reticuloendotheliosis virus (strain T) in chicken embryo cell culture. *J. Virol.* **1:** 1117–1121.

Boss, M., M. Greaves, and N. Teich. 1979. Abelson virus transformed haematopoietic cell lines with pre-B-cell characteristics. *Nature* **278:** 551–553.

Bosselman, R.A., L.J.L.D. Van Griensven, M. Vogt, and I.M. Verma. 1979. Genome organization of retroviruses. VI. Heteroduplex analysis of ecotropic and xenotropic sequences of Moloney mink cell focus-inducing viral RNA obtained from either a cloned isolate or a thymoma cell line. *J. Virol.* **32:** 968–978.

Bostock, D.E. and L.N. Owen. 1973. Porcine and ovine lymphosarcoma. A review. *J. Natl. Cancer Inst.* **50:** 933–939.

Bouillant, A.M.P., A.S. Greig, M.M. Lieber, and G.J. Todaro. 1975. Type C virus production by a continuous line of pig oviduct cells (PFT). *J. Gen. Virol.* **27:** 173–180.

Brahic, M. and A.T. Haase. 1981. Lentivirinae: Maedi/visna group infections. Comparative aspects and diagnosis. In *Comparative diagnosis of viral diseases* (ed. E. Kurstak), vol. 3. Academic Press, New York. (In press.)

Brahic, M., J. Tamalet, and C. Chippaux-Hyppolite. 1971. Virus Visna: Isolement d'une molecule d'acide ribonucleique de haut poids moleculaire. *C. R. Acad. Sci.* (Ser. D) **272:** 2115–2118.

Brahic, M., P. Filippi, R. Vigne, and A.T. Haase. 1977. Visna virus RNA synthesis. *J. Virol.* **24:** 74–81.

Brahic, M., J. Tamalet, P. Filippi, and L. Delbecchi. 1973. The high molecular weight RNA of Visna virus. *Biochimie* **55:** 885–891.

Breese, S.S., Jr. 1970. Virus-like particles occurring in cultures of stable pig kidney cell lines. *Arch. Gesamte Virusforsch.* **30:** 401–404.

Breitman, M.L., M.M.C. Lai, and P.K. Vogt. 1980. Attenuation of avian reticuloendotheliosis virus: Loss of the defective transforming component during serial passage of oncogenic virus in fibroblasts. *Virology* **101:** 304–306.

Brodey, R.S., S.M. McDonough, F.L. Frye, and W.D. Hardy, Jr. 1970. Epidemiology of feline leukemia (lymphosarcoma). In *Comparative leukemia research 1969* (ed. R.M. Dutcher), pp. 333–342. Karger, Basel.

Brown, E.R., L. Keith, J.J. Hazdra, and T. Arndt. 1975. Tumors in fish caught in polluted waters: Possible explanations. In *Comparative leukemia research 1973* (ed. Y. Ito and R.M. Dutcher), pp. 47–57. Karger, Basel.

Brown, E.R., J.J. Hazdra, L. Keith, I. Greenspan, J.B.G. Kwapinski, and P. Beamer. 1973. Frequency of fish tumors found in a polluted watershed as compared to nonpolluted Canadian waters. *Cancer Res.* **33:** 189–198.

Brown, E.R., W.C. Dolowy, T. Sinclair, L.Keith, S. Greenberg, J.J. Hazdra, P. Beamer, and O. Callaghan. 1976. Enhancement of lymphosarcoma transmission in *Esox lucius* and its epidemiologic relationship to pollution. In *Comparative leukemia research 1975* (ed. J. Clemmesen and D.S. Yohn), pp. 245–251. Karger, Basel.

Brown, H.R. and H. Thormar. 1975. Persistence of visna virus in murine and hamster cell cultures without the appearance of cell transformation. *Microbios* **13:** 51–60.

Brown, P., G. Nemo, and D.C. Gajdusek. 1978. Human foamy virus: Further characterization, seroepidemiology, and relationship to the chimpanzee foamy viruses. *J. Infect. Dis.* **137:** 421–427.

Bruns, M. and B. Frenzel. 1979. Isolation of a glycoprotein and two structural proteins of maedi-visna virus. *Virology* **97:** 207–211.

Bryan, W.R. 1958. Biological studies on the Rous sarcoma virus. I. General introduction. II. Review of sources of experimental variation and of methods for their control. *J. Natl. Cancer Inst.* **12:** 55–58.

Bryant, M.L. and V. Klement. 1976. Clonal heterogeneity of wild mouse leukemia viruses: Host range and antigenicity. *Virology* **73:** 532–536.

Bryant, M.L., B.K. Pal, M.B. Gardner, J.H. Elder, F.C. Jensen, and R.A. Lerner. 1978. Structural analysis of the major envelope glycoprotein (gp70) of the amphotropic and ecotropic type C viruses of wild mice. *Virology* **84:** 348–358.

Buchhagen, D.L., F.S. Pedersen, R.L. Crowther, and W.A. Haseltine. 1980. Most sequence differences between the genomes of the Akv virus and a leukemogenic Gross A virus passaged *in vitro* are located near the 3′ terminus. *Proc. Natl. Acad. Sci.* **77:** 4359–4363.

Burmester, B.R., R.F. Gentry, and N.F. Waters. 1955. The presence of the virus of visceral lymphomatosis in embryonated eggs of normal appearing hens. *Poultry Sci.* **34:** 609–617.

Burmester, B.R., C.O. Prickett, and T.C. Belding. 1946. A filtrable agent producing lymphoid tumors and osteopetrosis in chickens. *Cancer Res.* **6:** 189–196.

Burny, A., C. Bruck, H. Chantrenne, Y. Cleuter, D. Dekegel,, J.Ghysdael, R. Kettmann, M. Leclercq, J. Leunen, M. Mammerickx, and D. Portetelle. 1980. Bovine leukemia virus: Molecular biology and epidemiology. In *Viral oncology* (ed. G. Klein), pp. 231–289. Raven Press, New York.

Calafat, J., P.C. Hageman, and A.A. Ressang. 1974. Structure of C-type virus particles in lymphocyte cultures of bovine origin. *J. Natl. Cancer Inst.* **52:** 1251–1257.

Callahan, R. and G.J. Todaro. 1978. Four major endogenous retrovirus classes each genetically transmitted in various species of *Mus*. In *Origins of inbred mice* (ed. H.C. Morse, III), pp. 689–713. Academic Press, New York.

Callahan, R., M.M. Lieber, and G.J. Todaro. 1975. Nucleic acid homology of murine xenotropic type C viruses. *J. Virol.* **15:** 1378–1384.

Callahan, R., C. Meade, and G.J. Todaro. 1979. Isolation of an endogenous type C virus related to the infectious primate type C viruses from the Asian rodent *Vandeleuria oleracea*. *J. Virol.* **30:** 124–131.

Callahan, R., C.J. Sherr, and G.J. Todaro. 1977. A new class of murine retroviruses: Immunological and biochemical comparison of novel isolates from *Mus cervicolor* and *Mus caroli*. *Virology* **80:** 401–416.

Callahan R., R.E. Benveniste, C.J. Sherr, G. Schidlovsky, and G.J. Todaro. 1976a. A new class of genetically transmitted retravirus isolated from *Mus cervicolor*. *Proc. Natl. Acad. Sci.* **73:** 3579–3583.

Callahan, R., M.M. Lieber, G.J. Todaro, D.C. Graves, and J.F. Ferrer. 1976b. Bovine leukemia virus genes in the DNA of leukemic cattle. *Science* **192:** 1005–1007.

Calnek, B.W. 1968. Lymphoid leukosis virus: A survey of commercial breeding flocks for genetic resistance and incidence of embryo infection. *Avian Dis.* **12:** 104–111.

Cameron, K.R., S.M. Birchall, and M.A. Moses. 1978. Isolation of foamy virus from patient with dialysis encephalopathy. *Lancet* **2:** 796.

Campbell, W.F., K.L. Baxter-Gabbard, and A.S. Levine. 1971. Avian reticuloendotheliosis virus (strain T). I. Virological characterization. *Avian Dis.* **15:** 837–849.

Carr, J.G. and J.G. Campbell. 1958. Three new virus-induced sarcomata. *Br. J. Cancer* **12:** 631–635.

Carski, T.R. 1960. A fluorescent antibody study of the simian foamy agent. *J. Immunol.* **84:** 426–433.

Chang, K.S.S., T. Aoki, and L.W. Law. 1975. Isolation of B-tropic type-C virus from reticulum cell neoplasms induced in BALB/c mice by SJL/J type-C virus. *J. Natl. Cancer Inst.* **54:** 83–87.

Charman, H.P., N. Kim, and R.V. Gilden. 1974. Radioimmunoassay for the major structural protein of hamster type C viruses. *J. Virol.* **14:** 910–917.

Charman, H.P., S. Bladen, R.V. Gilden, and L. Coggins. 1976a. Equine infectious anemia virus: Evidence favoring classification as a retravirus. *J. Virol.* **19:** 1073–1079.

Charman, H.P., M.H. White, R. Rahman, and R.V. Gilden. 1976b. Species and interspecies radioimmunoassays for rat type C virus p30: Interviral comparisons and assay of human tumor extracts. *J. Virol.* **17:** 51–59.

Chatterjee, S. and E. Hunter. 1980. Fusion of normal primate cells: A common biological property of the D-type retroviruses. *Virology* **107:** 100–108.

Chattopadhyay, S.K., M.R. Lander, and W.P. Rowe. 1980a. Close similarity between endogenous ecotropic virus of *Mus musculus molossinus* and AKR virus. *J. Virol.* **36:** 499–505.

Chattopadhyay, S.K., M.R. Lander, E. Rands, and D.R. Lowy. 1980b. Structure of endogenous murine leukemia virus DNA in mouse genomes. *Proc. Natl. Acad. Sci.* **77:** 5774–5778.

Chattopadhyay, S.K., J.W. Hartley, M.R. Lander, B.S. Kramer, and W.P. Rowe. 1978. Biochemical characterization of the amphotropic group of murine leukemia viruses. *J. Virol.* **26:** 29–39.

Cheevers, W.P., B.G. Archer, and T.B. Crawford. 1977. Characterization of RNA from equine infectious anemia virus. *J. Virol.* **24:** 489–497.

Cheevers, W.P., C.M. Ackley, and T.B. Crawford. 1978. Structural proteins of equine infectious anemia virus. *J. Virol.* **28:** 997–1001.

Chen, Y.C. and P.K. Vogt. 1977. Endogenous leukosis viruses in the avian family *Phasianidae*. *Virology* **76:** 740–750.

Chien, Y.-H., I.M. Verma, T.Y. Shih, E.M. Scolnick, and N. Davidson. 1978. Heteroduplex analysis of the sequence relations between RNAs of mink cell focus-inducing and murine leukemia viruses. *J. Virol.* **28:** 352–360.

Chippaux-Hyppolite, C., C. Taranger, J. Tamalet, G. Pautrat, and M. Brahic. 1972. Aspects ultrastructuraux du virus visna en cultures cellularies. *Ann. Inst. Pasteur* **123:** 409–420.

Chirigos, M.A., D. Scott, W. Turner, and K. Perk. 1968. Biological, pathological and physical characterization of a possible variant of a murine sarcoma virus (Moloney). *Int. J. Cancer* **3:** 223–237.

Chiswell, D.J. and C.R. Pringle. 1977. Infectious DNA from cells infected with feline syncytium-forming virus (Spumavirinae). *J. Gen. Virol.* **36:** 551–555.

———. 1978. Feline syncytium-forming virus proviral DNA. Time of synthesis and relationship to the host genome. *Virology* **90:** 344–350.

———. 1979a. Feline syncytium-forming virus: Identification of a virion associated reverse transcriptase and electron microscopical observations of infected cells. *J. Gen. Virol.* **43:** 429–434.

———. 1979b. Feline syncytium-forming virus: DNA provirus size and structure. *J. Gen. Virol.* **44:** 145–152.

Chopra, H.C. and M.M. Mason. 1970. A new virus in a spontaneous mammary tumor of a rhesus monkey. *Cancer Res.* **30:** 2081–2086.

Chopra, H.C. and D.J. Taylor. 1970. Virus particles in rat mammary tumor of varying origin. *J. Natl. Cancer Inst.* **44:** 1141–1147.

Chopra, H.C., N.J. Woodside and A.E. Bogden. 1970a. Virus particles in rat leukemias. *Cancer Res.* **30:** 1544–1547.

Chopra, H.C., A.E. Bogden, I. Zelljadt, and E.M. Jensen. 1970b. Virus particles in a transplantable rat mammary tumor of spontaneous origin. *Eur. J. Cancer* **6:** 287–290.

Chopra, H.C., J.J. Hooks, M.J. Walling, and C.J. Gibbs, Jr. 1972. Morphology of simian foamy viruses, with particular reference to virus isolated from spontaneous tumor of a rhesus monkey. *J. Natl. Cancer Inst.* **48:** 451–463.

Chused, T.M. and H.C. Morse, III. 1978. Expression of XenCSA, a cell surface antigen related to the major glycoprotein (gp70) of xenotropic murine leukemia virus, by lymphocytes of inbred mouse strains. In *Origin of inbred mice* (ed. H.C. Morse, III), pp. 297–319. Academic Press, New York.

Clark, H.F., P.R. Andersen, and P.D. Lunger. 1979. Propagation and characterization of a C-type virus from a rhabdomyosarcoma of a corn snake. *J. Gen. Virol.* **43:** 673–683.

Clarke, J.K. and J.T. Attridge. 1968. The morphology of simian foamy agents. *J. Gen. Virol.* **3:** 185–190.

Clarke, J.K. and J.B. McFerran. 1970. The morphology of bovine syncytial virus. *J. Gen. Virol.* **9:** 155–157.

Clarke, J.K., J.T. Attridge, and F.W. Gay. 1969a. The morphogenesis of simian foamy agents. *J. Gen. Virol.* **4:** 183–188.

Clarke, J.K., F.W. Gay, and J.J. Attridge. 1969b. Replication of simian foamy virus in monkey kidney cells. *J. Virol.* **3:** 358–362.

Clarke, J.K., J.T. Attridge, D.S. Dane, and M. Briggs. 1967. A simian virus of new morphology. *J. Gen. Virol.* **1:** 565–566.

Clarke, J.K., J. Samuels, E. Dermott, and F.W. Gay. 1970. Carrier cultures of simian foamy virus. *J. Virol.* **5:** 624–631.

Clements, J.E., O. Narayan, D.E. Griffin, and R.T. Johnson. 1979. The synthesis and structure of visna virus DNA. *Virology* **93:** 377–386.

Cloyd, M.W., J.W. Hartley, and W.P. Rowe. 1979. Cell-surface antigens associated with recombinant mink cell focus-inducing murine leukemia viruses. *J. Exp. Med.* **149:** 702–712.

———. 1980. Lymphomagenicity of recombinant mink cell focus-inducing murine leukemia viruses. *J. Exp. Med.* **151:** 542–552.

Coggins, L. and N.L. Norcross. 1970. Immunodiffusion reaction in equine infectious anemia. *Cornell Vet.* **60:** 330–335.

Coggins, L., N.L. Norcross, and S.R. Nusbaum. 1972. Diagnosis of equine infectious anemia by immunodiffusion test. *Am. J. Vet. Res.* **33:** 11–18.

Cohen, J.C. and H.E. Varmus. 1979. Endogenous mammary tumour virus DNA varies among wild mice and segregates during inbreeding. *Nature* **278:** 418–423.

Colcher, D., Y.A. Teramoto, and J. Schlom. 1977a. Interspecies radioimmunoassay for the major structural proteins of primate type-D retroviruses. *Proc. Natl. Acad. Sci.* **74:** 5739–5743.

———. 1978. Immunological and structural relationships between langur virus and other primate type-D retroviruses. *Virology* **88:** 384–388.

Colcher, D., R.L. Heberling, S.S. Kalter, and J. Schlom. 1977b. Squirrel monkey retrovirus: An endogenous virus of a new world primate. *J. Virol.* **23:** 294–301.

Congdon, C.C. and E. Lorenz. 1954. Leukemia in guinea pigs. *Am. J. Pathol.* **30:** 337–359.

Cook, M.K. 1969. Cultivation of a filterable agent associated with Marek's disease. *J. Natl. Cancer Inst.* **43:** 203–212.

Cork, L.C. and O. Narayan. 1980. The pathogenesis of viral leukoencephalomyelitis-arthritis of goats. I. Persistent viral infection with progressive pathologic changes. *Lab. Invest.* **42:** 596–602.

Cork, L.C., W.J. Hadlow, T.B. Crawford, J.R. Gorham, and R.C. Piper. 1974. Infectious leukoencephalomyelitis of young goats. *J. Infect. Dis.* **129:** 134–141.

Crawford, D.H., B.G. Achong, N.M. Teich, S. Finerty, J.L. Thompson, M.A. Epstein, and B.C. Giovanella. 1979. Identification of murine endogenous xenotropic retrovirus in cultured multicellular tumour spheroids from nude-mouse-passaged nasopharyngeal carcinoma. *Int. J. Cancer* **23:** 1–7.

Crawford, T.B., T.C. McGuire, and J.B. Henson. 1971. Detection of equine infectious anemia virus *in vitro* by immunofluorescence. *Arch. Gesamte Virusforsch.* **34:** 332–339.

Crawford, T.C, D.S. Adams, W.P. Cheevers, and L.C. Cork. 1980. Chronic arthritis in goats caused by a retrovirus. *Science* **207:** 997–999.

Daams, J.H., P. Hageman, J. Calafat, and P. Bentvelzen. 1973. Antigenic structure of murine mammary tumour viruses. *Eur. J. Cancer* **9:** 567–572.

Dahlberg, J.E., K. Perk, and A.J. Dalton. 1974. Virus-like particles induced in guinea pig cells by 5-bromo-2′-deoxyuridine are morphologically similar to murine B-type virus. *Nature* **249:** 828–830.

Daly, J.J., C.N. Sun, A.L. Barron, and H.J. White. 1975. C-type viruslike particles in a nonproliferating sparganum of human host origin. *J. Parasitol.* **61:** 775–777.

Datta, S.K. and R.S Schwartz. 1976. Genetics of expression of xenotropic virus and autoimmunity in NZB mice. *Nature* **263:** 412–415.

———. 1977. Mendelian segregation of loci controlling xenotropic virus production in NZB crosses. *Virology* **83:** 449–452.

———. 1978. Restricted expression of ecotropic virus by thymocytes of leukemia-resistant (AKR x NZB)F_1 mice. *J. Exp. Med.* **148:** 329–334.

Dawson, P.J., W.M. Rose, and A.H. Fieldsteel. 1966. Lymphatic leukaemia in rats and mice inoculated with Friend virus. *Br. J. Cancer* **20:** 114–121.

Dawson, P.J., S.L. Dresler, and A.H. Fieldsteel. 1979. Erythroid leukemia induced by Friend lymphatic leukemia virus in T-cell-depleted mice. *Cancer Res.* **39:** 1611–1615.

De Boer, G.F. 1975. Zwoegerziekte virus, the causative agent for progressive interstitial pneumonia (maedi) and meningo-leucoencephalitis (visna) in sheep. *Res. Vet. Sci.* **18:** 15–25.

De Boer, G.F. and D.J. Houwers. 1979. Epizootiology of maedi/visna in sheep. In *Aspects of slow and persistent virus infections* (ed. D.A.J. Tyrrell) pp. 198–220. Martinus Nijhoff, The Hague.

Decleve, A., M. Lieberman, J.N. Ihle, and H.S. Kaplan. 1976. Biological and serological characterization of radiation leukemia virus. *Proc. Natl. Acad. Sci.* **73:** 4675–4679.

Decleve, A., O. Niwa, E. Gelmann, and H.S. Kaplan. 1975. Replication kinetics of N- and B-tropic murine leukemia viruses on permissive and nonpermissive cells *in vitro*. *Virology* **65:** 320–332.

Decleve, A., M. Lieberman, and H.S. Kaplan. 1977. *In vivo* interaction between RNA viruses isolated from the C57BL/Ka strain of mice. *Virology* **81:** 270–283.

Decleve, A., M. Lieberman, J.N. Ihle, P.N. Rosenthal, M.L. Lung, and H.S. Kaplan. 1978. Physiochemical, biological and serological properties of a leukemogenic virus isolated from cultured RadLV-induced lymphomas of C57BL/Ka mice. *Virology* **90:** 23–25.

Dienhardt, F., L. Wolfe, R. Northrop, B. Marczynska, J. Ogden, R. McDonald, L. Falk, G. Shramek, R. Smith, and J. Deinhardt. 1972. Induction of neoplasms by viruses in marmoset monkeys. *J. Med. Primatol.* **1:** 29–50.

Deinhardt, F., L. Wolfe, R. Massey, J. Hoekstra, and R. McDonald. 1973. Simian sarcoma virus: Oncogenicity, focus assay, presence of associated virus, and comparison with avian and feline sarcoma virus-induced neoplasia in marmoset monkeys. In *Unifying concepts of leukemia* (ed. R.M. Dutcher and L. Chieco-Bianchi), pp. 258–262, Karger, Basel.

Deng, C.-T. and E. Wimmer. 1978. Two different murine sarcoma virus isolates have homologous genome sequences: Implications for their origin. *Virology* **89:** 309–313.

De Paoli, A., D.O. Johnsen, and W.W. Noll. 1973. Granulocytic leukemia in whitehanded gibbons. *J. Am. Vet. Med. Assoc.* **163:** 624–628.

Dermott, E. and J. Samuels. 1973a. Electron microscopic observations on the mechanisms of entry of simian foamy virus in HEp-2 cells. *J. Gen. Virol.* **19:** 135–139.

———. 1973b. Intrachromosomal location of MK5, a foamy type 1 virus. *J. Gen. Virol.* **19:** 141–143.

Dermott, E., J.K. Clarke, and J. Samuels. 1971. The morphogenesis and classification of bovine syncytial virus. *J. Gen. Virol.* **12:** 105–119.

de Thé, G., C. Becker, and J.W. Beard. 1964. Virus of avian myeloblastosis (BAI strain A). XXV. Ultracytochemical study of virus and myeloblast phosphatase activity. *J. Natl. Cancer Inst.* **32:** 201–235.

Devare, S.G., R.E. Hanson, Jr. and J.R. Stephenson. 1978a. Primate retroviruses: Envelope glycoproteins of endogenous type C and type D viruses possess common interspecies antigenic determinants. *J. Virol.* **26:** 316–324.

Devare, S.G., L.O. Arthur, D.L. Fine, and J.R. Stephenson. 1978b. Primate retroviruses: Immunological cross-reactivity between major structural proteins of New and Old World primate virus isolates. *J. Virol.* **25:** 797–805.

Devare, S.G., J.R. Stephenson, P.S. Sarma, S.A. Aaronson, and S. Chander. 1976. Bovine lymphosarcoma: Development of a radioimmunologic technique for detection of the etiologic agent. *Science* **194:** 1428–1430.

Dietz, M., S.P. Fouchey, C. Longley, M.A. Rich, and P. Furmanski. 1977. Spontaneous regression of Friend virus-induced erythroleukemia. I. The role of the helper murine leukemia virus component. *J. Exp. Med.* **145:** 594–606.

Diglio, C.A. and J.F. Ferrer. 1976. Induction of syncytia by the bovine C-type leukemia virus. *Cancer Res.* **36:** 1056–1067.

Di Stefano, H.S. and R.M. Dougherty. 1966. Mechanisms for congenital transmission of avian leukosis virus. *J. Natl. Cancer Inst.* **37:** 869–883.

Donoghue, D.J., P.A. Sharp, and R.A. Weinberg. 1979. Comparative study of different isolates of murine sarcoma virus. *J. Virol.* **32:** 1015–1027.

Donoghue, D.J., E. Rothenberg, N. Hopkins, D. Baltimore, and P.A. Sharp. 1978. Heteroduplex analysis of the nonhomology region between Moloney MuLV and the dual host range derivative HIX virus. *Cell* **14:** 959–970.

Dougherty, R.M., H. Di Stefano, U. Feller, and J.F. Mueller. 1975. On the nature of particles lining the excretory ducts of pseudophyllidean cestodes. *J. Parasitol.* **61:** 1006–1015.

Dresler, S., M. Ruta, M.J. Murray, and D. Kabat. 1979. Glycoprotein encoded by the Friend spleen focus-forming virus. *J. Virol.* **30:** 564–575.

Drohan, W., D. Colcher, G. Schochetman, and J. Schlom. 1976. Distribution of Mason-Pfizer virus-specific sequences in the DNA of primates. *J. Virol.* **23:** 36–43.

Drohan, W., R. Kettmann, D. Colcher, and J. Schlom. 1977. Isolation of the mouse mammary tumor virus sequences not transmitted as germinal provirus in the C3H and RIII mouse strains. *J. Virol.* **21:** 986–995.

Dubois-Dalcq, M., T.S. Reese, and O. Narayan. 1976. Membrane changes associated with assembly of visna virus. *Virology* **74:** 520–530.

Duncan, I.B. 1978. Evidence for an oncovirus in swimbladder fibrosarcoma of Atlantic salmon *Salmo salar* L. *J. Fish Dis.* **1:** 127–131.

Dunkel, V.C., R.C. Bast, B.I. Gerwin, U. Heine, M. Cottler-Fox, and T. Boros. 1974. Presence of A-type and absence of C-type virus particles in a chemically induced guinea pig hepatoma. *J. Natl. Cancer Inst.* **53:** 591–593.

Dutcher, R.M., E.P. Larkin, and R.R. Marshak. 1964. Virus-like particles in cow's milk from a herd with a high incidence of lymphosarcoma. *J. Natl. Cancer Inst.* **33:** 1055–1064.

Dutta, S.K., V.L. Larson, D.K. Sorenson, A. Perman, A.F. Weber, R.F. Hammer, and R.E. Shope. 1970. Isolation of C-type virus particles from leukemic and lymphocytotic cattle. In *Comparative leukemia research 1969* (ed. R.M. Dutcher), pp. 538–544. Karger, Basel.

Eckert, E.A., D. Beard, and J.W. Beard. 1951. Dose-response relations in experimental transmission of avian erythromyeloblastic leukosis. I. Host-response to the virus. *J. Natl. Cancer Inst.* **12:** 447–463.

East, J., M.A.B. De Sousa, P.R. Prosser, and H. Jaquet. 1976a. Malignant changes in New Zealand Black mice. *Clin. Exp. Immunol.* **2:** 427–443.

East, J.L., J.E. Knesek, P.T. Allen, and L. Dmochowski. 1973. Structural characteristics and nucleotide sequence analysis of genomic RNA from RD-114 virus and feline RNA tumor viruses. *J. Virol.* **12:** 1085–1091.

East, J., P.R. Prosser, E.J. Holborow, and H. Jaquet. 1967b. Autoimmune reactions and virus-like particles in germ-free NZB mice. *Lancet* **1:** 755–757.

Eckert, E.A., R. Rott, and W. Schafer. 1963. Myxovirus-like structure of avian myeloblastosis virus. *Z. Natursforsch.* **18b:** 339–000.

Elder, J.H., F.C. Jensen, M.L. Bryant, and R.A. Lerner. 1977a. Polymorphism of the major envelope gylcoprotein (gp70) of murine C-type viruses: Virion associated and differentiation antigens encoded by a multi-gene family. *Nature* **267:** 23–28.

Elder, J.H., J.W. Gautsch, F.C. Jensen, R.A. Lerner, J.W. Hartley, and W.P. Rowe. 1977b. Biochemical evidence that MCF murine leukemia viruses are envelope (*env*) gene recombinants. *Proc. Natl. Acad. Sci.* **74:** 4676–4680.

Elder, J.H., J.W. Gautsch, F.C. Jensen, R.A. Lerner, T.M. Chused, H.C. Morse, J.W. Hartley, and W.P. Rowe. 1980. Differential expression of two distinct xenotropic viruses in NZB mice. *Clin. Immunol. Immunopathol.* **15:** 493–501.

Ellermann, V. and O. Bang. 1908. Experimentelle Leukamie bei Huhnern. *Zentral. Bakteriol.* **46:** 595–609.

Engle, G.C., S. Shirahama, and R.M. Dutcher. 1969. Preliminary report on virus-like particles in a transplantable rat mammary carcinoma. *Cancer Res.* **29:** 603–609.

Engelbreth-Holm, J. and A. Rothe Meyer. 1932. Bericht uber neue Erfahrungen mit einem Stamm Huhner-Erythroleukose. *Acta Pathol. Microbiol. Scand.* **9:** 293–332.

Enke, K.H. 1964. Vermutlicher Ubertragungsweg der Leukose vom Rind auf das Schaf. *Monatsshr. Veterinaermed. Sonderhft.* **19:** 45–00.

Enke, K.H., M. Jungnitz, and M. Rossger. 1961. Ein Kasuistischer Beitrag zur lymphatischer Leukose des Schafes. *Dtsch. Tieraerztl. Wochenschr.* **68:** 359–364.

Epstein, M.A., B.G. Achong, and G. Ball. 1974. Further observations on a human syncytial virus from a nasopharyngeal carcinoma. *J. Natl. Cancer Inst.* **53:** 681–688.

Erfle, V., R. Hehlmann, H. Schetters, A. Meier, and A. Luz. 1980. Time course of C-type retrovirus expression in mice submitted to osteosarcomagenic doses of ^{224}radium. *Int. J. Cancer* **26:** 107–113.

Erfle, V., S. Schulte-Overberg, K.-H. Marquart, I.-D. Adler, and A. Luz. 1979. Establishment and characterization of C-type RNA virus-producing cell lines from radiation-induced murine osteosarcoma. *J. Cancer Res. Clin. Oncol.* **94:** 149–162.

Essex, M. 1975. Horizontally and vertically transmitted oncornaviruses of cats. *Adv. Cancer Res.* **21:** 175–248.

Essex, M. and S.P. Snyder. 1973. Feline oncornavirus-associated cell membrane antigen. I. Serologic studies with kittens exposed to cell-free materials from various feline fibrosarcomas. *J. Natl. Cancer Inst.* **51:** 1007–1012.

Essex, M., G. Klein, S.P. Snyder, and J.B. Harrold. 1971a. Antibody to feline oncornavirus-associated cell membrane antigen in neonatal cats. *Int. J. Cancer* **8:** 384–390.

———. 1971b. Correlation between humoral antibody and regression of tumours induced by feline sarcoma virus. *Nature* **233:** 195–196.

Essex, M., C.K. Grant, S.M. Cotter, A.H. Sliski, and W.D. Hardy, Jr. 1979. Leukemia specific antigens: FOCMA and immune surveillance. In *Modern trends in human leukemia III* (ed. R. Neth et al.), pp. 453–467. Springer Verlag, Berlin.

Essex, M., A.H. Sliski, W.D. Hardy, Jr., F. deNoronha, and S.M. Cotter. 1978. Feline oncornavirus associated cell membrane antigen: A tumor specific cell surface marker. In *Advances in comparative leukemia research 1977* (ed. P. Bentvelzen et al.), pp. 337–340. Elsevier/North Holland, Amsterdam.

Fabisch, P.H., K.K. Takemoto, and J.F. Hruska. 1973. Characterization of a hamster "foamy" virus. In *Annual Meeting of American Society for Microbiology* **365:** 255. (Abstr.).

Fabricant, C.G., L.J. Rich, and J.H. Gillespie. 1969. Feline viruses. XI. Isolation of a virus similar to a myxovirus from cats in which urolithiasis was experimentally induced. *Cornell Vet.* **59:** 667–672.

Faller, D.V., J. Rommelaere, and N. Hopkins. 1978. Large T1 oligonucleotides of Moloney leukemia virus missing in an *env* gene recombinant, HIX, are present on an intracellular 21S Moloney viral RNA species. *Proc. Natl. Acad. Sci.* **75:** 2964–2968.

Feldman, D.G. and L. Gross. 1970. Electron microscopic study of guinea pig leukemia virus. *Cancer Res.* **30:** 2702–2711.

Feldman, D.G., T. Ehrenreich, and L. Gross. 1974. Type-C virus particles in a feline angioma: A case report. *J. Natl. Cancer Inst.* **53:** 1843–1846.

Fenner, F. 1975. The classification and nomenclature of viruses. *Intervirology* **6:** 1–12.

Ferrer, J.F. 1972. Antigenic comparison of bovine type C virus with murine and feline leukemia viruses. *Cancer Res.* **32:** 1871–1877.

Fey, F. and A. Graffi. 1965. Erythroblasten-Leukamie nach Injektion von Virus der myeloischen Leukamie der Maus. *Z. Krebsforsch.* **67:** 145–151.

Filippi, P., M. Brahic, R. Vigne, and J. Tamalet. 1979. Characterization of visna virus mRNA. *J. Virol.* **31:** 25–30.

Fine, D. and G. Schochetman. 1978. Type D primate retroviruses: A review. *Cancer Res.* **38:** 3123–3139.

Fine, D.L., L.O. Arthur, and G. Schochetman. 1980. Functionally conserved determinants on gp70s of endogenous primate retroviruses. *Virology* **101:** 176–184.

Fine, D.L., J.C. Landon, and M. Kubicek. 1971. Simian tumor virus isolate: Demonstration of cytopathic effects in vitro. *Science* **174:** 420–421.

Fine, D.L., E.W. Kingsbury, M.G. Valerio, M.T. Kubicek, J.C. Landon, and H.C. Chopra. 1972. Simian tumor virus proliferation in inoculated *Macaca mulatta. Nat. New Biol.* **238:** 191–192.

Fine, D.L., J.C. Landon, R.J. Pienta, M.T. Kubicek, M.J. Valerio, W.F. Loeb, and H.C. Chopra. 1975. Responses of infant rhesus monkeys to inoculation with Mason-Pfizer monkey virus materials. *J. Natl. Cancer Inst.* **54:** 651–658.

Fine, D.L., R.J. Pienta, L.B. Malan, M.T. Kubicek, D.G. Bennett, J.C. Landon, M.G. Valerio, D.M. West, D.A. Fabrizio, and H.C. Chopra. 1974. Biologic characteristics of transformed rhesus foreskin cells infected with Mason-Pfizer monkey virus. *J. Natl. Cancer Inst.* **52:** 1135–1142.

Finkel, M.P., B.O. Biskis, and P.B. Jinkins. 1966a. Virus induction of osteosarcomas in mice. *Science* **151:** 698–701.

Finkel, M.P., C.A. Reilly, Jr., and B.O. Biskis. 1975. Viral etiology of bone cancer. *Front. Radiat. Ther. Oncol.* **10:** 28–39.

———. 1976. Pathogenesis of radiation and virus-induced bone tumors. *Recent Results Cancer Res.* **54:** 92–103.

Finkel, M.P., P.B. Jinkins, J. Tolle, and B.O. Biskis. 1966b. Serial radiography of virus-induced osteosarcomas in mice. *Radiology* **87:** 333–339.

Finkel, M.P., C.A. Reilly, Jr., B.O. Biskis, and I.L. Greco. 1973. Bone tumor viruses. In *Bone—Certain aspects of neoplasia* (ed. C.H.G. Price and F.G.M. Ross), pp. 353–366. Butterworths, London.

Fischinger, P.J., S. Nomura, and D.P. Bolognesi. 1975. A novel murine oncornavirus with dual eco- and xenotropic properties. *Proc. Natl. Acad. Sci.* **72:** 5150–5155.

Fischinger, P.J., P.T. Peebles, S. Nomura, and D.K. Haapala. 1973. Isolation of an RD-114-like oncornavirus from a cat cell line. *J. Virol.* **11:** 978–985.

Fischinger, P.J., A.E. Frankel, J.H. Elder, R.A. Lerner, J.N. Ihle, and D.P. Bolognesi. 1978. Biological, immunological, and biochemical evidence that HIX virus is a recombinant between Moloney leukemia virus and a murine xenotropic C type virus. *Virology* **90:** 241–254.

Flavell, A.J. and D. Ish-Horowicz. 1981. Extrachromosomal circular copies of the eukaryotic transposable element *copia* in cultured *Drosophila* cells. *Nature* **292:** 591–595.

Fleming, W.A. and J.K. Clarke. 1970. Fluorescence assay of foamy virus. *J. Gen. Virol.* **6:** 277–284.

Flugel, R.M., H. Zentgraf, K. Munk, and G. Darai. 1978. Activation of an endogenous retrovirus from *Tupaia* (tree shrew). *Nature* **271:** 543–545.

Fong, C.K.Y. and G.D. Hsiung. 1976. Oncornavirus of guinea pigs. I. Morphology and distribution in normal and leukemic guinea pig cells. *Virology* **70:** 385–398.

Franklin, R.B., R.L. Maldonado, and H.R. Bose. 1974. Isolation and characterization of reticuloendotheliosis virus transformed bone marrow cells. *Intervirology* **3:** 342–352.

Frederickson, T.N., H.G. Purchase, and B.R. Burmester. 1964. Transmission of virus from field cases of avian lymphomatosis. III. Variation in the oncogenic spectra of passaged virus isolates. *Natl. Cancer Inst. Monogr.* **17:** 1–29.

Freeman, A.E., R.V. Gilden, M.L. Vernon, R.G. Wolford, P.E. Hugunin, and R.J. Huebner. 1973. 5-bromo-2′-deoxyuridine potentiation of transformation of rat-embryo cells induced *in vitro* by 3-methylcholanthrene: Induction of rat leukemia virus gs antigen in transformed cells. *Proc. Natl. Acad. Sci.* **70:** 2415–2419.

Freeman, A.E., G.J. Kelloff, R.V. Gilden, W.T. Lane, A.P. Swain, and R.J. Huebner. 1971. Activation and isolation of hamster-specific C-type RNA viruses from tumors induced by cell cultures transformed by chemical carcinogens. *Proc. Natl. Acad. Sci.* **68:** 2386–2390.

Freeman, A.E., G.J. Kelloff, M.L. Vernon, W.T. Lane, W.I. Capps, S. Bumgarner, H.C. Turner, and R.J. Huebner. 1974. Prevalence of endogenous type-C virus in normal hamster tissues and hamster tumors induced by chemical carcinogens, simian virus 40, and polyoma virus. *J. Natl. Cancer Inst.* **52:** 1469–1476.

Friedrich, R., V.L. Morris, H.M. Goodman, J.M. Bishop, and H.E. Varmus. 1976. Differences between genomes of two strains of mouse mammary tumor virus as shown by partial RNA sequence analysis. *Virology* **72:** 330–340.

Friend, C. 1957. Cell-free transmission in adult Swiss mice of a disease having the character of a leukemia. *J. Exp. Med.* **105:** 307–318.

Frisby, D.P., R. MacCormick, and R. Weiss. 1980. Origin of RAV-0, the endogenous retrovirus of chickens. *Cold Spring Harbor Conf. Cell Proliferation* **7:** 509–517.

Frisby, D.P., R.A. Weiss, M. Roussel, and D. Stehelin. 1979. The distribution of endogenous chicken retrovirus sequences in the DNA of galliform birds does not coincide with avian phylogenetic relationships. *Cell* **17:** 623–634.

Fritsch, E. and H.M. Temin. 1977. Formation and structure of infectious DNA of spleen necrosis virus. *J. Virol.* **21:** 119–130.

Fujinaga, K., A. Rankin, H. Yamazaki, K. Sekikawa, J. Bragdon, and M. Green. 1973. RD-114 virus: Analysis of viral gene sequences in feline and human cells by DNA-DNA reassociation kinetics and RNA-DNA hybridization. *Virology* **56:** 484–495.

Fujinami, A. and K. Inamoto. 1914. Ueber Geswulste bei japanishen Haushuhnern insbesondere uber einen transplantablen Tumor. *Z. Krebsforsch.* **14:** 94–119.

Fujita, D.J., Y.C. Chen, R.R. Friis, and P.K. Vogt. 1974. RNA tumor viruses of pheasants: Characterization of avian leukosis subgroups F and G. *Virology* **60:** 558–571.

Fujita, D.J., J. Tal, H.E. Varmus, and J.M. Bishop. 1978. *env* gene of chicken RNA tumor viruses: Extent of conservation in cellular and viral genomes. *J. Virol.* **27:** 465–474.

Gajdusek, D.C., N.G. Rogers, M. Basnight, C.J. Gibbs, Jr., and M. Alpers. 1969. Transmission experiments with kuru in chimpanzees and the isolation of latent viruses from the explanted tissues of infected animals. *Ann. N.Y. Acad. Sci.* **162:** 529–550.

Gallo, R.C., R.E. Gallagher, F. Wong-Staal, T. Aoki, P.D. Markham, H. Schetters, F. Ruscetti, M. Valero, M.J. Walling, R.T. O'Keeffe, W.C. Saxinger, R.G. Smith, D.H. Gillespie, and M.S. Reitz, Jr. 1978. Isolation and tissue distribution of type-C virus and viral components from a gibbon ape (*Hylobates lar*) with lymphocytic leukemia. *Virology* **84:** 359–373.

Gardner, M.B. 1978. Type C viruses of wild mice: Characterization and natural history of amphotropic, ecotropic and xenotropic MuLV. *Curr. Top. Microbiol. Immunol.* **79:** 215–259.

Gardner, M.B., B.E. Henderson, J.D. Estes, H. Menck, J.C. Parker, and R.J. Huebner. 1973a. Unusually high incidence of spontaneous lymphomas in wild house mice. *J. Natl. Cancer Inst.* **50:** 1571–1575.

Gardner, M.B., B.E. Henderson, J.D. Estes, R.W. Rongey, J. Casagrande, M. Pike, and R.J. Huebner. 1976. The epidemiology and virology of C-type virus-associated hematological cancers and related diseases in wild mice. *Cancer Res.* **36:** 574–581.

Gardner, M.B., R.W. Rongey, P. Arnstein, J.D. Estes, P. Sarma, R.J. Huebner, and C.G. Rickard. 1970. Experimental transmission of feline fibrosarcoma to cats and dogs. *Nature* **226:** 807–809.

Gardner, M.B., B.E. Henderson, J.E. Officer, R.W. Rongey, J.C. Parker, C. Oliver, J.D. Estes, and R.J. Huebner. 1973b. A spontaneous motor neuron disease apparently caused by indigenous type-C RNA virus in wild mice. *J. Natl. Cancer Inst.* **51:** 1243–1249.

Gaskin, J.M. and J.H. Gillespie. 1972. Detection of feline syncytium-inducing virus carrier state with a microimmunodiffusion test. *Am J. Vet. Res.* **34:** 245–247.

Gautsch, J.W., J.H. Elder, J. Schindler, F.C. Jensen, and R.A. Lerner. 1978a. Structural markers on core protein p30 of murine leukemia virus: Functional correlation with *Fv-1* tropism. *Proc. Natl. Acad. Sci.* **75:** 4170–4174.

Gautsch, J.W., R. Lerner, D. Howard, Y.A. Teramoto, and J. Schlom. 1978b. Strain-specific markers for the major structural proteins of highly oncogenic murine mammary tumor viruses by tryptic peptide analyses. *J. Virol.* **27:** 688–699.

Gazdar, A.F., H.C. Chopra, and P.S. Sarma. 1972a. Properties of a murine sarcoma virus isolated from a tumor arising in an NZW/NZB F_1 hybrid mouse. I. Isolation and pathology of tumors induced in rodents. *Int. J. Cancer* **9:** 219–233.

Gazdar, A.F., P.S. Sarma, and R.H. Bassin. 1972b. Properties of a murine sarcoma virus isolated from a tumor arising in an NZW/NZB F_1 hybrid mouse. II. Physical and biological characteristics. *Int. J. Cancer.* **9:** 234–241.

Gazdar, A.F., L.A. Phillips, P.S. Sarma, P.T. Peebles, and H.C. Chopra. 1971. Presence of sarcoma genome in a "non-infectious" mammalian virus. *Nat. New Biol.* **234:** 69–72.

Gazit, A., A. Yaniv, M. Ianconescu, K. Perk, B. Aizenberg, and A. Zimber. 1979. Molecular evidence for a type C retrovirus etiology of the lymphoproliferative disease of turkeys. *J. Virol.* **31:** 639–644.

Gazzolo, L., D. Simkovic, and M.C. Martin-Berthelon. 1971. The presence of C-type RNA virus particles in a rat embryo cell line spontaneously transformed in tissue culture. *J. Gen. Virol.* **12:** 303–311.

Geering, G., L.J. Old, and E.A. Boyse. 1966. Antigens of leukemias induced by naturally occurring murine leukemia virus: Their relation to the antigens of Gross virus and other murine leukemia viruses. *J. Exp. Med.* **124:** 753–772.

Gelmann, E.P., A. Decleve, and H.S. Kaplan. 1978. Biological and biochemical differences among ecotropic C-type RNA viral isolates chemically induced from C57BL/Ka mouse embryo cells *in vitro. Virology* **85:** 198–210.

Gilden, R.V., S. Oroszlan, and R.J. Huebner. 1971. Antigenic differentiation of M-MSV(O) from mouse, hamster, cat C-type viruses. *Virology* **43:** 722–724.

Gilden, R., Y.K. Lee, S. Oroszlan, J.L. Walker, and R.J. Huebner. 1970. Reptilian C-type virus: Biophysical, biological, and immunological properties. *Virology* **41:** 187–190.

Gilden, R.V., R. Toni, M. Hanson, D. Bova, H.P. Charman, and S. Oroszlan. 1974. Immunochemical studies of the major internal polypeptide of woolly monkey and gibbon ape type C viruses. *J. Immunol.* **112:** 1250–1254.

Gilden, R.V., C.W. Long, M. Hanson, R. Toni, H.P. Charman, S. Oroszlan, J.M. Miller, and M.J. Van Der Maaten. 1975. Characteristics of the major internal protein and RNA-dependent DNA polymerase of bovine leukaemia virus. *J. Gen. Virol.* **29:** 305–314.

Gillespie, D., S. Marshall, and R.C. Gallo. 1972. RNA of RNA tumour viruses contains poly A. *Nat. New Biol.* **236:** 227–231.

Gillespie, D., S. Gillespie, R.C. Gallo, J.L. East, and L. Dmochowski. 1973. Genetic origin of RD114 and other RNA tumour viruses assayed by molecular hybridization. *Nat. New Biol.* **244:** 51–54.

Gillespie, J.H. and F.W. Scott. 1973. Feline viral infections. *Adv. Vet. Sci. Comp. Med.* **17:** 164–195.

Gisselbrecht, S., R.H. Bassin, B.I. Gerwin, and A. Rein. 1974. Dual susceptibility of a 3T3 mouse cell line to infection by N- and B-tropic murine leukemia virus: Apparent lack of expression of the Fv-1 gene. *Int. J. Cancer* **14:** 106–113.

Goff. S.P., E. Gilboa, O.N. Witte, and D. Baltimore. 1980. Structure of the Abelson murine leukemia virus genome and the homologous cellular gene: Studies with cloned viral DNA. *Cell* **22:** 777–785.

Goldberg, R.J., E.M. Scolnick, W.P. Parks, L.A. Yakovleva, and B.A. Lapin. 1974. Isolation of a primate type-C virus from a lymphomatous baboon. *Int. J. Cancer* **14:** 722–730.

Gonda, M.A., N.R. Rice, and R.V. Gilden. 1980. Avian reticuloendotheliosis virus: Characterization of the high-molecular-weight viral RNA in transforming and helper virus populations. *J. Virol.* **34:** 743–751.

Gould, E.A. and J. Hartley. 1979. Comparison of the antigens produced by foamy virus in a cytolytic and persistent infection of HEp2 cells. *J. Gen. Virol.* **44:** 235–239.

Gould, E.A., G.M. Allan, E.F. Logan, and J.B. McFerran. 1978. Detection of antibody to bovine syncytial virus and respiratory syncytial virus in bovine fetal serum. *J. Clin. Microbiol.* **8:** 233–237.

Graf, T. and H. Beug. 1978. Avian leukemia viruses. Interaction with their target cells in vivo and in vitro. *Biochim. Biophys. Acta* **516:** 269–299.

Graffi, A. 1957. Chloroleukemia of mice. *Ann. N.Y. Acad. Sci.* **68:** 540–558.

Graffi, A., F. Fey, and T. Schramm. 1966. Experiments on the hematological diversification of viral mouse leukemias. *Natl. Cancer Inst. Monogr.* **22:** 21–31.

Graffi, A., T. Schramm, E. Bender, I. Graffi, K.H. Horn, and D. Bierwolf. 1968. Cell free transmissible leukosis in syrian hamster, probably of viral aetiology. *Br. J. Cancer* **22:** 577–581.

Graves, D.C. and J.F. Ferrer. 1976 *In vitro* transmission and propagation of the bovine leukemia virus in monolayer cell cultures. *Cancer Res.* **36:** 4152–4159.

Green, N., H. Hiai, J.H. Elder, R.S. Schwartz, R.H. Khiroya, C.Y. Thomas, P.N. Tsichlis, and J.M. Coffin. 1980. Expression of leukemogenic recombinant viruses associated with a recessive gene in HRS/J mice. *J. Exp. Med.* **152:** 249–264.

Grolle, P.F., P. Bentvelzen, and M.J. Van Noord. 1973. Activation of endogenous C-type oncornavirus by 5-bromodeoxyuridine in cultured embryonic rat fibroblasts. *Biomedicine* **19:** 148–151.

Gross, L. 1944. Is cancer a communicable disease? *Cancer Res.* **4:** 293–303.

———. 1951. "Spontaneous" leukemia developing in C3H mice following inoculation in infancy, with A-K leukemic extracts, or AK embryos. *Proc. Soc. Exp. Biol. Med.* **76:** 27–32.

———. 1959. Serial cell-free passage of a radiation-activated mouse leukemia agent. *Proc. Soc. Exp. Biol. Med.* **100:** 102–105.

———. 1960. Development of myeloid (chloro-) leukemia in thymectomized C3H mice following inoculation of lymphatic leukemia virus. *Proc. Soc. Exp. Biol. Med.* **103:** 509–514.

———. 1970. *Oncogenic viruses,* 2nd edition. Pergamon Press, Oxford.

Gross, L., G. Schidlovsky, D. Feldman, Y. Dreyfuss and L.A. Moore. 1975. C-type virus particles in placenta of normal healthy Sprague-Dawley rats. *Proc. Natl. Acad. Sci.* **72:** 3240–3244.

Gross, M.A., B.R. Burmester, and W.G. Walter. 1959. Pathogenicity of a viral strain (RPL12) causing avian visceral lymphomatosis and related neoplasms. I. Nature of the lesions. *J. Natl. Cancer Inst.* **22:** 83–101.

Gross, P.A., C.K.Y. Fong and G.D. Hsiung. 1973. Characterization of guinea pig C-type virus. *Proc. Soc. Exp. Biol. Med.* **143:** 367–370.

Gudnadottir, M. 1974. Visna-maedi in sheep. *Prog. Med. Virol.* **18:** 336–349.

Gudnadottir, M. and P.A. Palsson. 1967. Transmission of maedi by inoculation of a virus grown in tissue culture from maedi-affected lungs. *J. Infect. Dis.* **117:** 1–6.

Haas, M. 1978. Leukemogenic activity of thymotropic, ecotropic, and xenotropic radiation leukemia virus isolates. *J. Virol.* **25:** 705–709.

Haas, M. and T. Rashef. 1980. Isolation of dualtropic reticulum cell neoplasm-inducing retroviruses from C57BL/6 hematopoietic stromal cell lines. *Eur. J. Cancer* **16:** 888–896.

Haas, M., T. Sher, and S. Smolinsky. 1977. Leukemogenesis *in vitro* induced by thymic epithelium reticulum cells transmitting murine leukemia viruses. *Cancer Res* **37:** 1800–1807.

Haase, A.T. 1975. The slow infection caused by visna virus. *Curr. Top. Microbiol. Immunol.* **72:** 101–156.

Haase, A.T. and J.R. Baringer. 1974. The structural polypeptides of slow viruses. *Virology* **57:** 238–250.

Haase, A.T. and W. Levinson. 1973. Inhibition of RNA slow viruses by thiosemicarbazones. *Biochem. Biophys. Res. Commun.* **51:** 875–880.

Haase, A.T. and H.E. Varmus. 1973. Demonstration of a DNA provirus in the lytic growth of visna virus. *Nat. New Biol.* **245:** 237–239.

Haase, A.T., A.C. Garapin, A.J. Faras, H.E. Varmus, and J.M. Bishop. 1974a. Characterization of the nucleic acid product of the visna virus RNA dependent DNA polymerase. *Virology* **57:** 251–258.

Haase, A.T., B.L. Traynor, P.E. Ventura, and D.W. Alling. 1976. Infectivity of visna virus DNA. *Virology* **70:** 65–79.

Haase, A.T., A.C. Garapin, A.J. Faras, J.M. Taylor, and J.M. Bishop. 1974b. A comparison of the high molecular weight RNAs of visna virus and Rous sarcoma virus. *Virology* **57:** 259–270.

Haase, A.T., L. Stowring, O. Narayan, D. Griffin, and D. Price. 1977. Slow persistent infection caused by visna virus: Role of host restriction. *Science* **195:** 175–177.

Haase, A.T., M. Brahic, D. Carroll, J. Scott, L. Stowring, B. Traynor, and P. Ventura. 1978. Visna: An animal model for studies of virus persistence. In *Persistent viruses* (ed. J.G. Stevens et al.), pp. 643–654. Academic Press, New York.

Hackett, A.J. and J.S. Manning. 1971. Comments on feline syncytia-forming virus. *J. Am. Vet. Med. Assoc.* **158:** 948–954.

Hackett, A.J., A. Pfiester, and P. Arnstein. 1970. Biological properties of a syncytia-forming agent isolated from domestic cats (feline syncytia-forming virus). *Proc. Soc. Exp. Biol. Med.* **135:** 899–904.

Hageman, P., J. Calafat, and J.H. Daams. 1972. The mouse mammary tumor viruses. In *RNA viruses and host genomes in oncogenesis* (ed. P. Emmelot and P. Bentvelzen), pp. 283–300. North-Holland, Amsterdam.

Hageman, P.C., J. Links, and P. Bentvelzen. 1968. Biological properties of B particles from C3H and C3Hf mouse milk. *J. Natl. Cancer Inst.* **40:** 1319–1324.

Halpern, M.S., E. Wade, E. Rucker, K.L. Baxter-Gabbard, A.S. Levine, and R.R. Friis. 1973. A study of the relationship of reticuloendotheliosis virus to the avian leukosis-sarcoma complex of viruses. *Virology* **53:** 287–299.

Hamilton, R.C., A. MacGregor, and D. Pye. 1979. A marsupial oncovirus? *J. Gen. Virol.* **44:** 535–539.

Hampar, B., K.H. Rand, R.A. Lerner, B.C. Del Villano, Jr., R.M. McAllister, L.M. Martos, J.G. Derge, C.W. Long, and R.V. Gilden. 1973. Formation of syncytia in human lymphoblastoid cells infected with type C viruses. *Virology* **55:** 453–463.

Hanafusa, H. and T. Hanafusa. 1971. Noninfectious RSV deficient in DNA polymerase. *Virology* **43:** 313–316.

Hanafusa, H., T. Hanafusa, and H. Rubin. 1963. The defectiveness of Rous sarcoma virus. *Proc. Natl. Acad. Sci.* **49:** 572–580.

Hanafusa, T. and H. Hanafusa. 1973. Isolation of leukosis-type virus from pheasant embryo cells: Possible presence of viral genes in cells. *Virology* **51:** 247–254.

Hanafusa, T., H. Hanafusa, C.E. Metroka, W.S. Hayward, C.W. Rettenmier, R.C. Sawyer, R.M. Dougherty, and H.S. Di Stefano. 1976. Pheasant viruses: A new class of ribodeoxyviruses. *Proc. Natl. Acad. Sci.* **73:** 1333–1337.

Hand, P.H., Y.A. Teramoto, R. Callahan, and J. Schlom. 1980. Interspecies radioimmunoassay for the major internal protein of mammary tumor viruses. *Virology* **101:** 61–71.

Hardy, W.D., Jr., M. Essex, and A.J. McClelland, eds. 1980. *Feline leukemia virus.* Elsevier/ North-Holland, New York.

Hardy, W.D., Jr., E.E. Zuckerman, M. Essex, E.G. MacEwen, and A.A. Hayes. 1978. Feline oncornavirus-associated cell-membrane antigen: An FeLV- and FeSV-induced tumor-specific antigen. *Cold Spring Harbor Conf. Cell Proliferation* **5:** 601.

Hardy, W.D., Jr., E.E. Zuckerman, E.G. MacEwen, A.A. Hayes, and M. Essex. 1977. A feline leukaemia virus- and sarcoma virus-induced tumour specific antigen. *Nature* **270:** 249–251.

Harewood, K. and M. Ahmed. 1977. Production of antiserum to the reverse transcriptase of Mason-Pfizer monkey virus. *J. Gen. Virol.* **36:** 227–235.

Harris, R.J.C. and F.C. Chesterman. 1964. Growth of Rous sarcoma in rats, ferrets, and hamsters. *Natl. Cancer Inst. Monogr.* **17:** 321–335.

Harter, D.H. and P.W. Choppin. 1967a. Cell-fusing activity of visna virus particles. *Virology* **31:** 279–288.

———. 1967b. Plaque assay of visna virus using a secondary cellular overlay as an indicator. *Virology* **31:** 176–178.

Harter, D.H., K.C. Hsu, and H.M. Rose. 1968. Multiplication of visna virus in bovine and porcine cell lines. *Proc. Soc. Exp. Biol. Med.* **129:** 295–300.

Harter, D.H., J. Schlom and H. Spiegelman. 1971. Characterization of visna virus nucleic acid. *Biochim. Biophys. Acta* **240:** 435–441.

Harter, D.H., R. Axel, A. Burny, S. Gulati, J. Schlom, and S. Spiegelman. 1973. The relationship of visna, maedi and RNA tumor viruses as studied by molecular hybridization. *Virology* **52:** 287–291.

Hartley, J.W. and W.P. Rowe. 1975. Clonal cell lines from a feral mouse embryo which lack host-range restrictions for murine leukemia viruses. *Virology* **65:** 128–134.

———. 1976. Naturally occurring murine leukemia viruses in wild mice: Characterization of a new "amphotropic" class. *J. Virol.* **19:** 19–25.

Hartley, J.W., W.P. Rowe, and R.J. Huebner. 1970. Host-range restrictions of murine leukemia viruses in mouse embryo cell cultures. *J. Virol.* **5:** 221–225.

Hartley, J.W., W.P. Rowe, W.I. Capps, and R.J. Huebner. 1969. Isolation of naturally occurring viruses of the murine leukemia virus group in tissue culture. *J. Virol.* **3:** 126–132.

Hartley, J.W., N.K. Wolford, L.J. Old, and W.P. Rowe. 1977. A new class of murine leukemia virus associated with development of spontaneous lymphomas. *Proc. Natl. Acad. Sci.* **74:** 789–792.

Harvey, J.J. 1964. An unidentified virus which causes the rapid production of tumours in mice. *Nature* **204:** 1104–1105.

Harvey, J.J., J. East, and F.E. Katz. 1979a. Azathioprine-induced lymphocytic neoplasms of NZB mice lack ecotropic murine leukaemia virus. *Int. J. Cancer* **23:** 217–223.

Harvey, J.J., M. Tuffrey, H.C. Holmes, and J. East. 1979b. Absence of ecotropic or recombinant murine leukaemia virus in preleukaemic and leukaemic X-irradiated NZB mice. *Int. J. Cancer* **24:** 373–376.

Hatanaka, M., R.J. Huebner, and R.V. Gilden. 1970. DNA polymerase activity associated with RNA tumor virus. *Proc. Natl. Acad. Sci.* **67:** 143–147.

Hays, E.F. and D.L. Vredevoe. 1977. A discrepancy in XC and oncogenicity assays for murine leukemia virus in AKR mice. *Cancer Res.* **37:** 726–730.

Heberling, R.L., S.S. Kalter, S.T. Barker, and O.S. Weislow. 1976. Isolation and biological properties of endogenous baboon (*Papio cynocephalus*) type C viruses. In *Comparative leukemia research 1975* (ed. J. Clemmesen and D.S. Yohn), pp. 158–160. Karger, Basel.

Heberling, R.L., S.T. Barker, S.S. Kalter, G.C. Smith, and R.J. Helmke. 1977. Oncornavirus: Isolation from a squirrel monkey (Saimiri sciureus) lung culture. *Science* **195:** 289–292.

Heine, C.W., D.C. Kelly, and R.J. Avery. 1980. The detection of intracellular retrovirus-like entities in *Drosophila melanogaster* cell cultures. *J. Gen. Virol.* **49:** 385–395.

Hellman, A., P.T. Peebles, J.E. Strickland, A.K. Fowler, S.S. Kalter, S. Oroszlan, and R.V. Gilden. 1974. Baboon virus isolate M-7 with properties similar to feline virus RD-114. *J. Virol.* **14:** 133–138.

Henson, J.B. and T.C. McGuire. 1974. Equine infectious anemia. *Prog. Med. Virol.* **18:** 143–159.

Henson, J.B., T.C McGuire, and J.R. Gorham. 1971. The detection of precipitating antibodies in equine infectious anemia and partial purification of the antigen. *Arch. Gesamte Virusforsch.* **35:** 385–391.

Henson, J.B., T.C. McGuire, K. Kobayashi, K.L. Banks, W.C. Davis, and J.R. Gorham. 1970. Recent research on the virology, serology and pathology of equine infectious anemia. In *Proceedings of the 2nd International Conference on Equine Infectious Disease,* pp. 178–199.

Hertz, A., G.H. Theilen, O.W. Schalm, and R.J. Munn. 1970. C-type virus in bone marrow cells of cats with myeloproliferative disorders. *J. Natl. Cancer Inst.* **44:** 339–348.

Hilgers, J. and P. Bentvelzen. 1978. Interaction between viral and genetic factors in murine mammary cancer. *Adv. Cancer Res.* **26:** 143–195.

Hino, S., J.R. Stephenson, and S.A. Aaronson. 1975. Antigenic determinants of the 70,000 molecular weight glycoprotein of woolly monkey type C RNA virus. *J. Immunol.* **115:** 922–927.

———. 1976. Radioimmunoassays for the 70,000-molecular-weight glycoproteins of endogenous mouse type C viruses: Viral antigen expression in normal mouse tissues and sera. *J. Virol.* **18:** 933–941.

Hino, S., S.R. Tronick, R.L. Heberling, S.S. Kalter, A. Hellman, and S.A. Aaronson. 1977. Endogenous New World primate retrovirus: Interspecies antigenic determinants shared with the major structural protein of type-D RNA viruses of Old World monkeys. *Proc. Natl. Acad. Sci.* **74:** 5734–5738.

Hoekstra, J. and F. Deinhardt. 1973. Simian sarcoma and feline leukemia virus antigens: Isolation of species- and interspecies-specific proteins. *Intervirology* **2:** 222–230.

Hoelzer, J.D., R.B. Franklin, and H.R. Bose, Jr. 1979. Transformation by reticuloendotheliosis virus: Development of a focus assay and isolation of a nontransforming virus. *Virology* **93:** 20–30.

Hoelzer, J.D., R.B. Lewis, C.R. Wasmuth, and H.R. Bose, Jr. 1980. Hematopoietic cell transformation by reticuloendotheliosis virus: Characterization of the genetic defect. *Virology* **100:** 462–474.

Hooks, J.J. and B. Detrick-Hooks. 1979. Simian foamy virus-induced immunosuppression in rabbits. *J. Gen. Virol.* **44:** 383–390.

Hooks, J.J. and C.J. Gibbs, Jr. 1975. The foamy viruses. *Bacteriol. Rev.* **39:** 169–185.

Hooks, J., C.J. Gibbs, Jr., S. Chou, R. Howk, M. Lewis, and D.C. Gajdusek. 1973. Isolation of a new simian foamy virus from a spider monkey brain culture. *Infect. Immun.* **8:** 804–813.

Hooks, J.J., C.J. Gibbs, Jr., E.C. Cutchins, N.G. Rogers, P. Lampert, and D.C. Gajdusek. 1972. Characterization and distribution of two new foamy viruses isolated from chimpanzees. *Arch. Gesamte Virusforsch.* **38:** 38–55.

Hoss, H.E. and C. Olson. 1974. Infectivity of bovine C-type (leukemia) virus for sheep and goats. *Am. J. Vet. Res.* **35:** 633–637.

Howard, E.B., W.J. Clark, and P.L. Hackett. 1968. Experimental myeloproliferative and lymphoproliferative diseases of swine. In *Leukaemia in animals and man* (ed. H.J. Bendixen), pp. 255–262.

Hruska, J.F. and K.K. Takemoto. 1975. Biochemical properties of a hamster syncytium-forming ("foamy") virus. *J. Natl. Cancer Inst.* **54:** 601–605.

Hsiung, G.D. 1972. Activation of a guinea pig C-type virus in cultured spleen cells by 5-bromo-2′-deoxyuridine. *J. Natl. Cancer Inst.* **49:** 567–570.

Hsiung, G.D., C.K.Y. Fong, and C.H. Evans. 1974. Prevalence of endogenous oncornavirus in guinea pigs. *Intervirology* **3:** 319–331.

Hsiung, G.D., C.K.Y. Fong, and P.A. Gross. 1973. Oncogenic potential of guinea pig herpes- and C-type viruses. *Cancer Res.* **33:** 1436–1442.

Hu, S.S.F., M.M.C. Lai, T.C. Wong, R.S. Cohen, and M. Sevoian. 1981. Avian reticuloendotheliosis virus: Characterization of genome structure by heteroduplex mapping. *J. Virol.* **37:** 899–907.

Hyslop, N.St.G. 1966. Equine infectious anemia (swamp fever). A review. *Vet. Rec.* **78:** 858–864.

Ishii, S. 1963. Equine infectious anemia or swamp fever. *Adv. Vet. Sci.* **8:** 263–298.

Ishii, S. and R. Ishitani. 1975. Equine infectious anemia. *Adv. Vet. Sci. Comp. Med.* **19:** 195–222.

Ishizaki, R., R.W. Green, and D.P. Bolognesi. 1978. The structural polypeptides of equine infectious anemia virus. *Intervirology* **9:** 286–294.

Ito, Y., Y. Kono, and K. Kobayashi. 1969. Electron microscopic observations of equine infectious anemia (EIA) virus in cultivated horse leukocytes. *Arch. Gesamte Virusforsch.* **28:** 411–414.

———. 1971. Comment: Presence of feline syncytial virus in 2 primary cultures of feline embryo cells. *J. Am. Vet. Med. Assoc.* **158:** 954.

Jarrett, O. 1980. Natural occurrence of subgroups of feline leukemia virus. Cold Spring Harbor *Conf. Cell Proliferation:* 603–612.

Jarrett, O., D. Hay and H.M. Laird. 1974. Infection by feline syncytium forming virus in Britain. *Vet. Rec.* **94:** 201.

Jarrett, O., H.M. Laird, and D. Hay. 1973. Determinants of the host range of feline leukaemia viruses. *J. Gen. Virol.* **20:** 169–175.

Jarrett, W.F.H. 1971. Feline leukemia. *Int. Rev. Exp. Pathol.* **10:** 243–263.

———. 1975. Cat leukemia and its viruses. *Adv. Vet. Med. Comp. Med.* **19:** 165–193.

Jarrett, W.F.H., E.M. Crawford, W.B. Martin, and F. Davie. 1964a. Leukaemia in the cat. A virus-like particle associated with leukaemia (lymphosarcoma). *Nature* **202:** 567–568.

Jarrett, W.F.H., W.B. Martin, G.W. Crighton, R.G. Dalton, and M.F. Stewart. 1964b. Leukaemia in the cat. Transmission experiments with leukaemia (lymphosarcoma). *Nature* **202:** 566–567.

Jarrett, W., O. Jarrett, L. Mackey, H. Laird, W. Hardy, Jr. and M. Essex. 1973. Horizontal transmission of leukemia virus and leukemia in the cat. *J. Natl. Cancer Inst.* **51:** 833–841.

Jenkins, V.K. and A.C. Upton. 1963. Cell-free transmission of radiogenic myeloid leukemia in the mouse. *Cancer Res.* **23:** 1748–1755.

Jensen, E.M., I. Zelljadt, H.C. Chopra, and M.M. Mason. 1970. Isolation and propagation of a virus from a spontaneous mammary carcinoma of a rhesus monkey. *Cancer Res.* **30:** 2388–2393.

Johnson, A.W. 1966. Equine infectious anemia. An annotation. *Vet. Bull.* **36:** 465–469.

Johnston, P. 1961. A second immunological type of simian foamy virus: Monkey throat infections and unmasking by both types. *J. Infect. Dis.* **109:** 1–9.

———. 1971. Taxonomic features of seven serotypes of simian and ape foamy viruses. *Infect. Immun.* **3:** 793–799.

Kalter, S.S., R.J. Helmke, M. Panigel, R.L. Heberling, P.J. Belsburg, and L.R. Axelrod. 1973. Observations of apparent C-type particles in baboon (Papio cynocephalus) placentas. *Science* **179:** 1332–1333.

Kalter, S.S., S.A. Shain, G.C. Smith, B. McCullough, R.L. Heberling, and A.J. Dalton. 1975a. Oncorna-like viruses in baboon prostate tissue. *J. Natl. Cancer Inst.* **55:** 1237–1241.

Kalter, S.S., R.L. Heberling, G.C. Smith, M. Panigel, D.C. Kraemer, R.J. Helmke, and A. Hellman. 1975b. Vertical transmission of C-type viruses: Their presence in baboon follicular oocytes and tubal ova. *J. Natl. Cancer Inst.* **54:** 1173–1176.

Kalter, S.S., M. Panigel, D.C. Kraemer, R.L. Herberling, R.J. Helmke, G.C. Smith, and K. Hellman. 1974. C-type particles in baboon (*Papio cynocephalus*) preimplantation embryos. *J. Natl. Cancer Inst.* **52:** 1927–1928.

Kang, C.-Y. and H.M. Temin. 1973. Lack of sequence homology among RNAs of avian leukosis-sarcoma viruses, reticuloendotheliosis viruses, and chicken endogenous RNA-directed DNA polymerase activity. *J. Virol.* **12:** 1314–1324.

———. 1974. Reticuloendotheliosis virus nucleic acid sequences in cellular DNA. *J. Virol.* **14:** 1179–1188.

Kang, C.-Y., T.C. Wong, and K.V. Holmes. 1975. Comparative ultrastructural study of four reticuloendotheliosis viruses. *J. Virol.* **16:** 1027–1038.

Karasaki, S. 1969. Virus particles associated with transplantable Novikoff hepatoma in the rat. *Cancer Res.* **29:** 1313–1315.

Kasza, L., A.H.S. Hayward, and A.O. Betts. 1969. Isolation of a virus from a cat sarcoma in an established canine melanoma cell line. *Res. Vet. Sci.* **10:** 216–218.

Kawai, S., M. Yoshida, K. Segawa, H. Sugiyama, K. Ishizaki, and K. Toyoshima. 1980. Characterization of Y73, an avian sarcoma virus: A unique transforming gene and its product, a phosphopolyprotein with protein kinase activity. *Proc. Natl. Acad. Sci.* **77:** 6199–6203.

Kawakami, T.G. and P.M. Buckley. 1974. Antigenic studies on gibbon type C viruses. *Transplant. Proc.* **6:** 193–196.

Kawakami, T.G., G.V. Kollias, Jr., and C. Holmberg. 1980. Oncogenicity of gibbon type-C myelogenous leukemia virus. *Int. J. Cancer* **25:** 641–646.

Kawakami, T.G., L. Sun, and T.S. McDowell. 1978. Natural transmission of gibbon leukemia virus. *J. Natl. Cancer Inst.* **61:** 1113–1115.

Kawakami, T.G., P.M. Buckley, T.S. McDowell, and A. DePaoli. 1973. Antibodies to simian C-type virus antigen in sera of gibbons (*Hylobates* sp.). *Nat. New Biol.* **246:** 105–107.

Kawakami, T.G., P.M. Buckley, A. DePaoli, W. Noll, and L.K. Bustad. 1975. Studies on the prevalence of type C virus associated with gibbon hematopoietic neoplasms. In *Comparative leukemia research 1973* (ed. Y. Ito and R.M. Dutcher), pp. 385–389. Karger, Basel.

Kawakami, T.G., G.H. Theilen, D.L. Dungworth, R.J. Munn, and S.F. Beall. 1967. "C"-type viral particles in plasma of cats with feline leukemia. *Science* **158:** 1049–1050.

Kawakami, T.G., S.D. Huff, P.M. Buckley, D.L. Dungworth, S.P. Snyder, and R.V. Gilden. 1972. C-type virus associated with gibbon lymphosarcoma. *Nat. New Biol.* **235:** 170–171.

Kelloff, G., R.J. Huebner, and R.V. Gilden. 1971. Isolation of hamster viruses from preparations of hamster-specific sarcoma viruses. *J. Gen. Virol.* **13:** 289–294.

———. 1973. Isolation and characterization of the hamster C-type viruses. In *Unifying concepts of leukemia* (ed. R.M. Dutcher and L. Chieco-Bianchi), pp. 61–68. Karger, Basel.

Kelloff, G.J., W.T. Lane, H.C. Turner, and R.J. Huebner. 1969. *In vivo* studies of the FBJ murine osteosarcoma virus. *Nature* **223:** 1379–1380.

Kelloff, G., R.J. Huebner, N.J. Chang, Y.K. Lee, and R.V. Gilden. 1970a. Envelope antigen relationships among three hamster-specific sarcoma viruses and a hamster-specific helper virus. *J. Gen. Virol.* **9:** 19–26.

Kelloff, G., R.J. Huebner, Y.K. Lee, R. Toni, and R.V. Gilden. 1970b. Hamster-tropic sarcomagenic and non-sarcomagenic viruses derived from hamster tumors induced by the Gross pseudotype of Moloney sarcoma virus. *Proc. Natl. Acad. Sci.* **65:** 310–317.

Kelloff, G., R.J. Huebner, S. Oroszlan, R. Toni, and R.V. Gilden. 1970c. Immunological identity of the group-specific antigen of hamster-specific C-type viruses and an indigenous hamster virus. *J. Gen. Virol.* **9:** 27–33.

Kemen, M.J. and L. Coggins. 1972. Equine infectious anemia: Transmission from infected mares to foals. *J. Am. Vet. Med. Assoc.* **161:** 496–499.

Kennedy, R.C., C.M. Eklund, C. Lopez, and W.J. Hadlow. 1968. Isolation of a virus from lungs of Montana sheep affected with progressive pneumonia. *Virology* **35:** 483–484.

Kettmann, R., Y. Cleuter, M. Mammerickx, M. Meunier-Rotival, G. Bernardi, A. Burny, and H. Chantrenne. 1980. Genomic integration of bovine leukemia provirus: Comparison of persistent lymphocytosis with lymph node tumor form of enzootic bovine leukosis. *Proc. Natl. Acad. Sci.* **77:** 2577–2581.

Kettmann, R., D. Portetelle, M. Mammerickx, Y. Cleuter, D. Dekegel, M. Galoux, J. Ghysdael, A. Burny, and H. Chantrenne. 1976. Bovine leukemia virus: An exogenous RNA oncogenic virus. *Proc. Natl. Acad. Sci.* **73:** 1014–1018.

Khan, A.S., D.N. Deobagkar, and J.R. Stephenson. 1978. Isolation and characterization of a feline sarcoma virus-coded precursor polyprotein. Competitive immunoassay for nonstructural component(s). *J. Biol. Chem.* **253:** 8894–8901.

Kirsten, W.H. and L.A. Mayer. 1967. Morphologic responses to a murine erythroblastosis virus. *J. Natl. Cancer Inst.* **39:** 311–335.

Kirsten, W.H., L.A. Mayer, R.L. Wollmann, and M.I. Pierce. 1967. Studies on a murine erythroblastosis virus. *J. Natl. Cancer Inst.* **38:** 117–139.

Klement, V. and R.M. McAllister. 1972. Syncytial cytopathic effect in KB cells of a C-type RNA virus isolated from human rhabdomyosarcoma. *Virology* **50:** 305–308.

Klement, V., M.O. Nicolson and R.J. Huebner. 1971. Rescue of the genome of focus forming virus from rat non-productive lines by 5′-bromodeoxyuridine. *Nat. New Biol.* **234:** 12–14.

Klement, V., J.W. Hartley, W.P. Rowe, and R.J. Huebner. 1969. Recovery of a hamster-specific focus forming and sarcomagenic virus from a "noninfectious" hamster tumor induced by the Kirsten mouse sarcoma virus. *J. Natl. Cancer Inst.* **43:** 925–933.

Klement, V., M.P. Nicolson, R.V. Gilden, S. Oroszlan, P.S. Sarma, R.W. Rongey, and M.B. Gardner. 1972. Rat C-type virus induced in rat sarcoma cells by 5-bromodeoxyuridine. *Nat. New Biol.* **238:** 234–236.

Klement, V., M.O. Nicolson, W. Nelson-Rees, R.V. Gilden, S. Oroszlan, R.W. Rongey, and M.B. Gardner. 1973. Spontaneous production of a C-type RNA virus in rat tissue culture lines. *Int. J. Cancer* **12:** 654–666.

Klement, V., M.F. Dougherty, P. Roy-Burman, B.K. Pal, C.S. Shimizu, R.W. Rongey, W. Nelson-Rees, and R.J. Huebner. 1978. Endogenous type C RNA virus of mink (*Mustela vison*). *Virology* **85:** 296–306.

Kobayashi, K. 1961a. Studies on the cultivation of equine infectious anemia virus *in vitro.* II. Propagation of the virus in horse bone marrow culture. *Virus* **11:** 189–201.

———. 1961b. Studies on the cultivation of equine infectious anemia virus *in vitro.* III. Propagation of the virus in leukocyte culture. *Virus* **11:** 249–256.

Kobayashi, K., J.B. Henson, and J.R. Gorham. 1969. Viral neutralizing antibodies in equine infectious anemia. *Fed. Proc.* **28:** 429.

Kono, Y. 1968. Characteristics of complement fixing antigen in equine infectious anemia. *Natl. Inst. Anim. Health Q.* **8:** 117–121.

Kono, Y. and K. Kobayashi. 1966. Complement fixation test of equine infectious anemia. II. Relationship between CF antibody and the disease. *Natl. Inst. Animal Health Q.* **6:** 204–207.

Kono, Y., K. Kobayashi, and Y. Fukanaga. 1970a. Immunization of horses against equine infectious anemia (EIA) with an attenuated EIA virus. *Natl. Inst. Anim. Health Q.* **10:** 113–122.

———. 1971. Serological comparison among various strains of equine infectious anemia virus. *Arch. Gesamte Virusforsch.* **34:** 202–208.

Kono, Y., T. Yoshino, and Y. Fukanaga. 1970b. Growth characteristics of equine infectious anemia virus in horse leukocyte cultures. *Arch. Gesamte Virusforsch.* **30:** 252–256.

Korteweg, R. 1934. Proefondervindelijke onderzoekingen aangaandre erfelijkheid van kander. *Neder. Tijdschr. Geneeskd.* **78:** 240–245.

———. 1936. On the manner in which the disposition to carcinoma of the mammary gland is inherited in mice. *Genetics* **18:** 350–371.

Koshy, R., R.C. Gallo, and F. Wong-Staal. 1980. Characterization of the endogenous feline leukemia virus-related DNA sequences in cats and attempts to identify exogenous viral sequences in tissues of virus-negative leukemic animals. Virology **103:** 434–445.

Kozak, C. and W.P. Rowe. 1978. Genetic mapping of xenotropic leukemia virus-inducing loci in two mouse strains. *Science* **199:** 1448–1449.

Krakower, J.M., S.R. Tronick, R.E. Gallagher, R.C. Gallo, and S.A. Aaronson. 1978. Antigenic characterization of a new gibbon ape leukemia virus isolate: Seroepidemiologic assessment of an outbreak of gibbon leukemia. *Int. J. Cancer* **22:** 715–720.

Kramarsky, B., N.H. Sarkar, and D.H. Moore. 1971. Ultrastructural comparison of a virus from a Rhesus-monkey mammary carcinoma with four oncogenic RNA viruses. *Proc. Natl. Acad. Sci.* **68:** 1603–1607.

Kuff, E.L., R. Callahan, and R.S. Howk. 1980. Immunological relationship between the structural proteins of intracisternal A-particles of *Mus musculus* and the M432 retrovirus of *Mus cervicolor. J. Virol.* **33:** 1211–1214.

Kuff, E.L., K.K. Lueders, and E.M. Scolnick. 1978. Nucleotide sequence relationship between intracisternal type A particles of *Mus musculus* and an endogenous retrovirus (M432) of *Mus cervicolor. J. Virol.* **28:** 66–74.

Kung, H-J., S. Hu, W. Bender, J.M. Bailey, N. Davidson, M.O. Nicolson, and R.M. McAllister. 1976. RD-114, baboon, and woolly monkey viral RNAs compared in size and structure. *Cell* **7:** 609–620.

Laird, H.M., W.F.H. Jarrett, O. Jarrett, and G.W. Crighton. 1967. Virus-like particles in three field cases of feline lymphosarcoma. *Vet. Rec.* **80:** 606.

Lapin, B.A. 1976. Epidemiology of leukemia among baboons of Sukhumi monkey colony. In *Comparative leukemia research 1975* (ed. J. Clemmesen and D.S. Yohn), pp. 212–215. Karger, Basel.

Lathrop, A.E.C. and L. Loeb. 1918. Further investigation on the origin of tumors in mice. V. The tumor rate in hybrid strains. *J. Exp. Med.* **28:** 475–500.

Le Bousse-Kerdiles, M.C., F. Smadja-Joffe, B. Klein, B. Caillou, and C. Jasmin. 1980. Study of a virus-induced myeloproliferative syndrome associated with tumor formation in mice. *Eur. J. Cancer* **16:** 43–51.

Lee, C.K., E.W. Chan, C.A. Reilly, Jr., V.A. Pahnke, G. Rockus, and M.P. Finkel. 1979. *In vitro* properties of FBR murine osteosarcoma virus. *Proc. Soc. Exp. Biol. Med.* **162:** 214–220.

Lerner, R.A., C.B. Wilson, B.C. Del Villano, P.J. McConahey, and F.J. Dixon. 1976. Endogenous oncornaviral gene expression in adult and fetal mice: Quantitative, histologic, and physiologic studies of the major viral glycoprotein, gp70. *J. Exp. Med.* **143:** 151–166.

Levy, J.A. 1973. Xenotropic viruses: Murine leukemia viruses associated with NIH Swiss, NZB, and other mouse strains. *Science* **182:** 1151–1153.

———. 1975. Xenotropic C-type viruses and autoimmune disease. *J. Rheumatol.* **2:** 135–148.

———. 1978. Xenotropic type C viruses. *Curr. Top. Microbiol. Immunol.* **79:** 109–213.

Levy, J.A. and T. Pincus. 1970. Demonstration of biological activity of a murine leukemia virus of New Zealand Black mice. *Science* **170:** 326–327.

Levy, J.A., J.W. Hartley, W.P. Rowe, and R.J. Huebner. 1973. Studies of FBJ osteosarcoma virus in tissue culture. I. Biologic characteristics of the "C"-type viruses. *J. Natl. Cancer Inst.* **51:** 525–539.

———. 1975. Studies of FBJ osteosarcoma virus in tissue culture. II. Autoinhibition of focus formation. *J. Natl. Cancer Inst.* **54:** 615–619.

Levy, J.A., J. Joyner, K.T. Nayar, and R.E. Kouri. 1979. Genetics of xenotropic virus expression in mice. I. Evidence for a single locus regulating spontaneous production of infectious virus in crosses involving NZB/B1NJ and 129/J strains of mice. *J. Virol.* **30:** 754–758.

Levy, J.A., P.L. Kazan, C.A. Reilly, Jr., and M.P. Finkel. 1978. FBJ osteosarcoma virus in tissue culture. III. Isolation and characterization of non-virus-producing FBJ-transformed cells. *J. Virol.* **26:** 11–15.

Lieber, M.M., R.E. Benveniste, D.M. Livingston, and G.J. Todaro. 1973. Mammalian cells in culture frequently release type C viruses. *Science* **182:** 56–58.

Lieber, M.M., R.E. Benveniste, C.J. Sherr, and G.J. Todaro. 1975a. Isolation of a type C virus (FS-1) from the European wildcat (*Felis sylvestris*). *Virology* **66:** 117–127.

Lieber, M.M., C.J. Sherr, R.E. Benveniste, and G.J. Todaro. 1975b. Biologic and immunologic properties of porcine type C viruses. *Virology* **66:** 616–619.

Lieber, M., C. Sherr, M. Potter, and G. Todaro. 1975c. Isolation of type-C viruses from the Asian feral mouse *Mus musculus molossinus*. *Int. J. Cancer* **15:** 211–220.

Lieber, M.M., C.J. Sherr, G.J. Todaro, R.E. Benveniste, R. Callahan, and H.G. Coon. 1975d. Isolation from the Asian mouse *Mus caroli* of an endogenous type C virus related to infectious primate type C viruses. *Proc. Natl. Acad. Sci.* **72:** 2315–2319.

Lieberman, M. and H.S. Kaplan. 1959. Leukemogenic activity of filtrates from radiation-induced lymphoid tumors of mice. *Science* **130:** 387–388.

Lilly, F. and T. Pincus. 1973. Genetic control of murine viral leukemogenesis. *Adv. Cancer. Res.* **17:** 231–277.

Lin, F.H. and M. Papini. 1978. Evidence for two forms of RNA-dependent DNA polymerase in visna virus. *Biochim. Biophys. Acta* **561:** 383–395.

Lin, F.H. and H.A. Thormar. 1970. Ribonucleic acid-dependent deoxyribonucleic acid polymerase in visna virus. *J. Virol.* **6:** 702–704.

———. 1971. Characterization of ribonucleic acid from visna virus. *J. Virol.* **7:** 582–587.

———. 1972. Properties of maedi nucleic acid and the presence of ribonucleic acid- and deoxyribonucleic acid-dependent deoxyribonucleic acid polymerase in the virions. *J. Virol.* **10:** 228–233.

———. 1973. Properties of maedi nucleic acid and the presence of ribonucleic acid- and deoxyribonucleic acid-dependent deoxyribonucleic acid polymerase in the virions. *J. Virol.* **10:** 228–233.

———. 1974. Substructures and polypeptides of visna virus. *J. Virol.* **14:** 782–790.

———. 1979. Precipitation of visna viral proteins by immune sera of rabbits and sheep. *J. Virol.* **29:** 536–539.

Lin, F.H., M. Genovese, and H. Thormar. 1973. Multiple activities of DNA polymerase from visna virus. *Prep. Biochem.* **3:** 525–539.

Little, C.C. 1947. The genetics of cancer in mice. *Biol. Rev.* **22:** 313–347.

Liu, W-T., T. Natori, K.S.S. Chang, and A.M. Wu. 1977. Reverse transcriptase of foamy virus. Purification of the enzyme and immunological identification. *Arch. Virol.* **55:** 187–200.

Livingston, D.M. and G.J. Todaro. 1973. Endogenous type C virus from a cat cell clone with properties distinct from previously described feline type C virus. *Virology* **53:** 142–151.

Ljungberg, O. and J. Lange. 1968. Skin tumours of northern pike (*Esox lucius* L.). I. Sarcoma in a Baltic pike population. *Bull. Off. Int. Epizoot.* **69:** 1007–1022.

Loh, P.C., B.C. Achong, and M.A. Epstein. 1977. Further biological properties of the human syncytial virus. *Intervirology* **8:** 204–217.

Loh, P.C., F. Matsuura, and C. Mizumoto. 1980. Seroepidemiology of human syncytial virus: Antibody prevalence in the Pacific. *Intervirology* **13:** 87–90.

Lowy, D.R., W.P. Rowe, N. Teich, and J.W. Hartley. 1971. Murine leukemia virus: High-frequency activation in vitro by 5-iododeoxyuridine and 5-bromodeoxyuridine. *Science* **174:** 155–156.

Lowy, D.R., S.K. Chattopadhyay, N.M. Teich, W.P. Rowe, and A.S. Levine. 1974. AKR murine leukemia virus genome: Frequency of sequences in DNA of high-, low-, and non-virus-yielding mouse strains. *Proc. Natl. Acad. Sci.* **71:** 3555–3559.

Ludford, C.G., H.G. Purchase, and H.W. Cox. 1972. Duck infectious anemia virus associated with *Plasmodium lophurae*. *Exp. Parasitol.* **31:** 29–38.

Lunger, P.D. and H.F. Clark. 1977. Intracytoplasmic type A particles in viper spleen cells. *J. Natl. Cancer Inst.* **58:** 809–811.

Lunger, P.D., W.D. Hardy, Jr., and H.F. Clark. 1974. C-type particles in a reptilian tumor. *J. Natl. Cancer Inst.* **52:** 1231–1235.

Ma, B.I., D.C. Swartzendruber, and W.H. Murphy. 1969. Detection of virus-like particles in germinal centers of normal guinea pigs. *Proc. Soc. Exp. Biol. Med.* **130:** 586–590.

MacDonald, M.E., T.W. Mak, and A. Bernstein. 1980a. Erythroleukemia induction by replication-competent type C viruses cloned from the anemia- and polycythemia-inducing isolates of Friend leukemia virus. *J. Exp. Med.* **151:** 1493–1503.

MacDonald, M.E., F.H. Reynolds, Jr., W.J.M. Van de Ven, J.R. Stephenson, T.W. Mak, and A. Bernstein. 1980b. Anemia- and polycythemia-inducing isolates of Friend spleen focus-forming virus. Biological and molecular evidence for two distinct viral genomes. *J. Exp. Med.* **151:** 1477–1492.

Macintyre, E.H., C.J. Wintersgill, and H. Thormar. 1972. Morphological transformation of human astrocytes by visna virus with complete virus production. *Nat. New Biol.* **237:** 111–113.

Maldonado, R.L. and H.R. Bose, Jr. 1973. Relationship of reticuloendotheliosis virus to the avian tumor viruses: Nucleic acid and polypeptide composition. *J. Virol.* **11:** 741–747.

———. 1975. Polypeptide and RNA composition of the reticuloendotheliosis viruses. *Intervirology* **5:** 194–204.

———. 1976. Group-specific antigen shared by the members of the reticuloendotheliosis virus complex. *J. Virol.* **17:** 983–990.

Malmquist, W.A., M.J. Van der Maaten, and A.D. Boothe. 1969. Isolation, immunodiffusion, immunofluorescence, and electron microscopy of a syncytial virus of lymphosarcomatous and apparently normal cattle. *Cancer Res.* **29:** 188–200.

Mammerickx, M. 1972. La transmission verticale et horizontale de la leucose bovine enzootique. Premiers resultats apres cinq ans d'experimentation. *Ann. Med. Vet.* **116:** 647–659.

Manning, J.S. and A.J. Hackett. 1972. Morphological and biophysical properties of the Mason-Pfizer monkey virus. *J. Natl. Cancer Inst.* **48:** 417–422.

Manteuil-Brutlag, S., S. Liu, and H.S. Kaplan. 1980. Radiation leukemia virus contains two distinct viral RNAs. *Cell* **19:** 643–652.

Mason, M.M., A.E. Bogden, V. Ilievski, H.J. Esber, J.R. Baker, and H.C. Chopra. 1972. History of a rhesus monkey adenocarcinoma containing virus particles resembling oncogenic RNA viruses. *J. Natl. Cancer Inst.* **48:** 1323–1331.

Massey, R.J., L.O. Arthur, R.C. Nowinski, and G. Schochetman. 1980. Monoclonal antibodies identify individual determinants on mouse mammary tumor virus glycoprotein gp52 with group, class, or type specificity. *J. Virol.* **34:** 635–643.

McAllister, R.M., M. Nicolson, M.B. Gardner, R.W. Rongey, S. Rasheed, P.S. Sarma, R.J. Huebner, M. Hatanaka, S. Oroszlan, R.V. Gilden, A. Kabigting and L. Vernon. 1972. C-type virus released from cultured human rhabdomyosarcoma cells. *Nat. New Biol.* **235:** 3–6.

McClintock, P.R., J.N. Ihle, and D.R. Joseph. 1977. Expression of AKR murine leukemia virus gp71-like and BALB(X) gp71-like antigens in normal mouse tissues in the absence of overt virus expression. *J. Exp. Med.* **146:** 422–434.

McClure, H.M., M.E. Keeling, R.P. Custer, R.R. Marshak, D.A. Abt, and J.F. Ferrer. 1974. Erythroleukemia in two infant chimpanzees fed milk from cows naturally infected with the bovine C-type virus. *Cancer Res.* **34:** 2745–2757.

McDonald, H.C. and J.F. Ferrer. 1976. Detection, quantitation, and characterization of the major virion antigen of the bovine leukemia virus by radioimmmunoassay. *J. Natl. Cancer Inst.* **57:** 875–882.

McDonald, H.C., D.C. Graves, and J.F. Ferrer. 1976. Isolation and characterization of an antigen of the bovine C-type virus. *Cancer Res.* **36:** 1251–1257.

McDonough, S.K., S. Larsen, R.S. Brodey, N.D. Stock, and W.D. Hardy, Jr. 1971. A transmissible feline fibrosarcoma of viral origin. *Cancer Res.* **31:** 953–956.

McDougall, J.S., P.M. Biggs, R.W. Shilleto, and B.S. Milne. 1978. Lymphoproliferative disease of turkeys. II. Experimental transmission and aetiology. *Avian Pathol.* **7:** 141–155.

McGarry, M.P., R.A. Steeves, R.J. Eckner, E.A. Mirand, and P.J. Trudel. 1974. Isolation of a myelogenous leukemia-inducing virus from mice infected with the Friend virus complex. *Int. J. Cancer* **13:** 867–878.

McGuire, T.C. and J.B. Henson. 1973. Equine infectious anemia - pathogenesis of persistent viral infection. *Perspect. Virol.* **8:** 229–247.

McGuire, T.C., T.B. Crawford, and J.B. Henson. 1971. Immunofluorescent localization of equine infectious anemia virus in tissues. *Am. J. Pathol.* **62:** 283–292.

———. 1972. Equine infectious anemia. Detection of infectious virus-antibody complexes in the serum. *Immunol. Commun.* **1:** 545–551.

McKissick, G.E. and P.H. Lamont. 1970. Characteristics of a virus isolated from a feline fibrosarcoma. *J. Virol.* **5:** 247–257.

Mellors, R.C. and C.Y. Huang. 1966. Immunopathology of NZB/BL mice. V. Viruslike (filtrable) agent separable from lymphoma cells and identifiable by electron microscopy. *J. Exp. Med.* **124:** 1031–1038.

Melnick, J.L., B. Altenburg, P. Arnstein, R. Mirkovic, and S.S. Tevethia. 1973. Transformation of baboon cells with feline sarcoma virus. *Intervirology* **1:** 386–398.

Menko, A.S., F. Sokol, H.F. Clark, and K.B. Tan. 1976. Structural and enzymatic characterization of viper C-type virus. *Arch. Virol.* **50:** 125–135.

Michalides, R. and J. Schlom. 1975. Relationship in nucleic acid sequences between mouse mammary tumor virus variants. *Proc. Natl. Acad. Sci.* **72:** 4635–4639.

Michalides, R., J. Schlom, J. Dahlberg, and K. Perk. 1975. Biochemical properties of the bromodeoxyuridine-induced guinea pig virus. *J. Virol.* **16:** 1039–1050.

Michalides, R., J. Schlom, J. Pearson, K. Perk, and J. Dahlberg. 1976. Characterization of the oncornavirus particles in the plasma of guinea pigs with L2C leukemia. *J. Virol.* **18:** 1120–1130.

Miller, J.M., L.D. Miller, C. Olson, and K.G. Gillette. 1969. Virus-like particles in phytohemagglutinin-stimulated lymphocyte cultures with reference to bovine lymphosarcoma. *J. Natl. Cancer Inst.* **43:** 1297–1305.

Miller, L.D., J.M. Miller, and C. Olson. 1972. Inoculation of calves with particles resembling C-type virus from cultures of bovine lymphosarcoma. *J. Natl. Cancer Inst.* **48:** 423–428.

Mirand, E.A. 1967. Virus-induced erythropoiesis in hypertransfused-polycythemic mice. *Science* **156:** 832–833.

Moennig, V., H. Frank, G. Hunsmann, P. Ohms, H. Schwarz, W. Schafer, and H. Strandstrom. 1974. C-type particles produced by a permanent cell line from a leukemic pig. II. Physical, chemical, and serological characterization of the particles. *Virology* **57:** 179–188.

Moll, B., J.W. Hartley, and W.P. Rowe. 1979. Induction of B-tropic and N-tropic murine leukemia virus from B10.BR/SgLi mouse embryo cell lines by 5-iodo-2′-deoxyuridine. *J. Natl. Cancer Inst.* **63:** 213–217.

Moloney, J.B. 1960a. Biological studies on a lymphoid-leukemia virus extracted from Sarcoma 37. I. Origin and introductory investigations. *J. Natl. Cancer Inst.* **24:** 933–951.

———. 1960b. Properties of a leukemic virus. *Natl. Cancer Inst. Monogr.* **4:** 7–38.

———. 1962. The murine leukemias. *Fed. Proc.* **21:** 19–31.

———. 1966. A virus-induced rhabdomyosarcoma of mice. *Natl. Cancer Instr. Monogr.* **22:** 139–142.

Moore, D.H., C.A. Long, A.B. Vaidya, J.B. Sheffield, A.S. Dion, and E.Y. Lasfargues. 1979. Mammary tumor viruses. *Adv. Cancer Res.* **29:** 347–418.

Morris, V.L., E. Medeiros, G.M. Ringold, J.M. Bishop, and H.E. Varmus. 1977. Comparison of mouse mammary tumor virus-specific DNA in inbred, wild and Asian mice, and in tumors and normal organs from inbred mice. *J. Mol. Biol.* **114:** 73–91.

Morse, H.C., III, T.M. Chused, S.O. Sharrow, and J.W. Hartley. 1979a. Variations in expression of xenotropic murine leukemia virus genomes in lymphoid tissues of NZB mice. *J. Immunol.* **122:** 2345–2348.

Morse, H.C., III, T.M. Chused, M. Boehm-Truitt, B.J. Mathieson, S.O. Sharrow, and J.W. Hartley. 1979b. XenCSA: Cell surface antigens related to the major glycoproteins (gp70) of xenotropic murine leukemia viruses. *J. Immunol.* **122:** 443–454.

Moscovici, C., D. Chi, L. Gazzolo, and M.G. Moscovici. 1976. A study of plaque formation with avian RNA tumor viruses. *Virology* **73:** 181–189.

Mountcastle, W.E., D.H. Harter, and P.W. Choppin. 1972. The proteins of visna virus. *Virology* **47:** 542–545.

Mueller, J.F. and A.J. Strano. 1974a. *Sparganum proliferum,* a sparaganum infected with a virus? *J. Parasitol.* **60:** 15–19.

———. 1974b. The ubiquity of type-C viruses in spargana of *Spirometra* spp. *J. Parasitol.* **60:** 398–000.

Mühlbock, O. 1965. Note on a new inbred mouse-strain GR/A. *Eur. J. Cancer* **1:** 123–124.

Mulcahy, M.F. 1963. Lymphosarcoma in the pike, *Esox lucius* L., (Pisces; Esocidae) in Ireland. *Proc. R. Ir. Acad.* **63:** 103–129.

Mulcahy, M.F. and A. O'Leary. 1970. Cell-free transmission of lymphosarcoma in the northern pike, *Esox lucius* L. (Pisces; Esocidae). *Experientia* **26:** 891.

Muller, H.K., G. Ball, M.A. Epstein, B.G. Achong, G. Lenoir, and A. Levin. 1980. The prevalence of naturally occurring antibodies to human syncytial virus in East African populations. *J. Gen. Virol.* **47:** 399–406.

Murray, P.R. and D.P. Nayak. 1974. Characterization of bromodeoxyuridine-induced endogenous ginuea pig virus. *J. Virol.* **14:** 679–688.

Nadel, E., W. Banfield, S. Burstein, and A.J. Tousimis. 1967. Virus particles associated with strain-2 guinea pig leukemia (L2C/N-B). *J. Natl. Cancer Inst.* **38:** 979–982.

Nakajima, H. and J. Obara. 1964. Ether sensitivity of equine infectious anemia virus. *Natl. Inst. Anim. Health Q.* **4:** 129–134.

Nakajima, H., S. Tanaka, and C. Ushimi. 1969a. Physicochemical studies of equine infectious anemia virus. I. Buoyant density of the virus. *Arch. Gesamte Virusforsch.* **26:** 389–394.

———. 1970. Physicochemical studies of equine infectious anemia virus. IV. Determination of the nucleic acid type in the virus. *Arch. Gesamte Virusforsch.* **30:** 273–280.

Nakajima, H., M. Tajima, S. Tanaka, and C. Ushimi. 1969b. Physicochemical studies of equine infectious anemia virus. III. Purification and electron microscopic observation of the virus. *Arch. Gesamte Virusforsch.* **28:** 348–360.

Narayan, O., J.E. Clements, J.D. Strandberg, L.C. Cork, and D.E. Griffin. 1980. Biological characterization of the virus causing leukoencephalitis and arthritis in goats. *J. Gen. Virol.* **50:** 69–79.

Nayak, D.P. 1974. Endogenous guinea pig virus: Equability of virus-specific DNA in normal, leukemic, and virus-producing cells. *Proc. Natl. Acad. Sci.* **71:** 1164–1168.

Nayak, D.P. and A.R. Davis. 1976. Endogenous oncornaviral DNA sequences: Evidence for two classes of viral DNA sequences in guinea pig cells. *J. Virol.* **17:** 745–755.

Nayak, D.P. and P.R. Murray. 1973. Induction of type C viruses in cultured guinea pig cells. *J. Virol.* **12:** 177–187.

Nayak, D.P., P. Murray, D. Goldblatt, and K. Karpov. 1975. An endogenous oncornavirus of guinea pigs: Its expression in leukemic cells. In *Comparative leukemia research 1973* (ed. Y. Ito and R.M. Dutcher), pp. 545–559. Karger, Basel.

Nazerian, K., W. Payne, and R.L. Witter. 1980. Establishment of a lymphoblastoid cell line from leucosis-like lymphoma in adult chickens inoculated with reticuloendotheliosis virus. In *Annual Meeting of American Society for Microbiology,* p. 243. (Abstr.).

Neiman, P.E. 1973a. Measurement of endogenous leukosis virus nucleotide sequences in the DNA of normal avian embryos by RNA-DNA hybridization. *Virology* **53:** 196–204.

———. 1973b. Measurement of RD114 virus nucleotide sequences in feline cellular DNA. *Nat. New Biol.* **244:** 62–64.

Nelson-Rees, W.A., V. Klement, W.D. Peterson, Jr., and J.F. Weaver. 1973. Comparative study of two RD 114 virus-indicator cell lines, KC and KB. *J. Natl. Cancer Inst.* **50:** 1129–1135.

Nemo, G.J., P.W. Brown, C.J. Gibbs, Jr., and D.C. Gajdusek. 1978. Antigenic relationship of human foamy virus to the simian foamy viruses. *Infect. Immun.* **20:** 69–72.

Nermut, M.V., F. Hermann, and W. Schafer. 1972. Properties of mouse leukemia viruses. III. Electron microscopic appearance as revealed after conventional preparation techniques as well as freeze-drying and freeze-etching. *Virology* **49:** 345–358.

Niman, H.L. and J.H. Elder. 1980. Molecular dissection of Rauscher virus gp70 by using monoclonal antibodies: Localization of acquired sequences of related envelope gene recombinants. *Proc. Natl. Acad. Sci.* **77:** 4524–4528.

Nooter, K. and P. Bentvelzen. 1976 *In vitro* growth characteristics of virally transformed murine myeloid cells. *Cancer Res.* **36:** 1246–1250.

Norcross, N.L. and L. Coggins. 1971. Characterization of an equine infectious anemia antigen extracted from infected horse spleen tissue. *Infect. Immun.* **4:** 528–531.

Nowinski, R.C., E. Edynak and N.H. Sarkar. 1971a. Serological and structural properties of Mason-Pfizer monkey virus isolated from the mammary tumor of a rhesus monkey. *Proc. Natl. Acad. Sci.* **68:** 1608–1612.

Nowinski, R.C., L.J. Old, P.V. O'Donnell and F.K. Sanders. 1971b. Serological identification of hamster oncornaviruses. *Nat. New Biol.* **230:** 282–284.

Nowinski, R.C., E.F. Hays, T. Doyle, S. Linkhart, E. Medeiros, and R. Pickering. 1977. Oncornaviruses produced by murine leukemia cells in culture. *Virology* **81:** 363–370.

O'Donnell, P.V. and R.C. Nowinski. 1980. Serological analysis of antigenic determinants on the *env* gene products of AKR dualtropic (MCF) murine leukemia viruses. *Virology* **107:** 81–88.

O'Donnell, P.V., C.J. Deitch, and T. Pincus. 1976. Multiplicity-dependent kinetics of murine leukemia virus infection in *Fv-1*-sensitive and *Fv-1*-resistant cells. *Virology* **73:** 23–35.

Ogura, H., J. Paulsen, and H. Bauer. 1977. Cross-neutralization of ovine and bovine C-type leukemia virus-induced syncytia formation. *Cancer Res.* **37:** 1486–1489.

Okabe, H., R.V. Gilden, and M. Hatanaka. 1973a. Extensive homology of RD114 virus DNA with RNA of feline cell origin. *Nat. New Biol.* **244:** 54–56.

———. 1973b. RD 114 virus-specific sequences in feline cellular RNA: Detection and characterization. *J. Virol.* **12:** 984–994.

———. 1974. Specificity of the DNA product of RNA-dependent DNA polymerase of type C viruses. III. Analysis of viruses derived from Syrian hamsters. *Proc. Natl. Acad. Sci.* **71:** 3278–3282.

Okabe, H., E. Twiddy, R.V. Gilden, M. Hatanaka, E.A. Hoover, and R.G. Olsen. 1976. FeLV-related sequences in DNA from a FeLV-free cat colony. *Virology* **69:** 798–801.

Old, L.J., E.A. Boyse, and E. Stockert. 1964. Typing of mouse leukaemias by serological methods. *Nature* **201:** 777–779.

———. 1965. The G (Gross) leukemia antigen. *Cancer Res.* **25:** 813–819.

Olson, C., Jr. 1941. A transmissible lymphoid tumor of the chicken. *Cancer Res.* **1:** 384–392.

Olson, C. and L.E. Baumgartener. 1976. Pathology of lymphosarcoma in sheep induced with bovine leukemia virus. *Cancer Res.* **36:** 2365–2373.

Olson, C., J.M. Miller, L.D. Miller, and K.G. Gillette. 1970. C-type virus and lymphocytotic nuclear projections in bovine lymphosarcoma. *J. Am. Vet. Med. Assoc.* **156:** 1880– 1883.

Onuma, M., C. Olson, and D.M. Driscoll. 1976. Properties of two isolated antigens associated with bovine leukemia virus infection. *J. Natl. Cancer Inst.* **57:** 571–578.

Opler, S.R. 1967. Observation of a new virus associated with guinea pig leukemia: Preliminary note. *J. Natl. Cancer Inst.* **38:** 797–800.

Oroszlan, S., C. Foreman, G. Kelloff, and R.V. Gilden. 1971. The group-specific antigen and other structural proteins of hamster and mouse C-type viruses. *Virology* **43:** 665–674.

Oroszlan, S., D. Bova, R.J. Huebner, and R.V. Gilden. 1972a. Major group specific protein of rat type C viruses. *J. Virol.* **10:** 746–750.

Oroszlan, S., T. Copeland, M.R. Summers, and R.V. Gilden. 1973. Feline leukemia and RD-114 virus group-specific proteins: Comparison of amino terminal sequence. *Science* **181:** 454–456.

Oroszlan, S., T.D. Copeland, G. Smythers, M.R. Summers, and R.V. Gilden. 1977. Comparative primary structure analysis of the p30 protein of wolly monkey and gibbon type C viruses. *Virology* **77:** 413–417.

Oroszlan, S., T. Copeland, M.R. Summers, G. Smythers, and R.V. Gilden. 1975. Amino acid sequence homology of mammalian type C RNA virus major internal proteins. *J. Biol. Chem.* **250:** 6232–6239.

Oroszlan, S., D. Bova, M.H.M. White, R. Toni, C. Foreman, and R.V. Gilden. 1972b. Purification and immunological characterization of the major internal protein of the RD-114 virus. *Proc. Natl. Acad. Sci.* **69:** 1211–1215.

Ostertag, W., K. Vehmeyer, B. Fagg, I.B. Pragnell, W. Paetz, M.C. Le Bousse, F. Smadja-Joffe, B. Klein, C. Jasmin, and H. Eisen. 1980. Myeloproliferative virus, a cloned murine sarcoma virus with spleen focus-forming properties in adult mice. *J. Virol.* **33:** 573–582.

Pal, B.K., R.M. McAllister, M.B. Gardner, and P. Roy-Burman. 1975. Comparative studies on the structural phosphoproteins of mammalian type C viruses. *J. Virol.* **16:** 123–131.

Pang, R.H.L., L.A. Phillips, and D.K. Haapala. 1977. Characterization of Gazdar murine sarcoma virus by nucleic acid hybridization and analysis of viral expression in cells. *J. Virol.* **24:** 551–556.

Papas, T.S., J.E. Dahlberg, and R.A. Sonstegard. 1976. Type C virus in lymphosarcoma in northern pike (*Esox lucius*). *Nature* **261:** 506–508.

Papas, T.S., T.W. Pry, M.P. Schafer, and R.A. Sonstegard. 1977. Presence of DNA polymerase in lymphosarcoma in northern pike (*Esox lucius*). *Cancer Res.* **37:** 3214–3217.

Parekh, B., C.J. Issel, and R.C. Montelaro. 1980. Equine infectious anemia virus, a putative lentivirus, contains polypeptides analogous to prototype-C oncornaviruses. *Virology* **107:** 520–525.

Parks, W.P. and E.M. Scolnick. 1972. Radioimmunoassay of mammalian type-C viral proteins: Interspecies antigenic reactivities of the major internal polypeptide. *Proc. Natl. Acad. Sci.* **69:** 1766–1770.

Parks, W. and G. Todaro. 1972. Biological properties of syncytium-forming ("foamy") viruses. *Virology* **47:** 673–683.

Parks, W.P., E.M. Scolnic, M.C. Noon, and C.J. Watson. 1974. Immunological cross-reactions between two low-molecular-weight polypeptides from a murine type C virus. *J. Virol.* **14:** 430–433.

Parks, W.P., G.J. Todaro, E.M. Scolnick, and S.A. Aaronson. 1971. RNA dependent DNA polymerase in primate syncytium-forming (foamy) viruses. *Nature* **229:** 258–260.

Parks, W.P., E.M. Scolnick, M.C. Noon, C.J. Watson, and T.G. Kawakami. 1973a. Radioimmunoassay of mammalian type-C polypeptides. IV. Characteristization of woolly monkey and gibbon viral antigens. *Int. J. Cancer* **12:** 129–137.

Parks, W.P., R.V. Gilden, A.F. Bykovsky, G.G. Miller, V.M. Zhdanov, V.O. Soloviev, and E.M. Scolnick. 1973b. Mason-Pfizer virus characterization: A similar virus in a human aminotic cell line. *J. Virol.* **12:** 1540–1547.

Pauli, G., W. Rohde, H. Ogura, E. Harms, H. Bauer, and J. Paulsen. 1977. Comparative immunological studies on bovine and ovine C-type particles. In *Bovine leucosis: various methods of molecular virology* (ed. A. Burny), pp. 45–55. Commission of European Communities, Luxembourg.

Paulsen, J., R. Rudolph, and J.M. Miller. 1974. Antibodies to common ovine and bovine C-type virus specific antigen in serum from sheep with spontaneous leukosis and from inoculated animals. *Med. Microbiol. Immunol.* **159:** 105–114.

Paulsen, J., R. Rudolph, and T. Schliesser. 1975. Experimentelle Ubertragung der lymphatischen Leukose des Schafes. *Zentralbl. Veterinaermed.* **22:** 737–748.

Paulsen, J., W. Rohde, G. Pauli, E. Harms, and H. Bauer. 1976. Comparative studies on ovine and bovine C-type particles. In *Comparative leukemia research 1975* (ed. J. Clemmesen and D.S. Yohn). pp. 190–192. Karger, Basel.

Paulsen, J., R. Rudolph, R. Hoffmann, E. Weiss, and T. Schliesser. 1972. C-type virus particles in phytohemagglutinin-stimulated lymphocyte cultures with reference to enzootic lymphatic leukosis in sheep. *Med. Microbiol. Immunol.* **158:** 105–112.

Pearson, G., T. Orr, L. Redmon, and V. Bergs. 1972. Membrane immunofluorescence studies on cells producing rat C-type virus particles. *Int. J. Cancer* **10:** 14–19.

Pedersen, S.K., R.L. Crowther, D.Y. Tenney, A.M. Reimold, and W.A. Haseltine. 1981. Novel leukaemogenic retroviruses isolated from cell line derived from spontaneous AKR tumour. *Nature* **292:** 167–170.

Perk, K., M.W. Viola, K.L. Smith, N.A. Wivel, and J.B. Moloney. 1969. Biologic studies on hamster tumors induced by the murine sarcoma virus (Mololey). *Cancer Res.* **29:** 1089–1095.

Peters, G.G. and C. Glover. 1980. Low-molecular-weight RNAs and initiation of RNA-directed DNA synthesis in avian reticuloendotheliosis virus. *J. Virol.* **33:** 708–716.

Peters, R.L., G.J. Spahn, L.S. Rabstein, G.J. Kelloff, and R.J. Huebner. 1973. Murine C-type RNA virus from spontaneous neoplasms: In vitro host range and oncogenic potential. *Science* **181:** 665–667.

Peters, R.L., L.S. Rabstein, R. VanVleck, G.J. Kelloff, and R.J. Huebner. 1974. Naturally occurring sarcoma virus of the BALB/cCr mouse. *J. Natl. Cancer Inst.* **53:** 1725–1729.

Petursson, G., J.R. Martin, G. Georgsson, N. Nathanson, and P.A. Palsson. 1979. Visna. The biology of the agent and the disease. In *Aspects of slow and persistent virus infections* (ed. D.A.J. Tyrrell), pp. 165–197. Martinus Nijhoff, The Hague.

Pienta, R.J., D.L. Fine, T. Hurt, C.K. Smith, J.C. Landon, and H.C. Chopra. 1972. *In vitro* transformation of rhesus foreskin cells by Mason-Pfizer monkey virus (M-PMV). *J. Natl. Cancer Inst.* **48:** 1910–1917.

Pincus, T. 1980. The endogenous murine type C viruses. In *Molecular biology of RNA tumor viruses* (ed. J.R. Stephenson), pp. 77–130. Academic Press, New York.

Pincus, T., J.W. Hartley, and W.P. Rowe. 1971b. A major genetic locus affecting resistance to infection with murine leukemia viruses. I. Tissue culture studies of naturally occurring viruses. *J. Exp. Med.* **133:** 1219–1233.

———. 1975. A major genetic locus affecting resistance to infection with murine leukemia viruses. IV. Dose-response relationships in *Fv-1*-sensitive and resistant cell cultures. *Virology* **65:** 333–342.

Pincus, T., W.P. Rowe, and F. Lilly. 1971a. A major genetic locus affecting resistance to infection with murine leukemia viruses. II. Apparent identity to a major locus described for resistance to Friend virus. *J. Exp. Med.* **133:** 1234–1241.

Piper, C.E., D.A. Abt, J.F. Ferrer, and R.R. Marshak. 1975. Seroepidemiological evidence for horizontal transmission of bovine C-type virus. *Cancer Res.* **35:** 2714–2716.

Pitelka, D.R., H.A. Bern, S. Nandi, and K.B. DeOme. 1964. On the significance of virus-like particles in mammary tissues of C3Hf mice. *J. Natl. Cancer Inst.* **33:** 867–885.

Pluznik, D.H. and L. Sachs. 1964. Quantitation of a murine leukemia virus with a spleen colony assay. *J. Natl. Cancer Inst.* **33:** 535–546.

Pope, J.H. 1961. Studies of a virus isolated from a wild house mouse, *Mus musculus*, and producing spenomegaly and lymph node enlargement in mice. *Aust. J. Exp. Biol. Med. Sci.* **39:** 521–536.

———. 1962. The isolation of a mouse leukaemia virus resembling Friend virus. *Aust. J. Exp. Biol. Med. Sci.* **40:** 263–276.

Porzig, K.J., M. Barbacid, and S.A. Aaronson. 1979. Biological properties and translational products of three independent isolates of feline sarcoma virus. *Virology* **92:** 91–107.

Pragnell, I.B., A. Fusco, C. Arbuthnott, F. Smadja-Joffe, B. Klein, C. Jasmin, and W. Ostertag. 1981. Analysis of the myeloproliferative sarcoma virus genome: Limited changes in the prototype lead to altered target cell specificity. *J. Virol.* **38:** 952–957.

Prosser, P.R. 1968. Particles resembling murine leukaemia virus in New Zealand Black mice. *Clin. Exp. Immunol.* **3:** 213–226.

Purchase, H.G. and B.R. Burmester. 1978. Leukosis/sarcoma group. In *Diseases of poultry* (ed. M.S. Hofstad et al.), pp. 502–568. Iowa State University Press, Ames.

Purchase, H.C. and R.L. Witter. 1975. The reticuloendotheliosis viruses. *Curr. Top. Microbiol. Immunol.* **71:** 103–124.

Purchase, H.G., C. Ludford, K. Nazerian, and H.W. Cox. 1973. A new group of oncogenic viruses: Reticuloendotheliosis, chick syncytial, duck infectious anemia, and spleen necrosis viruses. *J. Natl. Cancer Inst.* **51:** 489–499.

Quigley, J.P., D.B. Rifkin, and E. Reich. 1971. Phospholipid composition of Rous sarcoma virus, host cell membranes and other enveloped RNA viruses. *Virology* **46:** 106–116.

Quintrell, N., H.E. Varmus, J.M. Bishop, M.O. Nicolson, and R.M. McAllister. 1974. Homologies among the nucleotide sequences of the genomes of C-type viruses. *Virology* **58:** 569–575.

Rabin, H. 1971. Assay and pathogenesis of oncogenic viruses in nonhuman primates. *Lab. Anim. Sci.* **21:** 1032–1049.

Rabin, H., C.V. Benton, M.A. Tainsky, N.R. Rice, and R.V. Gilden. 1979. Isolation and characterization of an endogenous type C virus of rhesus monkeys. *Science* **204:** 841–842.

Rabin, H., R.H. Neubauer, N.J. Woodside, J.L. Cicmanec, W.C. Wallen, B.A. Lapin, V.A. Agrba, L.A. Yakoleva, and G.N. Chuvirov. 1976. Virological studies of baboon (Papio hamadryas) lymphoma: Isolation and characterization of foamy viruses. *J. Med. Primatol.* **5:** 12–22.

Racevskis, J. and G. Koch. 1977. Viral protein synthesis in Friend erythroleukemia cell lines. *J. Virol.* **21:** 328–337.

Rand, K.H. and C. Long. 1972. Syncytial assay for the putative human C-type virus, RD-114, utilizing human cells transformed by Rous sarcoma virus. *Nat. New Biol.* **240:** 187–190.

———. 1973. Fusion of a Rous sarcoma virus transformed human cell line, KC, by RD-114 virus. *J. Gen. Virol.* **21:** 523–532.

Rand, K.H., C.W. Long, T.T. Wei, R.V. Gilden. 1974. Plaque assay for the Mason-Pfizer monkey virus. *J. Natl. Cancer Inst.* **53:** 449–452.

Rand, K., J. Davis, R.V. Gilden, S. Oroszlan, and C.W. Long. 1975. Fusion inhibition: Bioassay of a type C viral protein. *Virology* **64:** 63–74.

Rands, E., D.R. Lowy, M.R. Lander, and S.K. Chattopadhyay. 1981. Restriction endonuclease mapping of ecotropic murine leukemia viral DNAs: Size and sequence heterogeneity of the long terminal repeat. *Virology* **108:** 445–452.

Rangan, S.R.S. 1974. Antigenic relatedness of simian C-type viruses. *Int. J. Cancer* **13:** 64–70.

Rangan, S.R.S., P.J. Ueberhorst, and M.C. Wong. 1973. Syncytial giant cell focus assay for viruses derived from feline leukemia and a simian sarcoma. *Proc. Soc. Exp. Biol. Med.* **142:** 1077–1082.

Rangan, S.R.S., M.C. Wong, P.J. Ueberhorst, and D.V. Ablashi. 1972. Mixed culture cytopathogenicity induced by virus preparations derived from simian sarcoma virus (SSV-1) infected cultures. *J. Natl. Cancer Inst.* **49:** 571–577.

Rao, P.R., R.A. Bonar, and J.W. Beard. 1966. Lipids of the BAI strain A avian tumor virus and of the myeloblast host cell. *Exp. Mol. Pathol.* **5:** 374–385.

Rapp, U.R. and R.C. Nowinski. 1976. Endogenous ecotropic mouse type C viruses deficient in replication and production of XC plaques. *J. Virol.* **18:** 411–417.

Rapp, U.R. and G.J. Todaro. 1978a. Generation of oncogenic type C viruses: Rapidly leukemogenic viruses derived from C3H mouse cells *in vivo* and *in vitro*. *Proc. Natl. Acad. Sci.* **75:** 2468–2472.

———. 1978b. Generation of new mouse sarcoma viruses in cell culture. *Science* **201:** 821–824.

———. 1980. Generation of oncogenic mouse type C viruses: *In vitro* selection of carcinoma-inducing variants. *Proc. Natl. Acad. Sci.* **77:** 624–628.

Rasheed, S. 1980. Endogenous virogenes and oncogenes in rat-cell transformation: A new model system. *Cold Spring Harbor Symp. Quant. Biol.* **44:** 779–786.

Rasheed, S., M.B. Gardner and E. Chan. 1976a. Amphotropic host range of naturally occurring wild mouse leukemia virus. *J. Virol.* **19:** 13–18.

Rasheed, S., M.B. Gardner, and R.J. Huebner. 1978. *In vitro* isolation of stable rat sarcoma viruses. *Proc. Natl. Acad. Sci.* **75:** 2972–2976.

Rasheed, S., E. Toth, and M.B. Gardner. 1977. Characterization of purely ecotropic and amphotropic naturally occurring wild mouse leukemia viruses. *Intervirology* **8:** 323–335.

Rasheed, S., A.E. Freeman, M.B. Gardner, and R.J. Huebner. 1976b. Acceleration of transformation of rat embryo cells by rat type C virus. *J. Virol.* **18:** 776–782.

Rasheed, S., J. Bruszewski, R.W. Rongey, P. Roy-Burman, H.P. Charman, and M.B. Gardner. 1976c. Spontaneous release of endogenous ecotropic type C virus from rat embryo cultures. *J. Virol.* **18:** 799–803.

Rauscher, F.J. 1962. A virus-induced disease of mice characterized by erthrocytopoiesis and lymphoid leukemia. *J. Natl. Cancer Inst.* **29:** 515–543.

Reilly, C.A., Jr. and M.P. Finkel. 1976. *In vivo* interference of virus-induced osteosarcomas by a benign bone tumor virus. In *Comparative leukemia research 1975* (ed. J. Clemmesen and D.S. Yohn), pp. 441–444. Karger, Basel.

Reitz, M.S., Jr., F. Wong-Staal, W.A. Haseltine, D.G. Kleid, C.D. Trainor, R.E. Gallagher, and R.C. Gallo. 1979. Gibbon ape leukemia virus-Hall's Island: New strain of gibbon ape leukemia virus. *J. Virol.* **29:** 395–400.

Reynolds, F.H., Jr., T.L. Sacks, D.N. Deobagkar, and J.R. Stephenson. 1978. Cells nonproductively transformed by Abelson murine leukemia virus express a high molecular weight polyprotein containing structural and nonstructural components. *Proc. Natl. Acad. Sci.* **75:** 3974–3978.

Rhim, J.S., M.L. Vernon, R.J. Huebner, and H.C. Turner. 1972. Spontaneous transformation of rat cells after long-term *in vitro* cultivation and the "switch-on" of a new complement fixing antigen. *Proc. Soc. Exp. Biol. Med.* **140:** 414–419.

Rhim, J.S., K.D. Wuu, M.L. Vernon, and R.J. Huebner. 1974. Induction of guinea pig leukemia-like virus from cultured guinea pig cells. *Proc. Soc. Exp. Biol. Med.* **147:** 323–330.

Rhim, J.S., F.G. Duh, H.Y. Cho, E. Elder, and M.L. Vernon. 1973a. Activation of a type-C RNA virus from tumors induced by rat kidney cells transformed by a chemical carcinogen. *J. Natl. Cancer Inst.* **50:** 255–261.

Rhim, J.S., F.G. Duh, H.Y. Cho, K.D. Wuu, and M.L. Vernon. 1973b. Activation by 5-bromodeoxyuridine of particles resembling guinea pig leukemia virus from guinea pig nonproducer cells. *J. Natl. Cancer Inst.* **51:** 1327–1331.

Rho, H.M. and R.C. Gallo. 1979. Characterization of reverse transcriptase from feline leukemia virus by radioimmunoassay. *Virology* **99:** 192–196.

Rice, N.R. and L. Coggins. 1979. Synthesis of long complementary DNA in the endogenous reaction by equine infectious anemia virus. *J. Virol.* **29:** 907–914.

Rice, N.R., S. Simek, O.A. Ryder, and L. Coggins. 1978. Detection of proviral DNA in horse cells infected with equine infectious anemia virus. *J. Virol.* **26:** 577–583.

Rich, M.A., R. Siegler, S. Karl, and R. Clymer. 1969. Spontaneous regression of virus induced murine leukemia. I. Host-virus system. *J. Natl. Cancer Inst.* **43:** 559–570.

Rickard, C.G., J.E. Post, F. Noronha, and L.M. Barr. 1969. A transmissible virus-induced lymphocytic leukemia of the cat. *J. Natl. Cancer Inst.* **42:** 987–1014.

Rickard, C.G., L.M. Barr, F. Noronha, E. Dougherty, III, and J.E. Post. 1967. C-type virus particles in spontaneous lymphocytic leukemia in a cat. *Cornell Vet.* **57:** 302–307.

Rifkin, D.B. and R.W. Compans. 1971. Identification of the spike proteins of Rous sarcoma virus. *Virology* **46:** 485–489.

Riggs, J.L., L.S. Oshiro, D.O.N. Taylor, and E.H. Lennette. 1969. Syncytium-forming agent isolated from domestic cats. *Nature* **222:** 1190–1191.

Robbins, K.C., C.D. Cabradilla, J.R. Stephenson, and S.A. Aaronson. 1977. Segregation of genetic information for a B-tropic leukemia virus with the structural locus for BALB: virus-1. *Proc. Natl. Acad. Sci.* **74:** 2953–2957.

Robinson, F.R. and M.J. Twiehaus. 1974. Isolation of the avian reticuloendotheliosis virus (strain T). *Avian Dis.* **18:** 278–288.

Rogers, N.G., M. Basnight, C.J. Gibbs, Jr., and D.C. Gajdusek. 1967. Latent viruses in chimpanzees with experimental kuru. *Nature* **216:** 446–449.

Rohde, W., G. Pauli, J. Paulsen, E. Harms, and H. Bauer. 1978. Bovine and ovine leukemia viruses. I. Characterization of viral antigens. *J. Virol.* **26:** 159–164.

Rommelaere, J., D.V. Faller, and N. Hopkins. 1978. Characterization and mapping of RNase T1-resistant oligonucleotides derived from the genomes of Akv and MCF murine leukemia viruses. *Proc. Natl. Acad. Sci.* **75:** 495–499.

Rosenberg, N., D. Baltimore, and C.D. Scher. 1975. *In vitro* transformation of lymphoid cells by Abelson murine leukemia virus. *Proc. Natl. Acad. Sci.* **72:** 1932–1936.

Rossignol, J-M., M. Kress, and C. de Vaux Saint Cyr. 1975. Induction, par la 5-bromo-2′-desoxyuridine, d'un virus de type "foamy" dans des cellules de hamster transformees par le SV40. *C. R. Acad. Sci. Ser. D* **281:** 1145–1148.

Rous, P. 1911. A sarcoma of the fowl transmissible by an agent separable from the tumor cells. *J. Exp. Med.* **13:** 397–411.

Rowe, W.P., W.E. Pugh, and J.W. Hartley. 1970. Plaque assay techniques for murine leukemia viruses. *Virology* **42:** 1136–1139.

Rubin, H. 1960. A virus in chick embryos which induces resistance in vitro to infection with Rous sarcoma virus. *Proc. Natl. Acad. Sci.* **46:** 1105–1119.

Rubin, H. and P.K. Vogt. 1962. An avian leukosis virus associated with stocks of Rous sarcoma virus. *Virology* **17:** 184–192.

Rubin, H., A. Cornelius, and L. Fanshier. 1961. The pattern of congenital transmission of an avian leukosis virus. *Proc. Natl. Acad. Sci.* **47:** 1058–1069.

Rubin, H., L. Fanshier, A. Cornelius, and W.F. Hughes. 1962. Tolerance and immunity in chickens after congenital and contact infection with an avian leukosis virus. *Virology* **17:** 143–156.

Ruckle, G. 1958a. Studies with the monkey-intranuclear agent (MINIA) and foamy-agent derived from spontaneously degenerating monkey kidney cultures. I. Isolation and tissue culture behavior of the agents and identification of MINIA as closely related to measles virus. *Arch. Gesamte Virusforsch.* **8:** 139–166.

———. 1958b. Studies with the monkey-intranuclear agent (MINIA) and foamy-agent derived from spontaneously degenerating monkey kidney cultures. II. Immunologic and epidemiologic observations in monkeys in a laboratory colony. *Arch. Gesamte Virusforsch.* **8:** 167–182.

Ruprecht, R.M., N.C. Goodman, and S. Spiegelman. 1973. Determination of natural host taxonomy of RNA tumor viruses by molecular hybridization: Application to RD-114, a candidate human virus. *Proc. Natl. Acad. Sci.* **70:** 1437–1441.

Ruscetti, S.K., D. Linemeyer, J. Feild, D. Troxler, and E.M. Scolnick. 1979. Characterization of a protein found in cells infected with the spleen focus-forming virus that shares immunological cross-reactivity with the gp70 found in mink cell focus-inducing virus particles. *J. Virol.* **30:** 787–798.

Russell, P.H. and O. Jarrett. 1978. The specificity of neutralizing antibodies to feline leukaemia viruses. *Int. J. Cancer* **21:** 768–778.

Rustigian, R., P. Johnston, and H. Reihart. 1955. Infection of monkey kidney tissue cultures with virus-like agents. *Proc. Soc. Exp. Biol. Med.* **88:** 8–16.

Sacks, T.L., S.G. Devare, G.R. Blennerhassett, and J.R. Stephenson. 1978. Nonconditional replication mutants of type C and type D retroviruses defecting in *gag* gene-coded polyprotein post-translational processing. *Virology* **91:** 352–363.

Sandolin, K. and T. Estola. 1974. Occurrence of different subgroups of avian leukosis in Finnish poultry. *Avian Pathol.* **3:** 159–168.

Sarkar, N.H., D.H. Moore, and R.C. Nowinski. 1972. Symmetry of the nucleocapsid of the oncornaviruses. In *RNA viruses and host genome in oncogenesis* (ed. P. Emmelot and P. Bentvelzen), pp. 71–79. North-Holland, Amsterdam.

Sarma, P.S. and T. Log. 1971. Viral interference in feline leukemia-sarcoma complex. *Virology* **44:** 352–358.

———. 1973. Subgroup classification of feline leukemia and sarcoma viruses by viral interference and neutralization tests. *Virology* **54:** 160–169.

Sarma, P., T. Log and R.V. Gilden. 1970a. Studies of hamster-specific virus derived from hamster tumors induced by Kirsten murine sarcoma virus. *Proc. Soc. Exp. Biol. Med.* **133:** 718–722.

Sarma, P.S., J. Tseng, Y.K. Lee, and R.V. Gilden. 1973. Virus similar to RD114 virus in cat cells. *Nat. New Biol.* **244:** 56–59.

Sarma, P.C., R.J. Huebner, J.F. Basker, L. Vernon and R.V. Gilden. 1970b. Feline leukemia and sarcoma viruses: Susceptibility of human cells to infection. *Science* **168:** 1098–1100.

Sarma, P.S., T. Log, D. Jain, P.R. Hill, and R.J. Huebner. 1975. Differential host range of viruses of feline leukemia-sarcoma complex. *Virology* **64:** 438–446.

Sarma, P.S., A. Sharar, J. Tseng, P.J. Price, and M. Gardner. 1974. Studies on the prevalence of endogenous type C virus RD 114 in cats. *Proc. Soc. Exp. Biol. Med.* **145:** 757–762.

Sawyer, R.C. and H. Hanafusa. 1977. Formation of reticuloendotheliosis virus pseudotypes of Rous sarcoma virus. *J. Virol.* **22:** 634–639.

Schafer, W., J. Lange, D.P. Bolognesi, F. de Noronha, J.E. Post, and C.G. Rickard. 1971. Isolation and characterization of two group-specific antigens from feline leukemia virus. *Virology* **44:** 73–82.

Scher, C.D. and R. Siegler. 1975. Direct transformation of 3T3 cells by Abelson murine leukaemia virus. *Nature* **253:** 729–731.

Scher, C.D., E.M. Scolnick, and R. Siegler. 1975. Induction of erythroid leukaemia by Harvey and Kirsten sarcoma viruses. *Nature* **256:** 225–226.

Schlom, J. and S. Spiegelman. 1971. DNA polymerase activities and nucleic acid components of virions isolated from a spontaneous mammary carcinoma from a rhesus monkey. *Proc. Natl. Acad. Sci.* **68:** 1613–1617.

Schlom, J., D. Colcher, W. Drohan, and G. Schochetman. 1976. Nucleic acid and protein studies of the Mason-Pfizer virus. In *Comparative leukemia research 1975* (ed. J. Clemmesen and D.S. Yohn), pp. 134–140. Karger, Basel.

Schlom, J., D.H. Harter, A. Burny, and S. Spiegelman. 1971. DNA polymerase activities in virions of visna virus, a causative agent of a "slow" neurological disease. *Proc. Natl. Acad. Sci.* **68:** 182–186.

Schlom, J., P.H. Hand, Y.A. Teramoto, R. Callahan, G. Todaro, and G. Schidlovsky. 1978. Characterization of a new virus from *Mus cervicolor* immunologically related to the mouse mammary tumor virus. *J. Natl. Cancer Inst.* **61:** 1509–1519.

Schmidt-Ruppin, K.H. 1964. Heterotransplantation of Rous sarcoma and Rous sarcoma virus to mammals. *Oncologia* **17:** 247–272.

Schochetman, G. and J. Schlom. 1975. RNA subunit structure of Mason-Pfizer monkey virus. *J. Virol.* **15:** 423–427.

Schochetman, G., M. Boehm-Truitt, and J. Schlom. 1976. Antigenic analysis of the major structural protein of the Mason-Pfizer monkey virus. *J. Immunol.* **117:** 168–173.

Schochetman, G., K. Kortright and J. Schlom. 1975. Mason-Pfizer monkey virus: Analysis and localization of virion proteins and glycoproteins. *J. Virol.* **16:** 1208–1219.

Schochetman, G., D. Fine, L. Arthur, R. Gilden, and R. Heberling. 1977. Characterization of a retravirus isolated from squirrel monkeys. *J. Virol.* **23:** 384–393.

Scolnick, E.M. and W.P. Parks. 1973. Isolation and characterization of a primate sarcoma virus: Mechanism of rescue. *Int. J. Cancer* **12:** 138–147.

———. 1974. Harvey sarcoma virus: A second murine type C sarcoma virus with rat genetic information. *J. Virol.* **13:** 1211–1219.

Scolnick, E.M., R.J. Goldberg, and D. Williams. 1976a. Characterization of rat genetic sequences of Kirsten sarcoma virus: Distinct class of endogenous rat type C viral sequences. *J. Virol.* **18:** 559–566.

Scolnick, E.M., J.M. Maryak, and W.P. Parks. 1974a. Levels of rat cellular RNA homologous to either Kirsten sarcoma virus or rat type-C virus in cell lines derived from Osborne-Mendel rats. *J. Virol.* **14:** 1435–1444.

Scolnick, E.M., W.P. Parks, and G.J. Todaro. 1972a. Reverse transcriptase of primate viruses as immunological markers. *Science* **177:** 1119–1121.

Scolnick, E.M., D. Williams, and W.P. Parks. 1976b. Purification and characterization of viral RNA of a sarcoma virus isolated from a woolly monkey. *Nature* **264:** 809–811.

Scolnick, E.M., W.P. Parks, G.J. Todaro, and S.A. Aaronson. 1972b. Immunological characterization of primate C-type reverse transcriptases. *Nat. New Biol.* **235:** 35–40.

Scolnick, E., E. Rands, S.A. Aaronson, and G.J. Todaro. 1970. RNA-dependent DNA polymerase activity in five RNA viruses: Divalent cation requirements. *Proc. Natl. Acad. Sci.* **67:** 1789–1796.

Scolnick, E.M., E. Rands, D. Williams, and W.P. Parks. 1973. Studies on the nucleic acid sequences of Kirsten sarcoma virus: A model for formation of a mammalian RNA-containing sarcoma virus. *J. Virol.* **12:** 458–463.

Scolnick, E.M., W. Parks, T. Kawakami, D. Kohne, H. Okabe, R. Gilden, and M. Hatanaka. 1974b. Primate and murine type-C viral nucleic acid association kinetics: Analysis of model systems and natural tissues. *J. Virol.* **13:** 363–369.

Scott, F.W., J.N. Shively, J. Gaskin, and J.H. Gillespie. 1973. Bovine syncytial virus isolations. *Arch. Virol.* **43:** 43–52.

Scott, J.V., L. Stowring, A.T. Haase, O. Narayan, and R. Vigne. 1979. Antigenic variation in visna virus. *Cell* **18:** 321–327.

Sen, A. and G.J. Todaro. 1976. Specificity of in vitro binding of primate type C viral RNA and binding of primate type C viral RNA and the homologous viral p12 core protein. *Science* **193:** 326–328.

Sen, A., C.J. Sherr, and G.J. Todaro. 1976. Specific binding of the type C viral core protein p12 with purified viral RNA. *Cell* **7:** 21–32.

Sharp, D.G., E.A. Eckert, D. Beard, and J.W. Beard. 1952. Morphology of the virus of avian erythromyeloblastic leucosis and a comparison with the agent of Newcastle disease. *J. Bacteriol.* **63:** 151–000.

Sherr, C.J. and C.J. Todaro. 1974. Radioimmunoassay of the major group specific protein of endogenous baboon type C viruses: Relation to the RD-114/CCC group and detection of antigen in normal baboon tissues. *Virology* **61:** 168–181.

Sherr, C.J., R.E. Benveniste and G.J. Todaro. 1974a. Type C viral expression in primate tissues. *Proc. Natl. Acad. Sci.* **71:** 3721–3725.

———. 1978a. Endogenous mink (*Mustela vison*) type C virus isolated from sarcoma virus-transformed mink cells. *J. Virol.* **25:** 738–749.

Sherr, C.J., L.A. Fedele, R.E. Benveniste, and G.J. Todaro. 1975. Interspecies antigenic determinants of the reverse transcriptases and p30 proteins of mammalian type C viruses. *J. Virol.* **15:** 1440–1448.

Sherr, C.J., M.M. Lieber, R.E. Benveniste, and G.J. Todaro. 1974b. Endogenous baboon type C virus (M7): Biochemical and immunologic characterization. *Virology* **58:** 492–503.

Sherr, C.J., G.J. Todaro, A. Sliski, and M. Essex. 1978b. Characterization of a feline sarcoma virus-coded antigen (FOCMA-S) by radioimmunoassay. *Proc. Natl. Acad. Sci.* **75:** 4489–4493.

Sherr, C.J., A. Sen, G.J. Todaro, A. Sliski, and M. Essex. 1978c. Pseudotypes of feline sarcoma virus contain an 85,000-dalton protein with feline oncornavirus-associated cell membrane antigen (FOCMA) activity. *Proc. Natl. Acad. Sci.* **75:** 1505–1509.

Sherwin, S.A. and G.J. Todaro. 1979. A new endogenous primate type C virus isolated from the Old World monkey *Colobus polykomos. Proc. Natl Acad. Sci.* **76:** 5041–5045.

Sherwin, S.A., T.I. Bonner, U. Heine, and G.J. Todaro. 1979. The isolation of an endogenous retrovirus from the New World rodent *Dasyprocta punctata (agouti). Virology* **94:** 409–416.

Shih, T.Y., M.O. Weeks, H.A. Young, and E.M. Scolnick. 1979. Identification of a sarcoma virus-coded phosphoprotein in nonproducer cells transformed by Kirsten or Harvey murine sarcoma virus. *Virology* **96:** 64–79.

Shih, T.Y., M.O. Weeks, D.H. Troxler, J.M. Coffin, and E.M. Scolnick. 1978. Mapping host range-specific oligonucleotides within genomes of the ecotropic and mink cell focus-inducing strains of Moloney murine leukemia virus. *J. Virol.* **26:** 71–83.

Siden, E.J., D. Baltimore, D. Clark, and N. Rosenberg. 1979. Immunoglobulin synthesis by lymphoid cells transformed in vitro by Abelson murine leukemia virus. *Cell* **16:** 389–396.

Sigurdsson, B. 1954a. Maedi, a slow progressive pneumonia of sheep: An epizoological and pathological study. *Br. Vet. J.* **110:** 255–270.

———. 1954b. Rida, a chronic encephalitis of sheep: With general remarks on infections which develop slowly and some of their special characteristics. *Br. Vet. J.* **110:** 341–354.

Sigurdsson, B., H. Thormar, and P.A. Palsson. 1960. Cultivation of visna virus in tissue culture. *Arch. Gesamte Virusforsch.* **10:** 368–381.

Simek, S. and N.R. Rice. 1980. Analysis of the nucleic acid components in reticuloendotheliosis virus. *J. Virol.* **33:** 320–329.

Simons, P.J. and R.M. Dougherty. 1963. Antigenic characteristics of three variants of Rous sarcoma virus. *J. Natl. Cancer Inst.* **31:** 1275–1283.

Sklar, M.D., B.J. White, and W.P. Rowe. 1974. Initiation of oncogenic transformation of mouse lymphocytes *in vitro* by Abelson leukemia virus. *Proc. Natl. Acad. Sci.* **71:** 4077–4081.

Sliski, A.H., M. Essex, C. Meyer, and G. Todaro. 1977. Feline oncornavirus-associated cell membrane antigen: Expression in transformed nonproducer mink cells. *Science* **196:** 1336-1339.

Smith, G.C., R.L. Heberling, R.J. Helmke, S.T. Barker, and S.S. Kalter. 1977. Oncornavirus-like particles in squirrel monkey (*Saimiri sciureus*) placenta and placenta culture. *J. Natl. Cancer Inst.* **59:** 975–979.

Smith, R. and C. Moscovici. 1969. The oncogenic effects of nontransforming viruses from avian myeloblastosis virus. *Cancer Res.* **29:** 1356–1366.

Snyder, H.W., Jr., W.D. Hardy, Jr., E.E. Zuckerman, and E. Fleissner. 1978. Characterisation of a tumour-specific antigen on the surface of feline lymphosarcoma cells. *Nature* **275:** 656–658.

Snyder, H.W., Jr., K.J. Phillips, W.D. Hardy, Jr., E.E. Zuckerman, M. Essex, A.H. Sliski, and J. Rhim. 1980. Isolation and characterization of proteins carrying the feline oncornavirus-associated cell-membrane antigen. *Cold Spring Harbor Symp. Quant. Biol.* **44:** 787–799.

Snyder, S.P. 1971. Spontaneous feline fibrosarcomas: Transmissibility and ultrastructure of associated virus-like particles. *J. Natl. Cancer Inst.* **47:** 1079–1085.

Snyder, S.P. and G.H. Theilen. 1969. Transmissible feline fibrosarcoma. *Nature* **221:** 1074–1075.

Snyder, S.P., D.L. Dungworth, T.G. Kawakami, E. Callaway and D.T.-L. Lau. 1973. Lymphosarcoma in two gibbons (*Hylobates lar*) with associated C-type virus. *J. Natl. Cancer Inst.* **51:** 89–94.

Somers, K.D., J.T. May, S. Kit, K.J. McCormick, G.G. Hatch, W.A. Stenback and J.J. Trentin. 1973. Biochemical properties of a defective hamster C-type oncornavirus. *Intervirology* **1:** 11–18.

Sonstegard, R. 1975. Lymphosarcoma in muskellunge. In *Pathology of fishes* (ed. W.E. Ribelin and C. Migaki), pp. 907–924. University of Wisconsin Press, Madison.

———. R.A. 1976. Studies of the etiology and epizootiology of lymphosarcoma in Esox (*Esox lucius* L. and *Esox masquinongy*). *Prog. Exp. Tumor Res.* **20:** 141–155.

Soule, H.D. and W.J. Arnold. 1970. Murine myeloproliferative virus in cell culture. *J. Natl. Cancer Inst.* **45:** 253–262.

Spriggs, D.R. and R.G. Krueger. 1980. BALB/c myeloma retroviruses: Peptide mapping and immunological analysis of the pp12 structural protein. *J. Virol.* **36:** 533–540.

———. 1981. Envelope proteins of the BALB/c myeloma mink cell focus-inducing (MCF) viruses. *Virology* **108:** 474–483.

Spriggs, D.R., M.A. Diebold, and R.G. Krueger. 1980. BALB/c myeloma retroviruses have mink cell focus-inducing activity. *J. Virol.* **36:** 541–546.

Squire, R.A. 1968. Equine infectious anemia. A model of immunoproliferative disease. *Blood* **32:** 157–169.

Staal, S.P., J.W. Hartley, and W.P. Rowe. 1977. Isolation of transforming murine leukemia viruses from mice with a high incidence of spontaneous lymphoma. *Proc. Natl. Acad. Sci.* **74:** 3065–3067.

Staff of Roscoe B. Jackson Memorial Laboratory. 1933. The existence of non-chromosomal influence in the incidence of mammary tumors in mice. *Science* **78:** 465–466.

Stancek, D. and M. Gressnerova. 1974. A viral agent isolated from a patient with subacute de Quervain type thyroiditis. *Acta Virol.* **18:** 365.

Stancek, D., M. Stancekova, M. Janotka, P. Hnilica, and D. Oravec. 1975. Isolation and some serological and epidemiological data on the viruses recovered from patients with subacute thyroiditis de Quervain. *Med. Microbiol. Immunol.* **161:** 133–144.

Stansly, P.G. and H.D. Soule. 1962. Transplantation and cell-free transmission of a reticulum-cell sarcoma in BALB/c mice. *J. Natl. Cancer Inst.* **29:** 1083–1105.

Steeves, R.A., E.A. Mirand, A. Bulba, and P.J. Trudel. 1970. Spleen foci and polycythemia in C57B1 mice infected with host-adapted Friend leukemia virus. *Int. J. Cancer* **5:** 346–356.

Steeves, R.A., R.J. Eckner, M. Bennett, E.A. Mirand, and P.J. Trudel. 1971. Isolation and characterization of a lymphatic leukemia virus in the Friend virus complex. *J. Natl. Cancer Inst.* **46:** 1209–1217.

Stein, C.D., C.J. Lotze, and L.O. Mott. 1972. Transmission of equine infectious anemia by the stablefly, *Stomoxys calcitrans,* the horsefly, *Tabanus sulcifrons* (Macquart) and by the injection of minute amounts of virus. *Am. J. Vet. Res.* **3:** 183–193.

Stein, C.D., O.L. Osteen, L.O. Mott, and M.S. Shahan. 1944. Experimental transmission of equine infectious anemia by contact and body secretions and excretions. *Vet. Med.* **39:** 46–52.

Stenback, W.A., G.L. Van Hoosier and J.J. Trentin. 1966. Virus particles in hamster tumors as revealed by electron microscopy. *Proc. Soc. Exp. Biol. Med.* **122:** 1219–1223.

Stephenson, J.R. and S.A. Aaronson. 1974. Demonstration of a genetic factor influencing spontaneous release of a xenotropic virus of mouse cells. *Proc. Natl. Acad. Sci.* **71:** 4925–4929.

———. 1976. Induction of an endogenous B-tropic type C RNA virus from SWR/J mouse embryo cells in tissue culture. *Virology* **70:** 352–359.

Stephenson, J.R., R.K. Reynolds, and S.A. Aaronson. 1976a. Comparisons of the immunological properties of two structural polypeptides of type C RNA viruses endogenous to Old World monkeys. *J. Virol.* **17:** 374–384.

Stephenson, J.R., S.R. Tronick, and S.A. Aaronson. 1974a. Analysis of type specific antigenic determinants of two structural polypeptides of mouse RNA C-type viruses. *Virology* **58:** 1–8.

Stephenson, J.R., S. Hino, E.W. Garrett, and S.A. Aaronson. 1976b. Immunological cross reactivity of Mason-Pfizer monkey virus with type C RNA viruses endogenous to primates. *Nature* **261:** 609–611.

Stephenson, J.R., A.S. Khan, A.H. Sliski, and M. Essex. 1977a. Feline oncornavirus-associated cell membrane antigen: Evidence from an immunologically crossreactive feline sarcoma virus-coded protein. *Proc. Natl. Acad. Sci.* **74:** 5608–5612.

Stephenson, J.R., R.K., Reynolds, S.G. Devare, and F.H. Reynolds. 1977b. Biochemical and immunological properties of *gag* gene-coded structural proteins of endogenous type C RNA tumor viruses of diverse mammalian species. *J. Biol. Chem.* **252:** 7818–7825.

Stephenson, J.R., R.K. Reynolds, S.R. Tronick, and S.A. Aaronson. 1975. Distribution of three classes of endogenous type-C viruses among inbred strains of mice. *Virology* **67:** 404–414.

Stephenson, J.R., S.A. Aaronson, P. Arnstein, R.J. Huebner, and S.R. Tronick. 1974b. Isolation and characterization of two immunologically distinct xenotropic type C RNA viruses of mouse cells. *Virology* **61:** 56–63.

Stiles, G.E. 1968. Serologic screening of rhesus and grivet monkeys for SV40 and the foamy viruses. *Proc. Soc. Exp. Biol. Med.* **127:** 225–230.

Stiles, G.E., J.L. Bittle, and V.J. Cabasso. 1964. Comparison of simian foamy virus strains including a new serological type. *Nature* **201:** 1350–1351.

Stockert, E., L.J. Old, and E.A. Boyse. 1971. The G_{IX} system. A cell surface allo-antigen associated with murine leukemia virus; Implications regarding chromosomal integration of the viral genome. *J. Exp. Med.* **133:** 1334–1355.

Stockert, E., A.B. DeLeo, P.V. O'Donnell, Y. Obata, and L.J. Law. 1979. $G_{(AKSL2)}$: A new cell surface antigen of the mouse related to the dualtropic mink cell focus-inducing class of murine leukemia virus detected by naturally occurring antibody. *J. Exp. Med.* **149:** 200–215.

Stockert, E., P.V. O'Donnell, Y. Obata, and L.J. Old. 1980. Inhibition of AKR leukemogenesis by SMX-1, a dualtropic murine leukemia virus. *Proc. Natl. Acad. Sci.* **77:** 3720–3724.

Stone, L.B., K.K. Takemoto, and M.A. Martin. 1971a. Physical and biochemical properties of progressive pneumonia virus. *J. Virol.* **8:** 573–578.

Stone, L.B., E. Scolnick, K.K. Takemoto, and S.A. Aaronson. 1971b. Visna virus: A slow virus with an RNA dependent DNA polymerase. *Nature* **229:** 257–258.

Stowring, L., A.T. Haase, and H.P. Charman. 1979. Serological definition of the lentivirus group of retroviruses. *J. Virol.* **29:** 523–528.

Strandstrom, H., P. Veijalainen, V. Moennig, G. Hunsmann, H. Schwarz, and W. Schafer. 1974. C-type particles produced by a permanent cell line from a leukemic pig. I. Origin and properties of the host cells and some evidence for the occurrence of C-type-like particles. *Virology* **57:** 175–178.

Strickland, J.E., A.K. Fowler, P.P. Kind, A. Hellman, S.S. Kalter, R.L. Heberling, and R.J. Helmke. 1973. Group specific antigen and RNA-directed DNA polymerase activity in normal baboon placenta. *Proc. Soc. Exp. Biol. Med.* **144:** 256–258.

Suzuki, T., K. Yanagihara, K. Yoshida, T. Seido, N. Kuga, Y. Shimosato, and S. Oboshi. 1977. Infectious murine type-C viruses released from human cancer cells transplanted into nude mice. *Gann* **68:** 99–106.

Svoboda, J. and J. Grozdanovic. 1959. Heterotransplantation of Rous sarcoma in young rats. *Folia Biol.* **5:** 46–50.

Swack, N.S. and G.D. Hsiung. 1975. Pathogenesis of simian foamy virus infection in natural and experimental hosts. *Infect. Immun.* **12:** 470–474.

Tajima, M., H. Nakajima, and Y. Ito. 1969. Electron microscopy of equine infectious anemia virus. *J. Virol.* **4:** 521–527.

Takeichi, N., H. Kaji, and J. Kodama. 1974. Breakdown of Friend virus induced tolerance and development of runting syndrome in mice. *Cancer Res.* **34:** 543–550.

Takemoto, K.K. and L.B. Stone. 1971. Transformation of murine cells by two "slow viruses", visna virus and progressive pneumonia virus. *J. Virol.* **7:** 770–775.

Takemoto, K.K., C.F.T. Mattern, L.B. Stone, J.E. Coe, and G. Lavelle. 1971. Antigenic and morphological similarities of progressive pneumonia virus, a recently isolated "slow virus" of sheep, to visna and maedi viruses. *J. Virol.* **7:** 301–308.

Tanaka, K. and K. Sakaki. 1962. Neutralization test on serum from horses infected with the virus of equine infectious anemia. *Natl. Inst. Anim. Health Q.* **2:** 128–139.

Teich, N.M., R.A. Weiss, S.Z. Salahuddin, R.E. Gallagher, D.H. Gillespie, and R.C. Gallo. 1975. Infective transmission and characterisation of a C-type virus released by cultured human myeloid leukaemia cells. *Nature* **256:** 551–555.

Teitz, Y., E.H. Lennette, L.S. Oshiro, and N.E. Cremer. 1971. Release of C-type particles from normal rat thymus cultures and those infected with Moloney leukemia virus. *J. Natl. Cancer Inst.* **46:** 11–23.

Temin, H.M. 1960. The control of cellular morphology in embryonic cells infected with Rous sarcoma virus *in vitro*. *Virology* **10:** 182–197.

———. 1963. Separation of morphological conversion and virus production in Rous sarcoma virus infection. *Cold Spring Harbor Symp. Quant. Biol.* **27:** 407–414.

Temin, H.M. and V.K. Kassner. 1974. Replication of reticuloendotheliosis viruses in cell culture: Acute infection. *J. Virol.* **13:** 291–297.

———. 1975. Replication of reticuloendotheliosis viruses in cell cultures: Chronic infection. *J. Gen. Virol.* **27:** 267–274.

Tennant, J.R. 1962. Derivation of a murine lymphoid leukemia virus. *J. Natl. Cancer Inst.* **28:** 1291–1303.

Teramoto, Y.A. and T. Schlom. 1978. Radioimmunoassays that demonstrate type-specific and group-specific antigenic reactivities for the major internal structural protein of mouse mammary tumor viruses. *Cancer Res.* **38:** 1990–1995.

Teramoto, Y.A., D. Kufe, and J. Schlom. 1977. Type-specific antigenic determinants on the major external glycoprotein of high- and low-oncogenic murine mammary tumor viruses. *J. Virol.* **24:** 525–533.

Teramoto, Y.A., P.H. Hand, R. Callahan, and J. Schlom. 1980. Detection of novel murine mammary tumor viruses by interspecies immunoassays. *J. Natl. Cancer Inst.* **64:** 967–975.

Tereba, A., L. Skoog, and P.K. Vogt. 1975. RNA tumor virus specific sequences in nuclear DNA of several avian species. *Virology* **65:** 524–534.

Theilen, G.H., R.F. Zeigel, and M.J. Twiehaus. 1966. Biological studies with RE virus (strain T) that induces reticuloendotheliosis in turkeys, chickens, and Japanese quail. *J. Natl. Cancer Inst.* **37:** 731–743.

Theilen, G.H., D. Gould, M. Fowler, and D.L. Dungworth. 1971. C-type virus in tumor tissue of a woolly monkey (*Lagothrix* spp.) with fibrosarcoma. *J. Natl. Cancer Inst.* **47:** 881–889.

Theilen, G.H., L.G. Wolfe, H. Rabin, F. Deinhardt, D.L. Dungworth, M.E. Fowler, D. Gould, and R. Cooper. 1973. Biological studies in four species of nonhuman primates with simian sarcoma virus (*Lagothrix*). In *Unifying concepts of leukemia* (ed. R.M. Dutcher and L. Chieco-Bianchi), pp. 251–257. Karger, Basel.

Thormar, H. 1961a. An electron microscope study of tissue cultures infected with visna virus. *Virology* **14:** 463–475.

———. 1961b. Stability of visna virus in infectious tissue culture fluid. *Arch. Gesamte Virusforsch.* **10:** 501–509.

———. 1965. A comparison of visna and maedi viruses. I. Physical, chemical and biological properties. *Res. Vet. Sci.* **6:** 117–129.

Thormar, H. and J.G. Cruickshank. 1965. The structure of visna virus studied by the negative staining technique. *Virology* **25:** 145–148.

Thormar, H. and H. Helgadottir. 1965. A comparison of visna and maedi viruses. II. Serological relationship. *Res. Vet. Sci.* **6:** 456–465.

Thormar, H. and B. Sigurdsardottir. 1962. Growth of visna virus in primary tissue cultures from various animal species. *Acta Pathol. Microbiol. Scand.* **55:** 180–186.

Thurzo, V., J. Smida, V. Smidova-Kovarova, and D. Simkovic. 1963. Some properties of the fowl virus tumor B77. *Acta Int. Union Against Cancer* **19:** 304–305.

Tihon, C. amd M. Green. 1973. Cyclic AMP-amplified replication of RNA tumour virus-like particles in Chinese hamster ovary cells. *Nat. New Biol.* **244:** 227–231.

Ting, R.C. 1968. Biological and serological properties of viral particles from a nonproducer rat neoplasm induced by a murine sarcoma virus (Moloney). *J. Virol.* **2:** 865–868.

Todaro, G.J. 1973. Detection and characterization of RNA tumor viruses in normal and transformed cells. *Perspect. Virol.* **8:** 81–101.

Todaro, G.J., C.J. Sherr, and R.E. Benveniste. 1976. Baboons and their close relatives are unusual among primates in their ability to release nondefective endogenous type C viruses. *Virology* **72:** 278–282.

Todaro, G.J., S.S. Tevethia, and J.L. Melnick. 1973a. Isolation of an RD-114 related cat type-C virus from feline sarcoma virus-transformed baboon cells. *Intervirology* **1:** 399–404.

Todaro, G.J., R.E. Benveniste, M.M. Lieber, and D.M. Livingston. 1973b. Infectious type C viruses released by normal cat embryo cells. *Virology* **55:** 506–515.

Todaro, G.J., R.E. Benveniste, M.M. Lieber, and C.J. Sherr. 1974a. Characterization of a type C virus released from the porcine cell line PK(15). *Virology* **58:** 65–74.

Todaro, G.J., R.E. Benveniste, S.A. Sherwin, and C.J. Sherr. 1978a. MAC-1, a new genetically transmitted type C virus of primates: "Low frequency" activation from stumptail monkey cell cultures. *Cell* **13:** 775–782.

Todaro, G.J., P. Arnstein, W.P. Parks, E.H. Lennette, and R.J. Huebner. 1973c. A type-C virus in human rhabdomyosarcoma cells after inoculation into NIH Swiss mice treated with anti-thymocyte serum. *Proc. Natl. Acad. Sci.* **70:** 859–862.

Todaro, G.J., R.E. Benveniste, R. Callahan, M.M. Lieber and C.J. Sherr. 1974b. Endogenous primate and feline type C viruses. *Cold Spring Harbor Symp. Quant. Biol.* **39:** 1159–1168.

Todaro, G.J., C.J. Sherr, R.E. Benveniste, M.M. Lieber, and J.L. Melnick. 1974c. Type C viruses of baboons: Isolation from normal cell cultures. *Cell* **2:** 55–61.

Todaro, G.J., R.E. Benveniste, C.J. Sherr, J. Schlom, G. Schidlovsky, and J.R. Stephenson. 1978b. Isolation and characterization of a new type C retrovirus from the Asian primate, *Presbytis obscurus* (spectacled langur). *Virology* **84:** 189–194.

Todaro, G.J., M.M. Lieber, R.E. Benveniste, C.J. Sherr, C.J. Gibbs, Jr., and D.C. Gajdusek. 1975. Infectious primate type C viruses: Three isolates belonging to a new subgroup from the brains of normal gibbons. *Virology* **67:** 335–343.

Todaro, G.J., C.J. Sherr, A. Sen, N. King, M.D. Daniel, and B. Fleckenstein. 1978c. Endogenous New World primate type C viruses isolated from owl monkey (*Aotus trivirgatus*) kidney cell lines. *Proc. Natl. Acad. Sci.* **75:** 1004–1008.

Tooze, J., ed. 1973. *The molecular biology of tumor viruses.* Cold Spring Harbor Laboratory, Cold Spring Harbor, New York.

———. 1980. *DNA tumor viruses.* Cold Spring Harbor Laboratory, Cold Spring Harbor, New York.

Trager, W. 1959. A new virus of ducks interfering with development of malaria parasite (*Plasmodium lophurae*). *Proc. Soc. Exp. Biol. Med.* **101:** 578–582.

Tronick, S.R., J.R. Stephenson and S.A. Aaronson. 1974a. Comparative immunological studies of RNA C-type viruses: Radioimmunoassay for a low molecular weight polypeptide of woolly monkey leukemia virus. *Virology* **57:** 347–356.

———. 1974b. Immunological properties of two polypeptides of Mason-Pfizer monkey virus. *J. Virol.* **14:** 125–132.

Tronick, S.R., M.M. Golub, J.R. Stephenson, and S.A. Aaronson. 1977. Distribution and expression in mammals of genes related to an endogenous type C RNA virus of *Odocoileus hemionus. J. Virol.* **23:** 1–9.

Tronick, S.R., J.R. Stephenson, S.A. Aaronson, and T.G. Kawakami. 1975. Antigenic characterization of type C RNA virus isolates of gibbon apes. *J. Virol.* **15:** 115–120.

Trowbridge, R.S. 1974. Evaluation of a plaque assay for the maedi-progressive pneumonia-visna viruses. *Appl. Microbiol.* **28:** 366–373.

Troxler, D.H. and E.M. Scolnick. 1978. Rapid leukemia induced by cloned Friend strain of replicating murine type-C virus. Association with induction of xenotropic-related RNA sequences contained in spleen focus-forming virus. *Virology* **85:** 17–27.

Troxler, D.H., J.K. Boyars, W.P. Parks, and E.M. Scolnick. 1977a. Friend strain of spleen focus-forming virus: A recombinant between mouse type C ecotropic viral sequences and sequences related to xenotropic virus. *J. Virol.* **22:** 361–372.

Troxler, D.H., S.K. Ruscetti, D.L. Linemeyer, and E.M. Scolnick. 1980. Helper-independent and replication defective erythroblastosis-inducing viruses contained within anemia-inducing Friend virus complex (FV-A). *Virology* **102:** 28–45.

Troxler, D.H., D. Lowy, R. Howk, H. Young, and E.M. Scolnick. 1977b. Friend strain of spleen focus-forming virus is a recombinant between ecotropic murine type C virus and the *env* gene region of xenotropic type C virus. *Proc. Natl. Acad. Sci.* **74:** 4671–4675.

Troxler, D.H., E. Yuan, D. Linemeyer, S. Ruscetti, and E.M. Scolnick. 1978. Helper-independent mink cell focus-inducing strains of Friend murine type-C virus: Potential relationship to the origin of the replication-defective spleen focus-forming virus. *J. Exp. Med.* **148:** 639–653.

Tsuchida, N., R.V. Gilden, M. Hatanaka, A.E. Freeman, and R.J. Huebner. 1975. Type-C virus-specific nucleic acid sequences in cultured rat cells. *Int. J. Cancer* **15:** 109–115.

Tung, [illegible]-S., E.S. Vitetta, E. Fleissner, and E.A. Boyse. 1975. Biochemical evidence linking the G_{IX} thymocyte surface antigen to the gp69/71 envelope glycoprotein of murine leukemia virus. *J. Exp. Med.* **141:** 198–205.

Twardzik, D.R., T.S. Papas, and F.H. Portugal. 1974. DNA polymerase in virions of a reptilian type C virus. *J. Virol.* **13:** 166–170.
Umphenour, N.W., M.J. Kemen, and L. Coggins. 1974. Equine infectious anemia: A retrospective study of an epizootic. *J. Am. Vet. Med. Assoc.* **164:** 66–69.
Upton, A.C., F.F. Wolff, J. Furth, and A.W. Kimball. 1958. A comparison of the induction of myeloid and lymphoid leukemias in X-radiated RF mice. *Cancer Res.* **18:** 842–848.
Ushimi, C., J.B. Henson, and J.R. Gorham. 1972. Immunofluorescent study of the one-step growth curve of equine infectious anemia virus. *Infect. Immun.* **5:** 890–895.
Ushimi, C., H. Nakajima, and S. Tanaka. 1970. Demonstration of equine infectious anemia viral antigen by immunofluorescence. *Natl. Inst. Anim. Health Q.* **10:** 90–91.
Vallee, H. and H. Carre. 1904. Nature infectieuse de l'anemie du cheval. *C. R. Acad. Sci.* **139:** 331–333.
Van Der Maaten, M.J. and J.M. Miller. 1976. Induction of lymphoid tumors in sheep with cell-free preparations of bovine leukemia virus. In *Comparative leukemia research 1975* (ed. J. Clemmesen and D.S. Yohn), pp. 377–379. Karger, Basel.
Van Der Maaten, M.J., A.D. Boothe, and C.L. Seger. 1972. Isolation of a virus from cattle with persistent lymphocytosis. *J. Natl. Cancer Inst.* **49:** 1649–1657.
Van Der Maaten, M.J., J.M. Miller, and A.D. Boothe. 1974. Replicating type-C virus particles in monolayer cell cultures of tissue from cattle with lymphosarcoma. *J. Natl. Cancer Inst.* **52:** 491–497.
Van Griensven, L.J.L.D. and M. Vogt. 1980. Rauscher "mink cell focus-inducing" (MCF) virus causes erythroleukemia in mice: Its isolation and properties. *Virology* **101:** 376–388.
Varmus, H.E., S. Heasley, and J.M. Bishop. 1974. Use of DNA-DNA annealing to detect new virus-specific DNA sequences in chicken embryo fibroblasts after infection by avian sarcoma virus. *J. Virol.* **14:** 895–903.
Velicer, L.F. and D.C. Graves. 1974. Properties of feline leukemia virus. II. In vitro labeling of the polypeptides. *J. Virol.* **14:** 700–703.
Verma, I.M., N.L. Meuth, H. Fan, and D. Baltimore. 1974. Hamster leukemia virus DNA polymerase: Unique structure and lack of demonstrable endogenous activity. *J. Virol.* **13:** 1075–1082.
Verwoerd, D.W. and P.S. Sarma. 1973. Induction of type C virus related functions in normal rat embryo fibroblasts by treatment with 5-iododeoxyuridine. *Int. J. Cancer* **12:** 551–562.
Vigier, P. 1970. RNA oncogenic viruses: Structure, replication, and oncogenicity. *Prog. Med. Virol.* **12:** 240–283.
Vigne, R., M. Brahic, P. Filippi, and J. Tamalet. 1977. Complexity and polyadenylic acid content of visna virus 60–70S RNA. *J. Virol.* **21:** 386–395.
Vigne, R., P. Filippi, M. Brahic, and J. Tamalet. 1978. Absence of circularly permuted and largely redundant sequences in the genome of visna virus. *J. Virol.* **28:** 543–550.
Vogt, M. 1979. Properties of "mink cell focus-inducing" (MCF) virus isolated from spontaneous lymphoma lines of BALB/c mice carrying Moloney leukemia virus as an endogenous virus. *Virology* **93:** 226–236.
Vogt, P.K. 1971a. Spontaneous segregation of nontransforming viruses from cloned sarcoma viruses. *Virology* **46:** 939–946.
———. 1971b. Genetically stable reassortment of markers during mixed infection with avian tumor viruses. *Virology* **46:** 947–952.
Vogt, P.K. and R.R. Friis. 1971. An avian leukosis virus related to RSV(O). Properties and evidence for helper activity. *Virology* **43:** 223–234.
Vogt, P.K., R.A. Weiss, and H. Hanafusa. 1974. Proposal for numbering mutants of avian leukosis and sarcoma viruses. *J. Virol.* **13:** 551–554.
Vogt, P.K., J.L. Spence, W. Okazaki, R.L. Witter, and L.B. Crittenden. 1977. Phenotypic

mixing between reticuloendotheliosis virus and avian sarcoma viruses. *Virology* **80:** 127–135.

Walker, R. 1969. Virus associated with epidermal hyperplasia in fish. *Natl. Cancer Inst. Monogr.* **31:** 195–207.

Wallbank, A.M., F.G. Sperling, K. Hubben, and E.L. Stubbs. 1966. Isolation of a tumour virus from a chicken submitted to a poultry diagnostic laboratory—Esh sarcoma virus. *Nature* **209:** 1265.

Ward, B.C. and N. Pederson. 1969. Infectious peritonitis in cats. *J. Am. Vet. Med. Assoc.* **154:** 26.

Waters, L.C. 1975. Transfer RNAs associated with the 70S RNA of AKR murine leukemia virus. *Biochem. Biophys. Res. Commun.* **65:** 1130–1136.

Weiland, F., S. Ueberschär, O.C. Straub, O.R. Kaaden, and B. Dietzschold. 1974. C-type particles in cultured lymphocytes from highly leukemic cattle. *Intervirology* **4:** 140–149.

Weinstein, I.B., R. Gebert, U.C. Stadler, J.M. Orenstein, and R. Axel. 1972. Type C virus from cell cultures of chemically induced rat hepatomas. *Science* **178:** 1098–1100.

Weislow, O.S., S. Schneider, R.L. Heberling, S.S. Kalter, and A. Hellman. 1976. Autogenous humoral immunity to baboon xenotropic endogenous type C virus. *J. Natl. Cancer Inst.* **57:** 561–565.

Weiss, M.J., S.C. Gulati, D.H. Harter, R.W. Sweet, S. Spiegelman, and C. Lopez. 1975. Unique virus-related DNA sequences in sheep progressive pneumonia lung. *J. Gen. Virol.* **29:** 335–339.

Weiss, R.A. and P.M. Biggs. 1972. Leukosis and Marek's disease viruses of feral red jungle fowl and domestic fowl in Malaya. *J. Natl. Cancer Inst.* **49:** 1713–1725.

Weiss, R.A. and A.L. Wong. 1977. Phenotypic mixing between avian and mammalian RNA tumor viruses. I. Envelope pseudotypes of Rous sarcoma virus. *Virology* **76:** 826– 834.

Weiss, R.A., W.S. Mason, and P.K. Vogt. 1973. Genetic recombinants and heterozygotes derived from endogenous and exogenous avian RNA tumor viruses. *Virology* **52:** 535–552.

Weiss, R.A., R.R. Friis, E. Katz, and P.K. Vogt. 1971. Induction of avian tumor viruses in normal cells by physical and chemical carcinogens. *Virology* **46:** 920–938.

Weiss, M.J., R.W. Sweet, S.C. Gulati, and D.H. Harter. 1976. Nucleic acid sequence relationships among "slow" viruses of sheep. *Virology* **71:** 395–401.

Werner, J. and H. Gelderblom. 1979. Isolation of foamy virus from patients with de Quervain thyroiditis. *Lancet* **2:** 258–259.

Winqvist, G., O. Ljungberg, and B. Hellstroem. 1968. Skin tumors of northern pike (*Esox lucius* L.). II. Viral particles in epidermal proliferations. *Bull. Off. Int. Epizoot.* **69:** 1023–1031.

Winqvist, G., O. Ljundberg, and B. Ivarsson. 1973. Electron microscopy of sarcoma of the northern pike (*Esox lucius* L.). In *Unifying concepts of leukemia* (ed. R.M. Dutcher and L. Chieco-Bianchi), pp. 26–30. Karger, Basel.

Witte, O.N., N. Rosenberg, M. Paskind, A. Shields, and D. Baltimore. 1978. Identification of an Abelson murine leukemia virus-encoded protein present in transformed fibroblast and lymphoid cells. *Proc. Natl. Acad. Sci.* **75:** 2488–2492.

Witter, R.L. and L.B. Crittenden. 1979. Lymphomas resembling lymphoid leukosis in chickens inoculated with reticuloendotheliosis virus. *Int. J. Cancer* **23:** 673–678.

Witter, R.L., H.G. Purchase, and G.H. Burgoyne. 1970. Peripheral nerve lesions similar to those of Marek's disease in chickens inoculated with reticuloendotheliosis virus. *J. Natl. Cancer Inst.* **45:** 567–577.

Wolfe, L.G. and F. Deinhardt. 1972. Oncornaviruses associated with spontaneous and experimentally induced neoplasia in nonhuman primates. In *Medical primatology* (ed.

E.I. Goldsmith and J. Moor-Jankowski), pp. 176–196. Karger, Basel.

Wolfe, L.G., R.K. Smith, and F. Deinhardt. 1972. Simian sarcoma virus, type 1 (*Lagothrix*). Focus assay and demonstration of nontransforming associated virus. *J. Natl. Cancer Inst.* **48:** 1905–1908.

Wolfe, L.G., F. Deinhardt, G.H. Theilen, H. Rabin, T. Kawakami, and L.K. Bustad. 1971. Induction of tumors in marmoset monkeys by simian sarcoma virus, type 1 (*Lagothrix*): A preliminary report. *J. Natl. Cancer Inst.* **47:** 1115–1120.

Wong-Staal, F. and S.F. Josephs. 1981. Baboon endogenous virus genomes in four species of baboons and five other genera of Old World monkeys: Evidence for infection postspeciation. *Virology* **112:** 289–295.

Wong-Staal, F., R.C. Gallo, and D. Gillespie. 1975. Genetic relationship of a primate RNA tumor virus genome to genes in normal mice. *Nature* **256:** 670–672.

Wong, T.C. and M.M.C. Lai. 1981. Avian reticuloendotheliosis virus contains a new class of oncogene of turkey origin. *Virology* **111:** 289–293.

Woods, W.A., T.S. Papas, H. Hirumi, and M.A. Chirigos. 1973. Antigenic and biochemical characterization of the C-type particle of the stable porcine kidney cell line PK-15. *J. Virol.* **12:** 1184–1186.

Wuu, K.D., D.C. Graves, and J.F. Ferrer. 1977. Inhibition of the reverse transcriptase of bovine leukemia virus by antibody in sera from leukemic cattle and immunological characterization of the enzyme. *Cancer Res.* **37:** 1438–1442.

Yamamoto, T., R.D. MacDonald, D.C. Gillespie, and R.K. Kelly. 1976. Viruses associated with lymphocystis and dermal sarcoma of walleye *(Stizostedion vitreum vitreum). J. Fish. Res. Board Can.* **33:** 2408–2419.

Yaniv, A., A. Gazit, M. Ianconescu, K. Perk, B. Aizenberg, and A. Zimber. 1979. Biochemical characterization of the type C retrovirus associated with lymphoproliferative disease of turkeys. *J. Virol.* **30:** 351–357.

Yaniv, A., T. Ohno, D. Kacian, D. Colcher, S. Witkin, J. Schlom, and S. Spiegelman. 1974. Serological analysis of reverse transcriptase of the Mason-Pfizer monkey virus. *Virology* **59:** 335–338.

Young, D., J. Samuels, and J.K. Clarke. 1973. A foamy virus of possible human origin isolated in BHK-21 cells. *Arch. Gesamte Virusforsch.* **42:** 228–234.

Yumoto, T. and L. Dmochowski. 1967. Light and electron microscope studies of organs and tissues of the New Zealand Black (NZB/BL) strain mice with lymphoid leukemia and autoimmune disease. *Cancer Res.* **27:** 2083–2097.

Yumoto, T., W.E. Poel, T. Kodama, and L. Dmochowski. 1970. Studies on FBJ virus-induced bone tumors in mice. *Tex. Rep. Biol. Med.* **28:** 145–165.

Zavada, J., C. Dickson, and R. Weiss. 1977. Pseudotypes of vesicular stomatitis virus with envelope antigens provided by murine mammary tumor virus. *Virology* **82:** 221–231.

Zavada, J., L. Cerny, A.D. Altstein, and Z. Zavadova. 1978. Pseudotype particles of vesicular stomatitis virus with surface antigens of bovine leukaemia virus—VSV(BLV)—as a sensitive probe for detecting antibodies in the sera of spontaneously infected cattle. *Acta Virol.* **22:** 91–96.

Zavada, J., L. Cerny, Z. Zavadova, J. Bozonva, and A.D. Altstein. 1979. A rapid neutralization test for antibodies to bovine leukemia virus, with the use of rhabdovirus pseudotypes. *J. Natl. Cancer Inst.* **62:** 95–101.

Zeigel, R.F. and H.F. Clark. 1969. Electron microscopic observations on a "C"-type virus in cell cultures derived from a tumor-bearing viper. *J. Natl. Cancer Inst.* **43:** 1097–1102.

———. 1971. Histologic and electron microscopic observations on a tumor-bearing viper: Establishment of a "C"-type virus-producing cell line. *J. Natl. Cancer Inst.* **46:** 309–321.

Zeigel, R.F., B.R. Burmester, and F.J. Rauscher. 1964. Comparative morphologic and biologic studies of natural and experimental transmission of avian tumor viruses. *Natl. Cancer Inst. Monogr.* **17:** 711–731.

———. 1961. Pathogenicity of Rous sarcoma virus for rats and rabbits. *J. Natl. Cancer Inst.* **26:** 1295–1309.

Zook, B.C., N.W. King, R.L. Robinson, and H.L. McCombs. 1968. Ultrastructural evidence for the viral etiology of feline infectious peritonitis. *Pathol. Vet.* **5:** 91–95.

3

Experimental Biology and Assay of Retroviruses

I. INTRODUCTION

As with other animal viruses, the molecular biology of retroviruses has depended on the use of experimental laboratory procedures for the isolation, propagation, assay, and cloning of biologically active virions. The development of monolayer and suspension cell-culture systems has played a crucial role in experimental biology of retroviruses.

The replication of retroviruses need not kill the host cell. The maturation of viral particles by budding from the plasma membrane does not usually cause cytopathic effects; therefore, an infected cell can become transformed and proliferate while producing virus progeny. However, as Temin (1963) first reported, virus replication is not necessary for cell transformation; neither is cell transformation necessary for virus replication (see Fig. 3.1). These phenomena are discussed in detail in later sections.

Originally, the retroviruses were classified according to the disease that they caused and were named after their discoverers. C-type RNA tumor viruses may be broadly divided into sarcoma and leukemia (leukosis) viruses. The division is not a clear one because some leukemia viruses can also produce a wide spectrum of solid tumors (see Chapter 8). Also, leukemia viruses are commonly present in

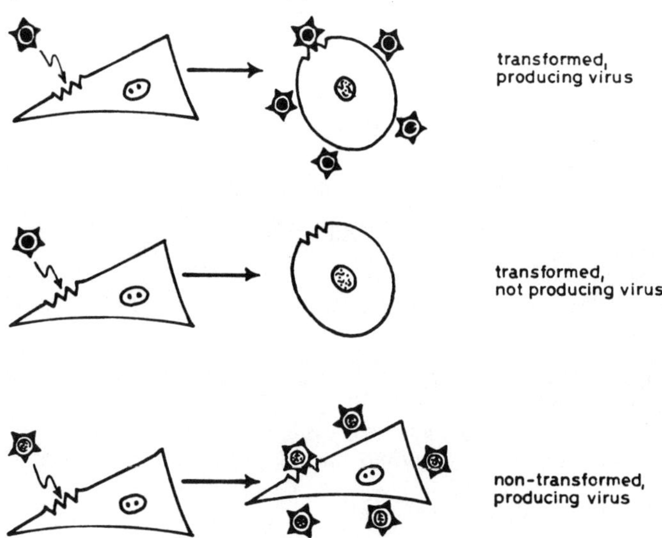

Figure 3.1 Schematic representation of the responses of fibroblasts to infection by retroviruses.

stocks of sarcoma viruses, and *src* deletion mutants (transformation-defective [*td*] viruses) of nondefective avian Rous sarcoma viruses (RSVs) are leukemogenic. Sarcoma viruses transform fibroblasts in culture, and cell transformation is the criterion by which these viruses are usually assayed. Avian leukemia viruses (ALVs) do not usually transform fibroblasts, although they readily infect and replicate in them. Some acute, defective leukemia viruses transform fibroblasts (e.g., avian erythroblastosis virus [AEV] and Abelson murine leukemia virus [Ab-MLV]), whereas others do not (e.g., avian myeloblastosis virus [AMV] and Friend spleen focus-forming virus [Fr-SFFV]). It is customary to refer to all C-type RNA viruses that fail to transform cultivated fibroblasts as leukemia viruses, irrespective of both their capacity to induce tumors in vivo and the type of tumors they may induce. Certain leukemia viruses may transform other kinds of cells in culture. For instance, chick embryo yolk-sac cells are susceptible to transformation by AMV but are not transformed by ALVs (Baluda and Goetz 1961; Smith and Moscovici 1969).

In general, a wider spectrum of cell types within the natural host species supports virus replication, rather than transformation. The specific interaction of transforming genes with differentiated cells is discussed later in this chapter (see Section III.C) and in Chapter 8. In contrast, infection of foreign species sometimes allows the expression of transforming genes in the absence of virus replication (e.g., infection of mammalian cells by avian sarcoma viruses [ASV]). Such cells are called nonpermissive for virus replication (see Section V.A.3).

The host range of RNA tumor viruses is complex and highly specific. It is controlled by virion structural gene products interacting with cell-surface and intracellular determinants (see Section V). Many RNA tumor viruses are defective and depend on helper viruses for the assembly of virion proteins (see Section IV.A and Chapter 7). Even with nondefective viruses, phenotypic mixing frequently occurs in mixed infections and can alter the host range and other biological properties of such virions.

II. REPLICATION ASSAYS

A variety of assay methods are used to detect and titrate virus production by infected cells. For retroviruses that transform cells in culture, quantitative focus assays can be used to titrate transforming units (see Section III). For nontransforming viruses, other methods of titration must be employed.

A. Immunological Assays of Viral Proteins

Most leukemia viruses are neither transforming nor cytopathic, so that morphological criteria cannot be exploited to detect virus infection. But immunological methods can be used to detect infected cells or tissues, usually with antisera reacting to the major *gag*-gene protein, p30. Complement fixation (CF) was first used to assay ALV infection (Sarma et al. 1964), and it is still used to detect leukosis virus infection of eggs in veterinary control. CF tests were subsequently developed for murine leukemia virus (MLV) (Hartley et al. 1965) and feline leukemia virus (FeLV) (Sarma et al. 1971). Radioimmunoassays (RIAs) (Strand et al. 1974) and enzyme-linked immunosorbent assays (ELISAs) (Clark and Dougherty 1980) are superseding CF assays in retrovirus laboratories owing to their greater sensitivity.

Quantitative assays of leukemia virus infectivity by CF or RIA employ end point-dilution titrations, but these are laborious. Immunocytological assays allowing the visualization of infected foci of cells were also developed but surprisingly little used. Vogt (1964) described a fluorescent-focus assay for ALV, and Nexo (1977) has developed an immunoperoxidase assay for MLV (see Fig. 3.2). These assays show that, as with transformation foci or cytopathic plaques, the number of immunologically detected foci of infection increases in linear proportion to the virus inoculum and therefore provides a simple method of titrating infectious units.

B. Plaque Assays

Some retroviruses cause cytopathic changes or induce syncytium (multinucleated giant cell) formation in certain types, and this phenomenon can be adapted for quantitative plaque assays.

As described in Chapter 2, cytopathic plaques develop in sheep choroid plexus cell cultures infected with visna virus. Foamy virus infection is visualized as vacuolation of glial cell cultures. Avian

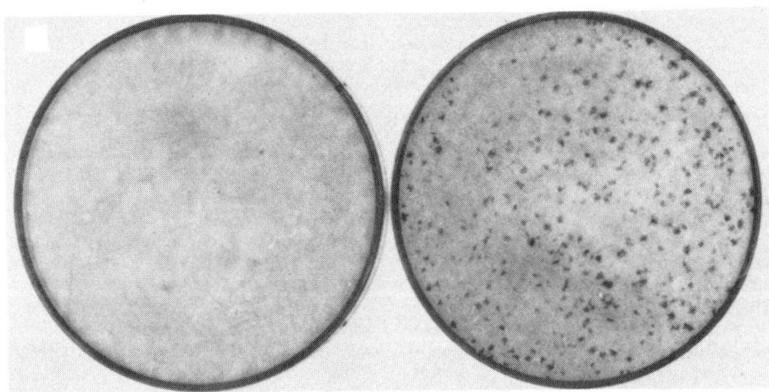

Figure 3.2 Immunoperoxidase focus assay for MLV. Two cultures of BALB/3T3 cells: (*left*) uninfected control; (*right*) infected with Mo-MLV. Cultures were stained 4 days after infection with peroxidase-coupled anti-Ra-MLV serum. (Reprinted, with permission, from Nexo 1977.)

reticuloendotheliosis-associated virus (REAV) is also cytopathic in avian fibroblasts early in infection and can be titrated in a plaque assay. Some ALVs are cytopathic under certain conditions. Kawai and Hanafusa (1972) and Wyke and Linial (1973) found that chick cells infected at the nonpermissive temperature with certain temperature-sensitive mutants of RSV failed to take up Neutral Red after superinfection with nontransforming viruses of envelope subgroups B and D (see below). This cytopathic effect (see Fig. 3.3) forms the basis of a plaque assay, because the number of plaques formed is linearly dependent on the dose of leukosis virus. Dougherty and Rasmussen (1964) and Graf (1972) have also described plaque assays in normal fibroblasts for ALVs belonging to subgroups B and D.

Some leukemia viruses induce syncytial plaques and the best known is the XC plaque assay for MLV. Klement et al. (1969) showed that when MLV-infected mouse cells were cocultivated with XC cells (derived from a rat tumor induced by RSV, Svoboda et al. 1963) in culture, the XC cells formed syncytia. This was developed into a sensitive plaque assay (Rowe et al. 1970), where focal areas of murine cells supporting the replication of some ecotropic strains of MLV are revealed by adding XC cells after UV-irradiation of the

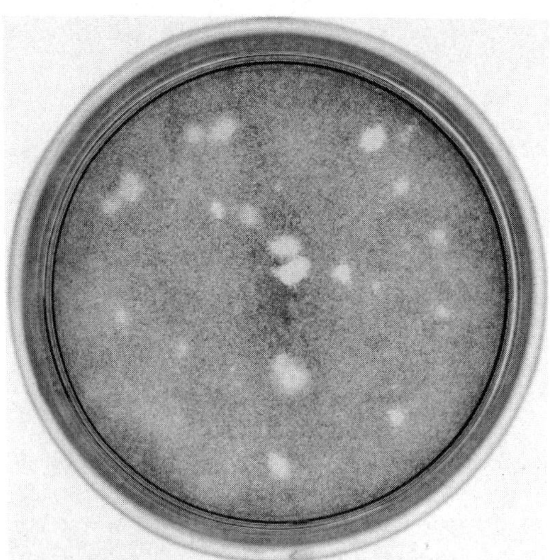

Figure 3.3 Plaques produced when chick fibroblasts infected by the PR-RSV mutant *ts* LA25 at 41°C are superinfected with Carr-Zilber avian leukosis virus. Cells stained with Neutral Red (J.A. Wyke.).

virus-producing cells. Plaques of multinucleated syncytia form where XC cells are in close contact with irradiated MLV-producing cells (see Fig. 3.4). The number of plaques is linearly related to the dilution of MLV, so that the XC plaque assay provides a sensitive assay of those strains of MLV that induce XC cell fusion. By harvesting the supernatant from a culture that subsequently proves to have only one XC plaque, MLV can be biologically cloned.

Primate leukemia viruses of the simian sarcoma-associated virus and gibbon ape leukemia virus (SSAV/GALV) group also induce syncytia in XC cells (Rangan et al. 1973), which can be exploited as a quantitative plaque assay (Teich et al. 1975). Bovine leukemia virus (BLV) induces syncytia in a variety of fibroblast strains, which also affords a plaque assay (Diglio and Ferrer 1976). Human KC cells are susceptible to syncytia formation by the endogenous cat virus (RD114), baboon endogenous virus (BaEV), and Mason-Pfizer monkey virus (MPMV) (Rand and Long 1972; Hellman et al. 1974; Ahmed et al. 1975), but these cells have not proved to be as reliable for syncytial plaque assays as have XC cells. Wong et al. (1977a,b) have described syncytial plaque formation following MLV infection of fu-1 cells, a nonfusing variant of L8 rat myoblasts.

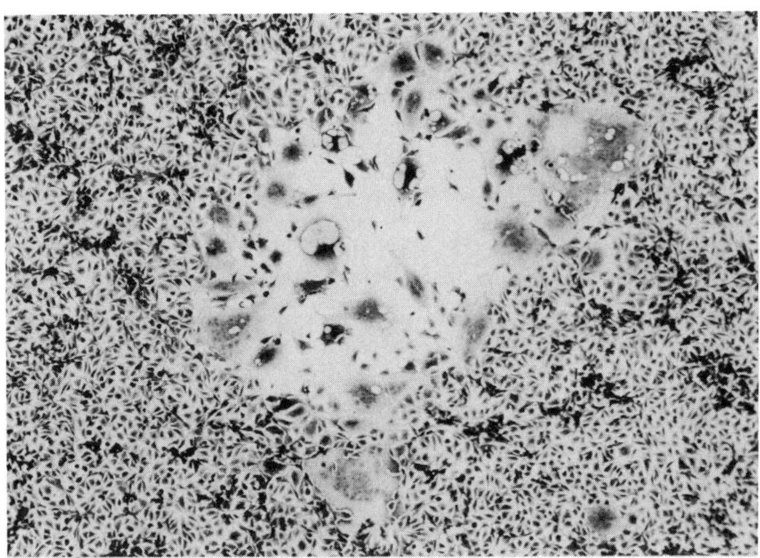

Fig 3.4 XC syncytial cell plaque assay. Syncytial plaques in an XC cell monolayer induced by MLV released by infected and irradiated mouse cells. The same assay can also be used for FeLV and SSAV/GALV (see text).

C. S^+L^- Focus Assay

Bassin et al. (1970, 1971a) observed that a revertant subline of 3T3 cells (sarcoma positive, leukemia-negative [S^+L^-]) originally transformed by Moloney murine sarcoma virus (Mo-MSV) would retransform when superinfected by MLV. The transformed, rounded cells tend to detach from the monolayer to leave plaques (where the MLV has replicated) that are easily enumerated. Using Mo-MLV, Bassin et al. (1971a) showed that the S^+L^- assay gave equivalent titrations to the XC plaque assay. The S^+L^- assay is also useful for titrating some ecotropic MLV strains that are not reactive in the XC plaque assay. A revertant, nonproducer mink line infected with S^+L^- MSV also retransforms upon infection with viruses such as xenotropic MLV or with primate and feline leukemia viruses, in this case yielding foci of transformed cells on the monolayer of revertant cells (Peebles 1975). Because mink cells are susceptible to infection with many strains of mammalian C-type viruses, this provides a simple focus assay for them.

The S^+L^- focus assay is not suitable for cloning leukemia viruses because MSV is rescued from the retransformed cells superinfected with the leukemia virus. A mouse cell subline, UC1B, of BALB/3T3 cells also forms foci after MLV infection (Hackett and Sylvester 1972) but has not been widely used.

D. Focus-interference Assays

Nontransforming viruses can also be titrated by the phenomenon of receptor interference (Rubin 1961) to infection by sarcoma viruses (see Section VI.A). When cultures are infected with leukemia viruses, the production of excess envelope glycoproteins by the leukemia virus blocks the receptors; thus, upon superinfection by a sarcoma virus with the same envelope specificity, the sarcoma virus cannot penetrate the cell surface. This phenomenon has been exploited as a "negative" focus assay for leukemia viruses. Cultures are infected with serial dilutions of leukemia virus and are passaged two to three times so that infection spreads to all cells. On subsequent challenge with a transforming sarcoma virus, foci will only appear in uninfected cultures, thus indicating an end point-dilution titer of the leukemia virus. Interference is most useful for defining receptor groups among retroviruses (see Sections V and VI.A).

E. Assays for Viral Particles

Replication of virus can be titrated by assays of physical particles. Although these methods do not have the sensitivity of assays based on infectivity, they are quicker to perform and may be suitable for the detection of noninfectious, defective particles. Virions released into the supernatant of infected cultures can be purified by sucrose gradient centrifugation or by other physical techniques and assayed by the following methods: (1) [^{3}H]uridine-labeling of virion RNA (Robinson et al. 1965), (2) molecular hybridization of virion RNA to cDNA probes (Ringold et al. 1975), (3) immunological assays for virion proteins, (4) enzymological assay of virion reverse transcriptase (Temin and Baltimore 1972), and (5) detection of particles by electron microscopy (Bernhard 1960).

Although the virions bear glycoprotein spikes in the envelope, hemagglutination assays have not been successfully developed for retroviruses. Some RNA tumor viruses assemble host proteins in the virions that can be used to assay for viral particles. For example, AMV grown in myeloblasts (but not in fibroblasts) has an envelope-associated ATPase (de Thé et al. 1964), and this enzyme activity was used in the first biochemical measure of viral particles in the plasma of infected chickens.

III. TRANSFORMATION ASSAYS

A. In Vivo Transformation

1. TD_{50} Assays

When Rous first discovered his sarcoma virus, it was titrated by injecting serial dilutions of virus into chickens to determine the end-point where 50% of the chickens developed tumors (TD_{50}). Virus is injected into the wing web because it is a suitable site for detecting the growth of even small tumors. TD_{50} assays have been used as the routine assay for neoplastic transformation in vivo; for RNA tumor viruses for which there are no in vitro transformation systems, it is the only way of titrating oncogenic potential, e.g., murine mammary tumor virus (MMTV) and some of the murine thymic lymphoma viruses.

Susceptibility to oncogenesis depends not only on the host strain, but also on the age of the host and the site of virus administration (see Chapter 8); thus, in vivo oncogenesis assays must be carefully standardized. For instance, in Gross's pioneering studies with AKR lymphoma, it took many years to prove a virus etiology, culminating in the discovery that newborn C3H mice were susceptible to infection. With the more recent isolation of recombinant, dualtropic murine lymphoma viruses (see Chapter 10), oncogenicity can be assayed in AKR mice destined to develop lymphoma in any case. Inoculation with dualtropic virus induces tumors to appear at an earlier age (Hartley et al. 1977), and hence the oncogenicity assay is known as a tumor-acceleration test.

2. Chorioallantoic Membrane Pocks

The first quantitative, focal transformation assay was developed for RSV on the chorioallantoic membrane (CAM) of embryonated eggs by Keogh (1938), who showed that discrete tumors or "pocks" develop on the CAM following inoculation with a suitable dilution of virus. This technique was refined by Rubin (1955, 1957) and by

Groupé et al. (1957), who used it to measure the production of virus by cultivated fibroblasts infected with RSV; the mean number of pocks per CAM was linearly related to the virus concentration. The CAM pock assay of RSV is still useful for screening the susceptibility of chick embryos to different strains of RSV (see, e.g., Payne et al. 1971; Pani 1976), but currently stocks of RSV are usually titrated by a focus assay in chick fibroblast cultures (see below). The pocks on the CAM are complex microtumors involving transformation of both the chorionic epithelium and the underlying mesenchyme.

The CAM can also be used as a culture vessel for the growth and migration of tumor cells (Poste and Flood 1979) or of retrovirus-infected cells in a transformation assay.

3. Spleen Colony Assays

In vivo focus assays have been successfully employed for murine erythroblastosis viruses, such as the defective transforming particles, Friend SFFV (Fr-SFFV) and Rauscher SFFV (Ra-SFFV). The rapid induction of splenomegaly in adult mice by Friend virus (Friend 1957; Rowe and Brodsky 1959) led to the development of a quantitative spleen focus assay (Axelrad and Steeves 1964; Pluznik and Sachs 1964). The spleen focus assay has been of great use for the analysis of genetic control of murine leukemogenesis, leading to the identification of the *Fv-1, Fv-2* series of host susceptibility genetic loci (Lilly and Pincus 1973). Susceptible mice show a one-hit dose response for spleen focus-forming units (Steeves et al. 1971), but it is still not clear whether helper-virus replication is necessary for the growth of spleen foci (see Chapter 8).

B. In Vitro Transformation of Fibroblasts

1. Focus Assay

Neoplastic transformation of cells in culture was first demonstrated by Halberstaedter et al. (1941), who observed morphological transformation of chick fibroblasts in explant cultures infected with RSV. With the use of dispersed, monolayer culture methods, discrete colonies of transformed cells could be observed following RSV infection (Manaker and Groupé 1956), leading to the design of a quantitative assay analogous to the CAM pocks (Temin and Rubin 1958; Vogt 1969).

Temin and Rubin (1958) showed that the number of discrete colonies or foci (see Fig. 3.5) of transformed cells in a culture of fibroblasts infected by RSV is, like the number of CAM pocks, linearly dependent on the dose of virus inoculated; this indicates that a single transforming RSV particle is sufficient to initiate a focus of transformed cells. The morphology of the transformed cells is governed by the virus strain or mutant used for infection (Ephrussi and Temin 1960; Temin 1960). Foci of rounded cells (morph r) and fusiform cells (morph f) transformed by Bryan high-titer RSV (BH-RSV) variants are shown in Figure 3.6. Experiments with X-irradiated feeder layers and X-irradiated transformants indicate that a focus grows both by mitosis of the transformed cells and by recruitment and transformation of neighboring cells by secondary infection with progeny RSV (Rubin 1960a).

Like the ASVs, mammalian sarcoma viruses can be assayed by focus formation on fibroblastic monolayers. Hartley and Rowe (1966) first described a focus assay for Moloney MSV (Mo-MSV) on mouse fibroblasts. In contrast to RSV focus assays on chick cells, a two-hit dose response was obtained, which was converted to a one-hit response when MSV stocks were titrated in the presence of excess MLV helper virus. It was concluded that focus formation depended on dual infection with MLV and MSV. Subsequent experiments, however, showed one-hit focus responses when MSV was

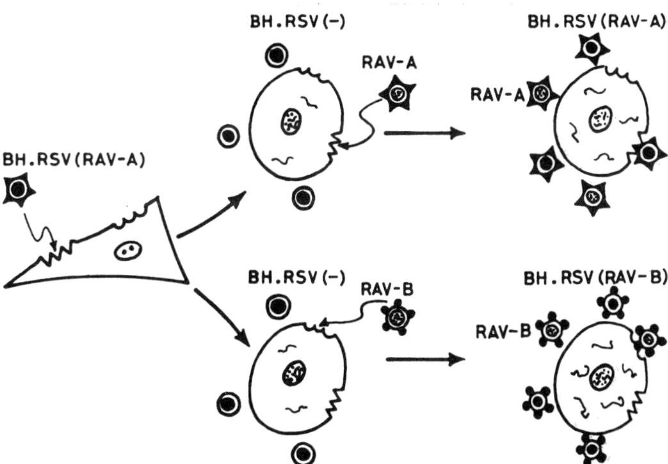

Figure 3.5 Diagram showing the rescue of the envelope-defective BH-RSV(−) strain by helper viruses of different subgroups.

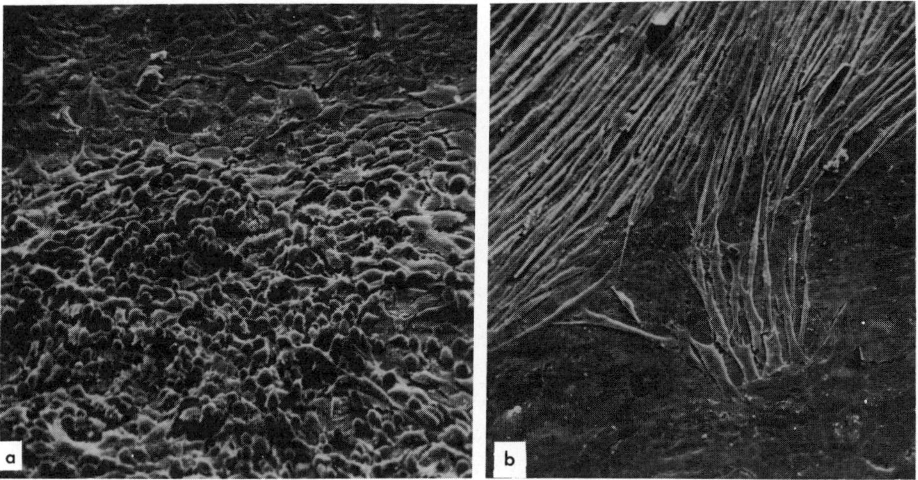

Figure 3.6 Transformed foci of quail cells infected with morphological variants of BH-RSV. (*a*) Round-cell (morph r) variant of BH-RSV; (*b*) fusiform-cell (morph f) variant of BH-RSV. (Scanning electron micrographs were provided by A. Boyde and R. Weiss.)

assayed on established cell lines, such as BALB/3T3 cells (Aaronson et al. 1970) or rat NRK cells (Parkman et al. 1970).

Other mammalian sarcoma viruses, such as simian sarcoma virus (SSV) and feline sarcoma virus (FeSV), can be assayed by focus formation similarly to MSV, using susceptible fibroblastic or epithelioid monolayers. Mink lung epithelial cells (Henderson et al. 1974) and feline embryo fibroblasts (Sarma and Law 1977; Markham et al. 1978) are particularly suitable for focus assays of SSV, FeSV, and MSV pseudotypes. Similarly, other ASVs, such as Fujinami virus (FuSV) and PRCII, are assayed as for RSV. The appearance of foci and the morphology of the transformed cells are characteristic for both the virus strain and the cell type used in the assay. The ASV assays on avian cells employ an agar gel overlay, which suppresses normal cell growth and retards secondary spread of virus. Agar overlays are not normally used for mammalian focus assays.

Some acute, defective leukemia viruses transform fibroblastic cells and can therefore be titrated in a focus assay: Ab-MLV forms foci on 3T3 cells and AEV forms foci on chick fibroblasts. However, murine Friend and Rauscher erythroblastosis viruses do not transform fibroblasts, nor does avian myeloblastosis virus (AMV), although focus assays in hematopoietic cell cultures have been devised (see below).

2. *Anchorage-independent Colonies*

The capacity of transformed cells to grow in a soft gel (Macpherson and Montagnier 1964; Sanders and Burford 1964; Stoker et al. 1968), such as agar or methylcellulose, has also been used as an assay of transformation by RSV (Rubin 1966; Weiss 1970; Wyke and Linial 1973) and by MSV (Bassin et al. 1970; Zavada and Macpherson 1970). The number of colonies obtained is linearly related to the infecting dose of virus, and cells from the transformed colonies can be isolated and cultivated as transformed cells. Anchorage-independent growth has been used as a method for selecting conditionally transformed mutants (Wyke 1973), and has proved very useful as a method for cloning both replicant-competent and defective transforming viruses.

3. *Plasmin Plaque Assays*

The enhanced release of plasminogen activator by RSV-transformed cells (Unkeless et al. 1973) has been exploited as a focal assay of transformation for RSV transformation and for other tumor cells. Plasminogen activator cleaves plasminogen to proteolytically active plasmin. When turbid casein (usually added as dried skimmed milk) is incorporated in an agar overlay on RSV-infected cells, clear plaques of digested casein appear above RSV-transformed colonies (Goldberg 1974; Balduzzi and Murphy 1975; Wolf and Goldberg 1976). In place of casein, fibrin has been used as a substrate and then stained with Coomassie blue to reveal the plaques (Jones et al. 1975). Some clones of RSV-transformed chick fibroblasts express very low levels of plasminogen activator, although they grow in soft agar and exhibit increased hexose transport (Wolf and Goldberg 1976).

4. *Hexose Transport*

Some cells transformed by sarcoma virus show an increased rate of uptake of hexose sugars (Hatanaka and Hanafusa 1970; Martin et al. 1971; Weber 1975; Wolf and Goldberg 1976), which can be used as an assay of the overall transformed state of a culture (see Chapter 8).

C. In Vitro Transformation of Other Cell Types

1. Sarcoma Viruses

Besides fibroblastic cells, a number of other cell types can be transformed by sarcoma viruses, including epithelial and mesenchymal cells. RSV-transformed epithelial cells include pigmented retinal cells (Ephrussi and Temin 1960; Boettiger et al. 1977) and neural retinal cells (Calothy and Pessac 1976), and MSV-transformed epithelial cells include kidney cells (Parkman et al. 1970) and lung cells (Henderson et al. 1974). Mesenchymal cells include myoblasts (Kaighn et al. 1966; Easton and Reich 1972), chondroblasts (Pacifici et al. 1977), glial cells, and hematopoietic cells, such as macrophages (Gazzolo et al. 1974). The specific differentiation of such cell types tends to be blocked or even reversed by RSV transformation (Fiszman and Fuchs 1975; Holtzer et al. 1975; Hynes et al. 1976; Boettiger et al. 1977; Pacifici et al. 1977); upon shift-up to the nonpermissive temperature of cells infected with temperature-sensitive RSV mutants, cellular differentiation resumes again (see Chapter 7). The interaction of viral transformation with cell-differentiation pathways is an active field of research which will benefit from the identification of oncogene products and the elucidation of their functions.

2. Acute Leukemia Viruses

The infection of hematopoietic cells with acute leukemia viruses is described in more detail in Chapter 8. Under appropriate conditions, focal transformation can be obtained and used as an assay of transforming virus. For instance, chick macrophages are susceptible to transformation by AMV and the avian myelocytomatosis virus, MC29. Baluda and Goetz (1961) first demonstrated in vitro transformation of chick egg yolk-sac macrophages by AMV, and this was later developed as a focus assay (Moscovici and Zanetti 1970; Moscovici et al. 1975). Graf (1973, 1975) has used chick bone marrow cultures to detect transformed cell colonies following infection with AMV, MC29, and AEV and has shown that different target cells are transformed in each case (see Chapter 8). A temperature-sensitive mutant of AEV transforms erythroblasts that differentiate to reticulocytes after shift to the nonpermissive temperature (Graf et al. 1978).

Ab-MLV can transform lymphoid cells in culture (Rosenberg et al. 1975). In the presence of mercaptoethanol, colonies of cells resembling pre-B cells proliferate in soft agar after Ab-MLV infection. In a series of studies, Dexter et al. (1977) have shown that long-term cultures of mouse bone marrow cells maintaining the proliferation of the hematopoietic stem cell, CFU-S, can be transformed and give rise to many kinds of cell lines following infection with a variety of MLVs, including Friend virus and Ab-MLV. With advances in the cultivation of special cell types, their transformation by specific strains of RNA tumor virus will be increasingly studied.

IV. PSEUDOTYPE VIRUSES

A. Propagation of Defective Viruses

Many strains of RNA tumor viruses are defective for replication owing to deletions in one or more genes. This is particularly frequent with sarcoma and acute leukemia viruses, where transforming oncogenes, often derived from host genes, are substituted in place of the virion structural genes, *gag, pol,* or *env.* Indeed, the only acutely transforming viruses that are known to be competent for replication are the Prague, Schmidt-Ruppin, Carr-Zilber, and B77 strains of ASV, which carry the *src* gene in addition to the three structural genes.

Defective viruses can be propagated in the presence of replication-competent helper viruses, which provide virion proteins for assembly, a process called phenotypic mixing. Helper viruses, usually lymphoid leukosis viruses (LLVs), are related RNA tumor viruses that do not transform cells in culture. The genetic analysis of defective viruses and their complementation by phenotypic mixing with helper viruses is described in Chapter 7.

The classic example of a defective RNA tumor virus is BH-RSV(−) (Hanafusa et al. 1963). Cells infected with BH-RSV(−), but not coinfected with the Rous-associated helper virus (RAV), do not produce infectious progeny and hence were called nonproducer cells. Subsequent studies, however, showed that noninfectious particles were released (Dougherty and Di Stefano 1965; Vogt 1967b; Weiss 1967, 1969a; T. Hanafusa et al. 1970) that lack envelope glycoproteins (Scheele and Hanafusa 1971). Mo-MSV-transformed cells may also release noninfectious particles in the absence of helper virus (Bassin et al. 1971b); such cells are called $S^{+}L^{-}$. Many other strains of defective viruses, e.g., Kirsten MSV (Ki-MSV) (Aaronson and Rowe 1970) and MC29 (Graf et al. 1979), produce no physical particles in the absence of helper virus, so that the transformed cells are genuine nonproducers. It appears that only *gag* proteins are necessary for virion budding (see Chapter 7).

The rescue of infectious progeny of defective viruses by helper viruses is due to the assembly of helper-virus proteins in virions carrying the defective viral genome. Such "wolves in sheep's clothing" are termed pseudotypes (Rubin 1965). The point of discussing defective/helper interactions here is to emphasize that many retrovirus populations are polymorphic and that some of the properties of the virus being assayed may be determined by another virus present in the mixed population. Many of the biological characteristics of viruses are, of course, functions of the virion proteins; therefore, properties such as antigenicity, host range, and interference patterns are determined by the helper virus, rather than by the defective genome, which determines oncogenicity. Thus, the replication properties of a defective virus may change according to the strain of helper virus with which it is propagated.

Phenotypic mixing also occurs between nondefective viruses (Vogt 1967a; Weiss and Bennett 1980), which may then exhibit dual properties. Phenotypic mixing should be distinguished from genetic recombination (see Chapter 7), as the phenotype of the virus does not breed true but is conferred only by the virion proteins.

B. Uses of Pseudotypes

Pseudotypes have proved to be important tools in the experimental manipulation of retroviruses. Phenotypic mixing has been used as a method to (1) rescue and propagate defective viruses (see above); (2) assign biological properties to virion proteins, e.g., host range determined by *env* proteins (Rubin 1965) and by *gag* proteins (Rein et al. 1976); (3) manipulate viruses to alter or broaden host range, e.g., the introduction of RSV into mammalian cells (Hanafusa and Hanafusa 1966; Levy 1977b; Weiss and Wong 1977; Quade 1979); (4) detect and analyze the genetics of cell-surface receptors for retroviruses (discussed in Section V); and (5) detect latent infections, e.g., the presence and expression of endogenous *env* genes, which was first observed in chick cells through the complementation of *env*⁻ RSV (Vogt 1967b; Weiss 1967, 1969b; H. Hanafusa et al. 1970).

C. Pseudotypes of Vesicular Stomatitis Virus

Phenotypic mixing of glycoproteins occurs widely among enveloped animal viruses (Zavadova et al. 1977; Boettiger 1979; Weiss 1980). Pseudotypes of vesicular stomatitis virus (VSV) bearing envelope proteins of retroviruses were first described by Zavada (1972a). In mixed infections of VSV and retroviruses, only the envelope glycoproteins are involved (Weiss et al. 1975, 1977; Livingston et al. 1976). The infectivity of VSV pseudotypes therefore distinguishes retroviral host-range specificities determined by cell-surface receptors for viral glycoproteins from those operating after virus penetration and uncoating, because the VSV pseudotype replicates as a vesicular stomatitis virion once uncoating has occurred.VSV pseudotype formation is also a sensitive method for detecting glycoprotein expression in the absence of retrovirus replication (Fig. 3.7).

VSV pseudotypes bearing retroviral glycoproteins are usually prepared with wild-type VSV (Zavada 1972a), but VSV mutants conditionally defective for glycoprotein assembly or function have also been used to advantage (Zavada 1972b; Boettiger et al. 1975; Weiss and Bennett 1980). With wild-type VSV, the nonpseudotype VSV progeny bearing VSV glycoproteins are neutralized by anti-VSV serum, leaving pseudotype particles as the only plaque-forming units that survive neutralization (see Fig. 3.8). These pseudotypes require retroviral receptors in order to penetrate cells, whereupon the VSV genome replicates to produce wild-type progeny and eventually a cytopathic plaque. Thus, a VSV plaque assay can be used in place of a sarcoma focus assay to detect cell-surface receptors for retroviruses.

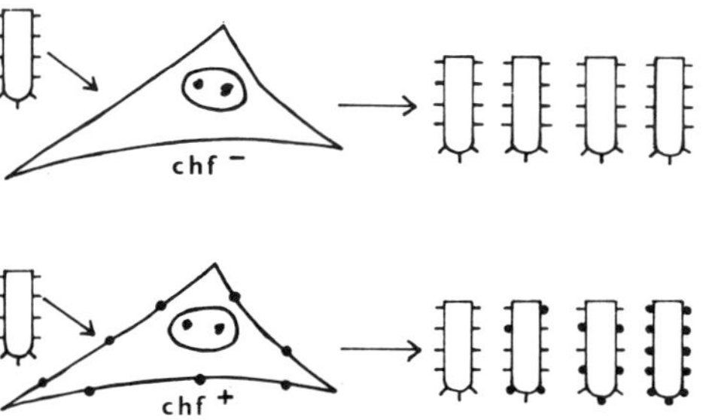

Figure 3.7 VSV pseudotypes are produced by propagation of VSV in cells expressing retroviral glycoproteins; chf⁻, chick cells not synthesizing endogenous gp85; chf⁺, chick cells synthesizing endogenous gp85. A proportion of the VSV progeny have envelopes in which the glycoprotein spikes are partially or wholly substituted by retroviral gp85.

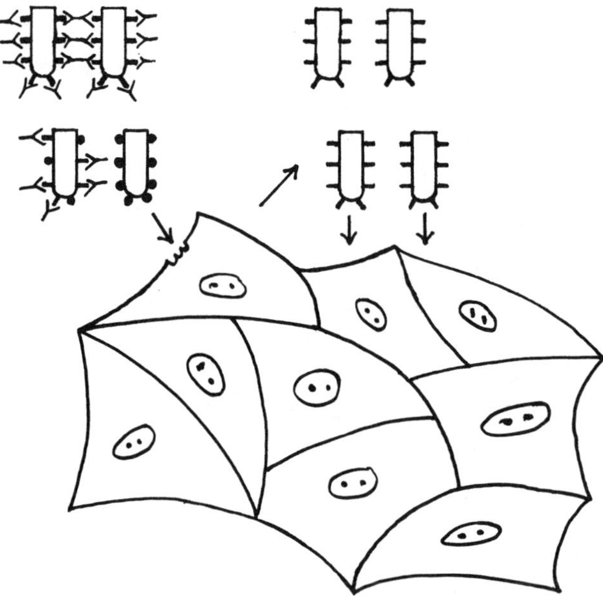

Figure 3.8 The use of retrovirus pseudotypes of VSV genomes for defining the presence or absence of cell-surface receptors for a particular retrovirus. Nonpseudotype VSV particles are efficiently neutralized by anti-VSV serum. Pseudotype VSV particles are not neutralized, can infect cells bearing the appropriate cell-surface receptors for the retroviral envelope proteins, and can initiate the formation of a lytic plaque. (Adapted from Weiss 1980.)

VSV pseudotypes have been extensively used for glycoprotein studies of MLV (Zavada 1972a; Huang et al. 1973; Krontiris et al. 1973), MMTV (Zavada et al. 1977), ALV (Zavada 1972a; Love and Weiss 1974; Boettiger et al. 1975), and primate retroviruses (Schnitzer et al. 1977; Thiry et al. 1978).

V. HOST SUSCEPTIBILITY AND RESISTANCE

RNA tumor viruses exhibit a high degree of host-range specificity. Virus replication is restricted to certain host strains or species and, to a lesser extent, to different cell types within those species. The spectrum of differentiated cell types susceptible to transformation is more restricted but may occur across many species, provided early steps in the replication cycle are satisfied. Restrictions on host range for replication can be broadly categorized as follows: (1) a bar to virus penetration because the appropriate cell-surface receptors are lacking (no infection), (2) a bar after penetration but before provirus integration (abortive infection), and (3) a bar after integration but before maturation of progeny virions (nonpermissive infection).

The most-detailed studies of host susceptibility and resistance have been made on avian and murine leukemia and sarcoma viruses. The host range of other C-type viruses has usually been studied by screening the in vitro infection of cell lines of a variety of host species. Productive infection by the B-type MMTV is not readily achieved in culture, as most cells become abortively or nonpermissively infected, although cell lines derived from mammary tumors produce substantial amounts of virus in culture. Thus, the infectibility of cells in culture does not necessarily reflect natural host range, since the cell lines tested are often broader (in numbers of species tested) or narrower (in cell types tested) than the host cells to which the viruses have access in nature.

Endogenous retroviruses (i.e., viruses derived from integrated genomes inherited through the host germ line) are frequently not able to reinfect cells of the species from which they have been activated. Levy (1973) coined the term xenotropism for such viruses. Most endogenous viruses are xenotropic, and it would appear that the hosts carrying genomes of endogenous viruses have evolved a variety of restriction mechanisms that suppress reinfection.

A major determinant of host susceptibility or resistance to retrovirus infection in vitro and in vivo is the interaction between the virion glycoproteins and specific cell-surface receptor sites. Viruses are divided into envelope glycoprotein classes according to their recognition of cellular receptors, and this frequently correlates with their classification by sensitivity to neutralizing antibodies. Cell-surface resistance to infection may occur because either there are no receptors (genetic or epigenetic resistance) or the receptors are saturated with glycoproteins already present in the cell, owing to existing exogenous or endogenous virus infection (receptor interference). Receptor phenomena are discussed in more detail after a survey of the host ranges of murine, avian, and feline retroviruses.

A. Host Range of Avian Retroviruses

1. ASLV in Birds

The avian sarcoma and leukosis virus (ASLV) strains show considerable diversity of host range within their natural host species at the level of envelope-glycoprotein-receptor specificity. The ASLVs have been divided into five "envelope" subgroups, A through E, on the basis of host range, cross-interference of receptors, and neutralization by antibodies (Payne and Biggs 1964, 1966; Hanafusa 1965; Rubin 1965; Vogt and Ishizaki 1965; Ishizaki and Vogt 1966; Duff and Vogt 1969; Weiss 1969a,b; T. Hanafusa et al. 1970). Further subgroups (F, G, etc.) have been identified among endogenous retroviruses of pheasant and quail species (Hanafusa and Hanafusa 1973; Fujita et al. 1974; Hanafusa et al. 1976; Chen and Vogt 1977).

The susceptibility of a cell to infection by a virus of a given subgroup depends on the presence of receptor sites specific for that subgroup (see Fig. 3.9). If receptors for a particular subgroup are lacking, the cell is resistant to infection by viruses of that subgroup; the efficiency of plating of a virus on resistant cells is 10^{-6} or less than the efficiency of plating on susceptible cells. Viral particles adsorb to both susceptible and resistant cells, but they penetrate only susceptible cells (Piraino 1967; Crittenden 1968). Resistance, however, may be overcome in two ways: (1) by forming a pseudotype with the envelope antigens of a virus of a subgroup to which the cell is susceptible (Hanafusa 1965; Vogt 1965; Crittenden 1968) or (2) by treating the resistant cells with inactivated Sendai virus or Newcastle disease virus (Robinson 1967; Weiss 1969a; T. Hanafusa et al. 1970) or polyethyleneglycol (Rohde et al. 1978), which probably works by causing fusion between the cellular and viral membranes. These findings showed that the viral receptors are located at the cell surface.

The phenotype of a cell is designated according to the virus subgroups that are excluded (Vogt and Ishizaki 1965); for example, C/AB signifies chick (C) cells resistant to (/) subgroup-A and subgroup-B viruses, whereas cells generally susceptible to all avian tumor viruses are designated C/O (resistant to no subgroup). This designation has certain disadvantages because it identifies resistance, which is a negative attribute. As new subgroups of viruses were identified (Duff and Vogt 1969; Weiss 1969a), some cells that were previously designated C/O with respect to viruses of subgroups A and B were found to be resistant to viruses of the new subgroups. Therefore, the designation C/O should be taken to signify susceptibility only to those subgroups under discussion.

Table 3.1 lists some chick-cell phenotypes and their responses to avian tumor viruses of different subgroups. Receptors for subgroups A, B, and C are independent, but a relationship exists between receptors for viruses of subgroups B, D, and E. Chick cells that are

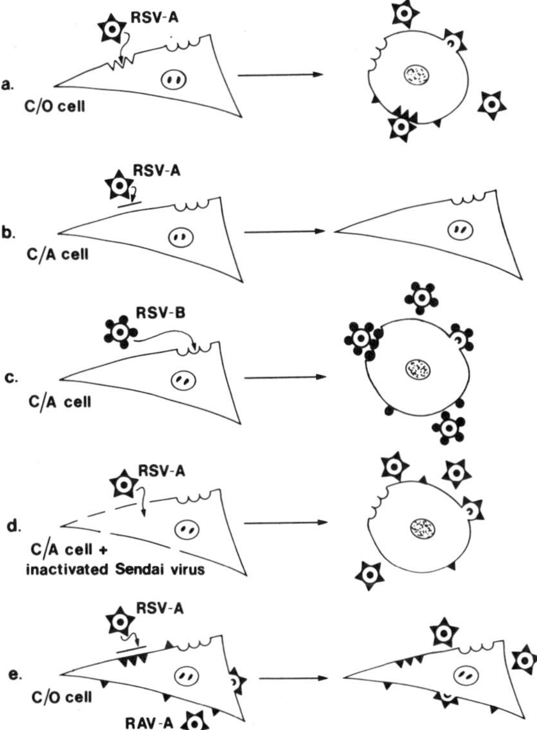

Figure 3.9 Receptor control of susceptibility to infection with RSV. (*a*) RSV-A enters a susceptible cell through a specific cell-surface receptor. As a consequence of infection, the virus replicates and the cell and its daughter cells become transformed. Progeny virus occupies the specific receptor sites. (*b*) RSV-A cannot enter a resistant cell because there is no compatible receptor. (*c*) RSV-B can enter a cell resistant to RSV-A provided there is a receptor specific to RSV-B. (*d*) RSV-A can enter a resistant cell that has been treated with inactivated Sendai virus, after which there is no further restriction to virus replication or cell transformation. (*e*) Preinfection of a C/O cell with a leukemia virus (RAV-A) interferes with subsequent infection by RSV-A, but not by RSV-B, because the appropriate receptors are specifically blocked by RAV-A gp85.

resistant to subgroup-B viruses show a 1000-fold to 100,000-fold reduction in efficiency of plating of subgroup-D viruses (Duff and Vogt 1969) and exclude subgroup-E viruses absolutely (Crittenden and Motta 1975). However, cells of most other galliform avian species, e.g., Japanese quail, ring-necked pheasant, and turkey, are resistant to viruses of subroup B but are susceptible to subgroup-E viruses.

Linial (1976) has reported that C/B chicken cells can be rendered

Table 3.1 Susceptibility and resistance of chick cells to RSV

Designated phenotype	Log$_{10}$ ffu/ml				
	RSV-A	RSV-B	RSV-C	RSV-D	RSV-E
C/0	7.2	6.6	7.4	6.8	6.1
C/E	7.2	6.6	7.3	6.8	1.3
C/AE	<0.4	6.5	7.2	6.7	<0.4
C/BE	7.2	<0.4	7.3	2.1	<0.4
C/ABE	<0.4	<0.4	6.7	2.0	<0.4
C/C	7.1	6.5	<0.4	6.6	6.4

Secondary cultures of secondary chick embryo fibroblasts were infected with serial dilutions of RSV of the subgroups indicated. After infection (18 hr), the cultures were overlaid with nutrient medium containing agar and were incubated for 7 days to allow the growth of foci of RSV-transformed cells. The foci at appropriate dilutions were enumerated and are expressed as infectious focus-forming units (ffu) per milliliter of undiluted virus. Data from Weiss (1981).

susceptible to RSV-B infection by trypsin treatment. Since genetic resistance is a recessive trait (see Section VI.D) indicative of the absence, rather than the masking, of receptors, the significance of Linial's finding is not clear. Further observations by Robinson (1976) and Linial and Neiman (1976) suggest a postreceptor host-range restriction in most chicken cells for the replication of RAV-0, the endogenous subgroup-E virus. Recombinant RSV-E viruses, selected for replication in chicken or quail cells (Weiss et al. 1973), are not sensitive to this restriction (Linial and Neiman 1976; see Chapter 10).

2. *Avian Sarcoma Viruses in Mammalian Hosts*

Infection of rats with avian tumor viruses was first reported by Svet-Moldavsky (1958) and by Zilber and Kryukova (see Zilber 1964). It was soon confirmed for a variety of other mammalian species (Schmidt-Ruppin 1959), including primates (Munroe and Windle 1963). Subsequently, Duff and Vogt (1969) showed that, with the exception of B77 RSV (subgroup C), only subgroup-D viruses infect mammals. Hanafusa and Hanafusa (1966) found that phenotypic mixing with RAV-50, a subgroup-D virus, conferred infectivity to RSV for mammalian cells, although at a lower efficiency than for chicken cells. Acute avian leukemia viruses can also be introduced into mammalian cells in this way (Quade 1979).

Altaner and Temin (1970) doubted that the envelope specificity of B77 virus (subgroup C) affected its oncogenicity for mammalian cells, since phenotypic mixing with RAV-1 (subgroup A) did not alter its plating efficiency on mammalian cells. However, Boettiger et al. (1975) using VSV pseudotypes showed that only those pseudotypes with B77 or subgroup-D envelopes plated on mammalian cells.

Mammalian cells transformed by RSV (Svoboda and Hlozanek 1970) truly appear to be nonproducer cells; no C-type particles are released. But certain strains of rat and hamster tumor cells infected with B77 virus (Klement and Vesely 1965; Altaner and Svec 1966; Simkovic et al. 1969) produce infectious transforming particles which preliminary evidence suggests may be recombinants between avian and mammalian retroviruses (M. Kotler; J. Svec; both pers. comm.).

RSV can be rescued by injecting the transformed mammalian cells into chickens or by cocultivating them with chicken cells (Svoboda 1960; Simkovic et al. 1962; Svoboda et al. 1963). Svoboda et al. (1967) and Shevliaghyn et al. (1969) showed that virus is rescued by fusing virogenic mammalian cells with permissive chick cells and that in some cases, virus synthesis commences in every heterokaryon (Machala et al. 1970). Chick cells other than fibroblasts are inefficient at rescue, but chick fibroblasts need not express endogenous viral genes to be permissive for rescue of RSV (Svoboda et al. 1971), nor need they be actively dividing (Coffin 1972).

Mammalian leukemia viruses do not rescue RSV from mammalian cells. However, phenotypic mixing with mammalian retroviruses able to replicate in avian cells aids infection and replication of RSV in mammalian cells (Levy 1977b; Weiss and Wong 1977).

The relative efficiency of transformation of mammalian cells, compared with chick cells, by B77 or RSV-D is considerably lower than that for the plating of VSV pseudotypes (Boettiger 1974a). Furthermore, mammalian cells transformed by RSV revert to a normal phenotype either spontaneously (Macpherson 1965; Boettiger 1974b; Deng et al. 1974; Wyke and Quade 1980) or after selection (Wyke et al. 1980; Varmus et al. 1981). Because mammalian cell lines, in contrast to chick cells, grow indefinitely and have a high plating efficiency for ease of cloning, the molecular analysis of avian tumor virus genetics has been aided by infection of such heterologous host cells.

The restrictions that render mammalian cells nonpermissive for

RSV replication are not understood. They occur late in the replication cycle and are readily complemented by fusion with chick cells, as described above. The mammalian cells express *gag* antigens (Bauer and Janda 1967) usually in the uncleaved, precursor form (Vogt et al. 1975), which may explain why budding virions are not seen. *pol* and *env* antigens are not usually expressed in ASLV-infected mammalian cells. Analysis of viral transcription indicates that *src* mRNA is the major transcript (Deng et al. 1977; Quintrell et al. 1980; Chiswell et al. 1982; see Chapter 5). It is noteworthy that only a small proportion of mammalian cells that acquire an RSV provirus become transformed (Boettinger 1974a). These, however, tend to express $pp60^{src}$ and become transformed spontaneously at a frequency of about 10^{-6} (Turek and Opperman 1980).

3. Avian Reticuloendotheliosis Virus

The lymphomatous helper virus, REAV, has probably evolved from a mammalian C-type virus (Charman et al. 1979), although its natural hosts are birds. REAV has a broad host range in birds and in avian cell cultures. Natural isolates of different strains were made from turkeys (Robinson and Twiehaus 1974) and ducks (Trager 1959), and each strain replicates in all the avian cells tested. REAV infection does not cross-interfere with ASLV infection and presumably utilizes different cell-surface receptors. Recent studies (R. Weiss and M. Harrison, pers. comm.) show that REAV replicates in dog and rat cell lines and can act as a helper virus for Mo-MSV.

B. Host Range of Murine Retroviruses

MLVs are classified into host-range subgroups known as tropisms. Restrictions at both surface reception and proviral synthesis define the tropism of MLV (see Fig. 3.10). As with other groups of C-type viruses, phenotypic mixing has been an important tool in determining mechanisms of host-range restriction of MLV. VSV pseudotypes with MLV *env* glycoproteins have helped to delineate envelope tropisms (Huang et al. 1973; Krontiris et al. 1973; Zavada et al. 1977), and phenotypic mixing between N-, B-, and NB-tropic MLVs (Rein et al. 1976) has indicated a role for *gag* proteins post-penetration restriction.

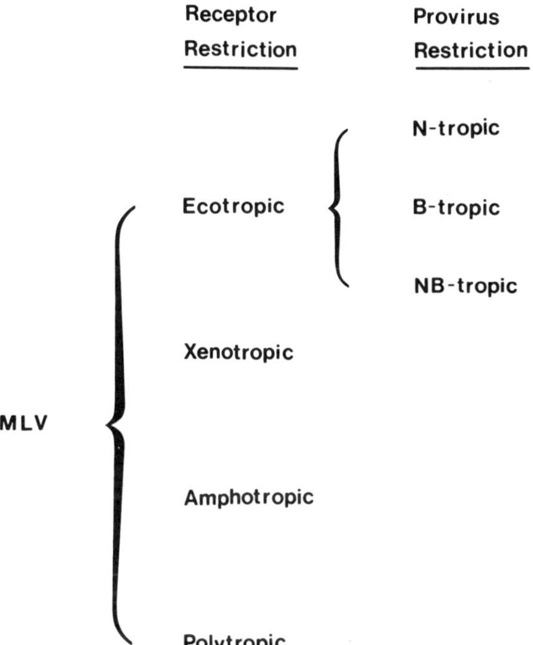

Figure 3.10 Classification of host-range categories of C-type murine retroviruses.

1. Receptor Restrictions

The MLV strains occurring spontaneously in laboratory mice are all endogenous. They have been classified by Levy (1973, 1974) into ecotropic and xenotropic host-range groups, respectively, according to infectivity for cells of the domestic species or of the foreign species. Thus, the efficient replication of ecotropic MLV strains is restricted to mouse cells, although some strains also replicate in rat cells. In contrast to what has been observed in chickens, no genetic polymorphism of cell-surface receptors for MLV has been observed in the laboratory mouse, despite the diversity of inbred strains studied. However, certain cell lines derived from feral mice do apparently contain receptors for xenotropic virus, suggesting at least some polymorphism in the species as a whole. Xenotropic MLV strains are unable to replicate in mouse cells, but they do infect a wide range of other species, such as rat, mink, human, and even quail cells (Levy 1975, 1978).

Certain recombinant viruses between ecotropic and xenotropic strains infect both murine and foreign cells (Hartley et al. 1977), and these are called dualtropic. These viruses utilize receptors for ecotropic MLV on mouse cells and for xenotropic MLV on foreign cells and are subject to cross-interference by ecotropic and xentropic viruses. Dualtropic viruses should not be confused with amphotropic viruses, which also replicate in both murine and foreign cells but utilize different sets of receptors. Amphotropic viruses are represented by some exogenous MLV strains isolated from feral mice in California (Hartley and Rowe 1976; Rasheed et al. 1976).

2. Postpenetration Restrictions

Although all ecotropic MLV strains interact with the same receptors on mouse cells, as ascertained by interference tests (Sarma et al. 1967), there is host-range diversity operating at an early stage of replication, probably during provirus synthesis (Jolicoeur and Baltimore 1976; Yang et al. 1980; Jolicoeur and Rassart 1981) (see Chapter 5). Hartley et al. (1970) first observed that different strains of ecotropic MLV could be divided into three categories according to their ability to replicate in NIH-Swiss (N) cells and BALB/c (B) cells. N-tropic viruses propagated more efficiently on N-type cells than on B-type cells, whereas B-tropic viruses showed a reciprocal pattern. In other words, B-type cells are relatively resistant to N-tropic viruses, and vice versa. Several strains of MLV that had been passaged in laboratories for many years, e.g., Mo-MLV and Ra-MLV, infected both cell types equally well and were designated NB tropic (Hartley et al. 1970). In contrast to host-range restrictions at the receptor level, the resistance of B-type cells to infection with N-tropic virus can be overcome by infection with higher doses of virus. In nonestablished mouse fibroblast strains, MLV titrates in the XC plaque assay on susceptible cells with single-hit kinetics and on resistant cells with two or more hits (Hartley et al. 1970; Pincus et al. 1971a; O'Donnell et al. 1976). However, the response of resistant cells does not follow a multihit pattern in all cell lines (Jolicoeur and Baltimore 1975; Schuh et al. 1976), and restriction is partially abrogated by the glucocorticoid hormone, dexamethasone (Blackstein and Kochman 1976).

Tests with F_1 hybrids between susceptible and resistant strains of mice (Pincus et al. 1971a) showed that resistance to infection was dominant for both types of virus. NB-tropic MLV, however, plated as well on F_1 hybrid cells as on parental N-type or B-type cells, showing that NB-MLV is not a mixture of N-tropic and B-tropic viral particles but possesses a distinct phenotype. Indeed, phenotypic mixing experiments between N-tropic and NB-tropic viruses (Rein et al. 1976) indicate that a viral component of N-tropic MLV can inhibit the plating of mixedly grown NB-tropic virus on B-type cells. This component is probably p30 (Gautsch et al. 1978; Tress et al. 1979). There is also some evidence that cellular extracts from resistant cells can affect the plating of MLV on susceptible cells (Tennant et al. 1974).

Further experiments by Pincus et al. (1971b) involving backcross matings showed that host susceptibility was determined by a single Mendelian locus. This gene proved to be identical with the *Fv-1* locus controlling susceptibility to Friend virus disease in vivo (Lilly 1967; Pincus et al. 1971b; Ware and Axelrad 1972; Lilly and Pincus 1973); the alleles for susceptibility to N-tropic and B-tropic MLV are called $Fv\text{-}1^{n}$ and $Fv\text{-}1^{b}$, respectively. The role of the *Fv-1* locus in controlling viral pathogenesis is discussed in Chapter 8.

Two mouse cell lines have been discovered to be equally susceptible to N-tropic and B-tropic viruses. The SC-1 cell line (Hartley and Rowe 1975) is derived from a feral mouse, and the 3T3FL line (Gisselbrecht et al. 1974) is derived from Swiss-3T3 cells. Presumably, these cells express neither $Fv\text{-}1^{n}$ nor $Fv\text{-}1^{b}$ gene products. Both lines are useful for propagating a wide range of ecotropic MLV strains.

As with avian viruses, envelope pseudotypes of MLV can be made in order to study the replication of MLV in cells lacking the appropriate surface receptors. Ecotropic MLV can be introduced into mink cells as a xenotropic pseudotype; it then replicates efficiently in the foreign cells (Besmer and Baltimore 1977; Ishimoto et al. 1977; Levy 1977a). On the other hand, when xenotropic MLV is introduced into mouse cells as an ecotropic pseudotype, there is still restriction on its replication (Ishimoto et al. 1977; Levy 1977a), which is not well understood.

C. Other Mammalian C-type Viruses

The host ranges of C-type viruses of mammals other than the murine viruses discussed above are described in Chapter 2. Only the feline viruses show a diversity of host-range patterns comparable to those of chicken or mouse viruses. FeLVs have been divided into envelope subgroups A, B, and C on the basis of host range, receptor interference, and cross-neutralization (Sarma and Log 1971, 1973; Jarrett et al. 1973); the endogenous feline C-type virus (RD114) differs from the FeLV subgroups. Where cells of a mammalian species are susceptible to infection with a wide variety of C-type viruses (e.g., human, mink, and bat cells), cross-interference tests can delineate which viruses use common receptor sites; this is discussed in the next section.

VI. GLYCOPROTEIN-RECEPTOR INTERACTIONS

A. Virus Interference

Susceptible cells can be rendered resistant to specific retrovirus infection by preinfection with a virus bearing the same viral glycoprotein specificity. This phenomenon is known as virus interference and is caused by blocking the cell receptor. Rubin (1960b) first observed interference to RSV infection in chick embryo fibroblast cultures derived from embryos that were congenitally infected with leukemia virus. Although leukemia viruses replicate efficiently in fibroblasts, they lack the capacity to transform these cells. As they are not cytocidal, they can persist as inapparent infections even when virus is released in high titer. Because leukemia virus particles bear envelope antigens similar to those of sarcoma viruses, excess production of leukemia virus envelope glycoprotein, gp85, competitively blocks the cell receptors that would otherwise be available for RSV infection. If the cells are treated with high concentrations of leukemia virus or gp85 at the same time they are infected with RSV, "early" interference is observed (Steck and Rubin 1966a; Tozawa et al. 1970). The interfering virus can be removed from some of the cell receptors by treatment with neutralizing antibodies or by elution at low pH (Steck and Rubin 1966b).

Cross-interference patterns among chicken retrovirus subgroups have been elucidated in cells initially infected with leukemia viruses and subsequently challenged by RSV pseudotypes bearing homologous or heterologous gp85 (see Figs. 3.9 and 3.11). As interference only occurs between viruses bearing related envelope glycoproteins, virus interference patterns can be used to characterize retrovirus strains into viral glycoprotein subgroups that correlate broadly with

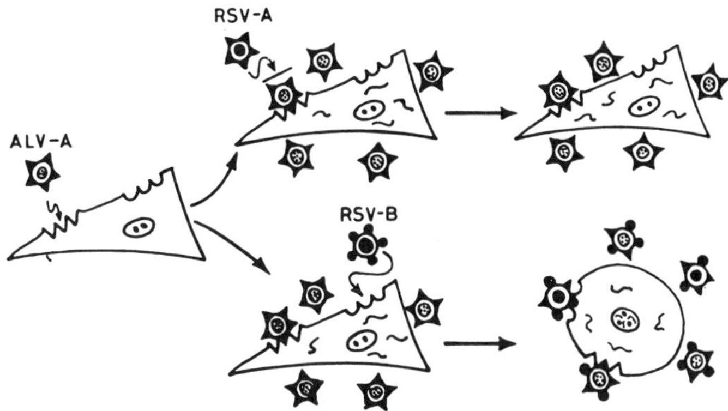

Figure 3.11 Schematic representation of interference to infection with RSV-A by preinfection with an avian leukosis virus of the same envelope subgroup specificity (ALV-A). The cells are, however, susceptible to infection and hence transformation with RSV-B via another receptor. The doubly-infected cells produce phenotypically mixed progeny particles.

the host range and neutralization classifications. Table 3.2 summarizes the interference patterns of chicken retroviruses, among which leukemia virus infection blocks superinfection of RSV bearing viral glycoproteins of the homologous subgroups (Ishizaki and Vogt 1966; Steck and Rubin 1966b; Duff and Vogt 1969; Weiss 1969b). It is notable that reciprocal interference is observed between subgroups B and D, indicating a relationship between the cell receptors of these subgroups; this is also reflected in the partial resistance of C/B cells to infection with subgroup-D viruses (see Table 3.1).

Another interesting feature is the nonreciprocal interference of subgroup-B and subgroup-D viruses with subgroup-E virus (the latter represents the viral glycoprotein specificity of the endogenous-retrovirus-related [*ev*] loci and of the endogenous chicken retrovirus, RAV-0) (see Chapter 10). Preinfection with subgroup-B or subgroup-D leukemia viruses blocks receptors for RSV-E, but preinfection with RAV-0 does not block receptors for RSV-B or RSV-D. It is possible that subgroup-B and subgroup-E viruses use the same cell receptors, but that subgroup-B viruses have a much stronger affinity for the cell receptors and thereby displace subgroup-E viral glycoprotein. A common cell receptor for these subgroups would also explain why all chicken cells that are genetically resistant to subgroup B are also resistant to subgroup E, but not vice versa. Several

Table 3.2 Receptor-interference patterns among chicken retroviruses

Subgroup of preinfecting interfering leukemia virus	Subgroup of challenging sarcoma virus				
	A	*B*	*C*	*D*	*E*
A	I[a]	–[b]	–	–	–
B	–	I	–	I	I
C	–	–	I	–	–
D	–	I	–	I	I
E	–	–	–	–	I

Interference patterns are discerned by preinfecting chick embryo fibroblasts bearing appropriate receptors with ALV of the envelope subgroups A–E. Two weeks later, the cultures are challenged with RSV of the same subgroups. In the infected cultures, ALV will block receptors for RSV bearing homologous *env* glycoprotein gp85; hence, there will be no infection by RSV, and no foci of RSV-transformed cells will develop. The absence of RSV foci in ALV-infected cells is called interference. Where the ALV interferes with infection by RSV, it may be assumed that viruses utilize the same cell-surface receptors.

[a]I indicates interference.

[b]– indicates no interference.

other species of galliform birds, however, are susceptible to RSV-E but resistant to RSV-B; the genetics of subgroup-E cell receptors is complex (see Section VI.D.). Cell-surface receptor sites probably consist of more than one protein subunit, in which case a model for nonreciprocal interference can be built upon viral glycoprotein interactions with homodimer and heterodimer receptors (Weiss 1981). Pseudotypes with the envelope antigens of endogenous pheasant viruses belonging to host-range subgroups F and G show distinct interference patterns, although cross-interference between subgroups E and F is found (Fujita et al. 1974).

An interesting phenomenon is that preinfection with ALVs of heterologous subgroups in some cases enhances, rather than interferes with, subsequent challenge by RSV (Hanafusa and Hanafusa

1968). In particular, this has been observed with interference to pseudotype infection by endogenous glycoprotein (chf) expression (Ishizaki and Shimizu 1970; Weiss 1973). The assembly of endogenous gp85 onto budding C-type particles of the heterologous virus may reduce the pool of gp85 molecules available at the cell surface, thus diminishing the degree of receptor interference.

Mammalian C-type viruses can also be classified on the basis of the host range determined by receptors. Thus, FeLVs are placed in subgroups A, B, and C by the same criteria of host-range, interference, and neutralization used for chicken viruses (Sarma and Log 1971; Jarrett et al. 1973; Russell and Jarrett 1978) (see Chapter 2). Similarly, ecotropic, xenotropic, and amphotropic MLVs belong to different interference groups. Studies with MSV (MLV) or VSV-(MLV) pseudotypes show that ecotropic and amphotropic viruses utilize different cell receptors on mouse cell surfaces and that ecotropic and xenotropic viruses recognize different receptors on rat cells (Besmer and Baltimore 1977; R. Weiss and M. Harrison, pers. comm.). The various strains of ecotropic MLV, however, apparently use the same receptors on mouse cells because they are subject to cross-interference (Sarma et al. 1967). Interference patterns have been elucidated for other mammalian and primate retroviruses using VSV pseudotypes (Schnitzer et al. 1977), as listed in Table 3.3.

Viruses with recombinant *env* genes have been described which express dualtropic host-range properties. For instance, MCF recombinants between xenotropic and ecotropic MLVs replicate in both

Table 3.3 Six distinct receptor-interference groups for retroviruses in human embryonic lung fibroblasts

Virus	Interference group
MLV-amphotropic	1
MLV-xenotropic	2
RD114, BaEV, MPMV	3
SSAV, GALV	4
FeLV-B	5
FeLV-C	6

Fibroblasts were infected with retroviruses and subsequently challenged with appropriate VSV pseudotypes. There was no cross-interference between groups (Schnitzer et al. 1977; R. Weiss, pers. comm.).

mouse and mink cells (Hartley et al. 1977), and avian subgroup-B and subgroup-E recombinants (Tsichlis et al. 1980) plate on both C/B and C/E cells. Such *env* recombinant viruses are subject to receptor interference by both parental virus strains.

B. Role of Cell-surface Receptors in Virion Adsorption and Penetration

The processes of adsorption to cells and penetration of cells by retroviruses are not well understood, but it appears that the major specificity of viral-glycoprotein–cell-receptor interaction may occur after the initial attachment of virions to the cell surface. The rate of adsorption of retroviral particles is considerably enhanced by pretreatment of the cells with polycations, such as DEAE-dextran or Polybrene (Duc-Nguyen 1968; Toyoshima and Vogt 1969), which probably act by decreasing the net negative charge on the cell surface and thus diminish repulsive forces between the cell and the negatively charged virions. This treatment is effective for all strains of retroviruses tested, with the exception of certain chicken subgroup-A viruses for which polycations weakly inhibit adsorption (Toyoshima and Vogt 1969).

RSV stocks that lack gp85, either as a result of a genetic defect (Scheele and Hanafusa 1971) or because they have been removed enzymically (Rifkin and Compans 1971), are not infectious. Nevertheless, it is evident that these "bald" particles adsorb to the cell surface (DeGiuli et al. 1975) and that adsorption is enhanced by polycations. Moreover, these adsorbed spikeless particles can functionally infect cells at low efficiency after treatment with inactivated Sendai virus (Weiss 1969a; T. Hanafusa et al. 1970).

Studies with RSV have shown that viral particles bind to genetically resistant cells as avidly as they bind to susceptible cells (Piraino 1967; Crittenden 1968). However, there is a recent report that small differences can be found (M. Notter et al., pers. comm.). Thus, the specificity of the cell receptor probably operates at the stage of virus penetration or uncoating, rather than adsorption, although neither process is understood at the molecular level. Electron microscopic studies (Dales and Hanafusa 1972) following adsorption of high multiplicities of RSV indicate that much virus becomes incorporated without uncoating into endocytotic vesicles, but it is not clear whether these particles represent the effective mode of penetration at lower multiplicities of infection and, if they do, how they eventually penetrate the vesicle membrane. An alternative hypothesis (Piraino 1967) is that the viral envelope fuses with the cell membrane and remains at the cell surface while the viral core is released directly into the cytoplasm. In that case, penetration and uncoating represent one process, which would be the specific function of the receptor site. It would also explain the function of inactivated Sendai virus in rendering cells susceptible despite the absence of receptors. Whereas RSV adsorbs to the cell surfaces effectively at 4°C, penetration appears to be a temperature-dependent event (Steck and Rubin 1966a; Piraino 1967; Dales and Hanafusa 1972). Whatever the mechanism of penetration proves to be, the event can be determined by monitoring when the infecting virus becomes insusceptible to the neutralizing effect of antibodies, i.e., when the eclipse period commences. The eclipse of RSV is apparent within 5 minutes of adsorption at 37°C but occurs much more slowly at 4°C (Steck and Rubin 1966b).

C. Binding of Purified Viral Glycoprotein to Cell Receptors

In contrast to the adsorption of whole virions to cells lacking cell receptors, binding of purified glycoprotein appears more specific. For example, iodinated preparations of the ecotropic MLV envelope glycoprotein, gp70, bind avidly to mouse cells but poorly, if at all, to cells of other mammalian species (DeLarco and Todaro 1976). Binding of gp70 to mouse cells is prevented if the cells are producing MLV, demonstrating that virus interference to binding of purified viral glycoprotein is effective. The reciprocal interference, that of adding purified viral glycoprotein to the cell surface in order to block infection by whole virions or binding of iodinated gp70, is less easily achieved (Tozawa et al. 1970; DeLarco and Todaro 1976). A study of RSV gp85 binding to genetically susceptible and resistant chicken cells indicates some specificity in binding kinetics, but this does not reflect the absolute resistance to infection exhibited by resistant cells (Moldow et al. 1979b). The initial attachment sites for gp85 may not necessarily be identical with the cell receptors identified genetically and in functional tests of infection.

With a variety of mammalian and avian retroviruses, viral glycoprotein binding shows single-order kinetics and is not markedly affected by temperature; binding occurs readily over a pH range from 6.0 to 8.0 and is optimal at pH 6.8 (DeLarco and Todaro 1976; Bishayee et al. 1978; Moldow et al. 1979a,b). The presence of calcium ions in the medium considerably enhances binding, but magnesium ions have little effect. Estimates of the number of cell receptors per cell have been made in terms of the number of viral glycoprotein molecules bound ($\sim 1 \times 10^5$ to 5×10^5 molecules/cell), but it is not yet known whether the cell receptors are clustered or randomly distributed over the cell surface.

Cross-interference studies involving productive infection of cell cultures followed by assays of binding of purified iodinated viral glycoprotein indicate that viral glycoprotein binding is specific and correlates well with interference patterns studied by challenge with viral pseudotypes. For example, amphotropic and ecotropic viral glycoproteins recognize different cell receptors on mouse cells (Hartley and Rowe 1976). On the other hand, the viral glycoproteins of the baboon C-type virus and those of the MPMV D-type viruses apparently recognize the same cell receptors (Moldow et al. 1979a); this may reflect a relationship between C-type and D-type viral glycoproteins, which has also been observed in immunological cross-reactions (Devare et al. 1978) (see Chapters 2 and 6).

The specificity of binding of purified viral glycoprotein to cell receptors should provide a means of isolating and purifying cell receptors, but thus far there have been few reports to this effect (Twardzik et al. 1979; Landen and Fox 1980). Moldow et al. (1977a,b) noted specific binding of solubilized chicken-cell-membrane components to RSV. However, it is not clear whether these components correlated with subgroup-specific cell receptors, as they appear to represent the initial attachment sites for RSV that are present on both susceptible and resistant cells. The chicken is the only host species studied that shows allelic polymorphism of cell receptors for retroviruses. It is conceivable that a single species of receptor molecule is responsible both for initial attachment and for penetration of a specific virus subgroup, in which case genetically resistant cells may have cell receptors that function well for initial attachment but not for subsequent processing of the virion. The initial attachment sites for subgroup-A chicken retroviruses can be solubilized either with trypsin (Moldow et al. 1977b) or with lithium diiodosalicylate (Moldow et al. 1977a). For chicken cells resistant to subgroup-B viruses, trypsin treatment renders the cells susceptible to infection (Linial 1976). This is a curious finding because resistance is genetically recessive to susceptibility (see below), which would not be expected for a trypsin-sensitive factor that exerted a masking or blocking function.

D. Genetics of Cell Receptors

The genetic basis of the specificity of retrovirus cell receptors was first studied in chickens using classic Mendelian methods (Payne and Biggs 1964, 1966; Rubin 1965; Vogt and Ishizaki 1965). Receptor alleles were identified at particular loci that govern susceptibility and resistance. In the mammalian species studied, there is no evident genetic diversity of cell-receptor loci within species; thus, most genetic studies have relied on an analysis of interspecies somatic-cell hybrids (Oie et al. 1978; Ruddle et al. 1978; Hilkens et al. 1979; Marshall and Rapp 1979; Schnitzer et al. 1980). The presence of cell receptors is assayed either by testing susceptibility to infection by pseudotypes of VSV or sarcoma viruses or by testing binding of iodinated viral glycoprotein.

In the chicken, four autosomal loci have been described which govern susceptibility to the leukosis virus subgroups A, B, C, and E; these are named *tv-a, tv-b, tv-c,* and *tv-e,* respectively, *tv* standing for tumor virus (Payne and Biggs 1964, 1966; Rubin 1965; Vogt and Ishizaki 1965; Crittenden et al. 1967; Duff and Vogt 1969; Payne et al. 1971; Motta et al. 1973). In each case, the resistance allele is recessive to the susceptibility allele, so that the C/A, C/B, C/C, and C/E resistance phenotypes described earlier occur only in animals homozygous for a particular resistance allele. A cell-receptor locus for subgroup-D chicken retroviruses has not been described, but the 10^5-fold resistance of C/B cells to subgroup-D viruses represents a degree of resistance regarded as partial only in comparison to the complete resistance of these cells to subgroup-B viruses, as shown in Table 3.1. Subgroup-D viral glycoproteins differ from those of subgroup B not only in recognizing cell receptors on C/B cells, but also in their capacity to interact with cell receptors on mammalian cells (Hanafusa and Hanafusa 1966; Boettiger et al. 1975). Subgroup-E viruses also depend on the presence of *tv-b* susceptibility alleles, and there is still some controversy whether *tv-e* is allelic to *tv-b* or whether components coded by independent *tv-e* and *tv-b* loci are required to form a functional cell receptor at the cell surface (Crittenden et al. 1973; Crittenden and Motta 1975; Pani 1976, 1977). The *tv-a, tv-b,* and *tv-c* loci code for independent cell receptors; *tv-a* and *tv-c* are genetically linked (Payne and Pani 1971) and may possibly have evolved by gene duplication, whereas *tv-b* alleles segregate independently of *tv-a* (Crittenden et al. 1967). The study of receptor genetics has been useful for the selection of leukosis-resistant chicken strains.

The genetics of susceptibility to the endogenous subgroup-E chicken viruses is more complicated, not only because of the unclear status of *tv-e* in regard to *tv-b,* but also because many chicken strains carry a third genetic locus, I^e, which confers a dominant resistance acting epistatically on the *tv-e* susceptibility allele (Payne et al. 1971). The effect of the I^e allele has been ascribed to blocking of subgroup-E cell receptors by synthesis of endogenous virus glycoprotein (Payne et al. 1971; Crittenden et al. 1973; Weiss 1973), as depicted in Figure 3.10. This has recently been confirmed in studies (H. Robinson, pers. comm.) showing that the I^e alleles segregate with the endogenous virus loci *ev*-3, *ev*-6, and *ev*-9, all of which are dominant for env^E gp85 expression (see Chapter 10) . The I^e alleles are the first example of dominant resistance in retrovirus cell-receptor studies. The replication of RAV-0 is also restricted in some C/O chicken cells by recessive alleles at a locus called *GR-E* (Robinson 1976). Not all subgroup-E viruses are restricted by this locus (Linial and Neiman 1976), and preliminary evidence suggests that it may be a post-penetration phenomenon. However, the restriction occurs before or during synthesis of viral DNA (Hughes et al. 1979).

Receptor genes for mammalian retroviruses have been assigned to particular chromosomes by analysis of segregating interspecies somatic-cell hybrids between susceptible and resistant species. Thus, the major cell-receptor gene for ecotropic MLV on murine cells has been assigned to chromosome 5 (Oie et al. 1978; Ruddle et al. 1978; Hilkens et al. 1979; Marshall and Rapp 1979), and the receptor on human cells for RD114 (the endogenous feline C-type virus) has been assigned to chromosome 19 (Schnitzer et al. 1980). Given the diversity of cell receptors for retroviruses and their assumed presence at the cell surface, one might expect cell receptors to act as histocompatibility antigens. However, with the exception of one of the chicken *tv-b* susceptibility alleles, which is genetically coupled with the R_1 erythrocyte antigen (Crittenden et al. 1970), cell receptors have not been identified immunologically. Cells that express specific viral receptors in the absence of major histocompatibility antigens, e.g., mouse embryonal carcinoma cells (Teich et al. 1977), may prove useful as immunogens for raising antibodies specific to cell receptors.

E. Tissue Distribution of Cell Receptors

Cell receptors for retroviruses are expressed on cells in culture that are not always related to the target cells for malignant transformation in vivo. Thus, leukemia viruses will readily replicate in fibroblastic and epithelial cells in vitro, and most cell-receptor studies have been carried out with fibroblasts. Early tests of cell-receptor genetics involved assays of RSV on the chorioallantoic membrane of chick eggs, in which the virus interacts first with cell receptors on epithelial cells.

Some diversity of cell-receptor expression has been discerned in cultured cells. Studies with VSV pseudotypes have also indicated differential cell-receptor expression of cells in culture. Thus, 3T3 cell lines derived from both BALB/c and NIH-Swiss mice are resistant to plating of pseudotypes of MMTV, whereas an epithelial cell line derived from the mouse mammary gland is highly susceptible (Zavada et al. 1977). However, primary fibroblast cultures are also susceptible to MMTV pseudotypes. These results indicate that expression of cell receptors for MMTV is not a specific marker for mammary gland cells or epithelial cells. It is not known whether 3T3 cells do not synthesize cell receptors for MMTV or whether the cell receptors are blocked by endogenous virus glycoprotein or other components. With chick embryonic cells, fibroblasts derived from C/E chick embryos are susceptible to infection by RSV of subgroups A, B, C, and D, but yolk-sac macrophages from the same eggs are selectively resistant to infection by subgroups A and D (Gazzolo et al. 1974). Another study (Teich et al. 1977) used VSV(MLV) pseudotypes to show that receptors for ecotropic MLV are expressed on undifferentiated teratocarcinoma cells in vitro, indicating that such receptors are assembled even in undifferentiated tissue. Thus, the cell receptors for retroviruses expressed on cells in culture have not proved to be particularly useful markers of cell-surface differentiation.

The distribution and expression of cell receptors on the cell surfaces of intact tissues in vivo appear, however, to be more restricted than those expressed in vitro. Binding studies with Ra-MLV (Fowler et al. 1977; DeLarco et al. 1978) indicate the presence of receptors mainly in lymphoid organs and brain. For recombinant thymic lymphoma viruses, receptors are restricted to a subset of thymocytes (McGrath et al. 1978; McGrath and Weissman 1979). These authors have postulated that each thymic lymphoma is a tumor clonally selected by a unique viral-glycoprotein–cell-receptor interaction between recombinant MLV and a cell receptor homologous or analogous to a T-cell immunological receptor. It is uncertain whether receptors defined in this way are the same as those used during infection. McGrath et al. (1980) have isolated monoclonal antibodies to T-cell lymphoma surface antigens that not only blockade virus binding, but also inhibit cell proliferation. If the specific interaction of virus with receptor is mitogenic and allows infection by the virus (and hence synthesis of more viral glycoprotein "mitogen"), then that infected cell and its progeny will proliferate indefinitely. According to this model, recombinant viral glycoproteins among MLVs act as viral transforming genes in cells with appropriate receptors.

Further biochemical characterization of receptors for retroviruses awaits their isolation through affinity with viral glycoproteins or the development of monoclonal antibodies. Such an approach has already been used to isolate a glycoprotein receptor for ecotropic MLV (Landen and Fox 1980). One may surmise that receptors have not evolved merely for the convenience of the infecting viruses but that they surely represent cell-surface moieties with presently undefined physiological roles.

F. Possible Roles of Endogenous Viral Glycoproteins as Cellular Glycoproteins

Many vertebrate species carry genetically transmitted retroviral genomes (see Chapter 10), and the viral glycoprotein coded by the *env* gene of these genomes is frequently expressed at the cell surface as if it were a host antigen. Indeed, the subgroup-E viral glycoprotein of the endogenous chicken virus, RAV-0, was first observed by its capacity to complement *env*-defective strains of RSV (Vogt

1967b; Weiss 1967, 1969a; H. Hanafusa et al. 1970). This viral glycoprotein is found on cultured fibroblasts and leukocytes of wild red jungle fowl as well as in domesticated chickens (Weiss and Biggs 1972); so its expression does not appear to be dependent on artificial breeding and may be advantageous under conditions of natural selection. However, other closely related species of jungle fowl do not carry the RAV-0 genome or related *ev* loci (Frisby et al. 1979), and chickens that lack any recognizable retrovirus-related sequences can also be bred (Astrin et al. 1979). The importance of *ev* loci in the development and life of the bird is therefore questionable, although endogenous *env* expression may affect the response to infection by exogenous ALVs (L. Crittenden et al., pers. comm.). Endogenous retroviruses frequently have a xenotropic host range, i.e., the species in which they are endogenous do not normally express cell receptors for these viral glycoproteins. However, it should be remembered that one must distinguish between a lack of cell receptors and the presence of cell receptors blocked by excess endogenous virus glycoprotein (Payne et al. 1971; Crittenden et al. 1973; Weiss 1973).

The viral glycoprotein gp70 of mouse endogenous retroviruses is commonly expressed on cell surfaces and also represents a major constituent of secretions, such as serum and seminal fluid (Elder et al. 1977). The serum gp70 is related to xenotropic MLV, whereas the seminal fluid gp70 more closely resembles that of Friend, Rauscher, and Moloney (FMR) ecotropic MLV strains. It has been postulated that endogenous virus glycoproteins may play important functions in cell-recognition phenomena during development and differentiation. For example, the viral glycoprotein in seminal fluid could conceivably play a role in the potentiation of sperm for recognizing and fertilizing ova. Moreover, the viral glycoproteins related to xenotropic and to FMR MLV appear to be specifically expressed in B-lymphocyte differentiation (Moroni and Schumann 1977; Moroni et al. 1980). Such functions remain speculative and await further analysis, particularly of host strains containing no endogenous *env* genes.

VII. CONCLUDING REMARKS

This chapter has surveyed the laboratory biology of retroviruses and has outlined methods of isolation and assay. Although retroviruses are relatively homogeneous in composition and genomic organization, they are surprisingly varied in their natural histories and experimental biologies. Their different modes of natural transmission (see Chapter 2), i.e., by horizontal infection, by congenital infection, and by Mendelian inheritance of integrated proviruses, compound the diversity of biological interactions between virus and host. Factors affecting virus replication have been studied genetically, especially the expression of specific cell-surface receptors recognized by the viral glycoproteins, which are necessary for virus entry into cells. The pathogenesis of retroviruses has not been discussed here but is reviewed in Chapter 8, and the molecular biology of transforming genes is presented in Chapter 9.

REFERENCES

Aaronson, S.A. and W.P. Rowe. 1970. Nonproducer clones of murine sarcoma virus transformed BALB/3T3 cells. *Virology* **42:**9–19.

Aaronson, S.A., J.L. Jainchill, and G.J. Todaro. 1970. Murine sarcoma virus transformation of BALB/3T3 cells: Lack of dependence on murine leukemia virus. *Proc. Natl. Acad. Sci.* **66:**1236–1243.

Ahmed, M., W. Korol, D.L. Larson, K.R. Harewood, and S.A. Mayyasi. 1975. Interactions between endogenous baboon type-C virus and oncogenic viruses. I. Syncytium induction and development of infectivity assay. *Int. J. Cancer* **16:**747–755.

Altaner, C. and F. Svec. 1966. Virus production in rat tumors induced by chicken sarcoma virus. *J. Natl. Cancer Inst.* **37:**745–752.

Altaner, C. and H.M. Temin. 1970. Carcinogenesis by RNA sarcoma viruses. XII. A quantitative study of infection of rat cells *in vitro* by avian sarcoma viruses. *Virology* **40:**118–134.

Astrin, S.M., E.G. Buss, and W.S. Hayward. 1979. Endogenous viral genes are non-essential in the chicken. *Nature* **282:**339–341.

Axelrad, A.A. and R.A. Steeves. 1964. Assay for Friend leukemia virus: Rapid quantitative method based on enumeration of macroscopic spleen foci in mice. *Virology* **24:**513–518.

Balduzzi, P.C. and H. Murphy. 1975. Plaque assay of avian sarcoma viruses using casein. *J. Virol.* **16:**707–711.

Baluda, M.A. and I.E. Goetz. 1961. Morphological conversion of cell cultures by avian myeloblastosis virus. *Virology* **15:**185–199.

Bassin, R.H., N. Tuttle, and P.J. Fischinger. 1970. Isolation of murine sarcoma virus-transformed cells which are negative for leukemia virus from agar suspension cultures. *Int. J. Cancer* **6:**95–107.

———. 1971a. Rapid cell culture assay technique for murine leukaemia viruses. *Nature* **229:**564–566.

Bassin, R.H., L.A. Phillips, M.J. Kramer, D.K. Haapala, P.T. Peebles, S. Nomura, and P.J. Fischinger. 1971b. Transformation of mouse 3T3 cells by murine sarcoma virus: Release of virus-like particles in the absence of replicating murine leukemia helper virus. *Proc. Natl. Acad. Sci.* **68:**1520–1524.

Bauer, H. and H.-G. Janda. 1967. Group-specific antigen of avian leukosis viruses. Virus specificity and relation to an antigen contained in Rous mammalian tumor cells. *Virology* **33:**483–490.

Bernhard, W. 1960. The detection and study of tumor viruses with the electron microscope. *Cancer Res.* **20:**712–727.

Besmer, P. and D. Baltimore. 1977. Mechanism of restriction of ecotropic and xenotropic murine leukemia viruses and formation of pseudotypes between the two viruses. *J. Virol.* **21:**965–973.

Bishayee, S., M. Strand, and J.T. August. 1978. Cellular membrane receptors for oncovirus envelope glycoprotein: Properties of the binding reaction and influence of different reagents on the substrate and the receptors. *Arch. Biochem. Biophys.* **189:**161–171.

Blackstein, M.E. and M.A. Kochman. 1976. Inherited resistance to N- and B-tropic murine leukemia viruses *in vitro:* Effect of dexamethasone on the expression of the Fv-1 gene in the congenic strains SIM and SIM.R. *Virology* **74:**252–255.

Boettiger, D. 1974a. Virogenic nontransformed cells isolated following infection of normal rat kidney cells with B77 strain Rous sarcoma virus. *Cell* **3:**71–76.

———. 1974b. Reversion and induction of Rous sarcoma virus expression in virus-transformed baby hamster kidney cells. *Virology* **62:**522–529.

———. 1979. Animal virus pseudotypes. *Prog. Med. Virol.* **25:**37–68.

Boettiger, D., D.N. Love, and R.A. Weiss. 1975. Virus envelope markers in mammalian tropism of avian RNA tumor viruses. *J. Virol.* **15:**108–114.

Boettiger, D., K. Roby, J. Brumbaugh, J. Biehl, and H. Holtzer. 1977. Transformation of chicken embryo retinal melanoblasts by a temperature-sensitive mutant of Rous sarcoma virus. *Cell* **11:**881–890.

Calothy, G. and B. Pessac. 1976. Growth stimulation of chick embryo neuroretinal cells infected with Rous sarcoma virus: Relationship to viral replication and morphological transformation. *Virology* **71:**336–345.

Charman, H.P., R.V. Gilden, and S. Oroszlan. 1979. Reticuloendotheliosis virus: Detection of immunological relationship to mammalian type C retroviruses. *J. Virol.* **29:**1221–1225.

Chen, Y.C. and P.K. Vogt. 1977. Endogenous leukosis viruses in the avian family *Phasianidae. Virology* **76:**740–750.

Chiswell, D.J., P.J. Enrietto, S. Evans, K. Quade, and J.A. Wyke. 1982. Molecular mechanisms involved in morphological variation of avian sarcoma virus-infected rat cells. *Virology* (in press).

Clark, D.P. and R.M. Dougherty. 1980. Detection of avian oncovirus group-specific antigens by the enzyme-linked immunosorbent assay. *J. Gen. Virol.* **47:**283–291.

Coffin, J.M. 1972. Rescue of Rous sarcoma virus from Rous sarcoma virus transformed cells. *J. Virol.* **10:**153–156.

Crittenden, L.B. 1968. Observations on the nature of a genetic cellular resistance to avian tumor viruses. *J. Natl. Cancer Inst.* **41:**145–153.

Crittenden, L.B. and J.V. Motta. 1975. The role of the *tvb* locus in genetic resistance to RSV(RAV-0). *Virology* **67:**327–334.

Crittenden, L.B., W.E. Briles, and H.A. Stone. 1970. Susceptibility to an avian leukosis-sarcoma virus: Close association with an erythrocyte isoantigen. *Science* **169:**1324–1325.

Crittenden, L.B., E.J. Wendel, and J.V. Motta. 1973. Interaction of genes controlling resistance to RSV(RAV-0). *Virology* **52:**373–384.

Crittenden, L.B., H.A. Stone, R.H. Reamer, and W. Okazaki. 1967. Two loci controlling genetic cellular resistance to avian leukosis-sarcoma viruses. *J. Virol.* **1:**898–904.

Dales, S. and H. Hanafusa. 1972. Penetration and intracellular release of the genomes of avian RNA tumor viruses. *Virology* **50:**440–458.

DeGiuli, C., S. Kawai, S. Dales, and H. Hanafusa. 1975. Absence of surface projections on some noninfectious forms of RSV. *Virology* **66:**253–260.

DeLarco, J. and G.J. Todaro. 1976. Membrane receptors for murine leukemia viruses: Characterization using purified viral envelope glycoprotein, gp71. *Cell* **8:**365–371.

DeLarco, J.E., U.R. Rapp, and G.J. Todaro. 1978. Cell surface receptors for ecotropic MuLV: Detection and tissue distribution of free receptors *in vivo*. *Int. J. Cancer* **21:**356–360.

Deng, C.-T., D. Boettiger, I. Macpherson, and H.E. Varmus. 1974. The persistence and expression of virus-specific DNA in revertants of Rous sarcoma virus-transformed BHK-21 cells. *Virology* **62:**512–521.

Deng, C.-T., D. Stehelin, J.M. Bishop, and H.E. Varmus. 1977. Characteristics of virus-specific RNA in avian sarcoma virus-transformed BHK-21 cells and revertants. *Virology* **76:**313–360.

de The, G., C. Becker, and J.W. Beard. 1964. Virus of avian myeloblastosis (BAI strain A). XXV. Ultracytochemical study of virus and myeloblast phosphatase activity. *J. Natl. Cancer Inst.* **32:**201–235.

Devare, S.G., R.E. Hanson, Jr., and J.R. Stephenson. 1978. Primate retroviruses: Envelope glycoproteins of endogenous type C and type D viruses possess common interspecies antigenic determinants. *J. Virol.* **26:**316–324.

Dexter, T.M., D. Scott, and N.M. Teich. 1977. Infection of bone marrow cells in vitro with FLV: Effects on stem cell proliferation, differentiation and leukemogenic capacity. *Cell* **12:**355–364.

Diglio, C.A. and J.F. Ferrer. 1976. Induction of syncytia by the bovine C-type leukemia virus. *Cancer Res.* **36:**1056–1067.

Dougherty, R.M. and H.S. Di Stefano. 1965. Virus particles associated with "nonproducer" Rous sarcoma cells. *Virology* **27:**351–359.

Dougherty, R.M. and R. Rasmussen. 1964. Properties of a strain of Rous sarcoma virus that infects mammals. *Natl. Cancer Inst. Monogr.* **17:**337–350.

Duc-Nguyen, H. 1968. Enhancing effect of diethylaminoethyl-dextran on the focus-forming titer of a murine sarcoma virus (Harvey strain). *J. Virol.* **2:**643–644.

Duff, R.G. and P.K. Vogt. 1969. Characteristics of two new avian tumor virus subgroups. *Virology* **39:**18–30.

Easton, T.G. and E. Reich. 1972. Muscle differentiation in cell culture. Effects of nucleoside inhibitors and Rous sarcoma virus. *J. Biol. Chem.* **247:**6420–6431.

Elder, J.H., F.C. Jensen, M.L. Bryant, and R.A. Lerner. 1977. Polymorphism of the major envelope glycoprotein (gp70) of murine C-type viruses: Virion associated and differentiation antigens encoded by a multi-gene family. *Nature* **267:**23–28.

Ephrussi, B. and H.M. Temin. 1960. Infection of chick iris epithelium with the Rous sarcoma virus *in vitro*. *Virology* **11:**547–552.

Fiszman, M.Y. and P. Fuchs. 1975. Temperature-sensitive expression of differentiation in transformed myoblasts. *Nature* **254:**429–431.

Fowler, A.K., D.R. Twardzik, C.D. Reed, O.S. Weislow, and A. Hellman. 1977. Binding characteristics of Rauscher leukemia virus envelope glycoprotein gp71 to murine lymphoid cells. *J. Virol.* **24:**729–735.

Friend, C. 1957. Cell-free transmission in adult Swiss mice of a disease having the character of a leukemia. *J. Exp. Med.* **105:**307–318.

Frisby, D.P., R.A. Weiss, M. Roussel, and D. Stehelin. 1979. The distribution of endogenous chicken retrovirus sequences in the DNA of galliform birds does not coincide with avian phylogenetic relationships. *Cell* **17:**623–634.

Fujita, D.J., Y.C. Chen, R.R. Friis, and P.K. Vogt. 1974. RNA tumor viruses of pheasants: Characterization of avian leukosis subgroups F and G. *Virology* **60:**558–571.

Gautsch, J.W., J.H. Elder, J. Schindler, F.C. Jensen, and R.A. Lerner. 1978. Structural markers on core protein p30 of murine leukemia virus: Functional correlation with *Fv-1* tropism. *Proc. Natl. Acad. Sci.* **75:**4170–4174.

Gazzolo, L., M.G. Moscovici, and C. Moscovici. 1974. Replication of avian sarcoma viruses in chicken macrophages. *Virology* **58:**514–525.

Gisselbrecht, S., R.H. Bassin, B.I. Gerwin, and A. Rein. 1974. Dual susceptibility of a 3T3 mouse cell line to infection by N- and B-tropic murine leukemia virus: Apparent lack of expression of the Fv-1 gene. *Int. J. Cancer* **14:** 106–113.

Goldberg, A.R. 1974. Increased protease levels in transformed cells: A casein overlay assay for the detection of plasminogen activator production. *Cell* **2:** 95–102.

Graf, T. 1972. A plaque assay for avian RNA tumor viruses. *Virology* **50:** 567–578.

———. 1973. Two types of target cells for transformation with avian myelocytomatosis virus. *Virology* **54:** 398–413.

———. 1975. *In vitro* transformation of chicken bone marrow cells with avian erythroblastosis virus. *Z. Naturforsch.* **30c:** 847–849.

Graf, T., N. Ade, and H. Beug. 1978. Temperature-sensitive mutant of avian erythroblastosis virus suggests a block of differentiation as mechanism of leukaemogenesis. *Nature* **275:** 496–501.

Graf, T., N. Oker-Blom, T.G. Todorov, and H. Beug. 1979. Transforming capacities and defectiveness of avian leukemia viruses OK10 and E26. *Virology* **99:** 431–436.

Groupé, V., V.C. Dunkel, and R.A. Manaker. 1957. Improved pock counting method for the titration of Rous sarcoma virus in embryonated eggs. *J. Bacteriol.* **74:** 409–410.

Hackett, A.J. and S.S. Sylvester. 1972. Cell line derived from Balb/3T3 that is transformed by murine leukaemia virus: A focus assay for leukaemia virus. *Nat. New Biol.* **239:** 164–166.

Halberstaedter, L., L. Doljanski, and E. Tenenbaum. 1941. Experiments on the cancerization of cells *in vitro* by means of Rous sarcoma agent. *Br. J. Exp. Pathol.* **22:** 179–187.

Hanafusa, H. 1965. Analysis of the defectiveness of Rous sarcoma virus. III. Determining influence of a new helper virus on the host range and susceptibility to interference of RSV. *Virology* **25:** 248–255.

Hanafusa, H. and T. Hanafusa. 1966. Determining factor in the capacity of Rous sarcoma virus to induce tumors in mammals. *Proc. Natl. Acad. Sci.* **55:** 532–538.

Hanafusa, H., T. Hanafusa, and H. Rubin. 1963. The defectiveness of Rous sarcoma virus. *Proc. Natl. Acad. Sci.* **49:** 572–580.

Hanafusa, H., T. Miyamoto, and T. Hanafusa. 1970. A cell-associated factor essential for formation of an infectious form of Rous sarcoma virus. *Proc. Natl. Acad. Sci.* **66:** 314–321.

Hanafusa, T. and H. Hanafusa. 1968. Interaction among avian tumor viruses giving enhanced infectivity. *Proc. Natl. Acad. Sci.* **58:** 818–825.

———. 1973. Isolation of a leukosis-type virus from pheasant embryo cells: Possible presence of viral genes in cells. *Virology* **51:** 247–251.

Hanafusa, T., T. Miyamoto, and H. Hanafusa. 1970. A type of chicken embryo cell that fails to support formation of infectious RSV. *Virology* **40:** 55–64.

Hanafusa, T., H. Hanafusa, C.E. Metroka, W.S. Hayward, C.W. Rettenmier, R.C. Sawyer, R.M. Dougherty, and H.S. DiStefano. 1976. Pheasant viruses: A new class of ribodeoxyviruses. *Proc. Natl. Acad. Sci.* **73:** 1333–1337.

Hartley, J.W. and W.P. Rowe. 1966. Production of altered cell foci in tissue culture by defective Moloney sarcoma virus particles. *Proc. Natl. Acad. Sci.* **55:** 780–786.

———. 1975. Clonal cell lines from a feral mouse embryo which lack host-range restrictions for murine leukemia viruses. *Virology* **65:** 128–134.

———. 1976. Naturally occurring murine leukemia viruses in wild mice: Characterization of a new "amphotropic" class. *J. Virol.* **19:** 19–25.

Hartley, J.W., W.P. Rowe, and R.J. Huebner. 1970. Host-range restrictions of murine leukemia viruses in mouse embryo cell cultures. *J. Virol.* **5:** 221–225.

Hartley, J.W., W.P. Rowe, W.I. Capps, and R.J. Huebner. 1965. Complement fixation and tissue culture assays for mouse leukemia viruses. *Proc. Natl. Acad. Sci.* **53:** 931–938.

Hartley, J.W., N.K. Wolford, L.J. Old, and W.P. Rowe. 1977. A new class of murine leukemia virus associated with development of spontaneous lymphomas. *Proc. Natl. Acad. Sci.* **74:** 789–792.

Hatanaka, M. and H. Hanafusa. 1970. Analysis of a functional change in membrane in the process of cell transformation by Rous sarcoma virus: Alteration in the characteristics of sugar transport. *Virology* **41:** 647–652.

Hellman, A., P.T. Peebles, J.E. Strickland, A.K. Fowler, S.S. Kalter, S. Oroszlan, and R.V. Gilden. 1974. Baboon virus isolate M-7 with properties similar to feline virus RD-114. *J. Virol.* **14:** 133–138.

Henderson, I.C., M.M. Lieber, and G.J. Todaro. 1974. Mink cell line MvlLu (CCL-64). Focus formation and the generation of "nonproducer" transformed cell lines with murine and feline sarcoma viruses. *Virology* **60:** 282–287.

Hilkens, J., A. Colombatti, M. Strand, E. Nichols, F. Ruddle, and J. Hilgers. 1979. Identification of a mouse gene required for binding of Rauscher MuLV envelope gp70. *Somat. Cell Genet.* **5:** 39–47.

Holtzer, H., J. Biehl, G. Yeoh, R. Meganathan, and A. Kaji. 1975. Effect of oncogenic virus on muscle differentiation. *Proc. Natl. Acad. Sci.* **72:** 4051–4055.

Huang, A.S., P. Besmer, L. Chu, and D. Baltimore. 1973. Growth of pseudotypes of vesicular stomatitis virus with N-tropic murine leukemia virus coats in cells resistant to N-tropic virus. *J. Virol.* **12:** 659–662.

Hughes, S.H., H.L. Robinson, J.M. Bishop, and H.E. Varmus. 1979. The replication of subgroup E avian retroviruses is blocked at or before viral DNA synthesis in restrictive chicken cells. *Virology* **99:** 437–442.

Hynes, R.O., G.S. Martin, M. Shearer, D.R. Critchley, and C.J. Epstein. 1976. Viral transformation of rat myoblasts: Effects on fusion and surface properties. *Dev. Biol.* **48:** 35–46.

Ishimoto, A., J.W. Hartley, and W.P. Rowe. 1977. Detection and quantitation of phenotypically mixed viruses: Mixing of ecotropic and xenotropic murine leukemia viruses. *Virology* **81:** 263–269.

Ishizaki, R. and T. Shimizu. 1970. Observations on the envelope properties of RSV(0). *Virology* **40:** 415–417.

Ishizaki, R. and P.K. Vogt. 1966. Immunological relationships among envelope antigens of avian tumor viruses. *Virology* **30:** 375–387.

Jarrett, O., H.M. Laird, and D. Hay. 1973. Determinants of the host range of feline leukaemia viruses. *J. Gen. Virol.* **20:** 169–175.

Jolicoeur, P. and D. Baltimore. 1975. Effect of the Fv-1 locus on the titration of murine leukemia viruses. *J. Virol.* **16:** 1593–1598.

———. 1976. Effect of *Fv-1* gene product on proviral DNA formation and integration in cells infected with murine leukemia viruses. *Proc. Natl. Acad. Sci.* **73:** 2236–2240.

Jolicoeur, P. and E. Rassart. 1981. Fate of unintegrated viral DNA in *Fv-1* permissive and resistant mouse cells infected with murine leukemia virus. *J. Virol.* **37:** 609–619.

Jones, P., W. Benedict, S. Strickland, and E. Reich. 1975. Fibrin overlay methods for the detection of single transformed cells and colonies of transformed cells. *Cell* **5:** 323–329.

Kaighn, M.E., J.D. Ebert, and P.M. Scott. 1966. The susceptibility of differentiating muscle clones to Rous sarcoma virus. *Proc. Natl. Acad. Sci.* **56:** 133–140.

Kawai, S. and H. Hanafusa. 1972. Genetic recombination with avian tumor virus. *Virology* **49:** 37–44.

Keogh, E.V. 1938. Ectodermal lesions produced by the virus of Rous sarcoma. *Br. J. Exp. Pathol.* **19:** 1–9.

Klement, V. and P. Vesely. 1965. Tumour induction with Rous sarcoma virus in hamsters and production of infectious Rous sarcoma virus in an heterologous host. *Neoplasma* **12:** 147–153.

Klement, V., W.P. Rowe, J.W. Hartley, and W.E. Pugh. 1969. Mixed culture cytopathogenicity: A new test for growth of murine leukemia viruses in tissue culture. *Proc. Natl. Acad. Sci.* **63:** 753–758.

Krontiris, T.G., R. Soeiro, and B.N. Fields. 1973. Host restriction of Friend leukemia virus. Role of the viral outer coat. *Proc. Natl. Acad. Sci.* **70:** 2549–2553.

Landen, B. and C.F. Fox. 1980. Isolation of BPgp70, a fibroblast receptor for the envelope antigen of Rauscher murine leukemia virus. *Proc. Natl. Acad. Sci.* **77:** 4988–4992.

Levy, J.A. 1973. Xenotropic viruses: Murine leukemia viruses associated with NIH Swiss, NZB, and other mouse strains. *Science* **182:** 1151–1153.

———. 1974. Autoimmunity and neoplasia: The possible role of C-type viruses. *Am. J. Clin. Pathol.* **62:** 258–280.

———. 1975. Host range of murine xenotropic virus: Replication in avian cells. *Nature* **253:** 140–142.

———. 1977a. Murine xenotropic type C viruses. II. Phenotypic mixing with mouse and rat ecotropic type C viruses. *Virology* **77:** 797–810.

———. 1977b. Murine xenotropic type C viruses. III. Phenotypic mixing with avian leukosis and sarcoma viruses. *Virology* **77:** 811–825.

———. Xenotropic type C viruses. *Curr. Top. Immunol.* **79:** 109–213.

Lilly, F. 1967. Susceptibility to two strains of Friend leukemia virus in mice. *Science* **155:** 461–462.

Lilly, F. and T. Pincus. 1973. Genetic control of murine viral leukemogenesis. *Adv. Cancer Res.* **17:** 231–277.

Linial, M. 1976. Infection of resistant avian cells by subgroup B Rous sarcoma virus. *J. Virol.* **20:** 384–390.

Linial, M. and P.E. Neiman. 1976. Infection of chick cells by subgroup E viruses. *Virology* **73:** 508–520.

Livingston, D.M., T. Howard, and C. Spence. 1976. Identification of infectious virions which are vesicular stomatitis virus pseudotypes of murine type C virus. *Virology* **70:** 432–439.

Love, D.N. and R.A. Weiss. 1974. Pseudotypes of vesicular stomatitis virus determined by exogenous and endogenous avian RNA tumor viruses. *Virology* **57:** 271–278.

Machala, O., L. Donner, and J. Svoboda. 1970. A full expression of the genome of Rous sarcoma virus in heterokaryons formed after fusion of virogenic mammalian cells and chicken fibroblasts. *J. Gen. Virol.* **8:** 219–229.

Macpherson, I. 1965. Reversion in hamster cells transformed by Rous sarcoma virus. *Science* **148:** 1731–1733.

Macpherson, I. and L. Montagnier. 1964. Agar suspension culture for the selective assay of cells transformed by polyoma virus. *Virology* **23:** 291–294.

Manaker, R.A. and V. Groupé. 1956. Discrete foci of altered chicken embryo cells associated with Rous sarcoma virus in tissue culture. *Virology* **2:** 838–840.

Markham, P.D., W. Dodge, S.Z. Salahuddin, and R.E. Gallagher. 1978. An *in vitro* transformation assay for SiSV-1 and HL23V using feline embryonic fibroblasts. *Proc. Soc. Exp. Biol. Med.* **157:** 312–318.

Marshall, T.H. and U.R. Rapp. 1979. Genes controlling receptors for ecotropic and xenotropic type C virus in *Mus cervicolor* and *Mus musculus*. *J. Virol.* **29:** 501–506.

Martin, G.S., S. Venuta, M. Weber, and H. Rubin. 1971. Temperature-dependent alterations in sugar transport in cells infected by a temperature-sensitive mutant of Rous sarcoma virus. *Proc. Natl. Acad. Sci.* **68:** 2739–2741.

McGrath, M.S. and I.L. Weissman. 1979. AKR leukemogenesis: Identification and biological significance of thymic lymphoma receptors for AKR retroviruses. *Cell* **17:** 65–75.

McGrath, M.S., E. Pillemer, and I.L. Weissman. 1980. Murine leukaemogenesis: Monoclonal antibodies to T-cell determinants arrest T-lymphoma cell proliferation. *Nature* **285:** 259–261.

McGrath, M.S., A. Decleve, M. Lieberman, H.S. Kaplan, and I.L. Weissman. 1978. Specificity of cell surface virus receptors on radiation leukemia virus and radiation-induced thymic lymphomas. *J. Virol.* **28:** 819–827.

Moldow, C.F., M. McGrath, and C. Peterson. 1977a. Solubilization of initial attachment site activity for avian tumour viruses with lithium diiodosalicylate. *Proc. Soc. Exp. Biol. Med.* **154:** 201–205.

Moldow, C.F., R.S. Kauffman, S.G. Devare, and J.R. Stephenson. 1979a. Type-C and type-D primate retrovirus envelope glycoproteins bind common cellular receptor sites. *Virology* **98:** 373–384.

Moldow, C.F., P. Volberding, M. McGrath, and J.J. Lee. 1977b. Avian tumour virus interactions with chicken fibroblast membranes: Partial characterization of initial attachment site activity. *J. Gen. Virol.* **37:** 385–398.

Moldow, C.F., F.H. Reynolds, Jr., J. Lake, K. Lundberg, and J.R. Stephenson. 1979b. Avian sarcoma virus envelope glycoprotein (gp85) specifically binds chick embryo fibroblasts. *Virology* **97:** 448–453.

Moroni, C. and G. Schumann. 1977. Are endogenous C-type viruses involved in the immune system? *Nature* **269:** 600–601.

Moroni, C., L. Forni, G. Hunsmann, and G. Schumann. 1980. Antibody directed against Friend leukemia virus stimulates DNA synthesis in a subpopulation of mouse B lymphocytes. *Proc. Natl. Acad. Sci.* **77:** 1486–1490.

Moscovici, C. and M. Zanetti. 1970. Studies on single foci of hematopoietic cells transformed by avian myeloblastosis virus. *Virology* **42:** 61–67.

Moscovici, C., L. Gazzolo, and M.G. Moscovici. 1975. Focus assay and defectiveness of avian myeloblastosis virus. *Virology* **68:** 173–181.

Motta, J.V., L.B. Crittenden, and W.O. Pollard. 1973. The inheritance of resistance to subgroup C leukosis-sarcoma virus in New Hampshire chickens. *Poultry Sci.* **52:** 578–586.

Munroe, J.S. and W.F. Windle. 1963. Tumors induced in primates by chicken sarcoma virus. *Science* **140:** 1415–1416.

Nexo, B.A. 1977. A plaque assay for murine leukemia virus using enzyme-coupled antibodies. *Virology* **77:** 849–852.

O'Donnell, P.V., C.J. Deitch, and T. Pincus. 1976. Multiplicity-dependent kinetics of murine leukemia virus infection in Fv-1-sensitive and Fv-1-resistant cells. *Virology* **73:** 23–35.

Oie, H.K., A.F. Gazdar, P.A. Lalley, E.K. Russell, J.D. Minna, J. DeLarco, G.J. Todaro, and U. Francke. 1978. Mouse chromosome 5 codes for ecotropic murine leukaemia virus cell-surface receptor. *Nature* **274:** 60–62.

Pacifici, M., D. Boettiger, K. Roby, and H. Holtzer. 1977. Transformation of chondroblasts by Rous sarcoma virus and synthesis of the sulfated proteoglycan matrix. *Cell* **11:** 891–899.

Pani, P.K. 1976. Further studies in genetic resistance of fowl to RSV(RAV 0): Evidence for interaction between independently segregating tumour virus *b* and tumour virus *e* genes. *J. Gen. Virol.* **32:** 441–453.

———. 1977. Evidence for complementary action of *tvb* and *tve* genes that control susceptibility to subgroup E RNA tumor virus in chickens. *J. Gen. Virol.* **37:** 639–646.

Parkman, R., J.A. Levy, and R.C. Ting. 1970. Murine sarcoma virus: The question of defectiveness. *Science* **168:** 387–389.

Payne, L.N. and P.M. Biggs. 1964. Differences between highly inbred lines of chickens in the response to Rous sarcoma virus of the chorioallantoic membrane and of embryonic cells in tissue culture. *Virology* **24:** 610–616.

———. 1966. Genetic basis of cellular susceptibility to the Schmidt-Ruppin and Harris strains of Rous sarcoma virus. *Virology* **29:** 190–198.

Payne, L.N. and P.K. Pani. 1971. Evidence for linkage between genetic loci controlling response of fowl to subgroup A and subgroup C sarcoma viruses. *J. Gen. Virol.* **13:**253–259.

Payne, L.N., P.K. Pani, and R.A. Weiss. 1971. A dominant epistatic gene which inhibits cellular susceptibility to RSV(RAV-0). *J. Gen. Virol.* **13:**455–462.

Peebles, P.T. 1975. An *in vitro* focus-induction assay for xenotropic murine leukemia virus, feline leukemia virus C, and the feline-primate viruses RD-114/CCC/M-7. *Virology* **67:**288–291.

Pincus, T., J.W. Hartley, and W.P. Rowe. 1971a. A major genetic locus affecting resistance to infection with murine leukemia viruses. I. Tissue culture studies of naturally occurring viruses. *J. Exp. Med.* **133:**1219–1233.

Pincus, T., W.P. Rowe, and F. Lilly. 1971b. A major genetic locus affecting resistance to infection with murine leukemia viruses. II. Apparent identity to a major locus described for resistance to Friend murine leukemia virus. *J. Exp. Med.* **133:**1234–1241.

Piraino, F. 1967. The mechanism of genetic resistance of chick embryo cells to infection by Rous sarcoma virus-Bryan strain (BS-RSV). *Virology* **32:**700–707.

Pluznik, D.H. and L. Sachs. 1964. Quantitation of a murine leukemia virus with a spleen colony assay. *J. Natl. Cancer Inst.* **33:**535–546.

Poste, G. and M.K. Flood. 1979. Cells transformed by temperature-sensitive mutants of avian sarcoma virus cause tumors in vivo at permissive and nonpermissive temperatures. *Cell* **17:**789–800.

Quade, K. 1979. Transformation of mammalian cells by avian myelocytomatosis virus and avian erythroblastosis virus. *Virology* **98:**461–465.

Quintrell, N., S.H. Hughes, H.E. Varmus, and J.M. Bishop. 1980. The structure of viral RNAs in mammalian cells infected with avian sarcoma virus. *J. Mol. Biol.* **143:** 363–393.

Rand, K.H. and C. Long. 1972. Syncytial assay for the putative human C-type virus, RD-114, utilizing human cells transformed by Rous sarcoma virus. *Nat. New Biol.* **240:** 187–190.

Rangan, S.R.S., P.J. Ueberhorst, and M.C. Wong. 1973. Syncytial giant cell focus assay for viruses derived from feline leukemia and a simian sarcoma. *Proc. Soc. Exp. Biol. Med.* **142:**1077–1082.

Rasheed, S., M.B. Gardner, and E. Chan. 1976. Amphotropic host range of naturally occurring wild mouse leukemia viruses. *J. Virol.* **19:**13–18.

Rein, A., S.V.S. Kashmiri, R.H. Bassin, B.I. Gerwin, and G. Duran-Troise. 1976. Phenotypic mixing between N- and B-tropic murine leukemia viruses: Infectious particles with dual sensitivity to Fv-1 restriction. *Cell* **7:**373–379.

Rifkin, D.B. and R.W. Compans. 1971. Identification of the spike proteins of Rous sarcoma virus. *Virology* **46:**485–489.

Ringold, G., E.Y. Lasfargues, J.M. Bishop, and H.E. Varmus. 1975. Production of mouse mammary tumor virus by cultured cells in the absence and presence of hormones: Assay by molecular hybridization. *Virology* **65:**135–147.

Robinson, F.R. and M.J. Twiehaus. 1974. Isolation of the avian reticuloendotheliosis virus (strain T). *Avian Dis.* **18:**278–288.

Robinson, H.L. 1967. Isolation of noninfectious particles containing Rous sarcoma virus RNA from the medium of Rous sarcoma virus-transformed nonproducer cells. *Proc. Natl. Acad. Sci.* **57:**1655–1662.

———. 1976. Intracellular restriction on the growth of induced subgroup E avian type C virus in chicken cells. *J. Virol.* **18:**856–866.

Robinson, W.S., A.P. Pitkanen, and H. Rubin. 1965. The nucleic acid of the Bryan strain of Rous sarcoma virus: Purification of the virus and isolation of the nucleic acid. *Proc. Natl. Acad. Sci.* **54:**137–144.

Rohde, W., G. Pauli, J. Henning, and R.R. Friis. 1978. Polyethylene glycol-mediated infection with avian sarcoma viruses. *Arch. Virol.* **58:** 55–59.

Rosenberg, N., D. Baltimore, and C.D. Scher. 1975. *In vitro* transformation of lymphoid cells by Abelson murine leukemia virus. *Proc. Natl. Acad. Sci.* **72:** 1932–1936.

Rowe, W.P. and I. Brodsky. 1959. A graded-response assay for the Friend leukemia virus. *J. Natl. Cancer Inst.* **23:** 1239–1248.

Rowe, W.P., W.E. Pugh, and J.W. Hartley. 1970. Plaque assay techniques for murine leukemia viruses. *Virology* **42:** 1136–1139.

Rubin, H. 1955. Quantitative relations between causative virus and cell in the Rous No. 1 chicken sarcoma. *Virology* **1:** 445–473.

———. 1957. The production of virus by Rous sarcoma cells. *Ann. N.Y. Acad. Sci.* **68:** 459–472.

———. 1960a. An analysis of the assay of Rous sarcoma cells *in vitro* by the infective center technique. *Virology* **10:** 29–49.

———. 1960b. A virus in chick embryos which induces resistance in vitro to infection with Rous sarcoma virus. *Proc. Natl. Acad. Sci.* **46:** 1105–1119.

———. 1961. The nature of a virus-induced cellular resistance to Rous sarcoma virus. *Virology* **13:** 200–206.

———. 1965. Genetic control of cellular susceptibility to pseudotypes of Rous sarcoma virus. *Virology* **26:** 270–276.

———. 1966. The inhibition of chick embryo cell growth by medium obtained from cultures of Rous sarcoma cells. *Exp. Cell Res.* **41:** 149–161.

Ruddle, N.H., B.S. Conta, L. Leinwand, C. Kozak, F. Ruddle, P. Besmer, and D. Baltimore. 1978. Assignment of the receptor for ecotropic murine leukemia virus to mouse chromosome 5. *J. Exp. Med.* **148:** 451–465.

Russell, P.H. and O. Jarrett. 1978. The specificity of neutralizing antibodies to feline leukaemia viruses. *Int. J. Cancer* **21:** 768–778.

Sanders, F.K. and B.O. Burford. 1964. Ascites tumours from *BHK*.21 cells transformed *in vitro* by polyoma virus. *Nature* **201:** 786–789.

Sarma, P.S. and M.J. Law. 1977. A comparison of cat and rat cultures for the assay of woolly monkey sarcoma and related viruses. *Proc. Soc. Exp. Biol. Med.* **156:** 480–484.

Sarma, P.S. and T. Log. 1971. Viral interference in feline leukemia-sarcoma complex. *Virology* **44:** 352–358.

———. 1973. Subgroup classification of feline leukemia and sarcoma viruses by viral interference and neutralization tests. *Virology* **54:** 160–169.

Sarma, P.S., R.V. Gilden, and R.J. Huebner. 1971. Complement-fixation test for feline leukemia and sarcoma viruses (the COCAL test). *Virology* **44:** 137–145.

Sarma, P.S., H.C. Turner, and R.J. Huebner. 1964. An avian leucosis group-specific complement fixation reaction. Application for the detection and assay of non-cytopathogenic leucosis viruses. *Virology* **23:** 313–321.

Sarma, P.S., M.P. Cheong, J.W. Hartley, and R.J. Huebner. 1967. A viral interference test for mouse leukemia viruses. *Virology* **33:** 180–184.

Scheele, C.M. and H. Hanafusa. 1971. Proteins of helper-dependent RSV. *Virology* **45:** 401–410.

Schmidt-Ruppin, K.N. 1959. Versuche zur heterologen Transplantation mit frischem und gefriergetrocknetem Material des Rous Sarcoms. *Z. Krebsforsch. Krebsbekampf.* **3:** 26–27.

Schnitzer, T.J., R.A. Weiss, and J. Zavada. 1977. Pseudotypes of vesicular stomatitis virus with the envelope properties of mammalian and primate retroviruses. *J. Virol.* **23:** 449–454.

Schnitzer, T.J., R.A. Weiss, D.K. Juricek, and F.H. Ruddle. 1980. Use of vesicular

stomatitis virus pseudotypes to map viral receptor genes: Assignment of RD114 virus receptor gene to human chromosome 19. *J. Virol.* **35:** 575–580.
Schuh, V., M.E. Blackstein, and A.A. Axelrad. 1976. Inherited resistance to N- and B-tropic murine leukemia viruses in vitro: Titration patterns in strains SIM and SIM.R congenic at the *Fv-1* locus. *J. Virol.* **18:** 473–480.
Shevliaghyn, V.J., T.I. Biryulina, Z.N. Tikhonova, and N.V. Karazas. 1969. Activation of Rous virus in the transplanted golden hamster tumour with the aid of artificial heterokaryon formation. *Int. J. Cancer* **4:** 42–46.
Simkovic, D., N. Valentova, and V. Thurzo. 1962. An in vitro system for the detection of the Rous sarcoma virus in the cells of the rat tumour X. *Neoplasma* **9:** 104–106.
Simkovic, D., M. Popovic, J. Svec, M. Grofova, and N. Valentova. 1969. Continuous production of avian sarcoma virus B77 by rat tumour cells in tissue culture. *Int. J. Cancer* **4:** 80–85.
Smith, R.E. and C. Moscovici. 1969. The oncogenic effects of nontransforming viruses from avian myeloblastosis virus. *Cancer Res.* **29:** 1356–1366.
Steck, F.T. and H. Rubin. 1966a. The mechanism of interference between an avian leukosis virus and Rous sarcoma virus. I. Establishment of interference. *Virology* **29:** 628–641.
———. 1966b. The mechanism of interference between an avian leukosis virus and Rous sarcoma virus. II. Early steps of infection by RSV of cells under conditions of interference. *Virology* **29:** 642–653.
Steeves, R.A., R.J. Eckner, E.A. Mirand, and R.L. Priore. 1971. Rapid assay of murine leukemia virus helper activity for Friend spleen focus-forming virus. *J. Natl. Cancer Inst.* **46:** 1219–1228.
Stoker, M., C. O'Neill, S. Berryman, and V. Waxman. 1968. Anchorage and growth regulation in normal and virus-transformed cells. *Int. J. Cancer* **3:** 683–693.
Strand, M., F. Lilly, and J.T. August. 1974. Host control of endogenous murine leukemia virus gene expression: Concentrations of viral proteins in high and low leukemia mouse strains. *Proc. Natl. Acad. Sci.* **71:** 3682–3686.
Svet-Moldavsky, G.J. 1958. Sarcoma in albino rats treated during the embryonic stage with Rous virus. *Nature* **182:** 1452–1453.
Svoboda, J. 1960. Presence of chicken tumour virus in the sarcoma of the adult rat inoculated after birth with Rous sarcoma tissue. *Nature* **186:** 980–981.
Svoboda, J. and I. Hlozanek. 1970. Role of cell association in virus infection and virus rescue. *Adv. Cancer Res.* **13:** 217–269.
Svoboda, J., O. Machala, and I. Hlozanek. 1967. Influence of Sendai virus on RSV formation in mixed culture of virogenic mammalian cells and chicken fibroblasts. *Folia Biol.* **13:** 155–157.
Svoboda, J., P. Chyle, D. Simkovic, and I. Hilgert. 1963. Demonstration of the absence of infectious Rous virus in rat tumor XC, whose structurally intact cells produce Rous sarcoma when transferred to chicks. *Folia Biol.* **9:** 77–81.
Svoboda, J., O. Machala, L. Donner, and V. Sovova. 1971. Comparative study of RSV rescue from RSV-transformed mammalian cells. *Int. J. Cancer* **8:** 391–400.
Teich, N.M., R.A. Weiss, S.Z. Salahuddin, R.E. Gallagher, and R.C. Gallo. 1975. Infective transmission and characterisation of a C-type virus released by cultured human myeloid leukaemia cells. *Nature* **256:** 551–555.
Teich, N.M., R.A. Weiss, G.R. Martin, and D.R. Lowy. 1977. Virus infection of murine teratocarcinoma stem cell lines. *Cell* **12:** 973–982.
Temin, H.M. 1960. The control of cellular morphology on embryonic cells infected with Rous sarcoma virus *in vitro*. *Virology* **10:** 182–197.
———. 1963. Separation of morphological conversion and virus production in Rous sarcoma virus infection. *Cold Spring Harbor Symp. Quant. Biol.* **27:** 407–414.

Temin, H.M. and D. Baltimore. 1972. RNA-directed DNA synthesis and RNA tumor viruses. *Adv. Virus Res.* **17:** 129–186.

Temin, H.M. and H. Rubin. 1958. Characteristics of an assay for Rous sarcoma virus and Rous sarcoma cells in tissue culture. *Virology* **6:** 669–688.

Tennant, R.W., B. Schluter, W.-K. Yang, and A. Brown. 1974. Reciprocal inhibition of mouse leukemia virus infection by *Fv-1* allele cell extracts. *Proc. Natl. Acad. Sci.* **71:** 4241–4245.

Thiry, L., S. Sprecher-Goldberger, M. Bossens, J. Cogniaux-Le Clerc, and P. Vereerstraeten. 1978. Neutralization of Mason-Pfizer virus by sera from patients treated for renal disease. *J. Gen. Virol.* **41:** 587–597.

Toyoshima, K. and P.K. Vogt. 1969. Enhancement and inhibition of avian sarcoma viruses by polycations and polyanions. *Virology* **38:** 414–426.

Tozawa, H., H. Bauer, T. Graf, and H. Gelderblom. 1970. Strain-specific antigen of the avian leukosis sarcoma virus group. I. Isolation and immunological characterization. *Virology* **40:** 530–539.

Trager, W. 1959. A new virus of ducks interfering with development of malaria parasite (*Plasmodium lophurae*). *Proc. Soc. Exp. Biol. Med.* **101:** 578–582.

Tress, E., P.V. O'Donnell, N. Famulari, R.W. Ellis, and E. Fleissner. 1979. Polymorphism of B-tropic leukemia viruses from BALB/c mice: Association of a p30 antigen with N-versus B-tropism. *J. Virol.* **32:** 350–355.

Tsichlis, P.N., K.F. Conklin, and J.M. Coffin. 1980. Mutant and recombinant avian retroviruses with extended host range. *Proc. Natl. Acad. Sci.* **77:** 536–540.

Turek, L.P. and H. Oppermann. 1980. Spontaneous conversion of nontransformed avian sarcoma virus-infected rat cells to the transformed phenotype. *J. Virol.* **35:** 466–478.

Twardzik, D.R., A.K. Fowler, O.S. Weislow, G.A. Hegamyer, and A. Hellman. 1979. Cell surface binding proteins for the major envelope glycoprotein of murine leukemia virus. *Proc. Soc. Exp. Biol. Med.* **162:** 304–309.

Unkeless, J.C., A. Tobia, L. Ossowski, J.P. Quigley, D.B. Rifkin, and E. Reich. 1973. An enzymatic function associated with transformation of fibroblasts by oncogenic viruses. I. Chick embryo fibroblast cultures transformed by avian RNA tumor viruses. *J. Exp. Med.* **137:** 85–111.

Varmus, H.E., N. Quintrell, and J.A. Wyke. 1981. Revertants of an ASV-transformed rat cell line have lost the complete provirus or sustained mutations in *src*. *Virology* **108:** 28–46.

Vogt, P.K. 1964. Fluorescence microscopic observations on the defectiveness of Rous sarcoma virus. *Natl. Cancer Inst. Monogr.* **17:** 523–541.

———. 1965. A heterogeneity of Rous sarcoma virus revealed by selectively resistant chick embryo cells. *Virology* **25:** 237–247.

———. 1967a. Phenotypic mixing in the avian tumor virus group. *Virology* **32:** 708–718.

———. 1967b. A virus released by "nonproducing" Rous sarcoma cells. *Proc. Natl. Acad. Sci.* **58:** 801–808.

———. 1969. Focus assay of Rous sarcoma virus. In *Fundamental techniques of virology* (ed. K. Habel and N.P. Salzman), pp. 198–211. Academic Press, New York.

Vogt, P.K. and R. Ishizaki. 1965. Reciprocal patterns of genetic resistance to avian tumor viruses in two lines of chickens. *Virology* **26:** 664–672.

Vogt, V.M., R. Eisenman, and H. Diggelmann. 1975. Generation of avian myeloblastosis virus structural proteins by proteolytic cleavage of a precursor polypeptide. *J. Mol. Biol.* **96:** 471–493.

Ware, L.M. and A.A. Axelrad. 1972. Inherited resistance to N- and B-tropic murine leukemia viruses in vitro: Evidence that congenic mouse strains SIM and SIM.R differ at the Fv-1 locus. *Virology* **50:** 339–348.

Weber, M.J. 1975. Inhibition of protease activity in cultures of Rous sarcoma virus-transformed cells: Effect on the transformed phenotype. *Cell* **5:**253–261.

Weiss, R. 1967. Spontaneous virus production from "non-virus producing" Rous sarcoma cells. *Virology* **32:**719–723.

———. 1969a. The host range of Bryan strain Rous sarcoma virus synthesized in the absence of helper virus. *J. Gen. Virol.* **5:**511–528.

———. 1969b. Interference and neutralization studies with Bryan strain Rous sarcoma virus synthesized in the absence of helper virus. *J. Gen. Virol.* **5:**529–539.

———. 1970. Studies on the loss of growth inhibition in cells infected with Rous sarcoma virus. *Int. J. Cancer* **6:**333–345.

———. 1973. Some interactions between endogenous and exogenous avian RNA tumor viruses. In *Virus research* (ed. C.F. Fox and W.S. Robinson), pp. 447–454. Academic Press, New York.

———. 1980. Rhabdovirus pseudotypes. In *Rhabdoviruses* (ed. D.H.L. Bishop), vol. 3, pp. 51–65. CRC Press, Boca Raton.

———. 1981. Retrovirus receptors. In *Virus receptors* (ed. K. Lonberg-Holm and L. Philipson), part 2, pp. 187–202. Chapman and Hall, London.

Weiss, R.A. and P.L.P. Bennett. 1980. Assembly of membrane glycoproteins studied by phenotypic mixing between mutants of vesicular stomatitis virus and retroviruses. *Virology* **100:**252–274.

Weiss, R.A. and P.M. Biggs. 1972. Leukosis and Marek's disease viruses of feral Red Jungle fowl and domestic fowl in Malaya. *J. Natl. Cancer Inst.* **49:**1713–1725.

Weiss, R.A. and A.L. Wong. 1977. Phenotypic mixing between avian and mammalian RNA tumor viruses. I. Envelope pseudotypes of Rous sarcoma virus. *Virology* **76:**826–834.

Weiss, R.A., D. Boettiger, and D.N. Love. 1975. Phenotypic mixing between vesicular stomatitis virus and avian RNA tumor viruses. *Cold Spring Harbor Symp. Quant. Biol.* **39:**913–918.

Weiss, R.A., D. Boettiger, and H.M. Murphy. 1977. Pseudotypes of avian sarcoma viruses with the envelope properties of vesicular stomatitis virus. *Virology* **76:**808–825.

Weiss, R.A., W.S. Mason, and P.K. Vogt. 1973. Genetic recombinants and heterozygotes derived from endogenous and exogenous avian RNA tumor viruses. *Virology* **52:**535–552.

Wolf, B.A. and A.R. Goldberg. 1976. Rous-sarcoma-virus-transformed fibroblasts having low levels of plasminogen activator. *Proc. Natl. Acad. Sci.* **73:**3613–3617.

Wong, P.K.Y., P.H. Yuen, and S. Kaufman. 1977a. Induction of syncytia by Moloney murine leukemia virus in myoblasts defective in differentiation. *J. Virol.* **21:**319–327.

———. 1977b. Mechanism of murine leukemia virus-induced fusion in rat myoblasts defective in differentiation. *J. Virol.* **23:**768–775.

Wyke, J.A. 1973. The selective isolation of temperature-sensitive mutants of Rous sarcoma virus. *Virology* **52:**587–590.

Wyke, J.A. and M. Linial. 1973. Temperature-sensitive avian sarcoma viruses: A physiological comparison of twenty mutants. *Virology* **53:** 152–161.

Wyke, J.A. and K. Quade. 1980. Infection of rat cells by avian sarcoma virus: Factors affecting transformation and subsequent reversion. *Virology* **106:**217–233.

Wyke, J.A., J.A. Beamand, and H.E. Varmus. 1980. Factors affecting phenotypic reversion of rat cells transformed by avian sarcoma virus. *Cold Spring Harbor Symp. Quant. Biol.* **44:** 1065–1075.

Yang, W.K., J.O. Kiggans, D.-M. Yang, C.-Y. Ou, R.W. Tennant, A. Brown, and R.H. Bassin. 1980. Synthesis and circularization of N- and B-tropic retroviral DNA in *Fv-1* permissive and restrictive mouse cells. *Proc. Natl. Acad. Sci.* **77:**2994–2998.

Zavada, J. 1972a. Pseudotypes of vesicular stomatitis virus with the coat of murine leukaemia and of avian myeloblastosis viruses. *J. Gen. Virol.* **15:** 183–191.

———. 1972b. VSV pseudotype particles with the coat of avian myeloblastosis virus. *Nat. New Biol.* **240:** 122–124.

Zavada, J. and I. Macpherson. 1970. Transformation of hamster cell lines *in vitro* by hamster sarcoma virus. *Nature* **225:** 24–26.

Zavada, J., C. Dickson, and R. Weiss. 1977. Pseudotypes of vesicular stomatitis virus with envelope antigens provided by murine mammary tumor virus. *Virology* **82:** 221–231.

Zavadova, Z., J. Zavada, and R. Weiss. 1977. Unilateral phenotypic mixing of envelope antigens between togaviruses and vesicular stomatitis or avian RNA tumour virus. *J. Gen. Virol.* **37:** 557–567.

Zilber, L.A. 1964. Some data on the interaction of Rous sarcoma virus with mammalian cells. *Natl. Cancer Inst. Monogr.* **17:** 261–275.

4

Structure of the Retroviral Genome

I. INTRODUCTION

At the time of the previous edition of this work (Tooze 1973), virtually nothing was known about the organization of the genomes of retroviruses; even their size was a matter of speculation. In the intervening years, a great deal of methodological power was brought to bear on this problem, with the result that we can now describe in great detail the arrangement of coding and noncoding sequences and, to a lesser extent, how they interact in virus replication and transformation. Because the most detailed information is available for the Rous sarcoma and avian leukosis viruses (RSV and ALV) and the murine leukemia viruses (MLV), this discussion will center on these groups, with other retroviruses introduced when appropriate for comparative purposes.

Ultimately, all effects of virus infection on a cell can be ascribed to interactions of the viral genome and its products with the machinery of the host cell. The genome of a retrovirus is relatively small, yet it displays a number of features unique to this virus group, including:

1. replication involving a proviral DNA intermediate, which subsequently becomes integrated into the host-cell genome and serves as a template for viral mRNA transcription by the host cell's RNA synthetic and processing systems;
2. a very high frequency of intermolecular recombination between related viruses;
3. an ability to acquire new genes that encode functions responsible for neoplastic transformation of the host cell; and
4. close relationship to endogenous proviruses in the cellular DNA of uninfected animals, which are passed from generation to generation by classical Mendelian inheritance.

It is therefore not surprising that the genomic RNA itself and its replicative intermediate forms also have a number of interesting sequence and structural features. These include (1) a dimeric or "diploid" structure, i.e., the presence in the virion of two identical subunits in a single complex; (2) a primer for DNA synthesis held in association with the genome by base pairing; (3) posttranscriptional modifications identical with those of eukaryotic-cell mRNA molecules; (4) a short terminally redundant sequence; and (5) the presence of sequences that presumably act as signals for recognition by host-cell transcriptional and RNA-processing systems.

In this chapter, the present state of knowledge concerning the various retroviral genomes is reviewed largely on a structural and comparative basis (Table 4.1). The sizes of viral nucleic acids in this and subsequent chapters are given in nucleotides or kilobases (kb) for single-stranded DNA or RNA and in kilobase pairs (kbp) for double-stranded DNA. Conversion factors to daltons depend on the exact base composition, but, in general, average values of 345 daltons and 330 daltons per nucleotide of RNA and DNA, respectively, give reasonable estimates. Thus:

10 kb = 3.45×10^6 daltons (RNA)
10 kb = 3.30×10^6 daltons (single-stranded DNA)
10 kbp = 6.60×10^6 daltons (double-stranded DNA)
10^6 daltons = 2.9 kb (RNA)
10^6 daltons = 1.5 kbp (double-stranded DNA)

The lengths of some regions have been estimated from the molecular weight of the protein, assuming an average of 110 daltons per amino acid, thus giving the conversion factors:

10 kilodaltons (protein) = 0.27 kb (RNA)
1 kb (RNA) = 37 kilodaltons (protein)

In mature viral particles of replication-competent retroviruses, the genome occurs as a dimer of apparently identical 8–10-kb RNA molecules. Each molecule contains a 5′-terminal m^7Gppp capping group, a 3′ poly(A) sequence, and some internal methyl groups. As with any viral genome, a retroviral genome contains nucleotide sequences with distinct functions, including coding for virus-specific proteins and recognition sites for the various enzyme systems involved in its replication and expression. Figure 4.1 shows these regions identified on scale maps of three studied retroviral genomes, nondefective RSV, Moloney MLV (Mo-MLV), and mouse mammary tumor virus (MMTV). As far as is known, the structure of RSV is unique; all other known replication-competent retroviruses have a structure and size similar to that of MLV, differing only in the lengths of certain regions. Maps like these will be used repeatedly in this and subsequent chapters. To begin, we present a brief glossary of the various regions of the genome:

R A short sequence (20–80 nucleotides) repeated at both ends of the genome. It is presumably used during replication to provide a means for the transfer of the nascent DNA chain

Table 4.1 Regions of retroviral genomes

Region	Function	primary gene product			Approximate coding requirement or size (kb)		
		RSV	MLV	MMTV	RSV	MLV	MMTV
gag	internal structure, assembly, and processing	Pr76	Pr65	Pr77	2.0	1.7	2.0
pol	DNA synthesis	Pr180	Pr180	Pr160	2.9	3.6	2.3
env	surface glycoprotein, cell recognition	gPr92 (Pr57)	gPr90 (Pr70)	gPr73 (Pr60)	1.7	1.9	1.7
src	transformation	pp60	—	—	2.0	—	—
U_3	transcription control?	—	—	—	0.24	0.45	1.165
R	transfer of DNA chain during synthesis	—	—	—	0.02	0.07	~0.02
U_5	?	—	—	—	0.08	0.08	<0.135
PB(−)	binding of tRNA primer	—	—	—	0.018	0.018	0.018
L	5′ untranslated sequence	—	—	—	0.25	0.06	0.16
Total					9.2	8.0	8.2

and DNA polymerase from the 5′ end to the 3′ end of the genome (see Chapter 5).

U_5 Defined as the region (80–100 nucleotides) of unique sequence separating R from the primer-binding site.

PB(−) The binding site of the tRNA primer for negative-strand DNA synthesis. It is complementary to the 3′-terminal 16–19

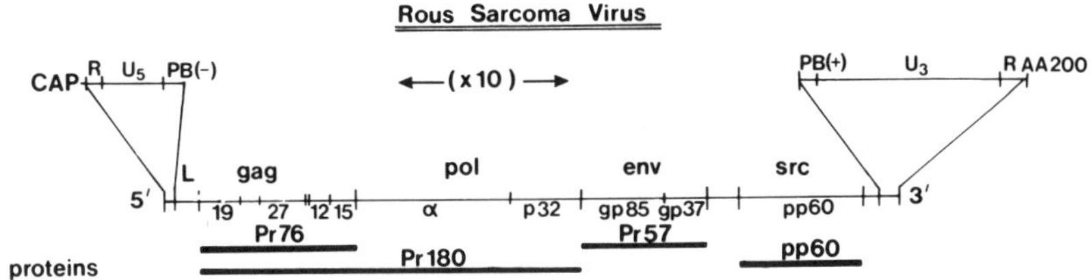

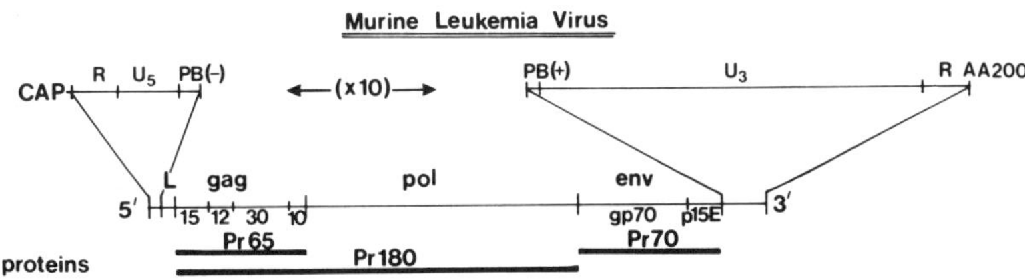

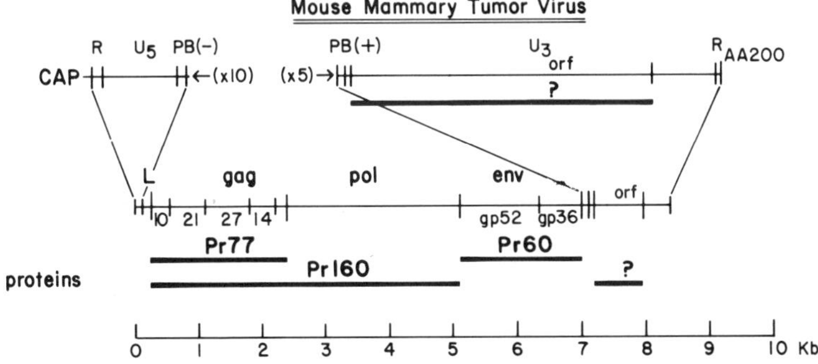

Figure 4.1 Genomes of nondefective RSV (*top*), and MLV (*middle*), and MMTV (*bottom*). The upper lines show the terminal regions expanded as indicated. The approximate molecular weights of the mature protein products are shown immediately below the genomes, with the precursor proteins as solid bars underneath. The various regions are defined in the text. The terminal regions of the genomes are based on their nucleotide sequences, as are the *gag* and *src* regions of RSV. The *orf* in the MMTV U_3 region indicates an open reading frame capable of encoding the protein shown.

nucleotides of the primer (see Chapter 5). For brevity, this will usually be cited simply as PB.

L An untranslated sequence (~250 nucleotides in the case of RSV) preceding the coding region for viral proteins. It may contain a sequence required for packaging of the genomic RNA into virions. R, U_5, PB(−), and most or all of L are part of a leader sequence that is ligated onto subgenomic mRNAs by splicing (e.g., for *env* and *src*) (see Chapter 5).

gag The region (~2 kb) encoding the internal structural proteins of the virion. Translation of this sequence results in a high-molecular-weight precursor polyprotein that is subsequently cleaved to give the mature proteins (see Chapter 6).

pol The region (~3 kb) encoding the virion RNA-dependent DNA polymerase (reverse transcriptase) with its various enzymic functions (see Chapter 5). Translation appears to occur as a readthrough of *gag* and *pol* sequences, resulting in the synthesis of a precursor of 180–200 kilodaltons that is subsequently processed into the one or two *pol* polypeptides (see Chapters 5 and 6).

env The region (~2 kb) encoding the proteins found on the surface of the virion envelope, at least one of which is a glycoprotein. Translation occurs from a spliced subgenomic-size mRNA giving rise to a glycosylated precursor that is subsequently cleaved, generally into two proteins (see Chapter 6).

src Found only in RSV. It is the region (2.0 kb) responsible for the rapid transformation of infected fibroblasts in vitro and is not required for replication. It is translated from a spliced subgenomic-size mRNA into a 60-kilodalton phosphoprotein that has protein kinase activity. Mutants that lack *src* function and most or all of the gene arise frequently during passage of the virus in cell culture and are referred to as transformation-defective (*td*) RSV (see Chapters 7 and 9).

PB(+) Formally defined as the region 5′ to the initiation site of positive-strand DNA synthesis, although the primer for this reaction is unknown. It is a purine-rich region and shows a high degree of sequence conservation among otherwise unrelated viruses.

U_3 The region between PB(+) and R near the 3′ end of the genome and present twice in unintegrated and integrated forms of viral DNA. It varies in length, from 0.2 kb to more than 1 kb in different viruses. One copy of U_3 is positioned to the 5′ side of the initiation site of transcription (see LTR below), and it is thought to contain the promoter for transcription of the genome.

U_5R Sometimes referred to as the "strong-stop" region because a major product of DNA-synthesis reactions in vitro, strong-stop DNA, is a copy of this part of the genome.

LTR The long terminal repeat of the combination U_3-R-U_5 that appears at each end of the unintegrated linear and proviral DNA forms.

onc Describes those sequences, found in some retroviruses, that are responsible for transformation of cells in culture and rapid induction of disease in animals. These sequences are not found in replication-competent nontransforming viruses (albeit these viruses may be quite oncogenic). At least 13 different *onc* sequences, including *src*, have been identified so far. With the exception of *src*, all other such genes are present only in replication-defective viruses, which, although they may lack substantial portions of *gag*, *pol*, and/or *env*, still retain the terminal noncoding regions. Many, if not all, *onc* sequences are closely related to sequences present in normal-cell DNA and are not associated in a linkage with any known endogenous virus. It is probable that *onc* sequences have become part of the viral genome through a recombinational event with normal-cell DNA. The origins and functions of *onc* genes are discussed in greater detail in Chapters 7 and 9.

II. VIRION NUCLEIC ACIDS

A. The Genome

All retroviruses contain a very similar complement of nucleic acids. Phenol extraction of purified virions yields two major size classes of RNA sedimenting at 60S–70S and 4S–5S, as well as small amounts of 18S and 28S ribosomal RNAs and traces of mRNA and DNA (Robinson and Baluda 1965; Robinson et al. 1965, 1967; Duesberg and Robinson 1966; Bishop et al. 1970a,b; Levinson et al. 1970; see also reviews by Duesberg 1970; Temin 1971). On the basis of several lines of evidence, the 60S–70S species has been identified as the viral genome. First, genetic variation in the virus is reflected by changes in the physical properties of the 60S–70S RNA. For example, the mutations giving rise to transformation-defective viruses result in a decrease of about 15–20% in the size of the subunits (Martin and

Duesberg 1972; Duesberg and Vogt 1973a). Second, the 60S–70S RNA of each strain of virus has unique and characteristic physical properties, such as the oligoribonucleotide fingerprint (Fig. 4.2, discussed later). Moreover, although this RNA is not itself infectious, complementary DNA (cDNA) copies of the 60S–70S RNA, obtained from infected cells (Hill and Hillova 1972; Cooper and Temin 1974), synthesized in vitro (Rothenberg et al. 1977; Lai and Verma 1980), or molecularly cloned (DeLorbe et al. 1980; Highfield et al. 1980; Lowy et al. 1980; Oliff et al. 1980; O'Rear et al. 1980), can give rise to fully infectious virus after "transfection" into appropriate host cells.

1. Complexity

When the 60S–70S RNA is gently heated or subjected to other denaturing treatments, the sedimentation coefficient changes to about 34S–38S, that of a molecule of about 8–10 kb (Duesberg 1968; Duesberg and Vogt 1973b). Thus, in its native state, the genome is a complex composed of a number of discrete subunits. For many years the nature of the complex remained obscure. Neither the number of subunits nor their total informational content was known. This lack of knowledge was a major impediment to the understanding of retrovirus biology, since the two possible models, that the genome was haploid (each subunit containing different genes) or polyploid (all subunits identical), had very different consequences for genetics and replication (Vogt 1973). For example, in the haploid model, the high frequency of recombination could have been explained by simple reassortment of subunits, analogous to the segmented RNA viruses. However, replication would have required the faithful assembly of the separate subunits into a complete functional genome complex. According to the polyploid model, replication would not require this additional step, whereas recombination would require physical separation and rejoining of pieces from different genomes. For reasons that are still obscure, approaches to this problem using hybridization kinetics yielded conflicting results, and values for the complexity of the viral genome ranged from 10×10^6 daltons (Fan and Paskind 1974; Taylor et al. 1974) to 3×10^6 daltons (Baluda et al. 1975). Similarly, genetic data could be interpreted in favor of either model. The observation that all subunits of nondefective transforming virus were altered in size by *td* mutations (Duesberg and Vogt 1973a) was most simply explained by the polyploid model. The unexpectedly high frequency of recombination (Vogt 1971; Kawai and Hanafusa 1972) and the absence of certain types of recombination, as between *env*⁻ Bryan high-titer strain, BH-RSV(−), and its helper to produce nondefective transforming virus, were most consistent with the haploid model.

Resolution of this issue came with the application of RNA-fingerprinting techniques. Digestion of an RNA molecule with RNase-T1 enzyme, which cleaves to the 3′ side of each G residue, yields a series of oligonucleotide digestion products, each terminating in Gp. Since the length of such products varies in a more or less random manner, some (representing 5–10% of the total RNA) will be long enough to be unique in the genome. Such oligonucleotides can be resolved by fingerprinting procedures, as shown in Figure 4.2. Because an oligonucleotide generated by RNase T1 can contain only one G residue, the length of such an oligonucleotide, uniformly labeled with ^{32}P, can be unambiguously determined from the ratio of its total radioactivity to the radioactivity isolated as Gp after complete hydrolysis. Similarly, if this oligonucleotide occurs only once in an RNA, the complexity of the complete RNA species can then be calculated from the length of this nucleotide and the ratio of total radioactivity in the RNA relative to that in the oligonucleotide; i.e.:

$$\begin{array}{c}\text{Total number of}\\ \text{nucleotides in RNA}\end{array} = \frac{\text{cpm } ^{32}\text{P in RNA}}{\text{cpm } ^{32}\text{P in oligonucleotide}} \times \begin{array}{c}\text{length of}\\ \text{oligonucleotide}\end{array}$$

Essentially simultaneous determinations of this sort for nondefective RSV gave nearly identical values: 9.8 ± 2.5 kb for the Schmidt-Ruppin (SR) strain (Billeter et al. 1974) and 10.7 ± 1.1 kb for the Prague (PR) strain (Beemon et al. 1974; Quade et al. 1974). Later determinations gave similar values for other retroviruses, such as MLV, reticuloendotheliosis-associated virus (REAV), and visna virus (Beemon et al. 1976; Vigne et al. 1977). Since these values correspond closely to the molecular weight of a 34S–38S subunit, each subunit must contain the entire genetic content of the virus and all subunits must be either identical in sequence or permutations of one another. Because the oligonucleotides have a unique map order with respect to the 3′-terminal poly(A) (Wang et al. 1975; Coffin and Billeter 1976), all subunits must be identical or nearly identical in sequence. These results have been amply confirmed by analysis of proviral DNA. Cooper and Temin (1974), by transfection with sheared DNA from RSV-infected chicken cells, showed that DNA of 6×10^6 daltons was sufficient to yield foci of transformed cells with single-hit kinetics, and therefore that a single 10-kb fragment contained all the necessary

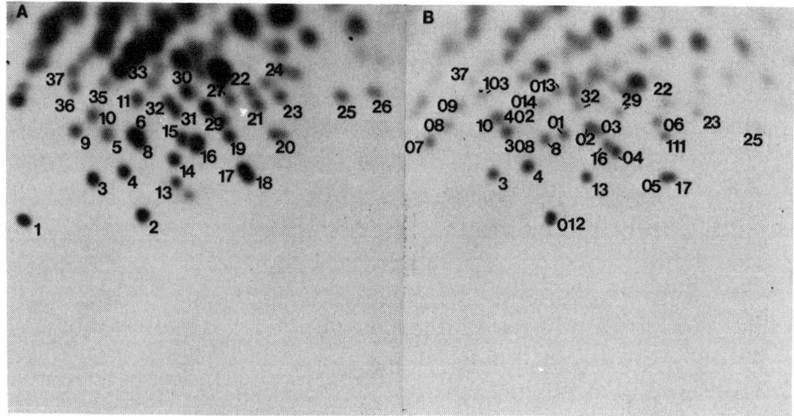

Figure 4.2 Oligoribonucleotide fingerprints of RSV and RAV-0 genomes. Large oligonucleotides derived from the genomes of Prague-RSV (subgroup B) (*A*) and RAV-0 (*B*) were separated by two-dimensional gel electrophoresis. Unique oligonucleotides are numbered, with identical numbers given to identical oligonucleotides. (Reprinted, with permission, from Coffin et al. 1978a.)

information to yield infectious virus. Identical results have been obtained more recently by numerous workers using molecularly cloned viral DNA with which it can be established with certainty that there is a single unique molecule 8–10 kb in length (DeLorbe et al. 1980; Highfield et al. 1980; Lowy et al. 1980; O'Rear et al. 1980). The maximum amount of protein that can be encoded in a single reading frame of a genome of 10,000 nucleotides is about 370,000 daltons, a value that is approximately the sum of the *gag-*, *pol-*, *env-*, and *src-*gene products. These proteins must represent all, or most, of the information encoded in the viral genome and all viral genetic phenomena should be attributable to these gene products alone.

The experiments described above set the size of the genome at about 10 kb but could not be used to provide a precise determination. Most other physical methods, such as electron microscopy of the RNA, are subject to errors of about 10%. Probably the most accurate measurement made directly on the genome is that of King (1976), who used a combination of sedimentation-velocity analysis and gel electrophoresis to arrive at values for a subunit of $3.3 \pm 0.1 \times 10^6$ daltons (9.6 ± 0.3 kb) for the RSV genome and $2.8 \pm 0.2 \times 10^6$ daltons (8.2 ± 0.6 kb) for the MLV genome. These values are very close to those of 9.4 kb and 8.2 kb determined from restriction endonuclease mapping of cloned infectious viral DNA (DeLorbe et al. 1980; Lowy et al. 1980; Shoemaker et al. 1980). Similar techniques have derived a value of 7.7 kb for the genome of spleen necrosis virus (SNV; a member of the REV group) (O'Rear et al. 1980), and a value of 7.4 kb can be estimated for *td* RSV (which should suffice for the Rous-associated viruses [RAV] and lymphoid leukosis viruses as well) by subtracting the length of the deletion from that of nondefective RSV, as described in a later section. These values are used throughout this chapter, and, where possible, previously published determinations have been adjusted accordingly. Precise information on the size of genomes will come from nucleotide-sequencing data as they become available. Some recently available nucleotide sequences (see Appendix E) give values of 9309 nucleotides for Pr-C RSV (D. Schwartz et al., pers. comm.), 8330 nucleotides for M-MLV (T. Shinnick et al., pers. comm.), and 5817 nucleotides for Moloney murine sarcoma virus (Mo-MSV) (strain 124) (E. Reddy et al.; C. Van Beveren et al.; both pers. comm.).

2. Dimer Structure of the Genome

As just described, application of standard formulas for determining the molecular weight of an RNA originally led to estimates of about 10^7 daltons for the 60S–70S RNA genome. However, molecular weights of single-stranded RNA molecules can only be determined accurately under conditions that minimize secondary structure, a clear impossibility in this case. As a result, sedimentation alone was not sufficiently accurate to allow estimation of the molecular weight of the genome complex and, therefore, of the number of subunits it contains. Several lines of evidence strongly favor the proposition that the 60S–70S retroviral genome is a dimer. First, careful determination of the weight of a virion combined with its average RNA content yielded an average value of about 5×10^6 daltons of genome per virion (Bellamy et al. 1974). Second, the combined data of sedimentation analysis and gel electrophoresis gave a value of 6.6×10^6 daltons (King 1976) and equilibrium sedimentation gave a value of 7.2×10^6 daltons (Riggin et al. 1975). The third line of evidence came from the visualization of dimer structures by electron microscopy. Spreading of 60S–70S RSV RNA using T4 gene-32 protein (Delius et al. 1973) showed complex structures consisting, on average, of two 10-kb molecules linked at multiple sites (Mangel et al. 1974; Weissmann et al. 1975). More detailed information concerning these structures comes from the work of Davidson and his colleagues (Kung et al. 1975, 1976; Bender and Davidson 1976; Bender et al. 1978; for review, see Chien et al. 1980). If carefully prepared 60S–70S RNA is subjected to partial denaturation by glyoxylation of G residues (to reduce G-C base pairing), a reproducible structure consisting of two RNA molecules linked by a single joining region near one end is often observed (see Fig. 4.3). The exact position of this joining region is difficult to ascertain, but it appears to be about 300 nucleotides from the end of each molecule. The arrangement of the molecule had a characteristic Y shape, which was originally referred to as rabbit ears. This euphemism has unfortunately lost favor, being replaced by the more prosaic term dimer-linkage structure. Other intramolecular secondary structure features, such as hairpins and loops, are also seen frequently. The arrangement of these features equidistant from the dimer-linkage structure suggested that the joining region occurred at the same end in both molecules. This conclusion was confirmed by

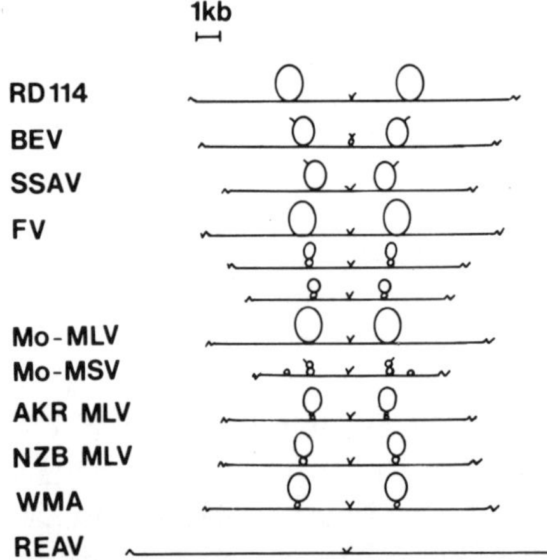

Figure 4.3 Dimer structures of some retroviral genomes. These schematic drawings represent structures visualized by electron microscopy after partial denaturation of genomic RNA with glyoxal and spreading. In each case, a dimer is shown with the 3′ ends at the outside margins and the 5′ ends at the center. Additional reproducible secondary structure features are also shown. (RD114) Endogenous cat virus; (BEV) endogenous baboon virus; (SSAV) simian sarcoma-associated virus; (FV) Friend erythroleukemia virus complex (containing the replication-competent Fr-MLV helper virus and the replication-defective spleen focus-forming virus, SFFV); (AKR MLV) endogenous ecotropic virus from the AKR mouse strain; (NZB MLV) endogenous xenotropic virus from the NZB mouse strain; (WMA) wild mouse amphotropic virus; (REAV) reticuloendotheliosis-associated helper virus. (Redrawn from Bender et al. 1978.)

annealing the viral RNA complexes with SV40 DNA molecules having poly(BrdU) tails to provide a visual marker for the retroviral 3′-terminal poly(A) region. The markers annealed to the RNA end farthest from the dimer-linkage structure; thus, the two molecules in the dimer must be joined near their 5′ ends. Similar types of dimer-linkage structures have been observed for all retroviruses examined, although that of the RSV genome has been difficult to obtain, presumably because it is not significantly more resistant to denaturation than other linkages in the molecules (Chien et al. 1980; Murti et al. 1981).

The nature of the dimer-linkage structure and how and why it is formed remain obscure. In the simplest model, the two identical subunits are joined by straightforward base pairing. If so, then the two subunits must contain a sequence at once identical and complementary. The only sort of sequence that satisfies these conditions is one that contains an inverted repeat, such as:

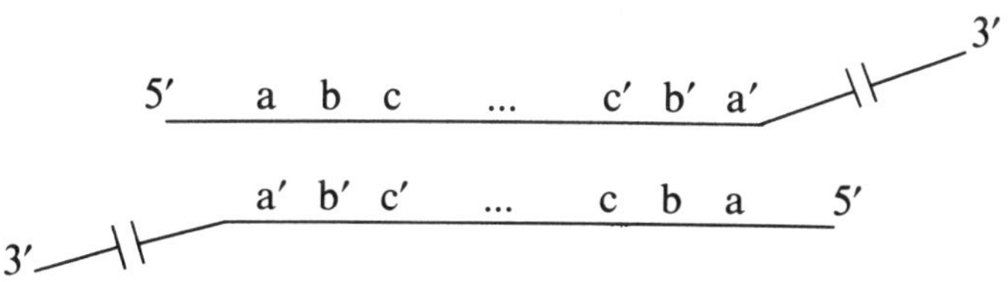

More complicated structures involving interlocked hairpins and small RNA bridges are also possible. From the sequences of PR-RSV-C strong-stop DNA and the $tRNA^{Trp}$ primer, Haseltine et al. (1977) proposed a rather complicated structure in which the tRNA primer could interact with both RNA strands and in which the two RNA subunits could also base pair with each other. A similar, although rather more extensive, structure can also be drawn on the basis of the nucleotide sequence of the 5′-terminal region of the Mo-MSV genome (W. McClements and G. Vande Woude, pers. comm.). These structures are shown in Figure 4.4, but it should be remembered that they are highly speculative and there is no independent evidence for their existence at this time. Another point to bear in mind is that polymerase-deficient mutants of RSV contain no tRNA primer but do contain 70S RNA molecules (Sawyer and Hanafusa 1979; Peters and Hu 1980) (see Section III.B.3).

It is important to point out that the dimer-linkage structure is not the only feature linking the two subunits, at least in phenol-extracted RNA. The 60S–70S RNA prepared from virus that has been aged (by

A. PR-RSV

3′ HO(N)10000
5′ m7G(N)60
tRNAtrp
AOH UUACUUCG
AAUGAAGC
CGAAGUAA
GCUUCAUU
tRNAtrp
5′
3′
10000
3′
L
PB
U5
5′
5′
U5
PB
L
3′

3′ OH(N)10000
5′ m7G(N)60
5′
OH 3′
10000
3′
L
PB
U5
5′
5′
U5
PB
L
3′

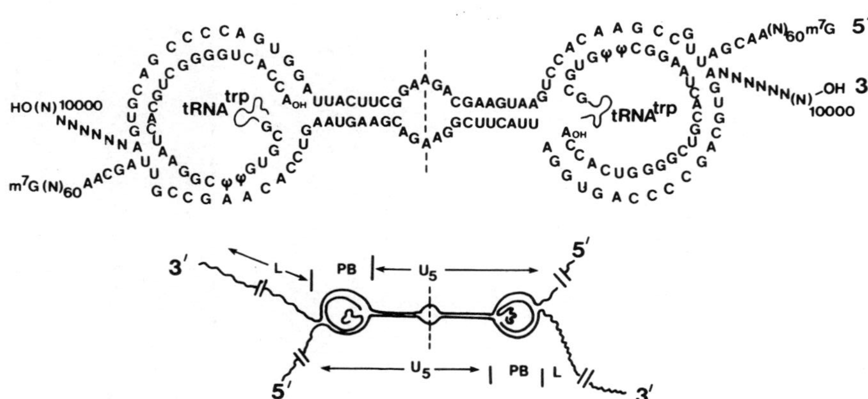

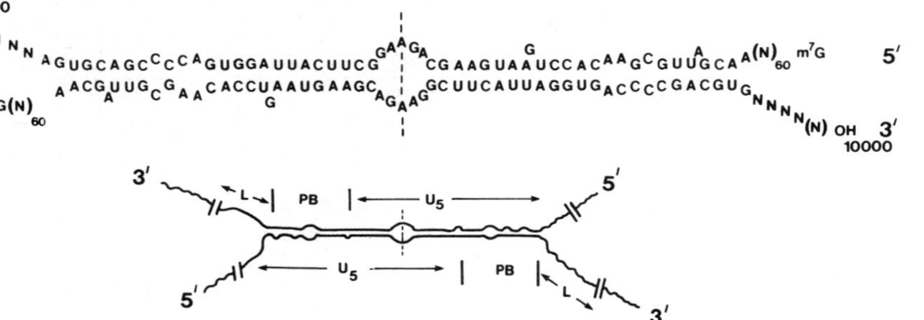

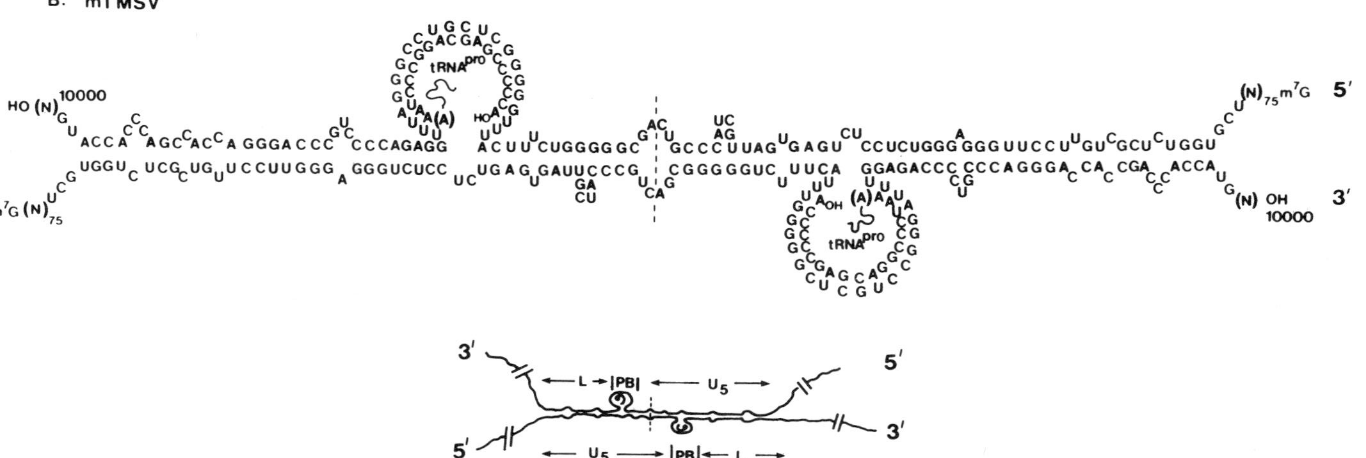

Figure 4.4 Possible dimer-linkage sequences. The configurations of these structures are based on (*A*) the nucleotide sequence of PR-RSV-C strong-stop DNA (Haseltine et al. 1977) and (*B*) the 5′-terminal region of the Mo-MSV genome (Dhar et al. 1980). The line drawings show schematic interpretations. The lower half of *A* shows the predicted RSV structure in the absence of $tRNA^{Trp}$ primer. (Part *A* was redrawn from Haseltine et al. [1977] and part *B* was provided by W. McClements and G. Vande Woude.)

harvesting at intervals of 1 day or more) has a sedimentation pattern indistinguishable from that of freshly prepared virus (harvested every 2 hours), yet is often found to be composed of "subunits" of no more than 8S–10S (Coffin 1979). Therefore, the RNA subunits must be linked at every few hundred nucleotides. Such a structure would be too complicated to analyze by electron microscopy, which requires partial denaturation before interpretable results are obtained.

The mechanism by which the dimer structure is formed has not been established. For several reasons it is currently thought to arise as virions assemble. Attempts to re-form the structure by annealing denatured subunits have not been successful. Also, the presence of 60S–70S RNA within cells has not been reported. Finally, Cheung et al. (1972) and Canaani et al. (1973) found that freshly budded virions of RSV contained 30S–40S RNA and that genomic-size 60S–70S RNA could be found only after incubating the virions for a few minutes. Thus, it seems that assembly of the subunits into the dimer complex is not a spontaneous process but probably involves active participation of some virion component during or shortly after release of the particles from the cells.

3. Significance of the Dimeric Genome

Retroviruses are unique among all virus families in having a diploid genome. The significance of such an unusual arrangement can be considered from several hypotheses. First, the complex series of jumps involved in the process of DNA synthesis may require that certain portions of the genome occur at least twice in order to conserve coding potential of the total genome in the progeny (see Chapter 5). Second, it is likely that recombination requires or is greatly enhanced by the formation of heterozygous virions (Wyke et al. 1975) (see Chapter 7). If so, then a diploid virus that could readily adapt by recombination might have a selective advantage over a haploid virus that could not recombine. Third, a "copy-choice" model for proviral DNA synthesis permits the repair of substantial damage to the genome if the polymerase transfers from one subunit to another as it encounters breaks in the RNA (Coffin 1979) (see Chapter 7). As virions with highly broken genomes are very common, such a mechanism would allow the synthesis of a complete provirus from a badly degraded parental genome. For example, Toyoshima et al. (1980) have shown that genomic RNA is more sensitive to degradation by γ-irradiation than is the infectivity of the virus, suggesting that some repair mechanisms operate.

The physically diploid nature of the genome suggests that the viruses may be genetically diploid. In principle, it would seem a simple matter to test this by infecting a cell with heterozygous virus and determining whether all genetic markers are transferred to the progeny particles. In practice, however, this is a very difficult experiment and there have been conflicting results. Weiss et al. (1973) observed a continued persistence of two *env* markers through several cycles when examining the progeny obtained from mixed infections with viruses of different subgroups. Also, McCarter (1977) found that cells doubly infected with MLV and a temperature-sensitive (*ts*) mutant produced progeny that, on subsequent infection, segregated both markers in the pattern expected for random synthesis of both parental and heterozygous particles. The opposite conclusion can be drawn from titration patterns of replication-defective transforming viruses, such as MSV or BH-RSV(−). If preparations of such viruses phenotypically mixed with helper viruses contain substantial amounts of heterozygous particles, and if both genomes are capable of being expressed after infection, then it should be possible to obtain clones of the infected cells that produce both viruses, detectable as cells releasing infectious focus-forming particles. However, when stocks of replication-defective RSV or MSV are assayed under conditions requiring formation of infectious progeny, two-hit kinetics are observed (Hartley and Rowe 1966; O'Connor and Fischinger 1969; Weiss et al. 1973), indicating that at best only a small minority of the virions are capable of expressing both genomes. Similarly, analysis of integrated proviruses in cells cloned shortly after infection does not support the idea that the virions contain two active genomes, since cells containing only one provirus are often found in such experiments, particularly under semipermissive conditions that limit the ability of the cell to be superinfected shortly after infection (Hughes et al. 1978, 1981b; Steffen and Weinberg 1978; Sabran et al. 1979).

The physical existence of heterozygotes has not been established unambiguously. In the case of a cell doubly infected with two closely related viruses, it is difficult to imagine a mechanism that would prevent heterozygote formation, unless the dimer structure is formed during or soon after RNA synthesis, which seems unlikely to be the case. High-molecular-weight genome complexes from cells coinfected with *td* RSV and a highly defective deletion mutant have sedimentation properties expected of heterodimeric molecules of one 34S subunit and one 24S subunit (J. Coffin et al., unpubl.). With mammalian viruses, however, electron microscopy, e.g., of virion

RNA from cells doubly infected with Mo-MSV and Mo-MLV, did not reveal the presence of heterodimers of one large subunit and one small subunit, although a single high-molecular-weight complex containing both subunits could be observed by gel electrophoresis (Maisel et al. 1978). It should be noted that there is as yet no evidence for recombination of MSV with its helper, and in the avian system where frequent recombination has been observed, heterodimers have not been observed by electron microscopy, since, as mentioned above, it has been repeatedly difficult to observe any dimer-linkage structures with avian viruses.

There is yet no clear resolution of this issue, but several possibilities arise. For example, virions with one complete subunit and one broken subunit should only be able to synthesize only one complete (although perhaps recombinant) provirus. In many preparations of virus, such virions might be quite frequent. Furthermore, their frequency could be quite variable, depending on the type of virus studied or its prior treatment; repeated freezing and thawing and long harvest intervals, for example, are likely to increase the proportion of degraded genomes. It is also possible that some pairs of viruses are capable of forming heterozygotes but that others are not. It could be imagined that it might be selectively advantageous for a replication-defective transforming virus like Mo-MSV not to recombine with its helper and therefore not to form heterozygotes.

4. *Resemblance of the Genome to mRNA Molecules*

The 34S–38S genomic subunits of retroviruses have several chemical modifications similar to those of eukaryotic-cell mRNA: (1) There is a poly(A) sequence of approximately 200 residues at the 3′ terminus (Gillespie et al. 1972; Horst et al. 1972; Lai and Duesberg 1972) and the exact 3′ terminus is A_{OH} (Keith et al. 1974). Since there is no corresponding A-T tract in the provirus, the addition of poly(A) must be posttranscriptional. (2) As with most eukaryotic mRNAs, the 5′ terminus of each molecule is modified with a typical capping group: the terminal virus-coded residue (G in both RSV and MLV) is methylated at the 2′ position of the ribose and 7-methyl GTP is added via a 5′-5′ triphosphate linkage, giving the structure $m^7G^{5'}ppp^{5'}Gm$ (Furuichi et al. 1975a; Keith and Fraenkel-Conrat 1975; Rose et al. 1976). As far as can be determined, all genomes in virions have both modifications. In cases (as in PR-RSV) where the capping group is found on a large RNase-T1-resistant oligonucleotide, no significant amount (less than 5%) of the corresponding uncapped oligonucleotide can be found; also, the 30–40% of apparently full-length genomes that do not bind to poly(U) or oligo(dT) columns can be attributed to genomes with breaks near the 3′ end (King and Wells 1976). (3) In addition to the terminal modifications, genomic RNA molecules contain internal methyl groups. In RSV RNA, all or nearly all are in 10–12 N^6-methyl adenosine (m^6A) residues (Furuichi et al. 1975a; Stoltzfus and Dimock 1976), which seem to be clustered in the 3′ third of the genome (Beemon and Keith 1976). Again, the presence of m^6A residues is a feature of eukaryotic RNAs and of mRNAs of DNA viruses that replicate in the nucleus (Furuichi et al. 1975b). As is the case with cellular mRNAs, the function of these modifications is not clearly understood, although it is generally believed that the capping group is essential for correct ribosome binding and is therefore a signal for the initiation of translation. Neither the terminal Gm nor the internal methylations are absolutely essential for replication, as growth of RSV-infected cells in cycloleucine, which inhibits these modifications (with the exception of m^7G addition), does not greatly reduce the yield of virus (Dimock and Stoltzfus 1978). As discussed below, the poly(A) and cap have proved to be very useful experimentally, providing specific markers and means of isolating 3′ and 5′ ends of the genome, respectively.

B. Other Virion RNAs

1. rRNA and tRNA Molecules

Even in highly purified virions, only about half the RNA by weight is in the genome. The remainder is in smaller species, most of which are host-specific (for review, see Taylor 1977). These include variable small amounts of 18S and 28S rRNAs (Bishop et al. 1970a,b), as well as 5S and 7S RNAs identical with species found in ribosomes from uninfected cells (Erikson et al. 1973; Walker et al. 1974). A small amount of host DNA can also be found (Levinson et al. 1970, 1972). In view of their low and variable amounts, it is unlikely that these molecules serve a function in the virus replicative cycle. In contrast, virions of Rous sarcoma and other retroviruses contain about 125 molecules of 4S RNA per virion, composed largely of host tRNA (Erikson and Erikson 1970, 1971; Faras et al. 1973). Most of the small RNAs do not cosediment with the genome; but about 20% of the 4S and 5S RNAs is found in weak association with the 60S–70S genome complex (Canaani and Duesberg 1972; Faras et al. 1973). Of the ten or so molecules of 70S-associated 4S and 5S RNAs, only one, the tRNA primer (see Section III.B.3), is known to play any significant role in the virus life cycle. The remainder of both the free and 70S-associated 4S RNAs seems to represent a collection of host tRNAs with no defined function for the virus and may merely be accidental inclusions in the virion. Some specificity exists, however, since the amino-acylation pattern of both total virion and 70S-associated tRNA (Waters et al. 1975) and the pattern of iso-accepting methionyl tRNA (Elder and Smith 1974) are quite different from those of the cell. The basis of such selectivity is not clear but may reflect fortuitous base pairing of tRNAs with complementary regions of the genome, the local tRNA composition in the cell near the site of budding, or the affinity of the tRNAs for some specific virion component, such as reverse transcriptase (Peters and Hu 1980). However, the phenomenon cannot be determined by the virion RNA per se, as MLV particles released from actinomycin-D-treated cells contain no 70S RNA but do contain small RNAs similar in composition to infectious MLV particles (Levin and Seidman 1979). Also, different viruses (e.g., REAV and RSV) grown in the same cell types show different and specific tRNA compositions (Sawyer and Hanafusa 1979; Peters and Glover 1980b). In the RSV and ALV systems, the selectivity of the free 4S RNA is apparently determined by the virion DNA polymerase (Sawyer and Hanafusa 1979; Peters and Hu 1980).

2. mRNA Molecules

RNAs with messenger activity of both cellular and viral origins can also be detected in virions. With the exception of *gag* and *gag-pol* mRNAs, which are similar to, or identical with, the genomes, such RNAs are in low amounts. For example, Ikawa et al. (1974) found that virus released from Friend erythroleukemia virus (FEV) tumor cells that had been induced to differentiate contained detectable globin mRNA both free and complexed with 60S–70S RNA. The amounts of this RNA were very small, about 1 copy per 10^3–10^4 genomes. A more abundant cell-derived mRNA species has been found in virions of RSV that can be translated into a protein of 34,000 daltons (Adkins and Hunter 1980). Furthermore, subgenomic

RNAs capable of directing the synthesis of authentic *env*-gene and *src*-gene products in vitro can also be detected in mature RSV particles (Purchio et al. 1977; Beemon and Hunter 1978; Pawson et al. 1980), as can species that direct the synthesis of presumably fragmentary proteins not found in infected cells (Beemon and Hunter 1977; Kamine et al. 1978). Since fragments derived by partial cleavage of full-length genomic RNA will also direct the synthesis of similar polypeptides (Purchio et al. 1978), it is likely that much of the activity detected is due to fragmented genomes that are present in virions. However, small amounts of authentic *env* mRNA are apparently present in virions; microinjection of 21S virion RNA into the cytoplasm of cells infected with *env*⁻ virus leads to the synthesis of biologically active *env*-gene product, whereas injection of 21S fragments of genomic RNA does not have any effect (Stacey and Hanafusa 1978; Stacey 1979). The active RNA is most likely present in association with the 60S–70S complex. The amount of such mRNA must be quite small, as it is not detected by physical techniques in RSV virions, in spite of the presence of abundant copies in the infected cell.

3. *tRNA Primer*

Of all the small 70S-associated RNA molecules, the one most tightly associated with the genome is a single molecule per genome of tRNA, which has been identified as the primer for DNA synthesis (see Chapter 5). The thermal stability of the association of primer tRNA with the genome is higher than those of the other 70S-associated tRNAs and of the 70S complex itself (Canaani and Duesberg 1972), a feature that has been used to purify and characterize the primer. Three primer tRNAs have now been identified, and their nucleotide sequences have been determined: $tRNA^{Trp}$ (in RSV and ALV), $tRNA^{Pro}_{1+2}$ (in MLV, REAV, and probably feline leukemia virus [FeLV], and simian sarcoma-associated virus [SSAV] as well), and $tRNA^{Lys}_{3}$ (in MMTV) (Dahlberg et al. 1974; Faras et al. 1974; Harada et al. 1975, 1979; Waters 1975; Waters et al. 1975; Peters et al. 1977; Waters and Mullin 1977; Peters and Glover 1980a,b). The nucleotide sequences of these primer tRNAs are shown in the Appendix.

Details of the interaction between the tRNA primer and the genome can be found in Chapter 5. Briefly, the tRNA molecules associate with the genomic RNA by base pairing of the 3′-terminal 16–19 nucleotides of the primer (Cordell et al. 1976; Eiden et al. 1976;

Peters et al. 1977) with a complementary sequence in the genome, referred to as the primer-binding site, PB(−), located 100–200 nucleotides from the 5′ end of the genome.

C. Specificity of Virion RNAs

The results described in the preceding sections imply that there must be a distinct selectivity of RNAs in the assembly of virions; genomic RNAs are strongly preferred over cellular RNAs and subgenomic viral mRNAs. This selectivity is not absolute, however. In at least two cases, viral particles that lack genomic RNA can be obtained. First, Levin et al. (1974) found that if MLV-infected cells were treated with actinomycin D to inhibit viral RNA synthesis, particles lacking genomes would be synthesized for some time. Second, Linial et al. (1978) obtained a mutant of RSV, SE21Q1b, that synthesizes particles with a full complement of viral proteins, yet the particles contain a collection of cellular RNAs and only about 1% genomic RNA (or about the same proportion as in the infected cell) (Gallis et al. 1979) (see Chapter 7). The genome of this mutant has a small deletion in the L region (Shank and Linial 1980), and it can be inferred that this region contains a site necessary for recognition of the genomic RNA by some virion structural element during the assembly process. It can be further concluded that the assembly of particles does not require the genome, and that in its absence, other RNA molecules may be substituted. Since genome-containing virions can be synthesized by cells infected with viruses like BH-RSV(−)α, which lacks both functional *env* and *pol* genes (Hanafusa and Hanafusa 1971; Hanafusa et al. 1972), the specificity for recognition of the genome most likely resides in one of the *gag*-gene products or the corresponding region of the *gag* precursor (Bolognesi et al. 1978; Wong et al. 1980), possibly p19 in RSV or p12 in MLV, both of which specifically bind to their respective genomes (Sen et al. 1976, 1978; Sen and Todaro 1977; Leis et al. 1978) (see Chapter 6).

In contrast to the genome, packaging of the specific tRNA primer into virions seems to involve the reverse transcriptase molecule. Sawyer and Hanafusa (1979) found that virions synthesized by cells infected with the *env⁻pol⁻* variant of BH-RSV contained the usual complement of low-molecular-weight RNAs, except that the $tRNA^{Trp}$ primer was absent. Also, the reverse transcriptase of avian myeloblastosis virus (AMV) specifically binds $tRNA^{Trp}$ with much higher affinity than other virion or cellular tRNAs (Panet et al. 1975; Peters and Hu 1980), although similar specificity has not been demonstrated for MLV reverse transcriptase (Panet and Berliner 1978). Nonetheless, it seems probable that binding to reverse transcriptase is an important mechanism for packaging of the tRNA primer, as well as other virion tRNAs (Peters and Hu 1980), but not the genome, at least with RSV. This specificity may account, in part, for observed complementation patterns between different retroviral groups. For example, REAV, which uses a $tRNA^{Pro}$ primer, can complement *env⁻* RSV but not *env⁻pol⁻* RSV (Sawyer and Hanafusa 1977) or the defective avian leukemia virus MC29 (Bister and Vogt 1978).

III. TERMINAL REGIONS OF RETROVIRAL GENOMES

The localization of the tRNA primer near the 5′ end of the genome brought to light the importance of 5′- and 3′-terminal regions in the replication of the virus. These regions are most accessible to direct nucleotide sequence determination by rapid sequencing techniques and were therefore the first regions for which exact sequences were available. The role of these regions in viral DNA synthesis is at least partially understood; the lack of genetic markers with characteristic phenotypes (except in the L and U_3 regions) has precluded an analysis of other possible functions for these regions. Portions of the 3′- and 5′-terminal regions of several retroviruses are shown schematically in Figure 4.5A.

The exact nucleotide sequences (see Appendix D) have been derived from molecular clones of viral DNA. A system for numbering of nucleotides in retroviral genomes has not yet been agreed upon; however, we will use the following convention. Position 1 in the sequence corresponds to the 5′ end of the genome (a G residue in all viruses examined to date) and therefore also corresponds to the most 5′ nucleotide in the repeat sequence (R) at the 3′ end of the genome. Numbering from the 5′ end to the 3′ terminus is positive; when a complete sequence is known, all nucleotides will have positive numbers. In the meantime, nucleotides near the 3′ end of the genome will be given negative numbers counting toward the 5′ terminus from the U_3-R junction. Note that a different convention is used for some of the sequences shown in the Appendix.

The 5′-terminal portion of any retroviral genome can be divided into four functional regions: the terminal redundancy (R), a unique

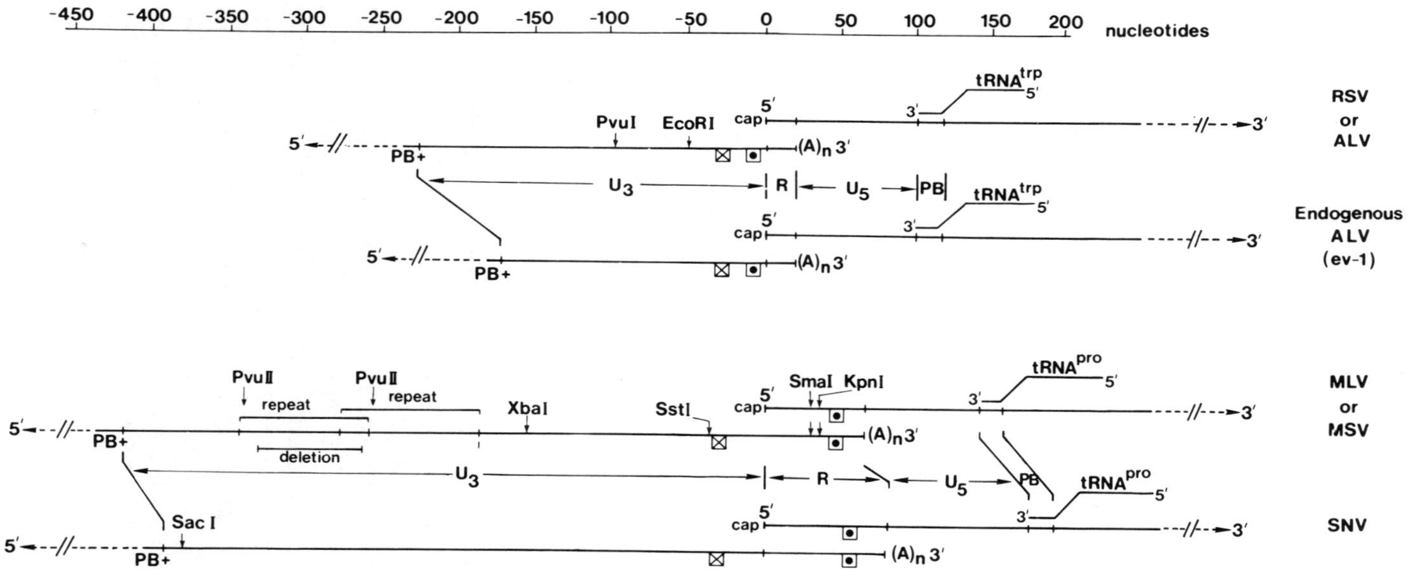

-450 -400 -350 -300 -250 -200 -150 -100 -50 0 50 100 150 200 nucleotides
RSV or ALV
Endogenous ALV (ev-1)
MLV or MSV
SNV
tRNA^trp
tRNA^pro
PvuI
EcoRI
PvuII
repeat
deletion
XbaI
SstI
SmaI
KpnI
Sac I
cap
PB+
PB
U3
R
U5
(A)n 3'
5'
3'

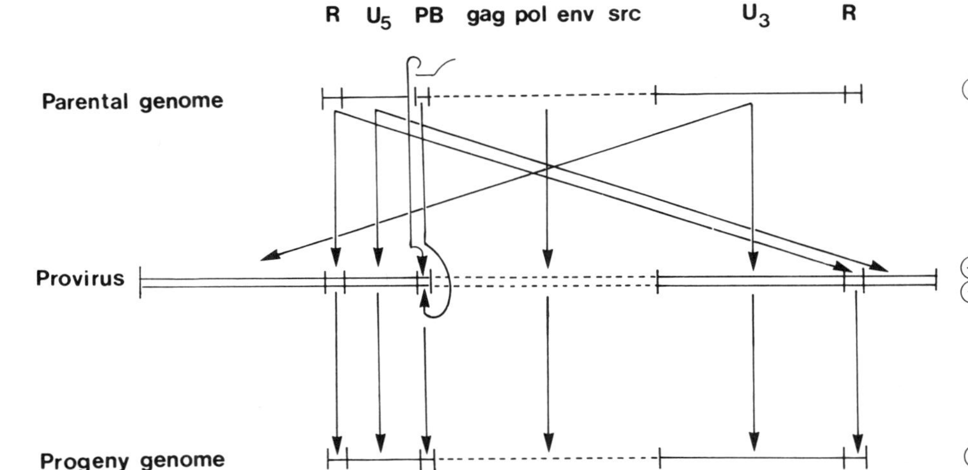

Figure 4.5 Terminal regions of some retroviral genomes. (*A*) The 5′ ends (top of each pair) and 3′ ends (bottom) of each genome with the redundant (R) sequences aligned. The small boxes indicate putative control sequences: the box with the X is the promoter or Hogness box, and the box with the circle represents the "polyadenylation" signal (AAUAAA). Useful restriction endonuclease cleavage sites in the DNA of each genome are indicated. All structures are derived from nucleotide-sequence data. ALV (or RSV) data were obtained from Haseltine et al. (1977), Schwartz et al. (1977), Shine et al. (1977), and Czernilofsky et al. (1980b). Information regarding the endogenous locus *ev*-1 (closely related to RAV-0) was obtained from Hishinuma et al. (1981). MLV or Mo-MSV drawings are based on data obtained from Dhar et al. (1980), Reddy et al. (1980), Sutcliffe et al. (1980a), and Van Beveren et al. (1980, 1981). The bars in the U_3 region of MLV/MSV indicate a repeated sequence, of which a portion is deleted in some strains (see text). The SNV sequence was obtained from Shimotohno et al. (1980). (*B*) Information flow of the terminal regions during replication (for further details, see Chapter 5). The genomes are not drawn to scale in *B*.

sequence (U_5), the primer-binding site (PB), and an untranslated sequence (L). The 3′-terminal region is divided into three regions: the primer-binding site for positive-strand DNA synthesis (PB[+]), a region unique to the 3′ end (U_3), and the other copy of the redundancy (R). All retroviral genomes contain these regions, no matter how defective they are in other functions. This conservation probably reflects the necessity of these seven regions to be present in a genome in order for it to be replicated, integrated, expressed, and packaged by systems that can be provided in *trans* by helper viruses or by the host. It is quite possible, although not yet demonstrated, that almost any sequence inserted between these terminal regions could be replicated and expressed as though it were a replication-defective retrovirus.

A. The Primer-binding Site

The recognition that there is a unique primer-binding site (PB) and its localization on the retroviral genome were of central importance to a more complete understanding of the mechanistic details of retrovirus replication. The key experiment was that of Taylor and Illmensee (1975), who hybridized labeled $tRNA^{Trp}$ to RSV RNA, partially fragmented the RNA, and isolated poly(A)-containing fragments. When these fragments were analyzed in a sucrose gradient or by gel electrophoresis, it was found that the labeled primer was associated only with essentially unbroken genome-length molecules. Since the poly(A) selection is specific for the 3′ end, this result located the primer-binding site to a region between 90% and 100% of the genome away from the 3′ end. In other words, the primer-binding site must be very near the 5′ end of the genome. A virtually identical result has been obtained for the $tRNA^{Pro}$ Mo-MLV primer (Peters and Dahlberg 1979).

The precise location of the primer-binding site in ALV and MLV has also been inferred from the length and sequence of strong-stop DNA, which is a major product of endogenous DNA polymerase reactions in vitro (Haseltine et al. 1976), especially those performed under less than ideal conditions (Novak et al. 1979). This DNA has a unique length and can be isolated with the primer attached at its 5′ end. Since it hybridizes to a 5′-terminal sequence containing the capping group (Cashion et al. 1976; Coffin and Haseltine 1977; Coffin et al. 1978b) and ends with a sequence consistent with the 5′-

terminal oligonucleotide (Haseltine et al. 1977; Shine et al. 1977; Stoll et al. 1977), the strong-stop DNA must be a copy of the sequence between the primer-binding site and the 5′ end of the genome. Given the length of strong-stop DNA in the different viruses examined, the primer-binding site is 101 nucleotides from the 5′ end of most or all RSV and ALV genomes, 140–146 nucleotides from the 5′ end of MLV and MSV, and 135 nucleotides from the 5′ end of MMTV (Lovinger and Schochetman 1979; G. Peters; G. Lovinger; J. Majors and H. Varmus; all pers. comm.). Judging from the DNA sequence, the strong-stop DNA of SNV must be about 176 nucleotides long (Shimotohno et al. 1980).

B. The Redundant Sequence

The finding of a 5′-proximal location for the tRNA primer led to a prediction that there would be a short sequence repeated at both ends of the genome to allow elongation of strong-stop DNA to continue using the 3′ end of the genome as a template (discussed further in Chapter 5). This prediction was quickly verified by direct sequence analysis of the region proximal to the poly(A) sequence of the ALV genome (Schwartz et al. 1977; Stoll et al. 1977) and by protection of this portion of both ALV and MLV genomes by hybridization to strong-stop DNA (Coffin and Haseltine 1977; Coffin et al. 1978b). There is still some uncertainty about the exact length of this sequence; in ALV it is estimated to be from 17 to 21 nucleotides, and it has been suggested that there may be a heterogeneity of a few nucleotides in length from one genome to another at the 3′ terminus (Schwartz et al. 1977; Stoll et al. 1977). A similar uncertainty exists in the precise location of the 3′ terminus of the Mo-MLV genome, where the redundancy is between 60 and 71 nucleotides in length. Because of this uncertainty and the possibility of genome heterogeneity, the 3′-terminal sequences of the viral genomes in Figure 4.5A are numbered from the junction of the U_3 and redundant sequences.

The mechanism of viral DNA synthesis implies that the redundant sequence has some interesting genetic properties. These properties can be easily studied in some ALV strains that have the convenient feature that this sequence contains no unmodified G residues, allowing examination of the 5′ copy of this sequence as a large oligonucleotide in a fingerprint of the total genome (this oligonucleotide is numbered 13 in the case of PR-RSV and RAV-0, as shown in

Figs. 4.2 and 4.6) (Beemon and Keith 1976; Cashion et al. 1976). The 3′ copy can be purified away from the rest of the genome by RNase-T1 digestion and isolation of the poly(A)-associated RNA. In this way, a number of slightly different redundant sequences have been characterized in different ALV strains (Wang et al. 1977; Joho et al. 1978). It can be predicted from the mechanism of replication (see Chapter 5) that the 3′ redundant sequence is not copied into DNA but merely serves as a bridge to facilitate elongation of nascent DNA chains and therefore that its genetic continuity resides in the 5′ sequence (see Fig. 4.5B). Thus, if a genome with different redundant sequences is generated by mutation or recombination, after one replication cycle the ends will again have the same sequence. Close examination of the redundant sequences of recombinant viruses (Wang et al. 1977; Joho et al. 1978) and of spontaneous mutants appearing after repeated passage of virus (J. Coffin et al., in prep.) bears out this prediction. In no case has a viral genome with differing terminal R sequences been found. In the same way, any variation in the length of the 3′ redundant sequence, by incorrect termination or processing, for example, would be corrected in the next round of replication.

A possible additional role for the R region in RSV is suggested by the results of Darlix et al. (1979), who found that the only significant region of the RSV genome that can be protected from ribonuclease digestion by binding to ribosomes is an oligonucleotide containing a portion of the R sequence, although the initiation site for translation is more than 300 nucleotides away. This result is consistent with the model of Kozak (1978, 1980) that ribosomes recognize and bind specifically only to 5′ ends of mRNAs and subsequently initiate translation at the first available AUG codons. The protection of the R sequence by ribosomes may thus reflect a specific affinity for this terminal sequence, or simply its proximity to the 5′ end of the genome.

C. The U_5 Region

Because strong-stop DNA containing the complement of R-U_5 is readily prepared in reasonable yield from endogenous DNA-polymerase reactions, this was the first significant region of many retroviral genomes to be sequenced (Haseltine et al. 1977; Shine et al.

1977; Stoll et al. 1977; Lovinger and Schochetman 1979, 1980). Some strong-stop sequences are shown in the Appendix D (as part of the LTR sequences).

Although the strong-stop sequences in distantly related viruses are quite different, there seem to be some conserved features. First, sequences of 9 nucleotides at the U_5-PB junctions are identical or very similar among different viruses (see Table 4.2). The meaning of this sequence identity is not obvious. The sequence immediately adjacent to the primer-binding site is the initiation site for replication and also contains one of the integration sites in the provirus (see Chapter 5). Second, the hexanucleotide AAUAAA is present in the redundant sequence of some viral genomes, such as MLV, MSV, and SNV. This sequence precedes the 3′ end of the genome (i.e., the beginning of the poly[A] region) by about 10–20 nucleotides. As the same sequence is found in the same location in virtually all eukaryotic viral and cellular mRNAs that become polyadenylated posttranscriptionally (Proudfoot and Brownlee 1976; Tooze 1980), it is presumed to form a signal for that system that adds poly(A) to mRNAs. The presence of this signal in R, and therefore near the 5′ end, as well as the 3′ end, of the genome, raises the unsolved question of how the system can distinguish the proper part of the genome for polyadenylation and not leave a genome consisting only of R, as would occur if polyadenylation occurred due to the signal in the 5′ LTR. In RSV and ALV genomes, the AAUAAA sequence is within U_3, rather than within R (see Section III.E). This difference in location is clearly related to the shorter redundant sequence in the avian tumor viruses. Oddly, this exact sequence does not seem to be present in those MMTV strains examined so far, although a related sequence AGUAAA is found (Donehower et al. 1981).

The strong-stop sequence is fairly highly conserved among related virus strains. Virtually complete cross-hybridization is observed between RSV strong-stop DNA and RNAs of all RSV and exogenous and endogenous ALV strains tested (Friedrich et al. 1977), and only a small number of differences are seen in their nucleotide sequences. For example, B77-RSV differs in sequence from PR-RSV-C in 3 positions out of the first 70 positions, from RAV-2 and the endogenous virus RAV-0 in 6 positions (R. Swanstrom, pers. comm.), and from AMV in 9 positions (Stoll et al. 1977). The length, however, is completely conserved; all RSV and ALV strong-stop DNAs are 101 nucleotides long. The nucleotide sequences of strong-

Table 4.2 Conserved nucleotide sequences in the terminal regions of retroviral genomes

Virus	PB(−)	PB(+)	Promoter box	Poly(A)
RSV and ALV	GCUUCAUUUGG (101)	CAUAGGGAGGGGGAAUGUAGUCU (−217)	UAUUUAAG (−23)	AAUAAA (−2)
MLV and MSV	CUUUCAUUUGG (146)	AGAAAAAGGGGGGAAUGAAAGAC (−373 or −445)	AAUAAAAG (−23)	AAUAAA (52)
SNV	ACAACAUUUGG (176)	AAGAGCAGUGGGGAAUGUGGGAG (−397)	UAUAUAAG (−23)	AAUAAA (58)
MMTV	GCGGCAUUGUA (133)	GAAAAAAGGGGGAAAUGCCGCGCC (−1190)	UAUAAAAG (−25)	AGUAAA (−4)

The sequence position indicated within parentheses denotes the location of the underlined nucleotide. SNV indicates spleen necrosis virus, a member of the avian reticuloendotheliosis virus group.

stop DNAs of mammalian C-type retroviruses have provided a useful basis of classification, either by length and oligopyrimidine patterns (Haseltine and Kleid 1978) or more recently by complete nucleotide sequence determination (Lovinger and Schochetman 1980). From this information, it is possible to draw relationship schemes that match closely those obtained by cross-hybridization or other criteria. For example, the RSV strong-stop sequence is not detectably related to that of the mammalian C-type viruses, whereas all of the latter show at least a small amount of relationship to one another. Thus, gibbon ape leukemia virus (GALV) and MLV are quite closely related, as are the baboon endogenous virus (BaEV) and cat virus (RD114). It is particularly interesing that this type of analysis reveals that REV (reticuloendotheliosis virus, an avian virus) is more closely related to CPC-1 and MAC-1 (two endogenous monkey viruses) than to any other avian or mammalian virus (G. G. Lovinger and L. Schochetman, pers. comm.).

At present, the U_5 region has no known functional role, except perhaps as a "spacer" between the sites of initiation of DNA synthesis and the redundant sequence. Although a role in translation is possible, it is improbable, as translation of all genes in RSV and ALV is apparently initiated about 270 nucleotides away from U_5 (G. Gasic and W. Hayward; R. Swanstrom et al.; both pers. comm.).

D. The L Region

Recent results suggest that retroviral genomes, by comparison with cellular mRNAs, have an unusually high amount of untranslated information at their 5′ ends. The nucleotide sequence of the 5′-terminal portion of the RSV genome does not coincide with the sequence predicted from the aminoterminal amino acid sequence of *gag* (Palmiter et al. 1978) until nucleotide 380 is reached (D. Schwartz et al.; R. Swanstrom et al.; both pers. comm.). Similarly, the nucleotide sequences of the 5′-terminal 225 nucleotides of Mo-MSV (Dhar et al. 1980), 300 nucleotides of MMTV (J. Majors, pers. comm.), and the 470 nucleotides of SNV (Shimotohno et al. 1980) reveal no AUG initiation codons. These sequences define that part of a leader region, L, that extends from the 3′ end of PB(−) to the initiation codon for *gag*. The length of L, obtained by subtracting the length of $R+U_5+PB$ from the position of the first translated codon, is therefore about 250 nucleotides in RSV and at least 61 nucleotides,

300 nucleotides, and 277 nucleotides in Mo-MSV, MMTV, and SNV, respectively. Possible functions for the L region include the following:

1. A splicing donor site for subgenomic mRNAs. The L regions of both Mo-MSV and SNV contain a sequence that matches 7 out of 8 nucleotides with a sequence, AGGUAAGU, that has been found at the donor splice junction of many eukaryotic mRNAs (Seif et al. 1979). Use of the sequence would result in a leader of about 206 nucleotides in Mo-MSV (and presumably MLV) RNA and 260 nucleotides in SNV subgenomic RNA. These predictions remain to be tested. In contrast, recent evidence from S1 mapping and nucleotide sequence analysis suggests that the splice donor for the RSV *env* and *src* mRNAs is probably within *gag* (P. Hackett et al.; D. Schwartz et al.; both pers. comm.).
2. Participation in the dimer-linkage structure of 70S RNA (see Fig. 4.4).
3. A recognition signal (or part of one) for packaging of genomic RNA into virions. Evidence for this function is provided by the RSV mutant SE21Q1b (Linial et al. 1978), which contains a small deletion in the L region (Shank and Linial 1980). Cells infected with this mutant synthesize an apparently normal complement of *gag-*, *pol-*, *env-*, and *src*-gene products, implying that the signals for mRNA processing (including the splice donor site) and protein synthesis (including the beginning of *gag*) are intact. The failure of this virus to package its own RNA effectively, then, implies the presence of a recognition signal for this purpose within L.

Other related, but more speculative, possibilities for functions of this region include a recognition sequence for some system that regulates splicing to maintain a proper balance between the concentrations of genomic RNA and mRNAs, and a region to allow distinction between these species to favor incorporation of genomic RNA into virions.

E. The U_3 Region

The portion of the genome immediately 5′ of the 3′ redundant sequence, originally referred to as the *c* region of RSV, has been defined in three different ways: (1) This region was originally defined on the basis of fingerprints of the 3′-terminal regions of the genomes of nondefective viruses and *td* deletion mutants of RSV (Wang et al. 1975; Perez-Bercoff and Billeter 1976), which revealed a short region 3′ to the *src* gene retained in the mutants. By heteroduplex mapping, this region was estimated to be 700–800 bases in length (Junghans et al. 1977; Hu et al. 1978a), and by restriction enzyme mapping, at about 500 bases (Shank et al. 1978). Nucleotide-sequence analysis suggests a length of 327 nucleotides between the 5′ end of R and the site of a *td* deletion (Yamamoto et al. 1980c). (2) Heteroduplex and fingerprint analysis of 3′-terminal regions of a number of avian oncoviruses showed that at least part of this region is highly, although not perfectly, conserved among otherwise rather divergent exogenous viruses (Wang et al. 1976b, 1977; Tal et al. 1977a). In particular, two oligonucleotides, one at position −1 through −11 (oligonucleotide C) and the other at position −23 through −30, have been found in all strains so far examined, including such diverse strains as PR-RSV-B, PR-RSV-C, RAV-1, RAV-2, and MC29 (Tsichlis and Coffin 1979; Robinson et al. 1980). (3) The mechanism of proviral DNA synthesis leads to a reiteration of the 3′-terminal 250 nucleotides at the 5′ end of RSV DNA (see Fig. 4.5B), about 445 nucleotides in MLV DNA, and as much as 1200 nucleotides in MMTV DNA (see Chapter 5). The region unique to the 3′ end of the viral RNA and present at both ends of viral DNA has also been referred to simply as 3′ (Shank et al. 1978) and as U_3 (Coffin et al. 1978b; Coffin 1979). The term U_3 is used here exclusively, noting that the RSV *c* region as originally defined exceeds U_3 by about 80 nucleotides of undetermined significance. The U_3 region is precisely defined as the portion of the sequence, repeated at both ends of linear unintegrated DNA, that is derived from information unique to the 3′-terminal region of the genomic RNA. It may thus be two nucleotides longer than the sequence that forms part of the LTR in the integrated provirus (see Chapter 5).

With the possible exception of MMTV (discussed in Section VII), the U_3 region seems to be noncoding. Although some early reports raised the possibility of a protein (Purchio et al. 1977) and of an mRNA (Krzyzek et al. 1978) encoded by this part of the RSV genome, nucleotide-sequence analysis does not reveal any large open reading frames. The longest possibility in the RSV genome, for example, could encode only 39 amino acids in a single reading frame (Czernilofsky et al. 1980b; Yamamoto et al. 1980c). Although the existence of such products has not been rigorously excluded, it is more likely that the primary and secondary structures of this region may function as signals for provirus integration and expression.

Two probable sequences with such functions are present in U_3 regions. One of these is the AAUAAA putative signal sequence for poly(A) addition at positions −2 through −7 in the RSV and ALV genomes and a related sequence at −4 through −9 of the MMTV genome (found also in the mammalian C-type viruses, but in the R region discussed in Section III.B; also see Table 4.2). Note that in the RSV genome this sequence forms part of an oligonucleotide (C) that was formerly used to define the commonness of the *c* region.

A second sequence, found in many eukaryotic genes and some viral genes, is the so-called Hogness box (Gannon et al. 1979). This sequence, usually of the form TAT (A or T)$_{3-4}$G, is located with the G residue 24 ± 1 nucleotides from the probable initiation site of RNA synthesis (i.e., the site that is capped in the finished mRNA). It is not universal; it is missing in some adenoviral and SV40 genes (Baker et al. 1979), and its precise role is in doubt, as it can be deleted from the early region of SV40 without greatly affecting expression in vivo (Benoist and Chambon 1980). This sequence bears a striking resemblance to the Pribnow box about 10 nucleotides upstream from the site of transcriptional initiation in many prokaryotes. In all retroviral genomes sequenced to date, such a sequence exists at positions −23 through −30 (see Table 4.2). The presence of this conserved sequence, within otherwise unrelated regions, supports the idea that the U_3 region contains the promoter for viral RNA synthesis.

The remaining identified sequence of probable functional significance in U_3 is within, and extends somewhat beyond, its 5′ end (see Table 4.2), where there is an identical 8-nucleotide sequence (GGGGAUG) in all retroviruses examined so far. Note that the AAUG (which probably forms the first 4 nucleotides copied into the positive strand of the provirus) is an inverted (complementary) repeat of the CAUU sequence within PB(−), the first 4 nucleotides copied into the negative strand of some viruses. This conservation could reflect either an initiation site for reverse transcription or a recognition signal for integration, or both.

The sequences just mentioned make up only a small fraction of the total length of the U_3 region. The remaining nucleotide sequences in this region show no obvious homologies between different retroviruses. However, it is highly improbable that the remaining sequence is without function, and it is interesting to speculate that it may play some as yet undiscovered role in controlling the expression of the viral genome.

Unlike the other terminal sequences, at least one phenotypic difference has been associated with sequence differences in the U_3 region. Endogenous avian retroviruses have a U_3 region substantially different from that of exogenous avian viruses, such that the two otherwise closely related groups share no common oligonucleotides (Coffin et al. 1978a) and little or no cross-hybridization can be detected (Hayward 1977; Neiman et al. 1977; Coffin et al. 1978a; Chien et al. 1980; Hishinuma et al. 1981; Hughes et al. 1981a; Shank et al. 1981), although some relationship has been found by nucleotide sequencing (see Chapter 10). Endogenous viruses of chickens also have a substantially reduced growth rate relative to exogenous viruses (Hanafusa et al. 1975; Linial and Neiman 1976; Robinson 1976). A direct correlation between these differences was found by Tsichlis and Coffin (1979, 1980a,b), who prepared recombinants between RAV-0 and a number of different exogenous viruses. Selection of the most rapidly growing recombinants was invariably accompanied by selection of the exogenous-type U_3 region, and no other part, of the exogenous viral genome. These results allow a genetic definition of two distinct alleles, U_3^x in exogenous viruses and U_3^n in endogenous viral genomes. It is likely that the difference in the U_3 region is, at least in part, responsible for the failure of endogenous viruses, such as RAV-0, to induce leukemia or other disease in chickens (Robinson et al. 1980).

An additional unusual feature has been found in the nucleotide sequence of the U_3 region of Mo-MSV (Dhar et al. 1980; Reddy et al. 1980; Van Beveren et al. 1981). There is an overlapping direct-repeat structure of the form "abcabca" that spans the 160 nucleotides between positions −183 and −343 (see Fig. 4.5A). The repeat unit "abc" is 69 nucleotides long, with nine mismatches. The overall length of U_3 synthesized in vitro and the presence of two *Pvu*II restriction enzyme sites in cloned proviral DNA (Gilboa et al. 1979; Shoemaker et al. 1980) indicate that the same feature is also present in Mo-MLV; however, two independently determined sequences of cloned in vitro synthesized or integrated proviral DNA do not have this feature (Sutcliffe et al. 1980a; Van Beveren et al. 1980). In the latter cases, the overall sequence is 69 nucleotides shorter, as though the repeat had been deleted by homologous recombination between the first two "a" segments, leaving the sequence "abca." Similarly, the U_3 region of SNV contains two such sequences and molecular clones of SNV DNA vary in length by the presence of one or two of each of these sequences with no apparent effect on biological activity (K. Shimotohno and H. Temin, pers. comm.). The significance of these findings remains to be elucidated.

IV. MAPPING RETROVIRAL GENES

With the knowledge that the coding capacity of most retroviral genomes is sufficient to code for only those proteins already identified as structural components of the virion, it became possible to identify and to localize the various genes on the genome. Thus, the three regions encoding virion proteins (*gag, pol,* and *env*) were formalized with names (Baltimore 1975). Since that time, no new structural genes have been identified, although the book is not yet closed.

Retroviral genes are most satisfactorily defined as the regions coding for the primary gene products, as described at the beginning of this chapter (see Table 4.1). Therefore, the translated sequence defines a gene. Eventually, precise assignment of gene boundaries will be based on the nucleotide sequences of the genome and mRNAs and on the amino acid sequences of the various proteins. Complete sequences of this sort are currently available for several viral genomes (see Appendix E), and sequence data are being generated rapidly due to new technological advances. Meanwhile, most of the available maps are based on physical and genetic approaches. For the purposes of genetic mapping, the general strategy has been to associate physical features of the genome with either deletion mutants, as in *td* RSV or *env*⁻ BH-RSV(−), or strain-specific markers such as host range, N tropism and B tropism, and *ts* mutations. The correlated physical features are then mapped on the genome, providing a genetic map. Detailed reviews of these approaches are available (Beemon 1978; Bishop 1978; Wang 1978; Chien et al. 1980; Coffin 1980; Hunter 1980) and are described in Chapter 7.

A. Genetic Mapping

When genetic recombination of retroviruses was first observed, there was some hope that classical techniques of genetic analysis developed in prokaryotic systems could be applied with similar success to developing genetic maps of retroviral genomes. For several reasons, however, this approach has not had great success. For one, recombination frequencies are extremely difficult to measure and compare in a meaningful way, since only in special cases can all markers be recovered, subtle selective effects are extremely difficult to control, and the number of rounds of recombination cannot be measured. Second, the recombinational frequency is so high that neighboring portions of the genome are essentially unlinked (Linial and Brown 1979; Tsichlis and Coffin 1980a). Third, there is a lack of markers sufficiently closely spaced to allow construction of recombinational frequency maps. Thus, although analysis of recombination frequencies seemed to yield a circular map of the correct gene order (*gag-pol-env-src*) (Hayman and Vogt 1976; Hunter 1978), this was probably a fortuitous result of selection (e.g., of a region in *gag* that is coselected with *src* in some crosses) (Tsichlis and Coffin 1980a). For these reasons, reliable genetic maps have been obtained only by working from physical maps generated by one of several techniques. A comparison of such maps is shown in Figure 4.6.

B. Oligonucleotide Mapping

Each large oligonucleotide in a fingerprint of viral RNA is a unique sequence from some region of the genome and can serve as a marker for that region. The positions of large oligonucleotides along the genome can be determined with reasonable accuracy relative to the 3′-terminal poly(A) (Wang et al. 1975; Coffin and Billeter 1976). To prepare such a map, viral RNA is partially fragmented by mild alkali treatment (or by aging the virus), and poly(A)-containing fragments of defined size are isolated by velocity sedimentation and chromatography on poly(U) or oligo(dT) affinity columns. A fingerprint of the poly(A)-containing fraction of each size of RNA is prepared. Those oligonucleotides closest to the 5′ end and farthest from the poly(A) end will be found only in the longest fragments, and those near the 3′ end will be found in all size classes; thus, one can place them in a relative linear order along the genome. Fingerprints of deletion mutants and recombinants can then be used to associate specific oligonucleotides with specific genes. Several features of this approach should be pointed out. For one, the position of an oligonucleotide in a fingerprint is very sensitive to its base composition, such that a single-base change within an oligonucleotide may often result in a

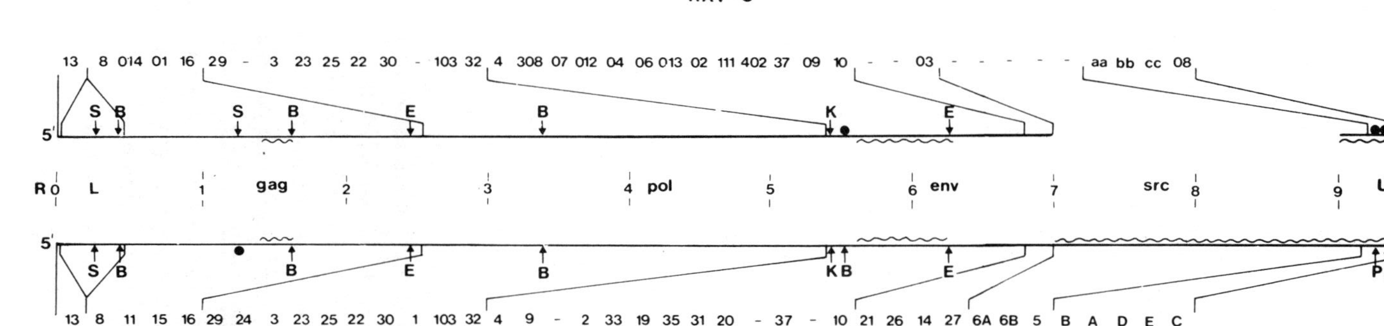

Figure 4.6 Comparative methods of physical mapping. The outer lines show oligonucleotide maps of PR-RSV-B and RAV-0 based on the fingerprints shown in Fig. 4.2. The inner lines show restriction maps of the same two genomes, with some cleavage sites and an indication of how the oligonucleotides align in the DNA. The wavy lines indicate regions of nonhomology determined by heteroduplex mapping. Note that the oligonucleotide maps are more sensitive to differences between the genomes, but that they are distorted due to uneven distribution along the genome of the large identifiable oligonucleotides. Restriction enzyme sites are denoted by the following code: (S) *Sst*I; (B) *Bam*HI; (E) *Eco*RI; (K) *Kpn*I; (P) *Pvu*I. The absence of a restriction enzyme site is indicated by solid circles.

change in mobility. Thus, different but related strains of viruses yield different fingerprints and hence different oligonucleotide maps as a consequence of single-base divergency. Despite this, comparison of maps of different strains can reveal regions of the genome more or less highly conserved in sequence (Joho et al. 1976; Coffin et al. 1978a). There are generally about 30–40 well-separated distinct oligonucleotides in a fingerprint, containing a total of some 600 nucleotides or about 6% of the genome. Thus, although only 1 of 16 base changes is detectable, a divergence of some 0.2% in sequence is detectable as a fingerprint difference. Recent technical improvements in resolution systems have increased the resolution to about 10% of the genome (Pedersen and Haseltine 1980). This technique has been valuable in analyzing relationships between different strains of viruses and their recombinants. The method is less sensitive for analysis of deletions, because an average of 300 nucleotides have to be removed to delete a single oligonucleotide. Furthermore, the oligonucleotides that can be resolved are distributed randomly, rather than at equal intervals along the genome.

C. Restriction Mapping

In principle, the same techniques developed for generating detailed restriction maps of DNA viruses (see Tooze 1980) can be applied directly to the viral DNA of retroviruses. In practice, the difficulty of obtaining pure viral DNA in sufficient quantity greatly delayed the application of this technique until the development of two techniques: DNA transfer or blotting (Southern 1975) and molecular cloning of viral DNAs. Restriction maps of retroviral genomes have proved most useful in analysis of replicative forms of viral DNA (see Chapter 5), in analysis of deletion and other replication-defective mutants (see Chapter 7), and in the study of endogenous viral genomes (see Chapter 10). A particular advantage of using restriction endonuclease digestion and DNA transfer hybridization in the latter two cases is that cells containing endogenous and defective proviruses often make little or no viral RNA to be analyzed by other methods, yet contain essentially the same amount of proviral DNA as cells infected with nondefective virus.

The general strategy for generating restriction maps of retroviral DNA is described in Chapter 5. As compared with oligonucleotide mapping, this kind of analysis is more sensitive to small deletions and insertions (a consequence of the high resolution of the electrophoretic systems employed) but less sensitive to the single-base differences that characterize different strains of virus, unless many enzymes are used to generate very detailed maps. As a result, many interesting genetic features are detectable in fingerprints but, at present, can be located only approximately in the genome; much of the discussion that follows will reflect this imprecision.

D. Heteroduplex Mapping

As with restriction mapping, localization of genetic features by visualization in the electron microscope of heteroduplexes between nucleic acids from different strains of viruses was applied to retroviruses relatively recently (Junghans et al. 1977). The principal obstacle to the use of this technique was the unavailability of DNA complementary to the viral genome of sufficient length, a situation finally resolved by the refinement of techniques of in vitro cDNA synthesis by the virion DNA polymerase (Junghans et al. 1975; Rothenberg and Baltimore 1977; for review, see Chien et al. 1980). With the availability of molecular clones of viral DNA, this type of analysis is becoming much more widely used. Under circumstances where cDNA and genomic RNA (or appropriate clones) are available, heteroduplex analysis is quite useful for localizing deletions and substitutions in two viral genomes relative to each other. Like restriction mapping, heteroduplex mapping is quite insensitive to differences in sequence due to base substitutions. Thus, for example, hybridization between cDNA and RNA of RSV strains of different subgroups frequently yields apparently perfect duplexes, even though there is significant sequence divergence.

E. Molecular Cloning

The application of recombinant DNA technology has become an important method for the analysis of the retroviral genome structure. The ability to obtain very large amounts of defined DNA of absolute purity as inserts in plasmid or bacteriophage genomes for analysis and manipulation offers substantial benefits. Because of the nature of the replication cycle, retroviruses offer a large selection of potentially clonable species, including cDNA copies of the genomic RNA and mRNAs synthesized in vitro and various DNA forms (linear, circular, and integrated) obtainable from exogenously infected cells or cells containing endogenous proviruses. All of these have been used in one instance or another. Although the method is very powerful, it cannot be assumed to be perfect, and a number of artifacts have already been observed.

1. Preexisting Mutants

The frequency of point and deletion mutations in retroviruses is sufficiently high ($\sim 10^{-3}$ to 10^{-4}) (Coffin et al. 1980) that any genome cloned from a population is likely to differ from the modal sequence by a significant number of nucleotide changes. Thus, a single cloned genome cannot be assumed to be that of the biologically active species unless tested appropriately. For example, O'Rear et al. (1980) found that out of eight clones of apparently normal SNV provirus, only four were infectious; apparently the noninfectious clones were due to defects in the proviruses themselves (J. O'Rear and H. Temin, pers. comm.). Similarly, Shoemaker et al. (1980) reported that three of six clones of Mo-MLV DNA were infectious.

This problem may be amplified by the use of cDNA synthesized in vitro by reverse transcriptase, as high misincorporation rates have been reported (see Chapter 5). The nucleotide sequences for the U_3 region of the Mo-MLV genome reported by Sutcliffe et al. (1980a) from cloned cDNA synthesized in vitro and by Van Beveren et al. (1980) from integrated DNA differ by three nucleotide changes, possibly due to errors introduced during reverse transcription or to some virus variation.

Deletion mutants, particularly of *src,* are also frequent in virus stocks. Of two clones obtained from cDNA copies of 21S *src* mRNA extracted from infected cells, one was apparently derived from the 21S *env* mRNA of *td* RSV contained in the stock (Yamamoto et al. 1980a,c).

2. Other Aberrant Forms

A number of structural variants apparently occur during the replication cycle and, although too low in frequency to be detected by examination of populations of infected cells, these can be isolated as viral DNA clones. Clones derived from circular Mo-MLV DNA contained several structures with a peculiar arrangement around the circle junction (Shoemaker et al. 1980). These structures had two copies of the LTR, but the sequence containing one of them was inverted with respect to its usual order, as though the DNA had integrated into itself. Other types of structures involving deletions corresponding to the 5′-terminal region of the MSV genome (Reddy et al. 1980) and the 3′-terminal region of the RSV and ALV genomes (Highfield et al. 1980; Ju and Skalka 1980; Ju et al. 1980) within the LTR have been found frequently in clones of circular viral DNA.

Besides peculiarities arising during DNA synthesis, there is at least one form that apparently results from atypical RNA synthesis or processing. Yamamoto et al. (1980a) obtained a cloned cDNA copy of the 3′-terminal region of 21S RNA from RSV-infected cells that had the sequence U_3-R-U_5 at its 3′ end, as though the usual polyadenylation site at the end of R had been ignored. Although it is possible that this structure represents a biologically active form, there is no independent evidence for its existence as a significant fraction of infected-cell virus-specific mRNA (see Chapter 5).A similar form is seen in virion RNA encoded by the *ev*-1 endogenous provirus of chickens (see Chapter 10).

Judging from the frequency with which structures such as these have been noted, it seems probable that various anomalous forms arise during the replication cycle, although each occurs at too low a frequency to be detected in mass cultures. Presumably most of these are of no consequence for virus replication.

3. *Variants Arising during Growth in Bacteria*

Although point mutations in cloned viral DNA do not occur with sufficiently high frequency to be bothersome, as judged from the stability of infectivity of the DNA to repeated passage, special kinds of rearrangements, particularly those involving the LTR, have been detected. Hager et al. (1979) cloned circular Harvey MSV (Ha-MSV) DNA with two copies of the LTR. After recloning, variants with one or three LTR copies were found (H. Chang et al. 1980). Similarly, McClements et al. (1980) isolated a variant of cloned integrated Mo-MSV in which virtually all of the provirus was deleted, leaving only a single copy of the LTR, i.e., this variant molecule seems to have undergone the transition from cell–U_3RU_5–(viral genes)–U_3RU_5–cell to cell–U_3RU_5–cell. These two types of variations may be a consequence of homologous recombinational events involving the repeated sequence.

4. Unclonable Sequences

Several groups have discovered that a complete genome of horizontally transmitted MMTV cannot be cloned in either plasmids or phage (Donehower et al. 1980; Majors and Varmus 1981; D. Ucker and K. Yamamoto, unpubl.). From the failure of repeated attempts to clone subgenomic restriction enzyme fragments of the 5′ region, it was concluded that there is a "poison" sequence somewhere in the *gag* region that is incompatible with the growth of a plasmid or phage containing it. This phenomenon may not be true of all MMTV strains, however, as Groner et al. (1980) have obtained apparently complete copies of an endogenous MMTV provirus in a cloned form. This difference may suggest a variation in *gag* sequences among the various MMTV strains.

The general conclusion from all these observations is that viral DNA clones must be carefully checked for biological activity before concluding that they are representative of the infectious viral genome.

V. GENOMES OF NONDEFECTIVE VIRUSES

Using the general strategies just described (and drawing on results from other methods as appropriate), the overall gene order and some structural details of individual genes have been deciphered. The overall structures of nondefective RSV and MLV are shown in Figure 4.7, along with sketches indicating relationships among the various strains. The complete nucleotide sequences of Pr-C RSV, Mo-MLV, and Mo-MSV can be found in Appendix E.

A. *gag-pol*

The *gag* and *pol* genes and their products are quite highly conserved among related strains of viruses. Until recently, mutants defective in these genes suitable for deletion mapping had not been isolated (see Chapter 7). For these reasons, most of the detailed information about the structure of *gag* and *pol* has been derived from studies of the proteins of nondefective and defective transforming viruses and, more recently, from nucleotide-sequence analysis. The details of the structure and functions of the virion proteins are presented in Chapter 6 and will not be repeated here, except as a reminder to the reader that the established order from 5′ to 3′ of the proteins in the

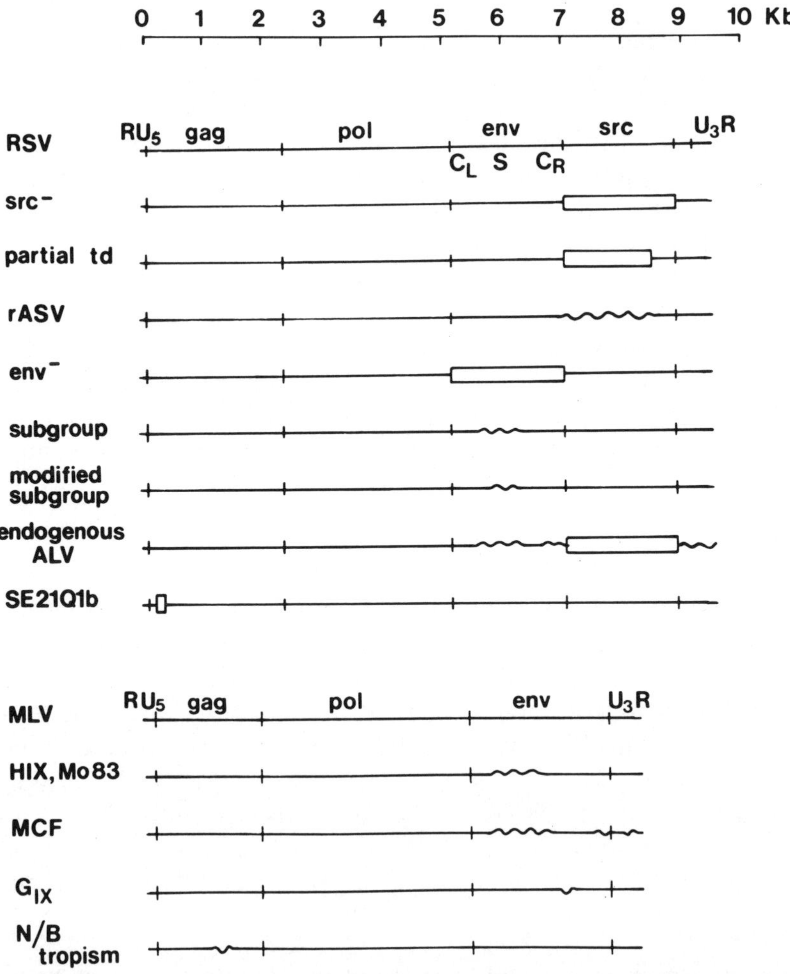

Figure 4.7 Maps of various RSV, ALV, and MLV strains used to localize genetic features on the genome. The RSV and MLV genomes are drawn to scale. A collection of variants with functionally important differences are indicated. An open box indicates a deletion; a wavy line indicates substitution of related, but functionally distinct, information (such as *env* genes of different subgroups). A full discussion of these viruses is presented in the text.

gag and *pol* precursors is NH_2-p19-p10-p27-p12-p15-*pol*-COOH for RSV and NH_2-p15-p12-p30-p10-*pol*-COOH for MLV (see Fig. 4.1). Since only genomic-size RNA directs the synthesis of *gag* and *gag-pol* precursors in vitro (von der Helm and Duesberg 1975; Pawson et al. 1976, 1977; Philipson et al. 1978) and in vivo (Fan and Verma 1978), these genes must occupy the 5′ half of the genome.

It has been possible to use a combination of genetic and physical analyses to identify and locate some markers in *gag* and *pol*. Joho et al. (1976) fingerprinted the RNA of a set of avian retroviral recombinants between *ts* LA337 PR-RSV-C ($pol^{ts}env^{C}src^{+}$) and RAV-6 ($pol^{+}env^{B}src^{-}$) (Mason et al. 1974). The unselected *ts* marker correlated with the region defined by one oligonucleotide specific for the *ts* LA337 parent, located approximately halfway between the 5′ end of the genome and *env*. This result allowed the localization of *pol* in the 5′ half of the RSV genome but, unfortunately, did not allow the relative order of *gag* and *pol* to be determined, since the *ts* marker could have been near either the amino terminus or the carboxyl terminus of the protein. Similar attempts to locate the gag^{ts} lesion in another avian mutant, *ts* LA334m, were unsuccessful, in that no oligonucleotide markers were linked to the *ts* phenotype (J. Coffin, M. Champion, and E. Hunter, cited in Coffin 1979). This result was probably a consequence of the very high frequency of recombination of avian tumor viruses, which has the effect of causing physically close markers in the genome to behave as independently segregating units (Linial and Brown 1979; Tsichlis and Coffin 1980a) (see Chapter 7). By analyzing another set of recombinants, Wang et al. (1976c) found that a set of oligonucleotides near the 5′ end was linked to electrophoretic mobility marker(s) in the *gag* proteins. Thus, the genetic map of RSV is in at least approximate concordance with the gene order inferred from protein studies. A similar concordance for MLV has been obtained in a detailed study of oligonucleotide maps and antigenic markers in recombinants between ecotropic and xenotropic viruses (Aaronson and Barbacid 1980).

The nucleotide sequence of the *gag-pol* region of the RSV genome (D. Schwartz et al., pers. comm.) (see Appendix E) is shown schematically in Figure 4.8. The composition and arrangement of the *gag*-gene products deduced from this sequence agree with the amino acid analysis of the proteins themselves (E. Hunter, pers. comm.) (see Chapter 6). In particular, p27 and p12, which had not previously been ordered, are found in the order NH_2-p27-p12-COOH. The most

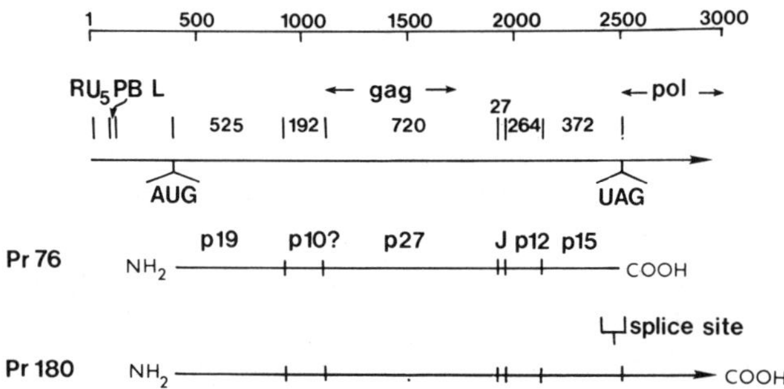

Figure 4.8 The *gag* region of RSV. The scheme is based on nucleotide-sequence data (D. Schwartz et al., pers. comm.) and partial amino acid sequence data (E. Hunter, pers. comm.). The lengths of the regions encoding the various *gag* proteins (in nucleotides) are shown above the genome. J is a small "joining" peptide predicted from the sequence. Note that the genome has a termination codon at the *gag-pol* boundary and that *pol* is in a different reading frame (see text).

interesting feature of the sequence is the region at the *gag-pol* boundary. As explained in greater detail in Chapters 5 and 6, both *gag* and *gag-pol* precursors are synthesized using apparently full-length genomic RNA as mRNA. In the case of RSV, the addition of amber termination suppressor tRNA to an in vitro translation reaction leads to a slightly longer product but does not allow readthrough synthesis of a complete *gag-pol* precursor (Weiss et al. 1978). The nucleotide sequence of this region shows that *gag* ends with an amber (UAG) codon immediately following the p15 sequence. Next are codons for amino acids identified as the amino terminus of the polymerase protein (the β and/or α subunit; see Chapter 6). These codons, however, are in a reading frame different from that of *gag*, so that readthrough of the termination codon would lead to missense translation of *pol*. The only reasonable hypothesis to explain the expression of *pol* is that there is a distinct mRNA that can be translated into the *gag-pol* precursor and that this mRNA is created by splicing around the UAG codon to shift the reading frame somewhere near the *gag-pol* boundary. Such a splicing event would have to remove 50–60 nucleotides in this region to avoid creating other termination codons and to provide the observed products. A similar situation has not been established for MLV, as amber suppressors do increase the amount of Mo-MLV *gag-pol* precursor at the expense of *gag* (Philipson et al. 1978). This result shows that the MLV *gag* and *pol* genes are in the same reading frame (as confirmed by the nucleotide sequence [T. Shinnick et al., pers. comm.]); it is still plausible that there are also two mRNAs, but this remains to be shown. A similar explanation could also account for the translation of two MMTV *gag*-related proteins and the *gag-pol* precursor from full-length mRNA (see Chapter 6 for further discussion). It is indeed possible that more than two full-length mRNA species exist, separately encoding the glycosylated and nonglycosylated *gag* precursors, as well as the *gag-pol* precursor in MLV (Murphy et al. 1980).

The nucleotide sequences of the 3′ end of *pol* of both RSV (D. Schwartz et al., pers. comm.) and MLV (T. Shinnick et al., pers. comm.) reveal a further interesting feature. In both cases, there is an overlap between the *pol* and *env* genes of about 113 nucleotides in RSV and 57 nucleotides in MLV. In both cases, the C-terminal amino acids of *pol* and the N-terminal amino acids of *env* are encoded in different reading frames.

The MLV *gag* marker that determines N tropism and B tropism has been localized by oligonucleotide mapping (see Fig. 4.7). Faller and Hopkins (1978c) analyzed the genomes of a set of recombinants that had been selected for N tropism and large-plaque morphology from a cross between a large-plaque-forming B-tropic virus and a small-plaque-forming N-tropic virus; only one oligonucleotide specific for the N-tropic parent was found in all recombinants. Also, one oligonucleotide specific for the B-tropic parent was missing. Both of these oligonucleotides were located at similar positions within the 5′-terminal 25% of the genome. These two oligonucleotides are closely related in nucleotide sequence, differing by 4 base changes out of 16 nucleotides (Rommelaere et al. 1979). Further experiments with NB-tropic viruses support the association between this oligonucleotide and tropism (Faller and Hopkins 1978b). NB-tropic variants arise at a reasonably high frequency from B-tropic viruses passaged in N-type ($Fv\text{-}1^{nn}$) cells but not from N-tropic viruses passaged in B-type ($Fv\text{-}1^{bb}$) cells. The genomes of NB-tropic viruses are identical with those of B-tropic viruses except that the B-specific oligonucleotide was replaced with another oligonucleotide, whose sequence differed by a single-base change from G to A (see Fig. 4.9) (Rommelaere et al. 1979). Although point mutations elsewhere in the genome could not be excluded, it seems as though one or a few base changes in this one oligonucleotide are necessary, and perhaps sufficient, to determine

```
N    GAUUACACCACCCAAAG
                ↕↕↕ ↕
B    GAUUACACCACUACAG
     ↕
NB   AAUUACACCACUACAG
```

Figure 4.9 Nucleotide sequences involved in N tropism and B tropism of MLV. Sequences of oligonucleotides in *gag* that segregate with N, B, or NB tropism were determined by oligonucleotide fingerprinting and sequencing. The NB-tropic oligonucleotide is from a spontaneous mutant from the B-tropic strain shown (Rommelaere et al. 1979). Arrows indicate base changes.

the tropism of MLV for N- and B-type mouse cells. This oligonucleotide is probably within the region that codes for p30, since (1) there is a small difference in electrophoretic mobility of the p30 proteins of the parental viruses, (2) all the N-tropic recombinants showed the N-type p30 mobility (Schindler et al. 1977; Gautsch et al. 1978), and (3) the electrophoretic mobility of p30 is altered in the NB-tropic variants (Hopkins et al. 1977b).

B. *env*

The *env* gene encodes the surface proteins of the virion that are required for recognition of specific cell-surface receptors early in infection. Because of their location and role, the *env*-gene products determine both host range (including subgroup specificity) and the neutralizing antigens of the virion. In both avian and murine viruses, the *env*-gene products are synthesized from a subgenomic-size mRNA as a high-molecular-weight glycosylated precursor ($gPr92^{env}$ in ALV and RSV, $gPr90^{env}$ or $gPr80^{env}$ in MLV, and $gPr73^{env}$ in MMTV). This precursor is subsequently cleaved into two polypeptides. In all three types of viruses, the larger aminoterminal polypeptide (gp85, gp70, and gp52, respectively) has been implicated in receptor recognition and the smaller carboxyterminal polypeptide (gp37, p15[E], and gp36, respectively), as a hydrophobic membrane "anchor" protein (see Chapter 6). Since there can be considerable variation in host range from one strain of virus to another (particularly in the avian subgroups), the *env* gene has provided very useful genetic markers and has been quite well characterized genetically and physically (see Chapter 7).

1. Avian Viruses

The map location of *env* was determined from analysis of both recombinants and deletion mutants. Fingerprints of *env*^{A}*src*$^{+}$ recombinants derived from a cross between RAV-1 (*env*^{A}*src*$^{-}$) and Pr-RSV-B (*env*^{B}*src*$^{+}$) show that a set of oligonucleotides always segregates with the subgroup-A host-range phenotype (Joho et al. 1975). These oligonucleotides map in a block roughly from the middle of the RSV genome to about halfway toward the *src* gene (Coffin and Billeter 1976; Wang et al. 1977). Replication-defective viruses that lack envelope glycoprotein, such as SR-RSV NY8 and BH-RSV(−) (Kawai and Hanafusa 1973), are missing a longer region, which includes the oligonucleotides that segregate with the subgroup (Wang et al. 1976a) (see Fig. 4.7). The *env* gene must therefore be located between the middle of the genome and *src* in nondefective RSV.

The location of *env* deletions and nonhomologies has been defined by other methods. As determined by restriction mapping, BH-RSV(−) lacks a region extending from about 2.4 kb to about 4.3 kb from the poly(A) region (Shank et al. 1978). By this analysis, the deletions seem to be close to one another or to overlap, i.e., no sequence between *env* and *src* of *td* RSV common to BH-RSV(−) RNA is detected (see Fig. 4.7). By heteroduplex mapping, the deletions in BH-RSV(−) and SR-RSV NY8 measure from 2.2 kb to 4.4 kb from the poly(A) end (Junghans et al. 1977). (Note that these values differ slightly from those presented in the original reports due to normalization to a total genomic length of 9.5 kb.) As with the restriction map, the *src* and *env* deletions seem to touch or overlap; heteroduplexes between *td* PR-RSV-B and BH-RSV(−) or NY8 contain the opposed nonhomologous regions of *src* and *env* with no detectable intervening homology (Junghans et al. 1977). Thus, as determined by deletion analysis, *src* and *env* directly adjoin each other. This structure could explain the failure of BH-RSV(−) and similar viruses to generate nondefective transforming viruses by recombination with helpers or with endogenous viruses, as there seems to be no homologous sequence that could mediate recombination (see Chapter 7). The size of the *env* deletion in these viruses (2 kb) is very close to the amount of genome required to encode the putative *env* precursor (the apoprotein is 57,000–62,000 daltons) (Diggelmann 1979; Stohrer and Hunter 1979). As with studies on *src*, this correspondence in size does not necessarily mean that the deletion exactly corresponds to the coding region for envelope glycoprotein.

The nucleotide sequence of Pr-RSV-C (D. Schwartz et al., pers. comm.) confirms the location and provides information concerning the internal structure and expression of *env*. The coding region encompasses 1785 nucleotides about 5.1–6.9 kb from the 5′ end of the genome. As noted above, there is an overlap, in a different reading frame, with the 3′ end of *pol*. A particularly interesting feature of *env* expression is revealed by nucleotide sequencing and S1 mapping (D. Schwartz et al.; R. Swanstrom et al.; both pers. comm.) As noted above, the splice donor site for the *env* (and *src*) leader sequence is 18 nucleotides 3′ of the *gag* N terminus, and the splice into *env* apparently preserves the reading frame, so that the first 6 amino acids are those encoded by the beginning of *gag*. The primary *env* gene product predicted thus consists of 601 amino acids, of which 62 can be assigned to the N-terminal signal peptide, 335 to gp85, and 198 to gp37, on the basis of partial amino acid sequence data (E. Hunter et al., pers. comm.) (see Chapter 6). There is also a short intervening peptide between gp85 and gp37.

Among different strains of nondefective ALV and RSV, the greatest sequence variation is found within the *env* gene, although even here substantial similarity is still detected. cDNA probes specific for the *env* gene, prepared by hybridizing total RSV cDNA with the RNA of the envelope deletion mutant SR-RSV NY8 and discarding the hybrid (Hayward 1977; Tal et al. 1977b), distinguish only slightly among subgroups A–E (Fujita et al. 1978). Subgroups A and C were indistinguishable by this test, and subgroups B, D, and E had homologies of 75–88% with a subgroup-A-specific or subgroup-C-specific probe. In no cases were differences in melting temperatures (T_m) of the hybrids detected, suggesting less than 1.5% divergence among the hybridizable sequences. Similarly, heteroduplexes between PR-RSV-B and PR-RSV-C formed under relatively nonstringent conditions did not have any mismatched regions in the *env* gene (Junghans et al. 1977); application of more stringent conditions, however, did reveal a region of partial nonhomology within *env* (Chien et al. 1980). By both methods, the subgroup-F and subgroup-G *env* genes of endogenous ring-necked and golden pheasant viruses (RPV and GPV) were substantially or completely unrelated to those of chicken subgroups A–E and to each other (Keshet and Temin 1977; Fujita et al. 1978; Hu et al. 1978a).

Oligonucleotide mapping of *env* genes of avian tumor viruses of subgroups A–E reveals more diversity than other techniques. For example, comparison of genomes of subgroups A, B, and C of PR-RSV by fingerprinting showed detectable sequence differences only within *env* (Joho et al. 1976). In a more extensive comparison, Coffin et al. (1980) found that different viruses of subgroups A–D contained between 1 and 6 of the 14 *env*^{E} oligonucleotides of RAV-0. Taken together, such structural comparisons show that the *env* genes of the various chicken viruses are probably derived from a common ancestor and presumably have diverged by mutation to encode proteins of distinct receptor specificity. Note that the subgroup of the ancestor virus cannot be determined from this analysis; in particular, there is no reason to assume that it was a subgroup-E endogenous virus (see Chapter 10).

Receptor specificity is encoded by only a portion of the total *env* gene. Recombinants selected for a specific subgroup inherit a subset of the oligonucleotides missing from *env*$^{-}$ mutants (Joho et al. 1975; Wang et al. 1976b). These subgroup-specific oligonucleotides map in a block toward the 5′ end of *env,* and some oligonucleotides on either side of these regions are either highly conserved in all strains or segregate independently of *env* in recombinants (Joho et al. 1975; Wang et al. 1976b; Tsichlis and Coffin 1980a,b). From these results, the *env* gene of avian oncoviruses can be divided into three regions: C_L, left common region; S, subgroup-coding region; and C_R, right common region (Coffin et al. 1978a) (Fig. 4.7). Not surprisingly, the greatest sequence divergence between subgroups is in the S region; oligonucleotides within this region of subgroup-B and subgroup-E viruses are not protected from RNase digestion by hybridization with cDNA from the other subgroup, and heteroduplexes between subgroup-B and -C or between subgroup-C and -E viruses are readily melted under relatively stringent conditions (Chien et al. 1980). Oligonucleotide mapping does not allow accurate estimates of the sizes of the various subregions of *env,* but heteroduplex maps suggest lengths of approximately 0.6 kb, 0.7 kb, and 0.8 kb for the C_L, S, and C_R regions, respectively. The length of the subgroup-coding region must be considered to be a minimum estimate, since sequences that segregate with the subgroup need not be sufficiently diverged to score as nonhomologous by this method.

The segregation of the S region of *env* with subgroup specificity seems invariant; large numbers of recombinants between different subgroups have been examined and, with one exception (described below), recombinants that join parts of the S regions of two subgroups have not been isolated as pure species (Joho et al. 1975, 1976; Wang et al. 1976b; Tsichlis and Coffin 1980a). The linkage of sequences in this region is in distinct contrast to most parts of *gag* and *pol* and to other parts of *env,* which, in general, segregate randomly among the progeny of such crosses (Galehouse and Duesberg 1978; Linial and Brown 1979). It is unlikely to be due to failure of recombination to occur within this region, since genomes with such crossovers can be detected in mixtures of recombinants (Tsichlis and Coffin 1980a). Most probably, crossovers within the S region between *env* genes of different subgroups give rise to noninfectious particles. Thus, the S region probably encodes a portion of the envelope glycoprotein that must be retained for proper receptor binding. The nucleotide sequence of Pr-RSV-C (D. Schwartz et al., pers. comm.) reveals that the S region occupies the central portion of the region encoding gp85.

There is one class in exception to this general rule (Tsichlis et al. 1980). Some recombinants formed between subgroup-E viruses and either subgroup-B or subgroup-D viruses have an intermediate host range in that they infect the respective nonpermissive avian cells, T/BD and C/E, with equal efficiency. Interference studies suggest that these viruses use the subgroup-E receptor on T/BD cells and the subgroup-B receptor on C/E cells. Fingerprint analysis of the genomes of two such recombinants shows a common feature: both have an S region derived largely from the subgroup-B or subgroup-D parent but contain a single subgroup-E-specific oligonucleotide. Such recombinants probably point to regions of the *env*-gene product directly involved in receptor binding.

2. *Mammalian Viruses*

A similar combination of genetic and physical analyses of *env* genes has been applied to some MLVs. Dualtropic (or polytropic) MLVs have been isolated both from stocks of MLV grown in culture and from certain strains of mice with a high incidence of leukemia (see Chapters 2, 8, and 10). These viruses have an extended host range in comparison with ecotropic MLV in that they can infect cells of many species as well as mice. Two such isolates, called HIX (Fischinger et al. 1975) and Mo-MLV$_{83}$ (Troxler et al. 1977b), were isolated from

Mo-MLV grown in cell culture. These variants appear to be *env* recombinants containing information related to endogenous xenotropic viruses, as the only difference in protein products is within gp70, where tryptic peptides resembling those of xenotropic MLV are present (Fischinger et al. 1978). Comparison of the HIX or Mo-MLV_{83} genomes with the parental virus by oligonucleotide mapping (Faller and Hopkins 1978a; Shih et al. 1978b) or by heteroduplex mapping (Chien et al. 1978; Donoghue et al. 1978) shows that a set of oligonucleotides mapping between 1.5 kb and 2.4 kb from the 3′ end has been replaced (see Fig. 4.7). Oligonucleotide mapping of the subgenomic 21S *env* mRNA of Mo-MLV shows that the 5′ end of this mRNA is very near the left end of the region that dualtropic viruses acquire by recombination (Faller et al. 1978). This mRNA species is about 2.8 kb in length (exclusive of the spliced leader derived from the 5′ end of the genome) (Rothenberg et al. 1978). Thus, recombinant maps and analysis of mRNA species suggest that the *env* gene must extend rightward from a point 2.8 kb from the 3′ end of the genome. Heteroduplex mapping of the substituted region in the 21S presumptive *env* mRNA of HIX and Mo-MLV_{83} suggests a structure for *env* analogous to that of RSV (Chien et al. 1978; Rothenberg et al. 1978): there is a common region of 0.33 kb at the left of *env,* followed by the nonhomologous region of about 0.9 kb, followed by complete homology with the 3′ end of the genome. The internal nonhomologous region presumably corresponds to a portion of gp70 involved in receptor binding and is detectable by differences in peptide maps. Detailed analysis of gp70 molecules of other recombinants by mapping the sites reactive with monoclonal antibodies (epitopes) is at least roughly consistent with this general structure. Niman and Elder (1980) mapped epitopes specific for polytropic recombinants at the carboxyterminal half of gp70. This location would place the nonhomology in the middle of the *env* gene or somewhat 3′ to the region suggested by structural studies.

The leukemogenic polytropic viruses, such as the mink-cell focus-inducing (MCF) viruses isolated from leukemic AKR and other mouse strains (Hartley et al. 1977), have *env* substitutions that vary from isolate to isolate but closely resemble those found in Mo-MLV_{83} and HIX viruses (Chien et al. 1978; Rommelaere et al. 1978). The roles of this substitution and of the altered host range it confers in the leukemogenic process are complex issues and will be considered in Chapters 8 and 10.

There are numerous isolates of polytropic *env*-gene recombinant viruses from many strains of mice, and although these have been intensively studied, the parental genome that donates the *env* substitution has not been identified. Analyses of the recombinant *env* gene by oligonucleotide mapping (Rommelaere et al. 1978; Green et al. 1980) and heteroduplex mapping (Bosselman et al. 1979) and of the gp70 by peptide mapping (Elder et al. 1977) have shown that the *env*-gene substitution is related to xenotropic viruses isolated from the same mouse strain. However, the genomes of polytropic viruses contain distinct oligonucleotides and tryptic peptides in *env* (Green et al. 1980) and in gp70 (Elder et al. 1977) not found in any of the common xenotropic viruses from the same mice. Thus, it cannot yet be determined whether the unique host range of the polytropic viruses is due to a preexisting parental *env* gene or is created by recombination between genes encoding ecotropic and xenotropic host ranges.

The additional MLV *env*-gene marker that has been identified and physically localized in the genome is a site that probably encodes G_{IX} antigen (see Chapter 6). The recombinants between N-tropic and B-tropic BALB/c endogenous viruses (discussed in Section V.A) also vary in G_{IX} antigenicity, since the B-tropic parent was G_{IX}^{+} and the N-tropic parent was G_{IX}^{-} (Hopkins et al. 1977a). In 16 recombinants examined, the presence of one oligonucleotide specific for the B-tropic parent correlated exactly with the G_{IX}^{+} phenotype (Faller and Hopkins 1978c). This oligonucleotide was mapped in the 3′ portion of *env*, to the right of the region associated with dualtropism (see Fig. 4.7). G_{IX} antigenicity correlates with a decreased apparent molecular weight of the gp70 (Hopkins et al. 1977a) and appears to be due to the absence of the asparagine-leucine-threonine glycosylation site (Donis-Keller et al. 1980; Rosner et al. 1980). Comparative sequence analysis of the G_{IX}-associated oligonucleotide and an allelic oligonucleotide from a G_{IX}^{-} strain (see Fig. 4.10) are consistent with a glycosylation site being removed due to the single-base change from G_{IX}^{-} to G_{IX}^{+} antigenicity (Donis-Keller et al. 1980).

Some additional insight into the structure of the MLV *env* gene and its relationship to the 3′ end of the genome has been obtained from the nucleotide sequence of a cloned in-vitro-synthesized cDNA copy of the 3′-terminal region of the Mo-MLV genome (Sutcliffe et al. 1980a). A schematic illustration of this region is shown in Figure 4.11. There is an open reading frame of 195 codons extending from the 5′ end of the sequenced portion to within 45 nucleotides of the beginning of U_3. Since the 5′ region of this sequence corresponds to the amino acid sequence near the amino terminus of p15(E) (S. Orozslan, pers. comm.), it must include all of p15(E) except the very amino terminus. The carboxyterminal amino acid predicted from this sequence is proline, whereas that of p15(E) is leucine; therefore, there must be an additional cleavage, probably during budding. It was originally suggested that a 95-amino-acid protein (the R or rightmost coding protein) was cleaved off (Sutcliffe et al. 1980b); however, it now seems more likely that this terminal cleavage removes only a small (16-amino-acid) peptide (S. Orozslan, pers. comm.).

The p15(E) coding region of the genome may also be important in leukemogenesis. F. Pedersen and W. Haseltine (pers. comm.) have obtained variants containing point mutations, detectable by oligonucleotide mapping, that distinguish highly leukemogenic strains from nonleukemogenic strains of MLV isolated from AKR mice. These oligonucleotides can be located in the p15(E) sequence. Additionally, N. Hopkins et al. (pers. comm.) have found a single AKR-MLV-specific oligonucleotide within this region whose presence correlates with oncogenicity of the AKR MCF viruses. The significance of these findings remains to be resolved (see Chapter 10).

C. *src*

Because *td* deletion mutants are readily isolated and replicate well, the RSV *src* gene was the first gene to be mapped on the genome. *td* PR-RSV lacks three large oligonucleotides (numbered 5, 6A, and 6B in Fig. 4.6) found in the nondefective parent; these must therefore be

G_{IX}^{-} UAUCUCAACCACCAUACUUAACCUCACCACYG

↕

G_{IX}^{+} UAUCUCAACCACCAUACUUG

G_{IX}^{-} ILE-SER-THR-THR-ILE-LEU-ASN-LEU-THR-THR

Figure 4.10 Nucleotide sequences involved in G_{IX} antigenicity of MLV. The sequence of two oligonucleotides in *env* that segregate with G_{IX} antigenicity are presented (Donis-Keller et al. 1980). The amino acid sequence at the bottom is inferred from the sequence of the G_{IX}^{-} oligonucleotide. The reading frame is inferred from the fact that the other two frames lead either to a termination codon (UAA) or to no change (UUA and UUG both code for leucine). The reading frame agrees with that found by T. Shinnick et al. (pers. comm.) in the complete Mo-MLV sequence. The underlined portion of the amino acid sequence is thought to be a glycosylation signal. Y indicates a pyrimidine. The arrow denotes the base change.

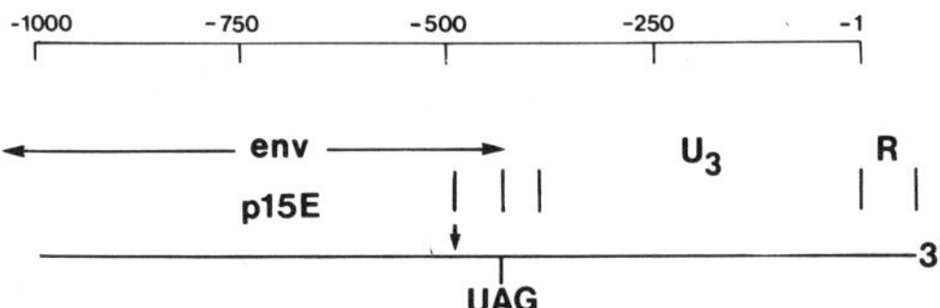

Figure 4.11 The 3′-terminal region of the Mo-MLV genome. The relative locations of the portion of the *env* gene that encodes p15(E) and the untranslated regions at the 3′ end of the genome are shown (Sutcliffe et al. 1980b). The upper line gives the scale in nucleotides. The small arrow indicates a site at which p15(E) is probably cleaved to yield the mature virion protein (S. Orozslan, pers. comm.).

within the *src* gene. Because these three, of all large nucleotides, are the nearest to the poly(A) region, the *src* gene must be near the 3′ end of the genome (Wang et al. 1975; Coffin and Billeter 1976). The association of the same oligonucleotides with *src* was also shown by using a series of $env^{A}src^{+}$ recombinants isolated from a cross between RAV-1 ($env^{A}src^{-}$) and PR-RSV-B ($env^{B}src^{+}$) (Joho et al. 1975). The two strains of viruses have rather different fingerprints, and thus analyses of the recombinants show which parts of the genome were inherited from each parent. The only region of all recombinants inherited from the src^{+} parent contained oligonucleotides 5, 6A, and 6B. Interestingly, some additional information to the 5′ side of *src* was also inherited by all transforming recombinants. This finding has recently been extended to a larger series of recombinants between PR-RSV-B and RAV-0 (Tsichlis and Coffin 1980a). Nucleotide-sequencing data indicate that this region to the left of *src* is not part of the coding region (Czernilofsky et al. 1980a; Yamamoto et al. 1980c; D. Schwartz et al., pers. comm.), yet it could contain some regulatory element or signal, such as a splice junction.

The *src* genes of different RSV strains (including some presumably independent isolates) are quite similar to, but not identical with, one another. Hybridization studies with $cDNA_{src}$ probes reveal no significant differences between strains (Stehelin et al. 1976). Detailed oligonucleotide mapping, however, does reveal small strain-specific sequence differences (Wang et al. 1980a,b), as do immunological and structural analyses of the *src*-gene product, $pp60^{src}$ (Brugge and Erikson 1977; Purchio et al. 1978) (see Chapter 9). Thus, all *src* genes of RSV must be derived from a common ancestor, most probably the related *c-src* sequence of the host cell.

The complete nucleotide sequence of a 3-kb region of the SR-RSV genome, containing *src,* has recently been determined by Czernilofsky et al. (1980a) and the complete sequence of Pr-C RSV, including *src,* has been determined by D. Schwartz et al. (pers. comm.) (see Appendix E). Schematic diagrams of the SR-D and Pr-C *src* regions are presented in Figure 4.12. Several interesting features have emerged: (1) The open reading frame in *src* is 1590 nucleotides in length; this is sufficient to code for a 530-amino-acid polypeptide with a molecular weight of 58,500, consistent with the 60,000-dalton estimate for $pp60^{src}$ (see Chapter 9). (2) The coding region is flanked by sequences with no substantial open reading frames. Between the potential *env* termination codon and the *src* initiation codon, there are about 400 nucleotides of apparently untranslated sequence; presumably the sequence between *env* and *src* contains sequences required for the expression of *src,* such as a splice-acceptor site, but these remain to be identified. Similarly, between the *src* termination codon and the U_3 region, there are 220 untranslated nucleotides. (3) The sequences flanking *src* contain a large direct repeat of 91 nucleotides, with only 13 mismatches (86% homology).

The Pr-C RSV *src* region is similar in general construction but has interesting differences in detail (Fig. 4.12). There are about 265 nucleotides between the end of the *env* and the initiation codon for *src* and about 350 nucleotides between the *src* termination codon and the beginning of U_3. There is also a directly repeated sequence flanking *src*, but it is rather differently arranged. The total length of repeated sequence is about 120 nucleotides and the copy 5′ of *src* is found in a single block. The copy 3′ of *src*, however, is divided into two regions, one of about 80 and the other of about 40 nucleotides, with a unique sequence of about 135 nucleotides intervening between the two. Although the 5′ end of the repeated sequence in Pr-C is in about the same place as that of Sr-RSV, the greater length of the Pr-C sequence results in the inclusion of the purine-rich PB+ sequence and a small portion of U_3 within the sequence 3′ of *src*. A probable splice-acceptor sequence (D. Schwartz et al.; R. Swanstom et al.; both pers. comm.) is found in the Pr-C sequence 14 nucleotides 3′ of the repeated sequence and about 70 nucleotides before the *src* initiation codon. Thus, although *src* apparently uses the same spliced leader as *env*, unlike *env*, *src* provides its own AUG.

As yet, nucleotide sequences of the corresponding region of nontransforming viruses have not been determined, and it is not

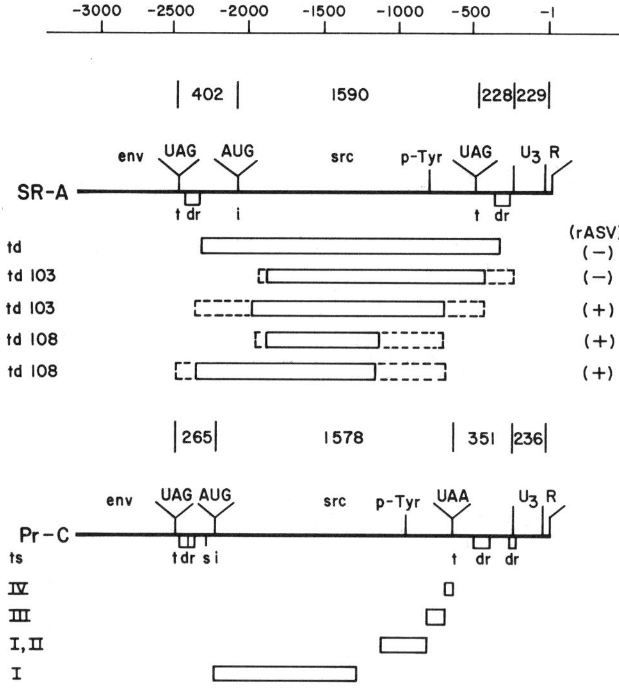

Figure 4.12 The *src* gene of RSV. Shown schematically are the nucleotide sequences of the 3′-terminal 3000 nucleotides of SR-RSV-A (Czernilofsky et al. 1980a) and Pr-RSV-C (D. Schwartz et al., pers. comm.). The top line shows the scale in nucleotides; the second line indicates the lengths of the various regions. i and t indicate initiation and termination codons, respectively, for translation. P-Tyr indicates the probable site of phosphotyrosine (see Chapter 9). The small boxes marked dr indicate a directly repeated sequence of about 91 nucleotides flanking *src*. In the lower part of the figure, the open boxes indicate the regions from which sequences are deleted from various transformation-defective mutants. The line marked td is a standard type of *td* deletion mutant sequenced by Yamamoto et al. (1980c). The lines following (*td* 103, *td* 105, *td* 108, and *td* 109) indicate partial deletion mutants (Wang et al. 1980b), with the position of the deletion (open box) inferred from the absence of specific large T1 oligonucleotides that define these regions. The dashed lines indicate uncertainty in the boundaries of the deletions. The column at the right indicates the ability of these viruses to give rise to recovered ASV (rASV) after injection into chickens (Halpern et al. 1979). The Pr-C *src* region is shown at the bottom with the same conventions. A candidate splice acceptor site is shown by S. The open boxes indicate the regions which contain the *src*^{ts} mutants of the four cooperative transformation groups shown (Wyke et al. 1975) (see Chapter 7), as inferred from recombination experiments with defined partial deletion mutants in *src* (V. Fincham et al., pers. comm.). Note that the last set (I, III) did not yield recombinants with any deletion tested and may include some double mutants.

known with certainty which parts of the flanking sequences are derived from virus information and which are required for replication or transformation. However, comparison of the sequence of the two RSV strains implies that the cellular *src* (*c-src*)-derived information is that which appears between the repeated sequences, and that the directly repeated sequences themselves were derived by a reduplication of virus information when *src* was acquired by the virus. It can be hypothesized that homologous recombination between the directly repeated sequences would result in deletion of *src* and most of the flanking sequences. Yamamoto et al. (1980a,c) reported the nucleotide sequence of the 3′-terminal region of a 21S RNA in RSV-infected cells, which seems to have been derived in this way. Comparison with the complete sequence of the *src* region shows that this RNA species is missing 2007 nucleotides (see Fig. 4.12), with the deletion extending from corresponding points in the direct repeats. This result is consistent with a deletion created by crossing-over in the homologous sequences on either side of *src*. It is likely that this deleted species was derived from *td* deletion mutants contaminating the RSV stock, but this point remains to be proved. Homologous crossing-over through this directly repeated sequence, e.g., by copy choice during reverse transcription (Coffin 1979), would explain the apparent uniformity in size of the genomes of many distinct *td* RSV isolates (Duesberg and Vogt 1973a; Bernstein et al. 1976). Crossing-over at this location cannot account for all *td* deletion mutants, however, as mutants with shorter deletions have been obtained from several RSV strains (Kawai et al. 1977; Lai et al. 1977; Yoshida et al. 1979; Fincham et al. 1980). These "partial" *td* deletion mutants have a genome size somewhat longer than standard *td* virus (see Fig. 4.7) and some are capable of recombining with *ts src* mutants to yield wild-type virus (Kawai and Hanafusa 1976; Fincham et al. 1980). The precise location of the deletions in some of these viruses has recently been determined and used to locate the regions containing some *ts* mutants (V. Fincham et al., pers. comm.), as shown in Fig. 4.12. Another interesting set has been subjected to detailed oligonucleotide mapping (Wang et al. 1978, 1980a,b; H. Hanafusa et al. 1980) and can be approximately mapped from the location of oligonucleotides missing from the *src* sequence (see Fig. 4.12).

Several partial *td* deletion mutants have the interesting property that they can give rise to transforming virus after injection into birds (Hanafusa et al. 1977; Halpern et al. 1979; Vigne et al. 1979). These transforming viruses, termed recovered ASV (rASV), are described in more detail in Chapters 7 and 9. Briefly, they appear to be recombinants between the viral genome and *c-src*-related information (see Chapter 9) endogenous to the host cell, a conclusion supported by fingerprint analysis of the rASV *src* gene (Wang et al. 1978, 1980a,b) and by analysis of its gene product (Karess et al. 1979). Not all partial *td* deletion mutants can give rise to rASV. Of the viruses shown in Figure 4.12, only those that retain a short region near the 3′ end of *src* can do so (H. Hanafusa et al. 1980; Wang et al. 1980b). The position of the 5′ end of the deletion seems to be immaterial. These results suggest either that some residual homology in the 3′ region with *c-src* is required to mediate the recombinational event or that the 3′ portion of *src* contains some functionally important sequence not found in *c-src*. A similar conclusion regarding the necessity of retained *src* sequences can be drawn from the results of Vigne et al. (1979). However, heteroduplex mapping studies suggested that retention of the 5′ region of *src* is necessary (Lai et al. 1977). Whether this discrepancy reflects strain differences, a requirement to retain at least one of the direct-repeat sequences, or a difference in techniques has not been resolved.

In most cases, the various rASV isolates are nondefective and identical with the starting RSV strain (except for the small differences in *src* that serve as markers) (Halpern et al. 1979; Vigne et al. 1979). However, several rASV strains derived from *td* NY109, which has a deletion extending to the 5′ side beyond the usual limit (see Fig. 4.12), are defective for replication, although *td* NY109 is not (H. Hanafusa et al. 1980). These defective viruses have a complete *src* gene, but large and variable deletions to the 5′ end of *src*. H. Hanafusa et al. (1980) have proposed that the 5′ sequences missing from *td* NY109 contain a region of homology with *c-src* necessary for recombination and that, in their absence, crossing-over occurs at other sites of random homology in the RSV genome, leading to a loss of sequences between *src* and the site of homology. Alternatively, it is possible that the region absent from *td* NY109 contains a sequence that must be adjacent to *src* for its expression and that this role can be filled by sequences in other locations of the genome.

VI. GENOMES OF DEFECTIVE TRANSFORMING VIRUSES

Many retroviruses capable of transforming appropriate tissue-culture cells and inducing rapid neoplastic disease in animals have been isolated. With the sole exception of the few strains of nondefective RSV, these viruses are defective for replication and require coinfection of the cell with a helper virus for the production of infectious virus. A number of defective transforming viruses have been associated with a wide variety of diseases, including sarcoma, carcinoma, and leukemia of various cell types. Details of the genomes of individual viruses are discussed below. In a stringent sense, neither FEV nor radiation leukemia virus (RadLV) (discussed in Sections VI.B.5 and VI.B.6) is known to transform cells in vitro as measured by the standard criteria for morphological conversion. Nevertheless, since they represent replication-defective oncogenic viruses, it is appropriate to discuss the structures of their genomes in this section. Many of the general features of this group of oncogenic defective viruses are summarized here (for reviews, see Hanafusa 1977; Vogt and Hu 1977; Bishop 1978; Graf and Beug 1978; Bishop et al. 1980; Bister and Duesberg 1980; Duesberg 1980; Sharp 1980):

1. Most isolates lack at least part of the *gag, pol,* and *env* genes and require that all three functions be provided by the helper for the rescue of the genome of the transforming virus. The 3′- and 5′-terminal noncoding regions are similar to or identical with the helper.
2. The genomes of defective transforming viruses are usually smaller than those of related replication-competent viruses.
3. In place of some of the deleted information, there is a specific sequence that is unrelated to the helper-virus genome. These sequences are generally called *onc* sequences (or, more loosely, *onc* genes) (Baltimore 1975; Duesberg 1980).
4. cDNA probes for the *onc* sequences are at least partially homologous to single-copy (unique) cellular DNA of the animal from which the virus was isolated. The related host DNA does not seem to be part of a discrete endogenous viral genome, but rather a normal host gene. In addition, probes for most *onc* genes detect at least a few copies per cell of related poly(A)-containing RNA in uninfected cells.

In many cases, a direct role for the *onc* sequence or its gene product in transformation by these viruses has not been rigorously established because of the lack of appropriate mutants. However, a few mutants or variants have been obtained and they do provide evidence for the role of *onc* sequences in vitro and in vivo (see Chapters 7 and 9). The similarity in structure of these viruses to one another, the analogy of the specific sequence to the *src* gene of RSV, and the presence of closely related sequences in independent isolates with similar biological properties provide compelling circumstantial evidence that transformation by the defective transforming viruses is due, at least in part, to the *onc* sequence in the genome. Although not proved directly, it is reasonable to hypothesize that these viruses arise as a result of recombination and deletion events that bring a normal host-cell gene under virus control and allow transcription and translation of the "cellular gene" insert at a high rate. Whether the higher rate of expression of some benign cell gene is in itself sufficient to induce transformation of the target cells or whether some additional alterations in the gene product are required pose questions that remain to be answered. These phenomena are discussed in greater detail in Chapter 9.

Many independent isolates of transforming viruses now exist and, in some cases, the same or a closely related *onc* sequence has been found in more than one isolate. So far, 13 distinct *onc* sequences have been identified. Although all of these sequences lead, in general terms, to the same effect (the transformation of a normal cell into a malignant one) they are unrelated to one another and may encode proteins with rather different functional properties. In the past, many of these *onc* sequences, now known to be unrelated to RSV *src,* have been called *src.* To avoid confusion arising from this ambiguous nomenclature, a proposal has been put forth to give names to the various *onc* sequences reminiscent of the prototype virus (J. Coffin et al., in prep.). These names (shown in Table 4.3, along with their probable *onc*-gene products and the names and abbreviations of the defective transforming viruses) will be used throughout the book. The complete guidelines for these names and their use are given in the Appendix A.

A. Transforming Viruses of Birds

1. Avian Myelocytomatosis Viruses

MC29, MH2, CMII, and OK10 viruses, although four independent isolates, form a related group in that they have similar pathogenicity in vivo, transform the same cell type in vitro (Beug et al. 1979), and have specific *onc* sequences with extensive homology to one another

Table 4.3 Suggested names for *onc* inserts in retroviral genomes

Name	Isolates	Prototype strain	Probable species of origin	Probable protein product
src		Rous sarcoma virus (RSV)	chicken	$pp60^{src}$
myb	AMV-*myb*	avian myeloblastosis virus (AMV-BAI/A)	chicken	$P35^{myb}$?
	E26-*myb*	avian myeloblastosis virus (E26)	chicken	$P150^{gag-myb}$
myc	MC29-*myc*	myelocytomatosis virus (MC29)	chicken	$P110^{gag-myc}$
	CMII-*myc*	myelocytomatosis virus (CMII)	chicken	$P90^{gag-myc}$
	OK10-*myc*	myelocytomatosis virus (OK10)	chicken	$P200^{gag-pol-myc}$
	MH2-*myc*	Mill Hill virus 2 (MH2)	chicken	$P100^{gag-myc}$
erb(A)		avian erythroblastosis virus (AEV)	chicken	$P75^{gag-erb\text{-}A}$
erb(B)		avian erythroblastosis virus (AEV)	chicken	$P40^{erb\text{-}B}$
ros		UR-2 virus	chicken	$p68^{gag-ros}$
fps	FuSV-*fps*	Fujinami sarcoma virus (FuSV)	chicken	$P140^{gag-fps}$
	PRCII-*fps*(P)	Poultry Research Centre virus 2 (PRCII)	chicken	$P105^{gag-fps}$
yes		Y73 avian sarcoma virus	chicken	$P90^{gag-yas}$
rel		reticuloendotheliosis virus strain T (REV-T)	turkey	?
abl		Abelson murine leukemia virus (Ab-MLV)	mouse	$P120^{gag-abl}$
mos	Mo-*mos*	Moloney murine sarcoma virus (Mo-MSV)	mouse	?
	Gz-*mos*	Gazdar murine sarcoma virus (Gz-MSV)	mouse	?
ras	Ra-*ras*	rat sarcoma virus (RaSV)	rat	$P29^{gag-ras}$
	Ki-*ras*	Kirsten murine sarcoma virus (Ki-MSV)	rat	$p21^{ras}$
	Ha-*ras*	Harvey murine sarcoma virus (Ha-MSV)	rat	$p21^{ras}$
fes	ST-*fes*	Snyder-Theilen feline sarcoma virus (ST-FeSV)	cat	$P85^{gag-fes}$
	GA-*fes*(GA)	Gardner-Arnstein feline sarcoma virus (GA-FeSV)	cat	$P95^{gag-fes}$
fms		McDonough feline sarcoma virus (SM-FeSV)	cat	$P180^{gag-fms}$
sis		Simian sarcoma virus (SSV)	woolly monkey	?

(Duesberg and Vogt 1979; Roussel et al. 1979; Sheiness et al. 1980b) (see Chapters 8 and 9). Nonproducer transformed fibroblast lines infected with MC29 or MH2 viruses (Bister et al. 1977; Hu and Vogt 1979; Quade 1979) are unable to complement ALV mutants containing lesions in *gag, pol,* or *env*. Therefore, MC29 and MH2 have defects in all three replicative genes. Immunoprecipitation of nonproducer cell proteins with antisera specific for the various helper-virus gene products reveals only one protein containing determinants related to *gag*-gene products (Bister et al. 1977; Hu et al. 1978b; Mellon et al. 1978; Hayman et al. 1979a; Kitchener and Hayman 1980; Ramsay et al. 1980) (see Chapters 7 and 9). This polyprotein has an apparent molecular weight of about 110,000 in MC29, 100,000 in MH2, 90,000 in CMII, and 200,000 in OK10-infected cells.

A direct role for the MC29 protein in transformation is implied by analysis of three mutants that have an altered transforming phenotype. These mutants encode *gag*-related proteins shorter than the "standard" P110 and which vary from 90,000 to 100,000 daltons (Ramsay et al. 1980). Preliminary evidence suggests that they might have arisen by replacement of some of the oncogene-specific sequences, *myc,* with additional *gag* information, perhaps by illegitimate recombination with the helper virus (G. Ramsay, K. Bister, P. Duesberg, and M. Hayman, pers. comm.).

Since cells infected with the transforming virus alone produce no virions (except in the case of OK10 virus, discussed below), analysis of the genomes of these viruses is always complicated by the presence of helper virus. Superinfection of nonproducer cells with nondefective ALV yields, in many cases, virions with a high proportion of transforming virus to helper virus. Such preparations contain two sizes of high-molecular-weight RNAs; one with the size and oligoribonucleotide fingerprint of the helper and a second smaller species. The smaller RNA can be identified as the genome of the transforming virus because (1) it is found only when biologically detectable transforming virus is present, (2) it contains nucleotide sequences not found in the helper alone, and (3) it can be translated in vitro to give a polyprotein indistinguishable from that found in infected nonproducer cells (Mellon et al. 1978). These small genomes have been studied extensively by oligonucleotide fingerprinting, heteroduplex mapping, and hybridization with specific cDNA probes, with good agreement among the various methods (although estimates of the exact sizes of the various regions vary somewhat).

The genome of MC29 is 5.0–5.5 kb, 65% of which is homologous with ALV (see Fig. 4.13) (Mellon et al. 1978; Sheiness et al. 1978, 1980b; Hu et al. 1979; Stehelin et al. 1980). The arrangement of sequences agrees with that expected from the protein studies. There is a region similar or identical in sequence to the helper of about 1.5–1.9 kb at the 5′ end, followed by the specific sequence of about 1.7 kb, followed by a 3′-terminal region of about 2 kb homologous to the 3′-terminal region of ALV (i.e., the 3′ end of *env* and the U_3R region). Thus, the P110 is most likely the translation product from the left-

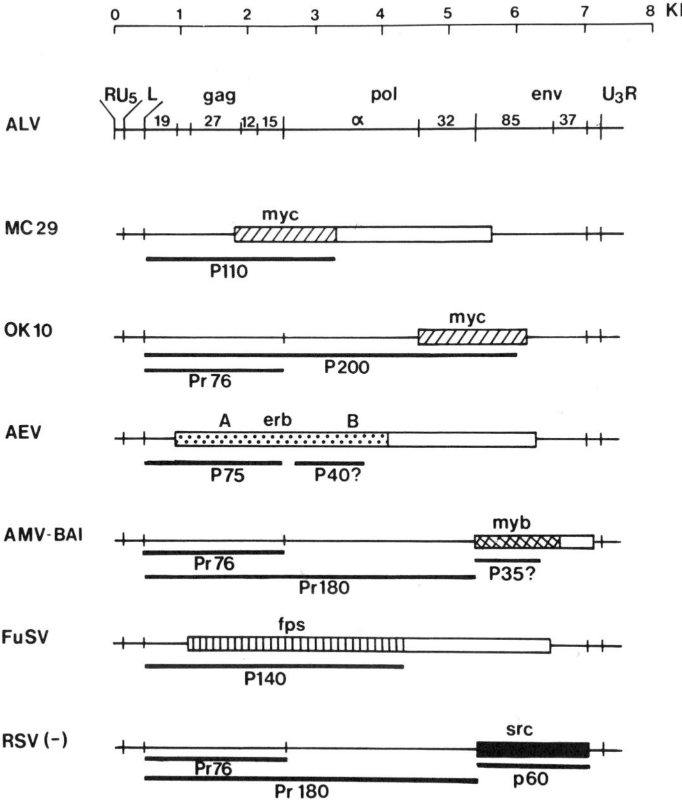

Figure 4.13 Defective transforming viruses of birds. Below the scale, the first line represents the genome of replication-competent ALV; the other lines show various isolates of transforming virus. The shaded boxes indicate *onc* inserts, with related inserts given the same shading, and the open boxes indicate deletions. The heavy bar(s) under each genome shows the size and probable location of the protein products encoded by each genome. Further discussion and references are presented in the text.

hand 3.3 kb or so of the MC29 genome, terminating near the end of the specific sequence. The genome contains ample capacity for an additional gene or genes (e.g., derived from the remaining *env* fragment), but no additional viral gene products have been detected in MC29 nonproducer cells and there is no detectable subgenomic mRNA (Bishop et al. 1980). The MC29 *onc* sequence has been called *mac* (Roussel et al. 1979), *mcv* (Duesberg and Bister 1981), and $onc_{\rm MCV}$ (Bishop et al. 1980). We will use the term *myc* (Table 4.3).

The *gag, env,* and U_3 sequences shared between MC29, CMII, OK10, or MH2 and their helpers are quite closely related, with a number of common oligonucleotides (Bister et al. 1979; Duesberg and Vogt 1979; Ramsay and Hayman 1980). At least part of the fragmentary *gag* and *env* genes of MC29 codes for functional polypeptide sequences, since replication-competent recombinants between MC29 and RAV-0 often contain oligonucleotides specific for these regions (Tsichlis and Coffin 1979). Such recombinants also contain the U_3 region of MC29, and often the terminally redundant sequence as well. Analogous to the situation described above with other exogenous viruses (see Section III.E), recombinants between MC29 and the endogenous RAV-0 that contain the MC29 U_3 region have a more rapid growth rate than RAV-0.

The *myc* sequence of MC29 has no detectable homology with any replication-competent viral genome. It is, however, closely related to the specific sequence of MH2, CMII, and OK10. An MC29-specific cDNA probe hybridizes essentially completely to CMII and OK10 RNAs and about 70% to MH2 RNA (Sheiness et al. 1978, 1980b; Duesberg and Vogt 1979; Roussel et al. 1979; Bister and Duesberg 1980), and the MC29, MH2, and CMII genomes have a number of identical oligonucleotides in their specific regions (Bister et al. 1979; Duesberg and Vogt 1979). As with $cDNA_{src}$, DNA complementary to the specific region of MC29 has extensive homology with single-copy cellular DNA of chickens, somewhat less homology with DNA of other birds, and a small, but detectable, homology with mammalian DNAs (Roussel et al. 1979; Sheiness and Bishop 1979; Sheiness et al. 1980a).

The genomes of CMII and MH2 have an overall structure very similar to that of MC29, with only small differences in size and position of the specific sequence (Bister et al. 1979; Roussel et al. 1979; Duesberg and Bister 1981). OK10, however, seems quite different. The genome of this virus is only slightly smaller than that of

ALV and it contains a complete *gag* gene and partial *pol* gene along with the *myc* sequences (Duesberg et al. 1980; Stehelin et al. 1980). Unlike the other viruses of this group, OK10-infected cells contain the *gag* precursor, $Pr76^{gag}$, as well as a 200,000-dalton protein (P200) that contains *gag, pol,* and *myc* peptides (Ramsay and Hayman 1980). Preliminary data suggest that there may be two virus-specific mRNA species produced by such cells (D. Chiswell, pers. comm.). Consistent with the presence of $Pr76^{gag}$ is the production by such cells of noninfectious particles containing the OK10 genome (Ramsay and Hayman 1980). Therefore, it seems probable that the *myc* sequence in OK10 is expressed by a mechanism involved in *pol* expression in ALV or RSV, rather than the mechanism involved in *gag*-gene expression, which is presumably the pathway used by MC29, CMII, and MH2 viruses.

2. Avian Erythroblastosis Virus

AEV induces erythroblastosis and sarcomas in chickens and transforms fibroblasts and erythroid cells in vitro (Graf and Beug 1978). It encodes a *gag*-related protein of about 75,000 daltons (P75) with determinants of the *gag* protein p19, but not p27 (Hayman et al. 1979b; Rettenmier et al. 1979). Evidence that this protein is involved in the oncogenicity of AEV has been provided by analysis of a mutant (*td* 359) that has lost the ability to transform erythroid cells, although it does transform fibroblasts (Royer-Pokora et al. 1979); this mutant has a P75 protein with decreased electrophoretic mobility (Beug et al. 1980a,b). The genome of AEV has been studied by oligonucleotide fingerprinting (Bister and Duesberg 1980), heteroduplex mapping (Lai et al. 1979), and hybridization with specific cDNA probes (Roussel et al. 1979; Bishop et al. 1980; Stehelin et al. 1980). Identity of the smaller genome as that of the transforming component has been confirmed by molecular cloning of the smaller species and rescue of transforming activity by transfection (Vennstrom et al. 1980). The overall structure of this genome is quite similar to MC29, although it is slightly shorter, with an estimated size of 4.9–5.5 kb. The specific sequence, however, is much larger (3.1–3.7 kb) and is unrelated to *src* or *myc,* as determined by hybridization or fingerprinting. It has been designated *erb* (see Table 4.3). The *erb* sequence is flanked by 0.75–1.1 kb of information related to the 5′-terminal region of the helper-virus genome on the 5′ side and 1–1.4 kb of *env* + U_3-related information on the 3′ side.

The size of the AEV genome is nearly three times that required to code for the P75. Furthermore, less than half the *erb* sequence would suffice to encode the 45,000-dalton non-*gag*-related sequences of P75. Recent evidence from a number of laboratories suggests the possibility that the AEV genome encodes a second, independently expressed protein. In vitro translation of RNA from AEV (plus helper virus) virions leads to the synthesis of a 40,000-dalton protein (P40), which is unrelated either to P75 or to any of the helper-virus proteins (Lai et al. 1980; Pawson and Martin 1980; Yoshida and Toyoshima 1980). This protein is apparently synthesized from a spliced subgenomic-size mRNA of about 3 kb (Anderson et al. 1980; D. Sheiness et al., pers. comm.) and contains no *gag*-related information. The presence of the same mRNA in AEV-infected nonproducer cells implies that such a protein is, in fact, a product of the AEV genome, but P40 has not yet been demonstrated in infected cells, due to the lack of an appropriate reagent for detection. If correct, this result implies that the *erb* sequence is actually two genes, tentatively designated *erb*-A and *erb*-B (see Fig. 4.13). The mode of *erb* expression implied by these results is unique; no other transforming retrovirus is yet known to encode two *onc*-gene products.

The *erb* insert seems to be derived from a normal-cell gene. DNA complementary to the AEV-specific sequence has homology with single-copy DNA of chickens and other birds (Roussel et al. 1979) and with a polyadenylated mRNA present in fibroblasts. This RNA, about 12 kb, is found at a level of 2–3 copies per cell (Bishop et al. 1980) and consists of several related species. The translation products of these RNAs have not been identified.

3. Avian Myeloblastosis Viruses

AMV strain BAI/A has a more limited target specificity than the preceding viruses, as it induces only myeloblastosis in animals and transforms only myeloid precursors and mature monocytes in culture (Baluda and Goetz 1961; Beug et al. 1979; Gazzolo et al. 1979; Durban and Boettiger 1981). Although very large amounts of this virus (plus helper) are grown for biochemical purposes, it is quite difficult to obtain nonproducer transformed cells and, therefore, relatively little work has been done on the structure of its genome. The structure of a presumptive AMV genome has been determined by molecular cloning and restriction and heteroduplex mapping in comparison to its associated helper virus (myeloblastosis-associated helper virus [MAV]) (Souza and Baluda 1980; Souza et al. 1980a,b). The genome is about 0.5 kb shorter than that of the helper, and the two are homologous for about 5 kb from the 5′ end, a length that should include the entire *gag* and *pol* genes. The putative *onc* sequence (*myb;* Table 4.3) (Roussel et al. 1979) is about 1.3 kb in length and appears to replace *env*. This overall structure is analogous to that of BH-RSV(−), with *myb* instead of *src* (see Fig. 4.13). Consistent with this structure, Duesberg et al. (1980) have found that AMV-infected cells (in the absence of helper-virus production) produce noninfectious particles and synthesize $Pr76^{gag}$. However, unlike BH-RSV(−), the particles contain no detectable reverse transcriptase activity and do not encode Pr180, in spite of the presence of an apparently complete *pol* region. Also consistent with the genomic structure is the presence in AMV-infected cells of a subgenomic-size spliced RNA of about 21S (about 2.3 kb) containing U_5, *myb,* and U_3 sequences (Chen et al. 1981; Gonda et al. 1981). It is therefore possible that the AMV genomic structure would require a mechanism for expression similar to that employed for *env* expression to synthesize a *myb*-specific mRNA. This situation contrasts with the MC29 and OK10 systems described above.

No gene product of *myb* has been definitively identified. Cells infected with AMV do not seem to produce any fusion proteins reactive with antisera against structural virion proteins (Silva and Baluda 1980). In vitro translation of 21S RNA from virions leads to a protein of about 35,000 daltons (Duesberg et al. 1980), but this protein has not yet been detected in infected cells. DNA complementary to the *myb* sequence hybridizes well to uninfected-chicken-cell DNA and somewhat to DNA of other birds (Roussel et al. 1979; Souza et al. 1980c). A related RNA species is found in uninfected chicken fibroblasts at about 1 copy per cell.

An independent AMV isolate, strain E26, has identical transforming and oncogenic properties (Beug et al. 1979) and a closely related *onc* sequence. Unlike AMV-BAI/A, however, the E26 *myb* sequence appears to replace *gag* (Graf et al. 1980; Stehelin et al. 1980). In addition, an apparent *gag-myb* fusion protein of about 150,000 daltons can be found in E26 virus-infected cells. Although a detailed analysis of this genome has not been reported, it probably resembles MC29 in structure. Thus, the two AMV isolates have closely related or identical *onc* genes, capable of functioning and leading to similar pathogenicity despite presumably different modes of expression.

4. Fujinami and PRCII Avian Sarcoma Viruses

FuSV is an independent strain of transforming virus isolated in Japan (Fujinami and Inamoto 1914) at about the same time as the discovery of RSV (Rous 1911). Since it has virtually identical transforming ability and pathogenicity as RSV, it was long thought to be a similar isolate, and indeed, at least some stocks recovered years later were quite similar to commonly used strains of RSV (Wang et al. 1980a). However, recent results, mainly from oligonucleotide mapping studies, have shown that FuSV is quite different from RSV, and its genome closely resembles that of some of the defective transforming viruses discussed above (T. Hanafusa et al. 1980; Lee et al. 1980). The genome is quite small (about 4.5–5.0 kb) and most of *gag, pol,* and *env* have been replaced by an *onc* sequence of about 3.2 kb unrelated to *src* or to any other avian *onc* gene (see Fig. 4.13); this sequence has been termed *fps* (see Table 4.3). As with other viruses of this general structure (cf. MC29 and AEV), FuSV encodes a *gag* fusion protein of about 140,000 daltons, a size that virtually exhausts the coding capacity of the genome. Thus, this structure (one that generates a *gag-x* fusion protein) is not limited to viruses that cause acute leukemia.

Another independent sarcoma virus, PRCII, isolated in Scotland (Carr and Campbell 1958), appears to be related to FuSV; there is considerable cross-hybridization of the *fps* sequence (Shibuya et al. 1980). PRCII encodes a related *gag* fusion protein (P105), which by peptide mapping shows no similarity to *myc, erb,* or *src* products (Breitman et al. 1981; Neil et al. 1981). A closely related specific sequence has also been recently described in another avian sarcoma virus, UR1, isolated in the United States (P. Balduzzi et al., pers. comm.).

A particularly interesting feature of the *fps* sequence is suggested by the results of Shibuya et al. (1980), who found a small, but significant, homology (25%) between a cDNA probe specific for *fps* and the genomes of the Gardner-Arnstein (GA) and Snyder-Theilen (ST) strains of feline sarcoma virus (FeSV). This result implies the independent acquisition of the same *onc* sequence from two very distantly related species, one a mammal and the other a bird.

5. Y73 Avian Sarcoma Virus

There is another strain of sarcoma virus of chickens, Y73 (Itohara et al. 1978), not yet very thoroughly studied. Its 4.8-kb (26S) genome contains neither *src-*, *erb-*, *myb-*, nor *fps*-related sequences (Kawai et al. 1980; Shibuya et al. 1980; Yoshida et al. 1980). A *gag*- related polyprotein (P90) has also been detected by analysis of infected-cell proteins and in vitro translation (Kawai et al. 1980). These data suggest that there is yet another avian *onc* gene, termed *yes* (Table 4.3), capable of conferring sarcomagenicity on the viruses that contain it. *yes*-specific cDNA probes detect a related sequence in uninfected-chicken-cell DNA structurally unrelated to *c-src* (Yoshida et al. 1980). An independent isolate, called Esh sarcoma virus has a similar *gag*-related polyprotein and presumably also has the *yes* sequence (Ghysdael et al. 1981).

6. Other ALV-related Transforming Viruses

UR2 virus was isolated in the United States in 1963 from a chicken sarcoma (P. Balduzzi et al., pers. comm.). The structure of its genome is similar to that of FuSV and Y73 in that it contains a specific *onc* sequence joined to part of *gag* and nonproducer cells contain a 68-kD *gag*-related fusion protein (L. Wang et al., pers. comm.). The specific sequence of UR2 seems to represent a new class, since it is unrelated to *onc* sequences from other avian transforming viruses.

Another set of defective transforming viruses, including SK770 and SK780, has been isolated from a stock of a *td* deletion mutant of B77-RSV after multiple passages in tissue culture (E. Stavnezer et al., pers. comm.). These viruses are also replication defective and their genomes apparently have a specific insert in *gag* and encode a *gag*-related fusion protein of about 125 kD. Again, the specific sequence on these viral genomes does not seem to be related to other avian *onc* genes. Although SK770 and SK780 transform fibroblasts efficiently, their pathogenicity in animals has not been demonstrated.

7. Reticuloendotheliosis Virus

REVs comprise a group of C-type viruses of birds that are unrelated to the RSV-ALV group, yet are detectably related to some mammalian viruses (see Chapters 2 and 6). Most viruses in this group, such as SNV, are nondefective viruses that do not transform cells in culture. The one exception is an REV strain that transforms cultured fibroblasts and lymphoid cells and induces a very rapid reticuloendothelial disease. Nonproducer transformed cells do not release particles, indicating that the genome of the transforming virus is defective and that the defectiveness probably represents extensive deletions (Hoelzer et al.

1979, 1980). The component responsible for transformation has been referred to as REV-T, and the helper virus in this particular strain has been referred to as REAV or REV-A (Robinson and Twiehaus 1974; Hoelzer et al. 1979).

Analysis of RNA monomers in particles released from virus-producing REV-T-transformed hematopoietic cells reveals two distinct RNA species (Breitman et al. 1980; Hoelzer et al. 1980; Simek and Rice 1980). The larger RNA species is presumably the genome of REV-A and has a length of approximately 8.7 kb (34S). The smaller RNA species, probably the genome of REV-T, has a length of 5.9 kb (28S). Therefore, it appears that the genome of REV-T, like other defective transforming viruses, contains an extensive deletion of replicative sequences. A third RNA species of 4.8 kb is also released from at least one REV-T-transformed clone (Simek and Rice 1980); since it contains only REAV-specific sequences, it may represent a defective REV-A genome (Gonda et al. 1980). Hybridization experiments indicate that 15–30% of the REV-T RNA consists of sequences not found in REV-A (Breitman et al. 1980; Gonda et al. 1980). These specific sequences may be the *onc* sequences of REV-T. REV-T shares 12–15 of 42 identifiable oligonucleotides with REAV (Breitman et al. 1980). REV-T does not contain the *myc*-specific oligonucleotides found in MC29, MH2, and CMII or the *src*-specific nucleotides of RSV. REV-T therefore appears to contain a unique class of *onc* gene, tentatively called *rel* (see Table 4.3). Restriction mapping and heteroduplex analysis indicate that *rel* consists of about 1.5 kb of sequence located about 1 kb from the 3′ end of the genome (probably in place of *env*) and may be expressed via a subgenomic mRNA. The REV-T genome also has a substantial deletion in the *gag-pol* region (M. Lai et al.; I. Ehen et al.; both pers. comm.). *rel*-specific probes detect unique related sequences in uninfected cells, with the most closely related sequences in turkeys, the species of origin of this virus.

B. Mammalian Viruses

1. Abelson Murine Leukemia Virus

Ab-MLV was isolated from a prednisolone-treated mouse infected with Mo-MLV (Abelson and Rabstein 1970) and has Mo-MLV as a helper. It induces a pre-B-cell lymphoma in mice and transforms some fibroblast lines and lymphoid cells in culture (Sklar et al. 1974; Rosenberg et al. 1975, 1980; Scher and Siegler 1975; Rosenberg and Baltimore 1976; Boss et al. 1979). Nonproducer Ab-MLV fibroblast or lymphoid cell lines are readily isolated. These produce no virions and the only detectable virus-related protein in the best-studied strain is a polyprotein of about 120,000 daltons (P120) containing determinants of the *gag* proteins p15, p12, and part of p30 (Reynolds et al. 1978; Witte et al. 1978). In addition to the helper-virus genome, virions rescued from nonproducer cells contain a 5.6-kb RNA species identified as the Ab-MLV genome, since it can be translated into an identical P120 polyprotein in vitro (Shields et al. 1979). Heteroduplex mapping of the RNA with Mo-MLV cDNA shows that about 1.25 kb at the 5′ end and 0.72 kb at the 3′ end of Mo-MLV are retained in the Ab-MLV genome and that the central 6.5-kb region of Mo-MLV has been replaced by 3.6 kb of Ab-MLV-specific (*abl*) sequence (see Fig. 4.14 and Table 4.3). More accurate estimates of 1320 bases and 730 bases for the lengths of the 5′- and 3′-terminal sequences, respectively, shared with Mo-MLV were obtained from the size of Mo-MLV cDNA fragments protected from nuclease-S1 digestion by hybridization to Ab-MLV RNA (Shields et al. 1979). Although it is not known exactly where translation of *gag* begins in the Mo-MLV genome, the 5′ shared region of Ab-MLV could encode, at most, about 300 amino acids, which should include all of p15 and p12 and less than half of p30, in good agreement with the inferred structure of P120.

As with some of the avian viruses, the Ab-MLV-specific region is much larger than the 2.4 kb needed to encode the *abl* portion of the P120 polyprotein. Several variants of Ab-MLV with different size polyproteins have been described (Rosenberg et al. 1980), one of which (perhaps the original progenitor strain) has a 160,000-dalton specific protein. The genome of this virus is about 1 kb larger than the P120 strain; thus, there is still the same discrepancy between genome and polyprotein size. Other variants, which have polyprotein sizes of 100,000, 90,000, and 85,000 daltons, have genomes indistinguishable from the P120 strain, indicating that the smaller polyproteins probably arise by nonsense or frameshift mutations (S. Goff et al., pers. comm.). These strains are capable of transforming fibroblasts but are reduced in their ability to (1) transform lymphocytes, (2) induce lymphoma, and (3) exhibit phosphokinase activity (Rosenberg et al. 1980). Some additional mutants of Ab-MLV lack kinase activity and

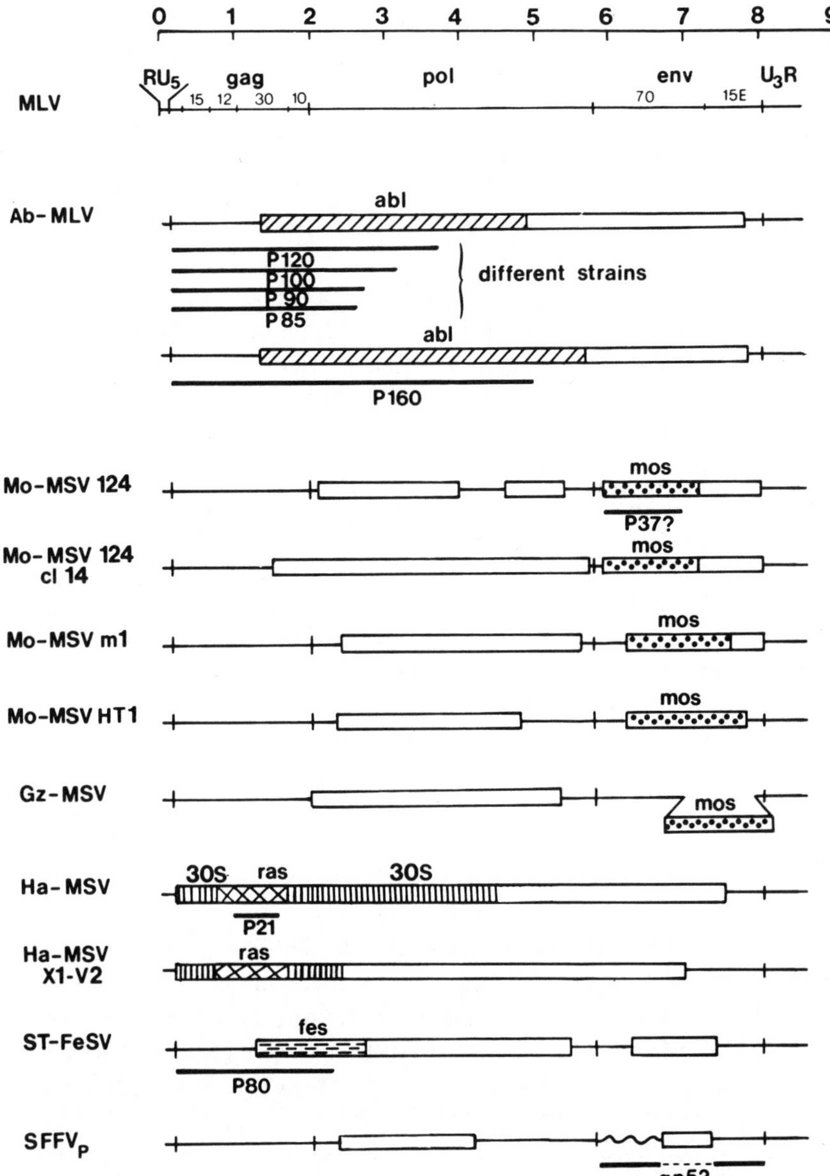

Figure 4.14 Defective transforming viruses of mammals. Conventions are given in Fig. 4.13. Wavy lines represent functionally related, but distinct, sequences. With the exception of FeSV, all the viruses shown were probably derived from MLV. ST-FeSV is most likely derived from FeLV; FeLV has a structure very similar to that of MLV (Sherr et al. 1980). Note that SFFV contains only virus-related information.

transforming activity entirely. One class of these has a normal-size P120 and may represent missense mutations (Reynolds et al. 1980), whereas one other mutant has a polyprotein of about 92,000 daltons and a small deletion (0.7 kb) in the *abl* sequence (Witte et al. 1980). Thus, unlike most other defective transforming viruses, there is genetic evidence for the role of *abl* and the enzymic activity of its gene product in transformation and leukemogenesis (see Chapter 7).

The Ab-MLV-specific sequence seems to be related to a cellular gene (Baltimore et al. 1980; Goff et al. 1980). The availability of an antiserum specific for the non-*gag*-related portion of P120 has made possible the detection of a related protein in uninfected cells (Witte et al. 1979). This protein is found predominantly in thymus cells and has a molecular weight of about 150,000 daltons. If this protein is the gene product of the endogenous cellular progenitor of the Ab-MLV-specific sequence, then only some 70% or less of its polypeptide sequence will appear in the Ab-MLV gene product.

2. Moloney Murine Sarcoma Virus

Mo-MSV was isolated from a sarcoma that appeared following injection of a BALB/c mouse with Mo-MLV (Moloney 1966). The viral complex consists of a replication-defective component and its helper virus. It induces fibrosarcomas in mice and transforms fibroblasts in culture. Several strains of this virus have been obtained from the original uncloned MSV stock and have somewhat different biochemical and biological properties. One cell line, G8-124 (Ball et al. 1973), has been intensively studied because it produces a very high ratio (about 30:1) of defective transforming virus, strain 124, to helper-virus genomes (Dina et al. 1976). The smaller genome released by these cells is 5.0–5.5 kb in length, of which 70% of the sequences are shared with Mo-MLV, whereas the remaining 30% consist of specific sequences (*mos*) (Dina et al. 1976). The organization of the MSV-124 genome has been examined by heteroduplex mapping (Hu et al. 1977; Donoghue et al. 1979a) and its complete nucleotide sequence has been determined (E. Reddy et al.; C. Van Beveren et al.; both pers. comm.) (see Appendix E). The *mos* sequence, approximately 1.2 kb in length, is inserted 3′ of the splice point for the 21S mRNA for *env* and replaces almost all of the *env* gene but retains about 10 nucleotides from the 5′ end of *env* that provide an apparent initiation sequence for *mos*. In strain HT-1 MSV, an early passage isolate from the uncloned MSV stock, *mos* appears to be substituted for a portion of the *env* gene of the same size as the insert, although the genome shows an extensive deletion in the *pol* region as well (Vande Woude et al. 1979). The m1 and 124 Mo-MSV strains, isolated from uncloned stocks after some 200 passages in BALB/c mice, have lost variable amounts of the Mo-MLV sequences at either side of the *mos* insert (Donoghue et al. 1979b; Vande Woude et al. 1979). The 5′ MSV-124 sequence derived from Mo-MLV has two large deletions, one between 2.7 kb and 4.3 kb from the 5′ end of Mo-MLV and one from about 4.9 kb to 6.1 kb (within *pol*) and three small deletions. In contrast, the m1 and HT-1 MSV isolates have deletions beginning about 2 kb from the 5′ end of each genome extending 3.2 kb and 2.4 kb, respectively, and probably map entirely within the *pol*-gene region (see Fig. 4.14). Comparison of the deleted regions in these three MSV isolates serves to exclude the entire *pol* gene from any transforming function. Further passaging of Mo-MSV 124 leads to selection of variants with additional deletions in the 5′ portion of the genome (Canaani and Aaronson 1980); one variant, clone 14, has lost the entire *pol* gene and the 3′ portion of *gag* (Canaani et al. 1979). Approximately 1.1 kb of Mo-MLV sequence is conserved at the 3′ end of the *mos* sequence in HT-1 MSV, whereas the other MSV isolates have conserved only 0.8 kb (Donoghue et al. 1979b; Vande Woude et al. 1979). Therefore, much of the *gag*-related and *pol*-related information in Mo-MSV does not seem to be required for transformation.

Although the *mos* regions of several MSV strains have been cloned (Tronick et al. 1979; Vande Woude et al. 1979; Verma et al. 1980) and sequenced (Reddy et al. 1980; Van Beveren et al. 1981), a protein product of the *mos* gene of Mo-MSV remains to be identified. In vitro translation of subgenomic-size RNA from Mo-MSV virions yields a series of products, the largest of which, about 37,000 daltons, is roughly consistent with the open reading frame predicted from the *mos* sequence (Papkoff et al. 1980), but no similar protein has been found in infected cells. Nevertheless, the *mos* sequence has been directly implicated in transformation by transfection with subgenomic fragments of Mo-MSV DNA. Andersson et al. (1979) found that a restriction fragment of MSV DNA synthesized in vitro, which includes the *mos* sequence and about 0.9 kb of the 5′ Mo-MLV sequence and little if any 3′ Mo-MLV sequences, efficiently transforms NIH-3T3 cells. Canaani et al. (1979) obtained similar results with a fragment of unintegrated linear DNA obtained from infected cells that included the specific *mos* sequence and 3′ Mo-MLV sequence. Direct DNA transfection with cloned genomic and subgenomic fragments of MSV (Vande Woude et al. 1979) showed that the 5′ end of the m1 MSV genome could be removed without markedly reducing the transforming activity of *mos;* however, the 3′ MLV-related sequences were essential for efficient transformation. These 3′ sequences were subsequently identified as containing the LTR region and could be placed at either the 3′ end or the 5′ end of *mos* in order to attain efficient transformation (Blair et al. 1980). Thus, very little more than the specific sequence appears to be required for transformation, but the LTR region is required both for efficient transformation by *mos* and for activation of the transforming potential of the related sequence in uninfected cells (see below). Not surprisingly, at least some of the shared sequences, although not required for transformation, are required for the virus to be replicated, since cells transformed by transfection with subgenomic Mo-MSV DNA fragments do not produce transforming virus after superinfection with MLV (Canaani et al. 1979).

The mode of expression of the MSV-specific sequence remains to be determined. A priori, it seems that there must be some sort of subgenomic-size mRNA if the MSV-specific sequence is to be translated, since the major product of m1 MSV in vivo is $P60^{gag}$ (Robey et al. 1977; Oskarsson et al. 1978); likewise, the in vitro translation products of MSV-124 viral RNA are 60,000-dalton and 72,000-dalton *gag*-related products (Philipson et al. 1978). Since the *gag*-related and *pol*-related sequences in the genome amount to some 2.5 kb (capable of encoding about 95,000 daltons of protein), these proteins cannot include information translated from the specific sequence. The preservation of the *pol-env* junction in all MSV strains would suggest that the *env* splicing site might be involved in generating a subgenomic-size mRNA, and a candidate splice-acceptor sequence can be found near the 5′ end of the *mos* sequence (Reddy et al. 1980). However, an mRNA with this structure has not yet been found. Instead, Donoghue et al. (1979a) have identified a subgenomic RNA in G8-124 cells that is about 2.1 kb shorter than the MSV genome. This small RNA is missing most of the *gag*-related information and contains about 0.44 kb of the 5′ end joined to the right-hand portion of the genome (as compared with about 0.17 kb for Mo-MLV). This species is found on polysomes and resembles a spliced retroviral mRNA, except that the usual splicing points for

Mo-MLV are apparently not used. Whether a similar RNA species exists for other Mo-MSV strains has not been determined, nor has it been demonstrated that this RNA is a spliced product of the MSV provirus, rather than a product of a deleted provirus present in the same cells. Clearly, the expression of *mos* is a major unresolved issue.

The *mos* sequences of the 124, HT-1, and m1 strains of MSV are closely related to one another (Donoghue et al. 1979a,b; Vande Woude et al. 1979) but not to the *onc* genes of other transforming viruses, except Gazdar (Gz)-MSV. Gz-MSV is an independent isolate (Gazdar et al. 1972) with a structure similar to that of m1 MSV, except that it retains much more of *env* (Donoghue et al. 1979b).

As expected, a DNA probe for the specific sequences hybridizes to a nonviral cellular sequence (termed *c-mos*) present in a unique 15-kb restriction fragment (and therefore presumably in single-copy DNA) of normal mouse DNA (Canaani et al. 1979, 1980; Tronick et al. 1979; Vande Woude et al. 1979); this fragment has been cloned molecularly (Jones et al. 1980; Oskarsson et al. 1980). The DNA fragment containing the *c-mos* sequence transforms cells if viral sequences are placed to the 5′ side of *c-mos* (Oskarsson et al. 1980). More specifically, if an MSV LTR is placed 0.6 kb to the 5′ side of *c-mos*, the gene can be activated to transform cells in a direct DNA transfection assay (W. McClements et al., pers. comm.). This result supports the idea that there are transcriptional control sequences within the LTR region (see Section III) (Dhar et al. 1980; Shimotohno et al. 1980; Sutcliffe et al. 1980a; Yamamoto et al. 1980b) and that integration of a proviral LTR upstream from, or within, a potentially transforming normal-cell sequence can activate or increase in vitro expression resulting in cell transformation.

3. Kirsten and Harvey Murine Sarcoma Viruses

Ki-MSV and Ha-MSV are closely related but independent isolates obtained from sarcomas that developed in rats following inoculation with Ki-MLV (Kirsten and Mayer 1967) or Mo-MLV (Harvey 1964), respectively. These viruses induce sarcomas and erythroleukemia in mice and transform mouse cells in culture but have genomes substantially different from that of Mo-MSV. The defective transforming genomes of Ki-MSV and Ha-MSV have been identified as species of about 7.5 kb and 5.5 kb, respectively (Chien et al. 1979) (see Fig. 4.14 for the structure of Ha-MSV). They have been compared with each other and with their presumptive ancestors by oligonucleotide mapping (Shih et al. 1978a,c) and by heteroduplexing mapping (Chien et al. 1979; Young et al. 1980), with similar results. Both viral genomes have relatively little homology to the helper virus, with a shared sequence of about 1 kb at the 3′ end. There is probably a short shared sequence at the 5′ end of both genomes, because Mo-MLV strong-stop DNA hybridizes with reasonable efficiency to both Ki-MSV and Ha-MSV genomes (Tronick et al. 1978), but heteroduplex and oligonucleotide maps are ambiguous on this point; the extent of such homology cannot exceed 200 bases. The specific sequences of Ki-MSV and Ha-MSV are closely related, with a number of shared oligonucleotides. They differ in the presence of two unrelated regions beginning about 0.7 kb from the 5′ end, with the greater length of these regions accounting for the greater size of the Ki-MSV genome.

The only protein known to be encoded by these two viral genomes is a phosphoprotein of about 21,000 daltons (p21) (Shih et al. 1978c, 1979a). The p21 proteins of Ki-MSV and Ha-MSV are antigenically related to each other and to a similarly sized protein in uninfected rat cells (Langbeheim et al. 1980; Scheinberg and Strand 1980) and do not contain helper-virus proteins. These proteins are biochemically distinct from other *onc*-gene products studied so far in that they have a guanine nucleotide-binding activity (Scolnick et al. 1979; Shih et al. 1980). Evidence for the role of this protein in transformation comes from mutants temperature-sensitive for the transformation phenotype in which the p21 is thermolabile (Shih et al. 1979b) (see Chapter 7). This protein is most likely translated from sequences near the 5′ end of the genome, since its synthesis in vitro can be directed only by full-length RNA, and no subgenomic mRNAs have been found for these viruses. Only about 600 nucleotides (or around 10%) of the specific sequences of Ki-MSV and Ha-MSV would be needed to encode this small protein. Consistent with this are several lines of evidence showing that the large majority of this sequences are nonessential. Goldfarb and Weinberg (1981) found, among a series of clones transformed by transfection with Ha-MSV DNA, a few clones that contained only a portion derived from the 5′ end of the genome. Transforming virus could be rescued from these clones at very low efficiency after superinfection with Mo-MLV. From a clone of cells transformed by the rescued virus, a recombinant (X1-V2) was obtained that both transformed cells and was rescuable with high efficiency. The genome of this virus was found to be quite small, consisting of 2.4 kb from the 5′ end of Ha-MSV joined to 1.6 kb of Mo-MLV-related sequence. Therefore, less than half of the specific sequence is nonessential for either transformation by Ha-MSV or its replication and packaging with the aid of a helper virus. Similar results have been obtained in transfection experiments with molecularly cloned Ha-MSV DNA (Hager et al. 1979; H. Chang et al. 1980). A 1.7-kb subgenomic fragment derived from the 5′ end of the clone is capable of transforming cells (E. Chang et al. 1980; Wei et al. 1980) (see below).

Like other transforming viruses, the specific sequence of these viruses is related to, and presumably derived from, sequences found in the genomes of uninfected rat cells (Scolnick et al. 1973). Unlike other such sequences, however, most of the cell information related to the specific sequence is not a single-copy gene, but rather the endogenous viruslike "30S" RNA of rats (Tsuchida et al. 1974; Scolnick et al. 1976). Such RNAs (discussed in more detail in Chapter 10) are unrelated to known viruses and have no known protein product; but they resemble viral genomes in that they are efficiently packaged into virions, they can be induced to high levels with halogenated pyrimidines, and related DNA is found in multiple copies (more than 20 per haploid genome) in the cell genome. The 30S RNA can be obtained as a pseudotype with SSAV and separated from the SSAV genome on the basis of size. As determined by fingerprinting (Shih et al. 1978a) and heteroduplex mapping (Chien et al. 1979), substantial homology of about 4 kb exists between 30S RNA and Ha-MSV or Ki-MSV (Young et al. 1980) (see Fig. 4.14).

The most detailed information comes from a direct comparison of molecularly cloned DNA copies of Ha-MSV and 30S RNA by restriction mapping and DNA-transfer hybridization (Ellis et al. 1980). These workers found that there was a region unrelated to the 30S RNA, and also unrelated to the helper-virus genome, spanning the region between about 750 nucleotides and 1650 nucleotides from the 5′ end. Furthermore, a probe specific for this region hybridized to single-copy DNA of uninfected rat cells. Clones of DNA that included all of this region could transform cells, whereas clones that included only a portion could not (E. Chang et al. 1980) and in-vitro-created insertion mutants within this region lost transforming ability (Wei et al. 1980). It was concluded that this region encoded p21 and is therefore the *onc* gene of Ha-MSV (*ras;* see Table 4.3). In summary, the Ha-MSV genome can be thought of as consisting of 5 parts: (1) a short 0.2-kb region at the 5′ end derived from the helper, (2) a region of about 0.5 kb from 30S RNA, (3) the 0.9-kb *ras* sequence, (4) about 2.9 kb of 30S sequence, and (5) the 3′-terminal 1 kb of helper-virus sequence (see Fig. 4.14). This structure suggests at least a two-step origin for this virus, involving recombination of *ras* with a 30S RNA genome and recombination with the helper, although no order for these events is implied. Oddly, the *ras* sequence of Ha-MSV is not closely related to that of Ki-MSV RNA by heteroduplex mapping (Chien et al. 1979), although the p21 proteins encoded by the two viruses seem immunologically and functionally identical. Furthermore, the Ki-MSV and Ha-MSV *ras* sequences are related to different sequences in the host cell (D. Lowy et al., pers. comm.) (see Chapter 9).

At least one more isolate of defective transforming virus also appears to contain the same *onc* sequence. Rasheed and her colleagues have obtained a rat cell line producing a replication-competent endogenous virus (SD-1), which yielded defective transforming virus after cocultivation with rat cell lines transformed chemically or by DNA tumor virus (Rasheed et al. 1978; Rasheed 1980). The genome of this virus (RaSV) has not been studied in detail, but it encodes a protein that is functionally and antigenically similar to p21, except that it has a molecular weight of about 29,000 daltons, and, unlike p21, it is precipitable with antibodies against virion structural proteins (Young et al. 1979). Thus, the same specific sequence, instead of being expressed more or less independently, seems to be expressed by this virus as a fusion protein, most likely with *gag*. Considering the apparent ease of isolation of this virus, it is possible that the *ras* sequence in the transformed rat embryo cell lines had already recombined with a 30S RNA genome, thus facilitating its rescue.

4. Feline Sarcoma Virus

Several isolates of FeSV have been obtained from cats infected with FeLV. Two such isolates, the ST (Snyder and Theilen 1969) and GA (Gardner et al. 1970) strains, have related polyproteins (Barbacid et al. 1980; Ruscetti et al. 1980; Van de Ven et al. 1980b) and therefore most likely related *onc* sequences, referred to as *fes* (Table 4.3). The only FeSV genome that has been studied in detail is that of the ST strain, which has been molecularly cloned and analyzed by restriction mapping and heteroduplex mapping with its helper virus (Sherr et al.

1979, 1980). The structure of the ST-FeSV genome is fairly usual for defective transforming viruses (see Fig. 4.14). It is about 4.5 kb in length, with a 1.6-kb specific *fes* sequence flanked by 1.3 kb and 1.6 kb of helper-related information to the 5′ and 3′ sides, respectively. The only known translation product of the ST-FeSV genome is a *gag*-related polyprotein of about 80,000 daltons containing determinants related to p15, p12, and possibly p30 (Porzig et al. 1979; Barbacid et al. 1980; Ruscetti et al. 1980). In contrast, the *gag*-related polyprotein encoded by GA-FeSV is about 100,000 daltons and has related, but distinct, antigenicity, and the specific sequence of the GA-FeSV genome has extensive homology with that of ST-FeSV (Frankel et al. 1980). Thus, although the organization of the GA-FeSV genome has not yet been examined, it seems also to contain *fes* sequences inserted into the *gag* gene. One further interesting observation is that both ST-FeSV and GA-FeSV contain sequences related to the *onc* gene (*fps*) of FuSV (Shibuya et al. 1980) (see Section VI.A.4).

The *onc* sequence of a third FeSV strain, SM-FeSV (McDonough et al. 1971; Sarma et al. 1972), is apparently unrelated to *fes* by hybridization analysis (Frankel et al. 1980) and its *gag*-related polyprotein of 180,000 daltons is unrelated antigenically and by tryptic mapping to the ST-FeSV and GA-FeSV polyproteins (Barbacid et al. 1980; Ruscetti et al. 1980; Van de Ven et al. 1980a,b). Although not well characterized, the *onc* gene of SM-FeSV has been tentatively named *fms* (see Table 4.3).

5. Simian Sarcoma Virus

SSV was isolated from a pet woolly monkey with a spontaneous sarcoma (Wolfe et al. 1971) and is the only transforming virus yet isolated from primates. SSV is a defective virus capable of transforming fibroblasts in culture and was isolated together with a helper virus, SSAV, which is closely related to gibbon ape leukemia virus (GALV) and may have derived from an infected gibbon sharing the same household (for review, see Gallo and Wong-Staal 1980). The genome of SSV has been studied by molecular cloning and analyzed by heteroduplex and restriction mapping (E. Gelman et al.; K. Robbins et al.; both pers. comm.). Its structure is highly reminiscent of Mo-MSV. Relative to SSAV, it contains deletions of part of *gag* and most of *pol*, and has a specific sequence (*sis*, Table 4.3) of about 1.1 kb that replaces most or all of *env* and is unrelated to other viral *onc* sequences. Like Mo-MSV, SSV encodes a *gag*-related protein, which does not contain peptides or antigens unique to SSV (H.-J. Thiel et al., pers. comm.), suggesting that *sis* may be expressed via a spliced mRNA. As with other *onc* genes, *sis*-specific probes detect related sequences in uninfected cell DNA, with the closest relationship to DNA from woolly monkeys (F. Wong-Staal et al., pers. comm.). This result combined with the history of the virus, suggests that SSV arose in the animal from which it was isolated.

6. Friend Erythroleukemia Virus

FEV (Friend 1957) induces a rapid erythroleukemia in mice and does not transform fibroblasts in culture (see Chapter 8). It is an exception to the general rule for the acute leukemia viruses in that no specific sequences or nonvirus-related gene products have been detected. There are two related strains of Friend virus: FV-A, which induces anemia, and FV-P, which induces polycythemia. Friend virus stocks are a mixture of two components, a nondefective leukemia virus helper (designated Fr-MLV) and a defective component (designated $SFFV_A$ and $SFFV_P$ for the spleen focus-forming virus of the anemia and polycythemia strains, respectively). The Fr-MLV genome is identical in size with that of Mo-MLV (Evans et al. 1979). Nonproducer rat and mouse cells infected with $SFFV_P$ and $SFFV_A$ have been isolated (Bernstein et al. 1977; Troxler et al. 1977a, 1980; MacDonald et al. 1980). Because these viruses do not cause transformation of cells in vitro, this was accomplished by cloning infected cells and testing whether virus rescued by superinfection could induce splenomegaly typical of Friend disease (for more details, see Chapter 8). Rescued virions contain two size classes of RNA, the smaller of which correlates strictly with disease induction. The conclusion that the smaller RNA species contains the transforming genome has been confirmed using a molecular clone of $SFFV_P$ DNA (Linemeyer et al. 1980) and $SFFV_A$ DNA (A. Bernstein et al., pers. comm.), since virus capable of inducing Friend disease could be recovered following transfection of the cloned SFFV into mouse cells, accompanied by superinfection or transfection with a cloned helper virus.

$SFFV_A$ and $SFFV_P$ genomes are about 6 kb. Their sequences have been compared with that of the helper by hybridization with specific cDNA probes (Troxler et al. 1977a,b; Mak et al. 1978; Bernstein et al. 1979) and by oligonucleotide mapping (Evans et al. 1979, 1980; Yoshida and Yoshikura 1980) with somewhat surprising results.

cDNA, prepared from a mixture of the ecotropic Fr-MLV and SFFV and made specific for the defective viral genome by hybridization with the helper, detects a sequence in $SFFV_A$ and $SFFV_P$ unrelated to the helper but present in normal mouse cells. However, such cDNA hybridizes extensively to the genomes of xenotropic and polytropic MCF MLVs. Similarly, the only oligonucleotides of the $SFFV_P$ genome not shared with or related by cross-hybridization to sequences of Fr-MLV are found in MCF viruses. Direct comparison of the $SFFV_P$ genome with a polytropic recombinant of Fr-MLV (Fr-MCF) shows that the only detectable difference is the presence of two deletions in the $SFFV_P$ RNA, one about 1.5–2.5 kb from the 3′ end (in the right end of *env*) and the other about 2.3–4.2 kb from the 5′ end (including most of *pol* and perhaps some of *gag*) (see Fig. 4.14). No oligonucleotides distinct from Fr-MLV and Fr-MCF could be detected. Heteroduplex mapping confirmed these results, although a slightly different pattern in *gag-pol* was observed for another SFFV strain (Bosselman et al. 1980). Thus, it has been suggested that the oncogenicity of these viruses is a result of an altered sequence of some viral gene product, rather than due to the acquisition of a new sequence. Consistent with the deletion in *env,* cells infected with $SFFV_A$ or $SFFV_P$ alone contain an *env*-related glycoprotein of about 52,000 daltons (Dresler et al. 1979; Ruscetti et al. 1979; Yoshida and Yoshikura 1980), which is immunologically related to the gp70 of polytropic viruses. $SFFV_A$ differs from $SFFV_P$ in the *env* region, as determined by oligonucleotide mapping (Evans et al. 1980) and tryptic peptide analysis of gp52 (MacDonald et al. 1980).

Further evidence for the role of the altered *env* gene and its product in spleen focus formation comes from the work of Linemeyer et al. (1980 and pers. comm.), who prepared a subgenomic fragment of the molecularly cloned SFFV genome derived from the 3′ end and containing the region encoding gp52. When this fragment is cotransfected into NIH-3T3 cells along with an Fr-MLV clone, a recombinant virus can be generated that is capable both of inducing typical spleen foci in mice and of inducing gp52 in cultured cells. Thus, the 5′ half of the genome is not required for spleen focus formation, and there is good correlation between gp52 and Friend erythroleukemia disease.

7. *Radiation Leukemia Virus*

It has long been known that T-cell lymphomas, induced by X-irradiation of certain strains of mice, release RadLV, which is capable of inducing similar disease relatively soon after inoculation into recipient mice (Lieberman and Kaplan 1959) (see Chapter 8). It has been suggested that RadLV may be an acutely transforming virus, although the latent period of the disease is relatively long (about 3 months) and transformation in vitro has not been demonstrated. Consistent with this idea, however, Manteuil-Brutlag et al. (1980) have demonstrated that one cell line, BL/VL3 (Lieberman et al. 1979), isolated from a RadLV-induced tumor, produces virions resembling those of defective transforming viruses. These virions contain two RNA species that sediment as distinct dimers of 70S and 54S. The former contains an 8-kb genome, presumably the helper virus, and the latter contains a genome of 5.6 kb. This smaller genome shows sequence homology to the 5′-terminal region of MLV and encodes a 100,000-dalton protein in vitro, with antigenic determinants of MLV p12 and p15, but not p30. These results are reminiscent of the structure of Ab-MLV. It must be emphasized, however, that although the cell line produces high titers of RadLV, the association of this defective genome and the protein it encodes with disease induction remains to be established.

VII. CONCLUSIONS AND OTHER POSSIBLE RETROVIRAL GENETIC FUNCTIONS

In the preceding sections, we have seen that the organization of retroviral genes encoding virion proteins and transforming functions has been deciphered in great detail, and, at least for some viruses, their modes of expression are fairly well understood. The major unanswered structural questions concerning transforming viruses revolve around the mechanism(s) by which they are generated and the detailed relationship between *onc* genes and their cellular relatives (see Chapter 9). Also, there are other phenomena to which no genes have been specifically assigned. In most cases, there is probably no additional sequence in the genome to encode another gene, and the characteristics are presumably attributable to some additional effect of known genes or regions.

Many questions remain to be answered; two of the most interesting and intensive areas of research concern the following:

1. Possible roles of regions of the genome in regulation of expression. A particularly interesting case is that of MMTV, whose transcription is under glucocorticoid hormone control (see Chapter 5) and which has an exceptionally long (about 1.2 kb) U_3

region (Majors and Varmus 1981). It is intriguing to speculate that these features are related in some way, but the connection remains to be made. Two groups have recently shown that the MMTV genome has potential protein-coding capacity within the U_3 region. The first approach involves in vitro translation of subgenomic-size poly(A)-containing RNA isolated from virions; this RNA directs the synthesis of a polypeptide of 36,000 daltons and three smaller related polypeptides (Dickson and Peters 1981). However, as these polypeptides are unrelated antigenically to any virion structural protein, it has not yet been possible to assay for their expression in infected cells. The same group also demonstrated synthesis of these polypeptides by translation of a bacterial plasmid containing only the MMTV LTR (C. Dickson et al., pers. comm.). Further evidence for a potential coding region in the MMTV LTR has appeared from nucleic acid sequencing, which shows that this region contains an open reading frame sufficient to encode a similar-sized protein (Donehower et al. 1981; J. Majors, pers. comm.). This region has been referred to as "orf" (for open reading frame). Since two additional strains of MMTV have also been found to have a similar open reading frame (H. Diggelman; G. Hager; both pers. comm.), it is highly probable that it has a functional significance. However, at the present time, no functional properties can be attributed to these polypeptides, although a role either in oncogenesis or in the response to glucocorticoid regulation can be considered an interesting possibility until proved otherwise. It is possible that similar regions may exist in other viruses, leading to more subtle effects, such as tissue specificity or pathogenicity.

2. The molecular basis of nonacute malignancies. Although many *onc*-gene sequences and their protein products have been identified, the biochemical mechanisms by which the *onc*-gene products function in cell transformation are unknown. However, viruses with the ability to induce disease rapidly are quite rare. The more common retroviruses induce either a cytopathic disease (such as visna virus) or a malignancy (usually leukemia) with long latency periods. Since these diseases are caused by nondefective viruses that seem to contain only replicative genes, they are most likely due to either a side effect of some normal replication process or a rare aberration of some such process. In general, the genetic and

structural bases of such effects are more difficult to elucidate because of the difficulty of separating effects that act directly on pathogenicity from those that affect replication only. Nevertheless, work on these areas is proceeding rapidly, and a number of viable models are being tested (see Chapter 8).

These phenomena include some of the most interesting unresolved aspects of retrovirus biology and will provide many of the objectives for further genetic and structural analyses in years to come.

REFERENCES

Aaronson, S.A. and M. Barbacid. 1980. Viral genes involved in leukemogenesis. I. Generation of recombinants between oncogenic and nononcogenic mouse type-C viruses in tissue culture. *J. Exp. Med.* **151:**467–480.

Abelson, H.T. and L.S. Rabstein. 1970. Lymphosarcoma: Virus induced thymic-independent disease in mice. *Cancer Res.* **30:**2213–2222.

Adkins, B. and T. Hunter. 1980. Packaging of an abundant host cell mRNA by Rous sarcoma virus. *J. Supramol. Struct.* (Suppl.) **4:**269.

Anderson, S.M., W.S. Hayward, B.G. Neel, and H. Hanafusa. 1980. Avian erythroblastosis virus produces two mRNA's. *J. Virol.* **36:**676–683.

Andersson, P., M.P. Goldfarb, and R.A. Weinberg. 1979. A defined subgenomic fragment of in vitro synthesized Moloney sarcoma virus DNA can induce cell transformation upon transfection. *Cell* **16:**63–75.

Baker, C.C., J. Herisse, G. Courtois, F. Galibert, and E. Ziff. 1979. Messenger RNA for the Ad2 DNA binding protein: DNA sequences encoding the first leader and heterogeneity at the mRNA 5′ end. *Cell* **18:**569–580.

Ball, J.K., J.A. McCarter, and S.M. Sunderland. 1973. Evidence for helper independent murine sarcoma virus. I. Segregation of replication-defective and transformation-defective viruses. *Virology* **56:**268–284.

Baltimore, D. 1975. Tumor viruses: 1974. *Cold Spring Harbor Symp. Quant. Biol.* **39:**1187–1200.

Baltimore, D., A. Shields, G. Otto, S. Goff, P. Besmer, O. Witte, and N. Rosenberg. 1980. Structure and expression of the Abelson murine leukemia virus genome and its relationship to a normal cell gene. *Cold Spring Harbor Symp. Quant. Biol.* **44:**849–854.

Baluda, M.A. and I.E. Goetz. 1961. Morphological conversion of cell cultures by avian myeloblastosis virus. *Virology* **15:**185–199.

Baluda, M.A., M. Shoyab, P.D. Markham, R.M. Evans, and W.N. Drohan. 1975. Base sequence complexity of 35S avian myeloblastosis virus RNA determined by molecular hybridization kinetics. *Cold Spring Harbor Symp. Quant. Biol.* **39:**869–874.

Barbacid, M., A.V. Lauver, and S.G. Devare. 1980. Biochemical and immunological characterization of polyproteins coded for by the McDonough, Gardner-Arnstein, and Snyder-Theilen strains of feline sarcoma virus. *J. Virol.* **33:**196–207.

Bassin, R.H., B.I. Gerwin, J.G. Levin, G. Duran-Troise, B.M. Benjers, and A. Rein. 1980. Macromolecular requirements for abrogation of *Fv-1* restriction by murine leukemia viruses. *J. Virol.* **35:**287–297.

Beemon, K.L. 1978. Oligonucleotide fingerprinting with RNA tumor virus RNA. *Curr. Top. Microbiol. Immunol.* **79:**73–110.

Beemon, K. and T. Hunter. 1977. *In vitro* translation yields a possible Rous sarcoma virus *src* gene product. *Proc. Natl. Acad. Sci.* **74:**3302–3306.

———. 1978. Characterization of Rous sarcoma virus *src* gene products synthesized in vitro. *J. Virol.* **28:**551–566.

Beemon, K.L. and J.M. Keith. 1976. Structure of Rous sarcoma virus RNA. 1. Localization of N^6-methyladenosine; 2. The sequence of 23 nucleotides following the 5′ capped terminus m^7GpppG^mp. In *Animal virology* (ed. D. Baltimore et al.), pp. 97–105. Academic Press, New York.

Beemon, K.L., P. Duesberg, and P. Vogt. 1974. Evidence for crossing-over between avian tumor viruses based on analysis of viral RNAs. *Proc. Natl. Acad. Sci.* **71:**4254–4258.

Beemon, K.L., A.J. Faras, A.T. Haase, P.H. Duesberg, and J.E. Maisel. 1976. Genome complexities of murine leukemia and sarcoma, reticuloendotheliosis, and visna viruses. *J. Virol* **17:**525–537.

Bellamy, A.R., S.C. Gillies, and J.D. Harvey. 1974. Molecular weight of two oncornavirus genomes: Derivation from particle molecular weights and RNA content. *J. Virol.* **14:**1388–1393.

Bender, W. and N. Davidson. 1976. Mapping of poly(A) sequences in the electron microscope reveals unusual structure of type C oncornavirus RNA molecules. *Cell* **7:**595–607.

Bender, W., Y.-H. Chien, S. Chattopadhyay, P.K. Vogt, M.B. Gardner, and N. Davidson. 1978. High-molecular-weight RNAs of AKR, NZB, and wild mouse viruses and avian reticuloendotheliosis virus all have similar dimer structures. *J. Virol.* **25:**888–896.

Benoist, C. and P. Chambon. 1980. Deletions covering the putative promoter region of early mRNAs of simian virus 40 do not abolish T-antigen expression. *Proc. Natl. Acad. Sci.* **77:**3865–3869.

Bernstein, A., R. MacCormick, and G.S. Martin. 1976. Transformation-defective mutants of avian sarcoma viruses: The genetic relationship between conditional and nonconditional mutants. *Virology* **70:**206–209.

Bernstein, A., T.W. Mak, and J.R. Stephenson. 1977. The Friend virus genome: Evidence for a stable association of MuLV sequences and sequences involved in erythroleukemic transformation. *Cell* **12:**287–294.

Bernstein, A., C. Gamble, D. Penrose, and T.W. Mak. 1979. Presence and expression of Friend erythroleukemia virus-related sequences in normal and leukemic mouse tissues. *Proc. Natl. Acad. Sci.* **76:**4455–4459.

Beug, H., G. Kitchener, G. Doederlein, T. Graf, and M.J. Hayman. 1980a. Mutant of avian erythroblastosis virus defective for erythroblast transformation: Deletion in the *erb* portion of p75 suggests function of the protein in leukemogenesis. *Proc. Natl. Acad. Sci.* **77:**6683–6686.

Beug, H., A. von Kirchbach, G. Doderlein, J.-F. Conscience, and T. Graf. 1979. Chicken hematopoietic cells transformed by seven strains of defective avian leukemia viruses display three distinct phenotypes of differentiation. *Cell* **18:**375–390.

Beug, H., G. Ramsay, S. Saule, D. Stehelin, M.J. Hayman, and T. Graf. 1980b. Transformation defective mutants of AEV and MC29 avian leukemia viruses synthesize smaller *gag*-related proteins with altered transformation specificity. In *Animal virus genetics* (ed. B. Fields et al.), pp. 551–567. Academic Press, New York.

Billeter, M.A., J.T. Parsons, and J.M. Coffin. 1974. The nucleotide sequence complexity of avian tumor virus RNA. *Proc. Natl. Acad. Sci.* **71:**3560–3564.

Bishop, J.M. 1978. Retroviruses. *Annu. Rev. Biochem.* **47:**35–88.

Bishop, J.M., W.E. Levinson, N. Quintrell, D. Sullivan, L. Fanshier, and J. Jackson. 1970a. The low molecular weight RNAs of Rous sarcoma virus. I. The 4 S RNA. *Virology* **42:**182–195.

Bishop, J.M., W.E. Levinson, D. Sullivan, L. Fanshier, N. Quintrell, and J. Jackson. 1970b. The low molecular weight RNAs of Rous sarcoma virus. II. The 7 S RNA. *Virology* **42:**927–937.

Bishop, J.M., S.A. Courtneidge, A.D. Levinson, H. Oppermann, N. Quintrell, D.K. Sheiness, S.R. Weiss, and H.E. Varmus. 1980. Origin and function of avian retrovirus transforming genes. *Cold Spring Harbor Symp. Quant. Biol.* **44:**919–930.

Bister, K. and P.H. Duesberg. 1980. Genetic structure of avian acute leukemia viruses. *Cold Spring Harbor Symp. Quant. Biol.* **44:**801–822.

Bister, K. and P.K. Vogt. 1978. Genetic analysis of the defectiveness in strain MC29 avian leukosis virus. *Virology* **88:**213–221.

Bister, K., M.J. Hayman, and P.K. Vogt. 1977. Defectiveness of avian myelocytomatosis virus MC29: Isolation of long-term nonproducer cultures and analysis of virus-specific polypeptide synthesis. *Virology* **82:**431–448.

Bister, K., H.-C. Löliger, and P.H. Duesberg. 1979. Oligoribonucleotide map and protein of CMII: Detection of conserved and nonconserved genetic elements in avian acute leukemia viruses CMII, MC29, and MH2. *J. Virol.* **32:**208–219.

Blair, D.G., W.L. McClements, M.K. Oskarsson, P.J. Fischinger, and G.F. Vande Woude. 1980. Biological activity of cloned Moloney sarcoma virus DNA: Terminally redundant sequences may enhance transformation efficiency. *Proc. Natl. Acad. Sci.* **77:**3504–3508.

Bolognesi, D.P., R.C. Montelaro, H. Frank, and W. Schäfer. 1978. Assembly of type C oncornaviruses: A model. *Science* **199:**183–186.

Boss, M., M. Greaves, and N. Teich. 1979. Abelson virus transformed haematopoietic cell lines with pre-B-cell characteristics. *Nature* **278:**551–553.

Bosselman, R.A., L.J.L.D. Van Griensven, M. Vogt, and I.M. Verma. 1979. Genome organization of retroviruses. VI. Heteroduplex analysis of ecotropic and xenotropic sequences of Moloney mink cell focus-inducing viral RNA obtained from either a cloned isolate or a thymoma cell line. *J. Virol.* **32:**968–978.

———. 1980. Genome organization of retroviruses. IX. Analysis of the genomes of Friend spleen focus-forming (F-SFFV) and helper murine leukemia viruses by heteroduplex-formation. *Virology* **102:**234–239.

Breitman, M.L., M.M.C. Lai, and P.K. Vogt. 1980. The genomic RNA of avian reticuloendotheliosis virus REV. *Virology* **100:**450–461.

Breitman, M.L., J.C. Neil, C. Moscovici, and P.K. Vogt. 1981. The pathogenicity and defectiveness of PRCII: A new type of avian sarcoma virus. *Virology* **108:**1–12.

Brugge, J.S. and R.L. Erikson. 1977. Identification of a transformation-specific antigen induced by an avian sarcoma virus. *Nature* **269:**346–348.

Canaani, E. and S.A. Aaronson. 1980. Isolation and characterization of naturally occurring deletion mutants of Moloney murine sarcoma virus. *Virology* **105:**456–466.

Canaani, E. and P. Duesberg. 1972. Role of subunits of 60 to 70S avian tumor virus ribonucleic acid in its template activity for the viral deoxyribonucleic acid polymerase. *J. Virol.* **10:**23–31.

Canaani, E., K.V.D. Helm, and P. Duesberg. 1973. Evidence for 30-40S RNA as precursor of the 60-70S RNA of Rous sarcoma virus. *Proc. Natl. Acad. Sci.* **70:**401–405.

Canaani, E., K.C. Robbins, and S.A. Aaronson. 1979. The transforming gene of Moloney murine sarcoma virus. *Nature* **282:**378–383.

Canaani, E., S.R. Tronick, K.C. Robbins, P.R. Andersen, and S.A. Aaronson. 1980. Cellular origin of the transforming gene of Moloney murine sarcoma virus. *Cold Spring Harbor Symp. Quant. Biol.* **44:**727–734.

Carr, J.G. and J.G. Campbell. 1958. Three new virus-induced fowl sarcomata. *Br. J. Cancer* **12:** 631–635.

Cashion, L., R.H. Joho, M.A. Planitz, M.A. Billeter, and C. Weissmann. 1976. Initiation sites of Rous sarcoma virus RNA-directed DNA synthesis *in vitro*. *Nature* **262:** 186–190.

Chang (sic), H.W., C.F. Garon, E.H. Chang, D.R. Lowy, G.L. Hager, E.M. Scolnick, R. Repaske, and M.A. Martin. 1980. Molecular cloning of the Harvey sarcoma virus circular DNA intermediates. II. Further structural analyses. *J. Virol.* **33:** 845–855.

Chang, E.H., J.M. Maryak, C.-M. Wei, T.Y. Shih, R. Shober, H.L. Cheung, R.W. Ellis, G.L. Hager, E.M. Scolnick, and D.R. Lowy. 1980. Functional organization of the Harvey murine sarcoma virus genome. *J. Virol.* **35:** 76–92.

Chen, J.H., W.S. Hayward, and C. Moscovici. 1981. Size and genetic content of virus-specific RNA in myeloblasts transformed by avian myeloblastosis virus (AMV). *Virology* **110:** 128–136.

Cheung, K.-S., R.E. Smith, M.P. Stone, and W.K. Joklik. 1972. Comparison of immature (rapid harvest) and mature Rous sarcoma virus particles. *Virology* **50:** 851–864.

Chien, Y.-H., R.P. Junghans, and N. Davidson. 1980. Electron microscopic analysis of the structure of RNA tumor virus nucleic acids. In *Molecular biology of RNA tumor viruses* (ed. J.R. Stephenson), p. 395–446. Academic Press, New York.

Chien, Y.-H., I.M. Verma, T.Y. Shih, E.M. Scolnick, and N. Davidson. 1978. Heteroduplex analysis of the sequence relations between RNAs of mink cell focus-inducing and murine leukemia viruses. *J. Virol.* **28:** 352–360.

Chien, Y.-H., M. Lai, T.Y. Shih, I.M. Verma, E.M. Scolnick, P. Roy-Burman, and N. Davidson. 1979. Heteroduplex analysis of the sequence relationships between the genomes of Kirsten and Harvey sarcoma viruses, their respective parental murine leukemia viruses, and the rat endogenous 30S RNA. *J. Virol.* **31:** 752–760.

Coffin, J.M. 1979. Structure, replication, and recombination of retrovirus genomes: Some unifying hypotheses. *J. Gen. Virol.* **42:** 1–26.

———. 1980. Structural analysis of retrovirus genomes. In *Molecular biology of RNA tumor viruses* (ed. J.R. Stephenson), pp. 199–243. Academic Press, New York.

Coffin, J.M. and M.A. Billeter. 1976. A physical map of the Rous sarcoma virus genome. *J. Mol. Biol.* **100:** 293–318.

Coffin, J.M. and W.A. Haseltine. 1977. Terminal redundancy and the origin of replication of Rous sarcoma virus RNA. *Proc. Natl. Acad. Sci.* **74:** 1908–1912.

Coffin, J.M., M. Champion, and F. Chabot. 1978a. Nucleotide sequence relationships between the genomes of an endogenous and an exogenous avian tumor virus. *J. Virol.* **28:** 972–991.

Coffin, J.M., T.C. Hageman, A.M. Maxam, and W.A. Haseltine. 1978b. Structure of the genome of Moloney murine leukemia virus: A terminally redundant sequence. *Cell* **13:** 761–773.

Coffin, J.M., P.N. Tsichlis, C.S. Barker, and S. Voynow. 1980. Variation in avian retrovirus genomes. *Ann. N.Y. Acad. Sci.* **354:** 410–425.

Cooper, G.M. and H.M. Temin. 1974. Infectious Rous sarcoma virus and reticuloendotheliosis virus DNAs. *J. Virol.* **14:** 1132–1141.

Cordell, B., E. Stavnezer, R. Friedrich, J.M. Bishop, and H.M. Goodman. 1976. Nucleotide sequence that binds primer for DNA synthesis to the avian sarcoma virus genome. *J. Virol* **19:** 548–558.

Czernilofsky, A.P., A.D. Levinson, H.E. Varmus, J.M. Bishop, E. Tischer, and H.M. Goodman. 1980a. Nucleotide sequence of an avian virus oncogene (*src*) and proposed amino acid sequence for gene product. *Nature* **287:** 198–203.

Czernilofsky, A.P., W. DeLorbe, R. Swanstrom, H.E. Varmus, J.M. Bishop, E. Tischer, and H.M. Goodman. 1980b. The nucleotide sequence of an untranslated but conserved domain at the 3′ end of the avian sarcoma virus genome. *Nucleic Acids Res.* **8:** 2967–2984.

Dahlberg, J.E., R.C. Sawyer, J.M. Taylor, A.J. Faras, W.E. Levinson, H.M. Goodman, and

J.M. Bishop. 1974. Transcription of DNA from the 70S RNA of Rous sarcoma virus. I. Identification of a specific 4S RNA which serves as primer. *J. Virol.* **13:** 1126–1133.

Darlix, J.-L., P.-F. Spahr, P.A. Bromley, and J.-C. Jaton. 1979. In vitro, the major ribosome binding site on Rous sarcoma virus RNA does not contain the nucleotide sequence coding for the N-terminal amino acids of the *gag* gene product. *J. Virol.* **29:** 597–611.

Delius, H., H. Westphal, and N. Axelrod. 1973. Length measurements of RNA synthesized *in vitro* by *Escherichia coli* RNA polymerase. *J. Mol. Biol.* **74:** 677–687.

DeLorbe, W.J., P.A. Luciw, H.M. Goodman, H.E. Varmus, and J.M. Bishop. 1980. Molecular cloning and characterization of avian sarcoma virus circular DNA molecules. *J. Virol.* **36:** 50–61.

Dhar, R., W.L. McClements, L.W. Enquist, and G.F. Vande Woude. 1980. Nucleotide sequences of integrated Moloney sarcoma provirus long terminal repeats and their host and viral junctions. *Proc. Natl. Acad. Sci.* **77:** 3937–3941.

Dickson, C. and G. Peters. 1981. Protein-coding potential of mouse mammary tumor virus genome RNA as examined by in vitro translation. *J. Virol.* **37:** 36–47.

Diggelmann, H. 1979. Biosynthesis of an unglycosylated envelope glycoprotein of Rous sarcoma virus in the presence of tunicamycin. *J. Virol.* **30:** 799–804.

Dimock, K. and C.M. Stoltzfus. 1978. Cycloleucine blocks 5′-terminal and internal methylations of avian sarcoma virus genome RNA. *Biochemistry* **17:** 3627–3632.

Dina, D., K. Beemon, and P. Duesberg. 1976. The 30S Moloney sarcoma virus RNA contains leukemia virus nucleotide sequences. *Cell* **9:** 299–309.

Donehower, L.A., A.L. Huang, and G.L. Hager. 1981. Regulatory and coding potential of the mouse mammary tumor virus long terminal redundancy. *J. Virol.* **37:** 226–238.

Donehower, L.A., J. Andre, O.S. Berard, R.G. Wolford, and G.L. Hager. 1980. Construction and characterization of molecular clones containing integrated mouse mammary tumor virus sequences. *Cold Spring Harbor Symp. Quant. Biol.* **44:** 1153–1159.

Donis-Keller, H., J. Rommelaere, R.W. Ellis, and N. Hopkins. 1980. Nucleotide sequences associated with differences in electrophoretic mobility of envelope glycoprotein gp70 and with G_{IX} antigen phenotype of certain murine leukemia viruses. *Proc. Natl. Acad. Sci.* **77:** 1642–1645.

Donoghue, D.J., P.A. Sharp, and R.A. Weinberg. 1979a. An MSV-specific subgenomic mRNA in MSV-transformed G8-124 cells. *Cell* **17:** 53–63.

———. 1979b. Comparative study of different isolates of murine sarcoma virus. *J. Virol.* **32:** 1015–1027.

Donoghue, D.J., E. Rothenberg, N. Hopkins, D. Baltimore, and P.A. Sharp. 1978. Heteroduplex analysis of the nonhomology region between Moloney MuLV and the dual host range derivative HIX virus. *Cell* **14:** 959–970.

Dresler, S., M. Ruta, M.J. Murray, and D. Kabat. 1979. Glycoprotein encoded by the Friend spleen focus-forming virus. *J. Virol.* **30:** 564–575.

Duesberg, P.H. 1968. Physical properties of Rous sarcoma virus RNA. *Proc. Natl. Acad. Sci.* **60:** 1511–1518.

———. 1970. On the structure of RNA tumor viruses. *Curr. Top. Microbiol. Immunol.* **51:** 79–104.

———. 1980. Transforming genes of retroviruses. *Cold Spring Harbor Symp. Quant. Biol.* **44:** 13–29.

Duesberg, P.H. and K. Bister. 1981. Transforming genes of retroviruses: Definition, specificity, and relation to cellular DNA. In *Feline leukemia virus* (ed. W.D. Hardy et. al.). Elsevier/North-Holland, New York. (In press.)

Duesberg, P.H. and W.S. Robinson. 1966. Nucleic acid and proteins isolated from the Rauscher mouse leukemia virus (MLV). *Proc. Natl. Acad. Sci.* **55:** 219–227.

Duesberg, and P.K. Vogt. 1973a. RNA species obtained from clonal lines of avian sarcoma and from avian leukosis virus. *Virology* **54:** 207–219.

———. 1973b. Gel electrophoresis of avian leukosis and sarcoma viral RNA in formamide: Comparison with other viral and cellular RNA species. *J. Virol.* **12:**594–599.

———. 1979. Avian acute leukemia viruses MC29 and MH2 share specific RNA sequences: Evidence for a second class of transforming genes. *Proc. Natl. Acad. Sci.* **76:**1633–1637.

Duesberg, P.H., K. Bister, and C. Moscovici. 1980. Genetic structure of avian myeloblastosis virus, released from transformed myeloblasts as a defective virus particle. *Proc. Natl. Acad. Sci.* **77:**5120–5124

Durban, E.M. and D. Boettiger. 1981. Replicating, differentiated macrophages can serve as in vitro targets for transformation by avian myeloblastosis virus. *J. Virol.* **37:**488–492.

Eiden, J.J., K. Quade, and J.L. Nichols. 1976. Interaction of tryptophan transfer RNA with Rous sarcoma virus 35S RNA. *Nature* **259:**245–247.

Elder, J.H., J.W. Gautsch, F.C. Jensen, R.A. Lerner, J.W. Hartley, and W.P. Rowe. 1977. Biochemical evidence that MCF murine leukemia viruses are envelope (*env*) gene recombinants. *Proc. Natl. Acad. Sci.* **74:**4676–4680.

Elder, K.T. and A.E. Smith. 1974. Methionine transfer RNAs associated with avian oncornavirus 70S RNA. *Nature* **247:**435–438.

Ellis, R.W., D. DeFeo, J.M. Maryak, H.A. Young, T.Y. Shih, E.H. Chang, D.R. Lowy, and E.M. Scolnick. 1980. Dual evolutionary origin for the rat genetic sequences of Harvey murine sarcoma virus. *J. Virol.* **36:**408–420.

Erikson, E. and R.L. Erikson. 1970. Isolation of amino acid acceptor RNA from purified avian myeloblastosis virus. *J. Mol. Biol.* **52:**387–390.

———. 1971. Association of 4S ribonucleic acid with oncornavirus ribonucleic acids. *J. Virol.* **8:**254–256.

Erikson, E., R.L. Erikson, B. Henry, and N.R. Pace. 1973. Comparison of oligonucleotides produced by RNase T1 digestion of 7 S RNA from avian and murine oncornaviruses and from uninfected cells. *Virology* **53:**40–46.

Evans, L.H., P.H. Duesberg, D.H. Troxler, and E.M. Scolnick. 1979. Spleen focus-forming Friend virus: Identification of genomic RNA and its relationship to helper virus RNA. *J. Virol.* **31:**133–146.

Evans, L.H., M. Nunn, P.H. Duesberg, D. Troxler, and E.M. Scolnick. 1980. RNAs of defective and nondefective components of Friend anemia and polycythemia virus strains identified and compared. *Cold Spring Harbor Symp. Quant. Biol.* **44:**823–835.

Faller, D.V. and N. Hopkins. 1978a. T1 oligonucleotide maps of Moloney and HIX murine leukemia viruses. *Virology* **90:**265–273.

———. 1978b. T1 oligonucleotide maps of N-, B-, and B → NB-tropic murine leukemia viruses derived from BALB/c. *J. Virol.* **26:**143–152.

———. 1978c. T1 oligonucleotides that segregate with tropism and with properties of gp70 in recombinants between N- and B-tropic murine leukemia viruses. *J. Virol.* **26:**153–158.

Faller, D.V., J. Rommelaere, and N. Hopkins. 1978. Large T1 oligonucleotides of Moloney leukemia virus missing in an *env* gene recombinant, HIX, are present on an intracellular 21S Moloney viral RNA species. *Proc. Natl. Acad. Sci.* **75:**2964–2968.

Fan, H. and M. Paskind. 1974. Measurement of the sequence complexity of cloned Moloney murine leukemia virus 60 to 70S RNA: Evidence for a haploid genome. *J. Virol.* **14:**421–429.

Fan, H. and I.M. Verma. 1978. Size analysis and relationship of murine leukemia virus-specific mRNA's: Evidence for transposition of sequences during synthesis and processing of subgenomic mRNA. *J. Virol.* **26:**468–478.

Faras, A.J., A.C. Garapin, W.E. Levinson, J.M. Bishop, and H.M. Goodman. 1973. Characterization of the low-molecular-weight RNAs associated with the 70S RNA of Rous sarcoma virus. *J. Virol.* **12:**334–342.

Faras, A.J., J.E. Dahlberg, R.C. Sawyer, F. Harada, J.M. Taylor, W.E. Levinson, J.M. Bishop, and H.M. Goodman. 1974. Transcription of DNA from the 70S RNA of Rous sarcoma virus. II. Structure of a 4S RNA primer. *J. Virol.* **13:**1134–1142.

Fincham, V.J., P.E. Neiman, and J.A. Wyke. 1980. Novel nonconditional mutants in the *src* gene of Rous sarcoma virus: Isolation and preliminary characterization. *Virology* **103:**99–111.

Fischinger, P.J., S. Nomura, and D.P. Bolognesi. 1975. A novel murine oncornavirus with dual eco- and xenotropic properties. *Proc. Natl. Acad. Sci.* **72:**5150–5155.

Fischinger, P.J., A.E. Frankel, J.H. Elder, R.A. Lerner, J.N. Ihle, and D.P. Bolognesi. 1978. Biological, immunological, and biochemical evidence that HIX virus is a recombinant between Moloney leukemia virus and a murine xenotropic C type virus. *Virology* **90:**241–254.

Frankel, A.E., J.H. Gilbert, K.J. Porzig, E.M. Scolnick, and S.A. Aaronson. 1980. Nature and distribution of feline sarcoma virus nucleotide sequences. *J. Virol.* **30:**821–827.

Friedrich, R., H.-J. Kung, B. Baker, H.E. Varmus, H.M. Goodman, and J.M. Bishop. 1977. Characterization of DNA complementary to nucleotide sequences at the 5′-terminus of the avian sarcoma virus genome. *Virology* **79:**198–215.

Friend, C. 1957. Cell-free transmission in adult Swiss mice of a disease having the character of a leukemia. *J. Exp. Med.* **105:**307–318.

Fujinami, A. and K. Inamoto. 1914. Ueber Geschwulste bei japanischen Haushuhnern insbesondere uber einen transplantablen Tumor. *Z. Krebsforsch.* **14:**94–119.

Fujita, D.J., J. Tal, H.E. Varmus, and J.M. Bishop. 1978. *env* gene of chicken RNA tumor viruses: Extent of conservation in cellular and viral genomes. *J. Virol.* **27:**465–474.

Furuichi, Y., A.J. Shatkin, E. Stavnezer, and J.M. Bishop. 1975a. Blocked, methylated 5′-terminal sequence in avian sarcoma virus RNA. *Nature* **257:**618–620.

Furuichi, Y., M. Morgan, A.J. Shatkin, W. Jelinik, M. Salditt-Georgieff, and J.E. Darnell. 1975b. Methylated, blocked 5′ termini in HeLa cell mRNA. *Proc. Natl. Acad. Sci.* **72:**1904–1908.

Galehouse, D.M and P.H. Duesberg. 1978. Glycoproteins of avian tumor virus recombinants: Evidence for intragenic crossing-over. *J. Virol.* **25:**86–96.

Gallis, B., M. Linial, and R. Eisenman. 1979. An avian oncovirus mutant deficient in genomic RNA: Characterization of the packaged RNA as cellular messenger RNA. *Virology* **94:**146–161.

Gallo, R.C. and F. Wong-Staal. 1980. Molecular biology of primate retroviruses. In *Viral oncology* (ed. G. Klein), pp. 399–431. Raven Press, New York.

Gannon, F., K. O'Hare, F. Perrin, J.P. LePennec, C. Benoist, M. Cochet, R. Breathnach, A. Royal, A. Garapin, B. Cami, and P. Chambon. 1979. Organisation and sequences at the 5′ end of a cloned complete ovalbumin gene. *Nature* **278:**428–434.

Gardner, M.B., R.W. Rongey, P. Arnstein, J.D. Estes, P. Sarma, R.J. Huebner, and C.G. Rickard. 1970. Experimental transmission of feline fibrosarcoma to cats and dogs. *Nature* **226:**807–809.

Gautsch, J.W., J.H. Elder, J. Schindler, F.C. Jensen, and R.A. Lerner. 1978. Structural markers on core protein p30 of murine leukemia virus: Functional correlation with *Fv-1* tropism. *Proc. Natl. Acad. Sci.* **75:**4170–4174.

Gazdar, A.F., H.C. Chopra, and P.S. Sarma. 1972. Properties of a murine sarcoma virus isolated from a tumor arising in an NZW/NZB F_1 hybrid mouse. I. Isolation and pathology of tumors induced in rodents. *Int. J. Cancer* **9:**219–233.

Gazzolo, L., C. Moscovici, M.G. Moscovici, and J. Samarut. 1979. Response of hemopoietic cells to avian acute leukemia virus: Effects on the differentiation of the target cells. *Cell* **16:**627–638.

Ghysdael, J., J.C. Neil, and P.K. Vogt. 1981. A third class of avian sarcoma viruses, defined by related transformation-specific proteins of Yamaguchi 73 and Esh sarcoma virus. *Proc. Natl. Acad. Sci.* **78:**2611–2615.

Gilboa, E., S. Goff, A. Shields, F. Yoshimura, S. Mitra, and D. Baltimore. 1979. In vitro synthesis of a 9 kbp terminally redundant DNA carrying the infectivity of Moloney murine leukemia virus. *Cell* **16:**863–874.

Gillespie, D., S. Marshall, and R.C. Gallo. 1972. RNA of RNA tumour viruses contains poly A. *Nat. New Biol.* **236:** 227–231.

Goff, S.P., E. Gilboa, O.N. Witte, and D. Baltimore. 1980. Structure of the Abelson murine leukemia virus genome and the homologous cellular gene: Studies with cloned viral DNA. *Cell* **22:** 777–785.

Goldfarb, M.P. and R.A. Weinberg. 1981. Generation of novel, biologically active Harvey sarcoma viruses via apparent illegitimate recombination. *J. Virol.* **38:** 136–150.

Gonda, M.A., N.R. Rice, and R.V. Gilden. 1980. Avian reticuloendotheliosis virus: Characterization of the high-molecular-weight viral RNA in transforming and helper virus populations. *J. Virol.* **34:** 743–751.

Gonda, T.J., D.K. Sheiness, L. Fanshier, J.M. Bishop, and C. Moscovici. 1981. The genome and the intracellular RNAs of avian myeloblastosis virus. *Cell* **23:** 279–290.

Graf, T. and H. Beug. 1978. Avian leukemia viruses. Interaction with their target cells in vivo and in vitro. *Biochim. Biophys. Acta* **516:** 269–299.

Graf, T., H. Beug, A. von Kirchbach, and M.J. Hayman. 1980. Three new types of viral oncogenes in defective avian leukemia viruses. II. Biological, genetic, and immunochemical evidence. *Cold Spring Harbor Symp. Quant. Biol.* **44:** 1225–1234.

Green, N., H. Hiai, J.H. Elder, R.S. Schwartz, R.H. Khiroya, C.Y. Thomas, P.N. Tsichlis, and J.M. Coffin. 1980. Expression of leukemogenic recombinant viruses associated with a recessive gene in HRS/J mice. *J. Exp. Med.* **152:** 249–264.

Groner, B., E. Buetti, H. Diggelmann, and N.E. Hynes. 1980. Characterization of endogenous and exogenous mouse mammary tumor virus proviral DNA with site-specific molecular clones. *J. Virol.* **36:** 734–745.

Hager, G.L., E.H. Chang, H.W. Chan, C.F. Garon, M.A. Israel, M.A. Martin, E.M. Scolnick, and D.R. Lowy. 1979. Molecular cloning of the Harvey sarcoma virus closed circular DNA intermediates: Initial structural and biological characterization. *J. Virol.* **31:** 795–809.

Halpern, C.C., W.S. Hayward, and H. Hanafusa. 1979. Characterization of some isolates of newly recovered avian sarcoma virus. *J. Virol.* **29:** 91–101.

Hanafusa, H. 1977. Cell transformation by RNA tumor viruses. In *Comprehensive virology* (ed. H. Fraenkel-Conrat and R.R. Wagner), vol. 10, p. 401–483. Plenum Press, New York.

Hanafusa, H. and T. Hanafusa. 1971. Noninfectious RSV deficient in DNA polymerase. *Virology* **43:** 313–316.

Hanafusa, H., C.C. Halpern, D.L. Buchhagen, and S. Kawai. 1977. Recovery of avian sarcoma virus from tumors induced by transformation-defective mutants. *J. Exp. Med.* **146:** 1735–1747.

Hanafusa, H., W.S. Hayward, J.H. Chen, and T. Hanafusa. 1975. Control of expression of tumor virus genes in uninfected chicken cells. *Cold Spring Harbor Symp. Quant. Biol.* **39:** 1139–1144.

Hanafusa, H., L.-H. Wang, S.M. Anderson, R.E. Karess, and W.S. Hayward. 1980. The nature and origin of the transforming gene of avian sarcoma virus. In *Animal virus genetics* (ed. B. Fields et al.), vol. 18, pp. 483–497. Academic Press, New York.

Hanafusa, H., D. Baltimore, D. Smoler, K.F. Watson, A. Yaniv, and S. Spiegelman. 1972. Absence of polymerase protein in virions of alpha-type Rous sarcoma virus. *Science* **177:** 1188–1191.

Hanafusa, T., L.-H. Wang, S.M. Anderson, R.E. Karess, W.S. Hayward, and H. Hanafusa. 1980. Characterization of the transforming gene of Fujinami sarcoma virus. *Proc. Natl. Acad. Sci.* **77:** 3009–3013.

Harada, F., G.G. Peters, and J.E. Dahlberg. 1979. The primer tRNA for Moloney murine leukemia virus DNA synthesis. Nucleotide sequence and aminoacylation of $tRNA^{Pro}$. *J. Biol. Chem.* **254:** 10979–10985.

Harada, F., R.C. Sawyer, and J.E. Dahlberg. 1975. A primer ribonucleic acid for initiation of *in vitro* Rous sarcoma virus deoxyribonucleic acid synthesis. Nucleotide sequence and amino acid acceptor activity. *J. Biol. Chem.* **250:** 3487–3497.

Hartley, J.W. and W.P. Rowe. 1966. Production of altered cell foci in tissue culture by defective Moloney murine sarcoma virus particles. *Proc. Natl. Acad. Sci.* **55:** 780–786.

Hartley, J.W., N.K. Wolford, L.J. Old, and W.P. Rowe. 1977. A new class of murine leukemia virus associated with development of spontaneous lymphomas. *Proc. Natl. Acad. Sci.* **74:** 789–792.

Harvey, J.J. 1964. An unidentified virus which causes the rapid production of tumours in mice. *Nature* **204:** 1104–1105.

Haseltine, W.A. and D.G. Kleid. 1978. A method for classification of 5′ termini of retroviruses. *Nature* **273:** 358–364.

Haseltine, W.A., A.M. Maxam, and W. Gilbert. 1977. Rous sarcoma virus genome is terminally redundant: The 5′ sequence. *Proc. Natl. Acad. Sci.* **74:** 989–993.

Haseltine, W.A., D.G. Kleid, A. Panet, E. Rothenberg, and D. Baltimore. 1976. Ordered transcription of RNA tumor virus genomes. *J. Mol. Biol.* **106:** 109–131.

Hayman, M.J. and P.K. Vogt. 1976. Subgroup-specific antigenic determinants of avian RNA tumor virus structural proteins: Analysis of virus recombinants. *Virology* **73:** 372–380.

Hayman, M.J., G. Kitchener, and T. Graf. 1979a. Cells transformed by avian myelocytomatosis virus strain CMII contain a 90K *gag*-related protein. *Virology* **98:** 191–199.

Hayman, M.J., B. Royer-Pokora, and T. Graf. 1979b. Defectiveness of avian erythroblastosis virus: Synthesis of a 75K *gag*-related protein. *Virology* **92:** 31–45.

Hayward, W.S. 1977. Size and genetic content of viral RNAs in avian oncovirus-infected cells. *J. Virol.* **24:** 47–63.

Highfield, P.E., L.F. Rafield, T.M. Gilmer, and J.T. Parsons. 1980. Molecular cloning of avian sarcoma virus closed circular DNA: Structural and biological characterization of three recombinant clones. *J. Virol.* **36:** 271–279.

Hill, M. and J. Hillova. 1972. Virus recovery in chicken cells tested with Rous sarcoma cell DNA. *Nat. New Biol.* **237:** 35–39.

Hishinuma, F., P.J. DeBona, S. Astrin, and A.M. Skalka. 1981. Nucleotide sequence of acceptor site and termini of integrated avian endogenous provirus *ev1*: Integration creates a 6 bp repeat of host DNA. *Cell* **23:** 155–164.

Hoelzer, J.D., R.B. Franklin, and H.R. Bose, Jr. 1979. Transformation by reticuloendotheliosis virus: Development of a focus assay and isolation of a nontransforming virus. *Virology* **93:** 20–30.

Hoelzer, J.D., R.B. Lewis, C.R. Wasmuth, and H.R. Bose, Jr. 1980. Hematopoietic cell transformation by reticuloendotheliosis virus: Characterization of the genetic defect. *Virology* **100:** 462–474.

Hopkins, N., J. Schindler, and P.D. Gottlieb. 1977a. Evidence for recombination between N- and B-tropic murine leukemia viruses. *J. Virol.* **21:** 1074–1078.

Hopkins, N., J. Schindler, and R. Hynes. 1977b. Six NB-tropic murine leukemia viruses derived from a B-tropic virus of BALB/c have altered p30. *J. Virol.* **21:** 309–318.

Horst, J., J. Keith, and H. Fraenkel-Conrat. 1972. Characteristic two-dimensional patterns of enzymatic digests of oncorna and other viral RNAs. *Nat. New Biol.* **240:** 105–109.

Hu, S.S.F. and P.K. Vogt. 1979. Avian oncovirus MH2 is defective in *gag, pol,* and *env*. *Virology* **92:** 278–284.

Hu, S.S.F., N. Davidson, and I.M. Verma. 1977. A heteroduplex study of the sequence relationships between the RNAs of M-MSV and M-MLV. *Cell* **10:** 469–477.

Hu, S.S.F., M.M.C. Lai, and P.K. Vogt. 1978a. Characterization of the *env* gene in avian oncoviruses by heteroduplex mapping. *J. Virol.* **27:** 667–676.

———. 1979. Genome of avian myelocytomatosis virus MC29: Analysis by heteroduplex mapping. *Proc. Natl. Acad. Sci.* **76:** 1265–1268.

Hu, S.S.F., C. Moscovici, and P.K. Vogt. 1978b. The defectiveness of Mill Hill 2, a carcinoma-inducing avian oncovirus. *Virology* **89:** 162–178.

Hughes, S.H., K. Toyoshima, J.M. Bishop, and H.E. Varmus. 1981a. Organization of the endogenous proviruses of chickens: Implications for origin and expression. *Virology* **108:** 189–207.

Hughes, S.H., P.K. Vogt, E. Stubblefield, J.M. Bishop, and H.E. Varmus. 1981b. Integration of avian sarcoma virus DNA in chicken cells. *Virology* **108:** 208–221.

Hughes, S.H., P.R. Shank, D.H. Spector, H.-J. Kung, J.M. Bishop, H.E. Varmus, P.K. Vogt, and M.L. Breitman. 1978. Proviruses of avian sarcoma viruses are terminally redundant, co-extensive with unintegrated linear DNA and integrated at many sites. *Cell* **15:** 1397–1410.

Hunter, E. 1978. The mechanism for genetic recombination in the avian retroviruses. *Curr. Top. Microbiol. Immunol.* **79:** 295–309.

———. 1980. Avian oncoviruses: Genetics. In *Viral oncology* (ed. G. Klein), p. 1–38. Raven Press, New York.

Ikawa, Y., J. Ross, and P. Leder. 1974. An association between globin messenger RNA and 60S RNA derived from Friend leukemia virus. *Proc. Natl. Acad. Sci.* **71:** 1154–1158.

Itohara, S., K. Hirata, M. Inoue, M. Hatsuoka, and A. Sato. 1978. Isolation of a sarcoma virus from a spontaneous chicken tumor. *Gann* **69:** 825–830.

Joho, R.H., M.A. Billeter, and C. Weissmann. 1975. Mapping of biological functions of RNA of avian tumor viruses: Location of regions required for transformation and determination of host range. *Proc. Natl. Acad. Sci.* **72:** 4772–4776.

———. 1978. Concordance of the RNA termini of recombinants from crosses between avian retroviruses with different termini. *Virology* **85:** 364–377.

Joho, R.H., E. Stoll, R.R. Friis, M.A. Billeter, and C. Weissmann. 1976. A partial genetic map of Rous sarcoma virus RNA: Location of polymerase, envelope and transformation markers. In *Animal virology* (ed. D. Baltimore et al.), vol. 4, pp. 127–145. Academic Press, New York.

Jones, M., R.A. Bosselman, F.A. v.d. Hoorn, A. Berns, H. Fan, and I.M. Verma. 1980. Identification and molecular cloning of Moloney mouse sarcoma virus-specific sequences from uninfected mouse cells. *Proc. Natl. Acad. Sci.* **77:** 2651–2655.

Ju, G. and A.M. Skalka. 1980. Nucleotide sequence analysis of the long terminal repeat (LTR) of avian retroviruses: Structural similarities with transposable elements. *Cell* **22:** 379–386.

Ju., G., L. Boone, and A.M. Skalka. 1980. Isolation and characterization of recombinant DNA clones of avian retroviruses: Size heterogeneity and instability of the direct repeat. *J. Virol.* **33:** 1026–1033.

Junghans, R.P., P.H. Duesberg, and C.A. Knight. 1975. *In vitro* synthesis of full-length DNA transcripts of Rous sarcoma virus RNA by viral DNA polymerase. *Proc. Natl. Acad. Sci.* **72:** 4895–4899.

Junghans, R.P., S. Hu, C.A. Knight, and N. Davidson. 1977. Heteroduplex analysis of avian RNA tumor viruses. *Proc. Natl. Acad. Sci.* **74:** 477–481.

Kamine, J., J.G. Burr, and J.M. Buchanan. 1978. Multiple forms of *sarc* gene proteins from Rous sarcoma virus RNA. *Proc. Natl. Acad. Sci.* **75:** 366–370.

Karess, R.E., W.S. Hayward, and H. Hanafusa. 1979. Cellular information in the genome of recovered avian sarcoma virus directs the synthesis of transforming protein. *Proc. Natl. Acad. Sci.* **76:** 3154–3158.

Kawai, S. and H. Hanafusa. 1972. Genetic recombination with avian tumor virus. *Virology* **49:** 37–44.

———. 1973. Isolation of defective mutant of avian sarcoma virus. *Proc. Natl. Acad. Sci.* **70:** 3493–3497.

———. 1976. Recombination between a temperature-sensitive mutant and a deletion mutant of Rous sarcoma virus. *J. Virol.* **19:**389–397.

Kawai, S., P.H. Duesberg, and H. Hanafusa. 1977. Transformation-defective mutants of Rous sarcoma virus with *src* gene deletions of varying length. *J. Virol.* **24:**910–914.

Kawai, S., M. Yoshida, K. Segawa, H. Sugiyama, K. Ishizaki, and K. Toyoshima. 1980. Characterization of Y73, an avian sarcoma virus: A unique transforming gene and its product, a phosphopolyprotein with protein kinase activity. *Proc. Natl. Acad. Sci.* **77:**6199–6203.

Keith, J. and H. Fraenkel-Conrat. 1975. Identification of the 5′ end of Rous sarcoma virus RNA. *Proc. Natl. Acad. Sci.* **72:**3347–3350.

Keith, J., M. Gleason, and H. Fraenkel-Conrat. 1974. Characterization of the end groups of RNA of Rous sarcoma virus. *Proc. Natl. Acad. Sci.* **71:**4371–4375.

Keshet, E. and H.M. Temin. 1977. Nucleotide sequences derived from pheasant DNA in the genome of recombinant avian leukosis viruses with subgroup F specificity. *J. Virol.* **24:**505–513.

King, A.M.Q. 1976. High molecular weight RNAs from Rous sarcoma virus and Moloney murine leukemia virus contain two subunits. *J. Biol. Chem.* **251:**141–149.

King, A.M.Q. and R.D. Wells. 1976. All intact subunit RNAs from Rous sarcoma virus contain poly(A). *J. Biol. Chem.* **251:**150–152.

Kirsten, W.H. and L.A. Mayer. 1967. Morphologic responses to a murine erythroblastosis virus. *J. Natl. Cancer Inst.* **39:**311–335.

Kitchener, G. and M.J. Hayman. 1980. Comparative tryptic peptide mapping studies suggest a role in cell transformation for the *gag*-related protein of avian erythroblastosis virus and avian myelocytomatosis virus strains CMII and MC29. *Proc. Natl. Acad. Sci.* **77:** 1637–1641.

Kozak, M. 1978. How do eucaryotic ribosomes select initiation regions in messenger RNA? *Cell* **15:**1109–1123.

———. 1980. Evaluation of the "scanning model" for initiation of protein synthesis in eucaryotes. *Cell* **22:**7–8.

Krzyzek, R.A., M.S. Collett, A.F. Lau, M.L. Perdue, J.P. Leis, and A.J. Faras. 1978. Evidence for splicing of avian sarcoma virus 5′-terminal genomic sequences onto viral-specific RNA in infected cells. *Proc. Natl. Acad. Sci.* **75:**1284–1288.

Kung, H.-J., J.M. Bailey, N. Davidson, P.K. Vogt, M.O. Nicolson, and R.M. McAllister. 1975. Electron microscope studies of tumor virus RNA. *Cold Spring Harbor Symp. Quant. Biol.* **39:**827–834.

Kung, H.-J., S. Hu, W. Bender, J.M. Bailey, N. Davidson, M.O. Nicolson, and R.M. McAllister. 1976. RD-114, baboon, and woolly monkey viral RNAs compared in size and structure. *Cell* **7:**609–620.

Lai, M.-H.T. and I.M. Verma. 1980. Genome organization of retroviruses. VII. Infection by double-stranded DNA synthesized *in vitro* from Moloney murine leukemia virus generates a virus indistinguishable from the original virus used in reverse transcription. *Virology* **100:**194–198.

Lai, M.M.C. and P.H. Duesberg. 1972. Adenylic acid-rich sequence in RNAs of Rous sarcoma virus and Rauscher mouse leukaemia virus. *Nature* **235:**383–386.

Lai, M.M.C, S.S.F. Hu, and P.K. Vogt. 1977. Occurrence of partial deletion and substitution of the *src* gene in the RNA genome of avian sarcoma virus. *Proc. Natl. Acad. Sci.* **74:**4781–4785.

———. 1979. Avian erythroblastosis virus: Transformation-specific sequences form a contiguous segment of 3.25 kb located in the middle of the 6-kb genome. *Virology* **97:**336–377.

Lai, M.M.C., J.C. Neil, and P.K. Vogt. 1980. Cell-free translation of avian erythroblastosis virus RNA yields two specific and distinct proteins with molecular weights of 75,000 and 40,000. *Virology* **100:**475–483.

Langbeheim, H., T.Y. Shih, and E.M. Scolnick. 1980. Identification of a normal vertebrate cell protein related to the p21 *src* of Harvey murine sarcoma virus. *Virology* **106:**292–300

Lee, W.-H., K. Bister, A. Pawson, T. Robins, C. Moscovici, and P.H. Duesberg. 1980. Fujinami sarcoma virus: An avian RNA tumor virus with a unique transforming gene. *Proc. Natl. Acad. Sci.* **77:**2018–2022.

Leis, J.P., J. McGinnis, and R.W. Green. 1978. Rous sarcoma virus p19 binds to specific double-stranded regions of viral RNA: Effects of p19 on cleavage of viral RNA by RNase III. *Virology* **84:**87–98.

Levin, J.G. and J.G. Seidman. 1979. Selective packaging of host tRNAs by murine leukemia virus particles does not require genomic RNA. *J. Virol.* **29:**328–335.

Levin, J.G., P.M. Grimley, J.M. Ramseur, and I.K. Berezesky. 1974. Deficiency of 60 to 70S RNA in murine leukemia virus particles assembled in cells treated with actinomycin D. *J. Virol.* **14:**152–161.

Levinson, W., J.M. Bishop, N. Quintrell, and J. Jackson. 1970. Presence of DNA in Rous sarcoma virus. *Nature* **227:**1023–1025.

Levinson, W.E., H.E. Varmus, A.-C. Garapin, and J.M. Bishop. 1972. DNA of Rous sarcoma virus: Its nature and significance. *Science* **175:**76–78.

Lieberman, M. and H.S. Kaplan. 1959. Leukemogenic activity of filtrates from radiation-induced lymphoid tumors of mice. *Science* **130:**387–388.

Lieberman, M., A. Decleve, P. Ricciardi-Castagnoli, J. Boniver, O.J. Finn, and H.S. Kaplan. 1979. Establishment, characterization and virus expression of cell lines derived from radiation- and virus-induced lymphomas of C57BL/Ka mice. *Int. J. Cancer* **24:**168–177.

Linemeyer, D.L., S.K. Ruscetti, J.G. Menke, and E.M. Scolnick. 1980. Recovery of biologically active spleen focus-forming virus from molecularly cloned spleen focus-forming virus-pBR322 circular DNA by cotransfection with infectious type C retroviral DNA. *J. Virol.* **35:**710–721.

Linial, M. and S. Brown. 1979. High frequency recombination within the *gag* gene of Rous sarcoma virus. *J. Virol.* **31:**257–260.

Linial, M. and P.E. Neiman. 1976. Infection of chick cells by subgroup E viruses. *Virology* **73:**508–520.

Linial, M., E. Medeiros, and W.S. Hayward. 1978. An avian oncovirus mutant (*SE* 21Q1b) deficient in genomic RNA: Biological and biochemical characterization. *Cell* **15:**1371–1381.

Lovinger, G.G. and G. Schochetman. 1979. 5′-terminal nucleotide sequences of the Rauscher leukemia virus and gibbon ape leukemia virus genomes exhibit a high degree of correspondence. *J. Virol.* **32:**803–811.

———. 1980. 5′ terminal nucleotide sequences of type C retroviruses: Features common to noncoding sequences of eucaryotic messenger RNAs. *Cell* **20:**441–449.

Lowy, D.R., E. Rands, S.K. Chattopadhyay, C.F. Garon, and G.L. Hager. 1980. Molecular cloning of infectious integrated murine leukemia virus DNA from infected mouse cells. *Proc. Natl. Acad. Sci.* **77:**614–618.

MacDonald, M.E., F.H. Reynolds, Jr., W.J.M. Van de Ven, J.R. Stephenson, T.W. Mak, and A. Bernstein. 1980. Anemia- and polycythemia-inducing isolates of Friend spleen focus-forming virus. Biological and molecular evidence for two distinct viral genomes. *J. Exp. Med.* **151:**1477–1492.

Maisel, J., W. Bender, S. Hu, P.H. Duesberg, and N. Davidson. 1978. Structure of 50 to 70S RNA from Moloney sarcoma viruses. *J. Virol.* **25:**384–394.

Majors, J.E. and H.E. Varmus. 1981. Nucleotide sequences at host-proviral junctions for mouse mammary tumour virus. *Nature* **289:**253–258.

Mak, T.W., D. Penrose, C. Gamble, and A. Bernstein. 1978. The Friend spleen focus-forming virus (SFFV) genome: Fractionation and analysis of SFFV and helper virus-related sequences. *Virology* **87:** 73–80.

Mangel, W.F., H. Delius, and P.H. Duesberg. 1974. Structure and molecular weight of the 60-70S RNA and the 30-40S RNA of the Rous sarcoma virus. *Proc. Natl. Acad. Sci.* **71:** 4541–4545.

Manteuil-Brutlag, S., S. Liu, and H.S. Kaplan. 1980. Radiation leukemia virus contains two distinct viral RNAs. *Cell* **19:** 643–652.

Martin, G.S. and P.H. Duesberg. 1972. The *a* subunit in the RNA of transforming avian tumor viruses. I. Occurrence in different virus strains. II. Spontaneous loss resulting in nontransforming variants. *Virology* **47:** 494–497.

Mason, W.S., R.R. Friis, M. Linial, and P.K. Vogt. 1974. Determination of the defective function in two mutants of Rous sarcoma virus. *Virology* **61:** 559–574.

McCarter, J.A. 1977. Genetic studies of the ploidy of Moloney murine leukemia virus. *J. Virol.* **22:** 9–15.

McClements, W.L., L.W. Enquist, M. Oskarsson, M. Sullivan, and G.F. Vande Woude. 1980. Frequent site specific deletion of coliphage λ murine sarcoma virus recombinants and its use in the identification of a retrovirus integration site. *J. Virol.* **35:** 488–497.

McDonough, S.K., S. Larsen, R.S. Brodey, N.D. Stock, and W.D. Hardy. 1971. A transmissible feline fibrosarcoma of viral origin. *Cancer Res.* **31:** 953–956.

Mellon, P., A. Pawson, K. Bister, G.S. Martin, and P.H. Duesberg. 1978. Specific RNA sequences and gene products of MC29 avian acute leukemia virus. *Proc. Natl. Acad. Sci.* **75:** 5874–5878.

Moloney, J.B. 1966. A virus-induced rhabdomyosarcoma of mice. *Natl. Cancer Inst. Monogr.* **22:** 139–142.

Murphy, E.C., Jr., N. Wills, and R.B. Arlinghaus. 1980. Suppression of murine retrovirus polypeptide termination: Effect of amber suppressor tRNA on the cell-free translation of Rauscher murine leukemia virus, Moloney murine leukemia virus, and Moloney murine sarcoma virus 124 RNA. *J. Virol.* **34:** 464–473.

Murti, K.G., M. Bondurant, and A. Tereba. 1981. Secondary structural features in the 70S RNAs of Moloney murine leukemia and Rous sarcoma viruses as observed by electron microscopy. *J. Virol.* **37:** 411–419.

Neil, J.C., M.L. Breitman, and P.K. Vogt. 1981. Characterization of a 105,000 molecular weight *gag*-related phosphoprotein from cells transformed by the defective avian sarcoma virus PRCII. *Virology* **108:** 98–110.

Neiman, P.E., S. Das, D. Macdonnell, and C. McMillin-Helsel. 1977. Organization of shared and unshared sequences in the genomes of chicken endogenous and sarcoma viruses. *Cell* **11:** 321–329.

Niman, H.L. and J.H. Elder. 1980. Molecular dissection of Rauscher virus gp70 by using monoclonal antibodies: Localization of acquired sequences of related envelope gene recombinants. *Proc. Natl. Acad. Sci.* **77:** 4524–4528.

Novak, U., R. Friedrich, and K. Moelling. 1979. Elongation of DNA complementary to the 5′ end of the avian sarcoma virus genome by the virion-associated RNA-directed DNA polymerase. *J. Virol.* **30:** 438–452.

O'Connor, T. and P.J. Fischinger. 1969. Physical properties of competent and defective states of a murine sarcoma (Moloney) virus. *J. Natl. Cancer Inst.* **43:** 487–497.

Oliff, A.I., G.L. Hager, E.H. Chang, E.M. Scolnick, H.W. Chan, and D.R. Lowy. 1980. Transfection of molecularly cloned Friend murine leukemia virus DNA yields a highly leukemogenic helper-independent type C virus. *J. Virol.* **33:** 475–486.

O'Rear, J.J., S. Mizutani, G. Hoffman, M. Fiandt, and H.M. Temin. 1980. Infectious and noninfectious recombinant clones of the provirus of SNV differ in cellular DNA and are apparently the same in viral DNA. *Cell* **20:** 423–430.

Oskarsson, N.K., J.H. Elder, J.W. Gautsch, R.A. Lerner, and G.F. Vande Woude. 1978.

Chemical determination of the ml Moloney sarcoma virus $pP60^{gag}$ gene order: Evidence for unique peptides in the carboxy terminus of the polyprotein. *Proc. Natl. Acad. Sci.* **75:** 4694–4698.

Oskarsson, M., W.L. McClements, D.G. Blair, J.V. Maizel, and G.F. Vande Woude. 1980. Properties of a normal mouse cell DNA sequence (*sarc*) homologous to the *src* sequence of Moloney sarcoma virus. *Science* **207:** 1222–1224.

Palmiter, R.D., J. Gagnon, V.M. Vogt, S. Ripley, and R.N. Eisenman. 1978. The NH_2-terminal sequence of the avian oncovirus *gag* precursor polyprotein ($Pr76^{gag}$). *Virology* **91:** 423–433.

Panet, A. and H. Berliner. 1978. Binding of tRNA to reverse transcriptase of RNA tumor viruses. *J. Virol.* **26:** 214–220.

Panet, A., W.A. Haseltine, D. Baltimore, G. Peters, F. Harada, and J.E. Dahlberg. 1975. Specific binding of tryptophan transfer RNA to avian myeloblastosis virus RNA-dependent DNA polymerase (reverse transcriptase). *Proc. Natl. Acad. Sci.* **72:** 2535–2539.

Papkoff, J., T. Hunter, and K. Beemon. 1980. *In vitro* translation of virion RNA from Moloney murine sarcoma virus. *Virology* **101:** 91–103.

Pawson, T. and G.S. Martin. 1980. Cell-free translation of avian erythroblastosis virus RNA. *J. Virol.* **34:** 280–284.

Pawson, T., R. Harvey, and A.E. Smith. 1977. The size of Rous sarcoma virus mRNAs active in cell-free translation. *Nature* **268:** 416–420.

Pawson, T., G.S. Martin, and A.E. Smith. 1976. Cell-free translation of virion RNA from nondefective and transformation-defective Rous sarcoma viruses. *J. Virol.* **19:** 950–967.

Pawson, T., P. Mellon, P.H. Duesberg, and G.S. Martin. 1980. *env* gene of Rous sarcoma virus: Identification of the gene product by cell-free translation. *J. Virol.* **33:** 993–1003.

Pedersen, F.S. and W.A. Haseltine. 1980. A micromethod for detailed characterization of high molecular weight RNA. *Methods Enzymol.* **65:** 680–687.

Perez-Bercoff, R. and M.A. Billeter. 1976. Characterization of the 3′-terminal region of the large molecular weight RNA subunits from normal and transformation-defective Rous sarcoma virus. *Biochim. Biophys. Acta* **454:** 383–388.

Peters, G. and J.E. Dahlberg. 1979. RNA-directed DNA synthesis in Moloney murine leukemia virus: Interaction between the primer tRNA and the genome RNA. *J. Virol.* **31:** 398–407.

Peters, G. and C. Glover. 1980a. Low-molecular-weight RNAs and initiation of RNA-directed DNA synthesis in avian reticuloendotheliosis virus. *J. Virol.* **33:** 708–716.

———. 1980b. tRNAs and priming of RNA-directed DNA synthesis in mouse mammary tumor virus. *J. Virol.* **35:** 31–40.

Peters, G.G. and J. Hu. 1980. Reverse transcriptase as the major determinant for selective packaging of tRNAs into avian sarcoma virus particles. *J. Virol.* **36:** 692–700.

Peters, G., F. Harada, J.E. Dahlberg, A. Panet, W.A. Haseltine, and D. Baltimore. 1977. Low-molecular-weight RNAs of Moloney murine leukemia virus: Identification of the primer for RNA-directed DNA synthesis. *J. Virol.* **21:** 1031–1041.

Philipson, L., P. Andersson, U. Olshevsky, R. Weinberg, D. Baltimore, and R. Gesteland. 1978. Translation of MuLV and MSV RNAs in nuclease-treated reticulocyte extracts: Enhancement of the *gag-pol* polypeptide with yeast suppressor tRNA. *Cell* **13:** 189–199.

Porzig, K.J., M. Barbacid, and S.A. Aaronson. 1979. Biological properties and translational products of three independent isolates of feline sarcoma virus. *Virology* **92:** 91–107.

Proudfoot, N.J. and G.G. Brownlee. 1976. 3′ non-coding region sequences in eukaryotic messenger RNA. *Nature* **263:** 211–214.

Purchio, A.F., E. Erikson, and R.L. Erikson. 1977. Translation of 35S and of subgenomic regions of avian sarcoma virus RNA. *Proc. Natl. Acad. Sci.* **74:** 4661–4665.

Purchio, A.F., E. Erikson, J.S. Brugge, and R.L. Erikson. 1978. Identification of a polypeptide encoded by the avian sarcoma virus *src* gene. *Proc. Natl. Acad. Sci.* **75:** 1567–1571.

Quade, K. 1979. Transformation of mammalian cells by avian myelocytomatosis virus and avian erythroblastosis virus. *Virology* **98:**461–465.

Quade, K., R.E. Smith, and J.L. Nichols. 1974. Evidence for common nucleotide sequences in the RNA subunits comprising Rous sarcoma virus 70 S RNA. *Virology* **61:**287–291.

Ramsay, G. and M.J. Hayman. 1980. Analysis of cells transformed by defective leukemia virus OK10: Production of noninfectious particles and synthesis of $Pr76^{gag}$ and an additional 200,000-dalton protein. *Virology* **106:**71–81.

Ramsay, G., T. Graf, and M.J. Hayman. 1980. Mutants of avian myelocytomatosis virus with smaller *gag* gene-related proteins have an altered transforming ability. *Nature* **288:**170–172.

Rasheed, S. 1980. Endogenous virogenes and oncogenes in rat-cell transformation: A new model system. *Cold Spring Harbor Symp. Quant. Biol.* **44:**779–786.

Rasheed, S., M.B. Gardner, and R.J. Huebner. 1978. *In vitro* isolation of stable rat sarcoma viruses. *Proc. Natl. Acad. Sci.* **75:**2972–2976.

Reddy, E.P., M.J. Smith, E. Canaani, K.C. Robbins, S.R. Tronick, S. Zain, and S.A. Aaronson. 1980. Nucleotide sequence analysis of the transforming region and large terminal redundancies of Moloney murine sarcoma virus. *Proc. Natl. Acad. Sci.* **77:**5234–5238.

Rettenmier, C.W., S.M. Anderson, M.W. Riemen, and H. Hanafusa. 1979. *gag*-related polypeptides encoded by replication-defective avian oncoviruses. *J. Virol.* **32:**749–761.

Reynolds, F.H., Jr., W.J.M. Van de Ven, and J.R. Stephenson. 1980. Abelson murine leukemia virus transformation-defective mutants with impaired P120-associated protein kinase activity. *J. Virol.* **36:**374–386.

Reynolds, F.H., Jr., T.L. Sacks, D.N. Deobagkar, and J.R. Stephenson. 1978. Cells nonproductively transformed by Abelson murine leukemia virus express a high molecular weight polyprotein containing structural and nonstructural components. *Proc. Natl. Acad. Sci.* **75:**3974–3978.

Riggin, C.H., M. Bondurant, and W.M. Mitchell. 1975. Physical properties of Moloney murine leukemia virus high-molecular-weight RNA: A two subunit structure. *J. Virol.* **16:**1528–1535.

Robey, W.G., M.K. Oskarsson, G.F. Vande Woude, R.B. Naso, R.B. Arlinghaus, D.K. Haapala, and P.J. Fischinger. 1977. Cells transformed by certain strains of Moloney sarcoma virus contain murine p60. *Cell* **10:**79–89.

Robinson, F.R. and M.J. Twiehaus. 1974. Isolation of the avian reticuloendotheliosis virus (strain T). *Avian Dis.* **18:**278–288.

Robinson, H.L. 1976. Intracellular restriction on the growth of induced subgroup E avian type C viruses in chicken cells. *J. Virol.* **18:**856–866.

Robinson, H.L., M.N. Pearson, D.W. DeSimone, P.N. Tsichlis, and J.M. Coffin. 1980. Subgroup-E avian-leukosis-virus-associated diseases in chickens. *Cold Spring Harbor Symp. Quant. Biol.* **44:**1133–1142.

Robinson, W.S. and M.A. Baluda. 1965. The nucleic acid from avian myeloblastosis virus compared with the RNA from the Bryan strain of Rous sarcoma virus. *Proc. Natl. Acad. Sci.* **54:**1686–1692.

Robinson, W.S., A. Pitkanen, and H. Rubin. 1965. The nucleic acid of the Bryan strain of Rous sarcoma virus: Purification of the virus and isolation of the nucleic acid. *Proc. Natl. Acad. Sci.* **54:**137–144.

Robinson, W.S, H.L. Robinson, and P.H. Duesberg. 1967. Tumor virus RNAs. *Proc. Natl. Acad. Sci.* **58:**825–834.

Rommelaere, J., H. Donis-Keller, and N. Hopkins. 1979. RNA sequencing provides evidence for allelism of determinants of the N-, B- or NB-tropism of murine leukemia viruses. *Cell* **16:**43–50.

Rommelaere, J., D.V. Faller, and N. Hopkins. 1978. Characterization and mapping of RNase T1-resistant oligonucleotides derived from the genomes of AKV and MCF murine leukemia viruses. *Proc. Natl. Acad. Sci.* **75:**495–499.

Rose, J.K., W.A. Haseltine, and D. Baltimore. 1976. 5′-terminus of Moloney murine leukemia virus 35S RNA is $m^7G^{5\prime}ppp^{5\prime}GmpCp$. *J. Virol.* **20:** 324–329.

Rosenberg, N. and D. Baltimore. 1976. A quantitative assay for transformation of bone marrow cells by Abelson murine leukemia virus. *J. Exp. Med.* **143:** 1453–1467.

Rosenberg, N., D. Baltimore, and C.D. Scher. 1975. *In vitro* transformation of lymphoid cells by Abelson murine leukemia virus. *Proc. Natl. Acad. Sci.* **72:** 1932–1936.

Rosenberg, N.E., D.R. Clark, and O.N. Witte. 1980. Abelson murine leukemia virus mutants deficient in kinase activity and lymphoid cell transformation. *J. Virol.* **36:** 766–774.

Rosner, M.R., J.-S. Tung, N. Hopkins, and P.W. Robbins. 1980. Relationship of G_{IX} antigen expression to the glycosylation of murine leukemia virus glycoprotein. *Proc. Natl. Acad. Sci.* **77:** 6420–6424.

Rothenberg, E. and D. Baltimore. 1977. Increased length of DNA made by virions of murine leukemia virus at limiting magnesium ion concentration. *J. Virol.* **21:** 168–178.

Rothenberg, E., D.J. Donoghue, and D. Baltimore. 1978. Analysis of a 5′ leader sequence on murine leukemia virus 21S RNA: Heteroduplex mapping with long reverse transcriptase products. *Cell* **13:** 435–451.

Rothenberg, E., D. Smotkin, D. Baltimore, and R.A. Weinberg. 1977. *In vitro* synthesis of infectious DNA of murine leukaemia virus. *Nature* **269:** 122–126.

Rous, P. 1911. A sarcoma of the fowl transmissible by an agent separable from the tumor cells. *J. Exp. Med.* **13:** 397–411.

Roussel, M., S. Saule, C. Lagrou, C. Rommens, H. Beug, T. Graf, and D. Stehelin. 1979. Three new types of viral oncogene of cellular origin specific for haematopoietic cell transformation. *Nature* **281:** 452–455.

Royer-Pokora, B., S. Grieser, H. Beug, and T. Graf. 1979. Mutant avian erythroblastosis virus with restricted target cell specificity. *Nature* **282:** 750–752.

Ruscetti, S.L., L.P. Turek, and C.J. Sherr. 1980. Three independent isolates of feline sarcoma virus code for three distinct *gag*-x polyproteins. *J. Virol.* **35:** 259–264.

Ruscetti, S.K., D. Linemeyer, J. Feild, D. Troxler, and E.M. Scolnick. 1979. Characterization of a protein found in cells infected with the spleen focus-forming virus that shares immunological cross-reactivity with the gp70 found in mink cell focus-inducing virus particles. *J. Virol.* **30:** 787–798.

Sabran, J.L., T.W. Hsu, C. Yeater, A. Kaji, W.S. Mason, and J.M. Taylor. 1979. Analysis of integrated avian RNA tumor virus DNA in transformed chicken, duck, and quail fibroblasts. *J. Virol.* **29:** 170–178.

Sarma, P.S., A.L. Sharar, and S. McDonough. 1972. The SM strain of feline sarcoma virus. Biologic and antigenic characterization of virus. *Proc. Soc. Exp. Biol. Med.* **140:** 1365–1368.

Sawyer, R.C. and H. Hanafusa. 1977. Formation of reticuloendotheliosis virus pseudotypes of Rous sarcoma virus. *J. Virol.* **22:** 634–639.

———. 1979. Comparison of the small RNAs of polymerase-deficient and polymerase-positive Rous sarcoma virus and another species of avian retrovirus. *J. Virol.* **29:** 863–871.

Scheinberg, D.A. and M. Strand. 1980. Transformation-related proteins associated with Kirsten sarcoma virus. *Virology* **106:** 335–348.

Scher, C.D. and R. Siegler. 1975. Direct transformation of 3T3 cells by Abelson murine leukaemia virus. *Nature* **253:** 729–731.

Schindler, J., R. Hynes, and N. Hopkins. 1977. Evidence for recombination between N- and B-tropic murine leukemia viruses: Analysis of three virion proteins by sodium dodecyl sulfate-polyacrylamide gel electrophoresis. *J. Virol.* **23:** 700–707.

Schwartz, D.E., P.C. Zamecnik, and H.L. Weith. 1977. Rous sarcoma virus genome is terminally redundant: The 3′ sequence. *Proc. Natl. Acad. Sci.* **74:** 994–998.

Scolnick, E.M., R.J. Goldberg, and D. Williams. 1976. Characterization of rat genetic sequences of Kirsten sarcoma virus: Distinct class of endogenous rat type C viral sequences. *J. Virol.* **18:** 559–566.

Scolnick, E.M., A.G. Papageorge, and T.Y. Shih. 1979. Guanine nucleotide-binding activity as an assay for *src* protein of rat-derived murine sarcoma viruses. *Proc. Natl. Acad. Sci.* **76:** 5355–5359.

Scolnick, E.M., E. Rands, D. Williams, and W.P. Parks. 1973. Studies on the nucleic acid sequences of Kirsten sarcoma virus: A model for formation of a mammalian RNA-containing sarcoma virus. *J. Virol.* **12:** 458–463.

Seif, I., G. Khoury, and R. Dhar. 1979. The genome of human papovavirus BKV. *Cell* **18:** 963–977.

Sen, A. and G.J. Todaro. 1977. The genome-associated, specific RNA binding proteins of avian and mammalian type C viruses. *Cell* **10:** 91–99.

Sen, A., C.J. Sherr, and G.J. Todaro. 1976. Specific binding of the type C viral core protein p12 with purified viral RNA. *Cell* **7:** 21–32.

———. 1978. Endogenous feline (RD-114) and baboon type C viruses have related specific RNA-binding proteins and genome binding sites. *Virology* **84:** 99–107.

Shank, P.R. and M. Linial. 1980. Avian oncovirus mutant (SE21Q1b) deficient in genomic RNA: Characterization of a deletion in the provirus. *J. Virol.* **36:** 450–456.

Shank, P.R., S.H. Hughes, and H.E. Varmus. 1981. Restriction endonuclease mapping of the DNA of Rous-associated virus 0 reveals extensive homology in structure and sequence with avian sarcoma virus DNA. *Virology* **108:** 177–188.

Shank, P.R., S.H. Hughes, H.-J. Kung, J.E. Majors, N. Quintrell, R.V. Guntaka, J.M. Bishop, and H.E. Varmus. 1978. Mapping unintegrated avian sarcoma virus DNA: Termini of linear DNA bear 300 nucleotides present once or twice in two species of circular DNA. *Cell* **15:** 1383–1395.

Sharp, P.A. 1980. Summary: Molecular biology of viral oncogenes. *Cold Spring Harbor Symp. Quant. Biol.* **44:** 1305–1322.

Sheiness, D. and J.M. Bishop. 1979. DNA and RNA from uninfected vertebrate cells contain nucleotide sequences related to the putative transforming gene of avian myelocytomatosis virus. *J. Virol.* **31:** 514–521.

Sheiness, D., L. Fanshier, and J.M. Bishop. 1978. Identification of nucleotide sequences which may encode the oncogenic capacity of avian retrovirus MC29. *J. Virol.* **28:** 600–610.

Sheiness, D.K., S.H. Hughes, H.E. Varmus, E. Stubblefield, and J.M. Bishop. 1980a. The vertebrate homolog of the putative transforming gene of avian myelocytomatosis virus: Characteristics of the DNA locus and its RNA transcript. *Virology* **105:** 415–424.

Sheiness, D., K. Bister, C. Moscovici, L. Fanshier, T. Gonda, and J.M. Bishop. 1980b. Avian retroviruses that cause carcinoma and leukemia: Identification of nucleotide sequences associated with pathogenicity. *J. Virol.* **33:** 962–968.

Sherr, C.J., L.A. Fedele, L. Donner, and L.P. Turek. 1979. Restriction endonuclease mapping of unintegrated proviral DNA of Snyder-Theilen feline sarcoma virus: Localization of sarcoma-specific sequences. *J. Virol.* **32:** 860–875.

Sherr, C.J., L.A. Fedele, M. Oskarsson, J. Maizel, and G. Vande Woude. 1980. Molecular cloning of Snyder-Theilen feline leukemia and sarcoma viruses: Comparative studies of feline sarcoma virus with its natural helper virus and with Moloney murine sarcoma virus. *J. Virol.* **34:** 200–212.

Shibuya, M., T. Hanafusa, H. Hanafusa, and J.R. Stephenson. 1980. Homology exists among the transforming sequences of avian and feline sarcoma viruses. *Proc. Natl. Acad. Sci.* **77:** 6536–6540.

Shields, A., S. Goff, M. Paskind, G. Otto, and D. Baltimore. 1979. Structure of the Abelson murine leukemia virus genome. *Cell* **18:** 955–962.

Shih, T.Y., M.O. Weeks, H.A. Young, and E.M. Scolnick. 1979a. Identification of a sarcoma virus-coded phosphoprotein in nonproducer cells transformed by Kirsten or Harvey murine sarcoma virus. *Virology* **96:** 64–79.

———. 1979b. p21 of Kirsten murine sarcoma virus is thermolabile in a viral mutant temperature sensitive for the maintenance of transformation. *J. Virol.* **31:** 546–556.

Shih, T.Y., H.A. Young, J.M. Coffin, and E.M. Scolnick. 1978a. Physical map of the Kirsten sarcoma virus genome as determined by fingerprinting RNase T1-resistant oligonucleotides. *J. Virol.* **25:**238–252.

Shih, T.Y., A.G. Papageorge, P.E. Stokes, M.O. Weeks, and E.M. Scolnick. 1980. Guanine nucleotide-binding and autophosphorylating activities associated with the p21^{src} protein of Harvey murine sarcoma virus. *Nature* **287:**686–691.

Shih, T.Y., M.O. Weeks, D.H. Troxler, J.M. Coffin, and E.M. Scolnick. 1978b. Mapping host range-specific oligonucleotides within genomes of the ecotropic and mink cell focus-inducing strains of Moloney murine leukemia virus. *J. Virol* **26:**71–83.

Shih, T.Y., D.R. Williams, M.O. Weeks, J.M. Maryak, W.C. Vass, and E.M. Scolnick. 1978c. Comparison of the genomic organization of Kirsten and Harvey sarcoma viruses. *J. Virol.* **27:**45–55.

Shimotohno, K., S. Mizutani, and H.M. Temin. 1980. Sequence of retrovirus provirus resembles that of bacterial transposable elements. *Nature* **285:**550–554.

Shine, J., A.P. Czernilofsky, R. Friedrich, J.M. Bishop, and H.M. Goodman. 1977. Nucleotide sequence at the 5′ terminus of the avian sarcoma virus genome. *Proc. Natl. Acad. Sci.* **74:**1473–1477.

Shoemaker, C., S. Goff, E. Gilboa, M. Paskind, S.W. Mitra, and D. Baltimore. 1980. Structure of a cloned circular Moloney murine leukemia virus DNA molecule containing an inverted segment: Implications for retrovirus integration. *Proc. Natl. Acad. Sci.* **77:**3932–3936.

Silva, R.F. and M.A. Baluda. 1980. Avian myeloblastosis virus proteins in leukemic chicken myeloblasts. *J. Virol.* **35:**766–774.

Simek, S. and N.R. Rice. 1980. Analysis of the nucleic acid components in reticuloendotheliosis virus. *J. Virol.* **33:**320–329.

Sklar, M.D., B.J. White, and W.P. Rowe. 1974. Initiation of oncogenic transformation of mouse lymphocytes *in vitro* by Abelson leukemia virus. *Proc. Natl. Acad. Sci.* **71:**4077–4081.

Snyder, S.P. and G.H. Theilen. 1969. Transmissible feline fibrosarcoma. *Nature* **221:**1074–1075.

Southern, E.M. 1975. Detection of specific sequences among DNA fragments separated by gel electrophoresis. *J. Mol. Biol.* **98:**503–517.

Souza, L.M. and M.A. Baluda. 1980. Identification of the avian myeloblastosis virus genome. I. Identification of restriction endonuclease fragments associated with acute myeloblastic leukemia. *J. Virol.* **36:**317–324.

Souza, L.M., M.C. Komaromy, and M.A. Baluda. 1980a. Identification of a proviral genome associated with avian myeloblastic leukemia. *Proc. Natl. Acad. Sci.* **77:**3004–3008.

Souza, L.M., M.J. Briskin, R.L. Hillyard, and M.A. Baluda. 1980b. Identification of the avian myeloblastosis virus genome. II. Restriction endonuclease analysis of DNA from λ proviral recombinants and leukemic myeloblast clones. *J. Virol.* **36:**325–336.

Souza, L.M., J.N. Strommer, R.L. Hillyard, M.C. Komaromy, and M.A. Baluda. 1980c. Cellular sequences are present in the presumptive avian myeloblastosis virus genome. *Proc. Natl. Acad. Sci.* **77:**5177–5181.

Stacey, D.W. 1979. Messenger activity of virion RNA for avian leukosis viral envelope glycoprotein. *J. Virol.* **29:**949–956.

Stacey, D.W. and H. Hanafusa. 1978. Nuclear conversion of microinjected avian leukosis virion RNA into an envelope-glycoprotein messenger. *Nature* **273:**779–782.

Steffen, D. and R.A. Weinberg. 1978. The integrated genome of murine leukemia virus. *Cell* **15:**1003–1010.

Stehelin, D., R.V. Guntaka, H.E. Varmus, and J.M. Bishop. 1976. Purification of cDNA complementary to nucleotide sequences required for neoplastic transformation of fibroblasts by avian sarcoma viruses. *J. Mol. Biol.* **101:**349–365.

Stehelin, D., S. Saule, M. Roussel, A. Sergeant, C. Lagrou, C. Rommens, and M.B. Raes. 1980. Three new types of viral oncogenes in defective avian leukemia viruses. I. Specific nucleotide sequences of cellular origin correlate with specific transformation. *Cold Spring Harbor Symp. Quant. Biol.* **44:** 1215–1223.

Stohrer, R. and E. Hunter. 1979. Inhibition of Rous sarcoma virus replication by 2-deoxyglucose and tunicamycin: Identification of an unglycosylated *env* gene product. *J. Virol.* **32:** 412–419.

Stoll, E., M.A. Billeter, A. Palmenberg, and C. Weissmann. 1977. Avian myeloblastosis virus RNA is terminally redundant: Implications for the mechanism of retrovirus replication. *Cell* **12:** 57–72.

Stoltzfus, C.M. and K. Dimock. 1976. Evidence for methylation of B77 avian sarcoma virus genome RNA subunits. *J. Virol.* **18:** 586–595.

Sutcliffe, J.G., T.M. Shinnick, I.M. Verma, and R.A. Lerner. 1980a. Nucleotide sequence of Moloney leukemia virus: 3′ end reveals details of replication, analogy to bacterial transposons, and an unexpected gene. *Proc. Natl. Acad. Sci.* **77:** 3302–3306.

Sutcliffe, J.G., T.M. Shinnick, N. Green, F.-T. Liu, H.L. Niman, and R.A. Lerner. 1980b. Chemical synthesis of a polypeptide predicted from nucleotide sequence allows detection of a new retroviral gene product. *Nature* **287:** 801–805.

Tal, J., H.-J. Kung, H.E. Varmus, and J.M. Bishop. 1977a. Characterization of DNA complementary to nucleotide sequences adjacent to poly(A) at the 3′-terminus of the avian sarcoma virus genome. *Virology* **79:** 183–197.

Tal, J., D.J. Fujita, S. Kawai, H.E. Varmus, and J.M. Bishop. 1977b. Purification of DNA complementary to the *env* gene of avian sarcoma virus and analysis of relationships among the *env* genes of avian leukosis-sarcoma viruses. *J. Virol.* **21:** 497–505.

Taylor, J.M. 1977. An analysis of the role of tRNA species as primers for the transcription into DNA of RNA tumor virus genomes. *Biochim. Biophys. Acta* **473:** 57–71.

Taylor, J.M. and R. Illmensee. 1975. Site on the RNA of an avian sarcoma virus at which primer is bound. *J. Virol.* **16:** 553–558.

Taylor, J.M., H.E. Varmus, A.J. Faras, W.E. Levinson, and J.M. Bishop. 1974. Evidence for non-repetitive subunits in the genome of Rous sarcoma virus. *J. Mol. Biol.* **84:** 217–221.

Temin, H.M. 1971. Mechanism of cell transformation by RNA tumor viruses. *Annu. Rev. Microbiol.* **25:** 609–648.

Tooze, J., ed. 1973. *The molecular biology of tumor viruses.* Cold Spring Harbor Laboratories, Cold Spring Harbor, New York.

———. 1980. *Molecular biology of tumor viruses.* 2nd Edition, part 2, *DNA tumor viruses.* Cold Spring Harbor Laboratories, Cold Spring Harbor, New York.

Toyoshima, K., O. Niwa, M. Yutsudo, H. Sugiyama, S. Tahara, and T. Sugahara. 1980. Sensitivity to γ rays of avian sarcoma and murine leukemia viruses. *Virology* **105:** 508–515.

Tronick, S.R., C.D. Cabradilla, S.A. Aaronson, and W.A. Haseltine. 1978. 5′-terminal nucleotide sequences of mammalian type C helper viruses are conserved in the genomes of replication-defective mammalian transforming viruses. *J. Virol.* **26:** 570–576.

Tronick, S.R., K.C. Robbins, E. Canaani, S.G. Devare, P.R. Andersen, and S.A. Aaronson. 1979. Molecular cloning of Moloney murine sarcoma virus: Arrangement of virus-related sequences within the normal mouse genome. *Proc. Natl. Acad. Sci.* **76:** 6314–6318.

Troxler, D.H., J.K. Boyars, W.P. Parks, and E.M. Scolnick. 1977a. Friend strain of spleen focus-forming virus: A recombinant between mouse type C ecotropic viral sequences and sequences related to xenotropic virus. *J. Virol.* **22:** 361–372.

Troxler, D.H., S.K. Ruscetti, D.L. Linemeyer, and E.M. Scolnick. 1980. Helper-independent and replication-defective erythroblastosis-inducing viruses contained within anemia-inducing Friend virus complex (FV-A). *Virology* **102:** 28–45.

Troxler, D.H., D. Lowy, R. Howk, H. Young, and E.M. Scolnick. 1977b. Friend strain of spleen focus-forming virus is a recombinant between ecotropic murine type C virus and the *env* gene region of xenotropic type C virus. *Proc. Natl. Acad. Sci.* **84:** 4671–4675.

Tsichlis, P.N. and J.M. Coffin. 1979. Recombination between the defective component of an acute leukemia virus and Rous associated virus 0, an endogenous virus of chickens. *Proc. Natl. Acad. Sci.* **76:** 3001–3005.

———. 1980a. Recombinants between endogenous and exogenous avian tumor viruses: Role of the C region and other portions of the genome in the control of replication and transformation. *J. Virol.* **33:** 238–249.

———. 1980b. Role of the *C* region in relative growth rates of endogenous and exogenous avian oncoviruses. *Cold Spring Harbor Symp. Quant. Biol.* **44:** 1123–1132.

Tsichlis, P.N., K.F. Conklin, and J.M. Coffin. 1980. Mutant and recombinant avian retroviruses with extended host range. *Proc. Natl. Acad. Sci.* **77:** 536–540.

Tsuchida, N., R.V. Gilden, and M. Hatanaka. 1974. Sarcoma-virus-related RNA sequences in normal rat cells. *Proc. Natl. Acad. Sci.* **71:** 4503–4507.

Van Beveren, C., J.G. Goddard, A. Berns, and I.M. Verma. 1980. Structure of Moloney murine leukemia viral DNA: Nucleotide sequence of the 5′ long terminal repeat and adjacent cellular sequences. *Proc. Natl. Acad. Sci.* **77:** 3307–3311.

Van Beveren C., J.A. Galleshaw, V. Jonas, A.J.M. Berns, R.F. Doolittle, D.J. Donoghue, and I.M. Verma. 1981. Nucleotide sequence and formation of the transforming gene of a mouse sarcoma virus. *Nature* **289:** 258–262.

Van de Ven, W.J.M., F.H. Reynolds, Jr., R.P. Nalewaik, and J.R. Stephenson. 1980a. Characterization of a 170,000-dalton polyprotein encoded by the McDonough strain of feline sarcoma virus. *J. Virol.* **35:** 165–175.

Van de Ven, W.J.M., A.S. Khan, F.H. Reynolds, Jr., K.T. Mason, and J.R. Stephenson. 1980b. Translational products encoded by newly acquired sequences of independently derived feline sarcoma virus isolates are structurally related. *J. Virol.* **33:** 1034–1045.

Vande Woude, G.F., M. Oskarsson, L.W. Enquist, S. Nomura, M. Sullivan, and P.J. Fischinger. 1979. Cloning of integrated Moloney sarcoma proviral DNA sequences in bacteriophage λ. *Proc. Natl. Acad. Sci.* **76:** 4464–4468.

Vennstrom, B., L. Fanshier, C. Moscovici, and J.M. Bishop. 1980. Molecular cloning of the avian erythroblastosis virus genome and recovery of oncogenic virus by transfection of chicken cells. *J. Virol.* **36:** 575–585.

Verma, I.M., M.-H.T. Lai, R.A. Bosselman, M.A. McKennett, H. Fan, and A. Berns. 1980. Molecular cloning of unintegrated Moloney mouse sarcoma virus DNA in bacteriophage λ. *Proc. Natl. Acad. Sci.* **77:** 1773–1777.

Vigne, R., M. Brahic, P. Filippi, and J. Tamalet. 1977. Complexity and polyadenylic acid content of visna virus 60-70S RNA. *J. Virol.* **21:** 386–395.

Vigne, R., M.L. Breitman, C. Moscovici, and P.K. Vogt. 1979. Restitution of fibroblast-transforming ability in *src* deletion mutants of avian sarcoma virus during animal passage. *Virology* **93:** 413–426.

Vogt, P.K. 1971. Genetically stable reassortment of markers during mixed infection with avian tumor viruses. *Virology* **46:** 947–952.

———. 1973. The genome of avian RNA tumor viruses: A discussion of four models. In *Possible episomes in eukaryotes* (ed. L.G. Silvestri), pp. 35–41. North-Holland, Amsterdam.

Vogt, P.K. and S.S.F. Hu. 1977. The genetic structure of RNA tumor viruses. *Annu. Rev. Genet.* **11:** 203–238.

von der Helm, K. and P.H. Duesberg. 1975. Translation of Rous sarcoma virus RNA in a cell-free system from ascites Krebs II cells. *Proc. Natl. Acad. Sci.* **72:** 614–618.

Walker, T.A., N.R. Pace, R.L. Erikson, E. Erikson, and F. Behr. 1974. The 7S RNA common to oncornaviruses and normal cells is associated with polyribosomes. *Proc. Natl. Acad. Sci.* **71:** 3390–3394.

Wang, L.-H. 1978. The gene order of avian RNA tumor viruses derived from biochemical analyses of deletion mutants and viral recombinants. *Annu. Rev. Microbiol.* **32:** 561–592.

Wang, L.-H., P. Duesberg, K. Beemon, and P.K. Vogt. 1975. Mapping RNase T1-resistant oligonucleotides of avian tumor virus RNAs: Sarcoma-specific oligonucleotides are near the poly(A) end and oligonucleotides common to sarcoma and transformation-defective viruses are at the poly(A) end. *J. Virol.* **161:** 1051–1070.

Wang, L.-H., P.H. Duesberg, S. Kawai, and H. Hanafusa. 1976a. Location of envelope-specific and sarcoma-specific oligonucleotides on RNA of Schmidt-Ruppin Rous sarcoma virus. *Proc. Natl. Acad. Sci.* **73:** 447–451.

Wang, L.-H., P.H. Duesberg, P. Mellon, and P.K. Vogt. 1976b. Distribution of envelope-specific and sarcoma-specific nucleotide sequences from different parents in the RNAs of avian tumor virus recombinants. *Proc. Natl. Acad. Sci.* **73:** 1073–1077.

Wang, L.-H., C.C. Halpern, M. Nadel, and H. Hanafusa. 1978. Recombination between viral and cellular sequences generates transforming sarcoma virus. *Proc. Natl. Acad. Sci.* **75:** 5812–5816.

Wang, L.-H., P. Snyder, T. Hanafusa, and H. Hanafusa. 1980a. Evidence for the common origin of viral and cellular sequences involved in sarcomagenic transformation. *J. Virol.* **35:** 52–64.

Wang, L.-H., P.H. Duesberg, T. Robins, H. Yokota, and P.K. Vogt. 1977. The terminal oligonucleotides of avian tumor virus RNAs are genetically linked. *Virology* **82:** 472–492.

Wang, L.-H., P. Snyder, T. Hanafusa, C. Moscovici, and H. Hanafusa. 1980b. Comparative analysis of cellular and viral sequences related to sarcomagenic cell transformation. *Cold Spring Harbor Symp. Quant. Biol.* **44:** 755–764.

Wang, L.-H., D. Galehouse, P. Mellon, P. Duesberg, W.S. Mason, and P.K. Vogt. 1976c. Mapping oligonucleotides of Rous sarcoma virus RNA that segregate with polymerase and group-specific antigen markers in recombinants. *Proc. Natl. Acad. Sci.* **73:** 3952–3956.

Waters, L.C. 1975. Transfer RNAs associated with the 70S RNA of AKR murine leukemia virus. *Biochem. Biophys. Res. Commun.* **65:** 1130–1136.

Waters, L.C. and B.C. Mullin. 1977. Transfer RNA in RNA tumor viruses. *Prog. Nucleic Acid Res. Mol. Biol.* **20:** 131–160.

Waters, L.C., B.C. Mullin, E.G. Bailiff, and R.A. Popp. 1975. tRNAs associated with the 70S RNA of avian myeloblastosis virus. *J. Virol.* **16:** 1608–1614.

Wei, C.-M., D.R. Lowy, and E.M. Scolnick. 1980. Mapping of transforming region of the Harvey murine sarcoma virus genome by using insertion-deletion mutants constructed *in vitro*. *Proc. Natl. Acad. Sci.* **77:** 4674–4678.

Weiss, R.A., W.S. Mason, and P.K. Vogt. 1973. Genetic recombinants and heterozygotes derived from endogenous and exogenous avian RNA tumor viruses. *Virology* **52:** 535–552.

Weiss, S.R., P.B. Hackett, H. Oppermann, A. Ullrich, L. Levintow, and J.M. Bishop. 1978. Cell-free translation of avian sarcoma virus RNA: Suppression of the *gag* termination codon does not augment synthesis of the joint *gag/pol* product. *Cell* **15:** 607–614.

Weissmann, C., J.T. Parsons, J.W. Coffin, L. Rymo, M.A. Billeter, and H. Hofstetter. 1975. Studies on the structure and synthesis of Rous sarcoma virus RNA. *Cold Spring Harbor Symp. Quant. Biol.* **39:** 1043–1056.

Witte, O.N., N.E. Rosenberg, and D. Baltimore. 1979. A normal cell protein cross-reactive to the major Abelson murine leukaemia virus gene product. *Nature* **281:** 396–398.

Witte, O.N., S. Goff, N. Rosenberg, and D. Baltimore. 1980. A transformation-defective mutant of Abelson murine leukemia virus lacks protein kinase activity. *Proc. Natl. Acad. Sci.* **77:** 4993–4997.

Witte, O.N., N. Rosenberg, M. Paskind, A. Shields, and D. Baltimore. 1978. Identification of an Abelson murine leukemia virus-encoded protein present in transformed fibroblast and lymphoid cells. *Proc. Natl. Acad. Sci.* **75:** 2488–2492.

Wolfe, L., F. Deinhardt, G. Theilen, T. Kawakami, and L. Bustad. 1971. Induction of tumors in marmoset monkeys by simian sarcoma virus type 1 (*Lagothrix*): A preliminary report. *J. Natl. Cancer Inst.* **47:**115–1120.

Wong, T.C., R.B. Lewis, H.R. Bose, Jr., and C.Y. Kang. 1980. Assembly of avian reticuloendotheliosis virus: Association of the core precursor polypeptide with the intracellular ribonucleoprotein complex. *J. Virol.* **34:**484–489.

Wyke, J.A., J.G. Bell, and J.A. Beamand. 1975. Genetic recombination among temperature-sensitive mutants of Rous sarcoma virus. *Cold Spring Harbor Symp. Quant. Biol.* **39:**897–905.

Yamamoto, T., G. Jay, and I. Pastan. 1980a. Unusual features in the nucleotide sequence of a cDNA clone derived from the common region of avian sarcoma virus messenger RNA. *Proc. Natl. Acad. Sci.* **77:**176–180.

Yamamoto, T., B. deCrombrugghe, and I. Pastan. 1980b. Identification of a functional promoter in the long terminal repeat of Rous sarcoma virus. *Cell* **22:**787–797.

Yamamoto, T., J.S. Tyagi, J.B. Fagan, G. Jay, B. deCrombrugghe, and I. Pastan. 1980c. Molecular mechanism for the capture and excision of the transforming gene of avian sarcoma virus as suggested by analysis of recombinant clones. *J. Virol.* **35:**436–443.

Yoshida, M. and K. Toyoshima. 1980. *In vitro* translation of avian erythroblastosis virus RNA: Identification of two major polypeptides. *Virology* **100:**484–487.

Yoshida, M. and H. Yoshikura. 1980. Analysis of spleen focus-forming virus-specific RNA sequences coding for spleen focus-forming virus-specific glycoprotein with a molecular weight of 55,000 (gp55). *J. Virol.* **33:**587–596.

Yoshida, M., S. Kawai, and K. Toyoshima. 1980. Uninfected avian cells contain structurally unrelated progenitors of viral sarcoma genes. *Nature* **287:**653–654.

Yoshida M., M. Yamashita, and A. Nomoto. 1979. Transformation-defective mutants of Rous sarcoma virus with longer sizes of genome RNA and their highly frequent occurrences. *J. Virol.* **30:**453–461.

Young, H.A., T.Y. Shih, E.M. Scolnick, S. Rasheed, and M.B. Gardner. 1979. Different rat-derived transforming retroviruses code for an immunologically related intracellular phosphoprotein. *Proc. Natl. Acad. Sci.* **76:**3523–3527.

Young, H.A., M.A. Gonda, D. De Feo, R.W. Ellis, K. Nagashima, and E.M. Scolnick. 1980. Heteroduplex analysis of cloned rat endogenous replication-defective (30 S) retrovirus and Harvey murine sarcoma virus. *Virology* **107:**89–99.

5

Replication of Retroviruses

I. INTRODUCTION TO THE REPLICATION CYCLE

Retroviruses are unified by the manner in which their genomes are replicated during infection. In its simplest form, replication can be envisioned as

$$\text{RNA} \rightarrow \text{DNA} \rightarrow \text{RNA}$$

with the first step mediated principally by a virus-coded, RNA-directed DNA polymerase (reverse transcriptase) carried in infectious particles, and the latter step mediated principally by host enzymes also responsible for expression of cellular genes.

Retroviruses commonly associate stably with the cells they infect. To perpetuate viral genes and provide a suitable template for synthesis of viral RNA, retroviral DNA generally integrates covalently into the chromosomal DNA of host cells and replicates with the host genome. Furthermore, production of virus requires the synthesis of proteins encoded in viral mRNAs. Hence, the replication cycle can be written in more complete form as

$$\text{RNA} \rightarrow \underset{\curvearrowleft}{\text{DNA}} \rightarrow \text{RNA} \rightarrow \text{protein.}$$

For the purposes of this chapter, it is convenient to partition the replicative cycle into two major phases: (1) the steps leading to the synthesis and integration of a complete DNA copy of viral RNA, i.e., adsorption to and penetration of the host cell, priming and polymerization of both strands of viral DNA leading to production of linear and circular forms, and linkage of viral DNA to host DNA, and (2) expression of viral genetic information, i.e., synthesis and processing of viral RNAs (both mRNAs and genomic RNA), synthesis of viral polypeptides, cleavage and modification of viral proteins, assembly of viral nucleocapsids, and budding and maturation of viral particles. The features of this scheme are considered in detail in this chapter and are outlined in Figure 5.1.

Three viral genes are required for the production of fully infectious progeny: *gag,* for the synthesis of nucleocapsid proteins; *pol,* for the

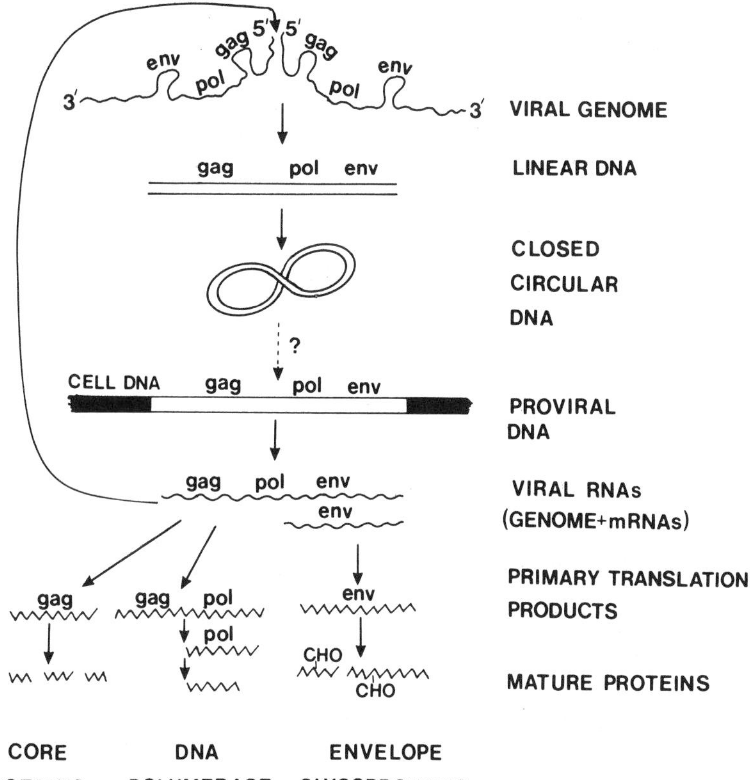

Figure 5.1 An overview of the replication cycle of retroviruses. A simplified schematic view of the major events in the life cycle of replication-competent retroviruses is shown, including regeneration of the viral RNA genome via DNA intermediates and production of viral structural proteins. The question mark indicates the uncertain role of closed circular DNA. Further uncertainties and details of each step are considered later in this chapter. (~~~) RNA; (═══) DNA; (ʌʌʌ) protein.

synthesis of reverse transcriptase; and *env*, for the synthesis of envelope glycoproteins. These three genes are arranged 5′-*gag-pol-env*-3′ in the RNA genomes of all the replication-competent retroviruses examined to date (see Chapter 4). Genomes that lack any of these three genes are defective for replication, but infectious pseudotypes can generally be produced in cells coinfected with defective viruses and competent helper viruses (see Chapter 3). Viral genes implicated in cellular transformation, e.g., the *src* gene of Rous sarcoma virus (RSV), do not appear to be necessary for viral replication (Chapter 9), although their expression is intimately linked to the replication pathway.

In the decade since it has become generally accepted that some RNA viruses replicate via DNA intermediates, an extraordinary amount of effort has been devoted to a complete description of this unusual sequence of events. Several aspects of the replication scheme have attracted investigators: the biochemical novelty of transcribing RNA into DNA, the broad genetic implications of integrating viral DNA into host-cell DNA, and the simplicity of studying eukaryotic gene expression with viral reagents.

In this chapter we review the experimental evidence supporting the still incomplete formulation of the replication cycle, and we summarize the prospects for new information in the near future. At the outset, however, we provide a brief history of the observations that led to the central theme of this chapter, the proposal that retroviruses replicate via a DNA intermediate called a provirus.

II. THE PROVIRUS HYPOTHESIS AND ITS ACCEPTANCE

There is now extensive direct evidence for the existence of the provirus, but up to 1970 it was only a hypothetical entity, proposed first by Temin as an explanation both for the results of a number of indirect experiments and for the remarkable stability of the transformed state of cells infected by RSV (for extensive discussions, see Temin 1964, 1971, 1974, 1976). Most of the indirect experiments involved the effect on virus multiplication of metabolic inhibitors that block selected aspects of cellular function. The results with inhibitors showed that retroviruses did not behave like any other RNA viruses. Compounds such as mitomycin C, actinomycin D, 5-bromodeoxyuridine (BrdU), cytosine arabinoside, and amethopterin, all of which interfere with the synthesis or expression of DNA, blocked retrovirus multiplication but not the multiplication of most other RNA viruses (Temin 1963, 1967; Bader 1965). To cite one illuminating example, when 12-hour pulses of cytosine arabinoside are added to a culture of stationary chicken cells starved of serum, a pulse beginning at the time of RSV infection can prevent infection as measured after the addition of serum, but pulses before infection or during the second 12 hours of infection produce little inhibition (Temin 1968; Murray and Temin 1970). Because serum-starved cells make little or no cellular DNA, this experiment suggests more strongly than most such experiments that virus-specific DNA synthesis is involved in retrovirus growth.

In 1970, a number of experiments were reported that made the existence of a provirus very likely. Among these was the demonstration by Boettiger and Temin (1970) and Balduzzi and Morgan (1970) that when chicken cells starved of serum are exposed to BrdU during the first 12 hours after their infection by RSV, subsequent exposure to light can abort the infection. Since DNA containing BrdU substituted for thymidine is light-sensitive and since synthesis of cellular DNA was arrested, these experiments suggested that viral genes must have entered a DNA form during infection. Another type of supportive experiment showed that when a cell infected by one avian tumor virus is superinfected by a second virus, successful superinfection depends on the occurrence of DNA synthesis after the second virus is added (Duesberg and Vogt 1969; Temin 1970).

The observation that convinced most workers that provirus formation was an integral part of the retrovirus life cycle was the discovery of an RNA-directed DNA-polymerase activity in virions of such viruses (Baltimore 1970, 1976; Temin and Mizutani 1970; Temin and Baltimore 1972; Temin 1976). Discovery of this enzyme provided biochemical proof that information encoded in RNA could be transcribed into DNA, thus removing the major objection to the provirus hypothesis, that no mechanism or precedent existed for such conversion.

Two other kinds of evidence provided strong support for the provirus hypothesis: virus-specific DNA was directly measured in infected cells by molecular hybridization, and DNA from infected cells was found to be infectious.

Identification of proviral DNA in infected cells by molecular hybridization is complicated by the technical difficulties of demonstrating a small number of viral sequences amid a vast excess of cellular DNA and by the presence of homologous virus-specific DNA endogenous to cells often used for the infection (see Chapter 10). For example, the first widely accepted hybridization experiments, those of Baluda and Nayak (1970), were compromised by the small fraction of radiolabeled RSV RNA that annealed to cellular DNA immobilized on filters and by the appreciable annealing to uninfected, as well as infected, chicken-cell DNA. Some of these problems were alleviated by the use of DNA-excess hybridization in solution to labeled RNA (Neiman 1972) and by the use of host cells that lacked sequences homologous to the virus-specific hybridization reagents prior to infection (Baluda 1972; Varmus et al. 1973a,b).

The most convincing evidence that a complete copy of the retroviral genome was present in the DNA of infected cells emerged from infectivity studies. Hill and Hillova (1972a) first demonstrated that the DNA of an infected cell could be used to infect other cells. They extracted DNA from rat cells that had been transformed by the Prague (PR) strain of RSV and from hamster cells that had been transformed by a temperature-sensitive mutant strain of RSV (Hill and Hillova 1972b). They then exposed susceptible chick cells to these DNAs in the presence of DEAE-dextran to facilitate uptake of the DNA. Within 8 to 20 days, foci of transformed chick fibroblasts appeared in the cultures that had been exposed to DNA from transformed cells but not in the cultures exposed to DNA from uninfected cells. The progeny RSV particles liberated by the transformed chick cells had the expected subgroup antigenicities and host ranges, and those stemming from the proviral DNA of the temperature-sensitive mutant were temperature-sensitive. A number of investigators had shown previously that retroviral genomes must persist in some form in transformed cells, even in those that failed to produce virus (nonpermissive cells), since fusion with permissive cells induced virus production (see, e.g., Svoboda and Dourmashkin 1969; Svoboda et al. 1972; Coffin 1972); however, the transfection experiments showed directly that the genome is perpetuated as DNA. Many investigators have subsequently shown that infectious DNA, both integrated and unintegrated, is present in cells infected with various retroviruses (Karpas and Milstein 1973; Svoboda et al. 1973; Cooper and Temin 1974; Smotkin et al. 1975; Haase et al. 1976; Chiswell and Pringle 1977, 1979; Fritsch and Temin 1977a; Lowy et al. 1978; Markham and Gallo 1978; Anderson et al. 1979; Canaani et al. 1979;

Copeland et al. 1979; Copeland and Cooper 1979, 1980; Goldfarb and Weinberg 1979; Sherr et al. 1979).

As we will show in the sections that follow, the provirus is no longer hypothetical. Viral DNA can be purified from infected cells, observed directly in the electron microscope, mapped physically with restriction endonucleases, and amplified by molecular cloning in prokaryotic host-vector systems. Even the DNA grown in bacteria has proved to be infectious (Hager et al. 1979; Blair et al. 1980; DeLorbe et al. 1980; Lowy et al. 1980; Oliff et al. 1980; O'Rear et al. 1980; Vande Woude et al. 1980; Mullins et al. 1981). Thus, there is no longer any doubt that retroviruses replicate via DNA intermediates. The major concerns in the field are now the precise mechanisms by which viral DNA is made, integrated, and expressed. It will be evident that the molecular hybridization and transfection techniques developed to test the provirus hypothesis are now central to efforts to provide a detailed description of the replicative cycle.

III. PHASE ONE: ESTABLISHMENT OF THE PROVIRAL STATE

The first half of the replication cycle is directed toward the integration of a complete DNA copy of viral genes, the provirus, into cellular DNA. To achieve the proviral state, an infecting virus must attach to and penetrate the host cell and synthesize a DNA product appropriate for insertion into the host genome. In the ensuing sections, we focus on the following questions: What is the structure of viral DNA synthesized in infected cells? What are the synthetic mechanisms required to generate the observed structures? How does viral DNA become covalently linked to the cellular genome?

Although complete answers to these questions are not yet available, we review a large body of experimental evidence that now supports several generalizations about the synthesis and integration of retroviral DNA. Synthesis is primed by a cellular tRNA species bound near the 5′ end of the 35S RNA template. The principal product of synthesis is a linear, duplex molecule with extensive terminal redundancies; this product can be synthesized either in the cytoplasm of infected cells or in detergent-disrupted virions, and the responsible enzymic activities are mostly, if not completely, encoded in the viral *pol* gene. The structure of the terminal redundancies implies that the nascent strand of DNA complementary to the viral genome is transferred twice between templates; likely mechanisms for these unusual events have been proposed and partially tested. In infected cells, linear DNA is converted to covalently closed circles after migration to the nucleus; both linear and circular DNAs are infectious, but the functional role for circular DNA is uncertain and is complicated by the existence of multiple forms. Integration of viral DNA can occur at any of a large number of sites in the host genome, though it is possible that the number of available sites is restricted. The structure of the provirus is highly uniform and virtually identical to the structure of unintegrated, linear DNA, with terminally repeated sequences flanking genes arranged as they are in viral RNA. As we shall see, this structure closely resembles that of transposable elements and fulfills important requirements for the expression of viral genes.

A. Early Events

The first step in the infection cycle is the adsorption of the virion to the cell. This is followed by steps that enable the virion or its internal components to penetrate the cell. Direct measurements of adsorption of avian viruses to chicken cells have shown that even cells totally resistant to infection can bind virus (Piraino 1967). However, measurement of virus adsorbed to single cells by laser-beam cytometry demonstrates that genetically susceptible cells also adsorb two- to tenfold more RSV than do resistant cells (M.F.D. Notter et al., in prep.). Measurements of penetration reveal a high degree of specificity (Steck and Rubin 1965; Piraino 1967), indicating that cellular genes encode structures that mediate the conversion of the extracellular form of the viruses to a form able to carry out reverse transcription (see Chapter 3). The site at which penetration takes place appears to be the site at which interference between viruses of like subgroups occurs, implying that cells (presumably plasma membranes) contain receptors that recognize glycoproteins in viral envelopes.

DeLarco and Todaro (1976) obtained direct experimental evidence for such receptors by measuring the binding of purified, radiolabeled murine leukemia virus (MLV) gp70 to intact mouse fibroblasts. Although the binding was independent of temperature, it exhibited specificity for certain virus strains (ecotropic, but not xenotropic, viruses competed for binding), and the binding sites could be saturated and counted (~2×10^5 sites/cell). Similar measurements have been made of binding sites for MLV glycoproteins on murine lymphocytes (Bishayee et al. 1978), for RSV gp85 on chicken fibroblasts (Moldow et al. 1979b), and for the envelope glycoproteins of primate viruses on various cell types (Moldow et al. 1979a). Nothing is known, however, about the biochemistry of these receptors or about the mechanism(s) by which they mediate penetration of retroviruses into host cells. The extensive studies of the host genes believed to encode the receptors are reviewed in another context (Chapter 3).

Virtually nothing is known about the structure of infectious particles as they enter cells and undergo DNA synthesis. Dales and Hanafusa (1972) have shown that after attachment to chicken cells many RSV virions are taken into the cell inside vacuoles and that labeled input RNA can be found in the nucleus within 10 minutes after attachment. However, in most retrovirus systems, the initial biochemical events in the replication of the genome appear to occur in the cytoplasm (Varmus et al. 1974) or possibly on plasma membranes (Kakefuda et al. 1974), so the significance of finding parental RNA in nuclei is uncertain.

The degree of uncoating that accompanies these initial events has not been established, in part because of the difficulty of distinguishing the excess of noninfectious particles that adsorb to cells from those particles that actually cause infection. There is indirect evidence to suggest that at least partial uncoating occurs within the cytoplasm during the first 1–2 hours after infection (Aboud et al. 1979).

B. Synthesis of Viral DNA

Synthesis of retroviral DNA from a template of genomic RNA is the first step in the virus life cycle, about which a great deal is known. The synthetic process has been approached from several experimental directions: using purified reverse transcriptase in "reconstructed" systems in which all the components are defined; following DNA synthesis in preparations of virions activated by detergents; and characterizing the products of synthesis in cells infected by retroviruses. Although the reconstructed systems permit the most refined enzymology, it has not been possible to recapitulate more than the initial steps in viral DNA synthesis, suggesting that the complete process is influenced by factors as yet poorly defined. (Examples of such factors might include conformation of the RNA template, interaction of RNA with viral proteins [e.g., *gag* products], cellular enzymes included in virions, and the environment of infected cells.) With careful attention to conditions of synthesis, however, detergent-activated virions are capable of producing complete or nearly complete species of viral DNA (Junghans et al. 1977; Rothenberg et al. 1977, 1978; Clayman et al. 1979a,b; Gilboa et al. 1979b; Boone and Skalka 1980; Bosselman and Verma 1980; Dina and Benz 1980; Guntaka 1980; Lai and Verma 1980). Studies of DNA synthesized in artificially disrupted particles must be interpreted with caution, since it is possible that the intracellular process is not faithfully recapitulated under these conditions. The preferable alternative, direct examination of viral DNA in infected cells, is complicated by the small amounts of product relative to the vast quantities of cellular DNA; under optimal conditions, the number of copies of viral DNA is still less than 10–100 per cell, i.e., less than 1 part in 10^4 or 10^5. Using molecular hybridization techniques, however, it is possible to follow the synthesis of each strand of viral DNA and to characterize the principal products. Molecular cloning of viral DNA from infected cells now permits detailed assessment of individual molecules.

Before embarking on a step-by-step account of how viral DNA is made, it is useful to consider the salient features of the viral DNA polymerase, its natural template and primer, and the major forms of viral DNA that appear in the infected cells.

1. Reverse Transcriptase

All replication-competent retroviruses carry a gene (*pol*) that encodes an enzyme capable of transcribing RNA into DNA (RNA-directed DNA polymerase, or reverse transcriptase, deoxynucleoside triphosphate: DNA deoxynucleotidyl transferase, E.C. 2.7.7.7). This activity is present in mature virions where it was initially discovered (Baltimore 1970; Temin and Mizutani 1970); unlike most other virus-associated polymerases, it can be readily dissociated from virions and purified to homogeneity for structural and enzymic investigation. Assays for the *pol* products have usually exploited their enzymic capacities to synthesize DNA from templates of RNA or DNA (RNA- and DNA-directed DNA-polymerase activities) and to hydrolyze RNA in an RNA:DNA hybrid (RNase-H activity). Anti-polymerase antisera, some of which are monospecific, have been developed and also have been used to assay retroviral polymerases by various immunological procedures, including immunoprecipitation of labeled *pol* products (Panet et al. 1975a; Oppermann et al. 1977) and inactivation of enzymic activity by antibody (Hanafusa et al. 1972).

Reverse transcriptase was first detected in virions of avian and murine viruses after partial disruption of the virions and incubation with deoxyribonucleoside triphosphates (dNTPs) (Baltimore 1970; Temin and Mizutani 1970). The reaction is sensitive to ribonuclease, indicating that RNA is required for DNA synthesis. Because the nascent DNA molecules can be recovered in association with 70S RNA and because the DNA can be hybridized to the 70S RNA, the template for DNA synthesis in the virions must be the 70S RNA (Garapin et al. 1970; Rokutanda et al. 1970; Spiegelman et al. 1970; Manly et al. 1971). This reaction, in which the DNA polymerase copies 70S RNA in disrupted virions, is called the endogenous reaction.

The viruses that contain reverse transcriptase include both the oncogenic and/or transforming retroviruses and the retroviruses that cause only nonneoplastic diseases or no known disease at all (e.g. Parks et al. 1973). Thus, reverse transcriptase is a characteristic of the family of retroviruses but does not imply oncogenicity of a virus that carries it.

a. Genetic Evidence for the Role of Reverse Transcriptase in the Virus Life Cycle. The discovery of an RNA-directed DNA polymerase fulfilled an important prediction of the provirus hypothesis and hence greatly accelerated its acceptance. The isolation of viral *pol* mutants has provided important support for the assumptions that viral DNA synthesis is, in fact, catalyzed by the virion-associated enzyme and that the enzyme is the product of a viral gene.

At least two kinds of mutants have been useful. Hanafusa and Hanafusa (1971) identified nonconditional replication-defective mutants of RSV, RSV(−)α, that fail to produce infectious progeny unless allowed to undergo phenotypic mixing with replication-competent virus. The noninfectious particles produced by cells infected with these mutants lack either enzymic or immunological evidence of reverse transcriptase (Hanafusa et al. 1972). Interestingly, these defective particles cannot be complemented by coinfection with replication-competent viruses, indicating that viral DNA polymerase needs to be introduced into the cell within the viral particle that contains the RNA it will use as template. Several other examples of nonconditional, replication-defective mutants of RSV and MLV, which produce altered or no DNA polymerase, have subsequently been identified (Linial et al. 1978a; Shields et al. 1978; Gerwin et al. 1979; see Chapter 7).

The isolation of temperature-sensitive *pol* mutants of both RSV and MLV has provided particularly strong evidence about the role of the viral polymerase. These mutants display the predicted phenotype, in that all the consequences of infection (replication and transformation) are aborted when the infection is initiated at the nonpermissive temperature (Linial and Mason 1973) (see Chapter 7). The enzymic activities of reverse transcriptase are temperature-sensitive in vitro, generally both before and after purification of the enzyme from viral particles (Verma et al. 1974a, 1976; Moelling and Friis 1979). Direct measurement of viral DNA in cells infected by these mutants demonstrates that synthesis of both strands is impaired at the nonpermissive temperature (Verma et al. 1976). These experiments show convincingly that the viral enzyme is required for synthesis of retroviral DNA, though they do not, of course, exclude the possibility that other factors may be important in the production of mature forms of DNA.

b. Biogenesis of Reverse Transcriptase. One conclusion drawn from the preceding genetic experiments, that reverse transcriptase is encoded in the viral genome, has been further confirmed by analysis of viral polyproteins synthesized both in vivo and in vitro. These studies, reviewed in greater detail in Chapter 6 and later in this chapter (Sections IV.B.4 and IV.C), have revealed that reverse transcriptase is generated from a large polyprotein of about 180,000 daltons translated from two adjacent genes: (5′) *gag-pol* (3′). It is not known whether the translational apparatus is guided past the termination signals for *gag* by a suppression event (Philipson et al. 1978) or by synthesis of a separate *gag-pol* mRNA that lacks the *gag* terminator codon (Weiss et al. 1978), although the latter now seems more likely (see Section IV.B.4.c and Chapter 6). The mature protein is presumably generated by cleavage of the *gag-pol* polyprotein, perhaps catalyzed, at least in part, by viral *gag*-gene products (e.g., p15 in the case of RSV) (Von der Helm 1977; Dittmar and Moelling 1978; Vogt et al. 1979; Moelling et al. 1980), but the cleavage reactions and their relationship to virus assembly are not well understood. It is likely, however, that cleavage occurs in assembled particles, during or after their exodus from the cell, implying that little or no mature polymerase is present within virus-producing cells (Oppermann et al. 1977; Witte and Baltimore 1978). It is doubtful that the precursor of the viral enzyme has the polymerizing activities found in the mature protein (Witte and Baltimore 1978).

c. Purification of Reverse Transcriptase. Virion-associated DNA-polymerase activities have been purified from several retroviruses. The purification has generally not been difficult, although absolute yields are compromised by the relatively small number of polymerase molecules (40–110) present per virion (Panet et al. 1975a; Krakower et al. 1977; Panet and Kra-Oz 1978; Bauer and Temin 1980a). Recovery of activity can be optimized by inclusion of a sulfhydryl reagent, glycerol, and a nonionic detergent at all steps during the purification.

Reverse-transcriptase activity is readily solubilized from the virion by treatment with a nonionic detergent. Only a small portion of the enzyme sediments with the detergent-resistant residue of the virions. The soluble enzyme can be purified by conventional methods: ion-exchange chromatography, gradient centrifugation, gel filtration, and affinity chromatography (Gerard and Grandgenett 1980). The last method exploits the affinity of reverse transcriptase for resin-bound polynucleotides (Kacian et al. 1971; Gerwin and Milstien 1972; Marcus et al. 1974; Grandgenett and Rho 1975; Grandgenett 1976; Hizi and Joklik 1977a) and several other ligands (pyran, dextran blue, and heparin) (Chirikjian et al. 1975; Moe 1978; Golomb et al. 1980). After purification, the polymerase activity is quite stable if stored at −70°C in an appropriate buffer.

Beard and his collaborators have developed a large-scale purification scheme for isolating reverse transcriptase from avian myeloblastosis virus (AMV) (Houts et al. 1979). This enzyme is widely used in contemporary biochemistry; for example, it has played a key role in the synthesis of hybridization probes and in the molecular cloning of DNA copies of mRNAs.

d. Structure of Reverse Transcriptase Isolated from Various Retroviruses. All retroviruses of the avian sarcoma-leukosis virus (ASLV) group have DNA polymerases that share common antigenic determinants (Nowinski et al. 1972; Parks et al. 1972; Mizutani and Temin 1974; Bauer and Temin 1979). The ASLV DNA polymerases are composed of two polypeptide subunits, one of about 92,000 daltons (β) and one of about 58,000 daltons (α) (Kacian et al. 1971; Faras et al. 1972; Grandgenett et al. 1973; Gibson and Verma 1974). Analysis of the peptides generated by limited protease digestion of isolated α and β subunits indicates that the subunits are homologous, suggesting that α is a proteolytic cleavage product of β (Gibson and Verma 1974; Rho et al. 1975). Amino acid sequence determinations have shown that α and β have a common amino terminus (T.D. Copeland et al. 1980). Most of the enzyme activity is associated with a structure that sediments as a globular protein of 170,000 daltons and is composed of equimolar amounts of α and β (Duesberg et al. 1971a; Hurwitz and Leis 1972; Grandgenett et al. 1973). Polymerizing activity is also associated with the monomeric form of α (Grandgenett et al. 1973). There are several lines of evidence indicating that one role of the β subunit is to augment the stability of enzyme-template interactions; for example, the $\alpha\beta$ form exhibits greater thermal stability than the α form of the polymerase in the presence of a template (Panet et al. 1975b). An enzymically active $\beta\beta$ dimer has been reported in virions of the B77 strain of RSV grown in duck embryo fibroblasts (Hizi and Joklik 1977a). The $\beta\beta$ dimer may represent an intermediate in the genesis of the $\alpha\beta$ form of the enzyme. A scheme outlining the generation of fragments, and associated activities of the β subunit, is shown in Figure 5.2. The cleavage of β to α and fragment B (p32; see Section III.B.1.e) may be mediated by the virus-coded protease, p15

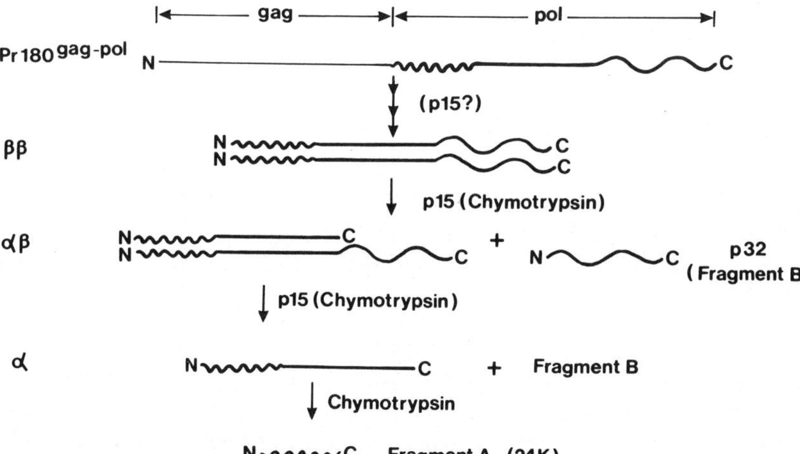

Figure 5.2 Biogenesis and components of reverse transcriptase of ALV and RSV. Different symbols are used to illustrate the functional domains in the primary translation product of *pol* (Pr180$^{gag\text{-}pol}$) and in products of natural and experimental cleavages.

(Moelling et al. 1980). Limited digestion with trypsin (Papas et al. 1976) or chymotrypsin catalyzes a similar cleavage, as well as another one that generates fragment A, a fragment containing only RNase-H activity (Lai and Verma 1978).

In vivo the β, but not the α, subunit of both the $\alpha\beta$ and $\beta\beta$ complexes can be phosphorylated (Hizi and Joklik 1977b). It is not known what role phosphorylation plays in the activity of the polymerase in vivo. It has been reported that phosphorylation of the polymerase in vitro increases its activity (Lee et al. 1975; Rokutanda et al. 1979), although this point is in dispute (Houts et al. 1978). The Zn^{++}-specific chelating agent, orthophenanthroline, inhibits polymerase activity, indicating that, like other DNA polymerases, reverse transcriptase is a zinc-metalloenzyme (Valenzuela et al. 1973; Auld et al. 1974; Poiesz et al. 1974).

The enzyme purified from MLV is a monomeric protein of 70,000–84,000 daltons (Ross et al. 1971; Hurwitz and Leis 1972; Tronick et al. 1972; Wang and Duesberg 1973; Moelling 1974; Gerard and Grandgenett 1975; Verma 1975a; Modak and Marcus 1977). Smaller proteins have been reported in MLV enzyme preparations, but these are present in submolar amounts and may represent degradation products (Gerard and Grandgenett 1975; Moelling 1976). Most of the other mammalian C-type retroviruses examined also contain a reverse transcriptase of approximately 70,000 daltons (Abrell and Gallo 1973; Gerwin et al. 1975; Sarin and Gallo 1976; Sarin et al. 1977). One exception is hamster leukemia virus, which appears to have an enzyme composed of two subunits (68,000 daltons and 58,000 daltons), although another hamster retrovirus has a polymerase with the more characteristic structure (Verma et al. 1974b; Gregerson et al. 1979). Another exception is an endogenous virus of mice, MOPC-315, which has a polymerase composed of two subunits, 28,000 daltons and 26,500 daltons (Hizi and Yaniv 1980). All of the mammalian C-type virus polymerases tested share antigenic determinants not found on the polymerases from the ASLV group or from the B-type or D-type viruses (Verma 1977; Krakower et al. 1977; Sarin et al. 1977; Krakower and Aaronson 1978; Panet and Kra-Oz 1978).

The DNA polymerase of the reticuloendotheliosis virus (REV) group of avian viruses is probably not related to the polymerase of the ASLV group (Nowinski et al. 1972; Mizutani and Temin 1973, 1974; Moelling et al. 1975; Bauer and Temin 1980a). The REV polymerase is composed of a single subunit of 70,000–84,000 daltons (Mizutani and Temin 1975; Moelling et al. 1975) and shares antigenic determinants with the polymerase from MLV (Bauer and Temin 1980b). The available evidence suggests that this class of viruses may be more closely related to the mammalian C-type viruses than to the ASLV group (see Chapter 2).

The DNA polymerases of murine mammary tumor virus (MMTV; single chain, 100,000 daltons) and of the Mason-Pfizer monkey virus (MPMV; single chain, 85,000–110,000 daltons) appear to be unrelated to the reverse transcriptases of C-type viruses and to each other by structural or immunological criteria (Abrell and Gallo 1973; Dion et al. 1974; Yaniv et al. 1974; Harewood and Ahmed 1977; Callahan et al. 1977; Colcher et al. 1977). In the several tested cases, there is little or no cross-reactivity between viral and cellular DNA polymerases (Ross et al. 1971; Nowinski et al. 1972; Long et al. 1973; Mizutani and Temin 1974).

There are several reports of a larger form of reverse transcriptase present in the cytoplasmic fraction of cells infected with certain mammalian C-type viruses (Gerwin et al. 1975; Marcus 1978; Rokutanda et al. 1978). In each case the polymerase activity is associated with proteins of between 95,000 and 110,000 daltons, whereas the activity in the mature virion is associated with proteins of about 70,000 daltons. It is possible that these larger forms are precursors to the smaller forms that are isolated from virions and thus analogous to the β form of ASLV enzymes. At present the larger species are poorly characterized.

e. Enzymic Activities Associated with Reverse Transcriptase. Two major enzymic activities have been definitively assigned to the *pol*-gene product: a DNA polymerase capable of copying RNA or DNA templates and a ribonuclease active on RNA:DNA hybrids.

(i) DNA POLYMERASE. *Template specificity.* The unique feature of this DNA polymerase is that RNA serves as its natural template (Temin and Baltimore 1972). In the detergent-disrupted virion reaction, the DNA product synthesized is complementary to and, at least initially, associated with the viral 70S RNA genome (Duesberg and Canaani 1970; Fujinaga et al. 1970; Garapin et al. 1970; Rokutanda et al. 1970; Spiegelman et al. 1970; Manly et al. 1971). The purified 70S RNA complex is also an effective template for purified reverse transcriptase in a reconstructed reaction. The template specificity of reverse transcriptase has been extensively studied using homopolymers (for review, see Temin and Baltimore 1972). Those studies can be summarized as follows: reverse transcriptase is active on a wide variety of RNA and DNA templates provided a complementary oligodeoxyribonucleotide primer is present. The level of activity is usually 10- to 1000-fold greater when a homopolymer, rather than viral RNA, is used as a template. The pattern of preferred, or most active, templates is characteristic for a specific polymerase, be it viral or cellular in origin. Finally, the unique ability of reverse transcriptase to use poly(rC)-oligo(dG) as a template primer can, in most cases, be used as a specific assay for this enzyme (Gerard et al. 1976; Kiessling and Goulian 1976). A divalent cation is required for activity, and the choice of Mg^{++} or Mn^{++} causes some variation in the level of activity on different templates. The activities of the MLV and RSV polymerases on a variety of templates have been reviewed by Verma (1977). In the few cases tested, a purified polymerase has been able to utilize heterologous, as well as homologous, 70S RNA as template (Haseltine et al. 1976).

Both the MLV and AMV polymerases efficiently transcribe the single-stranded regions of heteropolymeric nucleic acids when provided with an appropriate primer. However, neither of the purified polymerases appears to be able to carry out strand-displacement synthesis to allow transcription of duplex DNA regions (Hurwitz and Leis 1972). This situation appears to conflict with our current understanding of how viral DNA is synthesized in vivo, since it seems likely that both RNA:RNA and DNA:DNA duplex regions are transcribed during infection (see Section III.B.4). Moreover, displacement synthesis has been observed during synthesis by mellitin-activated ASLV polymerase in whole virions (Boone and Skalka 1981b; R. Junghans, pers. comm.). Other factors may be involved in displacement synthesis, but these have not yet been identified.

Primer requirement. Like all other known DNA polymerases, reverse transcriptase is primer-dependent (Baltimore and Smoler 1971; Goodman and Spiegelman 1971; Smoler et al. 1971; Hurwitz and Leis 1972; Leis and Hurwitz 1972a; Wells et al. 1972). The role of the primer during synthesis of poly(dT) by the AMV reverse transcriptase has been directly examined. When poly(A) is used as a template, the oligo(dT) primer is physically incorporated into the 5′ end of the poly(dT) product, indicating that synthesis occurs only by adding onto preformed chains (Smoler et al. 1971). When using homopolymer templates, oligodeoxyribonucleotides are the most efficient primers (Goodman and Spiegelman 1971; Hurwitz and Leis 1972; Leis and Hurwitz 1972a; Wells et al. 1972). This specificity is surprising since the natural primer is a tRNA (see Section III.B.2.b).

Two approaches have been used to develop convenient primers for copying heteropolymeric regions of specific templates. Naturally occurring homopolymeric tracts have been exploited to bind complementary homopolymer primers. The region next to the 3′ poly(A) tract of eukaryotic mRNAs can be specifically transcribed using an oligo(dT) primer (Kacian et al. 1972; Ross et al. 1972; Verma et al. 1972a). A similar strategy employing oligo(dC) has been used to transcribe an internal region of RSV RNA (Duesberg et al. 1971b; Collett et al. 1979). The second approach employs high-complexity DNA, degraded to oligonucleotides, to serve as "random primers" capable of priming synthesis on any heteropolymer template (Taylor et al. 1976a). Although the products of such a reaction are generally short, unique fragments can be isolated after cleavage with restriction endonucleases (D. Schwartz and W. Gilbert, pers. comm.).

DNA products synthesized in vitro. When native viral RNA is used in either the endogenous or reconstructed reactions, the major product is a short DNA transcript initiated on the tRNA primer and terminated at the 5′ end of the template (Cashion et al. 1976; Haseltine et al. 1976, 1977a; Taylor et al. 1976b; Coffin and Haseltine 1977a; Collett et al. 1977; Shine et al. 1977; Stoll et al. 1977). The length of this product varies from 100 to 180 bases, depending on the virus (Haseltine and Kleid 1978; Peters and Glover 1980a). The initial DNA strand synthesized, complementary to the RNA template, is called the minus strand. From the 5′ end of the template, minus-strand synthesis continues from a point near the 3′ end of the template (Junghans et al. 1977; Haseltine et al. 1979). The novel mechanism by which the growing DNA chain moves from the 5′ end of the template to copy sequences at the 3′ end of the template is discussed in Section III.B.4.b.

Once transcription has moved to the 3′ end of the template, the entire genome can be copied. Synthesis of the full-length minus strand, representative of the entire genome, has been accomplished in the endogenous, but not the reconstructed, reaction, and even under optimal conditions, this product is only a minor species (Junghans et al. 1975; Rothenberg and Baltimore 1977; Lai and Hu 1978). Mature viral DNA synthesized in vivo contains a large direct terminal repeat

(LTR). Only the MLV and murine sarcoma virus (MSV) endogenous reactions have conclusively been shown to produce duplex linear DNA containing the terminal repeat (Benz and Dina 1979; Gilboa et al. 1979b; Bosselman and Verma 1980; Dina and Benz 1980), although recent evidence suggests that this species of DNA can also be synthesized in the avian leukosis virus (ALV) endogenous reaction when the virions are disrupted with the detergent mellitin (Boone and Skalka 1981a). A detailed model describing how linear viral DNA may be synthesized is presented in Section III.B.4.

Much of the viral DNA synthesized in vitro is short and represents a limited portion of the genome (Temin and Baltimore 1972; Collett and Faras 1975; Haseltine et al. 1976; Taylor et al. 1976b). Yet, even these short products contain sequences transcribed from the entire genome at low frequency (Duesberg and Canaani 1970). Some of these short, high-complexity transcripts may arise by incorrect extension of the initial DNA transcript beyond the 5′ end of the template (Novak et al. 1979; Bunte et al. 1980). The presence of short DNA transcripts representing the entire template has been useful in isolating hybridization probes specific for defined regions of the viral genome (Stehelin et al. 1976).

Duplex DNA is also synthesized in vitro. The duplex DNA is a significant fraction of the total DNA product, but for the most part its sequence complexity is low (Gelb et al. 1971; Varmus et al. 1971; Taylor et al. 1972). Recently, full-length transcripts have been identified that appear to be duplex over their entire length (Benz and Dina 1979; Gilboa et al. 1979b; Bosselman and Verma 1980). Since we do not yet know for certain how the second strand of DNA is synthesized in vivo, it is difficult to assess the significance of the duplex molecules synthesized in vitro (see Section IV.B.4.d).

A class of duplex transcripts generated in vitro reanneals with zero-order kinetics (Fujinaga et al. 1970; Leis and Hurwitz 1972a; Taylor et al. 1972). These transcripts contain extensive regions of self-complementarity, or hairpins. In most of these cases, the mechanism of hairpin formation has not been fully explored. However, one hairpin species, synthesized using purified polymerase and RSV RNA as template (Collett and Faras 1978), has been studied in detail (Swanstrom et al. 1981a). After the RNA template has been copied to the 5′ terminus, the DNA transcript folds back on itself, forming a 5-base duplex between the 3′ end of the DNA and a complementary sequence internal to the transcript. In the process a 35-base loop is formed. The base-paired terminus then acts as a primer for further synthesis of duplex DNA. The proclivity of reverse transcriptase to synthesize duplex molecules by a hairpin mechanism has been particularly useful during synthesis of DNA complements of cellular mRNAs. Many investigators have exploited this tendency to generate duplex molecules, which, after treatment with nuclease S1, are often suitable substrates for molecular cloning (see, e.g., Efstratiatis et al. 1976; Maniatis et al. 1976).

The use of reverse transcriptase to synthesize cDNA copies of mRNAs has been an important biochemical tool. The most common strategy has been to use oligo(dT) to prime on the poly(A) tract of the mRNA. Generally, the transcripts are short (300–500 bases in length). Great efforts have been made to increase the length of the cDNA (for review, see Friedman and Rosbach 1977; Myers et al. 1977). To date the most important factors appear to be the integrity of the template, the absence of ribonuclease from the polymerase preparation, and the concentration of each dNTP (above 50 μM). One approach used to remove the secondary structure from the template prior to DNA synthesis is to treat the RNA with methylmercury hydroxide (Payvar and Schimke 1979). Several reports have suggested that the presence of sodium pyrophosphate during DNA synthesis increases the length of the DNA product. It was thought that this additive suppressed the synthesis of short second strands of DNA by inhibiting the polymerase-associated RNase-H activity (Kacian and Myers 1976; Myers and Spiegelman 1978). However, sodium pyrophosphate has no inhibitory effect on RNase H, and the observed effect on DNA synthesis may be attributable to inhibition of contaminating nucleases (Srivastaa and Modak 1979).

Rate of synthesis and misincorporation. The rates of retroviral DNA synthesis in vivo and in the endogenous reaction are significantly slower (30 nucleotides/min) than the rates of other cellular and viral reactions (Rothenberg and Baltimore 1977; Varmus et al. 1978), although improved conditions may increase the rate in the endogenous reaction (Boone and Skalka 1980, 1981a). In the reconstructed reaction, the rate of polymerization by reverse transcriptase is nearly equal to *Escherichia coli* DNA polymerase I on some templates but still generally slower than observed in vivo rates for other systems (Dube and Loeb 1976; Travaglini et al. 1976). It is not clear whether the slower rate is intrinsic for reverse transcriptase or whether other rate-limiting steps account for this observation.

The AMV polymerase has been reported to exhibit a high error rate under certain conditions when transcribing homopolymeric RNA and DNA templates or a single-stranded phage DNA template (Battula and Loeb 1974; Mizutani and Temin 1976; Gopinathan et al. 1979). Under certain conditions, the rate of improper incorporation is about ten times higher than that of *E. coli* DNA polymerase I. This observation has led to the suggestion that reverse transcription promotes a high mutation rate, although the error rate on viral RNA is not known. During passage of a clonal stock of MLV, mutants were observed at a relatively high frequency, perhaps due to misincorporation during reverse transcription (Shields et al. 1978). A high mutation rate may be a feature of an RNA template or the lack of a polymerase-associated editing function, but it is a feature shared by other RNA viruses (Weissmann et al. 1973; Tsipis and Bratt 1976).

The natural viral RNA template contains five to ten N^6-methyladenines per subunit (Furuichi et al. 1975; Beemon and Keith 1976). Since full-length viral DNA is synthesized, the N^6-methyladenine must be transcribed, and it is possible that copying of methylated bases is error-prone. Transcription of N^2-methylguanine has been reported to involve a pause, with synthesis then continuing beyond the site of the modified base (Youvan and Hearst 1979). However, not all methylated bases can be transcribed. It has recently been shown that the AMV polymerase cannot transcribe through a N^6-dimethyladenine (Hagenbuchle et al. 1978). There is circumstantial evidence that viral DNA synthesis in vivo terminates at an N^1-methyladenine and that this termination plays a role in the strategy of virus replication (see Section III.B.4.d).

Inhibitors of DNA synthesis. DNA polymerase activity can be inhibited by a variety of agents (for review, see Verma 1977). One general class of inhibitors covalently attaches to functional groups of the polymerase (e.g., pyridoxal 5′-phosphate and *N*-ethylmaleimide) (Modak 1976; Papas et al. 1977; Gorecki and Panet 1978). Another general class of inhibitors binds to templates. An important member of this class, actinomycin D, has the useful property of binding more tightly to DNA than to RNA, permitting a distinction between DNA and RNA templated reactions (McDonnell et al. 1970; Manly et al. 1971). A third class of inhibitors competes either for the template or primer (e.g., polynucleotide derivatives) or for the substrate. These types of inhibitors lack adequate specificity in discriminating between reverse transcriptase and other polymerizing activities, although the K_m values for these compounds may vary among cellular and viral polymerases. The most extensively studied compounds are the rifamycin SV derivatives (DiCioccio and Srivastava 1978). However, no derivative with satisfactory specificity has yet been identified. An inhibitor of cellular DNA synthesis, aphidocolin, is interesting because of its lack of effect on reverse transcriptase. Aphidocolin specifically inhibits cellular DNA polymerase α (Pedrali-Noy and Spadari 1979; Wist and Prydz 1979) but not the RSV polymerase. Full-length viral DNA can be made in infected cells in the presence of this inhibitor, suggesting that cellular polymerase α plays no role in the synthesis of viral DNA (H.-J. Kung and J. M. Taylor, pers. comm.).

Factors affecting DNA synthesis. Some aspects of the endogenous reaction have been shown to have a reproducible effect on the quality of the DNA product. Only when the concentrations of the nonionic detergent, dNTP, and the divalent cation are carefully controlled is a DNA product synthesized that resembles the viral DNA made in vivo (Junghans et al. 1975; Rothenberg and Baltimore 1976, 1977; Lai and Hu 1978; Verma 1978; Gilboa et al. 1979b; Novak et al. 1979; Van Beveren and Goulian 1979; Boone and Skalka 1980, 1981a). When these parameters are carefully controlled, infectious DNA can be synthesized (Rothenberg et al. 1977; Clayman et al. 1979a; Boone and Skalka 1980; Lai and Verma 1980).

Several other factors have been reported to improve DNA synthesis in either endogenous or reconstructed reactions: a virion-associated stimulatory protein (Leis and Hurwitz 1972b), a cellular nucleic-acid-binding protein (Lee and Hung 1977), a plasma-membrane fraction (Padhy et al. 1976), and a specific virion structural protein (p30 in the case of MLV [Bandyopadhyay 1977]). So far none of these have gained wide acceptance. All the steps involved in the synthesis of viral DNA are not understood, and some of these or other factors may yet be shown to have an important role.

(ii) RIBONUCLEASE H. Hausen and Stein (1970) first demonstrated that cells contain RNase H, an enzyme that degrades the RNA strand of a DNA:RNA hybrid but does not degrade either free RNA or double-stranded RNA. Moelling et al. (1971) found that virions of AMV contain RNase H and that, unlike other nucleases in the virion, RNase-H activity cannot be separated from the AMV DNA polymerase during purification. Since then, RNase-H activity has been found as constituent of the virions of all retroviruses tested (Grandgenett et al. 1972; Verma 1977).

There is convincing evidence that RNase H is covalently associated with DNA-polymerase activity. During all steps of purification, DNA-polymerase activity and RNase-H activity copurify (Moelling et al. 1971; Baltimore and Smoler 1972; Grandgenett et al. 1972; Keller and Crouch 1972; Moelling 1974; Gerard and Grandgenett 1975; Verma 1975a; Dion et al. 1977). In the case of the ASLVs, the $\alpha\beta$, $\beta\beta$, and α forms of enzyme contain both DNA-polymerase activity and RNase-H activity (Grandgenett et al. 1973; Hizi and Joklik 1977a). For the MLV enzyme, the single subunit has both activities (Moelling 1974; Verma 1975a). The most direct evidence that RNase H and DNA polymerase are part of the same protein is that a temperature-sensitive lesion renders both activities thermolabile. This observation has been made for both the RSV and MLV polymerases (Verma et al. 1974a; Tronick et al. 1975; Verma 1975b; Lai et al. 1978). Finally, a 24,000-dalton peptide containing only RNase-H activity can be generated from the purified β subunit by limited digestion with the protease chymotrypsin (Lai and Verma 1978). Although the DNA-polymerase and RNase-H activities reside on the same polypeptide, they probably have different active sites. The two activities also show differential sensitivity to thermal inactivation and the RNase H is more sensitive than the polymerase activity to inhibition by NaF, pyridoxal 5′-phosphate, and *N*-ethylmaleimide (Brewer and Wells 1974; Verma et al. 1974a; Modak 1976; Gorecki and Panet 1978). Another difference between the two activities is that chelation of the polymerase-bound zinc inhibits DNA synthesis but not RNase-H activity (Modak and Srivastava 1979).

The AMV RNase H degrades poly(A) of a poly(A)-poly(dT) hybrid mainly to oligonucleotides, most of which are at least 6 bases in length; the termini at the points of scission are 3′-hydroxyl and 5′-phosphoryl (Baltimore and Smoler 1972; Keller and Crouch 1972; Leis et al. 1973; Verma 1975a). It requires a free end in order to initiate degradation (Keller and Crouch 1972; Leis et al. 1973; Grandgenett and Green 1974; Moelling 1974; Verma 1975a); therefore, topologically it is an exonuclease. The $\alpha\beta$ form of the AMV polymerase has an RNase-H activity that is processive in its mode of action, whereas the α form is random (Keller and Crouch 1972; Leis et al. 1973; Grandgenett and Green 1974; Gerard 1981). The MLV RNase-H activity is also processive (Gerard 1981).

To date there is conflicting evidence about the role of RNase H in viral DNA synthesis. Studies with an inhibitor of RNase H have failed to affect synthesis of double-stranded DNA in vitro (Collett and Faras 1976). However, when viral RNA is used as a template, DNA synthesis appears to be followed by the loss of certain regions of the RNA template, presumably by the action of RNase H (Darlix et al. 1977a; Collett et al. 1978a; Friedrich and Moelling 1979). Recently, a model system employing RNA homopolymers has been used to show a need for RNase-H activity in second-strand synthesis (Watson et al. 1979). Furthermore, this study showed that oligoribonucleotides generated from a DNA:RNA hybrid by RNase H can serve as primers for the synthesis of second-strand DNA. A similar conclusion has been reached using viral RNA as template (Myers et al. 1980; Olsen and Watson 1980). It is not known whether this mechanism for priming second-strand synthesis is used in vivo. Some of the substrates envisioned for RNase H during the synthesis of viral DNA have only one free end and that end is a single-stranded tail (see Section III.B.4.d). Homopolymer hybrids have been constructed mimicking these structures, and it has been shown that RNase H is active on this type of substrate (Gerard 1981).

f. Other Enzymic Activities of the Virion. Three virus-coded enzymic activities, other than the DNA polymerase and RNase H of reverse transcriptase, have been found in virions: an endonuclease associated with a cleavage product of the β subunit of ASLV polymerases, a protease associated with an ASLV *gag*-gene product (p15; see Chapter 6), and a protein kinase that may be a product of the Moloney murine sarcoma virus (Mo-MSV) *onc* gene (see Chapter 9). Only the first of these appears to be relevant in the present context.

AMV contains an endonuclease of 32,000 daltons (p32) associated with the virion core (Grandgenett et al. 1978). Analysis of partial protease-digestion products indicates that p32 shares peptides with the β, but not with the α, subunit of the AMV polymerase (Schiff and Grandgenett 1978). Like α, the p32 can be generated from β by partial digestion with chymotrypsin (Grandgenett et al. 1980). Thus a single processing event may generate α and p32 from the β protein (see Fig. 5.2 and Section III.B.1.b). In the presence of Mg^{++}, p32 showed some site specificity in nicking ColE1 DNA (Grandgenett et al. 1978). p32 also binds efficiently to nucleic acids (Grandgenett et al. 1978). Recent studies with fragments of cloned RSV DNA suggest the binding exhibits specificity for sequences from the termini of viral

DNA and RNA, implying a possible role for this protein in provirus integration (D. Grandgenett, pers. comm.).

The $\alpha\beta$, but not the α, polymerase has a related endonuclease activity (Golomb and Grandgenett 1979; Samuel et al. 1979). Presumably, the activity associated with the $\alpha\beta$ enzyme lies in the p32 portion of the β subunit. The polymerase-associated endonuclease is active in the presence of Mn^{++} on single-stranded RNA and DNA and on double-stranded DNA but shows a preference for nicking supercoiled DNA (Golomb and Grandgenett 1979). An endonuclease also has been found associated with MLV (Nissen-Meyer and Nes 1980; Kopchick et al. 1981). Another activity associated with the α and $\alpha\beta$ forms of the ALSV polymerase has been reported to render duplex regions of DNA partially sensitive to the single-stranded nuclease S1 (Collett et al. 1978b). It is not clear what roles these activities may play in virus replication.

Numerous other enzymic activities have been identified in virions, but it is believed that most of these are cellular contaminants (Temin and Baltimore 1972). For example, a virion-associated DNA-ligase activity could be imagined to participate in the synthesis, circularization, or integration of viral DNA, but there is so much ligase in cells that the small amount provided by the virions is unlikely to be significant. Contaminating cellular enzymes are frequently observed with enveloped viruses.

One enzyme activity that has received considerable attention is protein kinase. This activity has been detected in, and in some cases purified from, a variety of retroviruses (Strand and August 1971; Hatanaka et al. 1972; Pal and Roy-Burman 1977; Houts et al. 1978; Blaas et al. 1979; Hizi et al. 1979; Rossok and Watson 1979). These studies showed that some virion structural proteins can serve as substrates for phosphorylation in vitro. It is not known whether these virion-associated kinase activities phosphorylate viral proteins in vivo.

2. *The Natural Template and Primer for Reverse Transcriptase*

a. Template. The central task of viral DNA polymerase is to convert all the genetic information of a subunit of viral RNA into DNA, which can, in turn, be used as a template to synthesize a subunit of viral RNA. Thus, the important templates for reverse transcription are single-stranded RNA subunits of about 5,000–10,000 bases, but the issue is complicated by two features. First, viral

RNA is present in viral particles as dimers of apparently identical subunits, with the subunits joined by uncertain means near or at their 5′ termini (see Chapter 4). Second, the final product of reverse transcription contains repeated sequences that are not repeated in a subunit of viral RNA. This implies that reverse transcriptase must either use more than one template to produce a completed molecule or copy repetitively certain portions of a single template. Mechanisms by which these possibilities could be accomplished are discussed below; it is sufficient at present to point out that the polymerase could use one or both of the subunits present in the dimer structure to generate a single product.

Several structural features of retroviral RNA are significant in relation to its role as a template for synthesis of DNA: (1) A short sequence (16–21 nucleotides for RSV; ~ 65 nucleotides for MLV) is repeated at the ends of the heteropolymeric portion of each RNA subunit. This sequence, called R, is essential to the early phases of DNA synthesis, allowing the polymerase to proceed beyond the 5′ end of a template to the 3′ end of another template (see below). (2) The RNAs generally have a high degree of secondary structure, which could pose impediments to the movement of the enzyme along the template. Thus far, there have been only modest attempts to correlate chain-termination points with highly base-paired regions of RNA (Darlix et al. 1977b). (3) Viral RNAs are polyadenylated at their 3′ termini (Chapter 4). Although reverse transcriptase is clearly capable of transcribing this homopolymer in vitro (see Section III.B.1.e), it does not appear to do so, either in vitro (Reitz et al. 1972) or in vivo (Varmus et al. 1978), unless synthesis is specifically primed with oligo(dT). (4) The 5′ termini of viral RNAs are capped by an inverted, methylated base (Furuichi et al. 1975; Keith and Fraenkel-Conrat 1975; Bondurant et al. 1976; Rose et al. 1976). The inverted nucleotide, like the poly(A) tract, is apparently added to viral RNA posttranscriptionally; thus, it need not be encoded in the provirus or copied during reverse transcription. (5) Some of the adenylate residues in heteropolymeric regions of viral RNA are methylated (Beemon and Keith 1976; Dimock and Stoltzfus 1978); it is not known whether such modifications affect reverse transcription in a significant fashion.

Some of these structural features also pose interesting problems for the RNase-H activity of the polymerase. It appears that RNA:DNA hybrids with a capped RNA terminus are subject to digestion by viral RNase H (Collett and Faras 1978; Darlix et al. 1978; Friedrich and

Moelling 1979); however, it is uncertain whether RNase H can function on an RNA:DNA hybrid terminated with an appreciable single-stranded tail of poly(A) (Leis et al. 1973). Nevertheless, removal of the RNA would seem to be a prerequisite for the synthesis of duplex DNA. This problem will be considered further in relation to synthesis of the second strand of viral DNA.

b. Primer. (i) IDENTIFICATION OF THE NATURAL PRIMER. Although reverse transcriptase appears to favor deoxyribonucleotide over ribonucleotide primers in reconstructed reactions using ribonucleotide homopolymers as templates (Goodman and Spiegelman 1971; Hurwitz and Leis 1972; Leis and Hurwitz 1972a; Wells et al. 1972), the "natural" primer for synthesis of the complement of viral RNA is a cellular tRNA. The primer in endogenous polymerase reactions was initially identified as RNA by centrifugation of nascent products, still attached to primer, in density gradients (Verma et al. 1971) and by the transfer of ^{32}P from the α position in dNTP substrates to ribonucleoside residues at the 3′ end of the primer (Flugel and Wells 1972; Verma et al. 1972a; Faras et al. 1973; Friedrich et al. 1977). Since a single dNTP acted as donor and a single ribonucleoside acted as recipient for ^{32}P in such experiments (e.g., ^{32}P is transferred from dATP to rA in RSV polymerase reactions), it seemed likely that a single primer was responsible for initiating synthesis.

To isolate the priming species, methods were developed for "tagging" the primer with only one or a few labeled deoxynucleotide residues (e.g., by omitting certain dNTPs from the reaction or by adding chain terminators) (Dahlberg et al. 1974; Faras et al. 1974). Primers were also isolated as RNA:DNA covalent hybrids and then released by digestion with DNase (Faras et al. 1973). The primer for RSV is similar in size to tRNA, comigrates in two-dimensional gel electrophoresis with one of the major species of cellular tRNA known to be present in viral particles, and has a simple oligonucleotide composition, suggesting that it is a single species (Sawyer and Dahlberg 1973). The identity of the RSV primer as a cellular tRNA was substantiated by showing that an appropriate tRNA species isolated from uninfected cells could be annealed to denatured viral RNA and function as primer (Sawyer et al. 1974; Faras and Dibble 1975; Taylor et al. 1975; Waters et al. 1975a; for review, see Taylor 1977).

The chromatographic properties, amino-acid-acceptor capacity, and sequence of the RSV primer identified it as $tRNA^{Trp}$ (Harada et al. 1975). Similar studies of the MLV and REV primers have identified them both as $tRNA^{Pro}_{1,2}$ (Peters et al. 1977; Harada et al. 1979; Peters and Dahlberg 1979; Peters and Glover 1980a), and the MMTV primer appears to be $tRNA^{Lys}_{3}$ (Peters and Glover 1980b). Identities of primers for other retroviruses are less certain.

Darlix et al. (1977a) have observed a short DNA primer that initiates synthesis near the middle of the viral genome in detergent-activated RSV. This finding has yet to be confirmed by other investigators, and there is no evidence for viral DNA initiated in this fashion in infected cells.

(ii) BINDING OF tRNAs TO DNA POLYMERASE. Although some primer tRNAs share some unusual features (e.g., the sequence Ψ-Ψ-C-G in loop IV of $tRNA^{Trp}$ and $tRNA^{Pro}$), there are no obvious characteristics that distinguish them as a class from other cellular tRNAs. The tRNAs found in retroviral particles are a nonrandom subset of the cellular species, and the priming species are generally dominant among those included in the particles (Sawyer and Dahlberg 1973). Avian viral polymerases have been shown to bind to the dominant tRNAs in avian viral particles ($tRNA^{Trp}$ and $tRNA^{Met}$) (Panet et al. 1975c, 1978a; Haseltine et al. 1977b; Cordell et al. 1978); thus, it seems likely that affinity for polymerase determines, at least in part, which tRNA species will be packaged. This idea is supported by the apparent absence of primer from RSV(-)α particles that lack polymerase (Sawyer and Hanafusa 1979; Peters and Hu 1980) and the inclusion of primer in particles that lack viral RNA but contain polymerase (Gerwin and Levin 1977; Levin and Seidman 1979). Little, if any, specificity for individual tRNA species has been observed in tests of mammalian reverse transcriptases, although these enzymes do bind tRNAs nonselectively (Panet and Berliner 1978). Recent observations with mutant MLV virions that lack the viral polymerase (Shields et al. 1978) indicate that the MLV enzyme is not required to bind the correct tRNA ($tRNA^{Pro}$) to viral RNA subunits, but the proportion of $tRNA^{Pro}$ among free tRNAs in mutant viral particles is markedly reduced (Levin and Seidman 1981). The somewhat different results with avian and mammalian polymerase mutants presumably reflect the differences in the binding affinities of the respective wild-type enzymes for tRNAs. Little is known about the manner in which primers (or other tRNAs) bind to polymerase, but an intact tRNA with normal conformation seems to be required (Cordell et al. 1978).

(iii) BINDING OF tRNA PRIMERS TO VIRAL RNA. Unlike several tRNAs that form unstable complexes with viral RNA, $tRNA^{Trp}$ or $tRNA^{Pro}$ can be dissociated from RSV or MLV RNA only by relatively rigorous denaturation procedures. When viral RNA is subjected to thermal denaturation, first nonpriming, low-molecular-weight RNAs dissociate from high-molecular-weight RNA; then the viral subunits disaggregate; and finally, the priming activity is lost, as the priming tRNA is removed from the viral subunits (Canaani and Duesberg 1972; Faras et al. 1973; Waters et al. 1975b; Peters and Dahlberg 1979). Conversely, $tRNA^{Trp}$ can be annealed to RSV RNA under relatively stringent conditions (Faras and Dibble 1975; Taylor et al. 1975). Approximately one $tRNA^{Trp}$ is bound per RNA subunit (Sawyer and Dahlberg 1973; Dahlberg et al. 1974), and these sites are mostly saturated in native 70S RNA (Taylor et al. 1975).

(iv) RNA-BINDING SITE IN tRNA. The portions of $tRNA^{Trp}$ and $tRNA^{Pro}$ that bind to RSV and MLV RNAs have been determined by analyzing the oligonucleotides of primer recovered from a duplex of labeled primer and template that resists digestion with ribonucleases (Eiden et al. 1975; Cordell et al. 1976; Peters and Dahlberg 1979). Sixteen bases at the 3′ terminus of $tRNA^{Trp}$ and 19 bases at the 3′ terminus of $tRNA^{Pro}$ were shown to be base-paired with their respective viral RNAs (see Chapter 4). In both cases, the 3′-terminal adenosine residue was released from the template-primer complex by pancreatic ribonuclease; this was surprising, since the first deoxynucleotide is added to this ribonucleotide. In addition, an important theoretical problem might be raised if the corresponding base in the genomic sequence were not complementary and if the 3′ end of the primer were copied during synthesis of plus strands of viral DNA (see below). In this case, reverse transcription would generate a heteroduplex. However, Coffin and Haseltine (1977b) have shown that the base at the 5′ boundary of the site to which the RSV primer binds is U; the susceptibility of the complementary rA residue to ribonuclease remains unexplained. Analysis of the DNA sequence of cloned RSV DNA has shown that the RNA^{Trp} binding site is actually 18 nucleotides long (Swanstrom et al. 1981b). Similarly sized potential binding sites for $tRNA^{Lys}$ in MMTV RNA and for $tRNA^{Pro}$ in REV RNA have been determined by direct sequencing of cloned viral DNA and by comparison with the known tRNA sequences (Majors and Varmus 1980, 1981; Shimotohno et al. 1980).

It is notable that, in these cases, the binding sites appear to end at positions corresponding to the first modified base (a l-methyladenosine residue) within the 3′ region of the tRNA. Reverse transcription of part of the primer during synthesis of viral DNA may have contributed to the development of such binding sites in the viral genomes, since the polymerase would be unlikely to copy the modified base (see Section III.B.1.f). (As discussed in Section III.B.4.e, transcription of the 3′ end of primer into plus-strand DNA appears to be central to the final phase of DNA synthesis.)

(v) BINDING SITE FOR tRNA PRIMERS ON VIRAL RNA. Taylor and Illmensee (1975) first determined the location of the site at which primer is bound to viral RNA. They isolated polyadenylated RSV RNA containing "tagged" primer and showed that only molecules of full genome length bore primer. This meant that the primer must be located close to the 5′ terminus of viral RNA, since the polyadenylated RNA of less than genome length is deficient at the 5′ terminus and not at the 3′ terminus. Similar results have been obtained for MLV by Peters and Dahlberg (1979) and for RSV by Staskus et al. (1976).

More precise localization of the primer-binding site became possible when it was recognized that a major product of synthesis during DNA-polymerase reactions in vitro was a short transcript (100–200 nucleotides) of the entire region of viral RNA lying between the end of the primer-binding site and the 5′ end of the genome (Haseltine et al. 1976). It was apparent that these so-called "strong-stop" DNAs were complements of the 5′ end of the genome, since they protected oligonucleotides mapped to the 5′ end of viral RNA from nuclease digestion after annealing (Coffin and Haseltine 1977a). In addition, the sequence of RSV strong-stop DNA is consistent with the composition of oligonucleotides derived from the capped 5′ terminus of RSV RNA (Haseltine et al. 1977a; Shine et al. 1977). Provided with the precedents of RSV and MLV, Haseltine and Kleid (1978) have estimated the positions of primers bound to RNAs of several retroviruses by determining the lengths of strong-stop DNAs. Thus far, most of the primers appear to initiate synthesis within 100 to 150 nucleotides of the 5′ terminus; the primer for REV appears to be about 180 nucleotides from the 5′ end of viral RNA (Peters and Glover 1980a; Shimotohno et al. 1980).

(vi) FUNCTIONS OF THE PRIMER. The principal function of the tRNA primers is to initiate the synthesis of minus-strand DNA. It is generally agreed to be the major, if not the sole, primer for minus strands active in reactions carried out with detergent-activated virions or with purified components; furthermore, the structure of viral DNA in infected cells indicates that it functions in a similar way in vivo (see below). A fragment of 27 nucleotides from the 3′ terminus of $tRNA^{Trp}$ is sufficient to initiate synthesis of DNA (Cordell et al. 1979). However, the remainder of the molecule may also have important functions. As suggested above, the concentration of primer tRNAs in the viral particles may depend on specific interactions with the viral polymerase; an intact tRNA appears to be necessary for such binding (Cordell et al. 1979). In addition, Haseltine et al. (1977a) have proposed that base pairing between the 5′ portion of $tRNA^{Trp}$ and the viral subunit to which its 3′ end is not bound could account for the dimeric form of the viral genome; however, virions depleted in $tRNA^{Trp}$ still contain 70S RNA (Peters and Hu 1980).

(vii) PRIMER(S) FOR PLUS STRANDS. The natural primers for plus strands have not yet been identified, although the probable site at which synthesis of the first plus strand is initiated has been sequenced for several retroviruses (Czernilofsky et al. 1980b; Dhar et al. 1980; Majors and Varmus 1980, 1981; Shimotohno et al. 1980; Sutcliffe et al. 1980; Swanstrom et al. 1981a). Features of this sequence are discussed in Section III.B.4.d.

3. Principal Products of Viral DNA Synthesis in Infected Cells

a. Introduction: Methodology and Physical Mapping with Restriction Endonucleases. Viral DNA comprises only a small fraction (0.001% or less) of the DNA in an infected cell, thus prohibiting reliable detection by direct labeling of newly synthesized DNA. However, the combination of molecular hybridization reagents of high specific activity and the techniques for fractionating DNA according to size and structure have permitted definition of three major forms of viral DNA in infected cells: linear duplexes, closed circular duplexes, and DNA covalently integrated into the host genome (Varmus et al. 1975; Weinberg 1977). These forms have also been identified by combining tests for infectious DNA with DNA fractionation procedures (see, e.g., Battula and Temin 1977, 1978; Fritsch and Temin 1977a).

The most useful hybridization reagents have been those that differentiate between strands, e.g., labeled viral RNA for detection of minus strands and labeled cDNAs synthesized in vitro for detection of plus strands, and those that differentiate among various regions of the viral genome, e.g., cDNAs specific for sequences unique to the 3′ and 5′ termini. The fractionation methods of particular importance have included rate-zonal sedimentation, equilibrium centrifugation in density gradients containing buoyant dyes, agarose gel electrophoresis, and preparative methods that separate high-molecular-weight cellular DNA from unintegrated viral DNA (NaCl-SDS precipitation, network formation, and subcellular fractionation).

For several years, most workers measured viral DNA by reacting unlabeled DNA from cells with labeled virus-specific reagents in solution and then determining the conversion of labeled probes from single-stranded forms to duplex forms by chromatographic or enzymic means. This approach, which was extremely laborious when applied to samples fractionated in gradients or gels, has been largely superseded by the DNA-transfer method (Southern 1975). It is now conventional practice to subject multiple samples to agarose gel electrophoresis, transfer the fractionated DNAs to nitrocellulose sheets, anneal with appropriate radioactive reagents, and then observe the positions of virus-specific molecules by autoradiography. These new methods permit more accurate analyses with much greater economy of materials than did previous procedures. Furthermore, since 1979, recombinant DNA methods have been widely applied to the study of retroviral DNA, permitting a complete analysis of the sequence of those species of viral DNAs amenable to cloning in available host-vector systems.

Among the most significant consequences of these improved methodologies for studying retroviral DNA has been the generation of physical maps based upon cleavage sites for restriction endonucleases. Most of the mapping was performed initially with minute amounts of completed linear or circular forms isolated from infected cells (Canaani et al. 1977; Hsu et al. 1978b; Shank et al. 1978a,b, 1981; Keshet et al. 1979; Sherr et al. 1979; Yoshimura and Weinberg 1979; Bergmann et al. 1980; Cohen et al. 1980; Mullins et al. 1980). Identification of digestion products required the use of virus-specific hybridization reagents that were annealed to DNA transferred to nitrocellulose filters. Organization of the fragments into physical maps was accomplished by the use of probes specific for various portions of the viral genome, by sequential digestions with two or more enzymes, by comparison of digestion products from linear and circular forms, and by the use of DNA from cells infected with deletion mutants (e.g., *env* or *src* deletion mutants of RSV). More detailed mapping has been possible using radiolabeled DNA synthesized in vitro; both incomplete and complete linear DNAs have been the source of considerable useful information (Taylor et al. 1976b, 1978; Benz and Dina 1979; Gilboa et al. 1979b; Verma 1979). Following the successful cloning of retroviral DNA in bacteria, large quantities of viral DNA, most of it thus far derived from circular or integrated forms in infected cells, have become available for mapping with restriction enzymes or heteroduplexing methods.

For most of the work alluded to in the ensuing sections, the pertinent restriction enzymes are those that recognize few (or no) sites in viral DNA. More detailed mapping with enzymes that cleave viral DNA into many fragments is a necessary prelude to sequencing viral genomes; these complex maps (see, e.g., Gilboa et al. 1979b; DeLorbe et al. 1980) are beyond the scope of the present discussion, but several are provided in Appendix B. Figure 5.3 summarizes several of the most useful restriction endonuclease sites that have been located on the linear DNA maps of extensively studied retroviruses—RSV, Rous-associated virus-0 (RAV-0), Mo-MLV, Mo-MSV, Harvey MSV (Ha-MSV), MMTV, spleen necrosis virus (SNV), and feline leukemia and sarcoma viruses (FeLV, FeSV). The sites included on these maps have been useful in several studies cited here and are generally common to the isolates of the indicated strains. However, it must be emphasized that different strains of closely related viruses (e.g., the several strains of RSV) have manifested surprisingly frequent differences in their restriction maps (Shank et al. 1978b), that strains may be mislabeled after long use without available tests for origin (cf. Studier 1979), and that genetic changes (recombination, deletion, and base substitution) during virus passage may result in the generation of viral DNA molecules that are heterogeneous with respect to their restriction maps (cf. Hughes et al. 1978; N.G. Copeland et al. 1980).

b. Linear Duplex DNA. (i) STRUCTURE AND TERMINAL REDUNDANCIES. The first and most abundant of the major species of viral DNA in infected cells is a double-stranded, linear molecule of approximately the same size as a subunit of viral RNA (i.e., 5–10 kb). When denatured, fractionated by size, and detected with radioactive probes specific for each strand, the linear DNA appears to be composed principally of a full-length minus strand and a heterogeneous

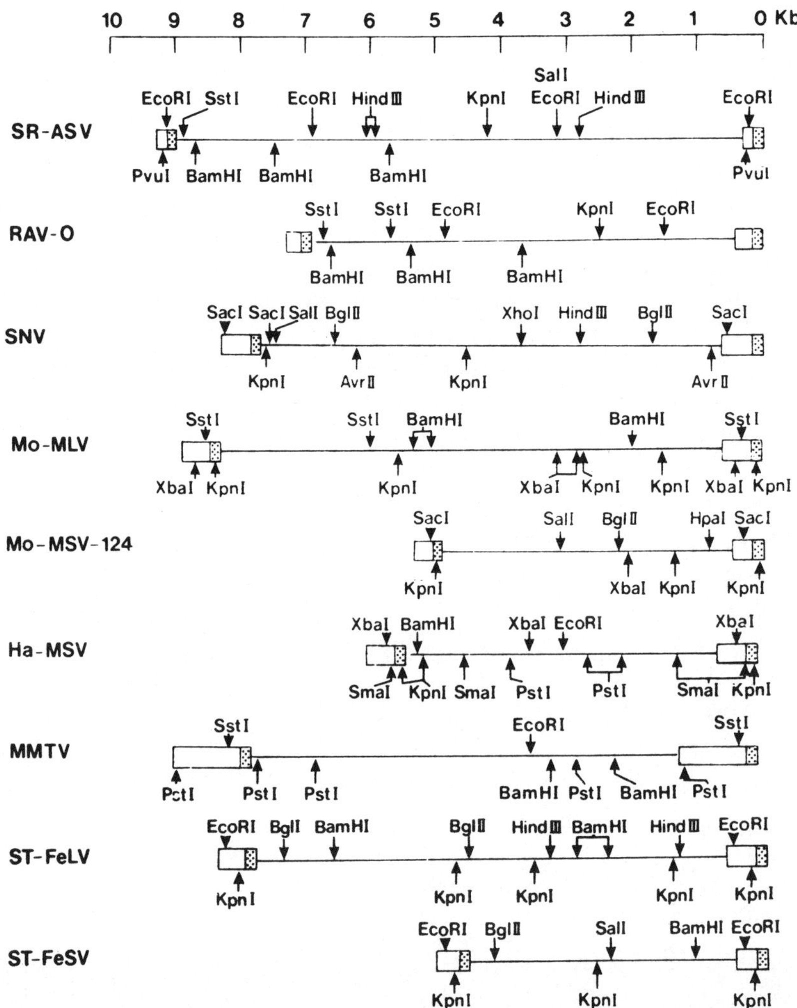

Figure 5.3 Physical maps of the unintegrated linear DNA synthesized by several important strains of retroviruses. The sequences directly repeated at the ends of linear DNA (LTRs) are denoted by boxes; a more detailed account of the composition of the repeated sequences is provided in the text and illustrated in Fig. 5.4. The positions of recognition sites for several commonly used restriction endonucleases are presented; more comprehensive restriction maps for these and other genomes can be found in Appendix B. Note particularly that restriction sites in one LTR are found in the predicted location in the other LTR. The maps are derived from published data for RSV DNA (Taylor et al. 1978; Shank et al. 1978b; DeLorbe et al. 1980), RAV-0 DNA (Shank et al. 1981), Mo-MLV DNA (Verma and McKennett 1978; Gilboa et al. 1979b; Yoshimura and Weinberg 1979), Ha-MSV DNA (Goldfarb and Weinberg 1979; Hager et al. 1979), Mo-MSV DNA (Verma et al. 1980), MMTV DNA (Shank et al. 1978a; Cohen et al. 1979b), SNV DNA (O'Rear et al. 1980), and Snyder-Theilen (ST) FeLV and FeSV DNAs (Sherr et al. 1980). The scale is in kilobases (kb).

collection of plus strands, ranging from a few hundred nucleotides to several thousand nucleotides in length (Gianni and Weinberg 1975; Varmus et al. 1976, 1978; Ringold et al. 1978). In some cases, the linear DNA has been shown to be partially or even principally single-stranded, due to the incompleteness of the plus-strand components (Gianni and Weinberg 1975), but in other cases some of the plus strands appear to be full length after synthesis in vitro or in vivo (Gilboa et al. 1979b; Chen and Temin 1980; Kung et al. 1981). It is not known whether the ends of the linear DNA are "blunt" or have single-stranded "tails"; the mechanistic importance of this issue will be apparent in later sections.

Several kinds of experimental evidence now support the fascinating proposal that a sequence of several hundred nucleotides is repeated in the same orientation at both termini of linear DNA; this LTR is composed of sequences derived from heteropolymeric regions at the 3′ and 5′ termini of viral RNA, in the manner illustrated in Figure 5.4. More specifically, the LTR contains about 250–1200 bp from a region unique to the 3′ terminus (the U_3 sequence), a single copy of the short sequence (R) present at both ends of the RNA, and about 80–120 bp from a region unique to the 5′ terminus (the U_5 sequence). Although the lengths of U_3 and U_5 vary among retroviruses (Appendix D), the lengths are determined by functionally homologous sites. U_5 is bounded on its 3′ side by the priming site for the minus strand and on its 5′ side by R; U_3 is bounded on its 5′ side by the presumptive priming site for the first plus strand and on its 3′ side by R (see Fig. 5.4). Sequencing studies of cloned DNA further indicate that LTRs conclude with short (5–22 bp) and often imperfect inverted repeats. These are discussed in greater detail below.

The unexpected structure of linear DNA was first suspected during efforts to prepare a physical map of linear RSV DNA with restriction endonucleases. Two enzymes (*Eco*RI and *Pvu*I), which recognize hexanucleotide sites encoded near the 3′ end of viral RNA (Taylor et al. 1976b, 1978; Varmus et al. 1978), cleaved viral DNA at both ends (Hsu et al. 1978b; Shank et al. 1978b). In addition, after limited digestion of linear DNA with exonuclease III, some of it formed circles, presumably as a consequence of exposure of complementary sequences at the redundant termini (Hsu et al. 1978b). In the most direct test of the proposed redundancies, cDNAs specific for sequences unique to the 3′ and 5′ ends of RNA annealed to restriction fragments generated from the two ends of linear DNA, as predicted from the model in Figure 5.5. Shank et al. (1978b) isolated *Bam*HI

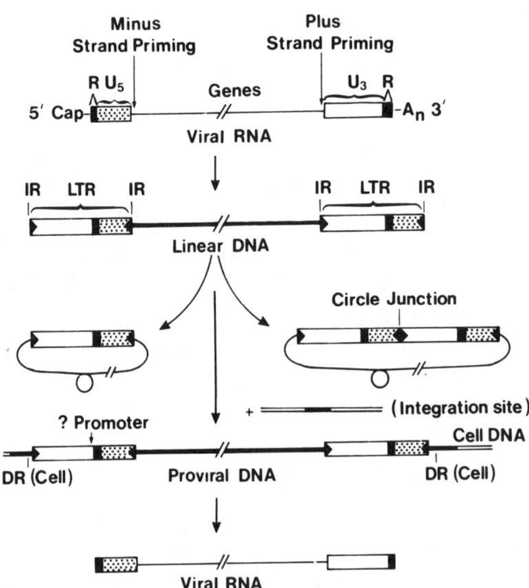

Figure 5.4 Role of repeated sequences in the replication of retroviruses. The top line shows several structural features of a subunit of viral RNA: the capped nucleotide at the 5′ terminus, the poly(A) tract at the 3′ terminus, and the site of binding of the cellular tRNA used to prime DNA synthesis. (■) Short sequence, R, which is present at both ends of viral RNA; (▦) U_5, which denotes the sequence unique to the 5′ terminus between the primer-binding site and R; (□) U_3, which denotes the sequence of several hundred bases unique to the 3′ terminus and repeated at both ends of unintegrated linear DNA. The subsequent lines show the organization of these repeated sequences as LTR units in linear DNA, the two forms of monomeric circular DNA, and proviral DNA, as determined from studies discussed in the text. (▶) Inverted repeats that terminate the LTR units; (▬▬), a direct repeat of a 4–6-bp cell sequence present once in the unoccupied integration site. For convenience, a subunit of viral RNA, the putative primary transcript of the provirus, is shown in the last line. To clarify the structural details, the figure is not drawn to scale. Variations among the lengths of the repeated components for several retroviruses are recorded in Appendix D.

fragments from both ends of RSV linear DNA and digested them with *Eco*RI (Fig. 5.5). The small *Eco*RI fragment from the right end of linear DNA annealed with both $cDNA_{5'}$ and $cDNA_{3'}$, whereas the large fragment from the internal region annealed only with $cDNA_{3'}$. The *Eco*RI fragment from the left end of linear DNA annealed only with $cDNA_{3'}$, whereas the penultimate *Eco*RI-*Bam*HI fragment annealed with both $cDNA_{3'}$ and $cDNA_{5'}$.

The generality of this structure for linear retroviral DNA is now

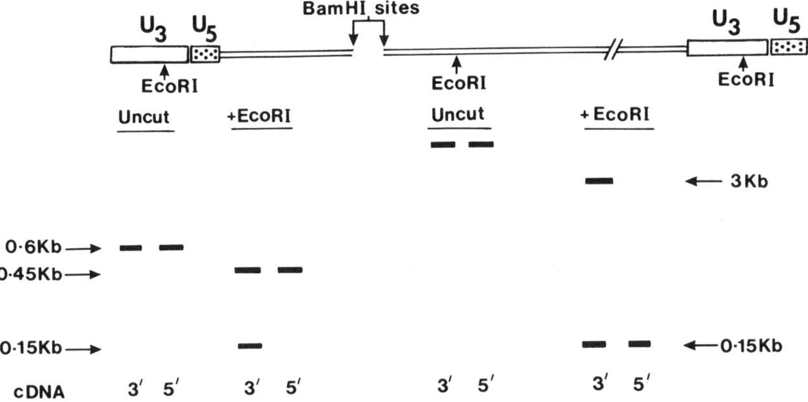

Figure 5.5 Strategy for definition of the terminal redundancies in linear DNA. Illustrated schematically is an experiment performed by Shank et al. (1978b) to characterize the sequences repeated at the ends of viral linear DNA isolated from the cytoplasm of cells acutely infected with RSV. *Bam*HI fragments from the left and right ends of linear DNA were isolated from slices of a preparative agarose gel, and each was subjected to a secondary digestion with *Eco*RI; the relevant sites are shown at the top of the figure (and in Fig. 5.3). The resulting fragments and the uncut *Bam*HI fragments were examined by gel electrophoresis, transfer to nitrocellulose paper, and hybridization with cDNAs specific for U_3 and U_5 ($cDNA_{3'}$ and $cDNA_{5'}$). The lower part of the figure shows a schematic version of the autoradiographs and the sizes of fragments represented by each band.

well established, based on restriction mapping studies of DNA from cells infected with MLV, MSV (Goldfarb and Weinberg 1979; Yoshimura and Weinberg 1979), MMTV (Shank et al. 1978a; Cohen et al. 1979b), REV (Keshet et al. 1979), FeLV, and FeSV (Sherr et al. 1979; Mullins et al. 1980). Moreover, terminally redundant duplexes have been synthesized in vitro using detergent-disrupted virions of MLV and MSV (Benz and Dina 1979; Gilboa et al. 1979b; Verma 1979; Bosselman and Verma 1980; Dina and Benz 1980). The abundance of the in vitro products has permitted a particularly satisfying validation of the structure proposed in Figure 5.4, using detailed mapping with restriction endonucleases and heteroduplex mapping with the 3′ terminus of viral RNA. Further validation of the direct repeats has come from analysis of cloned viral DNA molecules from several sources (Hager et al. 1979; Tronick et al. 1979; Vande Woude et al. 1979, 1981; DeLorbe et al. 1980; Dhar et al. 1980; Ju et al. 1980; Ju and Skalka 1980; Majors and Varmus 1980; Shimotohno et al.

1980; Sutcliffe et al. 1980; Van Beveren et al. 1980; Mullins et al. 1981; Swanstrom et al. 1981), although the linear species itself has only recently been cloned intact from infected cells (Scott et al. 1981).

By sequencing LTRs cloned as part of circular or integrated species of viral DNA, it has been found that the unit contains short repeated sequences in an inverted orientation (inverted repeats) near or at its ends. These inverted repeats vary in length among virus strains and are not always perfect repeats. Moreover, interpretation of the sequencing data must take into account the material used for the analysis. For example, it is now generally agreed that a small number of base pairs, usually two, are missing from each end of integrated viral DNA (see Section III.C.2), and circular DNA frequently exhibits significant heterogeneity in the region in which the two copies of the LTR have been joined (the "circle junction"; see Section III.B.3.c). An assessment of the true limits of the LTR will depend ultimately on direct inspection of the ends of linear DNA. Until linear DNA has been fully analyzed, provisional predictions must be made. The U_5 sequence at the right end is almost certain to terminate with the first base added to the tRNA primer; the identity of this terminus can thus be inferred from the sequence of short in vitro transcripts (e.g., strong-stop minus strands). The boundary of the U_3 sequence (i.e., the left end) is more difficult to predict. Arguments to date have been based largely on symmetry: circles that bear the entire U_5 sequence at the circle junction are likely to bear the entire U_3 sequence at the junction; proviruses that lack 2 bp of the U_5 sequence on the right end are likely to lack 2 bp of the U_3 sequence on the left; inverted repeat sequences are unlikely to extend beyond the ends of U_3 or U_5; and different retroviruses probably initiate plus-strand synthesis (thereby determining the end of U_3) at the same position within the highly homologous polypurine tracts which seem to encompass the 5′ boundary of the U_3 region. On the basis of such considerations, it has been estimated that an inverted repeat at the ends of the RSV LTR is 15 bases long, with 3 bases mismatched (Swanstrom et al. 1981b); the inverted repeats of Mo-MSV or MLV DNA comprise 13 bases of perfectly matched sequence or 23 bases, of which 18 are matched (Dhar et al. 1980; Shoemaker et al. 1980; Sutcliffe et al. 1980; Van Beveren et al. 1980); the inverted repeats of SNV DNA are only 5 bases in length (Shimotohno et al. 1980); and the inverted repeats of MMTV DNA are 6 bases long and are exceptional in that they begin with the third base from the probable ends of the LTR (Majors and Varmus 1980, 1981; Donehower et al. 1981).

Although the functional significance of the inverted repeats is unknown, they could be important in either circularization or integration of viral DNA, as discussed below. Furthermore, they suggest that viral DNA is closely related in structural organization to certain transposable elements of bacteria. Tn*9*, for example, is terminated by direct repeats of IS*1*, an element that contains an imperfect inverted repeat (18 of 25 bases) at its ends (MacHattie and Jackowski 1977; Ohtsubo and Ohtsubo 1978). The analogy with transposable elements is strengthened by recent evidence that a short cellular sequence at the integration site is duplicated during insertion of proviral DNA (see Section III.C).

(ii) LOCATION. Linear duplex DNA can generally be detected in the cytoplasm of infected cells within a few hours after infection. The most compelling evidence in favor of the cytoplasm as the site of synthesis comes from studies in which enucleated avian cells were infected with RSV; both strands of linear DNA were synthesized at about equal efficiency in enucleated and whole cells (Varmus et al. 1974, 1975). Additional support for this conclusion has come from measurement of viral DNA in the cytoplasmic fraction of whole cells (Varmus et al. 1974, 1978; Guntaka et al. 1976; Fritsch and Temin 1977a; Shank and Varmus 1978) and perhaps specifically in the plasma-membrane portion (Kakefuda et al. 1974). Approaches to this question, which have used labeled parental RNA (Dales and Hanafusa 1972; Sveda et al. 1974, 1976; Leis et al. 1975; Takano and Hatanaka 1975) or direct labeling of viral DNA (Hatanaka et al. 1971; Robin et al. 1974; Lovinger et al. 1975), have provided uncertain and, in some cases, conflicting results; these experiments are difficult to interpret in view of the large number of irrelevant (noninfectious) parental particles and the small amount of viral DNA synthesized relative to nuclear and mitochondrial DNAs. The cytoplasm, however, may not be an obligatory site of DNA synthesis for all retroviruses; visna virus DNA appears to be made in the nucleus, though perhaps initiated in the cytoplasm (A. Haase, unpubl.).

(iii) FUNCTION. The precise role of the linear duplex DNA in the life cycle of retroviruses has yet to be determined. There is substantial evidence that linear DNA is infectious in transfection experiments (Smotkin et al. 1975, 1976; Fritsch and Temin 1977a; Copeland et al. 1981), although it is unlikely that transfection resembles natural infection. Perhaps more tellingly, linear DNA has been shown to migrate from the cytoplasm to the nucleus, where it forms covalently closed circles (Shank and Varmus 1978). This was done by labeling cytoplasmic linear RSV DNA in both strands with BrdU, then following the migration of dense DNA into the nucleus and its conversion into closed circular forms during a subsequent chase with thymidine. However, only a minority of linear cytoplasmic molecules followed this course; it is not known whether the molecules that do circularize have special structural features.

As discussed in a later section, it is possible that linear DNA is integrated directly into host-cell DNA; certainly, the structural similarities between unintegrated linear duplexes and proviruses are striking (Fig. 5.4). It is also possible that these unintegrated species might be able to serve as template for the synthesis of viral RNA, but there is no direct evidence for this (see Section IV.B.1.a for further discussion). It is, however, very unlikely that unintegrated linear DNA ever serves as a template for DNA replication; even in chronically infected cells, which sometimes contain significant amounts of free DNA (Guntaka et al. 1976; Varmus and Shank 1976; Ringold et al. 1977c, 1978; B. Traynor and A. Haase, unpubl.), the DNA always seems to be transcribed from a template of RNA, as in acute infection.

Accumulation of up to 100–200 copies of free linear DNA in avian cells infected by SNV or certain cytopathic strains of RAV has been correlated with cell death, but the pathogenic mechanism is not known (Keshet and Temin 1979; Weller et al. 1980). One additional possible function for linear DNA warrants mention: the multiple plus strands present in some of these molecules could facilitate virus recombination according to certain models (Hunter 1978).

c. Circular DNA. (i) STRUCTURE. Closed circular retroviral DNA was first identified in acutely infected cells, using radioactive probes to measure small amounts of DNA that banded in dense regions of equilibrium gradients containing buoyant dyes and sedimented rapidly in rate-zonal gradients of alkaline sucrose (Gianni et al. 1975; Guntaka et al. 1975). Most of the circular molecules appear to be approximately the same size as linear DNA (i.e., about the length of an RNA subunit). The closed circular forms have subsequently been documented by migration in agarose gels, enzymic conversion to open circular and linear forms, mapping with restriction endonucleases, and direct visualization in the electron microscope after purification (Gianni et al. 1976; Guntaka et al. 1976; Fritsch and Temin 1977a; Kakefuda et al. 1977; Ringold et al. 1977c; Hsu et al. 1978a,b; Shank et al. 1978a,b; Clements et al. 1979). In addition, circular DNA has been amplified in bacterial host-vector systems after linearization with restriction endonucleases, and the cloned molecules were usually found to exhibit the expected permutation of sequence in relation to the natural linear DNA (Hager et al. 1979; DeLorbe et al. 1980; Ju et al. 1980; Ju and Skalka 1980; Shoemaker et al. 1980; Verma et al. 1980; Buetti and Diggelmann 1981).

However, as in the case of linear DNA, attempts to generate restriction maps of circular DNA from infected cells produced some intriguing anomalies. These were explained by proposing that some (usually most) circles have one copy, and some have two copies, of the LTR sequence (U_3RU_5) terminally repeated in linear DNA (Hsu et al. 1978b; Shank et al. 1978b; Taylor 1979; Varmus et al. 1979b). This formulation was consistent with several unexpected observations: (1) Two species of circular DNA that migrate closely in agarose gels can be recovered from cells infected by several retroviruses (Hsu et al. 1978b; Shank et al. 1978a,b, 1981; Yoshimura and Weinberg 1979), (2) these species differ in size by the length of the LTR sequence in each type of linear DNA, (3) restriction enzymes that cleave outside the repeated sequence generate two fragments that differ by the length of the repeat unit, and (4) restriction enzymes that cleave once within the LTR (e.g., *Pvu*I and *Eco*RI for RSV DNA) produce a fragment that is equal in size to the LTR and anneals with probes specific for U_3 and U_5 sequences (Shank et al. 1978b).

Recent studies of cloned circular DNA have substantiated this model. Most of the cloned molecules bear one or two copies of the LTR, and the two copies are generally found as a direct tandem repeat (Hager et al. 1979; DeLorbe et al. 1980; Ju et al. 1980; Shoemaker et al. 1980; Swanstrom et al. 1981b). The cloning experiments have also produced molecules with three, as well as two or one, copies of the LTR, but it is likely that such molecules are generated during the cloning procedures (Hager et al. 1979; Tronick et al. 1979; Chan et al. 1980; S. Hughes, unpubl.). Many of the cloned circular molecules with two LTRs manifest atypical features that probably reflect various mechanisms for circularization; these are considered in Section III.B.4.f.

Although the vast majority of circular DNA can be considered monomeric (i.e., the same length as linear DNA or smaller by the length of one LTR sequence), small quantities of dimeric and even trimeric closed circular species can be recovered from RSV-infected cells (Goubin and Hill 1979; Kung et al. 1980). These oligomers are composed of monomeric units linked head-to-tail, rather than head-to-head (Kung et al. 1980). Closed circles of considerably less than monomeric size have also been identified in cells infected with certain strains of RSV (Guntaka et al. 1976). The detailed structure of these molecules has not been determined; they may be derived from deletion mutants in the infecting stocks.

(ii) LOCATION. Circular DNA has been recovered only from the nuclear fraction of infected cells (Guntaka et al. 1976; Fritsch and Temin 1977a) and only after sufficient time has elapsed for linear DNA to be synthesized and transported to the nucleus (Shank and Varmus 1978). It is possible that the nucleus provides functions essential for correct circularization of linear DNA (see III.B.4.f).

(iii) FUNCTION. The discovery of closed circular forms of retroviral DNA excited speculation about the similarities of these viruses to well-studied DNA viruses (such as papovaviruses and lambdoid phages) for which genomic circles appear essential for replication and (at least in the case of phage λ) for integration into host chromosomes. However, to date there is no evidence that unintegrated retroviral DNA (circular or linear) constitutes a replicon capable of semiconservative replication, and it is unknown whether circular DNA serves as a substrate for integrative recombination during natural infection. Circular DNA is known to be infectious when administered directly to cells, but the specific infectivity appears to be modestly reduced relative to that of linear DNA (Smotkin et al. 1976; Fritsch and Temin 1977a). Moreover, the structure of proviruses acquired after transfection with circular DNA appears to differ from that of naturally acquired proviruses: no specificity for sites in viral DNA has been observed during integration of transfecting circular RSV DNA (P. Luciw, pers. comm.), whereas natural proviruses are always linked to cellular DNA via the terminal redundancies (cf. Fig. 5.4). Transfection remains a poorly defined process that may not accurately recapitulate natural infection; hence it is difficult to predict the role of circular DNA in the replication cycle from these experiments. Circular forms, particularly the oligomers, are candidates for roles in interviral recombination as well as integration, but no direct evidence is available.

4. Mechanisms Involved in the Synthesis of Retroviral DNA

The major product of viral DNA synthesis is the linear duplex molecule described above. In the following sections, we outline the steps involved in the synthesis of this molecule and its conversion to circular forms.

a. Initiation of the First (Minus) Strand of Viral DNA. The first step in the synthesis of viral DNA involves the addition of deoxynucleotides to the 3′ end of a cellular tRNA species positioned 100–200 nucleotides from the 5′ terminus of viral RNA. This step has been examined in particular detail in vitro, using either endogenous or reconstructed reactions (cf. Section III.B.2), but the structure of viral DNA from infected cells confirms that DNA synthesis is initiated near the 5′ end of the viral genome, almost certainly by the same mechanism.

The position of the primer poses an immediate obstacle to the polymerase's effort to elongate the newly initiated strand: template RNA is exhausted within 100–200 bases from the initiation point. On one hand, this dictates the accumulation in vitro of a useful short intermediate (strong-stop DNA) complementary to the entire sequence from the end of the primer-binding site to the end of the genome. The length of this species provides a fairly reliable estimate of the position of the tRNA primer for each retrovirus (Haseltine and Kleid 1978). The abundance of strong-stop DNA also permitted the first determination of interesting sequences from retroviral genomes (Haseltine et al. 1977a; Shine et al. 1977). On the other hand, the exhaustion of template implies that retroviruses must have developed a special mechanism for transferring the growing DNA chain from the finished template to a new one in order to complete transcription of the viral genome. It is worth noting that this requirement for transfer of nascent DNA chains between templates is not a consequence of the observed position of the primer. Any heteropolymeric primer base-paired with genomic RNA—i.e., any primer other than oligo(dT) base-paired with poly(A) at the 3′ end—would present the problem of preserving the primer-binding site and any genomic sequences to the 3′ side of it.

b. First Transfer between Templates. It is logical to assume that the polymerization of DNA would be relocated from the exhausted 5′ terminus to a 3′ terminus of viral RNA. The first sequencing studies of RSV cDNAs indicated that an identical sequence of 16–21 nucleotides was present at both the 3′ and 5′ termini of viral RNA (Haseltine et al. 1977a; Schwartz et al. 1977; Stoll et al. 1977). Similarly, an apparently identical sequence of about 50–60 nucleotides was found at both the 3′ and 5′ ends of Mo-MLV RNA (Coffin et al. 1978). The repeated sequence (R) is located immediately adjacent to the poly(A) tract at the 3′ end, and the inverted, capped nucleotide is located at the 5′ end. Since the poly(A) and "cap" residues are not copied into viral DNA (Reitz et al. 1972; Varmus et al. 1978) (they are presumably added to viral RNA posttranscriptionally), it seemed likely that the R sequence could be used to construct a bridge between the first and second templates (Coffin and Haseltine 1977a; Collett et al. 1977; Junghans et al. 1977; Stoll et al. 1977).

Figure 5.6 diagrams the manner in which this construction is cur-

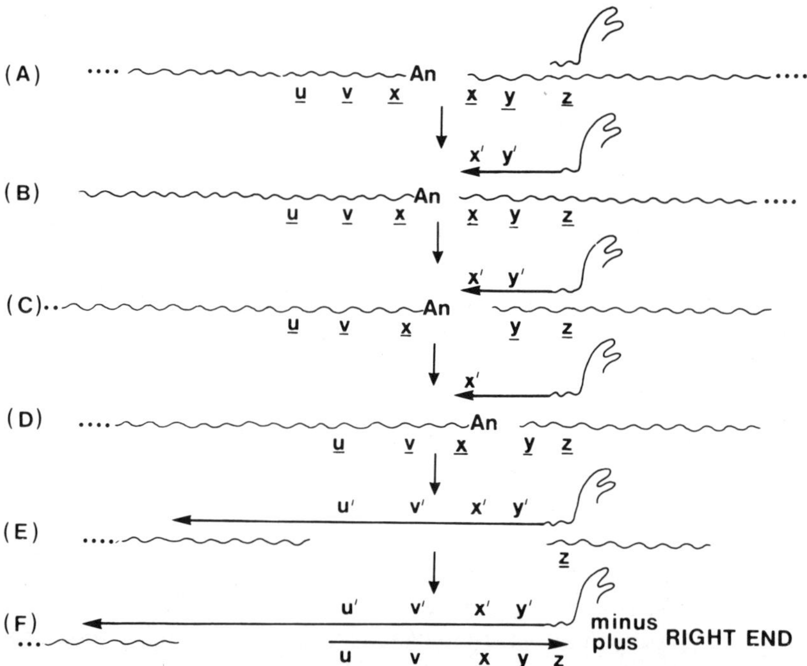

Figure 5.6 Mechanism for the first transfer between templates. The proposed sequence of events by which a nascent minus strand is transposed from the 5′ end of an exhausted template to a heteropolymeric region at a 3′ terminus is shown in schematic form. (u, v) Sequences unique to the 3′ terminus (U_3); (x) sequence (R) repeated at the ends of the RNA; (y) sequence unique to the 5′ terminus on the 5′ side of the primer-binding site (U_5); (z) primer-binding site. Details of the model are discussed in the text. (∼∼∼) RNA; (———) DNA. Arrows indicate the direction of synthesis (5′→3′). The diagram is intentionally ambiguous about whether one or two subunits of the viral genome are employed in these steps. If the ends belong to a single subunit, the intermediates shown in D and E will be circular.

rently envisioned. The model requires the following steps: (1) completion of strong-stop DNA, (2) displacement or digestion of a portion of the 5′ end of the RNA template, (3) base pairing between the R sequence at the 3′ end of strong-stop DNA and its complement adjacent to poly(A) at the 3′ end of a viral RNA subunit, and (4) continued DNA-polymerizing activity to extend the 3′ end of the minus strand on the new template.

There are several clear predictions of this model, most of which have now been validated. First, the RNA:DNA hybrid that results from the completion of strong-stop DNA should be susceptible to strand displacement or to the action of viral or cellular RNase H. Particularly under conditions that promote correct transfer between templates, the 5′ terminus of viral RNA is, in fact, digested during polymerase reactions in vitro, presumably by viral RNase H, despite the presence of the cap nucleotide (Darlix et al. 1977a; Collett et al. 1978a; Friedrich and Moelling 1979). Second, the predicted base pairing should generate an intermediate composed of one DNA strand linking two ends of viral RNA; if the ends of viral RNA belong to the same subunit, a circle will be formed. Although circles of this type have not been observed directly, they can be formed by annealing extended cDNA to viral RNA (Junghans et al. 1977; Rothenberg et al. 1978). Third, minus strands extended in this manner should contain only a single copy of the sequence (R) repeated at the ends of the RNA. This prediction has been validated for cDNA synthesized in vitro by detergent-disrupted virions of MLV (Haseltine et al. 1979; I. Verma, unpubl.) and RSV (Amer et al. 1981; Swanstrom et al. 1981b) and for DNA from infected cells by sequencing of DNA amplified in bacteria (Dhar et al. 1980; Sutcliffe et al. 1980; Van Beveren et al. 1980; Swanstrom et al. 1981a,b).

The sacrifice of one of the two copies of R in viral RNA during the initial phase of reverse transcription poses an important theoretical problem: How is the second copy regenerated? Although many interesting solutions were advanced (Haseltine and Baltimore 1976a; Bishop 1978), retroviruses appear to have engineered the most curious. Sequences from the termini of viral RNA are present at both ends of the linear product of DNA synthesis; hence, R is present at each end of linear DNA (Fig. 5.4). The genesis of this structure requires a second transfer between templates; the mechanism for the second transfer is less completely understood and is considered later in this section.

One important aspect of the first transfer remains obscure: Does the "jump" occur only between ends of the same subunit, only between the two RNA subunits present in each dimeric genome, or can either occur? The answer would be helpful to an understanding of the structure and function of the dimer and would have implications for models for genetic recombination (see Chapter 7). Recent experiments by R. Friedrich (unpubl.) using detergent-activated virions argue that the first jump occurs principally between two ends of the same subunit.

c. Elongation of the Minus Strand. DNA synthesis resumes after the first jump by elongation of strong-stop DNA along an extensive template of viral RNA. Compared to examples of DNA synthesis in other contexts, there are several notable features of the polymerization: it may be relatively slow, it is error-prone, and it is probably continuous. The rate has been measured in several ways: by determining the average length of minus strands at various times after infection by RSV (Varmus et al. 1978; Boone and Skalka 1981a), and by measuring the time required to transcribe templates of known length by MLV, MSV, RAV, and AMV polymerases in vitro (Dube and Loeb 1976; Rothenberg and Baltimore 1977; Dina and Benz 1980; Boone and Skalka 1981a). According to most of these estimates, nucleotides are added at a rate of about 0.5–1 per second; thus, about 3 hours is required to synthesize a complete copy of viral RNA in vivo or in vitro. However, a 5- to 10-fold more rapid rate was observed with mellitin-treated RAV particles (Boone and Skalka 1981a). Most known DNA polymerases work 10- to 1000-fold faster than reverse transcriptase (Edenberg and Huberman 1975). It is not known whether the relatively slow rate observed for reverse transcription is an inherent property of the viral enzyme or consequent to structural features of its template. The fidelity of retroviral polymerase is also less than that exhibited by other DNA polymerases (Battula and Loeb 1974; Weymouth and Loeb 1978; Gopinathan et al. 1979), despite its slow rate of elongation. The genetic implications of this observation are considered elsewhere (Chapter 4). Finally, it appears likely that extension of the minus strand occurs continuously, without additional independent priming events, for as many as 10,000 nucleotides; however, the possibility that elongation occurs by discontinuous synthesis has not been rigorously excluded.

d. Synthesis of Plus Strands. Much less is known about the manner in which the second (plus) strands are initiated and extended either in vivo or in vitro, although provocative clues have emerged from some recent studies.

(i) TEMPLATE:PRIMER. It is generally assumed that the second strand is templated by the first strand and that viral RNA is removed prior to synthesis of plus-strand DNA, but it is less obvious how plus strands are initiated. There is evidence from in vitro studies (described in Section III.B.1.e) to support the reasonable presumption that plus-strand synthesis depends on hydrolysis of viral RNA by the RNase-H activity of the viral polymerase, once an RNA:DNA hybrid has been formed by synthesis of the first strand. However, the existence of such hybrids has yet to be demonstrated convincingly in infected cells, and it remains possible that nascent minus-strand DNA is in a single-stranded form. There is, moreover, an additional unexplained difficulty. The poly(A) tract at the 3′ end of viral RNA is ignored during reverse transcription (Reitz et al. 1972; Varmus et al. 1978) and, hence, is not converted into a hybrid form acceptable to the RNase-H activity; nevertheless, the poly(A) sequence may need to be removed from any hybrid structure, since RNase H is an exonuclease apparently unable to attack a hybrid with a tail of single-stranded RNA (Leis et al. 1973; Verma 1975a). Despite this problem, the proposal that RNase H removes the used RNA template to make way for synthesis of plus strands has a particularly attractive feature: RNase H reduces RNA to oligomers, rather than to single nucleotides (Leis et al. 1973), and these might be appropriate for use as primers for plus strands. Furthermore, the viral nuclease might preserve the specificity necessary to produce efficient primers at certain points along the genome, thereby accounting for discrete species of subgenomic plus strands (see below). As noted in the following section, plus strands appear prior to completion of minus strands in infected cells (Varmus et al. 1978); hence, it is highly unlikely that the second strand is normally primed by formation of a self-complementary hairpin at the end of the first strand. (This is known, however, to occur during the copying of certain templates in vitro by reverse transcriptase; see Section III.B.1.e).

(ii) LENGTHS OF PLUS STRANDS AND KINETICS OF APPEARANCE. Although initially considered to be mainly heterogeneous and small (4S–10S) after synthesis either in vivo or in vitro (see, e.g., Gianni and Weinberg 1975; Varmus et al. 1976; Verma 1978), plus strands have recently been found to include some uniformly sized components that are likely to be important to the mode of synthesis of linear DNA. The first indication that this might be so emerged from studies of RSV DNA in acutely infected quail cells (Varmus et al. 1978). The first plus strands to appear after infection comprised a homogeneous class with the length (~300–350 nucleotides) and sequence content of the LTR unit (U_3RU_5) repeated at both ends of linear DNA. These strands were first detected by annealing cDNA probes specific for the 3′ and 5′ termini of viral RNA to denatured DNA fractionated in sucrose gradients or polyacrylamide gels after isolation from cells infected for 1 to 3 hours. Analogous plus strands have subsequently been identified in the products of in vitro synthesis by MLV and MSV polymerases (~600 nucleotides) (Mitra et al. 1979; Dina and Benz 1980) and in cells infected by MLV (~600 nucleotides) (H.J. Kung, unpubl.) or by MMTV (~1200 nucleotides) (Kung et al. 1981). This class of plus strand appears prior to completion of the minus strand and has been mapped to the right end of the intermediates in DNA synthesis; hence, it is primed at a relatively restricted site near the 5′ end of the minus strand.

For mechanistic reasons that will be described below, it is extremely likely that the initiation site for this plus strand defines the boundary of the U_3 component of the LTR unit. Since the complete repeat unit is terminated by short inverted repeats, it is possible to predict the start point for plus-strand synthesis to within a few bases. Sequencing studies of cloned DNA from this region of the genome have revealed a striking degree of similarity among several retroviruses. In all cases examined, the inverted repeat in U_3 is flanked by a run of purines; MMTV and RSV DNAs have an identical 10-base sequence (AG_5AATG) spanning the putative priming site (Czernilofsky et al. 1980b; Majors and Varmus 1980, 1981; Swanstrom et al. 1981), and the homologous regions of Mo-MLV and MSV DNAs (AG_6AATG) and of SNV DNA (TG_4AATG) are very similar (Dhar et al. 1980; Shimotohno et al. 1980; Sutcliffe et al. 1980; see Appendix D and E). On the basis of sequence analysis of circular and integrated DNAs, the 5′ end of the plus strand initiated near the U_3 boundary probably begins with the sequence AATG. This prediction has recently been validated in studies of MLV DNA synthesized in vitro (S. Mitra et al., pers. comm.). The elongation of this plus strand must soon be impeded by exhaustion of the minus-strand DNA template. (The possibility that a portion of the tRNA primer for the minus strand is used as template for the end of this plus strand will be considered in a later section.)

The initial synthesis of plus-strand DNA obviously resembles, in some features, the initial synthesis of the minus strand; by analogy, the product has been called plus-strand strong stop (Gilboa et al. 1979a; Mitra et al. 1979). A model in which the plus-strand strong stop is used to prime synthesis of longer plus strands, including full-length plus strands, is discussed in Section III.B.4.

Following synthesis of the plus-strand strong stop, a more heterogeneous collection of plus-strand DNAs appears in RSV-infected cells (Varmus et al. 1978). These strands represent most of the RSV genome and have been found to include several discrete size classes that anneal with cDNAs specific for various regions of the genome (Kung et al. 1981). These results indicate the existence of multiple sites for preferential priming of RSV plus strands; however, similar discrete species of subgenomic plus-strand DNAs other than plus-strand strong stop have not been observed in the DNAs of other retroviruses (Mitra et al. 1979; Chen and Temin 1980; Kung et al. 1981).

Plus strands equivalent in length to linear DNA are rare in RSV-infected cells (Shank and Varmus 1978; Varmus et al. 1978; Kung et al. 1981) but have been found in MLV DNA synthesized in vitro (Gilboa et al. 1979a) and in vivo (H.J. Kung, unpubl.) and in MMTV DNA and SNV DNA synthesized in vivo (Chen and Temin 1980; Kung et al. 1981). The plus strands of SNV DNA contain occasional ribonucleotides; these seem likely to result from misincorporation, rather than failure to remove vestiges of plus-strand primers, since ribonucleotides are also found in the minus strand, which is probably synthesized continuously (Chen and Temin 1980). The mechanism for synthesis of full-length plus strands is considered below.

e. Second Transfer between Templates. The mechanisms discussed thus far account for a linear molecule that can be represented as ———U_3RU_5, with synthesis of the first strand proceeding from right to left; but structural studies of completed linear DNA have demonstrated that the termini are redundant: U_3RU_5———U_3RU_5. This means that the polymerase must synthesize a copy of the tRNA primer-binding site preceding the U_5 sequence, the U_5 sequence, R, and a sequence of a few hundred nucleotides derived from the 3′ terminus (U_3) of viral RNA. It is obvious that more than one template is required to complete these steps, and at least two kinds of mechanisms can be envisioned (Fig. 5.7). In the first model (Fig. 5.7a), the polymerase would read to the end of the RNA template from which most of the minus strand has been transcribed; then the growing DNA chain would be transferred to a 3′ terminus of viral RNA, much in the fashion proposed for the first "jump." One obvious problem with this mechanism is that the polymerase must terminate synthesis of the minus strand at a defined point in the 3′ sequence previously copied without cessation. In addition, the model does not conform to recent experimental observations discussed below.

In the second model (Fig. 5.7b), the jump would be made from an RNA template to a DNA template, rather than between RNA templates. Proposal of this mechanism (Shank et al. 1978b; Baltimore et al. 1979; Varmus et al. 1979b) was initially stimulated by two findings: (1) Rothenberg et al. (1977, 1978) had shown that in vitro synthesis of the final 600 nucleotides of the MLV minus strand did not occur in the presence of actinomycin D, and (2) Varmus et al. (1978) had identified the short plus strand in RSV-infected cells (plus-strand strong stop) that would constitute an appropriate template for completing the minus strands. The use of plus strands of this type as templates would explain the abrupt termination of linear DNA within the viral 3′ sequence, and DNA-directed synthesis of minus-strand DNA would explain the observed sensitivity to actinomycin D. To permit the minus strand to form a bridge between the RNA and DNA templates, the minus strand would have to be extended into or beyond the primer-binding site, and the plus-strand strong stop would have to include at least a short sequence complementary to the 3′ end of the growing minus strand. The former

Figure 5.7 Alternative mechanisms for the second transfer of reverse transcriptase between templates. (*a*) Model I illustrates a mechanism similar to that proposed for the first transfer (cf. Fig. 5.6); (*b*) model II shows the currently favored mechanism for the second transfer, using plus-strand strong stop as the final template. (〰〰) RNA; (———) DNA. For both models, the diagrams are again intentionally ambiguous about whether one or two subunits of viral RNA are involved in the generation of a single molecule of linear DNA. It is possible to draw models in which two molecules of linear DNA are derived from a single dimeric genome; for simplicity, these possibilities are not illustrated. The dashed line representing primer tRNA in Model II (line A) implies that the primer may or may not remain base-paired with the genomic subunit, depending on whether it has been used as a primer. For discussion of these models, see text.

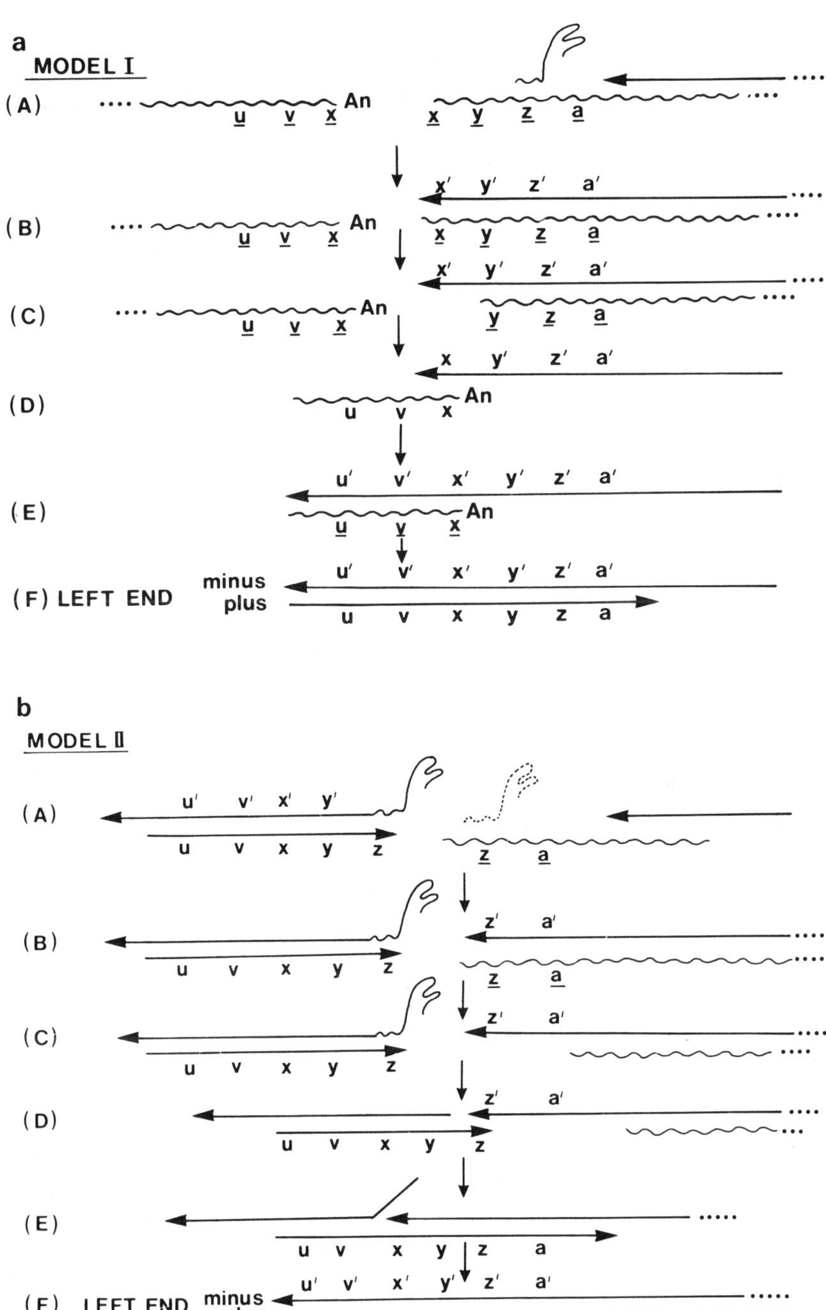

Figure 5.7 (See facing page.)

requirement probably involves displacement of the tRNA primer from its binding site on genomic RNA, a feat that may require factors in addition to the viral polymerase. The latter requirement could be achieved by extension of the plus-strand strong stop beyond the initiation point for minus-strand strong stop, using the 3′ terminus of primer tRNA as template. In this way, a bridge could be constructed, using the sequence of the primer-binding site in the manner illustrated in Figure 5.7b. Once transferred to the plus-strand template, the minus strand would be extended to the point within the 3′ sequence at which plus-strand strong stop was initiated. In addition, the plus strand could then be extended, using the minus strand as template, to generate long, even genome-length, plus strands.

This model makes several predictions, some of which have recently been validated experimentally.

1. Prior to the second jump, the minus strand need not contain a copy of the U_5 sequence. Gilboa et al. (1979a) prepared a physical map of the 3′ end of MLV minus strands synthesized in vitro in the presence of actinomycin D and showed that the unfinished minus strand includes little, if any, sequence complementary to viral RNA beyond the primer-binding site. This result implies that the minus strand would be unable to form the bridge required for the model in Figure 5.7a and thus favors the second model.
2. Plus-strand strong stop with the size and genetic content of the redundant U_3RU_5 sequences should be found in early DNA intermediates of all retroviruses. Thus far, this prediction has been confirmed for RSV (Varmus et al. 1978; Kung et al. 1981), MLV (Gilboa et al. 1979a; Mitra et al. 1979; Dina and Benz 1980; H.J. Kung, unpubl.), and MMTV (Kung et al. 1981) (see above).
3. Plus-strand strong stop should be extended at its 3′ end to include a partial copy of the tRNA primer for the minus strand. The experiments of Gilboa et al. (1979a) and of Taylor and Hsu (1980) indicate that the right end of linear MLV DNA or RSV DNA synthesized in vitro contains a single-stranded tail of about 15–20 nucleotides; indirect evidence strongly suggests that the tail is composed of plus strand. Similar results have been obtained with an early intermediate of RSV DNA from infected cells (R. Swanstrom, unpubl.). These presumed copies of the 3′ end of primer tRNAs are striking in a number of ways: their lengths

are similar, if not identical, to those of the primer-binding sites, and they may therefore terminate (as do the primer-binding sites) adjacent to the first base (m_1A), unacceptable as a template for DNA synthesis.

4. Following the second jump, long plus strands may be synthesized by extension of the plus-strand strong stop. Plus strands as long as minus strands have been produced during synthesis of MLV DNA in vitro (Gilboa et al. 1979a; Bosselman and Verma 1980; Dina and Benz 1980) and may result from extension of the preexisting plus-strand strong stop. The rarity of full-length plus strands in RSV linear DNA need not be incompatible with this model. The differences may simply reflect the extent to which primers are generated for synthesis of plus strands. If several are generated, as during synthesis of RSV DNA, the second strands may be largely "filled in" with subgenomic plus strands by the time of the second jump; if few are generated, as may be the case during synthesis of MLV DNA (Gianni and Weinberg 1975; Gilboa et al. 1979a), or MMTV DNA (Kung et al. 1981), then the relocated plus strands could be fully extended by the gap-filling activity of the viral polymerase. However, there has as yet been no direct demonstration that plus-strand strong stop positioned initially at the right end of early DNA intermediates is later transferred to the left end of linear DNA or that this molecule is the primer for longer plus strands.
5. The completed linear molecule should have at least one fully duplex terminus, and perhaps two. Sequences from the only cloned linear DNA suggest both ends are flush (Scott et al. 1981).

The second model for the second jump, despite its attractions, leaves some questions open. It does not, for example, provide an explanation for the necessary displacement of the plus strand from its original template of minus-strand DNA. Purified reverse transcriptase appears unable to effect displacement synthesis using gapped template:primers in vitro (Hurwitz and Leis 1972). On the other hand, duplex DNA bearing multiple, short, single-stranded tails has been identified biochemically and microscopically among products of synthesis by mellitin-activated RAV virions (Boone and Skalka 1981b; R. Junghans, unpubl.); these findings suggest that the virion-associated polymerase can effect strand displacement during synthesis of plus strands. The model is also ambiguous about whether one or two copies of plus-strand strong stop (each encoded by one or both subunits of viral RNA) figure(s) in the generation of a single linear molecule. Synthesis of two plus-strand strong-stop molecules would, of course, demand the prior synthesis of two extended minus strands. The use of both subunits would have interesting implications for viral genetics, since heterozygotic dimers could then produce viral DNA with differing termini, possibly including different R sequences (Wang et al. 1977). This could affect the infectivity of viral progeny if the R sequences were not sufficiently homologous to permit the first jump (Joho et al. 1978); in any case, genomes with different termini would be unlikely to persist, since the R sequence at the 3′ end is silent (i.e., not transcribed into DNA).

f. Conversion of Linear DNA to Circular Forms. A portion of the linear duplexes is transported to the nucleus and is converted to covalently closed, circular DNA (Shank and Varmus 1978). There is little or no evidence about the biochemistry of these steps, but it seems possible that host factors, perhaps some confined to the nucleus, are involved. On the other hand, small amounts of MLV and MSV open circular DNA bearing a single copy of the LTR have been synthesized in vitro by detergent-disrupted virions (Gilboa et al. 1979b; Dina and Benz 1980), and closed circles have been observed among the products of in vitro synthesis of RSV DNA (Clayman et al. 1979b; Guntaka 1980).

It is not known whether some of the linear molecules are favored for circularization. To form a closed circular duplex, of course, the plus strand must either be full length in the linear DNA (an apparently uncommon occurrence at least for RSV DNA) or gaps and nicks in the second strand must be repaired.

Joining of the ends of linear DNA to form circular species is likely to proceed in more than one way: homologous recombination between the redundant ends could produce the circle bearing a single copy of the LTR, and direct joining of the ends could produce the circle bearing two copies. The circularization step could be expedited by the existence of inverted repeats at the ends of linear DNA; base pairing between the 3′ and 5′ ends of each strand in the linear duplex would produce a cruciform structure at the joining point of a molecule that is, in effect, an open circle.

Comparisons of cloned circular molecules with two copies of the LTR indicate that circles differ with respect to the length of the U_3 and/or U_5 portions of the repeated sequence at the circle junctions (Highfield et al. 1980; Ju et al. 1980; Ju and Skalka 1980; Shoemaker et al. 1980; Swanstrom et al. 1981b). For example, one cloned RSV molecule retains the complete U_5 sequence and probably the complete U_3 sequence, judging from the inverted repeat at the junction point (Appendix D) but another molecule lacks 2 bases from the U_5 sequence and 61 bases from the U_3 sequence present in the first molecule (DeLorbe et al. 1980; Swanstrom et al. 1981b). The loss of 2 bp from U_5 suggests that a pseudointegration event, in which the right end of linear DNA has inserted near its own left end (in the U_3 region), may account for circles of this type. Shoemaker et al. (1980) have also observed circular molecules in which the LTRs are inverted and separated by an inverted unique sequence. Certain features of these molecules (a short [4 bp] duplication of unique sequence and a loss of 2 bp from the LTRs) suggest that they arise by the mechanism operative during integration into the host chromosome (see below). However, it is not known whether linear DNA or circles with one or two copies of the LTR are immediate precursors to the circles bearing these inversions. Heterogeneity among cloned circular DNAs is probably caused by differences in circularization in the infected cells, since similar aberrations have not arisen during growth of normal circular DNA in bacteria.

It is premature to speculate about the mechanism(s) by which dimeric and trimeric circles are formed.

C. Integration of Viral DNA into Host Chromosomes

Cells chronically infected with retroviruses carry anywhere from 1 to 20 copies of viral DNA covalently linked to the host genome. Association of viral DNA with high-molecular-weight cellular DNA has been shown using restriction enzymes to identify fragments of viral DNA joined to cellular DNA (see below), alkaline sucrose gradients to demonstrate viral sequences in strands much longer than the viral genome (Khoury and Hanafusa 1976; Varmus et al. 1976), and the network method to show viral DNA linked to cellular DNA containing reiterated sequences (Varmus et al. 1973b). For convenience, less rigorous methods (e.g., the SDS-NaCl precipitation method of Hirt [1967]) have also been used to assess integration. Integrated DNA has been observed within 9 hours after infection, prior to detectable synthesis of viral RNA (Varmus et al. 1973b; Ali and Baluda 1974), but the time course of integration has yet to be carefully defined. Likewise, there exist only crude estimates of the efficiency of integration; somewhere between a few percent and most of the newly synthesized DNA may be integrated (Varmus et al. 1973b, 1976; Khoury and Hanafusa 1976). In some cases, as many as 100 copies of unintegrated DNA have been observed in cells that ultimately acquire only a few copies of integrated DNA (Khoury and Hanafusa 1976), but it is not known whether this excess of unintegrated forms reflects inefficient transport to the nucleus, inefficient integration in some or all cells, or an abundance of DNA defective for integrative recombination. It is unlikely, however, to reflect saturation of integration sites (see below).

All chronically infected cells appear to contain integrated (proviral) DNA, often in the absence of detectable unintegrated DNA, suggesting that the integrated species is essential to perpetuation of the genome and its transcription into RNA. In a few cases, however, chronically infected cells contain unintegrated, as well as integrated, forms of viral DNA (Guntaka et al. 1976; Varmus and Shank 1976; Ringold et al. 1977c, 1978); the structure of this DNA (Varmus and Shank 1976) and the relationship of its synthesis to synthesis of viral RNA (Ringold et al. 1978) indicate that the unintegrated DNA is copied from RNA, rather than replicated by a semiconservative mechanism.

Technical advances in the study of viral DNA have revealed two cardinal characteristics of proviruses: (1) they are homogeneously organized, with a gene order colinear with that in viral RNA, and terminated on both sides by the U_3RU_5 sequence also redundant in linear and circular DNAs and (2) they may be accommodated at many different regions of host genomes.

1. Sites of Integration in the Host Genome

Several investigators have recently used restriction endonucleases to demonstrate that many sites in host DNA are able to accommodate a provirus (Battula and Temin 1977, 1978; Hughes et al. 1978, 1981c; Steffen and Weinberg 1978; Bacheler and Fan 1979, 1980; Canaani and Aaronson 1979; Cohen et al. 1979b; Gilmer and Parsons 1979; Keshet and Temin 1979; Ringold et al. 1979; Sabran et al. 1979; Jenkins and Cooper 1980). The strategy for these experiments was first employed by Botchan and his colleagues for the study of papovavirus DNA (Botchan and McKenna 1974; Botchan et al. 1976; Ketner and Kelly 1976). DNA from infected cells is digested with enzymes that cleave viral DNA at few or no sites (cf. Fig. 5.8), and the digestion products are analyzed by gel electrophoresis and molecular hybridization after transfer to nitrocellulose sheets. The distance between the ends of the provirus and the proximal restriction sites in host DNA can be determined from the sizes of fragments bearing viral DNA linked to host DNA.

The simplest strategy is to use an enzyme that fails to cleave viral DNA, e.g., *Eco*RI for proviruses of Mo-MLV; differences in *Eco*RI fragments bearing an MLV provirus imply that each copy of viral DNA is located at different positions in the host genome (Steffen and Weinberg 1978; Bacheler and Fan 1979, 1980; Canaani and Aaronson 1979; Van der Putten et al. 1979; Jahner et al. 1980). It is also possible to use enzymes that cleave viral DNA one or more times to characterize the integration site, provided that the internal structure of each provirus is analyzed. The latter strategy, though more formidable, yields smaller, more accurately measured fragments and can be used to develop a physical map of the region of cellular DNA into which a provirus has been inserted. For example,

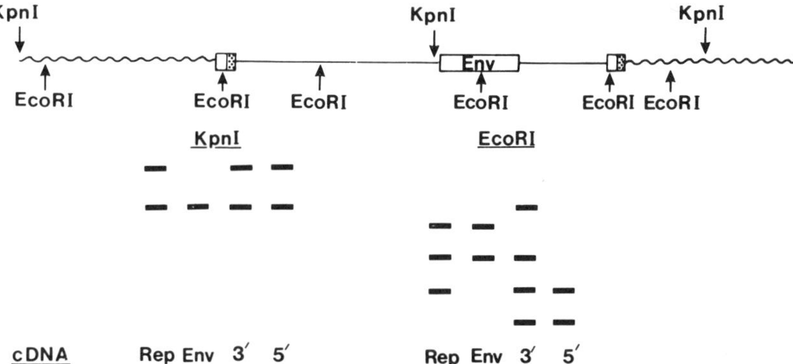

Figure 5.8 Strategy for determining the structure and location of proviral DNA with restriction endonucleases. The diagram illustrates with a single fictional provirus the strategy used by Hughes et al. (1978) to map RSV proviruses in clones of transformed rat cells. The top part shows proviral DNA (———) with terminal redundancies linked to cellular DNA (~~~~) with the relevant restriction sites. The lower part shows the predicted pattern of virus-specific bands on autoradiograms after DNA digested with *Kpn*I or *Eco*RI has been subjected to electrophoresis in agarose gels, transferred to nitrocellulose filters, and annealed with the indicated cDNAs labeled with ^{32}P. The region of the genome detected by $cDNA_{env}$ is shown in the top section. For a detailed picture of the terminal repetitions of RSV and their relationship to the *Eco*RI sites, see Fig. 5.3 through 5.5.

Hughes et al. (1978) used *Kpn*I, *Bam*HI, and *Eco*RI, which cleave RSV DNA one, three, and four times, respectively (cf. Fig. 5.3), to produce maps of integration sites of single proviruses in six clonal lines of RSV-transformed rat cells. An example of this strategy is diagrammed in Figure 5.8. In all cases, the maps of flanking host-cell DNA were completely unrelated, proving that six distinct regions of the host genome were employed as integration sites. A simple mathematical argument based on these and other clones suggested that there was a greater than 75% chance that more than 40 integration sites for RSV DNA exist in the rat genome (Hughes et al. 1978).

A wide range of biological materials has now been tested by such methods, e.g., clones and mass cultures of avian cells infected by RSV (Gilmer and Parsons 1979; Martin et al. 1979; Sabran et al. 1979; Hughes et al. 1981c); clones of mammalian (nonpermissive) cells transformed by RSV (Hughes et al. 1978; Collins et al. 1980; Quintrell et al. 1980); clones of mouse and rat cells infected by MLV (Steffen and Weinberg 1978; Bacheler and Fan 1979, 1980); clones of rat and mink cells infected by MMTV (Ringold et al. 1979; Majors and Varmus 1981); mass cultures of avian cells and clonal rat cells infected by SNV (Keshet and Temin 1978, 1979); and tissue infected by and tumors induced by ALVs (Neiman et al. 1980; Neel et al. 1981; Payne et al. 1981; H.J. Kung, unpubl.), MLV (Steffen and Weinberg 1978; Canaani and Aaronson 1979; Van der Putten et al. 1979; Jahner et al. 1980), MMTV (Cohen et al. 1979b; Cohen and Varmus 1980; Groner and Hynes 1980), and bovine leukemia virus (BLV) (Kettmann et al. 1979, 1980) and REV (H.J. Kung, unpubl.). In most cases, there was clear evidence that proviruses inhabited different sites after independent infections. Moreover, there was no evidence for tandem integration of new proviruses or for integration of a new provirus within virus-specific DNA endogenous to the host cell. Thus, the results argue against the existence of a small number of preferred sites for integration and against homologous recombination as a mechanism of integration. (The finding that a single region of the chicken genome is used as an integration site for at least one provirus in most tumors induced by ALV [Hayward et al. 1981; Neel et al. 1981; Payne et al. 1981] or by REV [H.J. Kung, unpubl.] probably reflects selection of cells with proviruses in that region rather than preferential integration; this problem is discussed in greater detail in Chapter 8 and in Section III.C.5.).

At least three qualifications should be placed upon these experiments: (1) Since eukaryotic cells contain over 10^9 possible integration sites, the method cannot exclude the existence of a large preferred subclass of sites; (2) since the nucleases cleave adjacent cellular DNA hundreds or thousands of nucleotides from the ends of the proviruses, the method defines the region of host DNA into which viral DNA was inserted, rather than the specific sequence to which it was joined; and (3) the procedure does not distinguish biologically active proviruses from inactive proviruses.

Despite these qualifications, the results cast serious doubt upon suggestions that the number of integration sites may be severely limited (Temin 1961; Khoury and Hanafusa 1976; Akiyami and Vogt 1979) or that integration occurs adjacent to homologous endogenous viral DNA (Shoyab et al. 1976). Some of these earlier observations may reflect the inadequacy of the technical procedures or other barriers to infection besides saturated integration sites (Khoury et al. 1979).

Other kinds of experimental approaches can be used to overcome the limitations of physical mapping with restriction enzymes alone.

1. Somatic-cell hybrids or physically fractionated chromosomes have been used to determine whether integration sites are distributed randomly among chromosomes. Proviruses acquired by infection with RSV have been found randomly distributed among fractionated chromosomes from infected chicken cells (Hughes et al. 1981c). On the other hand, provisional evidence from infected hybrid cells implicates human chromosome 6 as a favored, if not exclusive, integration locus for baboon endogenous virus (BaEV) DNA (Lemons et al. 1977, 1978).
2. Kettmann et al. (1979) fractionated DNA from bovine leukemia cells according to buoyant density and implicated a subpopulation of cellular DNA as possible sites for integration. However, the number of proviruses examined was small (four) in a selected population of cells, and this approach requires validation with a larger population of proviruses in a nonselected population of infected cells.
3. Prokaryotic cloning of restriction fragments containing ends of proviruses joined to host DNA allows sequencing of integration sites for several proviruses. In addition, DNA from flanking regions of cellular DNA can be used as a probe in tests of other integration sites or for heteroduplexing studies. Such tests indi-

cate little or no homology among sites for individual viruses (Vande Woude et al. 1979, 1980; Hager and Donehower 1980; Lowy et al. 1980; O'Rear et al. 1980; Shimotohno and Temin 1980; Shimotohno et al. 1980; Bacheler and Fan 1981; Majors and Varmus 1981; Hughes et al. 1981a).

4. Restriction fragments containing intact proviral DNA can be assayed by infectivity tests as well as physical tests. Studies of DNA from avian cells chronically infected by REVs indicate that biologically active proviruses may be present in only a limited number of sites, since a narrowly defined size class of infectious DNA fragments can be generated with an enzyme that does not cleave REV DNA (*Eco*RI) (Battula and Temin 1977, 1978; Keshet and Temin 1978). Similar tests of acutely infected cells, however, or physical measurements of proviruses in either acutely or chronically infected cells demonstrate that many sites can accommodate an REV provirus (Keshet and Temin 1978; Keshet et al. 1979). These results may mean that a large, but not unlimited, set of sites can acquire a provirus and that integration at different sites has different biological consequences (e.g., no viral gene expression, expression leading to cell death in the acute phase, or expression without toxic consequences). However, the infectious proviruses cloned from cells chronically infected with SNV have nonhomologous flanking sequences, despite the roughly similar sizes of the cloned *Eco*RI fragments (O'Rear et al. 1980).

2. *Structure of Proviral DNA*

In general, proviruses acquired by infection appear from restriction mapping to be colinear with unintegrated linear DNA and can be denoted cell DNA–U_3RU_5–(genes)–U_3RU_5–cell DNA (Hughes et al. 1978; Cohen et al. 1979b; Keshet et al. 1979; Ringold et al. 1979; Sabran et al. 1979). The principal exceptions to this rule are proviruses deleted for large regions of the genome, but these also appear in most cases to bear LTRs of U_3RU_5 (Hughes et al. 1978; Martin et al. 1979; Mason et al. 1979; Majors and Varmus 1980, 1981). This means that the provirus is linked to cellular DNA in a severely limited region of viral DNA, that viral genes are arranged in DNA as they are in viral RNA, and that a complete copy of viral RNA is flanked on both sides by extra sequences (U_3 and U_5) derived from the ends of viral RNA. (Proviral DNA lacking an LTR has been found in ALV-induced bursal lymphomas [Payne et al. 1981], but defective proviruses of this type may arise by deletion subsequent to integration [see Section III.C.5.f]).

The basis for these conclusions can be appreciated by reference to the restriction maps shown in Figure 5.3 and the structural model shown in Figure 5.4. Restriction endonucleases that cleave within linear viral DNA always generate the same internal fragments from nondeleted proviral DNA, even when they recognize sites close to the ends of linear DNA (e.g., *Pvu*I and *Eco*RI for RSV DNA or *Pst*I and *Sst*I for MMTV DNA). Similarly, viral sequences present in fragments from the ends of unintegrated linear DNA are found in fragments containing the ends of proviral DNA joined to host DNA. Prior to molecular cloning and sequencing, the structure of proviral DNA was best documented by the use of cDNAs specific for the 3′ and 5′ termini of viral DNA to detect fragments containing the ends of RSV proviral DNA (Hughes et al. 1978, 1981c; Martin et al. 1979; Quintrell et al. 1980). As predicted, fragments containing either end of a provirus could be detected with both $cDNA_{3'}$ and $cDNA_{5'}$ when the restriction enzyme (e.g., *Kpn*I or *Bam*HI) cleaved the provirus internally (Fig. 5.8). Cleavage within the U_3 sequence with *Eco*RI generated "joint fragments" that annealed either with $cDNA_{3'}$ only (left end) or with both $cDNA_{3'}$ and $cDNA_{5'}$ (right end) and internal fragments that anneal either with $cDNA_{3'}$ only (from the right side of the internal region) or with both probes (from the left side of the internal region) (Figure 5.8). Of the 20 proviruses examined with these techniques in 15 clones of RSV-transformed rat cells, at least 19 were shown to have the structure: cell DNA–U_3RU_5———U_3RU_5 –cell DNA, including several that displayed large deletions affecting genes required for virus replication (Hughes et al. 1978).

Definite confirmation of the structure proposed for proviral DNA has recently emerged from determinations of the sequences at the ends of proviruses cloned in bacteria. With mapping techniques alone, it was possible to estimate only that at least 200–250 nucleotides of the ~300-nucleotide U_3RU_5 repeat are maintained at both ends of RSV proviruses (Hughes et al. 1978; Sabran et al. 1979). Direct sequencing through the ends of cloned proviruses of many types into flanking host DNA has revealed that no more than a few base pairs (generally two) from the U_5 sequence are lacking on the right side of the provirus. Furthermore, the short inverted repeat sequence within the LTR unit appears to be retained in the U_3

sequence at the left end, again implying that no more than a few bases (again probably two) can be lost from unintegrated DNA during integration (Dhar et al. 1980; Hager and Donehower 1980; Shimotohno and Temin 1980; Shimotohno et al. 1980; Van Beveren et al. 1980; Majors and Varmus 1980, 1981; Hughes et al. 1981a).

In the few cases in which the junctions of viral and host DNAs have been sequenced, a provocative phenomenon has been observed: the same short sequence of host DNA (4–6 bases) is found at both ends of each provirus. Dhar et al. (1980) found the sequences AACG and CCCC flanking both sides of two MSV proviruses; Shimotohno et al. (1980) found the sequence AAAAT at both ends of an SNV provirus, and then reported five different 5-bp repeats flanking five other SNV proviruses (Shimotohno and Temin 1980); Majors and Varmus (1980, 1981) found the sequence GTAAGG at both ends of one MMTV provirus and the sequence GAGGTT at both ends of another provirus; and Hughes et al. (1981a) found the sequence CTGTGG flanking the ends of an RSV provirus in rat cells. Majors and Varmus (1980, 1981), Hughes et al. (1981a), R. Dhar (pers. comm.), and I. Verma (pers. comm.) also determined the sequence of the cellular site at which integration had occurred; the sequence repeated at the ends of the provirus was present only once in the unoccupied site, indicating that the duplication was generated during integration. Analogous observations have been made by Shoemaker et al. (1980) using a cloned circular species of Mo-MLV DNA, described earlier (Section III.B.4.f), in which the LTRs were inverted, reduced by 2 bp, and separated by nonrepeated DNA, as though the molecule had used itself as an integration site. A 4-base sequence (CTGA) present once at the putative integration site in Mo-MLV DNA was repeated at the ends of the LTRs in a manner expected from results with proviral DNA.

It has been widely recognized that the structure of proviral DNA closely resembles that of certain transposable elements of bacteria (Bukhari et al. 1977; Kleckner 1977; Calos and Miller 1980), yeast (Cameron et al. 1979), and *Drosophila* (Finnegan et al. 1978; Potter et al. 1979; Strobel et al. 1979). (For a recent survey of such elements, see *Cold Spring Harbor Symp. Quant. Biol.,* Vol. 45 [1981].) In most of these genetic units, a few thousand bases of nonrepeated sequences, generally encoding structural genes, are terminated by direct and/or inverted repeat sequences up to several hundred bases long. The case of the bacterial transposable element Tn*9* is particularly striking in relation to proviruses: structural information of more than 1000 bases is flanked by a direct repeat of 800 bases, which itself is terminated by an imperfect inverted repeat of 18 out of 25 bases (MacHattie and Jackowski 1977; Ohtsubo and Ohtsubo 1978). The analogy with transposons is greatly strengthened by the recent finding that insertion of retroviral DNA generates a direct duplication of a short sequence from the insertion site. Essentially the same phenomenon was described earlier for bacterial transposable elements: direct flanking repeats usually of 5 bp or 9 bp are generated from the insertion site during transposition (Calos et al. 1978; Grindley 1978; Johnsrud et al. 1978; Kleckner 1979; for reviews, see Grindley and Sherratt 1979; and Calos and Miller 1980). Similar short duplications occur during transposition of elements in yeast (Farabaugh and Fink 1980; Gafner and Phillipsen 1980) and *Drosophila* (Dunsmuir et al. 1980).

Transposable elements, like proviruses, can be found at many apparently nonhomologous sites in host genomes (Kleckner 1977), indicating that they transpose by mechanisms inherently different from the mechanism employed during the integration of a circular form of phage λ DNA into a homologous site on the bacterial chromosome (Landy and Ross 1977). It is not yet certain whether classes of preferred integration sites exist for retroviral DNA, as have been documented for some bacterial transposons (Calos and Miller 1980); evidence on this issue was discussed in Section III.C.1. It is conceivable that some feature of LTR sequences may be recognized by bacterial systems involved in transposition of insertion sequences: deletion of a cloned, integrated MSV provirus has been shown to occur in *recA*-deficient strains of *E. coli* via recombination between its LTRs (McClements et al. 1980), a reaction similar to that reported for deletions of Tn*9* in lambda phage (Shapiro and MacHattie 1979).

3. *Endogenous Proviruses*

Although the origins and functions of endogenous proviruses are more fully considered in Chapter 10, it is pertinent to note here that the structure of several genetically transmitted proviruses of birds and mice conforms to the structure deduced for proviruses acquired by infection (Cohen et al. 1979a; Hughes et al. 1979b, 1981b; McClements et al. 1979; Hayward et al. 1980). This has been most convincingly demonstrated by sequencing the ends of an endogenous provirus of chickens, called *ev*-1 (Hishinuma et al. 1981). *ev*-1 concludes with a 273-bp LTR, containing a 7-bp inverted repeat, and it is flanked by a 6-bp duplication of a sequence present once in the unoccupied integration site.

Endogenous proviruses are found in varying numbers and are situated at different sites in the genomes of outbred individuals or different inbred strains (Astrin 1978; Steffen and Weinberg 1978; Cohen and Varmus 1979; Hughes et al. 1979b; Humphries et al. 1979; Steffen et al. 1979). They may also be found on multiple chromosomes (Chattopadhyay et al. 1975; Morris et al. 1979; Jolicoeur et al. 1980; A. Tereba, unpubl.). In sum, these findings provide support for the notion that endogenous proviruses of several types have been acquired by relatively recent (postspeciation) infection of germ-line cells by retroviruses (Todaro et al. 1975; Astrin et al. 1979; Cohen and Varmus 1979; Frisby et al. 1979; Hughes et al. 1979b).

4. Mechanism of Integration

At present there is more speculation than fact about the mechanisms used for integrative recombination of retroviral DNA. It is apparent from the foregoing discussion that, in contrast to the integration of papovavirus DNA, which appears to occur randomly on both viral and host DNAs (Botchan et al. 1976; Ketner and Kelly 1976), integration of retroviral DNA is under some constraints to join specific sequences in viral DNA to host DNA (cf. Weinberg 1980). To establish a provirus that is colinear with unintegrated linear DNA, either the linear DNA itself must be used as a substrate for recombination or there must be a mechanism for orienting circular DNA during its insertion into the host genome.

There have been several traditional and circumstantial reasons for favoring integration of circular DNA: the simplicity of the Campbell model, which allows insertion of a circular duplex with a single crossing-over event (Campbell 1962); the analogies with other viruses, which integrate their genomes via circular intermediates (e.g., lambdoid phages); the demonstrated infectivity of circular retroviral DNA (Smotkin et al. 1975; Guntaka et al. 1976; Fritsch and Temin 1977a); and the correlations between production of circular intermediates and establishment of the provirus (Guntaka et al. 1975; Jolicoeur and Baltimore 1976a; Sveda and Soeiro 1976; Jolicoeur and Rassart 1980; Yang et al. 1980a,b). The required orientation of circular intermediates might be achieved by structural features, rather than specific sequences; for example, Hsu et al. (1978a) have claimed that the single-strand-specific nuclease S1 attacks RSV closed circular DNA at a preferred site near the LTR.

The recent definition of host-virus junctions, described in the preceding section, has established a number of guidelines that should be met by any tenable integrative mechanism: (1) The mechanism must exhibit a high degree of precision with respect to the viral sequence joined to cellular DNA, since there is little, if any, variation in the ultimate viral nucleotide pairs at the ends of each provirus. (2) The mechanism must include a device for eliminating a few base pairs (usually two) from the ends of both LTRs at some point prior to, or during, integration. (3) The mechanism should not depend on homologous recombination with host DNA; if certain sites in host DNA are preferred targets for integration, the recognition signals are likely to be subtle. (4) Integration must generate a duplication of 4, 5, or 6 bases at the host site, presumably by use of a nuclease that makes staggered cuts in the manner proposed for transposable elements (Grindley and Sherratt 1979; Shapiro 1979). (5) It is attractive to assume that the short inverted repeats found at the ends of all proviruses thus far are instrumental in the integration process.

Despite these stipulations, it is still possible to devise models for integration that can accommodate any of the following three candidate precursors to the provirus: (1) Linear DNA has the advantages of abundance, existence of free ends needed for insertion, and ready-made colinearity with the provirus. It is necessary to consider some means of bringing the ends of linear DNA into proximity to facilitate insertion without deletion of host DNA. This could conceivably be accomplished by base pairing between the ends of the same strand in the regions of the inverted repeats. It is also necessary to posit some activity that can remove a small number of base pairs from the ends of linear DNA. (2) Circular DNA bearing one LTR unit could be the substrate for integrative recombination provided that a mechanism existed for generating a second copy of the LTR. The example of replicon fusion in prokaryotes suggests such a mechanism (cf. Shapiro 1979), as illustrated by Shoemaker et al. (1980). One advantage of this model is that staggered cleavages on opposite strands, 2 bases within the ends of the single LTR, lead to an apparent loss of 2 bases from each of the LTRs at the ends of the inserted provirus. However, the mechanism does not explain why retroviruses would bother to synthesize linear DNA with two copies of the

LTR unit, if it were possible to generate the second copy at a later stage. Moreover, the endonucleases required to make the staggered scissions would be predicted to attack circles bearing two LTRs in a manner that should produce proviruses with three or four copies of the LTR. Such proviruses have not, however, been observed. (3) Circular DNAs with two copies of the LTR have generally been considered to be the most likely candidates for integrative substrates. They require enzymes that recognize the circle-junction region and can eliminate bases from the ends of the LTRs. Of course, the circles themselves should lack no more than 2 bases from each LTR at the circle junction. As noted earlier, cloned molecules with two copies of the LTR frequently display aberrancies at the circle junction and would not appear to be suitable for integration.

Two kinds of questions have been asked in attempting to identify the immediate precursor to the provirus: Which unintegrated forms of viral DNA are infectious in transfection tests? Which forms fail to accumulate under conditions that impair the frequency of integration? To date, both approaches have failed to identify the precursor unambiguously.

First, both linear and circular DNAs prepared from infected cells are infectious (Guntaka et al. 1976; Smotkin et al. 1976; Fritsch and Temin 1977a). Most tests for the infectivity of both forms of DNA have been done in permissive hosts, so that the vast majority of cells ultimately contain proviruses acquired by virus spread; hence, the manner in which the delivered molecules were expressed has generally not been examined. In some recent experiments, cloned circular RSV DNA bearing two complete LTRs has been recircularized in vitro and used for transfection of nonpermissive (mouse) cells (P. Luciw, unpubl.). The resulting transformed cells carried proviruses joined to cellular DNA at many different sites within viral DNA, indicating that transfection with this form of viral DNA does not recapitulate natural infection. There may, however, be trivial reasons for this: the delivered molecules may have had the wrong superhelical density or may have been degraded during the manipulations. Alternatively, viral proteins may be required to facilitate proper integration of circular DNA. Microinjection into mammalian cells of closed circular DNA containing RSV LTRs likewise does not result in integration at the predicted site within the LTR (P. Luciw and M. Capecchi, unpubl.). Copeland et al. (1981) have recently examined the structure of viral DNA integrated into nonpermissive cells transformed with unintegrated linear DNA. Most of the proviruses contained an appreciable portion of both LTRs and appeared to be colinear with the unintegrated form by restriction mapping. However, it was not possible to conclude whether the linear DNA was integrated via mechanisms operative during natural infection, since the host-virus junctions were not sequenced. The approximate colinearity of integrated DNA with delivered DNA may simply reflect the manner in which transfecting DNA is assimilated and the selection for cells with expressed proviruses.

Second, certain mouse cells that restrict replication of MLV by the action of alleles at the *Fv-1* locus appear to restrict the appearance of both circular and proviral DNAs (Jolicoeur and Baltimore 1976a; Sveda and Soeiro 1976; Rassart and Jolicoeur 1980; Yang et al. 1980a; Jolicoeur and Rassart 1981) (see Section V.B.2). However, it does not necessarily follow that circular DNA is required for integration. Instead, the observations may reflect the defectiveness of the linear DNA for both circularization and integration. Similar arguments may apply to the observation that ethidium bromide and cycloheximide depress the accumulation of both circular and integrated DNAs (Guntaka et al. 1975; Yang et al. 1980b) (see Section VI.).

The very existence of circular DNA has been considered an argument in favor of its role in integration. However, it is possible that the circular forms are accidental consequences of the properties of linear DNA. The redundant termini of linear DNA could promote homologous recombination to generate circles with one LTR sequence, whereas the free ends of linear DNA may be efficiently joined to produce the circles with two copies of the LTR. Both forms, in this view, would be functionally void.

The structural homogeneity of proviruses examined in infected cells suggests that the U_3RU_5 sequence may be intimately involved in the recombinational events during natural infection. However, the sequence is neither absolutely required nor preferentially used for integration of retroviral DNA delivered by transfection. This has been shown most simply by transformation of cells with subgenomic fragments of viral DNA that lack an LTR unit (Andersson et al. 1979; Canaani et al. 1979; Blair et al. 1980; N.G. Copeland et al. 1980; Oskarsson et al. 1980; P. Luciw, unpubl.). In addition, cells have been transfected with permuted RSV DNA that, after cloning in bacteria, contains two adjacent copies of the LTR at an internal position in a linear structure. In most cases, the viral DNA is perpetuated in the transformed cells as an integrated species colinear with the permuted, transfecting DNA. In other words, the U_3RU_5 sequence was not preferentially joined to host DNA, at least when delivered either as part of a permuted DNA molecule or as part of a circular species formed in vitro (see above). Although it may not facilitate integration of transfecting DNA, the LTR sequence can markedly augment the efficiency of successful transfection, presumably by supplying a promoter for expression of viral genes (Blair et al. 1980; Oskarsson et al. 1980; P. Luciw, unpubl.).

As yet, no host or virus functions have been genetically or biochemically defined as part of the mechanism of integrative recombination. The viral *pol* gene is, of course, required for production of an appropriate substrate, and it is probable that cellular nuclease(s) and ligase(s) are involved in the recombinational steps. For example, cellular DNA gyrase might be used to produce a staggered cleavage at the integration site (Peebles et al. 1979). On the other hand, available results are also consistent with the possibility that the size of the duplicated cellular sequence is determined by the infecting virus; if so, a viral protein, perhaps the nucleic acid binding and endonuclease activities encoded in *pol* (see III.B.1.f), might be involved in the cleavage of viral or host DNAs, or both. Varmus et al. (1977) showed that RSV proviruses entered only cellular DNA that replicated during infection; however, it is not known whether cellular DNA synthesis is required for completion of viral DNA, whether the topology of replicating DNA enhances its activity in integrative recombination, or whether the integration event promotes local replication. Efforts to show that DNA repair processes augment integration of proviruses have been unsuccessful (Tsuruo and Baluda 1977).

5. *Unusual Functions of the Provirus*

The central function of the provirus is to act as a template, both for the replication of viral DNA and for the synthesis of viral RNA, the initial step in expression of the viral genome. The manner in which the viral genome is expressed is considered in detail later in this chapter. In this section, we explore briefly some possible additional functions and consequences of the integration of viral DNA.

a. Mutagenesis. Elements capable of being inserted into many regions of host DNA are theoretically capable of affecting host genes, either by disrupting them physically or by influencing their expression from a proximal position. Well-studied examples of such phenomena are found among mutator phages and other transposable elements of prokaryotes (Bukhari et al. 1977; Kleckner 1977; Ross et al. 1979; Calos and Miller 1980). Varmus et al. (1981b) have demonstrated the mutational capacity of retroviruses by superinfecting an RSV-transformed rat cell with a nontransforming MLV. Two morphological revertants carried MLV proviruses inserted within RSV DNA on the 5′ side of *src*, producing polar effects on *src* expression by affecting processing and/or termination of transcripts initiated in the RSV LTR. Preliminary results of M. Capecchi (unpubl.) also suggest that infection with MLV may interrupt host genes that synthesize selectable markers.

As discussed below and in Chapter 8, insertion of ALV proviruses in the vicinity of a cellular progenitor of a viral transforming sequence may alter the regulation of the cellular gene (Hayward et al. 1981).

b. Promotion of Transcription of Cellular DNA. Transcription of host DNA positioned "downstream" from viral DNA and under the influence of viral LTRs has been observed both in occasional mammalian cells transformed by RSV (Quintrell et al. 1980) and in tumors induced by ALVs (Neel et al. 1981; Payne et al. 1981). These instances are discussed more fully in the ensuing section and in Section IV.B.4.c.

c. Oncogenesis. In most cases, proviruses appear to function in oncogenesis or transformation primarily by encoding a responsible gene product (cf. Chapters 8 and 9). However, in the several cases in which no viral genes or nucleotide sequences have been implicated in oncogenesis, it is possible that the position of the provirus within the host genome has a determining effect. This idea has been most dramatically supported by the finding of Hayward et al. (1981) that the great majority of ALV-induced bursal lymphomas carry a proviral insertion near the cellular progenitor (*c-myc*) of the putative transforming sequence (*v-myc*) of MC29 virus. In these tumors, a new ALV provirus is generally positioned upstream from *c-myc* and expression of *c-myc* appears to be enhanced via transcripts bearing both U_5 and *c-myc* sequences. The significance of the insertion site is emphasized by the findings that the proviruses themselves are frequently defective and are not expressed (Neel et al. 1981; Payne et al.

1981). However, the activation of *c-myc* may not always proceed through a "promoter insertion" mechanism, since some tumors contain proviruses in the incorrect transcriptional orientation to *c-myc* or on the 3′ side of c-*myc* (Payne et al. 1981, and unpubl.). The role of these insertions in the pathogenesis of lymphomas is considered in greater detail in Chapter 8.

It is unclear whether other viruses lacking *onc* sequences initiate tumors by integration of viral DNA at certain sites in host genomes. A wide variety of tumors induced by such viruses—lymphoproliferative tumors induced by MLV (Steffen and Weinberg 1978; Canaani and Aaronson 1979; Van der Putten et al. 1979; Jahner et al. 1980), mammary carcinomas induced by MMTV (Cohen et al. 1979b; Groner and Hynes 1980), leukosis induced by bovine leukemia virus (Kettman et al. 1979, 1980), lymphomas induced by chicken syncytial virus (CSV) (H. J. Kung, pers. comm.), as well as ALV-induced bursal lymphomas and nephroblastomas (Neiman et al. 1980; Neel et al. 1981; Payne et al. 1981; T. Fung and H. J. Kung, pers. comm.)—are composed largely or exclusively of the descendants of one or a few infected cells. The evidence for the clonal, or quasi-clonal, nature of such tumors comes from analysis of newly acquired proviruses with restriction enzymes. Although proviruses are distributed at many different sites in the many independently infected cells in preneoplastic tissues (e.g., mammary glands infected with MMTV) (Cohen et al. 1979b), only one or a few integration sites are occupied in the cells present in each tumor. Although the sites usually appear to vary from tumor to tumor within each study population, further work is required to determine whether certain regions of the host genome related or analogous to *c-myc* are occupied by at least one of the often multiple proviruses in each tumor. Preliminary results with CSV-induced bursal lymphomas, for example, indicate that a provirus occupies the *c-myc* locus (H.J. Kung, pers. comm.).

d. Transduction. There are substantial reasons for believing that retroviruses can acquire cellular sequences during passage through certain hosts. For example, rare events of this sort appear to be responsible for the presence of transforming genes in many viruses (see Chapter 9). From what is known of the structure of proviral DNA, however, it seems unlikely that cellular sequences at or adjacent to integration sites are commonly transduced, e.g., by extended transcription beyond viral DNA into host sequences. (Such transcripts would be unlikely to be perpetuated by reverse transcription during the next round of infection.) However, there are claims that such transduction events can occur at relatively high frequency when RSV is passaged through duck cells (Shoyab et al. 1975) or rat cells (Baxt and Meinkoth 1978).

e. Transposition. As discussed above, the structure of proviral DNA resembles that of transposable elements of prokaryotes in certain respects. This similarity raises the as yet unsupported possibility that proviruses can be transposed to new sites by mechanisms akin to those operative in bacteria. (In a strict sense, of course, proviruses behave as transposable elements, since their genes can be moved to a new site by synthesis of viral RNA, reverse transcription of viral RNA into DNA, and integration of the new viral DNA into the host genome.) Examination of proviruses in multiple subclones of infected cells (Steffen and Weinberg 1978; Bacheler and Fan 1979; Collins et al. 1980; Quintrell et al. 1980; S. Hughes, unpubl.) and in multiple related individuals bearing the same endogenous proviruses (Astrin 1978; Cohen and Varmus 1979; Hughes et al. 1979b; Humphries et al. 1979) argues thus far for stability. Genetic selection, however, may be required to detect rare transpositions of the classical type.

f. Deletion Formation and Excision. Transposable elements of bacteria can be precisely or imprecisely deleted and can generate deletions in flanking DNA (see, e.g., Ross et al. 1979; Calos and Miller 1980). Deletions removing LTRs, usually the left-hand LTR, have been observed among endogenous proviruses of chickens (Hayward et al. 1980; Hughes et al. 1981c), ALV proviruses in bursal tumors (Neel et al. 1981; Payne et al. 1981; T. Fung and H.J. Kung, unpubl.), and in an RSV provirus after reversion of a transformed rat cell (Varmus et al. 1981a). However, the mechanisms responsible for these deletions are not known.

Excision of most of a provirus could theoretically occur via homologous recombination or unequal crossing-over between LTRs. The former mechanism may explain the loss of all but one LTR from the MLV provirus inserted in an RSV provirus (Varmus et al. 1981a), the presence in white leghorn chickens of endogenous elements annealing only with reagents specific for LTR sequences (Hughes et al. 1981c), and the elimination of most of a provirus in a spontaneous revertant of an FeSV-transformed mink cell (Donner et al. 1980). Unequal crossing-over, on the other hand, could explain the generation of a duplicated provirus (cell DNA–U_3RU_5–genes

-U_3RU_5–genes–U_3RU_5–cell DNA) from a normal RSV provirus in a cultured cell line (Hsu et al. 1981).

In a few cases, reversion of virus-transformed cells to a normal phenotype can be explained by loss of proviral DNA (Frankel et al. 1976; Nomura 1978; Trainor and Reitz 1979; Yang et al. 1979; Varmus et al. 1981b); in several clones examined by restriction mapping, the entire provirus, including both copies of the direct terminal repeat, was missing (Varmus et al. 1981b). It is not known whether such events reflect a loss of chromosomes or mechanisms more specifically directed toward proviral DNA.

IV. PHASE TWO: EXPRESSION OF THE VIRAL GENOME

A. An Overview of the Strategy of Expression

The first phase of the virus life cycle ends with the establishment of the provirus and is dominated by the action of a viral gene product, reverse transcriptase. The second phase begins with the expression of the genes encoded in the provirus and ends, in most cases, with the production of viral particles; the dominant tools in this process are supplied by the host cell. Host factors are responsible for the synthesis and processing of viral RNA, for the maintenance of a template by replication of proviral DNA, for the synthesis of viral proteins from viral mRNAs, and for at least certain aspects of the processing of viral proteins.

Retroviruses have adopted a combination of devices to facilitate expression in host cells that normally deal with a different pattern of genetic organization. In eukaryotic cells, genes appear to be arranged principally as single cistrons interrupted by noncoding regions (intervening sequences or introns). Proviruses are, in contrast, multicistronic genetic units in which individual cistrons do not seem to be interrupted by noncoding regions.[1] Since animal cells are presumably not equipped to translate several genes independently from a single mRNA, animal viruses have generally depended on two kinds of strategy for gene expression: production of multiple mRNAs from either segmented or nonsegmented genomes, or cleav-

[1]There is still insufficient evidence from sequencing of retroviral DNA to be certain of this statement, but the notion is strongly supported by translation of virion RNAs in vitro (see, e.g., Beemon and Hunter 1978; Purchio et al. 1978) and by sequencing of selected viral genes (see Appendix E).

age of primary translation products (polyproteins) to generate multiple proteins. Retroviruses employ both of these mechanisms. Subgenomic mRNAs direct the synthesis of proteins encoded at internal positions in the viral genome, and multiple mature proteins are generated by cleavage of primary products of translation (see Eisenman and Vogt 1978 and Chapter 6).

As discussed in Chapter 4, the common gene order of replication-competent retroviruses, from the 5′ end to the 3′ end of viral RNA, is *gag-pol-env* (or *gag-pol-env-src,* in the case of RSV). The *gag*-gene product is a polyprotein of approximately 65,000–80,000 daltons synthesized from an mRNA indistinguishable from genomic subunits; the *gag* polyprotein is modified (e.g., phosphorylated) and cleaved to yield the small core proteins (10,000–30,000 daltons) found in mature viral particles (Vogt and Eisenman 1973; Vogt et al. 1975). The primary translation product of *pol* is a large polyprotein (160,000–180,000 daltons) containing *gag* as well as *pol* peptides (Jamjoon et al. 1977; Oppermann et al. 1977). The mRNA for the precursor to DNA polymerase has thus far not been distinguished structurally from *gag* mRNA, although the mechanism by which the *gag* termination codon is bypassed probably involves its elimination from the RNA by splicing. Production of functional reverse transcriptase involves cleavage and modification of the *gag-pol* polyprotein. The *env* gene is expressed via a subgenomic mRNA that is almost certainly generated by the processing of RNA of genomic size; sequences that are not contiguous in genomic RNA (or in proviral DNA) are joined in the subgenomic mRNAs, presumably by the mechanisms used to splice cellular mRNAs from larger precursors (Abelson 1979). The primary translation product of *env* mRNA is presumably inserted into cell membranes during synthesis and is subsequently glycosylated and cleaved to generate the envelope glycoproteins present in viral particles (England et al. 1977; Hayman 1978; Diggelmann 1979). Certain *onc* genes, at least the *src* gene of RSV, may also be expressed by spliced subgenomic mRNA. The protein product of *src,* which is not required for replication and is not readily found in viral progeny, is phosphorylated and inserted into the plasma membrane (cf. Chapter 9).

Virus-producing cells must generate viral RNA that can be packaged into progeny virions as well as viral RNA that serves messenger functions. Thus far, no structural differences have been perceived between the subunit-size species that appear in particles and those that perform as mRNAs for *gag* (or *gag-pol*) polyproteins. Genomic RNA and mRNA, however, can be distinguished functionally. If MLV RNA synthesis is inhibited by actinomycin D, viral proteins continue to be synthesized, and particles are assembled with cellular, rather than viral, RNA (Levin et al. 1974; Levin and Rosenak 1976). These results indicate that genomic RNA and mRNA comprise distinct pools and that the half-life of the mRNA pool is greater. It is not known how or when viral transcripts are assigned to these two pools, but it is possible that a specific sequence near the 5′ end of viral RNA is required for entry into particles. Linial and her associates have described a deletion mutant of RSV that produces functional mRNAs for *gag* and *pol* but fails to package genomic RNA into particles, even when cells containing the mutant provirus have been superinfected with helper virus (Linial et al. 1978b; Gallis et al. 1979). This mutant lacks about 150 nucleotides in a noncoding region near the 5′ end of the genome (Shank and Linial 1980).

Although the central outlines of the strategy of retroviral gene expression are now apparent, the ensuing discussion reveals several unanswered questions of considerable import: What are the promoters for transcription of proviral DNA? How is transcriptional activity regulated? What is the primary product of transcription and how is it processed? What is the precise composition of viral mRNAs? Is there a distinct *pol* mRNA? What are the signals for translation of viral mRNAs and where are they located?

B. Transcription

1. Mechanisms of Synthesis of Viral RNA

There remains considerable uncertainty about the mechanisms required to generate the species of viral RNA discussed in the following sections. Most, if not all, viral RNA is probably transcribed from a template of integrated (proviral) DNA by host RNA polymerase II, processed by a variety of cellular enzymes, and transported to the cytoplasm where it associates either with polyribosomes (to serve as mRNA) or with structural polyproteins (to serve as genomic RNA). The size of the primary transcript has not been determined unambiguously by direct measurement, but has been predicted to be the same as genomic RNA, based upon identification of probable signals within the LTRs for initiation and polyadenylation of transcripts.

Only the rudimentry aspects of the processing and modification of various species of viral RNA and of the determinants of viral RNA concentrations are now known.

a. The Template. The structure of viral DNA suggests that it was designed to serve as a template for the synthesis of viral RNA. As pointed out earlier, the DNA contains a complete copy of a subunit of viral RNA, including two copies of the short sequence (R) repeated at the ends of the viral RNA, plus extra sequences from the 3′ end of the RNA (the U_3 region) positioned upstream and extra sequences from the 5′ end (the U_5 region) positioned downstream (cf. Fig. 5.4). This structure has prompted suggestions that viral DNA might carry its own regulatory apparatus for initiation and termination of transcription (Hughes et al. 1978; Shank et al. 1978b; Sabran et al. 1979; Taylor 1979). If so, then both integrated and unintegrated forms of viral DNA might serve as templates for synthesis of viral RNA. In most chronically infected cells, only integrated forms of viral DNA have been detected; in those cases in which free DNA is present as well, it has not been possible to determine whether both forms are utilized as templates for RNA synthesis.

The kinetics of appearance of newly synthesized viral RNA and of integrated DNA are too poorly defined to determine whether viral DNA is ever copied into RNA prior to its integration. The transfection experiments of Cooper and his colleagues offer one possible instance in which viral DNA may be transcribed in an unintegrated state (Cooper and Okenquist 1978). They found that transfection of chicken cells with proviral or unintegrated viral DNA required recruitment (virus spread). This result implies (but does not prove) that stable association of the transfecting DNA and the initially transfected cell did not occur and that the presumably unintegrated DNA was transcribed to generate viral progeny. Recent work with visna virus also suggests that unintegrated DNA is transcribed, since the concentration of viral RNA appears to be directly proportional to the amount of unintegrated DNA and since little or no integrated DNA can be found in these acutely infected cultures (J. Harris et al., unpubl.). However, the issue of whether unintegrated DNA can be transcribed has yet to be settled by a direct test.

b. The Enzyme. Retroviral RNA appears to be synthesized by the cellular RNA polymerase(s) (generally known as RNA polymerase II) responsible for the synthesis of cellular mRNAs. Evidence for this view comes entirely from experiments with the drug α-amanitin, which inhibits RNA polymerase II at low concentrations relative to concentrations required for inhibition of other RNA polymerases (Lindell et al. 1970). Administration of the drug to intact virus-producing cells (Dinowitz 1975; Bishop et al. 1976), to nuclei or chromatin isolated from infected cells (Jaquet et al. 1974; Rymo et al. 1974; Stallcup et al. 1978), or to an in vitro transcription system (Manley et al. 1980) programmed with cloned RSV DNA (Yamamoto et al. 1980a; W. DeLorbe, unpubl.) inhibits synthesis of retroviral RNA at doses inhibitory to RNA polymerase II.

c. Promoters and Primary Transcripts. Several investigators have pointed out features of the available sequence from U_3 regions that resemble potentially important features of other putative promoters (Taylor 1979; Czernilofsky et al. 1980b; Dhar et al. 1980; Hager and Donehower 1980; Majors and Varmus 1980; Shimotohno et al. 1980; Sutcliffe et al. 1980; Swanstrom et al. 1981b; Yamamoto et al. 1980b; Van Beveren et al. 1980). Sequences closely related to the "canonical" sequence TATAAAA, frequently observed around 24–31 nucleotides on the 5′ side of the initiation sites for many viral and cellular RNAs (e.g., Ziff and Evans 1978), have been found in all retroviral LTRs sequenced to date at an appropriate distance from the predicted initiation site (cf. Appendix E). Examination of the consequences of defined mutations in the U_3 region and direct study of the RNA polymerase with this region will be required to define the viral promoter with precision. The behavior of recombinant viruses differing in the U_3 region also favors the notion that U_3 encodes a promoter (Tsichlis and Coffin 1980).

Two pieces of direct evidence indicate that the U_3 region lies immediately to the 5′ side of the initiation site for RNA synthesis and that transcription initiates with the capped nucleotide within the R sequence encoded in the LTR: (1) the composition of nascent MLV transcripts from nuclei from infected cells (Benz et al. 1980) and (2) the size and oligonucleotide composition of transcripts synthesized in vitro from cloned RSV DNA (Yamamoto et al. 1980a). In addition, there is increasing evidence that RNA synthesis from eukaryotic genes is generally initiated with the nucleotide that is capped in mature cytoplasmic RNA (see, e.g., Ziff and Evans 1978). Three indirect experimental results also bear on this question.

1. If the U_3 sequence at the upstream end of the provirus serves as a promoter, the primary transcript is unlikely to be longer than a subunit of virion RNA (unless termination is not effected within the provirus). Thus far, efforts to detect viral RNA of greater than subunit size, which serves as precursor to mature forms, have been generally unsuccessful (Fan 1977). Small quantities of RNA slightly larger than virion subunits have been observed in MLV-producing cells (Haseltine and Baltimore 1976b; Fan 1977), but the significance of these species is uncertain in the absence of evidence that they are processed to smaller size.
2. Since the provirus is terminally redundant, both ends should be able to promote transcription of DNA positioned downstream. Therefore infected cells should contain RNA species linking the RU_5 sequence from the right end of the provirus with cellular sequences from flanking DNA. Candidate species of this type have been identified by Quintrell et al. (1980) in clones of mammalian cells transformed by RSV and by Neel et al. (1981) and Payne et al. (1981) in ALV-induced tumor cells. As discussed elsewhere (Chapter 8), in the latter case the viral promoter is frequently positioned upstream from the cellular homolog of a virus transforming gene (*c-myc*), producing augmented expression by a mechanism referred to as "promoter insertion" (Hayward et al. 1981).
3. If the viral promoter is encoded within U_3, efficient transfection should depend on the presence of an LTR unit upstream from the viral genes for which the assay scores. Several groups have found that restriction fragments bearing viral transforming genes, but lacking LTRs, transform cells at low frequency (Andersson et al. 1979; Canaani et al. 1979; Blair et al. 1980; Chang et al. 1980; N.G. Copeland et al. 1980; P. Luciw, unpubl.). In these cases, it is likely that successful transfection depends on insertion downstream from an effective cellular promoter. This idea is supported by the augmented efficiency of "secondary" transfection, using DNA from cells successfully transformed by restriction fragments lacking LTRs (N.G. Copeland et al. 1980). The ligation of fragments containing an LTR to fragments bearing an *onc* gene can dramatically enhance the efficiency of transformation, in some cases by a factor of as much as 3000 (Blair et al. 1980; Chang et al. 1980; Oskarsson et al. 1980). Recent studies

of the structure of the integrated recombinant DNA and its transcripts support the conclusion that the LTR promotes transcription (T. Wood et al., pers. comm.).

Although the promoter sequences have yet to be precisely located, there are several reasons to believe that at least the major species of viral RNA are transcribed from a single initiation site: (1) Subgenomic mRNAs are generally spliced (see below), and the 5′ ends of the spliced mRNAs are identical to the 5′ ends of virion RNA (Mellon and Duesberg 1977; Cordell et al. 1978). This observation implies that internal promoters within the provirus are not commonly used to generate subgenomic mRNAs. (2) Studies with the UV mapping technique of Hackett and Sauerbier (1975) indicate that all three major species of RSV RNA have similar target sizes, again suggesting that they are produced under the influence of a single promoter (Hackett et al. 1981). (3) The use of a single promoter to produce multiple species of RNA is also consistent with evidence for coordinate regulation of viral RNA concentrations. For example, expression of the genes of MMTV appears to be coordinately regulated by glucocorticoid hormones (for review, see Varmus et al. 1979a), and modulation of RNA levels in sibling clones of RSV-infected hamster cells affects multiple species in coordinate fashion (Deng et al. 1977; Quintrell et al. 1980).

The evidence cited in a later section for variable amounts of viral RNA transcribed from proviruses of the same type under different conditions or in different cells is most simply explained by variations in the rate of initiation or extension of RNA. Mechanisms by which such control might be exerted have not been defined. Possibly, the pattern of methylation of proviral DNA is implicated in some cases (Humphries et al. 1979; Cohen 1980; Guntaka et al. 1980). The influence of chromosome structure (Panet and Cedar 1977; Groudine et al. 1978; Cedar and Panet 1979; Breindl et al. 1980; Stalder et al. 1980) or the secondary structure of proviral DNA (Leibovitch et al. 1977) upon the efficiency of transcription has yet to be fully assessed.

d. Termination of Transcription. It is attractive to speculate that transcription terminates near the right end of proviral DNA, at the end of the U_3R sequence found adjacent to poly(A) at the 3′ terminus of virion RNA. Although this scheme has the virtue of simplicity, there is as yet no direct evidence for it. Conversely, Yamamoto et al. (1980b) determined the sequence near the 3′ terminus of a single molecule of subgenomic RSV mRNA after cloning cDNA transcribed from 21S RNA and found that all but 2 bases of the U_5 sequences and 18 bases of unrecognizable sequence were positioned downstream from the U_3R sequence. These results suggested that transcription continued through the entire LTR and past at least 18 bases of flanking cellular DNA prior to termination. However, the generality of this observation needs to be tested by the cloning and sequencing of multiple examples. Studies of heteroduplexes formed between viral subgenomic mRNA and cDNA do not reveal evidence for mRNA species with the U_5 sequence at both ends (Donoghue et al. 1978, 1979; Panet et al. 1978b; Rothenberg et al. 1978). However, it is plausible that readthrough of the U_5 sequence in the right LTR occurs commonly, but that processing events usually remove this sequence, in the manner elucidated for late mRNAs of adenovirus (Fraser et al. 1979). In other words, the clone described by Yamamoto et al. (1980b) could reflect an error of either termination or processing.

e. Possible Additional Effects of LTRs upon Transcriptional Activity. It is apparent from the preceeding sections that LTRs probably provide explicit signals for the initiation, polyadenylation, and perhaps termination of viral RNA. The LTR, in particular the U_3 region, is also likely to determine, in part, the level of transcriptional activity of a provirus, either by providing a promoter sequence recognized efficiently by host polymerase or by serving as a site at which modulating factors act. For example, the difference in replication activity between RAV-0 and RSV in most chicken cells has been attributed to a difference in the U_3 regions of their genomes (Tsichlis and Coffin 1980; Chapters 4 and 7), and the regulation of MMTV gene expression by glucocorticoid hormones is likely to be mediated through interactions involving an LTR (see Section IV.B.3). LTRs may also have less well-defined influences upon the transcriptional activity of surrounding regions of DNA. This hypothesis receives support from at least two recent observations: (1) an LTR positioned only on the 3′ side of a cloned viral transforming gene (*v-mos*) markedly enhances the efficiency of DNA transformation (Oskarsson et al. 1980; T. Wood et al., pers. comm.) and (2) augmented expression of *c-myc* occurs in ALV-induced bursal lymphomas when an ALV provirus is inserted on the 3′ side of *c-myc* or on the 5′ side of *c-myc* in the transcriptional orientation opposite to that of cellular genes (G. Payne et al., pers. comm.), as well as by the "promoter insertion" mechanism.

f. Processing of Viral RNA. Structural studies of viral mRNAs and genomic RNAs have indicated requirements for multiple processing events during the generation of mature species: addition of inverted, methylated nucleotides (caps) at the 5′ termini (Furuichi et al. 1975; Keith and Fraenkel-Conrat 1975; Bondurant et al. 1976; Rose et al. 1976); covalent joining of sequences noncontiguous in the provirus to form subgenomic species (splicing) (see Section IV.B.4.b); methylation of adenylate residues (Beemon and Keith 1976; Dimock and Stoltzfus 1978); and polyadenylation of the 3′ termini. However, there is little available information about the manner in which processing is effected or regulated.

Sequencing of RSV, MLV, MSV, and SNV DNAs has revealed that the 3′ ends of the RNAs of these viruses include the hexanucleotide, AAUAAA (Czernilofsky et al. 1980b; Dhar et al. 1980; Shimotohno et al. 1980; Sutcliffe et al. 1980; Swanstrom et al. 1981b); this sequence is commonly found 10–20 nucleotides from the start of the poly(A) tract at the 3′ ends of eukaryotic mRNAs (Proudfoot and Brownlee 1974) and may provide a signal for polyadenylation (Fitzgerald and Shenk 1980). However, the experiments of Yamamoto et al. (1980b) question whether polyadenylation of mRNA occurs regularly at the predicted site. In addition, the internal methylations do not appear necessary for efficient production of virus (Dimock and Stoltzfus 1978; see also Section VI).

Stacey and Hanafusa (1978) have used microinjection techniques to show that the conversion of genomic RNA to functional subgenomic mRNA involves a nuclear step. Employing a sensitive biological assay for synthesis of envelope glycoproteins—the production of infectious pseudotypes of RSV (−)—they showed that injection of RAV-2 virion RNA into the nucleus of RSV(−)-transformed chick cells led to production of glycoproteins, as did injection of subgenomic mRNA into the cytoplasm, whereas injection of virion subunits into the cytoplasm was without effect. These experiments also support the notion that a single, primary, subunit-size transcript serves as a precursor to subgenomic mRNAs.

The proportions of viral RNA species vary among types of host cells (see Section IV.B.2), presumably as a consequence of alterations in the regulation of processing reactions. Little is known, however, about the nature of these reactions or the manner in which they are regulated. Leis et al. (1978) have suggested that the nucleic-acid-binding properties of viral structural proteins (such as RSV pp19) might modulate processing. There is, however, only indirect support for this view.

2. *Measurement of Viral RNA in Infected Cells*

Most retroviruses are not detrimental to the growth of cultured cells; hence, the vast majority of RNA synthesized in infected cells is cellular in origin. Although this complicates the measurement and characterization of viral RNA, many investigators have successfully used molecular hybridization methods to determine the concentration of unlabeled viral RNA or the accumulation of labeled viral RNA in such cells. In the most widely used method, a comparison is made of the kinetics of annealing of radioactive, virus-specific cDNA with pure viral RNA and with unlabeled RNA from infected cells (see, e.g., Leong et al. 1972b; Fan and Baltimore 1973). Results are plotted as a function of RNA concentration × time ($C_r t$), and the values at which half-maximal annealing is achieved ($C_r t_{1/2}$) are indicative of the concentration of viral RNA in the sample of cellular RNA. For example, if 1000-fold more cellular RNA than viral RNA is required to obtain half-maximal hybridization, then 0.1% of the cellular RNA must be virus-specific. In other words, the $C_r t_{1/2}$ is proportional to the complexity of the RNA; annealing of cDNA to pure retroviral RNA usually occurs with a $C_r t_{1/2}$ of about 2×10^{-2} mole · sec/liter; RNA from cells in which 0.1% of the RNA was virus-specific would appear more complex, with a $C_r t_{1/2}$ of 2×10^{1} mole · sec/liter.

Several methods have been devised for measuring newly labeled viral RNA from infected cells (Parsons et al. 1973; Coffin et al. 1974; Fan 1977; Ringold et al. 1977b; Young et al. 1977; Bromley et al. 1979). In general, these depend on hybridizing radiolabeled RNA to an excess of unlabeled virus-specific DNA. Such assays are cumbersome and have required exorbitant amounts of viral DNA synthesized in vitro; the availability of cloned viral DNA should now make such assays more attractive. Thus far, methods that measure newly synthesized viral RNA have proved less sensitive than methods that determine the concentration of unlabeled viral RNA. The latter methods can detect less than one viral RNA molecule per cell.

Methods for hybridization to viral RNA in situ have recently been developed (Brahic and Haase 1978; Godard and Jones 1979; Kaufman et al. 1979); although difficult to execute, these techniques are potentially useful for gauging cell-to-cell variations in gene expression.

3. Amounts of Viral RNA in Infected Cells: Variation and Regulation

Investigators too numerous to mention have generally found that approximately 0.1–1% of the RNA is virus-specific in a permissive cell producing high titers of retroviruses (for reviews, see Fan 1977; Bishop 1978). Since most, if not all, species of retroviral RNA are polyadenylated (see below), viral RNA may comprise as much as 20% of the polyadenylated RNA in an infected cell. Similarly, since a substantial fraction of the viral RNA is mRNA, as opposed to RNA destined to be packaged in progeny virions (Fan and Baltimore 1973; Lee et al. 1979), up to 5–10% of the mRNA in a virus-producing cell may be virus-specific. As discussed earlier, infected cells usually contain between 1 and 20 copies of proviral DNA; the synthesis of several thousand copies of viral RNA per cell thus represents a major amplification of viral genetic information.

The kinetics of appearance of newly synthesized RNA after infection has been difficult to measure in the face of a large excess of parental virion RNA. However, Schincariol and Joklik (1973) were able to measure a twofold increment in RSV-specific RNA in whole cells within 24 hours after infection. Similar results were obtained by Salzberg et al. (1973), using MSV-infected cells. The initial increases appeared to reflect synthesis in the nucleus, consistent with observations that newly labeled viral RNA in chronically infected cells is first detected in nuclei (Parsons et al. 1973) and that viral RNA synthesis can be performed by nuclei isolated from such cells (Jaquet et al. 1974; Rymo et al. 1974). These findings are compatible with the generally held view that viral RNA is synthesized in the nucleus from a template of integrated viral DNA, but a complete analysis of the kinetics of viral DNA synthesis, integration, and viral RNA synthesis after a single highly synchronous infection is not available.

Despite the presence of large amounts of viral RNA in infected mass cultures of permissive cells, it should be stressed that the efficiency of expression at the transcriptional level may vary considerably from cell to cell, from provirus to provirus, and even for a single provirus under varied conditions. Several types of differences have been documented.

1. Viral gene expression can be markedly influenced by the nature of the host cell. For instance, the amount of RSV-specific RNA is generally 2–3 logs greater in permissive (avian) cells than in nonpermissive (mammalian) cells, although the amounts of proviral DNA per cell are similar (Coffin and Temin 1972; Bishop et al. 1976; Quintrell et al. 1980).
2. Expression of apparently similar proviruses in parallel clones of infected cells can vary dramatically. For example, clones of rat hepatoma cells infected with MMTV may contain no viral RNA or up to thousands of copies (Ringold et al. 1979); clones of RSV-transformed rat cells may differ by 1–2 logs with respect to viral RNA concentrations (Quintrell et al. 1980); Friend-virus-induced erythroleukemia cell lines may have markedly different amounts of viral RNA (Berkower et al. 1980); and clones of infected cells bearing similar MLV proviruses exhibit varying levels of viral RNA (Fan et al. 1978).
3. Different proviruses in the same cells may be differentially expressed. For example, the amounts of MLV and MSV RNAs in infected mouse cells containing similar numbers of both proviruses can differ by 1–2 logs (Dina and Penhoet 1978). Similarly, endogenous and newly acquired proviruses may be expressed at independent rates in the same cells (Hayward and Hanafusa 1976).
4. A viral genome may be more efficiently expressed when its provirus is located at a new site. For example, the endogenous provirus of RAV-0 in line-100 chicken cells (*ev*-2) is inefficiently expressed; but superinfection of the same cells with RAV-0 results in heightened virus production, presumably as a result of efficient transcription of the newly inserted RAV-0 provirus (Crittenden et al. 1974). These differences have been ascribed to a *cis*-acting regulator of transcription of the endogenous provirus (Cooper and Temin 1976; Cooper and Silverman 1978).
5. Single proviruses in clonal cell populations may exhibit radical changes in the level of expression. This has been most readily observed in transformed cells that revert to a normal phenotype as a consequence of a reduction in viral RNA (and hence a reduction in transforming proteins). In the most extensively studied example of this phenomenon, RSV-transformed baby hamster kidney (BHK) cells undergo morphological reversion at high frequency (Macpherson 1965; Boettiger 1974a). The revertant cells contain as little as 1% as much viral RNA as do transformed

cells of siblings, despite the persistence of a single, nondefective provirus at an unaltered site in the host genome (Deng et al. 1974, 1977; Bondurant et al. 1979; also see Porzig et al. 1979; Quintrell et al. 1980). In a similar case, there is preliminary evidence for a *cis*-acting regulator close to the provirus in the cells with low levels of expression (Catala and Vigier 1979), but, in general, the mechanism of this type of regulation is considered unknown. Halogenated pyrimidines such as BrdU can stimulate transcription from proviruses in the revertant cells (Deng et al. 1974; N. Quintrell, unpubl.), but again the mechanism is unknown.

6. Expression of proviruses may be affected by a variety of chemical or hormonal agents. The most striking example of this sort of phenomenon is the stimulation of MMTV RNA synthesis by glucocorticoid hormones (for review, see Varmus et al. 1979a). Physiological doses of dexamethasone, a potent glucocorticoid, augment the concentration of viral RNA by 10- to 1000-fold in infected mouse, rat, cat, and mink cells (McGrath et al. 1972; Parks et al. 1974; Ringold et al. 1975a,b, 1977a; Vaidya et al. 1976; Robertson and Varmus 1979). The response appears to be a primary effect of the hormone, since a markedly altered rate of accumulation of labeled viral RNA can be detected within 15 minutes (Ringold et al. 1977b; Young et al. 1977) and synthesis of proteins or DNA is not required for the response (Ringold et al. 1975b). In addition, augmented synthesis of labeled MMTV RNA is observed in nuclei isolated from hormone-treated cells (Stallcup et al. 1978). Dexamethasone generally stimulates MMTV gene expression above a preexisting constitutive level, rather than inducing expression of silent proviruses (Scolnick et al. 1976). Since the majority of transcribed proviruses in several different hosts are hormone-sensitive, either MMTV proviruses are preferentially inserted into steroid-responsive regions of host DNA or, more likely, the proviruses themselves carry sequences (e.g., within U_3) that respond to complexes of hormone and hormone-binding proteins in several animals. The latter interpretation is favored by recent studies of the transcriptional activity of an integration site for a steroid-responsive provirus in rat hepatoma cells (D. Ucker and K. Yamamoto, in prep.) and by studies of expression of viral and cellular genes recombined in vitro with an MMTV LTR (F. Lee and G. Ringold; G. Hager; J. Majors; all pers. comm.).

The expression of other retroviruses may also be modestly regulated at the transcriptional level by glucocorticoids (Lowy and Scolnick 1978). As considered elsewhere (Chapter 10), transcription of endogenous proviruses may be enhanced by glucocorticoids, halogenated pyrimidines, or other inducers of endogenous viruses.

4. Structure and Function of Intracellular Viral RNAs

Early efforts to determine the sizes of intracellular viral RNAs, particularly mRNAs associated with polyribosomes, suggested that subgenomic species of about half genomic size were present, in addition to RNA of genomic size (Fan and Baltimore 1973; Gielkens et al. 1974; Shanmugan et al. 1974; Tsuchida and Green 1974). Satisfying evidence that these represent discrete forms of viral RNA, rather than degradation products of genome-sized RNA, is now available as a result of several technical advances: the preparation of hybridization probes specific for defined portions of the genome, the purification of intracellular RNA for oligonucleotide fingerprinting, the synthesis of long viral cDNA for heteroduplex studies with viral mRNA, and the development of high-resolution methods for gel electrophoresis and hybridization of viral RNA transferred to filter paper (Alwine et al. 1977).

a. Genetic Composition and Size of Subgenomic RNAs. Weiss et al. (1977) and Hayward (1977) used hybridization reagents specific for several regions of the genome to define the size and genetic composition of the major cytoplasmic species of RSV RNA in infected chicken cells. Denatured RNA from cells infected with wild-type virus or with mutants deleted for *env* or *src* was subjected to rate-zonal sedimentation in sucrose gradients. Virus-specific RNA in each gradient fraction was then detected by annealing with several cDNAs, including cDNAs specific for the 3′ terminus of viral RNA and for internal regions corresponding approximately to the *gag, pol, env,* and *src* genes (Fig. 5.9). Three species of viral RNA (with sedimentation coefficients of 38S, 28S, and 21S and lengths of about 9 kb, 5.4 kb, and 3.3 kb) were identified in cells infected with wild-type RSV. All three species annealed with cDNA for the 3′ terminus and for the 3′ proximal gene (*src*); however, only the largest species (38S) annealed with probes for the 5′ half of the genome (*gag* and *pol*), and the smallest species (21S) did not anneal with cDNA for the *env* region. Cells infected with *env* deletion mutants lacked the

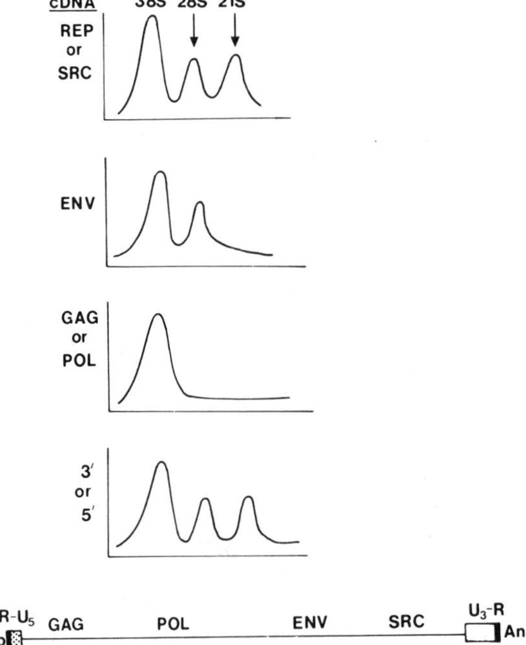

Figure 5.9 Strategy used to define the major species of intracellular RSV RNA. The figure approximates the results of the experiments of Hayward (1977) and of Weiss et al. (1977) establishing the size and genetic content of the principal species of RSV RNA in transformed chicken cells. Whole-cell RNA or cytoplasmic RNA was sedimented (from right to left) in rate-zonal sucrose gradients, and each gradient fraction was tested for viral RNA by hybridization with cDNAs specific for the indicated regions of the genome. The extent of hybridization is plotted on the vertical axes against fraction number on the horizontal axes. Locations of the tested genetic components of the genome are indicated at the bottom.

28S species, and cells infected with *src* deletion mutants replaced the usual 21S species with an RNA of similar size that annealed with cDNA for the *env* region. In their studies, Weiss et al. (1977) encountered a curious finding: all three species of RSV RNA annealed with cDNA specific for the 5′ terminus of viral RNA (cf. Fig. 5.8). Although other explanations were plausible, it was suggested that sequences from the 5′ end of viral RNA might have been joined to sequences near the *env* or *src* genes by a mechanism previously postulated to explain the joining of RNA sequences from noncontiguous regions of adenovirus and papovavirus genomes (for review, see Abelson 1979; Tooze 1980).

b. Structure and function of viral mRNAs. The proposal stimulated by these data was that genes located in the 3′ half of retroviral genomes (e.g., *env* and *src*) are expressed via spliced subgenomic mRNAs, whereas *gag* and *pol* are translated from mRNAs of subunit size. This proposal is now supported by studies of several retroviruses in various hosts, using tests of both structure and function (Fig. 5.10).

(i) RSV. All three species of viral RNA observed in the cytoplasm of permissive cells infected by RSV (Brugge et al. 1977a; Hayward 1977; Weiss et al. 1977; Krzyzek et al. 1978; Parsons et al. 1978; Martin et al. 1979) have also been observed in nonpermissive (mammalian) cells (Quintrell et al. 1980). As noted earlier, the concentration of viral RNA is considerably lower in the nonpermissive cells than in the permissive cells. In addition, the relative concentrations of the three major species are different in the two cell types. In the permissive cells, the 38S species, representing genomic RNA as well as *gag* and *pol* mRNAs, is dominant, whereas in the nonpermissive cells, the 21S species is the most abundant. The very low concentrations of the larger species, particularly the 28S species, probably

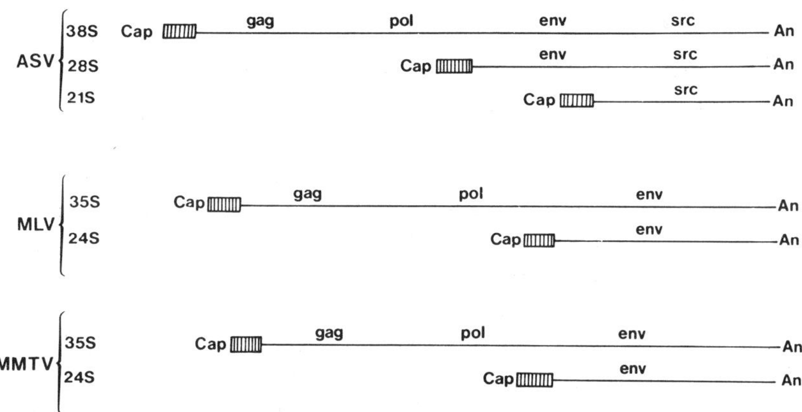

Figure 5.10 The major spliced mRNAs of several retroviruses are depicted schematically. Hatched boxes at the 5′ termini represent the region transposed to internal sequences during processing, but the size is only an approximation. The presence of capped 5′ ends on subgenomic mRNAs has been shown directly only for RSV (Mellon and Duesberg 1977; Cordell et al. 1978); the other capped ends are presumptive. The sizes of the RNAs are drawn in approximate accord with results for each virus (see text).

accounts for the failure of several investigators to detect one or both of them (Bishop et al. 1976; Brugge et al. 1977b; Deng et al. 1977; Krzyzek et al. 1979), until methods were developed for transferring RNA from agarose gels and binding it to chemically activated paper for hybridization (Alwine et al. 1977). The introduction of this procedure also sharpened the resolution of viral RNAs but failed to reveal additional major species in most cases. However, in some clonal lines of mammalian cells, minor variations in the sizes of the major RNAs have been observed (e.g., *env* mRNA of 5.7 kb, instead of 5.4 kb, and *src* mRNAs ranging from 3.0 kb to 3.6 kb) (Quintrell et al. 1980).

Several anomalous viral RNAs have also been observed in RSV-infected cells. In some cases, these are associated with proviruses bearing large deletions and presumably reflect alterations in the template or the primary transcript (Martin et al. 1979). The low-molecular-weight RNAs (~14S) observed in RSV-transformed chicken cells by Brugge et al. (1977a) may be analogous to similarly sized species in MLV-infected and MMTV-infected cells (Gielkens et al. 1974; Robertson and Varmus 1979; Sen et al. 1979); however, their significance is uncertain, since other investigators have failed to find them in RSV-infected cells or have considered them to be products of degradation (cf. Krzyzek et al. 1979; Yamamoto et al. 1980b).

The functions of the three major size classes of RSV RNA have been assessed principally by translation in vitro; the results conform to predictions based on the genetic content of each species. Thus, 38S RNA isolated either from virions or infected cells directs the synthesis of the *gag* and *pol* precursor proteins ($Pr76^{gag}$ and $Pr180^{pol}$, respectively) in several translational systems (Von der Helm and Duesberg 1975; Pawson et al. 1976; Patterson et al. 1977; Purchio et al. 1977; McGinnis et al. 1978; Weiss et al. 1978), including *Xenopus* oocytes (Katz et al. 1979). A subgenomic RNA species, presumably 28S, elicits synthesis of the *env* precursor protein in vitro (Pawson et al. 1977, 1980), and microinjection of 21S RNA from cells infected with a transformation-defective deletion mutant of RSV into chicken cells infected with an *env*-defective deletion mutant induces synthesis of complementing envelope glycoprotein (Stacey et al. 1977). Lastly, addition of 21S RSV RNA from transformed chicken cells to a lysate of rabbit reticulocytes promotes the synthesis of $p60^{src}$ (Yamamoto et al. 1980; Weiss et al. 1981).

Consistent with these findings, all three species of RSV RNA are associated with polyribosomes in a form releasable with ethylenediaminetetraacetic acid (EDTA) (Deng et al. 1977; Krzyzek et al. 1979; Lee et al. 1979; Quintrell et al. 1980). Membrane-bound polyribosomes are enriched for the presumptive *env* mRNA, 28S RNA (Lee et al. 1979), as might be expected for mRNA engaged in the synthesis of a protein to be inserted into membranes. 38S and 21S RNAs are found principally on free polyribosomes, although the protein product of *src* is localized in plasma membranes (Willingham et al. 1979; Courtneidge et al. 1980; Krueger et al. 1980).

(ii) MLV. Two major species of viral RNA, genome-size 35S and spliced 22S–24S, are agreed to be present in MLV-infected cells (Fan and Baltimore 1973; Gielkens et al. 1974; Shanmugan et al. 1974; van Zaane et al. 1977; Fan and Verma 1978; Rothenberg et al. 1978); in addition, some investigators have detected smaller species of about 12S–14S (Gielkens et al. 1974). As in the case of RSV RNA, genome-size species from virions or infected cells direct the synthesis of *gag* and *pol* precursor proteins in vitro or in *Xenopus* oocytes (Gielkens et al. 1974; Kerr et al. 1976; van Zaane et al. 1977; Murphy and Arlinghaus 1978; Philipson et al. 1978; Murphy et al. 1979). In addition, antibodies against *gag* proteins specifically immunoprecipitate polyribosomes containing 35S RNA (Mueller-Lantzsch and Fan 1976). 22S–24S RNA is found mainly on membrane-bound polyribosomes, as expected for an *env* mRNA (van Zaane et al. 1977), and RNA of this size prompts the synthesis of precursors to envelope glycoproteins in vitro (Murphy et al. 1979). No function has yet been assigned to the smallest RNAs.

(iii) DEFECTIVE TRANSFORMING VIRUSES. Several defective sarcoma viruses and acute leukemia viruses of mammals and birds appear to have a single genome-size mRNA that directs the synthesis of a single polyprotein containing fused products of *gag* and *onc* (Mellon et al. 1978; Reynolds et al. 1978; Shields et al. 1979; Sheiness et al. 1981). Avian erythroblastosis virus (AEV), on the other hand, may encode two proteins in the region believed to be responsible for its oncogenic activity (Lai et al. 1980; Pawson and Martin 1980; Yoshida and Toyoshima 1980), and these proteins may be synthesized via two mRNAs, the smaller of which is spliced (Anderson et al. 1980; Sheiness et al. 1981). AMV also appears to produce a subgenomic mRNA of 2.3 kb, in addition to a genomic RNA of 8.0 kb (Gonda et al. 1981; M. Roussel and D. Stehelin, unpubl.); similar findings have been made with the defective leukemia virus, OK-10 (D. Chiswell, pers. comm.). Cells transformed by the 124 strain of Mo-MSV contain two MSV-specific RNAs, one of genome length (~28S or 5.2 kb) and a spliced RNA of 23S or 3.1 kb (Donoghue et al. 1979). Direct evidence for the messenger activity of the latter species is not yet available, and it has only been identified in a single cell line. These issues are considered in greater detail in Chapters 4 and 9.

(iv) MMTV. In agreement with the general scheme for gene expression by replication-competent retroviruses, two predominant MMTV RNA species have been found in virus-producing cells by several investigators (Groner et al. 1979; Robertson and Varmus 1979, 1981; Sen et al. 1979; Buetti and Diggelmann 1981; Dudley and Varmus 1981). Again, the genome-size species (36S) is responsible for synthesis of *gag* and *pol* precursor proteins in vitro (Nusse et al. 1978; Sen et al. 1979; Dahl and Dickson 1979; D. Robertson, unpubl.), and a subgenomic spliced species (24S) directs synthesis of the *env* precursor (Robertson and Varmus 1979; Sen et al. 1979; Dudley and Varmus 1981). The existence of separate mRNAs for *gag* and *env* proteins was predicted by the salt-shift experiments of Schochetman and Schlom (1976); the kinetics of appearance of *gag* and *env* proteins were differentially affected by alterations in the NaCl concentrations in growth medium, indicating different initiation sites for translation (Saborio et al. 1974).

Additional RNA species of uncertain significance have also been observed in MMTV-producing cells. Robertson and Varmus (1979) reported a discrete species of 13S RNA in a wide variety of cells, but subsequent experiments with cloned viral DNA as probes revealed the 13S species to be cellular in origin (Robertson and Varmus 1981). Sen et al. (1979) found a heterogeneous collection of 12S–16S RNAs in mammary tumor cells, and Groner et al. (1979) detected in cultured tumor cells a species about 1.2 kb smaller than genomic RNA. Although these species appeared to be associated with polyribosomes, their functions are not known. More recently, a 20S species containing sequences from U_5, *env*, and U_3, and thus probably spliced, has been identified in MMTV-infected rat cells transiently during steroid induction; no protein product has been unambiguously assigned to this species, although there is a concurrent synthesis of small, aberrant *env*-related proteins (Robertson and Varmus 1981). As yet there is no well-characterized RNA species likely to serve as mRNA for intracellular synthesis of proteins produced in vitro from a large open reading frame in the U_3 region of the MMTV LTR (Dickson and Peters 1981) (cf. Chapter 4).

(v) OTHER VIRUSES. Subgenomic RNAs have been identified in cells producing FeLV (Conley and Velicer 1978) and visna virus (Filippi et al. 1979), but their sizes and genetic content have yet to be precisely defined.

c. Further Evidence That Subgenomic mRNAs Are Spliced. Several kinds of experiments have provided rigorous confirmation of the proposal that subgenomic mRNAs are spliced:

1. Mellon and Duesberg (1977) isolated ^{32}P-labeled 38S, 28S, and 21S RSV RNAs from infected chicken cells and found that all three species terminated with the large, capped oligonucleotide present at the 5′ terminus of genomic RNA. In agreement with the hybridization studies of Hayward (1977) and Weiss et al. (1977), the subgenomic RNAs also contained subsets of oligonucleotides mapped to the 3′ end of the viral genome. Hence, a sequence of at least 25 nucleotides from the 5′ end of 38S RNA must have been joined to sequences from the *env* and *src* regions during the generation of subgenomic RNAs. Similarly, Faller et al. (1978) showed that subgenomic (21S) RNA of Mo-MLV contained two copies of an oligonucleotide previously assigned to the R sequence (Coffin et al. 1978).
2. A variation of this approach was used by Cordell et al. (1978) to obtain a longer minimum length for the transposed sequence. ^{32}P-labeled 38S, 28S, and 21S RSV RNAs were annealed to strong-stop cDNA (101 nucleotides in length). The T1 oligonucleotides from hybrids formed with all three species of RNA indicated that at least 104 nucleotides must be transposed from the 5′ end of 38S RNA and joined to internal regions of the genome during the production of subgenomic species. Confirmatory results have been reported by Stoltzfus and Kuhnert (1979).
3. A vivid display of the structure of subgenomic mRNAs was achieved by annealing long Mo-MLV cDNA, synthesized in vitro, with 24S RNA (the putative *env* mRNA) from Mo-MLV-infected cells (Panet et al. 1978b; Rothenberg et al. 1978). Observation of the resulting heteroduplexes in the electron microscope revealed the several structures predicted for spliced RNA annealed with cDNAs of full and almost full length. However, the

initial estimate of the length of the transposed sequence (~600 nucleotides) may have been exaggerated, since the structure of completed cDNA, with U_3RU_5 sequences at both ends (Gilboa et al. 1979b), was not known at the time. Heteroduplexing methods have also been used to demonstrate the splicing of subgenomic RNAs of the HIX strain of MLV (Donoghue et al. 1978) and the 124 strain of MSV (Donoghue et al. 1979).

4. The nuclease-S1 mapping technique of Berk and Sharp (1977) has been recently employed to gauge the size of the sequence transposed to the 5′ ends of RSV subgenomic mRNAs. 28S and 21S RNAs from RSV-infected cells were used to protect labeled restriction fragments of cloned RSV DNA from nuclease digestion. From the size of the protected fragments, it was estimated that about 390 nucleotides from the 5′ end of the genome were joined to internal coding sequences during RNA processing (P. Hackett et al.; D. Schwartz et al.; both pers. comm.).
5. Direct sequencing of part of the 5′ terminus of the *env* mRNA of RAV-2 indicates that at least 340 bases from the 5′ end of the genomic RNA are transferred to this subgenomic mRNA (G. Gasic and W. Hayward, unpubl.).
6. A truncated MMTV provirus cloned and analyzed by Majors and Varmus (1980, 1981) appears to be a reverse transcript of an *env* mRNA, confirming the predictions of Stacey (1980) that subgenomic mRNAs can be packaged, copied by reverse transcriptase, and represented in the host genome as stably integrated DNA. Nucleotide sequencing of portions of this provirus and of wild-type MMTV DNA indicates that the *env* mRNA has a leader sequence of ~290 bases from the 5′ terminus of viral RNA (J. Majors, pers. comm.). In this instance, the sites used for splicing conform to donor and acceptor sites in a large number of other viral genomes and cellular genes (Lerner et al. 1980).

Precise definition of transposed (leader) sequences and the points at which splicing occurs will require the cloning and sequencing of cDNAs transcribed from various mRNAs. However, several additional observations are informative about the structure of spliced mRNAs and the function of the transposed sequences.

1. Quintrell et al. (1980) have examined the structure of the 21S *src* mRNA in RSV-transformed mammalian cells and have shown that at least two regions not coding for the *src* protein must be

positioned on the 5′ side of the gene: the approximately 390-base sequence transposed from the 5′ end of the genome and a sequence derived from the region of the genome deleted in certain *env* mutants of RSV. Interestingly, *src* mRNA from cells transformed by such *env* deletion mutants appears to be identical in size to wild-type *src* mRNA (Lee et al. 1979; Quintrell et al. 1980). In this case, sequences transposed from the 5′ end of the genome are presumably joined to an alternative splice point on the 5′ side of the *env* deletion.

2. Quail cells bearing single RSV proviruses with deletions encompassing most or all of *gag, pol,* and *env* have anomalous RNA species capable of directing synthesis of *src* protein of normal size (Martin et al. 1979). The predominant RNAs in these clones are moderately larger than wild-type *src* mRNAs and may not be spliced.
3. A hamster cell transformed by a single RSV provirus contains two anomalous *src* mRNAs (3.0 kb and 3.6 kb) in the absence of the usual species, yet normal *src* protein is made (Quintrell et al. 1980). The anomalous RNAs appear to reflect properties of the template, rather than the host cell, since chicken cells propagating virus rescued from the hamster cell also contain the two anomalous *src* mRNAs.
4. Cells have been transformed, albeit at low efficiency, by subgenomic restriction fragments of RSV and MSV DNAs (Andersson et al. 1979; Canaani et al. 1979; Blair et al. 1980; Chang et al. 1980; N.G. Copeland et al. 1980; P. Luciw, unpubl.). In these instances, the normal virus-coded RNA-processing signals are unlikely to be present, yet functional transforming proteins are apparently synthesized.
5. Sequences from the 5′ end of viral RNA may not be absolutely required for translation of internal cistrons, at least in vitro. This has been illustrated by the synthesis of RSV *src* protein from fragments of genomic RNA (Purchio et al. 1977; Beemon and Hunter 1978; Kamine et al. 1978), even when precautions were taken to remove any *src* mRNA that might have been packaged in the virion (Purchio et al. 1978).

d. Some Leading but Unanswered Questions. Several unresolved issues about the structure and significance of viral mRNAs should be briefly addressed.

(i) ARE THERE STRUCTURAL DIFFERENCES BETWEEN SUBUNITS OF THE VIRAL GENOME AND GENOME-SIZE mRNAs? Despite the evidence noted above for independent pools of pregenome RNA and *gag* mRNA (Levin and Rosenak 1976), no structural distinctions between these species have yet been made. RNA prepared from virions is capable of directing synthesis of *gag* and *pol* precursor proteins in vitro; however, it is not certain that the messenger activities are present in infectious particles, since a high percentage of particles in retrovirus stocks is noninfectious. Moreover, it has been shown that subgenomic mRNAs are occasionally packaged in mature virions (Stacey 1979); hence genome-size mRNAs might also be packaged. Many eukaryotic mRNAs are spliced, and there is experimental evidence favoring the idea that splicing may be required, in at least some situations, to effect the transfer of RNA from nucleus to cytoplasm (Hamer and Leder 1979). But subunit-size retroviral RNA may have special features that ensure its stability and transport in the absence of splicing. Certainly pregenome RNA cannot be spliced, in the conventional sense, and still retain the full complement of viral sequences. Perhaps the RNA used for synthesis of *gag* is indistinguishable from pregenome RNA until association with polyribosomes confers a prolonged half-life.

Structural differences between *gag* mRNA and genomic RNA would create an additional problem unless the mRNA were inefficiently packaged: *gag* mRNA should be transcribed into DNA in ensuing rounds of infection, producing deleted (and presumably defective) proviruses.

(ii) IS THERE MORE THAN ONE mRNA FOR *gag* PROTEINS? Edwards and Fan (1979) and Ledbetter et al. (1978) have identified two species of MLV *gag* products: one is glycosylated, but not cleaved, and is detected in cell membranes, and the other is cleaved, but not glycosylated, and is found ultimately in viral particles. The former appears to have a primary sequence longer at the amino terminus (Schultz and Oroszlan 1978), and both are synthesized during translation of genome-size RNA in vitro (Edwards and Fan 1979). One explanation of these observations would be the existence of two *gag* mRNAs, perhaps differing by virtue of splicing events that generate intact coding regions of two lengths.

(iii) IS THERE A UNIQUE mRNA FOR *pol*? As yet, there is no definite answer to the question of how the termination signal in *gag* is bypassed to permit the synthesis of the *gag-pol* polyprotein that serves as a precursor to reverse transcriptase (Oppermann et al. 1977; Kopchick et al. 1978). Philipson et al. (1978) found that yeast tRNA, which suppresses amber termination codons (UGA), increased the synthesis of $Pr180^{gag\text{-}pol}$ at the expense of $Pr65^{gag}$ in reticulocyte lysates programmed by Mo-MLV 35S RNA. In similar experiments, Murphy et al. (1980) used an amber-suppressor tRNA to boost the synthesis of $Pr180^{gag\text{-}pol}$ of Rauscher MLV (Ra-MLV) at the expense of $Pr65^{gag}$. Although these results indicated that the *gag* polyprotein was terminated by a single UGA and that *pol* was coded in phase with *gag* (conclusions now confirmed by DNA sequencing [T. Shinnick et al., pers. comm.; Appendix E]), a different result was obtained when the same experiment was performed with 38S RSV RNA (Weiss et al. 1978). In this case, $Pr76^{gag}$ was suppressed in favor of a *gag* protein about 40 amino acids longer at its carboxyl terminus, but without augmented synthesis of $Pr180^{gag\text{-}pol}$. Thus, RSV *gag,* like MLV *gag,* terminates with UGA, but another termination codon is present in phase about 120 nucleotides downstream. This result strongly implied that a different mechanism must be responsible for production of $Pr180^{gag\text{-}pol}$. The most obvious possibility is the production of an mRNA specifically designed for *pol,* lacking the *gag* termination signals. Little structural information could be eliminated from the *gag* region, judging from tryptic peptides of *gag* and *gag-pol* polyproteins (Hizi et al. 1978; Rettenmier et al. 1979).

Confirmation of the predictions of Weiss et al. (1978) has recently emerged from sequencing studies of the amino terminus of the β subunit of AMV polymerase (T.D. Copeland et al. 1980) and of the *gag-pol* boundary region in PR-C-RSV RNA (D. Schwartz et al., pers. comm.). The *gag* termination codon is, in fact, UGA, and it is followed by another amber codon in phase about 114 bases downstream. Further reading in that frame appears to be blocked by multiple termination codons. On the other hand, a shift into a new reading frame beginning 20 bases from the *gag* terminator permits translation of the RNA into the 17 amino acids identified at the amino terminus of the polymerase. Thus, a splicing event that removes (or inactivates) the *gag* terminator and shifts the reading frame by 1 base should generate an appropriate mRNA for *pol.* This could conceivably be effected by elimination of as few as two or as many as several hundred nucleotides.

The predicted *pol* mRNA has not yet been physically identified. This may be due to inherent experimental difficulties in detecting it: its low abundance relative to *gag* mRNA (generally only 1–10% as much *gag-pol* as *gag* polyprotein is made either in vivo or in vitro) and the subtle differences between two very large RNAs.

(iv) ARE THERE OTHER mRNAs AND GENES TO BE DISCOVERED? Thus far, there is a general consensus that the genes required to account for the structural proteins of retroviruses have been identified, but only in a few cases have the products of genes encoding nonstructural proteins been characterized (Chapter 9). Some of the orphan viral RNAs without assigned functions (see above) may be responsible for synthesis of nonstructural (or structural) viral proteins as yet unknown. This seems unlikely in the case of small RNAs occasionally found in RSV-infected cells, since the RNA appears to represent the 3′ region of the genome, which is well endowed with termination codons in all three reading frames (Czernilofsky et al. 1980b; Yamamoto et al. 1980b). On the other hand, nucleotide sequencing has revealed a long open reading frame in the LTRs of several strains of MMTV (Donehower et al. 1981; H. Diggelmann et al.; J. Majors; both pers. comm.). This open frame was predicted from the in vitro translation studies of Dickson and Peters (1981), but neither the expected proteins nor a suitable mRNA have been observed in infected cells.

(v) WHAT IS THE ORIGIN AND ROLE OF MINUS-STRAND RNA? Although the possibility that retroviruses replicate via RNA intermediates has been abandoned, Stavnezer et al. (1976) have detected small amounts of RNA complementary to a substantial portion of RSV and MMTV genomes in the nucleus and cytoplasm of infected cells and in viral particles. The negative-strand RNA constitutes about 1% of total viral RNA and appears to exist in duplex form with plus-strand RNA. Similar observations have been made with cells infected with Mo-MSV (MLV) (Biswal and Benyesh-Melnick 1969; Knesek et al. 1980). Nothing is known about the mechanism of synthesis or the functional role of these unusual species of RNA.

C. Translation of Viral RNA

Although a great deal is now known about the completed products of translation of retroviral mRNAs (cf. Chapter 6), there remain many unanswered questions about the mechanism of translation, the structure of the primary products, and the processing of those products.

Until recently, a major deficiency in our knowledge about translation of viral proteins was the lack of a precise definition of gene boundaries. This situation is now being rectified by the sequencing of cloned DNA and the correlation of sequences with known properties of viral proteins. For example, the *gag* gene of RSV, long known to be encoded near the 5′ end of viral RNA, begins about 370 bases from the 5′ end, despite the presence of several possible initiation codons closer to the 5′ terminus (Haseltine et al. 1977a; Shine et al. 1977; Palmiter et al. 1978; R. Swanstrom; D. Schwartz et al.; both pers.comm.). The sequence transposed to the 5′ end of RSV mRNAs includes three AUG codons that appear to be ignored in the synthesis of $Pr76^{gag}$ and probably the *gag* initiation codon as well (P. Hackett et al.; D. Schwartz et al.; both pers. comm.). However, in the case of *env* mRNA, the *gag* AUG probably initiates translation of *env* protein, whereas it does not function in *src* mRNA, as judged from probable splice-acceptor sites (D. Schwartz et al., pers.comm.). Thus, all RSV mRNAs seem likely to violate the hypothesis that ribosomes attach to eukaryotic mRNAs near or at their 5′ termini and begin reading upon encountering the first codon for methionine (Kozak 1978).

Only fragmentary information is available about the functional significance of noncoding regions of viral mRNA. Darlix et al. (1979) have identified a ribosome-binding site approximately 9–51 nucleotides from the 5′ terminus of 38S RSV RNA; since this site is upstream from methionine codons that are apparently not used for synthesis of $Pr76^{gag}$, the role of this binding site is uncertain. Beemon and Hunter (1977) have shown that translation of 38S RNA to produce $Pr76^{gag}$ in vitro is sensitive to addition of 7-methyl-G, implying that the cap structure at the 5′ end of 38S RNA promotes efficient translation. However, it has also been demonstrated that retroviral genes can be translated in vitro from RNA species that presumably lack both the cap structure and the leader sequences normally present at the 5′ terminus. For example, Purchio et al. (1978) prepared subgenomic, polyadenylated fragments of 38S RSV RNA and showed that the fragments could direct the synthesis of the protein product of *src* in vitro. In similar experiments, Beemon and Hunter (1978) found that synthesis of $p60^{src}$ from fragmented viral RNA was resistant to addition of 7-methyl-G, an inhibitor of translation of capped mRNAs. In addition, several investigators have observed proteins apparently initiated in vitro at multiple sites within viral genes (Beemon and Hunter 1977, 1978; Kamine et al. 1978; Papkoff et al. 1980; Dickson and Peters 1981).

The mechanisms that govern the assignment of RNA species to polyribosomes, either free or membrane-bound, are not known. It is possible that structural differences, perhaps sensed by ribosomes, differentiate 35S–38S RNAs destined to serve as progeny RNA or mRNA. Envelope glycoproteins appear to be synthesized on membrane-bound polyribosomes, whereas the products of *gag* and *pol* (and probably *src*) are produced on free polyribosomes (van Zaane et al. 1977; Lee et al. 1979; Purchio et al. 1980; D. Robertson, unpubl.); however, the manner in which these associations occur is not known. Judging from studies with other viruses, insertion of hydrophobic amino termini of the primary products of *env* into membranes may mediate the attachment of polyribosomes synthesizing *env* products to membranes (Rothman and Lodish 1977).

Synthesis of viral proteins is generally considered to occur mainly in the final stages of virus replication, followed by cleavage and modification of polyproteins and by assembly and maturation of particles. At present, there is little reason to suppose that translation of RNA from input virions early in the life cycle plays an essential role in virus replication. All the proteins known to be encoded by most replication-competent viruses are carried into the cell as structural components of the virus, and mutants temperature-sensitive during early steps in the life cycle are defective either for glycoprotein-mediated entry into cells or for reverse transcription (see Chapter 7). However, a functional role for translation of viral RNA at an early phase of the life cycle has not been rigorously excluded. Gallis et al. (1976) have found that infection of chicken cells with high multiplicities of AMV is followed by the rapid appearance of $Pr76^{gag}$, even when RNA synthesis is blocked by actinomycin D. Since subgenomic mRNAs are sometimes packaged in viral particles (Stacey 1979), it is also possible to envision synthesis of *env*-gene or *src*-gene products during the early phase of infection, though such events have not been reported. However, Shurtz et al. (1979) have demonstrated association of MLV 38S and 23S RNAs with polyribosomes early after infection. Brief administration of inhibitors of protein synthesis early after infection by MLV has been claimed to impair infection (Salzberg et al. 1977; D. Smotkin and R. Weinberg, pers. comm.); it is not known whether this phenomenon applies to other retroviruses or whether cellular or viral proteins are implicated.

D. Final Steps in the Replicative Cycle

The virus life cycle does not end with the synthesis of viral proteins; these must be modified (by glycosylation, phosphorylation, and cleavage) and assembled into particles containing viral RNA. Virions then exit from the cell by budding from the plasma membrane and undergo maturation after release. The details of these events are considered in Chapter 6.

V. INFLUENCE OF HOST CELLS ON THE REPLICATION CYCLE

Throughout this chapter, many host-cell functions have been assumed to assist events in virus replication, including the circularization, integration, and replication of viral DNA, as well as the transcription and translation of viral genes and the processing of viral gene products. In this section, we consider supporting evidence for the roles of host functions in both major phases of the replicative cycle. This evidence comes principally from two experimental perspectives: attempts to determine the relationship of the virus life cycle to events in the cell cycle and attempts to identify host cells that prohibit some specific step in the virus life cycle.

A. Retrovirus Replication and the Cell Cycle

Cultured cells have been manipulated in two ways to examine the relationship of the cell cycle to the virus life cycle. First, by withdrawal of serum from culture media, cells can be placed in a stationary phase at a point in the cell cycle near G_1 (sometimes called G_0). Second, by using a variety of means to place cells at the same point in the cell cycle, cells can be induced to cycle synchronously for one to three generations.

1. Starved Stationary Cells Do Not Support Normal Synthesis of Viral DNA

There is a plethora of evidence indicating that replication of retroviruses proceeds more efficiently if cells are cycling, particularly through S phase, at the time of infection (Bader 1965, 1966; Temin 1965, 1967; Nakata and Bader 1968a,b; Hobom-Schnegg et al. 1970; Yoshikura 1970a,b; Baker and Simons 1971; Weiss 1971; Humphries and Temin 1972, 1974). Investigators in two laboratories have attempted to define the effect of the cell cycle on the initiation of infection by measuring and characterizing the viral DNA synthesized in cells held in the stationary phase by depletion of the culture medium.

Fritsch and Temin (1977b) found that chicken cells in the G_0 state supported the synthesis of less than 10% as much RSV DNA of normal size as found in growing cells. Since normal quantities of viral DNA were made when the starved, infected cells were replenished with serum, some early replicative intermediate was presumed to be preserved in a stable form during starvation. Earlier experiments of Boettiger and Temin (1970) indicated that this intermediate included newly synthesized DNA, since addition of BrdU rendered the provirus light-sensitive, but the nature of the presumed stationary phase intermediate has not been defined. Varmus et al. (1977) performed similar experiments in stationary quail cells and observed marked retardation of elongation of both plus and minus strands. Little or no full-size DNA was present, but atypically short strands were made in the starved cells. Thus, both experimental systems showed that cells removed from the cell cycle supported the synthesis of viral DNA poorly, but the nature of the defect in G_0 cells has not been further defined.

Interestingly, all retroviruses may not be subject to these constraints. Viral DNA is synthesized normally in stationary cultures of sheep choroid plexus cells after infection by visna virus (A. Haase, unpubl.). It may be significant that visna virus DNA, unlike other retroviral DNA, is synthesized principally in the nucleus (A. Haase, unpubl.).

2. Cellular DNA Synthesis Is Required for Integration

Varmus et al. (1977, 1979b) have exploited density-labeling techniques to determine whether viral DNA integrates into recently replicated cellular DNA. Randomly growing cultures of chicken or quail cells were infected with RSV in the presence of BrdU for several hours; then high-molecular-weight DNA was banded in density gradients of CsCl. Unintegrated viral DNA banded in the high-density region as expected, but integrated DNA linked to high-molecular-weight cellular DNA was found only at intermediate regions and not at light-density regions. This finding indicated that viral DNA entered only the cellular DNA that had replicated during the infection. However, the basis of this result is not known. Competent viral DNA might not be synthesized in cells that have not traversed the S phase; some feature of DNA replication (e.g., an enzyme specific to the S phase or the topology of replicating DNA) might be required for integration; or the integrative events themselves might initiate replication of adjacent cellular DNA.

3. Virus Production Is Impaired in Stationary Cells

Several groups have shown that virus production by cells chronically infected with retroviruses is markedly reduced when the cells are placed in stationary phase by serum deprivation or thymidine block (Leong et al. 1972a; Panem and Kirsten 1973; Paskind et al. 1975). In some cases, a pool of competent precursor RNA appeared to be present in the arrested cells. Leong et al. (1972a) found that virus production resumed promptly (before entry into the S phase) after serum replacement, but radiolabeled uridine appeared in viral particles only several hours later. Similarly, Paskind et al. (1975) showed that the initial wave of virus production after serum replacement was sensitive to cycloheximide, but not to actinomycin D. However, a second wave of virus production was sensitive to actinomycin D. In contrast to these findings with RSV-infected chick cells and MLV-infected mouse cells, Panem and Kirsten (1973) found that virus production in MLV-infected rat cells resumed only after passage through mitosis. Furthermore, Humphries and Coffin (1976) could detect no changes in the rate of viral RNA synthesis related to the cell cycle in synchronized cells producing ALVs. The significance of these apparently conflicting results is not known. Humphries and Temin (1974) have argued that one round of mitosis is required to initiate virus production after acute infection, measuring either the kinetics of virus production after release from the stationary phase or the effects of metaphase arrest induced by Colcemid. The delayed appearance of virus after restoration of serum to starved cultures probably reflects the time required to synthesize, integrate, and transcribe viral DNA; the modest effects of the mitotic inhibitor may, however, indicate a specific requirement for a cellular function supplied during or after mitosis to establish efficient virus production (Humphries et al. 1981).

B. Host Cells Can Affect Virus Replication at Stages Subsequent to Virus Entry

Most restrictions on virus host range appear to be imposed by surface interactions: cells lacking receptors for viral envelope glycoproteins cannot be penetrated by those viruses. Such determinants of host range are discussed more fully in Chapter 3. For several combinations of cells and viruses, however, there is evidence for a block to replication at some point following virus entry.

1. Mammalian Cells Are Nonpermissive for Replication of RSV

Although mammalian cells resist the entry of most strains of RSV (Altaner and Temin 1970; Boettiger et al. 1975), viral DNA can be synthesized and integrated with moderate efficiency after infection with certain RSV stocks able to infect mammalian cells (Varmus et al. 1973b). Nevertheless, the frequency of transformation appears to be low; virus is seldom, if ever, produced (Altaner and Temin 1970); and infected, nontransformed cells, capable of releasing transforming virus after fusion with chick cells, can be isolated from RSV-infected mammalian cell cultures (Boettiger 1974b; Turek and Oppermann 1980). The blocks to viral gene expression probably occur at transcriptional and other levels: one to three logs less viral RNA is present in mammalian cells, as compared with avian cells (Bishop et al. 1976); the processing of viral RNA favors 21S mRNA over 38S RNA (Quintrell et al. 1980); viral polyproteins are synthesized but not cleaved (Vogt et al. 1975); and viral particles are generally not detected. The reduction in viral RNA is not adequate to account for the complete absence of viral particles, but it is not known whether the failure to cleave viral polyproteins in the nonpermissive cells is responsible for the nonpermissiveness or is a consequence of the failure to assemble particles in which cleavage can occur.

2. Alleles at the Fv-1 Locus Restrict Replication of MLV

The step in the virus life cycle at which the products of *Fv-1* alleles block replication of certain strains of MLV falls somewhere between virus entry and synthesis of viral RNA (Huang et al. 1973; Krontiris et al. 1973; Jolicoeur and Baltimore 1976b; Jolicoeur 1979). Integration of MLV DNA does not seem to occur during infection under restrictive conditions (Jolicoeur and Baltimore 1976a; Sveda and Soeiro 1976), but it has yet to be established whether the block specifically affects integration of competent viral DNA or whether it impairs the synthesis of competent DNA. Recent reports that viral DNA synthesized in restrictive hosts may be less infectious than DNA synthesized in permissive hosts (see Yang et al. 1980a) and that the amount of closed circular DNA is reduced in at least some restrictive hosts (Jolicoeur and Rassart 1980; Yang et al. 1980a) suggest that the restriction may be directed at the synthesis of linear DNA competent to circularize and/or integrate. Linear DNA synthesized in a restrictive host is transferred normally to the nucleus, although it fails to circularize (Jolicoeur and Rassart 1981). The evidence linking MLV p30 to N and B tropisms (Hopkins et al. 1977; Schindler et al. 1977; Gautsch et al. 1978; Tress et al. 1979) may be related to evidence that p30 associates with and stimulates reverse transcriptase (Bandyopadhyay and Levy 1978). Alternatively, the mechanism might specifically affect circularization.

3. Other Examples

There are several additional interesting instances in which cells restrict the replication of retroviruses by mechanisms that may be intracellular.

1. Robinson (1976) and Linial and Neiman (1976) have found that cells from many types of chicken embryos fail to support the efficient replication of subgroup-E ALV or RSV. Hughes et al. (1979a) have measured viral DNA synthesis in restrictive and permissive hosts and have found excellent correlations between the amounts of linear viral DNA made and the titers of virus produced. Hence, the restriction must operate before or during reverse transcription; impaired entry of virus particles has not been rigorously excluded as an explanation.
2. Peries et al. (1977) and Teich et al. (1977) were unable to establish a productive infection of teratocarcinoma cells with MLV, although the same cells appeared fully susceptible to replication of some other RNA and DNA viruses and differentiated descendants supported at least a low level of production of MLV. The nature of the block has not been fully defined, but it appears to differ between nullipotent and pluripotent cell types. Both nullipotent and pluripotent cells permitted entry of MLV pseudotypes of vesicular stomatitis virus (VSV), but in nullipotent cells, new viral DNA was either not synthesized or not integrated and, in pluripotent cells, viral DNA persisted but was not expressed

(Teich et al. 1977). It is possible that impaired expression reflects an incapacity of these cells to process (splice) viral RNA, as observed after SV40 infection of one teratocarcinoma line (Segal et al. 1979). Fusion of acutely infected embryonal carcinoma cells with cells permissive for virus production restores permissivity, suggesting that the immature cells lack a function necessary for virus growth (Gautsch 1980). The block to replication may not be absolute, since it can be overcome by infection at extremely high multiplicities (J. Levy, unpubl.).

The situation with cultured pluripotent stem cells appears to mimic the resistance of preimplantation embryos to productive infection by MLV, since adult mice derived from infected blastocysts contained viral DNA and expressed it in at least some tissues (Jaenisch 1976). By injection of postimplantation embryos, Jaenisch (1980) has recently found that the embryo may be particularly receptive to infection by MLV about 8 to 10 days after fertilization.

3. A lymphoblastoid line derived from a chicken with the herpesvirus-induced Marek's disease has been shown to restrict the propagation of some strains of RSV but not of *src* deletion mutants of RSV (Neiman et al. 1978). Since viral DNA appears to be made in similar amounts shortly after infection by the two types of agents, the authors proposed that viral DNA containing *src* fails to integrate, perhaps as a consequence of site-specific degradation. Direct evidence concerning the mechanism of restriction is not yet available.
4. Fully differentiated cells no longer capable of entering the cell cycle may prove to be resistant to infection if some component of the cell cycle is required for early events in virus replication. This possibility has yet to be explored.
5. A variety of other poorly defined host factors appears to influence the replication of retroviruses. This view is based on evidence that certain chromosomes are required for replication of MLVs (Gazdar et al. 1977) or BaEV (Brown et al. 1979), on observations suggesting that certain types of cells are particularly suited to support replication of certain viruses (see, e.g., Gazzolo et al. 1974; Hu et al. 1979; Shimakage et al. 1979; Yoshikura et al. 1979; Breitman et al. 1980; Graf et al. 1980), and on the possibility that genetic loci that determine resistance to virus-induced disease may (as in the well-studied case of *Fv*-1) mediate their

effects by impairing virus replication (see, e.g., Mak et al. 1979; Evans et al. 1980; Gardner et al. 1980; Suzuki and Axelrad 1980).

VI. INHIBITORS OF REPLICATION

The dependence of retroviruses on many components and functions of host cells suggests that their growth will be affected by inhibitors of host macromolecular synthesis. This prediction has been frequently documented for inhibitors of the synthesis of DNA, RNA, and protein (for review, see Bader 1975). In addition, replication is usually inhibited by agents that inhibit the action of reverse transcriptase (see Section III.B.1.f), although only in a few cases have the molecular consequences of the inhibitors been directly assessed in infected cells (Lovinger et al. 1978). Treatment of viral particles with UV-irradiation affects replication at an early step, apparently independent of its mutagenic effects. The lesions are believed to impair the capacity of reverse transcriptase to synthesize full-size DNA (Lovinger et al. 1975; Owada et al. 1976; Bister et al. 1977; Martin et al. 1979).

The most attractive inhibitors are those that may specifically affect virus functions, without major detriment to host functions:

1. Production of infectious virus can be severely inhibited by the use of drugs (tunicamycin or glucosamine) that interfere with glycosylation of envelope glycoproteins (see, e.g., Lewandowski et al. 1975; Schwarz et al. 1976; Diggelmann 1979; Schultz and Oroszlan 1979; Stohrer and Hunter 1979).
2. Low doses of ethidium bromide have been shown by several investigators to have inhibitory effects on retrovirus replication, particularly when administered prior to or early in the life cycle (Richert and Hare 1972; Guntaka et al. 1975; Avery and Levy 1979). One mechanism of inhibition has been claimed to involve reduced accumulation of closed circular DNA and proviral DNA (Guntaka et al. 1975), but the modest differences observed have yet to be confirmed with more recently developed techniques. Effects of ethidium bromide on mitochondrial function have also been proposed to account for the inhibition (Richert and Hare 1972), but there is no evidence that the mitochondria are directly involved in the replicative cycle (Bader 1973; Guntaka et al. 1975; Leblond-Larouche et al. 1979).

3. Drugs that inhibit the methylation of viral (and cellular) RNAs have been reported to interfere with the replication of RSV in the absence of appreciable cellular toxicity (Robert-Gero et al. 1975; Bader et al. 1978). On the other hand, Dimock and Stoltzfus (1978) used cycloleucine to inhibit methylation of internal adenosines and the penultimate nucleotide at the 5′ terminus of RSV RNA, and they observed no significant effect on virus production. Since this agent does not impair formation of a methylated cap nucleotide, it was proposed that more general inhibitors of methylation may be effective because of their ability to interfere with production of capped mRNAs. On the other hand, cycloleucine appears to have a modest inhibitory effect on the production of spliced mRNAs (M. Stoltzfus, unpubl.).
4. Zamecnik and Stephenson (1978) have shown that a chemically synthesized 13-nucleotide complement of part of the sequence redundant at the termini of viral RNA can inhibit RSV replication in chicken cells. The mechanism of inhibition has not been established.
5. Guntaka et al. (1979) have observed a striking inhibition of replication of RSV in chicken cells treated with 5-methylcytidine; again the mechanism is not known.
6. Ascorbic acid has been reported to affect both replication of RSV and RSV-induced transformation by uncertain mechanisms (Bissell et al. 1980).
7. Several investigators have shown that interferon can depress the replication of murine retroviruses (Friedman 1977). In relatively high doses, interferon may block the establishment of the proviral state after infection with MSV (Morris and Burke 1979), but in conventional doses, it appears primarily to perturb the assembly and/or release of infectious particles by chronically infected cells (Friedman et al. 1975; Strauchen et al. 1977; Salzberg et al. 1978; Pitha et al. 1979; Sen and Sarkar 1980). Studies with an MLV mutant temperature sensitive for virus assembly suggest that the major effect is on a relatively early step in assembly (Chang et al. 1977). No direct effects on synthesis of viral RNA have been observed (Fan and MacIsaac 1978).
8. Cycloheximide has recently been reported to depress the accumulation of closed circular DNA, without appreciable effects upon the synthesis of linear DNA, when administered early during infection (Yang et al. 1980b).

VII. REPRISE

The story that has unfolded about the replication of retroviruses in the decade since the discovery of reverse transcriptase has been full of the ingenuities of nature. Repetitions are prominent in this story: The genome, being diploid, is itself redundant, and each subunit ends with a short repeat required for an early step in DNA synthesis. The major product of DNA synthesis has long terminal redundancies that are themselves terminated by inverted repeats, perhaps instrumental during integration; and the process of integration generates a new repeat from a cellular sequence that then flanks both sides of the new provirus. Although the implications of these symmetries are not yet apparent, one of the benefits of the structure of proviruses may be the self-provision of regulatory signals for promotion, processing, and perhaps termination of viral RNA. The rationale for a diploid genome is less evident: structural stability, facilitation of DNA synthesis, and genetic flexibility are among the possible advantages. Coffin (1979) has proposed that the high frequency of genetic recombination observed during retrovirus replication might be linked to the ability to transfer nascent DNA strands between templates; heterozygotic dimers would then be obligatory intermediates in recombination.

Another striking feature of the replication pathway is the balance achieved between virus and host functions during the life cycle. In the early phases, the virus provides most of the ingredients—at least template and DNA polymerase—although the cell has supplied the first primer during a previous round of replication. Among the subtleties yet to be elucidated are the functions supplied by the cell during the final stages of viral DNA synthesis and during integration. The integrative mechanism, in particular, may have far-reaching implications, since it is possible that similar mechanisms underlie other events involving the incorporation of foreign DNA into eukaryotic genomes or transposition within them. During the late phase of the replicative cycle, retroviruses employ strategies for gene expression that reflect the successful adaptation of a compact genetic unit to the capabilities of host cells. To synthesize proteins encoded by internal cistrons in this polycistronic unit, subgenomic mRNAs are produced by the processing of a single primary transcript. It appears that a single set of signals, supplied by viral DNA itself, directs the synthesis of the minimal effective transcript by a host RNA polymerase. This transcript can be used as genomic subunits, as mRNA, or as a precursor to subgenomic mRNAs. A similar conservatism is evident in the primary products of translation. These are generally polyproteins from which several end products are derived by cleavage and modification, using, it appears, both viral and host machineries. Still uncertain are the ways in which the host cell modulates expression of viral genes in several instances. Elucidation of such mechanisms could help to shape our sense of the possibilities for more general control of eukaryotic genes.

REFERENCES

Abelson, J. 1979. RNA processing and the intervening sequence problem. *Annu. Rev. Biochem.* **48:**1035–1069.

Aboud, M., R. Shoor, and S. Salzberg. 1979. Adsorption, penetration, and uncoating of murine leukemia virus studied by using its reverse transcriptase. *J. Virol.* **30:**32–37.

Abrell, J.W. and R.C. Gallo. 1973. Purification, characterization, and comparison of the DNA polymerases, from two primate RNA tumor viruses. *J. Virol.* **12:**431–439.

Akiyama, Y. and P.K. Vogt. 1979. Integration of different sarcoma virus genomes into host DNA: Evidence against tandem arrangement and for shared-integration sites. *Proc. Natl. Acad. Sci.* **76:**2465–2469.

Ali, M. and M.A. Baluda. 1974. Synthesis of avian oncornavirus DNA in infected chicken cells. *J. Virol.* **13:**1005–1013.

Altaner, C. and H.M. Temin. 1970. Carcinogenesis by RNA sarcoma viruses. XII. A quantitative study of infection of rat cells *in vitro* by avian sarcoma viruses. *Virology* **40:**118–134.

Alwine, J.C., D.J. Kemp, and G.R. Stark. 1977. Method for detection of specific RNAs in agarose gels by transfer to diazobenzyloxymethyl-paper and hybridization with DNA probes. *Proc. Natl. Acad. Sci.* **74:**5350–5354.

Amer, C.A., J.T. Parsons, and A.J. Faras. 1981. Direct proof of the 5′ to 3′ transcriptional jump during reverse transcription of the avian retrovirus genome by DNA sequencing. *J. Virol.* **38:**398–402.

Anderson, S.M., W.S. Hayward, B.G. Neel, and H. Hanafusa. 1980. Avian erythroblastosis virus produces two mRNAs. *J. Virol.* **36:**676–683.

Andersson, P., M.P. Goldfarb, and R.A. Weinberg. 1979. A defined subgenomic fragment of in vitro synthesized Moloney sarcoma virus DNA can induce cell transformation upon transfection. *Cell* **16:**63–75.

Astrin, S.M. 1978. Endogenous viral genes of the White Leghorn chicken: Common site of residence and sites associated with specific phenotypes of viral gene expression. *Proc. Natl. Acad. Sci.* **75:**5941–5945.

Astrin, S.M., E.G. Buss, and W.S. Hayward. 1979. Endogenous viral genes are non-essential in the chicken. *Nature* **282:**339–341.

Auld, D.S., H. Kawaguchi, D.M. Livingston, and B.L. Vallee. 1974. Reverse transcriptase from avian myeloblastosis virus: A zinc metalloenzyme. *Biochem. Biophys. Res. Commun.* **57:**967–972.

Avery, R.J. and J.A. Levy. 1979. The effect of ethidium bromide on C type virus production and induction. *Virology* **95:**277–284.

Bacheler, L.T. and H. Fan. 1979. Multiple integration sites for Moloney murine leukemia virus in productively infected mouse fibroblasts. *J. Virol.* **30:**657–667.

———. 1980. Integrated Moloney murine leukemia virus DNA studied by using complementary DNA which does not recognize endogenous related sequences. *J. Virol.* **33:** 1074–1082.

———. 1981. Isolation of recombinant DNA clones carrying complete integrated proviruses of Moloney murine leukemia virus. *J. Virol.* **37:**181–190.

Bader, A.V. 1973. Role of mitochondria in the production of RNA-containing tumor viruses. *J. Virol.* **11:**314–324.

Bader, J.P. 1965. The requirement for DNA synthesis in the growth of Rous sarcoma and Rous-associated viruses. *Virology* **26:**253–261.

———. 1966. Metabolic requirements for infection by Rous sarcoma virus. II. The participation of cellular DNA. *Virology* **29:**452–461.

———. 1975. Reproduction of RNA tumor viruses. In *Comprehensive virology* (ed. H. Fraenkel and R.R. Wagner), vol. 4, pp. 253–332. Plenum Press, New York.

Bader, J.P., N.R. Brown, P.K. Chiang, and G.L. Cantoni. 1978. 3-diazoadenosine, an inhibitor of adenosylhomocysteine hydrolase, inhibits reproduction of Rous sarcoma virus and transformation of chick embryo cells. *Virology* **89:**494–505.

Baker, R.S. and P.J. Simons. 1971. Alterations in the susceptibility of cultured mouse cells to transformation by murine sarcoma virus (Harvey). *J. Gen. Virol.* **12:**95–104.

Balduzzi, P. and H.R. Morgan. 1970. Mechanisms of oncogenic transformation by Rous sarcoma virus. I. Intracellular inactivation of cell-transforming ability of Rous sarcoma virus by 5-bromodeoxyuridine and light. *J. Virol.* **5:**470–477.

Baltimore, D. 1970. RNA-dependent DNA polymerase in virions of RNA tumour viruses. *Nature* **226:**1209–1211.

———. 1976. Viruses, polymerases, and cancer. *Science* **192:**632–636.

Baltimore, D. and D. Smoler. 1971. Primer requirement and template specificity of the DNA polymerase of RNA tumor viruses. *Proc. Natl. Acad. Sci.* **68:**1507–1511.

———. 1972. Association of an endoribonuclease with the avian myeloblastosis virus deoxyribonucleic acid polymerase. *J. Biol. Chem.* **247:**7282–7287.

Baltimore, D., E. Gilboa, E. Rothenberg, and F. Yoshimura. 1979. Production of a discrete, infectious double-stranded DNA by reverse transcription in virions of Moloney murine leukemia virus. *Cold Spring Harbor Symp. Quant. Biol.* **43:**869–874.

Baluda, M.A. 1972. Widespread presence, in chickens, of DNA complementary to the RNA genome of avian leukosis viruses. *Proc. Natl. Acad. Sci.* **69:**576–580.

Baluda, M. and D.P. Nayak. 1970. DNA complementary to viral RNA in leukemic cells induced by avian myeloblastosis virus. *Proc. Natl. Acad. Sci.* **67:**329–336.

Bandyopadhyay, A.K. 1977. Effect of Rauscher leukemia virus-specific proteins on reverse transcriptase. Binding between reverse transcriptase and p30. *J. Biol. Chem.* **252:**5883–5887.

Bandyopadhyay, A.K. and C.C. Levy. 1978. Effect of RNA tumor virus-specific protein p30 on reverse transcriptase. Intraspecies and interspecies interaction between reverse transcriptase and p30. *J. Biol. Chem.* **253:**8285–8290.

Battula, N. and L.A. Loeb. 1974. The infidelity of avian myeloblastosis virus deoxyribonucleic acid polymerase in polynucleotide replication. *J. Biol. Chem* **249:**4086–4093.

Battula, N. and H.M. Temin. 1977. Infectious DNA of spleen necrosis virus is integrated at a single site in the DNA of chronically infected chicken fibroblasts. *Proc. Natl. Acad. Sci.* **74:**281–285.

———. 1978. Sites of integration of infectious DNA of avian reticuloendotheliosis viruses in different avian cellular DNAs. *Cell* **13:**387–398.

Bauer, G. and H.M. Temin. 1979. Pheasant virus DNA polymerase is related to avian leukosis virus DNA polymerase at the active site. *J. Virol.* **32:**78–90.

———. 1980a. Radioimmunological comparison of the DNA polymerases of avian retroviruses. *J. Virol.* **33:**1046–1057.

———. 1980b. Specific antigenic relationships between the RNA-dependent DNA polymerases of avian reticuloendotheliosis viruses and mammalian type C retroviruses. *J. Virol.* **34:**168–177.

Baxt, W.G. and J.L. Meinkoth. 1978. Transfer of duck cell DNA sequences to nucleus of 3T3 cells by Rous sarcoma virus. *Proc. Natl. Acad. Sci.* **75:**4252–4256.

Beemon, K. and T. Hunter. 1977. *In vitro* translation yields a possible Rous sarcoma virus *src* gene product. *Proc. Natl. Acad. Sci.* **74:**3302–3306.

———. 1978. Characterization of Rous sarcoma virus *src* gene products synthesized in vitro. *J. Virol.* **28:**551–566.

Beemon, K.L. and J.M. Keith. 1976. Structure of Rous sarcoma virus RNA. 1. Localization of N^6-methyladenosine; 2. the sequence of 23 nucleotides following the 5′ capped terminus in m^7GpppG^mp. In *Animal virology* (ed. D. Baltimore et al.), vol. 4, pp. 95–105. Academic Press, New York.

Benz, E.W., Jr. and D. Dina. 1979. Moloney murine sarcoma virions synthesize full-genome-length double-stranded DNA *in vitro. Proc. Natl. Acad. Sci.* **76:**3294–3298.

Benz, E.W., Jr., R.W. Wydro, B. Nadal-Ginard, and D. Dina. 1980. Moloney murine sarcoma proviral DNA is a transcriptional unit. *Nature* **288:**665–669.

Bergmann, D.G., L.M. Souza, and M.A. Baluda. 1980. Characterization of avian myeloblastosis-associated virus DNA intermediates. *J. Virol.* **34:**366–372.

Berk, A.J. and P.A. Sharp. 1977. Sizing and mapping of early adenovirus mRNAs by gel electrophoresis of Sl endonuclease-digested hybrids. *Cell* **12:**721–732.

Berkower, A.S., F. Lilly, and R. Soeiro. 1980. Expression of viral RNA in Friend virus-induced erythroleukemia cells. *Cell* **19:**637–642.

Bishayee, S., M. Strand, and J.T. August. 1978. Cellular membrane receptors for oncovirus envelope glycoprotein: Properties of the binding reaction and influence of different reagents on the substrate and the receptors. *Arch. Biochem. Biophys.* **189:**161–171.

Bishop, J.M. 1978. Retroviruses. *Annu. Rev. Biochem.* **47:**35–88.

Bishop, J.M., C.-T. Deng, B.W.J. Mahy, N. Quintrell, E. Stavnezer, and H.E. Varmus. 1976. Synthesis of viral RNA in cells infected by avian sarcoma viruses. In *Animal virology* (ed. D. Baltimore et al.), vol. 4, pp. 1–20. Academic Press, New York.

Bissell, M.J., C. Hatie, D.A. Farson, R.I. Schwartz, and W.-J. Soo. 1980. Ascorbic acid inhibits replication and infectivity of avian RNA tumor virus. *Proc. Natl. Acad. Sci.* **77:**2711–2715.

Bister, K., H.E. Varmus, E. Stavnezer, E. Hunter, and P.K. Vogt. 1977. Biological and biochemical studies on the inactivation of avian oncoviruses by ultraviolet irradiation. *Virology* **77:**689–704.

Biswal, N. and M. Benyesh-Melnick. 1969. Complementary nuclear RNAs of murine sarcoma-leukemia virus complex in transformed cells. *Proc. Natl. Acad. Sci.* **64:** 1372–1379.

Blaas, D., M. Rucheton, and P. Jeanteur. 1979. Characterization and properties of a protein kinase associated with murine sarcoma-leukemia virus (MSV-MuLV). Endogenous phosphorylation of a unique p10 polypeptide. *Biochem. Biophys. Res. Commun.* **87:**272–280.

Blair, D.G., W.L. McClements, M.K. Oskarsson, P.J. Fischinger, and G.F. Vande Woude. 1980. Biological activity of cloned Moloney sarcoma virus DNA: Terminally redundant sequences may enhance transformation efficiency. *Proc. Natl. Acad. Sci.* **77:**3504–3508.

Boettiger, D. 1974a. Reversion and induction of Rous sarcoma virus expression in virus-transformed baby hamster kidney cells. *Virology* **62:**522–529.

———. 1974b. Virogenic, nontransformed cells isolated following infection of normal rat kidney cells with B77 strain Rous sarcoma virus. *Cell* **3:**71–76.

Boettiger, D. and H.M. Temin. 1970. Light inactivation of focus formation by chicken embryo fibroblasts infected with avian sarcoma virus in the presence of 5-bromodeoxyuridine. *Nature* **228:**622–624.

Boettiger, D., D.N. Love, and R.A. Weiss. 1975. Virus envelope markers in mammalian tropism of avian RNA tumor viruses. *J. Virol.* **15:**108–114.

Bondurant, M., S.-I. Hashimoto, and M. Green. 1976. Methylation pattern of genomic RNA from Moloney murine leukemia virus. *J. Virol.* **19:**998–1005.

Bondurant, M., R. Ramabhadran, M. Green, and W.S.M. Wold. 1979. "*sarc*" sequence transcription in Moloney sarcoma virus-transformed nonproducer cell lines. *J. Virol.* **29:**76–82.

Boone, L.R. and A. Skalka. 1980. Two species of full-length cDNA are synthesized in high yield by mellitin-treated avian retrovirus particles. *Proc. Natl. Acad. Sci.* **77:**847–851.

———. 1981a. Viral DNA synthesized in vitro by avian retrovirus particles permeabilized with melittin. I. Kinetics of synthesis and size of minus- and plus-strand transcripts. *J. Virol.* **37:**109–116.

———. 1981b. Viral DNA synthesized in vitro by avian retrovirus particles permeabilized with melittin. II. Evidence for a strand displacement mechanism in plus-strand synthesis. *J. Virol.* **37:**117–126.

Bosselman, R.A. and I.M. Verma. 1980. Genome organization of retroviruses. V. In vitro-synthesized Moloney murine leukemia viral DNA has long terminal redundancy. *J. Virol.* **33:**487–493.

Botchan, M. and G. McKenna. 1974. Appendix. Cleavage of integrated SV40 by RI restriction endonuclease. *Cold Spring Harbor Symp. Quant. Biol.* **38:**391–395.

Botchan, M., W. Topp, and J. Sambrook. 1976. The arrangement of simian virus 40 sequences in the DNA of transformed cells. *Cell* **9:**269–285.

Brahic, M. and A.T. Haase. 1978. Detection of viral sequences of low reiteration frequency by *in situ* hybridization. *Proc. Natl. Acad. Sci.* **75:**6125–6129.

Breindl, M., L. Bacheler, H. Fan, and R. Jaenisch. 1980. Chromatin conformation of integrated Moloney leukemia virus DNA sequences in tissues of BALB/Mo mice and in virus-infected cell lines. *J. Virol.* **34:**373–382.

Breitman, M.L., M.M.C. Lai, and P.K. Vogt. 1980. Attenuation of avian reticuloendotheliosis virus: Loss of the defective transforming component during serial passage of oncogenic virus in fibroblasts. *Virology* **101:**304–306.

Brewer, L.C. and R.D. Wells. 1974. Mechanistic independence of avian myeloblastosis virus DNA polymerase and ribonuclease H. *J. Virol.* **14:**1494–1502.

Bromley, P.A., P.-F. Spahr, and J.-L. Darlix. 1979. New procedure for isolation of Rous sarcoma virus-specific RNA from infected cells. *J. Virol.* **31:**86–93.

Brown, S., H.K. Oie, A.F. Gazdar, J.D. Minna, and U. Francke. 1979. Requirement of human chromosomes 19, 6 and possibly 3 for infection of hamster X human hybrid cells with baboon M7 type C virus. *Cell* **18:**135–143.

Brugge, J.S., A.F. Purchio, and R.L. Erikson. 1977a. Virus-specific RNA species present in the cytoplasm of Rous sarcoma virus-infected chicken cells. *Virology* **83:**16–26.

———. 1977b. The distribution of virus-specific RNA in Rous sarcoma virus-induced hamster tumor cells. *Virology* **83:**27–33.

Buetti, E. and H. Diggelmann. 1981. Cloned mouse mammary tumor virus DNA is biologically active in transfected mouse cells and its expression is stimulated by glucocorticoid hormones. *Cell* **23:**335–345.

Bukhari, A.T., J.A. Shapiro, and S.L. Adhya, eds. 1977. *DNA insertion elements, plasmids, and episomes.* Cold Spring Harbor Laboratory, Cold Spring Harbor, New York.

Bunte, T., U. Novak, R. Friedrich, and K. Moelling. 1980. Effect of actinomycin D on nucleic acid hybridization. The cause of erroneous DNA elongation during DNA synthesis of RNA tumor viruses in vitro. *Biochim. Biophys. Acta* **610:**241–247.

Callahan, R., C.J. Sherr, and G.J. Todaro. 1977. A new class of murine retroviruses: Immunological and biochemical comparison of novel isolates from *Mus cervicolor* and *Mus caroli. Virology* **80:**401–416.

Calos, M.P. and J.H. Miller. 1980. Transposable elements. *Cell* **20:**579–595.

Calos, M.P., L. Johnsrud, and J.H. Miller. 1978. DNA sequence at the integration sites of the insertion element IS1. *Cell* **13:**411–418.

Cameron, J.R., E.Y. Loh, and R.W. Davis. 1979. Evidence for transposition of dispersed repetitive DNA families in yeast. *Cell* **16:**739–751.

Campbell, A. 1962. Episomes. *Adv. Genet.* **11:**101–145.

Canaani, E. and S.A. Aaronson. 1979. Restriction enzyme analysis of mouse cellular type C viral DNA: Emergence of new viral sequences in spontaneous AKR/J lymphomas. *Proc. Natl. Acad. Sci.* **76:**1677–1681.

Canaani, E. and P. Duesberg. 1972. Role of subunits of 60 to 70 S avian tumor virus ribonucleic acid in its template activity for the viral deoxyribonucleic acid polymerase. *J. Virol.* **10:**23–31.

Canaani, E., P. Duesberg, and D. Dina. 1977. Cleavage map of linear mouse sarcoma virus DNA. *Proc. Natl. Acad. Sci.* **74:**29–33.

Canaani, E., K.C. Robbins, and S.A. Aaronson. 1979. The transforming gene of Moloney murine sarcoma virus. *Nature* **282:**378–383.

Cashion, L.M., R.H. Joho, M.A. Planitz, M.A. Billeter, and C. Weissmann. 1976. Initiation sites of Rous sarcoma virus RNA-directed DNA synthesis *in vitro*. *Nature* **262:**186–190.

Catala, F. and P. Vigier. 1979. Infectivity of proviral DNA from avian sarcoma virus-transformed mammalian cells. *J. Virol.* **29:**833–839.

Cedar, H. and A. Panet. 1979. Activation of the endogenous proviral genes in mouse cells is not followed by increased sensitivity to deoxyribonuclease I digestion. *J. Gen. Virol.* **45:**765–769.

Chan, H.W., C.F. Garon, E.H. Chang, D.R. Lowy, G.L. Hager, E.M. Scolnick, R. Repaske, and M.A. Martin. 1980. Molecular cloning of the Harvey sarcoma virus circular DNA intermediates. II. Further structural analyses. *J. Virol.* **33:**845–855.

Chang, E.H., M.W. Myers, P.K.Y. Wong, and R.M. Friedman. 1977. The inhibitory effect of interferon on a temperature-sensitive mutant of Moloney murine leukemia virus. *Virology* **77:**625–636.

Chang, E.H., J.M. Maryak, C.-M. Wei, T.Y. Shih, R. Shober, H.L. Cheung, R.W. Ellis, G.L. Hager, E.M. Scolnick, and D.R. Lowy. 1980. Functional organization of the Harvey murine sarcoma virus genome. *J. Virol.* **35:**76–92.

Chattopadhyay, S.K., W.P. Rowe, N.M. Teich, and D.R. Lowy. 1975. Definitive evidence that the murine C-type virus inducing locus *Akv-1* is viral genetic material. *Proc. Natl. Acad. Sci.* **72:**906–910.

Chen, I.S.Y. and H.M. Temin. 1980. Ribonucleotides in unintegrated linear spleen necrosis virus DNA. *J. Virol.* **33:**1058–1073.

Chirikjian, J.G., L. Rye, and T.S. Papas. 1975. Affinity chromatography of viral DNA polymerases on pyran-sepharose. *Proc. Natl. Acad. Sci.* **72:**1142–1146.

Chiswell, D.J. and C.R. Pringle. 1977. Infectious DNA from cells infected with feline syncytium-forming virus (Spumaviridae). *J. Gen. Virol.* **36:**551–555.

———. 1979. Feline syncytium-forming virus: DNA provirus size and structure. *J. Gen. Virol.* **44:**145–152.

Clayman, C.H., E. Mosharrafa, and A.J. Faras. 1979a. In vitro synthesis of infectious transforming DNA by the avian sarcoma virus reverse transcriptase. *J. Virol.* **29:**242–249.

Clayman, C.H., E.T. Mosharrafa, D.L. Anderson, and A.J. Faras. 1979b. Circular forms of DNA synthesized by Rous sarcoma virus in vitro. *Science* **206:**582–584.

Clements, J.E., O. Narayan, D.E. Griffin, and R.T. Johnson. 1979. The synthesis and structure of visna virus DNA. *Virology* **93:**377–386.

Coffin, J.M. 1972. Rescue of Rous sarcoma virus from Rous sarcoma virus-transformed mammalian cells. *J. Virol.* **10:**153–156.

———. 1979. Structure, replication, and recombination of retrovirus genomes: Some unifying hypotheses. *J. Gen. Virol.* **42:**1–26.

Coffin, J.M. and W.A. Haseltine. 1977a. Terminal redundancy and the origin of replication of Rous sarcoma virus RNA. *Proc. Natl. Acad. Sci.* **74**:1908–1912.

———. 1977b. Nucleotide sequence of Rous sarcoma virus RNA at the initiation site of DNA synthesis. The 102nd nucleotide is U. *J. Mol. Biol.* **117**:805–814.

Coffin J.M. and H.M. Temin. 1972. Hybridization of Rous sarcoma virus deoxyribonucleic acid polymerase product and ribonucleic acids from chicken and rat cells infected with Rous sarcoma virus. *J. Virol.* **9**:766–775.

Coffin, J.M., T.C. Hageman, A.M. Maxam, and W.A. Haseltine. 1978. Structure of the genome of Moloney murine leukemia virus: A terminally redundant sequence. *Cell* **13**:761–773.

Coffin, J.M. J.T. Parsons, L. Rymo, R.K. Haroz, and C. Weissmann. 1974. A new approach to the isolation of RNA-DNA hybrids and its application to the quantitative determination of labeled tumor virus RNA. *J. Mol. Biol.* **86**:373–396.

Cohen, J.C. 1980. Methylation of milk-borne and genetically transmitted mouse mammary tumor virus proviral DNA. *Cell* **19**:653–662.

Cohen, J.C. and H.E. Varmus. 1979. Endogenous mammary tumour virus DNA varies among wild mice and segregates during inbreeding. *Nature* **278**:418–423.

———. 1980. Proviruses of mouse mammary tumor virus in normal and neoplastic tissues from GR and C3Hf mouse strains. *J. Virol.* **35**:298–305.

Cohen J.C., J.E. Majors, and H.E. Varmus. 1979a. Organization of mouse mammary tumor virus-specific DNA endogenous to BALB/c mice. *J. Virol.* **32**:483–496.

Cohen, J.C., P.R. Shank, V.L. Morris, R. Cardiff, and H.E. Varmus. 1979b. Integration of the DNA of mouse mammary tumor virus in virus-infected normal and neoplastic tissue of the mouse. *Cell* **16**:333–346.

Cohen, M., M.O. Nicolson, R.M. McAllister, M. Shure, N. Davidson, N. Rice, and R.V. Gilden. 1980. Baboon endogenous virus genome. I. Restriction enzyme map of the unintegrated DNA genome of a primate retrovirus. *J. Virol.* **34**:28–29.

Colcher, D., R.L. Heberling, S.S. Kalter, and J. Schlom. 1977. Squirrel monkey retrovirus: An endogenous virus of a new world primate. *J. Virol.* **23**:294–301.

Collett, M.S. and A.J. Faras. 1975. In vitro transcription of DNA from the 70S RNA of Rous sarcoma virus: Identification and characterization of various size classes of DNA transcripts. *J. Virol.* **16**:1220–1228.

———. 1976. In vitro transcription of 70S RNA by the RNA-directed DNA polymerase of Rous sarcoma virus: Lack of influence of RNase H. *J. Virol.* **17**:291–295.

———. 1978. Avian retrovirus RNA-directed DNA synthesis: Transcription at the 5′ terminus of the viral genome and the functional role for the viral terminal redundancy. *Virology* **86**:297–311.

Collett, M.S., M.L. Perdue, and A.J. Faras. 1979. Initiation of DNA synthesis by the avian retrovirus reverse transcriptase in vitro: Nature and location of the oligodeoxycytidylic acid primer binding site. *J. Virol.* **30**:319–338.

Collett, M.S., P. Dierks, J.T. Parsons, and A.J. Faras. 1978a. RNase H hydrolysis of the 5′ terminus of the avian sarcoma virus genome during reverse transcription. *Nature* **272**:181–183.

Collett, M.S., J.P. Leis, M.S. Smith, and A.J. Faras. 1978b. Unwinding-like activity associated with avian retrovirus RNA-directed DNA polymerase. *J. Virol.* **26**:498–509.

Collett, M.S., P. Dierks, J.F. Cahill, A.J. Faras, and J.T. Parsons. 1977. Terminally repeated sequences in the avian sarcoma virus RNA genome. *Proc. Natl. Acad. Sci.* **74**:2389–2393.

Collins, C.J., D. Boettiger, T.L. Green, M.B. Burgess, B.H. Devlin, and J.T. Parsons. 1980. Arrangement of integrated avian sarcoma virus DNA sequences within the cellular genomes of transformed and revertant mammalian cells. *J. Virol.* **33**:760–768.

Conley, A.J. and L.F. Velicer. 1978. Analysis of cytoplasmic RNA and polyribosomes from feline leukemia virus-infected cells. *J. Virol.* **25**:750–763.

Cooper, G.M. and S. Okenquist. 1978. Mechanism of transfection of chicken embryo fibroblasts by Rous sarcoma virus DNA. *J. Virol.* **28:**45–52.

Cooper, G.M. and L. Silverman. 1978. Linkage of the endogenous avian leukosis virus genome of virus-producing chicken cells to inhibitory cellular DNA sequences. *Cell* **15:**573–577.

Cooper, G.M. and H.M. Temin. 1974. Infectious Rous sarcoma virus and reticuloendotheliosis virus DNAs. *J. Virol.* **14:**1132–1141.

———. 1976. Lack of infectivity of the endogenous avian leukosis virus-related genes in the DNA of uninfected chicken cells. *J. Virol.* **17:**422–430.

Copeland, N.G. and G.M. Cooper. 1979. Transfection by exogenous and endogenous murine retrovirus DNAs. *Cell* **16:**347–356.

———. 1980. Transfection by DNAs of avian erythroblastosis virus and avian myelocytomatosis virus strain MC29. *J. Virol.* **33:**1199–1202.

Copeland, N.G., N.A. Jenkins, and G.M. Cooper. 1981. Integration of Rous sarcoma virus DNA during transfection. *Cell* **23:**51–60.

Copeland, N.G., A.D. Zelenetz, and G.M. Cooper. 1979. Transformation of NIH/3T3 mouse cells by DNA of Rous sarcoma virus. *Cell* **17:**993–1002.

———. 1980. Transformation by subgenomic fragments of Rous sarcoma virus DNA. *Cell* **19:** 863–870.

Copeland, T.D., D.P. Grandgenett, and S. Oroszlan. 1980. Amino acid sequence analysis of reverse transcriptase subunits from avian myeloblastosis virus. *J. Virol.* **36:**115–119.

Cordell, B., R. Swanstrom, H.M. Goodman, and J.M. Bishop. 1979. $tRNA^{Trp}$ as primer for RNA-directed DNA polymerase: Structural determinants of function. *J. Biol. Chem.* **254:**1866–1874.

Cordell, B., S.R. Weiss, H.E. Varmus, and J.M. Bishop. 1978. At least 104 nucleotides are transposed from the 5′ terminus of the avian sarcoma virus genome to the 5′ termini of smaller viral mRNAs. *Cell* **15:**79–91.

Cordell, B., E. Stavnezer, R. Friedrich, J.M. Bishop, and H.M. Goodman. 1976. The nucleotide sequence that binds primer for DNA synthesis to the avian sarcoma virus genome. *J. Virol.* **19:**548–558.

Courtneidge, S.A., A.D. Levinson, and J.M. Bishop. 1980. The protein encoded by the transforming gene of avian sarcoma virus ($pp60^{src}$) and a homologous protein in normal cells ($pp60^{proto-src}$) are associated with the plasma membrane. *Proc. Natl. Acad. Sci.* **77:**3783–3787.

Crittenden, L.B., E.J. Smith, R.A. Weiss, and P.S. Sarma. 1974. Host gene control of endogenous avian leukosis virus production. *Virology* **57:**128–138.

Czernilofsky, A.P., A.D. Levinson, H.E. Varmus, J.M. Bishop, E. Tischer, and H.M. Goodman. 1980a. Nucleotide sequence of an avian sarcoma virus oncogene (*src*) and proposed amino acid sequence for gene product. *Nature* **287:**198–203.

Czernilofsky, A.P. W. DeLorbe, R. Swanstrom, H.E. Varmus, J.M. Bishop, E. Tischer, and H.M. Goodman. 1980b. The nucleotide sequence of an untranslated but conserved domain at the 3′ end of the avian sarcoma virus genome. *Nucleic Acids Res.* **8:** 2967–2984.

Dahl, H.-H.M. and C. Dickson. 1979. Cell-free synthesis of mouse mammary tumor virus Pr77 from virion and intracellular mRNA. *J. Virol.* **29:**1131–1141.

Dahlberg, J.E., R.C. Saywer, J.M. Taylor, A.J. Faras, W.E. Levinson, H.M. Goodman, and J.M. Bishop. 1974. Transcription of DNA from the 70S RNA of Rous sarcoma virus. I. Identification of a specific 4S RNA which serves as primer. *J. Virol.* **13:**1126–1133.

Dales, S. and H. Hanafusa. 1972. Penetration and intracellular release of the genomes of avian RNA tumor viruses. *Virology* **50:**440–458.

Darlix, J.-L., P.A. Bromley, and P.-F. Spahr. 1977a. Extensive in vitro transcription of Rous sarcoma virus RNA by avian myeloblastosis virus DNA polymerase and concurrent activation of the associated RNase H. *J. Virol.* **23:**659–668.

———. 1977b. New procedure for the direct analysis of in vitro reverse transcription of Rous sarcoma virus RNA. *J. Virol.* **22:**118–129.

Darlix, J.-L., P.-F. Spahr, and P.A. Bromley. 1978. Analysis of Rous sarcoma virus (RSV) RNA structure by means of specific nucleases. *Virology* **90:**317–329.

Darlix, J.-L., P.-F. Spahr, P.A. Bromley, and J.-C. Jaton. 1979. In vitro, the major ribosome binding site on Rous sarcoma virus RNA does not contain the nucleotide sequence coding for the N-terminal amino acids of the *gag* gene product. *J. Virol.* **29:**597–611.

DeLarco, J. and G.J. Todaro. 1976. Membrane receptors for murine leukemia viruses: Characterization using the purified viral envelope glycoprotein, gp71. *Cell* **8:**365–371.

DeLorbe, W.J., P.A. Luciw, H.M. Goodman, H.E. Varmus, and J.M. Bishop. 1980. Molecular cloning and characterization of avian sarcoma virus circular DNA molecules. *J. Virol.* **36:**50–61.

Deng, C.T., D. Boettiger, I. Macpherson, and H.E. Varmus. 1974. The persistance and expression of virus-specific DNA in revertants of Rous sarcoma virus-transformed BHK-21 cells. *Virology* **62:**512–521.

Deng, C.-T., D. Stehelin, J.M. Bishop, and H.E. Varmus. 1977. Characteristics of virus-specific RNA in avian sarcoma virus-transformed BHK-21 cells and revertants. *Virology* **76:**313–330.

Dhar, R., W.L. McClements, L.W. Enquist, and G.F. Vande Woude. 1980. Nucleotide sequences of integrated Moloney sarcoma provirus long terminal repeats and their host and viral junctions. *Proc. Natl. Acad. Sci.* **77:**3937–3941.

DiCioccio, R.A. and B.I. Srivastava. 1978. Structure-activity relationships and specificity of inhibition of DNA polymerases from normal and leukemia cells of man and from simian sarcoma virus by rifamycin derivatives. *J. Natl. Cancer Inst.* **61:**1187–1194.

Dickson, C. and G. Peters. 1981. Protein-coding potential of mouse mammary tumor virus genome RNA as examined by in vitro translation. *J. Virol.* **37:**36–47.

Diggelmann, H. 1979. Biosynthesis of an unglycosylated envelope glycoprotein of Rous sarcoma virus in the presence of tunicamycin. *J. Virol.* **30:**799–804.

Dimock, K. and C.M. Stoltzfus. 1978. Cycloleucine blocks 5′-terminal and internal methylations of avian sarcoma virus genome RNA. *Biochemistry* **17:**3627–3632.

Dina, D. and E.M. Benz, Jr. 1980. Structure of murine sarcoma virus DNA replicative intermediates synthesized in vitro. *J. Virol.* **33:**377–389.

Dina, D. and E.E. Penhoet. 1978. Viral gene expression in murine sarcoma virus (murine leukemia virus)-infected cells. *J. Virol.* **27:**768–775.

Dinowitz, M. 1975. Inhibition of Rous sarcoma virus by α-amanitin: Possible role of cell DNA-dependent RNA polymerase form II. *Virology* **66:**1–9.

Dion, A.S., C.J. Williams, and D.H. Moore. 1977. RNase H and RNA-directed DNA polymerase: Associated enzymatic activities of murine mammary tumor virus. *J. Virol.* **22:**187–193.

Dion, A.S., A.B. Vaidya, G.S. Fout, and D.H. Moore. 1974. Isolation and characterization of RNA-directed DNA polymerase from a B-type RNA tumor virus. *J. Virol.* **14:**40–46.

Dittmar, K.J. and K. Moelling. 1978. Biochemical properties of p15-associated protease in an avian RNA tumor virus. *J. Virol.* **28:**106–118.

Donehower, L.A., A.L. Huang, and G.L. Hager. 1981. Regulatory and coding potential of the mouse mammary tumor virus long terminal redundancy. *J. Virol.* **37:**226–238.

Donner, L., L.P. Turek, S.K. Ruscetti, L.A. Fedele, and C.J. Sherr. 1980. Transformation-defective mutants of feline sarcoma virus which express a product of the viral *src* gene. *J. Virol.* **35:**129–140.

Donoghue, D.J. P.A. Sharp, and R.A. Weinberg. 1979. An MSV-specific subgenomic mRNA in MSV-transformed G8-124 cells. *Cell* **17:**53–63.

Donoghue, D.J., E. Rothenberg, N. Hopkins, D. Baltimore, and P.A. Sharp. 1978. Heteroduplex analysis of the nonhomology region between Moloney MuLV and the dual host range derivative HIX virus. *Cell* **14:**959–970.

Dube, D.K. and L.A. Loeb. 1976. On the association of reverse transcriptase with polynucleotide templates during catalysis. *Biochemistry* **15:**3605–3611.

Dudley, J.P. and H.E. Varmus. 1981. Purification and translation of murine mammary tumor virus messenger RNAs. *J. Virol.* **39:**207–218.

Duesberg, P.H. and E. Canaani. 1970. Complementarity between Rous sarcoma virus (RSV) RNA and the *in vitro*-synthesized DNA of the virus-associated DNA polymerase. *Virology* **42:**783–783.

Duesberg, P.H. and P.K. Vogt. 1969. On the role of DNA synthesis in avian tumor virus infection. *Proc. Natl. Acad. Sci.* **64:**939–946.

Duesberg, P., K.V.D. Helm, and E. Canaani. 1971a. Properties of a soluble DNA polymerase isolated from Rous sarcoma virus. *Proc. Natl. Acad. Sci.* **68:**747–751.

———. 1971b. Comparative properties of RNA and DNA templates for the DNA polymerase of Rous sarcoma virus. *Proc. Natl. Acad. Sci.* **68:**2505–2509.

Dunsmuir, P., W.J. Brorein, Jr., M.A. Simon, and G.M. Rubin. 1980. Insertion of the *Drosophila* transposable element *copia* generates a 5 base pair duplication. *Cell* **21:** 575–579.

Edenberg, H.J. and J.A. Huberman. 1975. Eukaryotic chromosome replication. *Annu. Rev. Genet.* **9:**245–284.

Edwards, S.A. and H. Fan. 1979. *gag*-related polyproteins of Moloney murine leukemia virus: Evidence for independent synthesis of glycosylated and unglycosylated forms. *J. Virol.* **30:**551–563.

Efstratiatis, A., F.C. Kafatos, A.M. Maxam, and T. Maniatis. 1976. Enzymatic in vitro synthesis of globin genes. *Cell* **7:**279–288.

Eiden, J.J., K. Quade, and J.L. Nichols. 1976. Interaction of tryptophan transfer RNA with Rous sarcoma virus 35S RNA. *Nature* **259:**245–247.

Eisenman, R.N. and V.M. Vogt. 1978. The biosynthesis of oncovirus proteins. *Biochim. Biophys. Acta* **473:**187–239.

England, J.M., D.P. Bolognesi, B. Dietzschold, and M.S. Halpern. 1977. Evidence that a precursor glycoprotein is cleaved to yield the major glycoprotein of avian tumor virus. *Virology* **21:**810–814.

Evans, L.H., P.H. Duesberg, and E.M. Scolnick. 1980. Replication of spleen focus-forming Friend virus in fibroblasts from C57BL mice that are genetically resistant to spleen focus formation. *Virology* **101:**534–539.

Faller, D.V., J. Rommelaere, and N. Hopkins. 1978. Large T1 oligonucleotides of Moloney leukemia virus missing in an *env* gene recombinant, HIX, are present on an intracellular 21S Moloney viral RNA species. *Proc. Natl. Acad. Sci.* **75:**2964–2968.

Fan, H. 1977. RNA metabolism of murine leukemia virus: Size analysis of nuclear pulse-labeled virus-specific RNA. *Cell* **11:**297–305.

Fan, H. and D. Baltimore. 1973. RNA metabolism of murine leukemia virus: Detection of virus-specific RNA sequences in infected and uninfected cells and identification of virus-specific messenger RNA. *J. Mol. Biol.* **80:**93–117.

Fan, H. and P. MacIsaac. 1978. Virus-specific RNA synthesis in interferon-treated mouse cells productively infected with Moloney murine leukemia virus. *J. Virol.* **27:**449–452.

Fan, H. and I.M. Verma. 1978. Size analysis and relationship of murine leukemia virus-specific mRNA's: Evidence for transposition of sequences during synthesis and processing of subgenomic mRNA. *J. Virol.* **26:**468–478.

Fan, H., R. Jaenisch, and P. MacIsaac. 1978. Low-multiplicity infection of Moloney murine leukemia virus in mouse cells: Effect on number of viral DNA copies and virus production in producer cells. *J. Virol.* **28:**802–809.

Farabaugh, P.J. and G.R. Fink. 1980. Insertion of the eukaryotic transposable element Ty1 creates a 5-base pair duplication. *Nature* **286:**352–356.

Faras, A.J. and N.A. Dibble. 1975. RNA-directed DNA synthesis by the DNA polymerase of Rous sarcoma virus: Structural and functional identification of 4S primer RNA in uninfected cells. *Proc. Natl. Acad. Sci.* **72:**859–863.

Faras, A.J., J.M. Taylor, J.P. McDonnell, W.E. Levinson, and J.M. Bishop. 1972. Purification and characterization of the deoxyribonucleic acid polymerase associated with Rous sarcoma virus. *Biochemistry* **11:**2334–2342.

Faras, A.J., J.M. Taylor, W.E. Levinson, H.M. Goodman, and J.M. Bishop. 1973. RNA-directed DNA polymerase of Rous sarcoma virus: Initiation of synthesis with 70 S viral RNA as template. *J. Mol. Biol.* **79:**163–183.

Faras, A.J., J.E. Dahlberg, R.C. Sawyer, F. Harada, J.M. Taylor, W.E. Levinson, J.M. Bishop, and H.M. Goodman. 1974. Transcription of DNA from the 70S RNA of Rous sarcoma virus. II. Structure of a 4S RNA primer. *J. Virol.* **13:**1134–1142.

Filippi, P., M. Brahic, R. Vigne, and J. Tamalet. 1979. Characterization of visna virus mRNA. *J. Virol.* **31:**25–30.

Finnegan, D.J., G.M. Rubin, M.W. Young, and D.S. Hogness. 1978. Repeated gene families in *Drosophila melanogaster. Cold Spring Harbor Symp. Quant. Biol.* **42:**1053– 1063.

Fitzgerald, M. and T. Shenk. 1980. The site at which late mRNA's are polyadenylated is altered in SV40 mutant dl 1882. *Ann. N.Y. Acad. Sci.* **354:**53.

Flugel, R.M. and R.D. Wells. 1972. Nucleotides at the RNA-DNA covalent bonds formed in the endogenous reaction by the avian myeloblastosis virus DNA polymerase. *Virology* **48:**394–401.

Frankel, A.E., D.K. Haapala, R.L. Neubauer, and P.J. Fischinger. 1976. Elimination of the sarcoma genome from murine sarcoma virus transformed cat cells. *Science* **191:**1264–1266.

Fraser, N., J.R. Nevins, E. Ziff, and J.E. Darnell. 1979. The major late adenovirus type-2 transcription unit: Termination is downstream from the last poly(A) site. *J. Mol. Biol.* **129:**643–656.

Friedman, E.Y. and M. Rosbach. 1977. The synthesis of high yields of full-length reverse transcripts of globin mRNA. *Nucleic Acids Res.* **4:**3455–3471.

Friedman, R.M. 1977. Antiviral activity of interferons. *Bacteriol. Rev.* **41:**543–567.

Friedman, R.M., E.H. Chang, J.M. Ramseur, and M.W. Myers. 1975. Interferon-directed inhibition of chronic murine leukemia virus production in cell cultures: Lack of effect on intracellular viral markers. *J. Virol.* **16:**569–574.

Friedrich, R., and K. Moelling. 1979. Effect of viral RNase H on the avian sarcoma viral genome during early transcription in vitro. *J. Virol.* **31:**630–638.

Friedrich, R., H.-J. Kung, B. Baker, H.E. Varmus, H.M. Goodman, and J.M. Bishop. 1977. Characterization of DNA complementary to nucleotide sequences at the 5′-terminus of the avian sarcoma virus genome. *Virology* **79:**198–215.

Frisby, D.P., R.A. Weiss, M. Roussel, and D. Stehelin. 1979. The distribution of endogenous chicken retrovirus sequences in the DNA of galliform birds does not coincide with avian phylogenetic relationships. *Cell* **17:**623–634.

Fritsch, E. and H.M. Temin. 1977a. Formation and structure of infectious DNA of spleen necrosis virus. *J. Virol.* **21:**119–130.

———. 1977b. Inhibition of viral DNA synthesis in stationary chicken embryo fibroblasts infected with avian retroviruses. *J. Virol.* **24:**461–469.

Fujinaga, K., J.T. Parsons, J.W. Beard, D. Beard, and M. Green. 1970. Mechanism of carcinogenesis by RNA tumor viruses. III. Formation of RNA-DNA complex and duplex DNA molecules by the DNA polymerase(s) of avian myeloblastosis virus. *Proc. Natl. Acad. Sci.* **67:**1432–1439.

Furuichi, Y., A.J. Shatkin, E. Stavnezer, and J.M. Bishop. 1975. Blocked, methylated 5′-terminal sequence in avian sarcoma virus RNA. *Nature* **257:**618–620.

Gafner, J. and P. Phillipsen. 1980. The yeast transposon Ty1 generates duplications of target DNA on insertion. *Nature* **286:**414–418.

Gallis, B.M., R.N. Eisenman, and H. Diggelmann. 1976. Synthesis of the precursor to avian RNA tumor virus internal structural proteins early after infection. *Virology* **74:**302–313.

Gallis, B., M. Linial, and R. Eisenmann. 1979. An avian oncovirus mutant deficient in genomic RNA: Characterization of the packaged RNA as cellular messenger RNA. *Virology* **94:**146–161.

Garapin, A.C., J.P. McDonnell, W.E. Levinson, N. Quintrell, L. Fanshier, and J.M. Bishop. 1970. Deoxyribonucleic acid polymerase associated with Rous sarcoma virus and avian myeloblastosis virus: Properties of the enzyme and its product. *J. Virol.* **6:**589–598.

Gardner, M.B., S. Rasheed, B.K. Pal, J.D. Estes, and S.J. O'Brien. 1980. *Akvr-1*, a dominant murine leukemia virus restriction gene, is polymorphic in leukemia-prone wild mice. *Proc. Natl. Acad. Sci.* **77:**531–535.

Gautsch, J.W. 1980. Embryonal carcinoma stem cells lack a function required for virus replication. *Nature* **285:**110–112.

Gautsch, J.W., J.H. Elder, J. Schindler, F.C. Jensen, and R.A. Lerner. 1978. Structural markers on core protein p30 of murine leukemia virus: Functional correlation with *Fv-1* tropism. *Proc. Natl. Acad. Sci.* **75:**4170–4174.

Gazdar, A.F., H. Oie, P. Lalley, W.W. Moss, J.D. Minna, and U. Francke. 1977. Identification of mouse chromosomes required for murine leukemia virus replication. *Cell* **11:**949–956.

Gazzolo, L., M.G. Moscovici, and C. Moscovici. 1974. Replication of avian sarcoma viruses in chicken macrophages. *Virology* **58:**514–525.

Gelb, L., S.A. Aaronson, and M. Martin. 1971. Heterogeneity of murine leukemia virus in vitro DNA; detection of viral DNA in mammalian cells. *Science* **172:**1353–1355.

Gerard, G.F. 1981. Mechanism of action of Moloney murine leukemia virus RNA-directed DNA polymerase associated RNase H (RNase H I). *Biochemistry* **20:**256–265.

Gerard, G.F. and D.P. Grandgenett. 1975. Purification and characterization of the DNA polymerase and RNase H activities in Moloney murine sarcoma-leukemia virus. *J. Virol.* **15:**785–797.

———. 1980. Retrovirus reverse transcriptase. In *Molecular biology of RNA tumor viruses* (ed. J. Stephenson), pp. 345–394. Academic Press, New York.

Gerard, G.F., F. Rottman, and M. Green. 1976. Poly (2′-*0*-methylcytidylate) oligodeoxyguanylate as a template for the ribonucleic acid directed deoxyribonucleic acid polymerase in ribonucleic acid tumor virus particles and a specific probe for the ribonucleic acid directed enzyme in transformed murine cells. *Biochemistry* **13:**1632–1641.

Gerwin, B. and J.G. Levin. 1977. Interactions of murine leukemia virus core components: Characterization of reverse transcriptase packaged in the absence of 70S genomic RNA. *J. Virol.* **24:**478–488.

Gerwin, B.I. and J.B. Milstien. 1972. An oligonucleotide affinity column for RNA-dependent DNA polymerase from RNA tumor viruses. *Proc. Natl. Acad. Sci.* **69:**2599–2603.

Gerwin, B.I., S.G. Smith and P.T. Peebles. 1975. Two active forms of RD-114 virus DNA polymerase in infected cells. *Cell* **6:**45–52.

Gerwin, B.I., A. Rein, J.G. Levin, R.H. Bassin, B.M. Benjers, S.V.S. Kashmiri, D. Hopkins, and B.J. O'Neill. 1979. Mutant of B-tropic murine leukemia virus synthesizing an altered polymerase molecule. *J. Virol.* **31:**741–751.

Gianni, A.M. and R.A. Weinberg. 1975. Partially single-stranded form of free Moloney viral DNA. *Nature* **255:**646–648.

Gianni, A.M., D. Smotkin, and R.A. Weinberg. 1975. Murine leukemia virus: Detection of unintegrated double-stranded DNA forms of the provirus. *Proc. Natl. Acad. Sci.* **72:**447–451.

Gianni, A.M., J.R. Hutton, D. Smotkin, and R.A. Weinberg. 1976. Proviral DNA of Moloney leukemia virus: Purification and visualization. *Science* **191**:569–571.

Gibson, W. and I.M. Verma. 1974. Studies on the reverse transcriptase of RNA tumor viruses. Structural relatedness of two subunits of avian RNA tumor viruses. *Proc. Natl. Acad. Sci.* **71**:4991–4994.

Gielkens, A.L.J., M.H.L. Salden, and H. Bloemendal. 1974. Virus-specific mesenger RNA on free and membrane-bound polyribosomes from cells infected with Rauscher leukemia virus. *Proc. Natl. Acad. Sci.* **71**:1093–1097.

Gilboa, E., S.W. Mitra, S. Goff, and D. Baltimore. 1979a. A detailed model of reverse transcription and tests of crucial aspects. *Cell* **18**:93–100.

Gilboa, E., S. Goff, A. Shields, F. Yoshimura, S. Mitra, and D. Baltimore. 1979b. In vitro synthesis of a 9-kbp terminally redundant DNA carrying the infectivity of Moloney murine leukemia virus. *Cell* **16**:863–874.

Gilmer, T.M. and J.T. Parsons. 1979. Analysis of cellular integration sites in avian sarcoma virus-infected duck embryo cells. *J. Virol.* **32**:762–769.

Godard, C. and K.W. Jones. 1979. Detection of AKR MuLV-specific RNA in AKR mouse cells by in situ hybridization. *Nucleic Acids Res.* **6**:2849–2861.

Goldfarb, M.P. and R.A. Weinberg. 1979. Physical map of biologically active Harvey sarcoma virus unintegrated linear DNA. *J. Virol.* **32**:30–39.

Golomb, M. and D.P. Grandgenett. 1979. Endonuclease activity of purified RNA-directed DNA polymerase from avian myeloblastosis virus. *J. Biol. Chem.* **254**:1606–1613.

Golomb, M., A.C. Vora, and D.P. Grandgenett. 1980. Purification of reverse transcriptase from avian retroviruses using affinity chromatography on heparin-sepharose. *J. Virol. Methods* **1**:157–165.

Gonda, T.J., D.K. Sheiness, L. Fanshier, J.M. Bishop, C. Moscovici, and M.G. Moscovici. 1981. The genome and the intracellular RNAs of avian myeloblastosis virus. *Cell* **23**:279–290.

Goodman, N.C. and S. Spiegelman. 1971. Distinguishing reverse transcriptase of an RNA tumor virus from other known DNA polymerases. *Proc. Natl. Acad. Sci.* **68**:2203–2206.

Gopinathan, K.P., L.A. Weymouth, T.A. Kunkel, and L.A. Loeb. 1979. Mutagenesis *in vitro* by DNA polymerase from an RNA tumor virus. *Nature* **278**:857–859.

Gorecki, M. and A. Panet. 1978. Discrimination of DNA polymerase and RNase H activities in reverse transcriptase of avian myeloblastosis virus. *Biochemistry* **17**:2438– 2442.

Goubin, G. and M. Hill. 1979. Monomer and multimer covalently closed circular forms of Rous sarcoma virus DNA. *J. Virol.* **29**:799–804.

Graf, T., H. Beug, and M.J. Hayman. 1980. Target cell specificity of defective avian leukemia viruses: Hematopoietic target cells for a given virus type can be infected but not transformed by strains of a different type. *Proc. Natl. Acad. Sci.* **77**:389–393.

Grandgenett, D.P. 1976. Purification of the α subunit of avian myeloblastosis virus DNA polymerase by polyuridylic acid-Sepharose. *J. Virol.* **20**:348–350.

Grandgenett, D.P. and M. Green. 1974. Different mode of action of ribonuclease H in purified α and $\alpha\beta$ ribonucleic acid-directed deoxyribonucleic acid polymerase from avian myeloblastosis virus. *J. Biol. Chem.* **294**:5148–5152.

Grandgenett, D.P. and H.M. Rho. 1975. Binding properties of avian myeloblastosis virus DNA polymerases to nucleic acid affinity columns. *J. Virol.* **15**:526–533.

Grandgenett, D.P. G.F. Gerard, and M. Green. 1972. Ribonuclease H: A ubiquitous activity in virions of ribonucleic acid tumor viruses. *J. Virol.* **10**:1136–1142.

———. 1973. A single subunit from avian myeloblastosis virus with both RNA-directed DNA polymerase and ribonuclease H activity. *Proc. Natl. Acad. Sci.* **70**:230–234.

Grandgenett, D.P., M. Golomb, and A.C. Vora. 1980. Activation of an Mg^{+2} -dependent DNA endonuclease of avian myeloblastosis virus $\alpha\beta$ DNA polymerase by *in vitro* proteolytic cleavage. *J. Virol.* **33**:264–271.

Grandgenett, D.P., A.C. Vora, and R.D. Schiff. 1978. A 32,000-dalton nucleic acid-binding protein from avian retrovirus cores possesses DNA endonuclease activity. *Virology* **89:**119–132.

Gregerson, D.S., P. Russell, and T.W. Reid. 1979. Biochemical and immunological properties of the reverse transcriptase associated with a hamster retrovirus. *J. Gen. Virol.* **43:**327–337.

Grindley, N.D.F. 1978. IS1 insertion generates duplication of a nine base pair sequence at its target site. *Cell* **13:**419–426.

Grindley, N.D.F. and D.J. Sherratt. 1979. Sequence analysis at IS1 insertion sites: Models for transposition. *Cold Spring Harbor Symp. Quant. Biol.* **43:**1257–1261.

Groner, B. and N.E. Hynes. 1980. Number and location of mouse mammary tumor virus proviral DNA in mouse DNA of normal tissue and of mammary tumors. *J. Virol.* **33:**1013–1025.

Groner, B., N.E. Hynes, and H. Diggelmann. 1979. Identification of mouse mammary tumor virus-specific mRNA. *J. Virol.* **30:**417–420.

Groudine, M., S. Das, P. Neiman, and H. Weintraub. 1978. Regulation of expression and chromosomal subunit conformation of avian retrovirus genomes. *Cell* **14:**865–878.

Guntaka, R.V. 1980. Synthesis of circular DNA in avian tumor virus particles. *Virology* **101:** 525–528.

Guntaka, R.V., R.A. Katz, A.J. Weiner, and M.M. Widman. 1979. Effect of 5-methylcytidine on virus production in avian sarcoma virus-infected chicken embryo cells. *J. Virol.* **29:**475–482.

Guntaka, R.V., B.W.J. Mahy, J.M. Bishop, and H.E. Varmus. 1975. Ethidium bromide inhibits the appearance of closed circular viral DNA and integration of virus-specific DNA in duck cells infected by avian sarcoma virus. *Nature* **253:**507–511.

Guntaka, R.V., P.Y. Rao, S.A. Mitsialis, and R. Katz. 1980. Modification of avian sarcoma proviral DNA sequences in nonpermissive XC cells but not in permissive chicken cells. *J. Virol.* **34:**569–572.

Guntaka, R.V., O.C. Richards, P.R. Shank, H.-J. Kung, N. Davidson, E. Fritsch, J.M. Bishop, and H.E. Varmus. 1976. Covalently closed circular DNA of avian sarcoma virus: Purification from nuclei of infected quail tumor cells and meaurement by electron microscopy and gel electrophoresis. *J. Mol. Biol.* **106:**337–357.

Haase, A.T., B.L. Traynor, P.E. Ventura, and D.W. Alling. 1976. Infectivity of visna virus DNA. *Virology* **70:**65–79.

Hackett, P.B. and W. Sauerbier. 1975. The transcriptional organization of the ribosomal RNA genes in mouse L cells. *J. Mol. Biol.* **91:**235–256.

Hackett, P.B., H.E. Varmus, and J.M. Bishop. 1981. The genesis of Rous sarcoma virus messenger RNAs. *Virology* **112:**714–728.

Hagenbuchle, O., M. Santer, J.A. Steitz, and R.J. Mans. 1978. Conservation of the primary structure at the 3′ end of 18S rRNA from eucaryotic cells. *Cell* **13:**551–563.

Hager, G.L. and L.A. Donehower. 1980. Observations on the DNA sequence of the extended terminal redundancy and adjacent host sequences for integrated mouse mammary tumor virus. *ICN-UCLA Symp. Mol. Cell. Biol.* **18:**255.

Hager, G.L., E.H. Chang, H.W. Chan, C.F. Garon, M.A. Israel, M.A. Martin, E.M. Scolnick, and D.R. Lowy. 1979. Molecular cloning of the Harvey sarcoma virus closed circular DNA intermediates: Initial structural and biological characterization. *J. Virol.* **31:**795–809.

Hamer, D. and P. Leder. 1979. Splicing and the formation of stable RNA. *Cell* **18:** 1299–1302.

Hanafusa, H. and T. Hanafusa. 1971. Noninfectious RSV deficient in DNA polymerase. *Virology* **43:**313–316.

Hanafusa, H., D. Baltimore, D. Smoler, K.F. Watson, A. Yaniv, and S. Spiegelman. 1972.

Absence of polymerase protein in virions of alpha-type Rous sarcoma virus. *Science* **177**:1188–1191.

Harada, F., G.G. Peters, and J.E. Dahlberg. 1979. The primer tRNA for Moloney murine leukemia virus DNA synthesis. Nucleotide sequence and aminoacylation of $tRNA^{Pro}$. *J. Biol. Chem.* **254**:10979–10985.

Harada, F., R.C. Sawyer, and J.E. Dahlberg. 1975. A primer ribonucleic acid for initiation of *in vitro* Rous sarcoma virus deoxyribonucleic acid synthesis. Nucleotide sequence and amino acid acceptor activity. *J. Biol. Chem.* **250**:3487–3497.

Harewood, K. and M. Ahmed. 1977. Production of antiserum to the reverse transcriptase of Mason-Pfizer monkey virus. *J. Gen. Virol.* **36**:227–235.

Haseltine, W.A. and D. Baltimore 1976a. *In vitro* replication of RNA tumor viruses. *ICN-UCLA Symp. Mol. Cell. Biol.* **4**:175–213.

———. 1976b. Size of murine RNA tumor virus-specific nuclear RNA molecules. *J. Virol.* **19**:331–337.

Haseltine, W.A. and D.G. Kleid. 1978. A method for classification of 5′ termini of retroviruses. *Nature* **273**:358–364.

Haseltine, W.A., J.M. Coffin, and T.C. Hageman. 1979. Structure of products of the Moloney murine leukemia virus endogenous DNA polymerase reaction. *J. Virol.* **30**:375–383.

Haseltine, W.A., A.M. Maxam, and W. Gilbert. 1977a. Rous sarcoma virus genome is terminally redundant: The 5′ sequence. *Proc. Natl. Acad. Sci.* **74**:989–993.

Haseltine, W.A., D.G. Kleid, A. Panet, E. Rothenberg, and D. Baltimore. 1976. Ordered transcription of RNA tumor virus genomes. *J. Mol. Biol.* **106**:109–131.

Haseltine, W.A., A. Panet, D. Smoler, D. Baltimore, G. Peters, F. Harada, and J.E. Dahlberg. 1977b. The interaction of tryptophan tRNA and avian myeloblastosis virus reverse transcriptase: Further characterization of the binding reaction. *Biochemistry* **16**:3625–3632.

Hatanaka, M., E. Twiddy, and R.V. Gilden. 1972. Protein kinase associated with RNA tumor viruses and other budding RNA viruses. *Virology* **47**:536–538.

Hatanaka, M., T. Kakefuda, R.V. Gilden, and E.A.O. Callan. 1971. Cytoplasmic DNA synthesis induced by RNA tumor viruses. *Proc. Natl. Acad. Sci.* **68**:1844–1847.

Hausen, P. and H. Stein. 1970. Ribonuclease H. An enzyme degrading the RNA moiety of DNA-RNA hybrids. *Eur. J. Biochem.* **14**:278–283.

Hayman, M. 1978. Synthesis and processing of avian sarcoma virus glycoproteins. *Virology* **85**:475–486.

Hayward, W.S. 1977. Size and genetic content of viral RNAs in avian oncovirus-infected cells. *J. Virol* **24**:47–63.

Hayward, W.S. and H. Hanafusa. 1976. Independent regulation of endogenous and exogenous avian RNA tumor virus genes. *Proc. Natl. Acad. Sci.* **73**:2259–2263.

Hayward, W., S.B. Braverman, and S.M. Astrin. 1980. Transcriptional products and DNA structure of endogenous avian proviruses. *Cold Spring Harbor Symp. Quant. Biol.* **44**:1111–1121.

Hayward, W.S., B.G. Neel, and S.M. Astrin. 1981. Activation of a cellular *onc* gene by promoter insertion in ALV-induced lymphoid leukosis. *Nature* **290**:475–480.

Highfield, P.E., L.F. Rafield, T.M. Gilmer, and J.T. Parsons. 1980. Molecular cloning of avian sarcoma virus closed circular DNA: Structural and biological characterization of three recombinant clones. *J. Virol.* **36**:271–279.

Hill, M. and J. Hillova. 1972a. Virus recovery in chicken cells tested with Rous sarcoma cell DNA. *Nat. New Biol.* **237**:35–39.

———. 1972b. Recovery of the temperature-sensitive mutant of Rous sarcoma virus from chicken cells exposed to DNA extracted from hamster cells transformed by the mutant. *Virology* **49**:309–313.

Hirt, B. 1967. Selective extraction of polyoma DNA from infected mouse cell cultures. *J. Mol. Biol.* **26:**365–369.

Hishinuma, F., P.J. DeBona, S. Astrin, and A.M. Skalka. 1981. Nucleotide sequence of acceptor site and termini of integrated avian endogenous provirus *ev-1:* Integration creates a 6 bp repeat of host DNA. *Cell* **23:**155–164.

Hizi, A. and W.K. Joklik. 1977a. RNA-dependent DNA polymerase of avian sarcoma virus B77. I. Isolation and partial characterization of the α, β_2, and $\alpha\beta$ forms of the enzyme. *J. Biol. Chem.* **252:**2281–2289.

——— 1977b. The β subunit of the DNA polymerase of avian sarcoma virus strain B77 is a phosphoprotein. *Virology* **78:**571–575.

Hizi, A. and A. Yaniv. 1980. RNA-dependent DNA polymerase of an endogenous type C virus of mice: Purification and partial characterization. *J. Virol.* **34:**795–801.

Hizi, A., M.A. McCrae, and W.K. Joklik. 1978. Studies on the amino acid sequence content of proteins specified by the *gag* and *pol* genes of avian sarcoma virus B77. *Virology* **89:**272–284.

Hizi, A., W. Wunderli, and W.K. Joklik. 1979. Purification and partial characterization of a protein kinase from the Prague-C strain of Rous sarcoma virus. *Virology* **93:**146–158.

Hobom-Schnegg, B., H.L. Robinson, and W.S. Robinson. 1970. Replication of Rous sarcoma virus in synchronized cells. *J. Gen. Virol.* **7:**85–93.

Hopkins, N., J. Schindler, and R. Hynes. 1977. Six NB-tropic murine leukemia viruses derived from a B-tropic virus of BALB/c have altered p30. *J. Virol.* **21:**309–318.

Houts, G.E., M. Miyagi, C. Ellis, D. Beard, and J.W. Beard. 1979. Reverse transcriptase from avian myeloblastosis virus. *J. Virol.* **29:**517–522.

Houts, G.E., M. Miyagi, C. Ellis, D. Beard, K.F. Watson, and J.W. Beard. 1978. Protein kinase from avian myeloblastosis virus. *J. Virol.* **25:**546–552.

Hsu, T.W., R.V. Guntaka, and J.M. Taylor. 1978a. Specific site of action for single-strand specific nuclease on the double-stranded circular DNA intermediates of an avian RNA tumor virus. *J. Virol.* **26:**1015–1017.

Hsu, T.W., J.L. Sabran, G.E. Mark, R.V. Guntaka, and J.M. Taylor. 1978b. Analysis of unintegrated avian RNA tumor virus double-stranded DNA intermediates. *J. Virol.* **28:**810–818.

Hsu, T.W., J.M. Taylor, C. Aldrich, J.B. Townsend, G. Seal, and W.S. Mason. 1981. Tandem duplication of the proviral DNA in avian sarcoma virus-transformed quail clone. *J. Virol.* **38:**219–223.

Hu, S.S.F., P.H. Duesberg, M.M.C. Lai, and P.K. Vogt. 1979. Avian oncovirus MH2: Preferential growth in macrophages and exact size of the genome. *Virology* **96:**302–306.

Huang, A.S., P. Besmer, L. Chu, and D. Baltimore. 1973. Growth of pseudotypes of vesicular stomatitis virus with N-tropic murine leukemia virus coats in cells resistant to N-tropic virus. *J. Virol.* **12:**659–662.

Hughes, S.H., H.L. Robinson, J.M. Bishop, and H.E. Varmus. 1979a. The replication of subgroup E avian retroviruses is blocked at or before viral DNA synthesis in restrictive chicken cells. *Virology* **99:**437–442.

Hughes, S.H., A. Mutschler, J.M. Bishop, and H.E. Varmus. 1981a. A. Rous sarcoma virus provirus is flanked by short direct repeats of a cellular DNA sequence present in only one copy prior to integration. *Proc. Natl. Acad. Sci.* **78:** (in press).

Hughes, S.H., K. Toyoshima, J.M. Bishop, and H.E. Varmus. 1981b. Organization of the endogenous proviruses of chickens: Implications for origin and expression. *Virology* **108:**189–207.

Hughes, S.H., P.K. Vogt, E. Stubblefield, J.M. Bishop, and H.E. Varmus. 1981c. Integration of avian sarcoma virus DNA in chicken cells. *Virology* **108:**208–221.

Hughes, S.H., F. Payvar, D. Spector, R.T. Schimke, H.L. Robinson, G.S. Payne, J.M. Bishop, and H.E. Varmus. 1979b. Heterogeneity of genetic loci in chickens: Analysis of endogenous viral and nonviral genes by cleavage of DNA with restriction endonucleases. *Cell* **18:**347–360.

Hughes, S.E., P.R. Shank, D.H. Spector, H.-J. Kung, J.M. Bishop, H.E. Varmus, P.K. Vogt, and M.L. Breitman. 1978. Proviruses of avian sarcoma virus are terminally redundant, co-extensive with unintegrated linear DNA and integrated at many sites. *Cell* **15:**1397–1410.

Humphries, E.H. and J.M. Coffin. 1976. Rate of virus-specific RNA synthesis in synchronized chicken embryo fibroblasts infected with avian leukosis virus. *J. Virol.* **17:**393–401.

Humphries, E.H. and H.M. Temin. 1972. Cell cycle-dependent activation of Rous sarcoma virus-infected stationary chicken cells: Avian leukosis virus group-specific antigens and ribonucleic acid. *J. Virol.* **10:**82–87.

———. 1974. Requirement for cell division for initiation of transcription of Rous sarcoma virus RNA. *J. Virol.* **14:**531–546.

Humphries, E.H., C. Glover, and M.E. Reichmann. 1981. Rous sarcoma virus infection of synchronized cells establishes provirus integration during S phase DNA synthesis prior to cell division. *Proc. Natl. Acad. Sci.* **78:**2601–2605.

Humphries, E.H., C. Glover, R.A. Weiss, and J.R. Arrand. 1979. Differences between the endogenous and exogenous DNA sequences of Rous-associated virus-0. *Cell* **18:**803–815.

Hunter, E. 1978. The mechanism for genetic recombination in the avian retroviruses. *Curr. Top. Microbiol. Immunol.* **79:**295–309.

Hurwitz, J. and J.P. Leis. 1972. RNA-dependent DNA polymerase activity of RNA tumor viruses. I. Directing influence of DNA in the reaction. *J. Virol.* **9:**116–129.

Jaenisch, R. 1976. Germ line integration and Mendelian transmission of the exogenous Moloney leukemia virus. *Proc. Natl. Acad. Sci.* **73:**1260–1264.

———. 1980. Retroviruses and embryogenesis: Microinjection of Moloney leukemia virus into midgestation mouse embryos. *Cell* **19:**181–188.

Jahner, D., H. Stuhlmann, and R. Jaenisch. 1980. Conformation of free and of integrated Moloney leukemia virus proviral DNA in preleukemic and leukemic BALB/Mo mice. *Virology* **101:**111–123.

Jamjoom, G.A., R.B. Naso, and R.B. Arlinghaus. 1977. Further characterization of intracellular precursor polypeptides of Rauscher leukemia virus. *Virology* **78:**11–34.

Jaquet, M., Y. Groner, G. Monroy, and J. Hurwitz. 1974. The *in vitro* synthesis of avian myeloblastosis viral RNA sequences. *Proc. Natl. Acad. Sci.* **71:**3045–3049.

Jenkins, N.A. and G.M. Cooper. 1980. Integration, expression, and infectivity of exogenously acquired proviruses of Rous-associated virus-0. *J. Virol.* **36:**684–691.

Johnsrud, L., M.P. Calos, and J.H. Miller. 1978. The transposon Tn9 generates a 9 bp repeated sequence during integration. *Cell* **15:**1209–1219.

Joho, R.H., M.A. Billeter, and C. Weissmann. 1978. Concordance of the RNA termini of recombinants from crosses between avian retroviruses with different termini. *Virology* **85:**364–377.

Jolicoeur, P. 1979. The *Fv*-1 gene of the mouse and its control of murine leukemia virus replication. *Curr. Top. Microbiol. Immunol.* **86:**67–122.

Jolicoeur, P. and D. Baltimore. 1976a. Effect of *Fv*-1 gene product on proviral DNA formation and integration in cells infected with murine leukemia viruses. *Proc. Natl. Acad. Sci.* **73:**2236–2240.

———. 1976b. Effect of *Fv*-1 gene product on synthesis of N-tropic and B-tropic murine leukemia viral RNA. *Cell* **7:**33–39.

Jolicoeur, P. and E. Rassart. 1980. Effect of Fv-1 gene product on synthesis of linear and supercoiled viral DNA in cells infected with murine leukemia virus. *J. Virol.* **33:**183–195.

———. 1981. Fate of unintegrated viral DNA in *Fv*-1 permissive and resistant mouse cells infected with murine leukemia virus. *J. Virol.* **37:**609–619.

Jolicoeur, P., E. Rassart, C. Kozak, F. Ruddle, and D. Baltimore. 1980. Distribution of endogenous murine leukemia virus DNA sequences among mouse chromosomes. *J. Virol.* **33:**1229–1235.

Ju, G. and A.M. Skalka. 1980. Nucleotide sequence analysis of the long terminal repeat (LTR) of avian retroviruses: Structural similarities with transposable elements. *Cell* **22:**379–386.

Ju, G., L. Boone, and A.M. Skalka. 1980. Isolation and characterization of recombinant DNA clones of avian retroviruses: Size heterogeneity and instability of the direct repeat. *J. Virol.* **33:**1026–1033.

Junghans, R.P., P.H. Duesberg, and C.A. Knight. 1975. *In vitro* synthesis of full-length DNA transcripts of Rous sarcoma virus RNA by viral DNA polymerase. *Proc. Natl. Acad. Sci.* **72:**4895–4899.

Junghans, R.P., S. Hu, C.A. Knight, and N. Davidson. 1977. Heteroduplex analysis of avian RNA tumor viruses. *Proc. Natl. Acad. Sci.* **74:**477–481.

Kacian, D.L. and J.C. Myers. 1976. Synthesis of extensive, possibly complete, DNA copies of poliovirus RNA in high yields and at high specific activities. *Proc. Natl. Acad. Sci.* **73:**2191–2195.

Kacian, D.L., K.F. Watson, A. Burny, and S. Spiegelman. 1971. Purification of the DNA polymerase of avian myeloblastosis virus. *Biochim. Biophys. Acta* **246:**365–383.

Kacian, D.L., S. Spiegelman, A. Bank, M. Terada, S. Metafora, L. Dow, and P.A. Marks. 1972. *In vitro* synthesis of DNA components of human genes for globins. *Nat. New Biol.* **235:**167–169.

Kakefuda, T., G.G. Lovinger, R.V. Gilden, and M. Hatanaka. 1977. Electron microscopic studies of circular DNA in mouse embryo fibroblasts infected by Rauscher leukemia virus. *J. Virol.* **21:**792–795.

Kakefuda, T., C.W. Dingman, T.M. Bak, M. Hatanaka, and Y. Kitano. 1974. Reverse transcription of the viral genome associated with the plasma membrane after infection with RNA tumor viruses. *Cancer Res.* **34:**679–688.

Kamine, J., J.G. Burr, and J.M. Buchanan. 1978. Multiple forms of *sarc* gene proteins from Rous sarcoma virus RNA. *Proc. Natl. Acad. Sci.* **75:**366–370.

Karpas, A. and C. Milstein. 1973. Recovery of the genome of murine sarcoma virus (MSV) after infection of cells with nuclear DNA from MSV transformed non-virus producing cells. *Eur. J. Cancer* **9:**295–299.

Katz, R.A., G.M. Maniatis, and R.V. Guntaka. 1979. Translation of avian sarcoma virus RNA in *Xenopus laevis* oocytes. *Biochem. Biophys. Res. Commun.* **86:**447–453.

Kaufman, S.L., R.C. Gallo, and N.R. Miller. 1979. Detection of virus-specific RNA in simian sarcoma-leukemia virus-infected cells by in situ hybridization to viral complementary DNA. *J. Virol.* **30:**637–641.

Keith, J. and H. Fraenkel-Conrat. 1975. Identification of the 5′ end of Rous sarcoma virus RNA. *Proc. Natl. Acad. Sci.* **72:**3347–3350.

Keller, W. and R. Crouch. 1972. Degradation of DNA RNA hybrids by ribonuclease H and DNA polymerases of cellular and viral origin. *Proc. Natl. Acad. Sci.* **69:**3360–3364.

Kerr, I.M., U. Olshevsky, H.F. Lodish, and D. Baltimore. 1976. Translation of murine leukemia virus RNA in cell-free systems from animal cells. *J. Virol.* **18:**627–635.

Keshet, E. and H.M. Temin. 1978. Sites of integration of reticuloendotheliosis virus in chicken DNA. *Proc. Natl. Acad. Sci.* **75:**3372–3376.

———. 1979. Cell killing by spleen necrosis virus is correlated with a transient accumulation of spleen necrosis virus DNA. *J. Virol.* **31:**376–386.

Keshet, E., J.J. O'Rear, and H.M. Temin. 1979. DNA of noninfectious and infectious integrated spleen necrosis virus (SNV) is colinear with unintegrated SNV DNA and not grossly abnormal. *Cell* **16:**51–61.

Ketner, G. and T.J. Kelly, Jr. 1976. Integrated simian virus 40 sequences in transformed cell DNA: Analysis using restriction endonucleases. *Proc. Natl. Acad. Sci.* **73:**1102–1106.

Kettmann, R., Y. Cleuter, M. Mammerickx, M. Meunier-Rotival, G. Bernardi, A. Burny, and H. Chantrenne. 1980. Genomic integration of bovine leukemia provirus: Comparison of persistent lymphocytosis with lymph node tumor form of enzootic bovine leukosis. *Proc. Natl. Acad. Sci.* **77**:2577–2581.

Kettmann, R., M. Meunier-Rotival, J. Cortadas, G. Cuny, J. Ghysdael, M. Mammerickx, A. Burny, and G. Bernardi. 1979. Integration of bovine leukemia virus DNA in the bovine genome. *Proc. Natl. Acad. Sci.* **76**:4822–4826.

Khoury, A.T. and H. Hanafusa. 1976. Synthesis and integration of viral DNA in chicken cells at different times after infection with various multiplicities of avian oncornavirus. *J. Virol.* **18**:383–400.

Khoury, A.T., H. Hanafusa, and C.A. Namy. 1979. Production of avian oncoviral subgroups after multiple infection. *J. Virol.* **29**:926–937.

Kiessling, A.A. and M. Goulian. 1976. A comparison of the enzymatic responses of the DNA polymerases from four RNA tumor viruses. *Biochem. Biophys. Res. Commun.* **71**: 1069–1077.

Kleckner, N. 1977. Translocatable elements in procaryotes. *Cell* **11**:11–23.

———. 1979. DNA sequence analysis of Tn10 insertions: Origin and role of 9 bp flanking repetitions during Tn10 translocation. *Cell* **16**:711–720.

Knesek, J.E., M.A. Nash, J.C. Chan, R.J. Bartlett, J.M. Bowen, and J.L. East. 1980. Intracellular RNA complementary to the RNA genome of the Moloney-murine sarcoma virus complex. *Virology* **100**:288–299.

Kopchick, J.J., G.A. Jamjoon, K.T. Watson, and R.B. Arlinghaus. 1978. Biosynthesis of reverse transcriptase from Rauscher murine leukemia virus by synthesis and cleavage of a *gag-pol* readthrough viral precursor polyprotein. *Proc. Natl. Acad. Sci.* **75**:2016–2020.

Kopchick, J.J., J. Harless, B.S. Geissner, R. Killam, R.R. Hewitt, and R.B. Arlinghaus. 1981. Endodeoxyribonuclease activity associated with Rauscher murine leukemia virus. *J. Virol.* **37**:274–283.

Kozak, M. 1978. How do eucaryotic ribosomes select initiation regions in messenger RNA? *Cell* **15**:1109–1123.

Krakower, J.M. and S.A. Aaronson. 1978. Radioimmunologic characterization of RD-114 reverse transcriptase: Evolutionary relatedness of mammalian type C viral *pol* gene products. *Virology* **86**:127–137.

Krakower, J.M., M. Barbacid, and S.A. Aaronson. 1977. Radioimmunoassay for mammalian type C viral reverse transcriptase. *J. Virol.* **22**:331–339.

Krontiris, T.G., R. Soiero, and B.N. Fields. 1973. Host restriction of Friend leukemia virus. Role of the viral outer coat. *Proc. Natl. Acad. Sci.* **70**:2549–2553.

Krueger, J.G., E. Wang, and A.R. Goldberg. 1980. Evidence that the *src* gene product of Rous sarcoma virus is membrane associated. *Virology* **101**:25–40.

Krzyzek, R.A., A.F. Lau, and A.J. Faras. 1979. Nature of Rous sarcoma virus-specific RNA in transformed and revertant field vole cells. *J. Virol.* **29**:507–516.

Krzyzek, R.A., M.S. Collett, A.F. Lau, M.L. Perdue, J.P. Leis, and A.J. Faras. 1978. Evidence for splicing of avian sarcoma virus 5′-terminal genomic sequences onto viral-specific RNA in infected cells. *Proc. Natl. Acad. Sci.* **75**:1284–1288.

Kung, H.-J., P.R. Shank, J.M. Bishop, and H.E. Varmus. 1980. Identification and characterization of dimeric and trimeric circular forms of avian sarcoma virus-specific DNA. *Virology* **103**:425–433.

Kung, H.J., Y.K. Fung, J.E. Majors, J.M. Bishop, and H.E. Varmus. 1981. Synthesis of plus strands of retroviral DNA in cells infected with avian sarcoma virus and mouse mammary tumor virus. *J. Virol.* **37**:127–138.

Lai, M.-H.T. and S.S.F. Hu. 1978. *In vitro* synthesis of full- and half-length complementary DNA from avian oncoviruses. *Nature* **271**:481–483

Lai, M.-H.T. and I.M. Verma. 1978. Reverse transcriptase of RNA tumor viruses. V. In vitro proteolysis of reverse transcriptase from avian myeloblastosis virus and isolation of a polypeptide manifesting only RNase H activity. *J. Virol.* **25:**652-663.

———. 1980. Genome organization of retroviruses. VII. Infection by double-stranded DNA synthesized *in vitro* from Moloney murine leukemia virus generates a virus indistinguishable from the original virus used in reverse transcription. *Virology* **100:**194–198.

Lai, M.-H.T., I.M. Verma, S.R. Tronick, and S.A. Aaronson. 1978. Mammalian retrovirus-associated RNase H is virus coded. *J. Virol.* **27:**823–825.

Lai, M.M.C. and S.S.F. Hu. 1978. *In vitro* synthesis and characterisation of full- and half-genome length complementary DNA from avian oncoviruses. *Nature* **271:**481–483.

Lai, M.M.C., J.C. Neil, and P.K. Vogt. 1980. Cell-free translation of avian erythroblastosis virus RNA yields two specific and distinct proteins with molecular weights of 75,000 and 40,000. *Virology* **100:**475–483.

Landy, A. and W. Ross. 1977. Viral integration and excision: Structure of the lambda *att* sites. *Science* **197:**1147–1160.

Leblond-Larouche, L., R. Morais, and M. Zollinger. 1979. Studies of the effect of chloramphenicol, ethidium bromide and camptothecin on the reproduction of Rous sarcoma virus in infected chick embryo cells. *J. Gen. Virol.* **44:**323–331.

Ledbetter, J.A., R.C. Nọwinski, and R.N. Eisenman. 1978. Biosynthesis and metabolism of viral proteins expressed on the surface of murine leukemia virus-infected cells. *Virology* **91:**116–129.

Lee, J.S., H.E. Varmus, and J.M. Bishop. 1979. Virus-specific messenger RNAs in permissive cells infected by avian sarcoma virus. *J. Biol. Chem.* **245:**8015–8022.

Lee, S.G. and P.P. Hung. 1977. Extensive reverse transcription of RSV genome by nucleic acid-binding protein. *Nature* **270:**336–368.

Lee, S.G., M.V. Miceli, R.A. Jungmann, and P.P. Hung. 1975. Protein kinase and its regulatory effect on reverse transcriptase activity of Rous sarcoma virus. *Proc. Natl. Acad. Sci.* **72:**2945–2949.

Leibovitch, S.A., H. Tapiero, and J. Harel. 1977. Single-stranded DNA from oncornavirus-infected cells enriched in virus-specific DNA sequences. *Proc. Natl. Acad. Sci.* **74:** 3720–3724.

Leis, J.P. and J. Hurwitz. 1972a. RNA-dependent DNA polymerase activity of RNA tumor viruses. II. Directing influence of RNA in the reaction. *J. Virol.* **9:**130–142.

———. 1972b. Isolation and characterization of a protein that stimulates DNA synthesis from avian myeloblastosis virus. *Proc. Natl. Acad. Sci.* **69:**2331–2335.

Leis, J.P., I. Berkower, and J. Hurwitz. 1973. Mechanism of action of ribonuclease H isolated from avian myeloblastosis virus and *Escherichia coli*. *Proc. Natl. Acad. Sci.* **70:**466–470.

Leis, J.P., J. McGinnis, and R.W. Green. 1978. Rous sarcoma virus p19 binds to specific double-stranded regions of viral RNA: Effect of p19 on cleavage of viral RNA by RNase III. *Virology* **84:**87–98.

Leis, J.P., A. Schincariol, R. Ishizaki, and J. Hurwitz. 1975. RNA-dependent DNA polymerase activity of RNA tumor viruses. V. Rous sarcoma virus single-stranded RNA-DNA covalent hybrids in infected chicken embryo fibroblast cells. *J. Virol.* **15:**484–489.

Lemons, R.S., S.J. O'Brien, and C.J. Sherr. 1977. A new genetic locus, *Bevi,* on human chromosome 6 which controls the replication of baboon type C virus in human cells. *Cell* **12:**251–262.

Lemons, R.S., W.G. Nash, S.J. O'Brien, R.E. Benveniste, and C.J. Sherr. 1978. A gene (*Bevi*) on human chromosome 6 is an integration site for baboon type C DNA provirus in human cells. *Cell* **14:**995–1005.

Leong, J.A., W. Levinson, and J.M. Bishop. 1972a. Synchronization of Rous sarcoma virus production in chick embryo cells. *Virology* **47:**133–144.

Leong, J.A., A.-C. Garapin, N. Jackson, L. Fanshier, W. Levinson, and J.M. Bishop. 1972b.

Virus-specific ribonucleic acid in cells producing Rous sarcoma virus: Detection and characterization. *J. Virol.* **9:**891–902.

Lerner, M.R., J.A. Boyle, S.M. Mount, S.L. Wolin, and J.A. Steitz. 1980. Are snRNPs involved in splicing? *Nature* **283:**220–224.

Levin, J.G. and M.J. Rosenak. 1976. Synthesis of murine leukemia virus proteins associated with virions assembled in actinomycin D-treated cells: Evidence for the persistence of viral messenger RNA. *Proc. Natl. Acad. Sci.* **73:**1154–1158.

Levin, J.G. and J.G. Seidman. 1979. Selective packaging of host tRNA's by murine leukemia virus particles does not require genomic RNA. *J. Virol.* **29:**328–335.

———. 1981. Effect of polymerase mutations on packaging of primer $tRNA^{Pro}$ during murine leukemia virus assembly. *J. Virol.* **38:**403–408.

Levin, J.G., P.M. Grimley, J.M. Ramseur, and I.K. Berezesky. 1974. Deficiency of 60 to 70S RNA in murine leukemia virus particles assembled in cells treated with actinomycin D. *J. Virol.* **14:**152–161.

Lewandowski, L.J., R.E. Smith, D.P. Bolognesi, and M.S. Halpern. 1975. Viral glycoprotein synthesis under conditions of glucosamine blocks in cells transformed by avian sarcoma viruses. *Virology* **66:**347–355.

Lindell, T.J., F. Weinberg, P.W. Morris, R.G. Roeder, and W.J. Rutter. 1970. Specific inhibition of nuclear RNA polymerase II by α-amanitin. *Science* **170:**447–449.

Linial, M. and W.S. Mason. 1973. Characterization of two conditional early mutants of Rous sarcoma virus. *Virology* **53:**258–273.

Linial, M. and P.E. Neiman. 1976. Infection of chick cells by subgroup E viruses. *Virology* **73:**508–520.

Linial, M., S. Brown, and P. Neiman. 1978a. A nonconditional mutant of Rous sarcoma virus containing defective polymerase. *Virology* **87:**130–141.

Linial, M., E. Medeiros, and W.S. Hayward. 1978b. An avian oncovirus mutant (SE 21Q1b) deficient in genomic RNA: Biological and biochemical characterization. *Cell* **15:**1371–1381.

Long, C., R. Sachs, J. Norvell, V. Huebner, M. Hatanaka, and R. Gilden. 1973. Specificity of antibody to the RD-114 viral polymerase. *Nat. New Biol.* **241:**147–149.

Lovinger, G.G., R.V. Gilden, and M. Hatanaka. 1978. Effects of hydroxyurea on murine type C virus-specific DNA synthesis in newly infected cells. *Cancer Res.* **38:**2112–2117.

Lovinger, G.G. H.P. Ling, R.V. Gilden, and M. Hatanaka. 1975. Effect of UV light on RNA-directed DNA polymerase activity of murine oncornaviruses. *J. Virol.* **15:**1273– 1275.

Lowy, D.R. and E.M. Scolnick. 1978. Glucocorticoids induce focus formation and increase sarcoma viral expression in a mink cell line that contains a murine sarcoma viral genome. *J. Virol.* **25:**157–163.

Lowy, D.R., E.M. Rands, and E.M. Scolnick. 1978. Helper-independent transformation by unintegrated Harvey sarcoma virus DNA. *J. Virol.* **26:**291–298.

Lowy, D.R., E. Rands, S.K. Chattopadhyay, C.F. Garon, and G.L. Hager. 1980. Molecular cloning of infectious integrated murine leukemia virus DNA from infected mouse cells. *Proc. Natl. Acad. Sci.* **77:**614–618.

MacHattie, L.A. and J.B. Jackowski. 1977. Physical structure and deletion effects of the chloramphenicol resistance element Tn9 in phage lambda. In *DNA insertion elements, plasmids and episomes* (ed. A.I. Bukhari et al.), pp.219–228. Cold Spring Harbor Laboratory, Cold Spring Harbor, New York.

Macpherson, I. 1965. Reversion in hamster cells transformed by Rous sarcoma virus. *Science* **148:**1731–1733.

Majors, J.E. and H.E. Varmus. 1980. Learning about the replication of retroviruses from a single cloned provirus of mouse mammary tumor virus. *ICN-UCLA Symp. Mol. Cell. Biol.* **18:**241–253.

———. 1981. Nucleotide sequences at host-proviral junctions for mouse mammary tumour virus. *Nature* **289:**253–258.

Mak, T.W., A.A. Axelrad, and A. Bernstein. 1979. *Fv-2* locus controls expression of Friend spleen focus-forming virus-specific sequences in normal and infected mice. *Proc. Natl. Acad. Sci.* **76:**5809–5812.

Maniatis, T., S.G. Kee, A. Efstratiadis, and F.C. Kafatos. 1976. Amplification and characterization of a β-globin gene synthesized in vitro. *Cell* **8:**163–182.

Manley, J.L., A. Fire, A. Cano, P.A. Sharp, and M.L. Gefter. 1980. DNA-dependent transcription of adenovirus genes in a soluble whole-cell extract. *Proc. Natl. Acad. Sci.* **77:**3855–3859.

Manly, K., D.F. Smoler, E. Bromfeld, and D. Baltimore. 1971. Forms of deoxyribonucleic acid produced by virions of the ribonucleic acid tumor viruses. *J. Virol.* **7:**106–111.

Marcus, S.L. 1978. Resolution and characterization of intracytoplasmic forms of reverse transcriptase from Rauscher leukemia virus-producing cells. *J. Virol.* **26:**1–10.

Marcus, S.L., M.J. Modak, and L.F. Cavalieri. 1974. Purification of avian myeloblastosis virus DNA polymerase by affinity chromatography on polycytidylate-agarose. *J. Virol.* **14:**853–859.

Markham, P.D. and R.C. Gallo. 1978. Infectious primate type C virus proviral DNA in productively infected cells. *J. Virol.* **25:**936–939.

Martin, G.S. K. Radke, S. Hughes, N. Quintrell, J.M. Bishop, and H.E. Varmus. 1979. Mutants of Rous sarcoma virus with extensive deletions of the viral genome. *Virology* **96:**530–546.

Mason, W.S., T.W. Hsu, C. Yeater, J.L. Sabran, G.E. Mark, A. Kaji, and J.M. Taylor. 1979. Avian sarcoma virus-transformed quail clones defective in the production of focus-forming virus. *J. Virol.* **30:**132–140.

McClements, W., H. Hanafusa, S. Tilghman, and A. Skalka. 1979. Structural studies on oncornavirus-related sequences in chicken genomic DNA: Two-step analyses of *Eco*RI and *Bgl*I restriction digests and tentative mapping of a ubiquitous endogenous provirus. *Proc. Natl. Acad. Sci.* **76:**2165–2169.

McClements, W.L., L. Enquist, M. Oskarsson, M. Sullivan, and G.F. Vande Woude. 1980. A frequent site specific deletion of coliphage lambda murine sarcoma virus recombinants and its use in the identification of a retrovirus integration site. *J. Virol.* **35:**488–497.

McDonnell, J.P., A.-C. Garapin, W.E. Levinson, N. Quintrell, L. Fanshier, and J.M. Bishop. 1970. DNA polymerases of Rous sarcoma virus: Delineation of two reactions with actinomycin. *Nature* **228:**433–435.

McGinnis, J., A. Hizi, R.E. Smith, and J.P. Leis. 1978. *In vitro* translation of a 180,000-dalton Rous sarcoma virus precursor polypeptide containing both the DNA polymerase and the group-specific antigens. *Virology* **84:**518–522.

McGrath, C.M., S. Nandi, and L. Young. 1972. Relationship between organization of mammary tumors and the ability of tumor cells to replicate mammary tumor virus and to recognize growth-inhibitory contact signals in vitro. *J. Virol.* **9:**367–376.

Mellon, P. and P.H. Duesberg. 1977. Subgenomic, cellular Rous sarcoma virus RNAs contain oligonucleotides from the 3′ half and the 5′ terminus of virion RNA. *Nature* **270:**631–634.

Mellon, P., A. Pawson, K. Bister, G.S. Martin, and P.H. Duesberg. 1978. Specific RNA sequences and gene products of MC29 avian acute leukemia virus. *Proc. Natl. Acad. Sci.* **75:**5874–5878.

Mitra, S.W., S. Goff, E. Gilboa, and D. Baltimore. 1979. Synthesis of a 600-nucleotide-long plus-strand DNA by virions of Moloney murine leukemia virus. *Proc. Natl. Acad. Sci.* **76:**4355–4359.

Mizutani, S. and H.M. Temin. 1973. Lack of serological relationship among DNA polymerases of avian leukosis-sarcoma viruses, reticuloendotheliosis viruses, and chicken cells. *J. Virol.* **12:**440–448.

———. 1974. Specific serological relationships among partially purified DNA polymerases of avian leukosis-sarcoma viruses, reticuloendotheliosis viruses, and avian cells. *J. Virol.* **13:**1020–1029.

———. 1975. Purification and properties of spleen necrosis virus DNA polymerase. *J. Virol.* **16:**797–806.

———. 1976. Incorporation of noncomplementary nucleotides at high frequencies by ribodeoxyvirus DNA polymerases and *Escherichia coli* DNA polymerase I. *Biochemistry* **15:**1510–1516.

Modak, M.J. 1976. Pyridoxal 5′ phosphate: A selective inhibitor of oncornaviral DNA polymerases. *Biochem. Biophys. Res. Commun.* **71:**180–187.

Modak, M.J. and S.L. Marcus. 1977. Purification and properties of Rauscher leukemia virus DNA polymerase and selective inhibition of mammalian viral reverse transcriptase by inorganic phosphate. *J. Biol. Chem.* **252:**11–19.

Modak, M.J. and A. Srivastava. 1979. Reverse transcriptase-associated ribonuclease H does not require zinc for catalysis. *J. Biol. Chem.* **254:**4756–4759.

Moe, J. 1978. "Isoleucyl tRNA synthetase: Purification and genetic analysis through interaction with blue dextran." Ph.D. thesis, University of California, Irvine.

Moelling, K. 1974. Characterization of reverse transcriptase and RNase H from Friend-murine leukemia virus. *Virology* **62:**46–59.

———. 1976. Further characterization of the Friend murine leukemia virus reverse transcriptase-RNase H complex. *J. Virol.* **18:**418–425.

Moelling, K. and R.R. Friis. 1979. Two avian sarcoma virus mutants with defects in the DNA polymerase-RNase H complex. *J. Virol.* **32:**370–378.

Moelling, K., A. Scott, K.E.J. Dittmar, and M. Owada. 1980. Effect of p15-associated protease from an avian RNA tumor virus on avian virus-specific polyprotein precursors. *J. Virol.* **33:**680–688.

Moelling, K., H. Gelderblom, G. Pauli, R. Friis, and H. Bauer. 1975. A comparative study of the avian reticuloendotheliosis virus: Relationship to murine leukemia virus and viruses of the avian sarcoma-leukosis complex. *Virology* **65:**546–557.

Moelling, K., D.P. Bolognesi, H. Bauer, W. Busen, H.W. Plassmann, and P. Hausen. 1971. Association of viral reverse transcriptase with an enzyme degrading the RNA moiety of RNA-DNA hybrids. *Nat. New Biol.* **234:**240–243.

Moldow, C.F., R.S. Kauffman, S.G. Devane, and J.R. Stephenson. 1979a. Type-C and type-D primate retrovirus envelope glycoproteins bind common cellular receptor sites. *Virology* **98:**373–384.

Moldow, C.F., F.H. Reynolds, Jr., J. Lake, K. Lundberg, and J.R. Stephenson. 1979b. Avian sarcoma virus envelope glycoprotein (gp85) specifically binds chick embryo fibroblasts. *Virology* **97:**448–453.

Morris, A.G. and D.C. Burke. 1979. An interferon-sensitive early step in the establishment of infection of murine cells by murine sarcoma/leukeamia virus. *J. Gen. Virol.* **43:**173–181.

Morris, V.L., C. Kozak, J.C. Cohen, P.R. Shank, P. Jolicoeur, F. Ruddle, and H.E. Varmus. 1979. Endogenous mouse mammary tumor virus DNA is distributed among multiple mouse chromosomes. *Virology* **92:**46–55.

Mueller-Lantzsch, N. and H. Fan. 1976. Monospecific immunoprecipitation of murine leukemia virus polyribosomes: Identification of p30 protein-specific messenger RNA. *Cell* **9:**579–588.

Mullins, J.I., J.W. Casey, M.O. Nicolson, and N. Davidson. 1980. Sequence organization of feline leukemia virus DNA in infected cells. *Nucleic Acids Res.* **8:**3287–3305.

Mullins, J.I., J. Casey, M.O. Nicolson, K.Bauman-Burck, and N. Davidson. 1981. Sequence arrangement and biological activity of cloned feline leukemia virus provirus from a virus-productive human cell line. *J. Virol.* **38:**688–703.

Murphy, E.C. and R.B. Arlinghaus. 1978. Cell-free synthesis of Rauscher murine leukemia virus *"gag"* and *"gag-pol"* precursor polypeptides from virion 35S RNA in a mRNA-dependent translation system derived from mouse tissue culture cells. *Virology* **86:** 329–343.

Murphy, E.C., Jr., D. Campos III, and R.B. Arlinghaus. 1979. Cell-free synthesis of Rauscher murine leukemia virus "*gag*" and "*env*" gene products from separate cellular mRNA species. *Virology* **93:**293–302.

Murphy, E.C., Jr., N. Wills, and R.B. Arlinghaus. 1980. Suppression of murine retrovirus polypeptide termination: Effect of amber suppressor tRNA on the cell-free translation of Rauscher murine leukemia virus, Moloney murine leukemia virus, and Moloney murine sarcoma virus 124 RNA. *J. Virol.* **34:**464–473.

Murray, R.K. and H.M. Temin. 1970. Carcinogenesis by RNA sarcoma viruses. XIV. Infection of stationary cultures with murine sarcoma virus (Harvey). *Int. J. Cancer* **5:**320–326.

Myers, J.C. and S. Spiegelman. 1978. Sodium pyrophosphate inhibition of RNA-DNA hybrid degradation by reverse transcriptase. *Proc. Natl. Acad. Sci.* **75:**5329–5333.

Myers, J.C., C. Dobkin, and S. Spiegelman. 1980. RNA primer used in synthesis of anticomplementary DNA by reverse transcriptase of avian myeloblastosis virus. *Proc. Natl. Acad. Sci.* **77:**1316–1320.

Myers, J.C., S. Spiegelman, and D.L. Kacian. 1977. Synthesis of full-length DNA copies of avian myeloblastosis virus RNA in high yields. *Proc. Natl. Acad. Sci.* **74:**2840–2843.

Nakata, Y. and J.P. Bader. 1968a. Studies on the fixation and development of cellular transformation by Rous sarcoma virus. *Virology* **36:**401–410.

———. 1968b. Transformation by murine sarcoma virus: Fixation (deoxyribonucleic acid synthesis) and development. *J. Virol.* **2:**1255–1261.

Neel, B.G., W.S. Hayward, H.L. Robinson, J. Fang, and S.M. Astrin. 1981. Avian leukosis virus-induced tumors have common proviral integration sites and synthesize discrete viral RNAs: Oncogenesis by promoter insertion. *Cell* **23:**323–334.

Neiman, P.E. 1972. Rous sarcoma virus nucleotide sequences in cellular DNA: Measurement by RNA-DNA hybridization. *Science* **178:**750–753.

Neiman, P.E., C. McMillin-Helsel, and G.M. Cooper. 1978. Specific restriction of avian sarcoma viruses by a line of transformed lymphoid cells. *Virology* **89:**360–371.

Neiman, P., L.N. Payne, and R.A. Weiss. 1980. Viral DNA in bursal lymphomas induced by avian leukosis viruses. *J. Virol.* **34:**178–186.

Nissen-Meyer, J. and I.F. Nes. 1980. Purification and properties of DNA endonuclease associated with Friend leukemia virus. *Nucleic Acids Res.* **8:**5043–5055.

Nomura, S. 1978. Revertants of mouse cells transformed by murine sarcoma virus. V. Loss of MSV-specific nucleotide sequences from cellular RNA. *Virology* **91:**444–452.

Novak, U., R. Friedrich, and K. Moelling. 1979. Elongation of DNA complementary to the 5′ end of the avian sarcoma virus genome by the virion-associated RNA-dependent DNA polymerase. *J. Virol.* **30:**438–452.

Nowinski, R.C., K.F. Watson, A. Yaniv, and S. Spiegelman. 1972. Serological analysis of the deoxyribonucleic acid polymerase of avian oncornaviruses. II. Comparison of avian deoxyribonucleic acid polymerases. *J. Virol.* **10:**959–964.

Nusse, R., F.A.M. Asselbergs, M.H.L. Salden, R.J.A.M. Michalides, and H. Bloemendal. 1978. Translation of mouse mammary tumor virus RNA: Precursor polypeptides are phosphorylated during processing. *Virology* **91:**106–115.

Ohtsubo, H. and E. Ohtsubo. 1978. Nucleotide sequence of an insertion element, IS1. *Proc. Natl. Acad. Sci.* **75:**615–619.

Oliff, A.I., G.L. Hager, E.H. Chang, E.M. Scolnick, H.W. Chan, and D.R. Lowy. 1980. Transfection of molecularly cloned Friend murine leukemia virus DNA yields a highly leukemogenic helper-independent type C virus. *J. Virol.* **33:**475–486.

Olsen, J.C. and K.F. Watson. 1980. Avian retrovirus RNA-directed DNA synthesis by purified reverse transcriptase. Covalent linkage of RNA to plus strand DNA. *Biochem. Biophys. Res. Commun.* **97:**1376–1383.

Oppermann, H., J.M. Bishop, H.E. Varmus, and L. Levintow. 1977. A joint product of the genes *gag* and *pol* of avian sarcoma virus: A possible precursor of reverse transcriptase. *Cell* **12:**993–1005.

O'Rear, J.J., S. Mizutani, G. Hoffman, M. Fiandt, and H.M. Temin. 1980. Infectious and noninfectious recombinant clones of the provirus of SNV differ in cellular DNA and are apparently the same in viral DNA. *Cell* **20:**423–430.

Oskarsson, M., W.L. McClements, D.G. Blair, J.V. Maizel, and G.F. Vande Woude. 1980. Properties of a normal mouse cell DNA sequence (*sarc*) homologous to the *src* sequence of Moloney sarcoma virus. *Science* **207:**1222–1224.

Owada, M., S. Ihara, K. Toyoshima, Y. Kozai, and Y. Sugino. 1976. Ultraviolet inactivation of avian sarcoma viruses: Biological and biochemical analysis. *Virology* **69:**710–718.

Padhy, L.C., S.K. Kar, K.K. Rao, and M.R. Das. 1976. Role of plasma membranes in stimulation of RNA-directed DNA synthesis. *Nature* **262:**805–807.

Pal, B.K. and P. Roy-Burman. 1977. RNA tumor virus phosphoproteins: Subvirion location of the multiple phosphorylated species. *Virology* **83:**423–427.

Palmiter, R.D., J. Gagnon, V.M. Vogt, S. Ripley, and R.N. Eisenman. 1978. The NH_2-terminal sequence of the avian oncovirus *gag* precursor polyprotein ($Pr76^{gag}$). *Virology* **91:**423–433.

Panem, S. and W.H. Kirsten. 1973. Release of mouse leukemia-sarcoma virus from synchronized cells. *J. Natl. Cancer. Inst.* **50:**563–566.

Panet, A. and H. Berliner. 1978. Binding of tRNA to reverse transcriptase of RNA tumor viruses. *J. Virol.* **26:**214–220.

Panet, A. and H. Cedar. 1977. Selective degradation of integrated murine leukemia proviral DNA by deoxyribonucleases. *Cell* **11:**933–940.

Panet, A. and Z. Kra-Oz. 1978. A competition immunoassay for characterizing the reverse transcriptase of mammalian RNA tumor viruses. *Virology* **89:**95–101.

Panet, A., D. Baltimore, and T. Hanafusa. 1975a. Quantitation of avian RNA tumor virus reverse transcriptase by radioimmunoassay. *J. Virol.* **16:**146–152.

Panet, A., I.M. Verma, and D. Baltimore. 1975b. Role of the subunits of the avian RNA tumor virus reverse transcriptase. *Cold Spring Harbor Symp. Quant. Biol.* **39:**919–923.

Panet, A., G. Weil, and R.R. Friis. 1978a. Binding of tryptophanyl-tRNA to the reverse transcriptase of replication-defective avian sarcoma viruses. *J. Virol.* **28:**434–443.

Panet, A., M. Gorecki, S. Bratosin, and Y. Aloni. 1978b. Electron microscopic evidence for splicing of Moloney murine leukemia virus RNAs. *Nucleic Acids Res.* **5:**3219–3230.

Panet, A., W.A. Haseltine, D. Baltimore, G. Peters, F. Harada, and J.E. Darlberg. 1975c. Specific binding of tryptophan transfer RNA to avian myeloblastosis virus RNA-dependent DNA polymerase (reverse transcriptase). *Proc. Natl. Acad. Sci.* **72:**2535–2539.

Papas, T.S., T.W. Pry, and D.J. Marciani. 1977. Inactivation of avian myeloblastosis virus DNA polymerase by specific binding of pyridoxal 5′-phosphate to deoxynucleoside triphosphate binding site. *J. Biol. Chem.* **252:**1425–1430.

Papas, T.S., D.J. Marciani, K. Samuel, and J.G. Chirikjian. 1976. Mechanism of release of active α subunit from dimeric $\alpha\beta$ avian myeloblastosis virus DNA polymerase. *J. Virol.* **18:**904–910.

Papkoff, J., T. Hunter, and J. Beemon. 1980. *In vitro* translation of virion RNA from Moloney murine sarcoma virus. *Virology* **101:**91–103.

Parks, W.P., E.M. Scolnick, and E.H. Kozikowski. 1974. Dexamethasone stimulation of murine mammary tumor virus expression: A tissue culture source of virus. *Science* **184:**158–160.

Parks, W.P., E.M. Scolnick, J. Ross, G.J. Todaro, and S.A. Aaronson. 1972. Immunological relationships of reverse transcriptases from ribonucleic acid tumor viruses. *J. Virol.* **9:**110–115.

Parks, W.P., R.V. Gilden, A.F. Bykovsky, G.G. Miller, V.M. Zhdanov, V.D. Soloviev, and

E.M. Scolnick. 1973. Mason-Pfizer virus characterization: A similar virus in a human amniotic cell line. *J. Virol.* **12:**1540–1547.

Parsons, J.T., P. Lewis, and P. Dierks. 1978. Purification of virus-specific RNA from chicken cells infected with avian sarcoma virus: Identification of genome-length and subgenomic-length viral RNAs. *J. Virol.* **27:**227–238.

Parsons, J.T., J.M. Coffin, R.K. Haroz, P.A. Bromley, and C. Weissmann. 1973. Quantitative determination and location of newly synthesized virus-specific ribonucleic acid in chicken cells infected with Rous sarcoma virus. *J. Virol.* **11:**761–774.

Paskind, M.P., R.A. Weinberg, and D. Baltimore. 1975. Dependence of Moloney murine leukemia virus on cell growth. *Virology* **67:**242–248.

Patterson, B.M., D.J. Marciani, and T.S. Papas. 1977. Cell-free synthesis of the precursor polypeptide for avian myeloblastosis virus DNA polymerase. *Proc. Natl. Acad. Sci.* **74:**4951–4954.

Pawson, T. and G.S. Martin. 1980. Cell-free translation of avian erythroblastosis virus RNA. *J. Virol.* **34:**280–284.

Pawson, T., R. Harvey, and A.E. Smith. 1977. The size of Rous sarcoma virus mRNAs active in cell-free translation. *Nature* **268:**416–420.

Pawson, T., G.S. Martin, and A.E. Smith. 1976. Cell-free translation of virion RNA from nondefective and transformation-defective Rous sarcoma viruses. *J. Virol.* **19:**950–967.

Pawson, T., P. Mellon, P.H. Duesberg, and G.S. Martin. 1980. *env* gene of Rous sarcoma virus: Identification of the gene product by cell-free translation. *J. Virol.* **33:**993–1003.

Payne, G.S., S.A. Courtneidge, L.B. Crittenden, A.M. Fadly, J.M. Bishop, and H.E. Varmus. 1981. Analysis of avian leukosis virus DNA and RNA in bursal tumors: Viral gene expression is not required for maintenance of the tumor state. *Cell* **23:**311–322.

Payvar, R. and R.T. Schimke. 1979. Methylmercury hydroxide enhancement of translation and transcription of ovalbumin and conalbumin mRNA's. *J. Biol. Chem.* **254:**7636–7642.

Pedrali-Noy, G. and S. Spadari. 1979. Effect of aphidicolin on viral and human DNA polymerases. *Biochem. Biophys. Res. Commun.* **88:**1194–1202.

Peebles, C.L., N.P. Higgins, K.N. Kreuzer, A. Morrison, P.O. Brown, A. Sugino, and N.R. Cozzarelli. 1979. Structure and activities of *Escherichia coli* DNA gyrase. *Cold Spring Harbor Symp. Quant. Biol.* **43:**41–52.

Peries, J., E. Alves-Cardoso, M. Canivet, M.C. Debons-Guillemin, and J. Lasneret. 1977. Lack of multiplication of ecotropic murine C-type viruses in mouse teratocarcinoma primitive cells. *J. Natl. Cancer Inst.* **59:**463–465.

Peters, G. and J.E. Dahlberg. 1979. RNA-directed DNA synthesis in Moloney murine leukemia virus: Interaction between the primer tRNA and the genome RNA. *J. Virol.* **31:**398–407.

Peters, G.G. and C. Glover. 1980a. Low-molecular-weight RNAs and initiation of RNA-directed DNA synthesis in avian reticuloendotheliosis virus. *J. Virol.* **33:**708–716.

———. 1980b. tRNA's and priming of RNA-directed DNA synthesis in mouse mammary tumor virus. *J. Virol.* **35:**31–40.

Peters, G.G. and J. Hu. 1980. Reverse transcriptase as the major determinant for selective packaging of tRNAs into avian sarcoma virus particles. *J. Virol.* **36:**692–700.

Peters, G., F. Harada, J.E. Dahlberg, A. Panet, W.A. Haseltine, and D. Baltimore. 1977. Low-molecular-weight RNAs of Moloney murine leukemia virus: Identification of the primer for RNA-directed DNA synthesis. *J. Virol.* **21:**1031–1041.

Philipson, L., P. Andersson, U. Olshevsky, R. Weinberg, D. Baltimore, and R. Gesteland. 1978. Translation of MuLV and MSV RNA's in nuclease-treated reticulocyte extracts: Enhancement of the *gag-pol* polypeptide with yeast suppressor tRNA. *Cell* **13:** 189–199.

Piraino, F. 1967. The mechanisms of genetic resistance of chick embryo cells to infection by Rous sarcoma virus—Bryan strain (BS-RSV). *Virology* **32:**700–707.

Pitha, P.M., N.A. Wivel, B.F. Fernie, and H.P. Harper. 1979. Effect of interferon on murine leukaemia virus infection. IV. Formation of non-infectious virus in chronically infected cells. *J. Gen. Virol.* **42**:467–480.

Poiesz, B.J., N. Battula, and L.A. Loeb. 1974. Zinc in reverse transcriptase. *Biochem. Biophys. Res. Commun.* **56**:959.

Porzig, K.J., K.C. Robbins, and S.A. Aaronson. 1979. Cellular regulation of mammalian sarcoma virus expression: A gene regulation model for oncogenesis. *Cell* **16**:875–884.

Potter, S.S., W.J. Brorein, Jr., P. Dunsmuir, and G.M. Rubin. 1979. Transposition of elements of the *412, copia,* and *297* dispersed repeated gene families in *Drosophila. Cell* **17**:415–427.

Proudfoot, N.J. and G.G. Brownlee. 1974. Sequence analysis at the 3′ end of globin mRNA shows homology with immunoglobulin light chain messenger mRNA. *Nature* **252**:359–362.

Purchio, A.F., E. Erikson, and R.L. Erikson. 1977. Translation of 35S and of subgenomic regions of avian sarcoma virus RNA. *Proc. Natl. Acad. Sci.* **74**:4661–4665.

Purchio, A.F., S. Jovanovich, and R.L. Erikson. 1980. Sites of synthesis of viral proteins in avian sarcoma virus-infected chicken cells. *J. Virol.* **35**:629–636.

Purchio, A.F., E. Erikson, J.S. Brugge, and R.L. Erikson. 1978. Identification of a polypeptide encoded by the avian sarcoma virus *src* gene. *Proc. Natl. Acad. Sci.* **75**: 1567–1571.

Quintrell, N., S.H. Hughes, H.E. Varmus, and J.M. Bishop. 1980. Structure of viral DNA and RNA in mammalian cells infected with avian sarcoma virus. *J. Mol. Biol.* **143**: 363–393.

Rassart, E. and P. Jolicoeur. 1980. Restriction endonuclease mapping of unintegrated viral DNA of B- and N-tropic BALB/c murine leukemia virus. *J. Virol.* **36**:812–823.

Reitz, M., D. Gillespie, W.C. Saxinger, M. Robert, and R.C. Gallo. 1972. Poly(rA) tracts of tumor virus 70S RNA are not transcribed in endogenous or reconstructed reactions of viral reverse transcriptase. *Biochem. Biophys. Res. Commun.* **49**:1216–1224.

Rettenmier, W., R.E. Karess, S.M. Anderson, and H. Hanafusa. 1979. Tryptic peptide analysis of avian oncovirus *gag* and *pol* gene products. *J. Virol.* **32**:102–113.

Reynolds, R.K., W.J.M. van de Ven, and J.R. Stephenson. 1978. Translation of type C viral RNA's in *Xenopus laevis* oocytes: Evidence that the 120,000-molecular-weight polyprotein expressed in Abelson leukemia virus-transformed cells is virus-coded. *J. Virol.* **28**:665–670.

Rho, H.M., D.P. Grandgenett and M. Green. 1975. Sequence relatedness between the subunits of avian myeloblastosis virus reverse transcriptase. *J. Biol. Chem.* **250**:5278–5280.

Richert, N.J. and J.D. Hare. 1972. Distinctive effects of inhibitors of mitochondrial function on Rous sarcoma virus replication and malignant transformation. *Biochem. Biophys. Res. Commun.* **46**:5–10.

Ringold, G.M., P.R. Shank, and K.R. Yamamoto. 1978. Production of unintegrated mouse mammary tumor virus DNA in infected rat hepatoma cells is a secondary action of dexamethasone. *J. Virol.* **26**:93–101.

Ringold, G.M., R.D. Cardiff, H.E. Varmus, and K.R. Yamamoto. 1977a. Infection of cultured rat hepatoma cells by mouse mammary tumor virus. *Cell* **10**:11–18.

Ringold, G., E.Y. Lasfargues, J.M. Bishop, and H.E. Varmus. 1975a. Production of mouse mammary tumor virus by cultured cells in the absence and presence of hormones: Assay by molecular hybridization. *Virology* **65**:135–147.

Ringold, G.M., K.R. Yamamoto, J.M. Bishop, and H.E. Varmus. 1977b. Glucocorticoid-stimulated accumulation of mouse mammary tumor virus RNA: Increased rate of synthesis of viral RNA. *Proc. Natl. Acad. Sci.* **74**:2879–2883.

Ringold, G.M., K.R. Yamamoto, P.R. Shank, and H.E. Varmus. 1977c. Mouse mammary tumor virus DNA in infected rat cells: Characterization of unintegrated forms. *Cell* **10**:19–26.

Ringold, G.M., P.R. Shank, H.E. Varmus, J. Ring, and K.R. Yamamoto. 1979. Integration and transcription of mouse mammary virus DNA in rat hepatoma cells. *Proc. Natl. Acad. Sci.* **76**:665–669.

Ringold, G.M., K.R. Yamamoto, G.M. Tomkins, J.M. Bishop, and H.E. Varmus. 1975b. Dexamethasone-mediated induction of mouse mammary tumor virus RNA: A system for studying glucocorticoid action. *Cell* **6**:299–305.

Robert-Gero, M., F. Lawrence, G. Farrugia, A. Berneman, P. Blanchard, P. Vigier, and E. Lederer. 1975. Inhibition of virus-induced cell transformation by synthetic analogues of S-adenosyl homocysteine. *Biochem. Biophys. Res. Commun.* **65**:1242–1249.

Robertson, D.L. and H.E. Varmus. 1979. Structural analysis of the intracellular RNAs of murine mammary tumor virus. *J. Virol.* **30**:576–589.

———. 1981. Dexamethasone induction of the intracellular RNAs of mouse mammary tumor virus. *J. Virol.* (in press).

Robin, M.S., S. Salzberg, and M. Green. 1974. Cytoplasmic synthesis of viral DNA early during infection and cell transformation by the murine sarcoma-leukemia virus. *Intervirology* **4**:268–278.

Robinson, H.L. 1976. Intracellular restriction on the growth of induced subgroup E avian type C viruses on chicken cells. *J. Virol.* **18**:856–866.

Rokutanda, M., Y.Y. Maeda, and S. Takahama. 1979. Purification of protein kinase of mouse sarcoma virus and its effect on reverse transcriptase activity. *Biochem. Biophys. Res. Commun.* **88**:1322–1328.

Rokutanda, M., Y. Maeda, and N. Watanabe. 1978. High molecular weight viral reverse transcriptase in Moloney sarcoma virus transformed cells. *Biochem. Biophys. Res. Commun.* **80**:729–734.

Rokutanda, M., H. Rokutanda, M. Green, K. Fujinaga, R.K. Ray, and C. Gurgo. 1970. Formation of viral RNA-DNA hybrid molecules by the DNA polymerase of sarcoma-leukaemia viruses. *Nature* **227**:1026–1028.

Rose, J.K., W.A. Haseltine, and D. Baltimore. 1976. 5′-terminus of Moloney murine leukemia virus 35S RNA is $m^7G^{5'}$ $ppp^{5'}$ GmpCp. *J. Virol.* **20**:324–329.

Rosok, M.J. and K.F. Watson. 1979. Fractionation of two protein kinases from avian myeloblastosis virus and characterization of the protein kinase activity preferring basic phosphoacceptor proteins. *J. Virol.* **29**:872–880.

Ross, J., H. Aviv, E. Scolnick, and P. Leder. 1972. *In vitro* synthesis of DNA complementary to purified rabbit globin mRNA. *Proc. Natl. Acad. Sci.* **69**:264–268.

Ross, J., E.M. Scolnick, G.J. Todaro, and S.A. Aaronson. 1971. Separation of murine cellular and murine leukaemia virus DNA polymerases. *Nat. New Biol.* **231**:163–167.

Ross, D.G., J. Swan, and N. Kleckner. 1979. Physical structures of Tn10-promoted deletions and inversions: Role of 1400 bp inverted repetitions. *Cell* **16**:721–731.

Rothenberg, E. and D. Baltimore. 1976. Synthesis of long, representative DNA copies of the murine RNA tumor virus genome. *J. Virol.* **17**:168–174.

———. 1977. Increased length of DNA made by virions of murine leukemia virus at limiting magnesium ion concentration. *J. Virol.* **21**:168–178.

Rothenberg, E., D.J. Donoghue, and D. Baltimore. 1978. Analysis of a 5′ leader sequence on murine leukemia virus 21S RNA: Heteroduplex mapping with long reverse transcriptase products. *Cell* **13**:435–451.

Rothenberg, E., D. Smotkin, D. Baltimore, and R.A. Weinberg. 1977. *In vitro* synthesis of infectious DNA of murine leukaemia virus. *Nature* **269**:122–126.

Rothman, J.E. and H.F. Lodish. 1977. Synchronised transmembrane insertion and glycosylation of a nascent membrane protein. *Nature* **269**:775–780.

Rymo, L., J.T. Parsons, J.M. Coffin, and C. Weissmann. 1974. *In vitro* synthesis of Rous sarcoma virus-specific RNA is catalyzed by a DNA-dependent RNA polymerase. *Proc. Natl. Acad. Sci.* **71**:2782–2786.

Saborio, J.L., S.-S. Pong, and G. Koch. 1974. Selective and reversible inhibition of initiation of protein synthesis in mammalian cells. *J. Mol. Biol.* **85**:195–211.

Sabran, J.L., T.W. Hsu, C. Yeater, A. Kaji, W.S. Mason, and J.M. Taylor. 1979. Analysis of integrated avian RNA tumor virus DNA in transformed chicken, duck, and quail fibroblasts. *J. Virol.* **29**:170–178.

Salzberg, S., M. Barkanashvili, and M. Aboud. 1978. Effect of interferon on mouse cells chronically infected with murine leukemia virus: Kinetic studies on virus production and virus RNA synthesis. *J. Gen. Virol.* **40**:121–130.

Salzberg, S., M.S. Robin, and M. Green. 1973. Appearance of virus-specific RNA, viral particles, and cell surface changes in cells rapidly transformed by the murine sarcoma virus. *Virology* **53**:186–195.

———. 1977. A possible requirement for protein synthesis early in the infectious cycle of the murine sarcoma-leukemia virus. *Virology* **76**:341–351.

Samuel, K.P., T.S. Papas, and J.G. Chirikjian. 1979. DNA endonucleases associated with the avian myeloblastosis virus DNA polymerase. *Proc. Natl. Acad. Sci.* **76**:2659–2663.

Sarin, P.S. and R.C. Gallo. 1976. Purification and characterization of gibbon ape leukemia virus DNA polymerase. *Biochim. Biophys. Acta* **454**:212–221.

Sarin, P.S., B. Friedman, and R.C. Gallo. 1977. Purification and characterization of baboon endogenous virus DNA polymerase. *Biochim. Biophys. Acta* **479**:198–206.

Sawyer, R.C. and J.E. Dahlberg. 1973. Small RNAs of Rous sarcoma virus: Characterization by two-dimensional polyacrylamide gel electrophoresis and fingerprint analysis. *J. Virol.* **12**:1226–1237.

Sawyer, R.C. and H. Hanafusa. 1979. Comparison of the small RNAs of polymerase-deficient and polymerase-positive Rous sarcoma virus and another species of avian retrovirus. *J. Virol.* **29**:863–871.

Sawyer, R.C., F. Harada, and J.E. Dahlberg. 1974. Virion-associated RNA primer for Rous sarcoma virus DNA synthesis: Isolation from uninfected cells. *J. Virol.* **13**:1302–1311.

Schiff, R.D. and D.P. Grandgenett. 1978. Virus-coded origin of a 32,000-dalton protein from avian retrovirus cores: Structural relatedness of p32 and the β polypeptide of the avian retrovirus DNA polymerase. *J. Virol.* **28**:279–291.

Schincariol, A.L. and W.K. Joklik. 1973. Early synthesis of virus-specific RNA and DNA in cells rapidly transformed with Rous sarcoma virus. *Virology* **56**:532–548.

Schindler, J., R. Hynes, and N. Hopkins. 1977. Evidence for recombination between N- and B-tropic murine leukemia viruses: Analysis of three virion proteins by sodium dodecyl sulfate-polyacrylamide gel electrophoresis. *J. Virol.* **23**:700–707.

Schochetman, G. and J. Schlom. 1976. Independent polypeptide chain initiation sites for the synthesis of different classes of proteins for a RNA tumor virus: Mouse mammary tumor virus. *Virology* **73**:431–441.

Schultz, A.M. and S. Oroszlan. 1978. Murine leukemia virus *gag* polyproteins: The peptide chain unique to Pr80 is located at the amino terminus. *Virology* **91**:481–486.

———. 1979. Tunicamycin inhibits glycosylation of precursor polyprotein encoded by *env* gene of Rauscher murine leukemia virus. *Biochem. Biophys. Res. Commun.* **86**:1206–1213.

Schwartz, D.E., P.C. Zamecnik, and H.L. Weith. 1977. Rous sarcoma virus genome is terminally redundant: The 3′ sequence. *Proc. Natl. Acad. Sci.* **74**:994–998.

Schwarz, R.T., J.M. Rohrschneider, and M.F.G. Schmidt. 1976. Suppression of glycoprotein formation by Semliki forest, influenza, and avian sarcoma virus by tunicamycin. *J. Virol.* **19**:782–791.

Scolnick, E.M., H.A. Young, and W.P. Parks. 1976. Biochemical and physiological mechanisms in glucocorticoid hormone induction of mouse mammary tumor virus. *Virology* **69**:148–156.

Scott, M.L., K. McKereghan, H.S. Kaplan, and K.E. Fry. 1981. Molecular cloning and partial characterization of unintegrated linear DNA from gibbon ape leukemia virus. *Proc. Natl. Acad. Sci.* **78:**4213–4217.

Segal, S., A.J. Levine, and G. Khoury. 1979. Evidence for non-spliced SV40 RNA in undifferentiated murine teratocarcinoma stem cells. *Nature* **280:**335–338.

Sen, G.C. and N.H. Sarkar. 1980. Effects of interferon on the production of murine mammary tumor virus by mammary tumor cells in culture. *Virology* **102:**431–443.

Sen, G.C., S.W. Smith, S.L. Marcus, and N.H. Sarkar. 1979. Identification of the messenger RNAs coding for the *gag* and *env* gene products of the murine mammary tumor virus. *Proc. Natl. Acad. Sci.* **76:**1736–1740.

Shank, P.R. and M. Linial. 1980. Avian oncornavirus mutant (*SE*21Q1b) deficient in genomic RNA: Characterization of a deletion in the provirus. *J. Virol.* **36:**450–456.

Shank, P.R. and H.E. Varmus. 1978. Virus-specific DNA in the cytoplasm of avian sarcoma virus-infected cells is a precursor to covalently closed circular viral DNA in the nucleus. *J. Virol.* **25:**104–114.

Shank, P.R., S.H. Hughes, and H.E. Varmus. 1981. Restriction endonuclease mapping of the DNA of Rous-associated virus-0 reveals extensive homology in structure and sequence with avian sarcoma virus DNA. *Virology* **108:**177–188.

Shank, P.R., J.C. Cohen, H.E. Varmus, K.R. Yamamoto, and G.M. Ringold. 1978a. Mapping of linear and circular forms of mouse mammary tumor virus DNA with restriction endonucleases: Evidence for a large specific deletion occurring at high frequency during circularization. *Proc. Natl. Acad. Sci.* **75:**2112–2116.

Shank, P.R., S.H. Hughes, H.-J. Kung, J.E. Majors, N. Quintrell, R.V. Guntaka, J.M. Bishop, and H.E. Varmus. 1978b. Mapping unintegrated avian sarcoma virus DNA: Termini of linear DNA bear 300 nucleotides present once or twice in two species of circular DNA. *Cell* **15:**1383–1395.

Shanmugan, G., S. Bhaduri, and M. Green. 1974. The virus-specific RNA species in free and membrane-bound polyribosomes of transformed cells replicating murine sarcoma-leukemia viruses. *Biochem. Biophys. Res. Commun.* **56:**697–702.

Shapiro, J.A. 1979. Molecular model for the transposition and replication of bacteriophage Mu and other transposable elements. *Proc. Natl. Acad. Sci.* **76:**1933–1937.

Shapiro, J.A. and L.A. MacHattie. 1979. Integration and excision of prophage λ mediated by the IS*1* element. *Cold Spring Harbor Symp. Quant. Biol.* **43:**1135–1142.

Sheiness, D., B. Vennstrom, and J.M. Bishop. 1981. Virus-specific RNAs in cells infected by avian myelocytomatosis virus and avian erythroblastosis virus: Modes of oncogene expression. *Cell* **23:**291–300.

Sherr, C.J., L.A. Fedele, L. Donner, and L.P. Turek. 1979. Restriction endonuclease mapping of unintegrated proviral DNA of Snyder-Theilen feline sarcoma virus: Localization of sarcoma-specific sequences. *J. Virol.* **32:**860–875.

Sherr, C.J., L.A. Fedele, M. Oskarsson, J. Maizel, and G. Vande Woude. 1980. Molecular cloning of Snyder-Theilen feline leukemia and sarcoma viruses: Comparative studies of feline sarcoma virus with its natural helper virus and with Moloney murine sarcoma virus. *J. Virol.* **34:**200–212.

Shields, A., O.N. Witte, E. Rothenberg, and D. Baltimore. 1978. High frequency of aberrant expression of Moloney murine leukemia virus in clonal infections. *Cell* **14:**601–609.

Shields, A., S. Goff, M. Paskind, G. Otto, and D. Baltimore. 1979. Structure of the Abelson murine leukemia virus genome. *Cell* **18:**955–962.

Shimakage, M.I., T. Kamahora, A. Hakura, and K. Toyoshima. 1979. Selective replication of transformation-defective avian sarcoma virus mutants in duck embryo fibroblasts. *J. Gen. Virol.* **45:**99–105.

Shimotohno, K. and H.M. Temin. 1980. No apparent nucleotide sequence specificity in cellular DNA juxtaposed to retrovirus proviruses. *Proc. Natl. Acad. Sci.* **77:**7357–7361.

Shimotohno, K., S. Mizutani, and H.M. Temin. 1980. Sequence of retrovirus provirus resembles that of bacterial transposable elements. *Nature* **285:**550–554.

Shine, J., A.P. Czernilofsky, R. Friedrich, J.M. Bishop, and H.M. Goodman. 1977. Nucleotide sequence at the 5′ terminus of the avian sarcoma virus genome. *Proc. Natl. Acad. Sci.* **74:**1473–1477.

Shoemaker, C., S. Goff, E. Gilboa, M. Paskind, S.W. Mitra, and D. Baltimore. 1980. Structure of a cloned circular Moloney murine leukemia virus molecule containing an inverted segment: Implications for retrovirus integration. *Proc. Natl. Acad. Sci.* **77:** 3932–3936.

Shoyab, M., M.N. Dastoor, and M.A. Baluda. 1976. Evidence for tandem integration of avian myeloblastosis virus DNA with endogenous provirus in leukemic chicken cells. *Proc. Natl. Acad. Sci.* **73:**1749–1753.

Shoyab, M., P.D. Markham, and M.A. Baluda. 1975. Host induced alteration of avian sarcoma virus B-77 genome. *Proc. Natl. Acad. Sci.* **72:**1031–1035.

Shurtz, R., S. Dolev, M. Aboud, and S. Salzberg. 1979. Viral genome RNA serves as messenger early in the infectious cycle of murine leukemia virus. *J. Virol.* **31:**668–676.

Smoler, D., I. Molineux, and D. Baltimore. 1971. Direction of polymerization by the avian myeloblastosis virus deoxyribonucleic acid polymerase. *J. Biol. Chem.* **246:**7697–7700.

Smotkin, D., F.K. Yoshimura, and R.A. Weinberg. 1976. Infectious, linear, unintegrated DNA of Moloney murine leukemia virus. *J. Virol.* **20:**621–626.

Smotkin, D., A.M. Gianni, S. Rozenblatt, and R.A. Weinberg. 1975. Infectious viral DNA of murine leukemia virus. *Proc. Natl. Acad. Sci.* **72:**4910–4913.

Southern, E.M. 1975. Detection of specific sequences among DNA fragments separated by gel electrophoresis. *J. Mol. Biol.* **98:**503–517.

Spiegelman, S., A. Burny, M.R. Das, J. Keydar, J. Schlom, M. Travnicek, and K. Watson. 1970. Characterization of the products of RNA-directed polymerases in oncogenic RNA viruses. *Nature* **227:**563–567.

Srivastava, A. and M.J. Modak. 1979. Reverse transcriptase-associated RNase H. IV. Pyrophosphate does not inhibit RNase H activity of AMV DNA polymerase. *Biochem. Biophys. Res. Commun.* **91:**892–899.

Stacey, D.W. 1979. Messenger activity of virion RNA for avian leukosis viral envelope glycoprotein. *J. Virol.* **29:**949–956.

———. 1980. Expression of a subgenomic retroviral messenger RNA. *Cell* **21:**811–820.

Stacey, D.W. and H. Hanafusa. 1978. Nuclear conversion of microinjected avian leukosis virion RNA into an envelope-glycoprotein messenger. *Nature* **273:**779–782.

Stacey, D.W., V.G. Allfrey, and H. Hanafusa. 1977. Microinjection analysis of envelope-glycoprotein messenger activities of avian leukosis viral RNAs. *Proc. Natl. Acad. Sci.* **74:**614–1618.

Stalder, J., M. Groudine, J.B. Dodgson, J.D. Engel, and H. Weintraub. 1980. Hb switching in chickens. *Cell* **19:**973–980.

Stallcup, M.R., J.R. Ring, and K.R. Yamamoto. 1978. Synthesis of mouse mammary tumor virus ribonucleic acid in isolated nuclei from cultured mammary tumor cells. *Biochemistry* **17:**1515–1521.

Staskus, K.A., M.S. Collett, and A.J. Faras. 1976. Initiation of DNA synthesis by the avian oncornavirus RNA-directed DNA polymerase: Structural and functional localization of the major species of primer RNA on the oncornavirus genome. *Virology* **71:**162–168.

Stavnezer, E., G. Ringold, H.E. Varmus, and J.M. Bishop. 1976. RNA complementary to the genome of RNA tumor viruses in virions and virus-producing cells. *J. Virol.* **20:**342–347.

Steck, F.T. and H. Rubin. 1965. The mechanism of interference between an avian leukosis virus and Rous sarcoma virus. II. Early steps of infection by RSV of cells under conditions of interference. *Virology* **29:**642–653.

Steffen, D. and R.A. Weinberg. 1978. The integrated genome of murine leukemia virus. *Cell* **15**:1003–1010.

Steffen, D., S. Bird, W.P. Rowe, and R.A. Weinberg. 1979. Identification of DNA fragments carrying ecotropic proviruses of AKR mice. *Proc. Natl. Acad. Sci.* **76**:4554–4558.

Stehelin, D., R.V. Guntaka, H.E. Varmus, and J.M. Bishop. 1976. Purification of DNA complementary to nucleotide sequences required for neoplastic transformation of fibroblasts by avian sarcoma viruses. *J. Mol. Biol.* **101**:349–365.

Stohrer, R. and E. Hunter. 1979. Inhibition of Rous sarcoma virus replication by 2-deoxyglucose and tunicamycin: Identification of an unglycosylated *env* gene product. *J. Virol.* **32**:412–419.

Stoll, E., M.A. Billeter, A. Palmenberg, and C. Weissmann. 1977. Avian myeloblastosis virus RNA is terminally redundant: Implications for the mechanism of retrovirus replication. *Cell* **12**:57–72.

Stoltzfus, C.M. and L.K. Kuhnert. 1979. Evidence for the identity of shared 5′-terminal sequences between genome RNA and subgenomic mRNA's of B77 avian sarcoma virus. *J. Virol.* **32**:536–545.

Strand, M. and J.T. August. 1971. Protein kinase and phosphate acceptor proteins in Rauscher murine leukaemia virus. *Nat. New Biol.* **233**:137–140.

Strauchen, J.A., N.A. Young, and R.M. Friedman. 1977. Interferon-mediated inhibition of mouse mammary tumor virus expression in cultured cells. *Virology* **82**:232–236.

Strobel, E., P. Dunsmuir, and G.M. Rubin. 1979. Polymorphisms in the chromosomal locations of elements in the *412*, *copia*, and *297* dispersed repeated gene families in *Drosophila*. *Cell* **17**:429–439.

Studier, F.W. 1979. Relationships among different strains of T7 and among T7-related bacteriophages. *Virology* **95**:70–84.

Sutcliffe, J.G., T.M. Shinnick, I.M. Verma, and R.A. Lerner. 1980. Nucleotide sequence of Moloney leukemia virus: 3′ end reveals details of replication, analogy to bacterial transposons, and an unexpected gene. *Proc. Natl. Acad. Sci.* **77**:3302–3306.

Suzuki, S. and A.A. Axelrad. 1980. *Fv-2* locus controls the proportion of erythropoietic progenitor cells (BFU-E) synthesizing DNA in normal mice. *Cell* **19**:225–236.

Sveda, M.M. and R. Soeiro. 1976. Host restriction of Friend leukemia virus: Synthesis and integration of the provirus. *Proc. Natl. Acad. Sci.* **73**:2356–2366.

Sveda, M.M., B.N. Fields, and R. Soeiro. 1974. Host restriction of Friend leukemia virus: Fate of input virion RNA. *Cell* **2**:271–277.

———. 1976. Fate of input oncornavirion RNA—Biological studies. *J. Virol.* **18**:85–91.

Svoboda, J. and J. Dourmashkin. 1969. Rescue of Rous sarcoma virus from virogenic mammalian cells associated with chicken cells and treated with Sendai virus. *J. Gen. Virol.* **4**:523–529.

Svoboda, J., I. Hlozanek, and O. Mach. 1972. Detection of chicken sarcoma virus after transfection of chicken fibroblasts with DNA isolated from mammalian cells transformed with Rous virus. *Folia Biol.* **18**:149.

Svoboda, J., I. Hlozanek, O. Mach, A. Michlova, J. Riman, and M. Urbankova. 1973. Transfection of chicken fibroblasts with single exposure to DNA from virogenic mammalian cells. *J. Gen. Virol.* **21**:47–55.

Swanstrom, R., H.E. Varmus, and J.M. Bishop. 1981a. The terminal redundancy of the retrovirus genome facilitates chain elongation by reverse transcriptase. *J. Biol. Chem.* **256**:1115–1121.

Swanstrom, R., W.J. DeLorbe, J.M. Bishop, and H.E. Varmus. 1981b. Nucleotide sequence of cloned unintegrated avian sarcoma virus DNA: Viral DNA contains direct and inverted repeats similar to those in transposable elements. *Proc. Natl. Acad. Sci.* **78**:124–128.

Takano, T. and M. Hatanaka. 1975. Fate of viral RNA of murine leukemia virus after infection. *Proc. Natl. Acad. Sci.* **72**:343–347.

Taylor, J.M. 1977. An analysis of the role of tRNA species as primers for the transcription into DNA of RNA tumor virus genomes. *Biochim. Biophys. Acta* **473:**57–71.

———. 1979. DNA intermediates of avian RNA tumor viruses. *Curr. Top. Microbiol. Immunol.* **87:**23–41.

Taylor, J.M. and T.W. Hsu. 1980. Reverse transcription of avian sarcoma virus RNA into DNA might involve copying of the tRNA primer. *J. Virol.* **33:**531–534.

Taylor, J.M. and R. Illmensee. 1975. Site on the RNA of an avian sarcoma virus at which primer is bound. *J. Virol.* **16:**553–558.

Taylor, J.M., T.W. Hsu, and M.M.C. Lai. 1978. Restriction enzyme sites on the avian RNA tumor virus genome. *J. Virol.* **26:**479–484.

Taylor, J.M., R. Illmensee, and J. Summers. 1976a. Efficient transcription of RNA into DNA by avian sarcoma virus polymerase. *Biochim. Biophys. Acta* **442:**324–330.

Taylor, J.M. R. Illmensee, L.R. Trusal, and J. Summers. 1976b. Transcription of avian sarcoma virus RNA. *In Animal virology* (ed. D. Baltimore et al.), vol. IV, p. 161–173. Academic Press, New York.

Taylor, J.M., B. Cordell-Stewart, W. Rohde, H.M. Goodman, and J.M. Bishop. 1975. Reassociation of 4 S and 5 S RNA's with the genome of avian sarcoma virus. *Virology* **65:**248–259.

Taylor, J.M., A.J. Faras, H.E. Varmus, W.E. Levinson, and J.M. Bishop. 1972. Ribonucleic acid directed deoxyribonucleic acid synthesis by the purified deoxyribonucleic acid polymerase of Rous sarcoma virus. Characterization of the enzymatic product. *Biochemistry* **11:**2343–2351.

Teich, N.M., R.A. Weiss, G.R. Martin, and D.R. Lowy. 1977. Virus infection of murine teratocarcinoma stem cell lines. *Cell* **12:**973–982.

Temin, H.M. 1961. Mixed infection with two types of Rous sarcoma virus. *Virology* **13:**158–163.

———.1963. The effects of actinomycin D on growth of Rous sarcoma virus *in vitro*. *Virology* **20:**577–582.

———. 1964. Nature of the provirus of Rous sarcoma. *Natl. Cancer. Inst. Monogr.* **17:**557–570.

———. 1965. The mechanism of carcinogenesis by avian sarcoma viruses. I. Cell multiplication and differentiation. *J. Natl. Cancer Inst.* **35:**679–693.

———. 1967. Studies on carcinogenesis by avian sarcoma virus. V. Requirement for new DNA synthesis and for cell division. *J. Cell. Physiol.* **69:**53–64.

———. 1968. Carcinogenesis by avian sarcoma viruses. *Cancer Res.* **28:**1835–1838.

———. 1970. Formation and activation of the provirus of RNA sarcoma virus. In *The biology of large RNA viruses* (ed. R.D. Barry and B.W. Mahy), pp. 233–249. Academic Press, London.

———. 1971. Mechanism of cell transformation by RNA tumor viruses. *Annu. Rev. Microbiol.* **25:**609–649.

———. 1974. The cellular and molecular biology of RNA tumor viruses, especially avian leukosis-sarcoma viruses and their relatives. *Adv. Cancer Res.* **19:**47–104.

———. 1976. The DNA provirus hypothesis: The establishment and implications of RNA-directed DNA synthesis. *Science* **192:**1075–1080.

Temin, H.M. and D. Baltimore. 1972. RNA-directed DNA synthesis and RNA tumor viruses. *Adv. Virus Res.* **17:**129–186.

Temin, H.M. and S. Mizutani. 1970. RNA-directed DNA polymerase in virions of Rous sarcoma virus. *Nature* **226:**1211–1213.

Todaro, G.J., R.E. Benveniste, R. Callahan, M.M. Lieber, and C.J. Sherr. 1975. Endogenous primate and feline type C viruses. *Cold Spring Harbor Symp. Quant. Biol.* **39:**1159–1168.

Tooze, J., ed. 1980. *Molecular biology of tumor viruses,* 2nd ed. *DNA Tumor Viruses.* Cold Spring Harbor Laboratory, Cold Spring Harbor, New York.

Trainor, C.D. and M.S. Reitz, Jr. 1979. Loss of proviral DNA sequences in a revertant of Kirsten sarcoma virus-transformed murine fibroblasts. *J. Gen. Virol.* **44:**245–249.

Travaglini, E.C., D.K. Dube, S. Surrey, and L.A. Loeb. 1976. Template recognition and chain elongation in DNA synthesis *in vitro*. *J. Mol. Biol.* **106:**605–621.

Tress, E., P.V. O'Donnell, N. Famulari, R.W. Ellis, and E. Fleissner. 1979. Polymorphism of B-tropic leukemia viruses from BALB/c mice: Association of a p30 antigen with N-versus B-tropism. *J. Virol.* **32:**350–355.

Tronick, S.R., E.M. Scolnick, and W.P. Parks. 1972. Reversible inactivation of the deoxyribonucleic acid polymerase of Rauscher leukemia virus. *J. Virol.* **10:**885–888.

Tronick, S.R., J.R. Stephenson, I.M. Verma, and S.A. Aaronson. 1975. Thermolabile reverse transcriptase of a mammalian leukemia virus mutant temperature sensitive in its replication and sarcoma virus helper functions. *J. Virol.* **16:**1476–1482.

Tronick, S.R., K.C. Robbins, E. Canaani, S.G. Devare, P.R. Anderson, and S.A. Aaronson. 1979. Molecular cloning of Moloney murine sarcoma virus: Arrangement of virus-related sequences within the normal mouse genome. *Proc. Natl. Acad. Sci.* **76:**6314–6318.

Tsichlis, P.N. and J.M. Coffin. 1980. Recombinants between endogenous and exogenous avian tumor viruses: Role of the C region and other portions of the genome in the control of replication and transformation. *J. Virol.* **33:**238–249.

Tsipis, J.E. and M.A. Bratt. 1976. Isolation and preliminary characterization of temperature sensitive mutants of Newcastle disease virus. *J. Virol.* **18:**848–855.

Tsuchida, N. and M. Green. 1974. Intracellular and virion 35 S RNA species of murine sarcoma and leukemia viruses. *Virology* **59:**258–265.

Tsuruo, T. and M.A. Baluda. 1977. Integration of proviral DNA in chicken cells infected with Schmidt-Ruppin Rous sarcoma virus is not enhanced by DNA repair. *J. Virol.* **23:**533–542.

Turek, L.P. and H. Oppermann. 1980. Spontaneous conversion of nontransformed avian sarcoma virus-infected rat cells to the transformed phenotype. *J. Virol.* **35:**466–478.

Vaidya, A.B., E.Y. Lasfargues, G. Heubel, J.C. Lasfargues, and D.H. Moore. 1976. Murine mammary tumor virus: Characterization of infection of nonmurine cells. *J. Virol.* **18:**911–917.

Valenzuela, P., R.M. Morris, A. Faras, W. Levinson, and W.J. Rutter. 1973. Are all nucleotidyl transferases metalloenzymes? *Biochem. Biophys. Res. Commun.* **53:**1036–1041.

Van Beveren, C. and M. Goulian. 1979. Optimal conditions for synthesis of long complementary DNA product with Moloney murine leukemia virus. *J. Virol.* **30:**951–954.

Van Beveren, C., J.G. Goddard, A. Berns, and I.M. Verma. 1980. Structure of Moloney murine leukemia viral DNA: Nucleotide sequence of the 5′ long terminal repeat and adjacent cellular sequence. *Proc. Natl. Acad. Sci.* **77:**3307–3311.

Van der Putten, H., E. Terwindt, A. Berns, and R. Jaenisch. 1979. The integration sites of endogenous and exogenous Moloney murine leukemia virus. *Cell* **18:**109–118.

Vande Woude, G.F., M. Oskarsson, L.W. Enquist, S. Nomura, M. Sullivan, and P.J. Fischinger. 1979. Cloning of integrated Moloney sarcoma proviral DNA sequences in bacteriophage λ. *Proc. Natl. Acad. Sci.* **76:**4464–4468.

Vande Woude, G.F., M. Oskarsson, W.L. McClements, L.W. Enquist, D.G. Blair, P.J. Fischinger, J. Maizel, and M. Sullivan. 1980. Characterization of integrated Moloney sarcoma provirus and flanking host sequences cloned in bacteriophage λ. *Cold Spring Harbor Symp. Quant. Biol.* **44:**735–748.

van Zaane, D., A.L.J. Gielkens, W.G. Hesselink, and H.P.J. Bloemers. 1977. Identification of Rauscher murine leukemia virus-specific mRNAs for synthesis of *gag*-and *env*-gene products. *Proc. Natl. Acad. Sci.* **74:**1855–1859.

Varmus, H.E. and P.R. Shank. 1976. Unintegrated viral DNA is synthesized in the cytoplasm of avian sarcoma virus-transformed duck cells by viral DNA polymerase. *J. Virol.* **18:**567–573.

Varmus, H.E. J.M. Bishop, and P.K. Vogt. 1973a. Appearance of virus-specific DNA in mammalian cells following transformation by Rous sarcoma virus. *J. Mol. Biol.* **74:**613–626.

Varmus, H.E., W.E. Levinson, and J.M. Bishop. 1971. Extent of transcription by the RNA-dependent DNA polymerase of Rous sarcoma virus. *Nat. New Biol.* **233:**19–21.

Varmus, H.E., N. Quintrell, and S. Oritz. 1981a. Retroviruses as mutagens: Insertion and excision of a nontransforming provirus alter expression of a resident transforming provirus. *Cell* **25:**23–36

Varmus, H.E., N. Quintrell, and J. Wyke. 1981b. Revertants of an ASV-transformed rat cell line have lost the complete provirus or sustained mutations in *src. Virology* **108:**28–46.

Varmus, H.E., G. Ringold, and K.R. Yamamoto. 1979a. Regulation of mouse mammary tumor virus gene expression by glucocorticoid hormones. In *Glucocorticoid hormone action* (ed. J. Baxter and G. Rousseau), pp. 253–278. Springer-Verlag, Berlin.

Varmus, H.E., P.K. Vogt, and J.M. Bishop. 1973b. Integration of deoxyribonucleic acid specific for Rous sarcoma virus after infection of permissive and nonpermissive hosts. *Proc. Natl. Acad. Sci.* **70:**3067–3071.

Varmus, H.E., R.V. Guntaka, C.T. Deng, and J.M. Bishop. 1975. Synthesis, structure, and function of avian sarcoma virus-specific DNA in permissive and nonpermissive cells. *Cold Spring Harbor Symp. Quant. Biol.* **39:**987–996.

Varmus, H.E., S. Heasley, J. Linn, and K. Wheeler. 1976. Use of alkaline sucrose gradients in a zonal rotor to detect integrated and unintegrated avian sarcoma virus-specific DNA in cells. *J. Virol.* **18:**574–585.

Varmus, H.E., R.V. Guntaka, W.J.W. Fan, S. Heasley, and J.M. Bishop. 1974. Synthesis of viral DNA in the cytoplasm of duck embryo fibroblasts and in enucleated cells after infection by avian sarcoma virus. *Proc. Natl. Acad. Sci.* **71:**3874–3878.

Varmus, H.E., T. Padgett, S. Heasley, G. Simon, and J.M. Bishop. 1977. Cellular functions are required for the synthesis and integration of avian sarcoma virus-specific DNA. *Cell* **11:**307–319.

Varmus, H.E., S. Heasley, H.-J. Kung, H. Oppermann, V.C. Smith, J.M. Bishop, and P.R. Shank. 1978. Kinetics of synthesis, structure and purification of avian sarcoma virus-specific DNA made in the cytoplasm of acutely infected cells. *J. Mol. Biol.* **120:**55–82.

Varmus, H.E., P.R. Shank, S.E. Hughes, H.-J. Kung, S. Heasley, J. Majors, P.K. Vogt, and J.M. Bishop. 1979b. Synthesis, structure, and integration of the DNA of RNA tumor viruses. *Cold Spring Harbor Symp. Quant. Biol.* **43:**851–864.

Verma, I.M. 1975a. Studies on reverse transcriptase of RNA tumor viruses. III. Properties of purified Moloney murine leukemia virus DNA polymerase and associated RNase H. *J. Virol.* **15:**843–854.

———. 1975b. Studies on reverse transcriptase of RNA tumor viruses. I. Localization of thermolabile DNA polymerase and RNase H activities on one polypeptide. *J. Virol.* **15:**121–126.

———. 1977. The reverse transcriptase. *Biochim. Biophys. Acta* **473:**1–38.

———. 1978. Genome organization of RNA tumor viruses. I. In vitro synthesis of full-genome-length single-stranded and double-stranded viral DNA transcripts. *J. Virol.* **26:**615–629.

———. 1979. Genome organization of retroviruses. III. Restriction endonuclease cleavage maps of mouse sarcoma virus double-stranded DNA synthesized in vitro. *Nucleic Acids Res.* **6:**1863–1867.

Verma, I.M. and M.A. McKennett. 1978. Genome organization of RNA tumor viruses. II. Physical maps of in vitro-synthesized Moloney leukemia virus double-stranded DNA by restriction endonucleases. *J. Virol.* **26:**630–645.

Verma, I.M., N.L. Meuth, and D. Baltimore. 1972a. Covalent linkage between ribonucleic acid primer and deoxyribonucleic acid product of the avian myeloblastosis virus deoxyribonucleic acid polymerase. *J. Virol.* **10:**622–627.

Verma, I.M., H.E. Varmus, and E. Hunter. 1976. Characterization of "early" temperature-sensitive mutants of avian sarcoma viruses: Biological properties, thermolability of reverse transcriptase *in vitro,* and synthesis of viral DNA in infected cells. *Virology* **74:**16–29.

Verma, I.M., W.S. Mason, S.D. Drost, and D. Baltimore. 1974a. DNA polymerase activity from two temperature-sensitive mutants of Rous sarcoma virus is thermolabile. *Nature* **251:**27–31.

Verma, I.M., N.L. Meuth, H. Fan, and D. Baltimore. 1974b. Hamster leukemia virus: Lack of endogenous DNA synthesis and unique structure of its DNA polymerase. *J. Virol.* **13:**1075–1082.

Verma, I.M., G.F. Temple, H. Fan, and D. Baltimore. 1972b. *In vitro* synthesis of DNA complementary to rabbit reticulocyte 10S RNA. *Nat. New Biol.* **235:**163–167.

Verma, I.M., N.L. Meuth, E. Bromfeld, K.F. Manly, and D. Baltimore. 1971. Covalently linked RNA-DNA molecule as initial product of the RNA tumour virus DNA polymerase. *Nat. New Biol.* **233:**131–134.

Verma, I.M., M.-H.T. Lai, R.A. Bosselman, M.A. McKennett, H. Fan, and A. Berns. 1980. Molecular cloning of unintegrated Moloney mouse sarcoma virus DNA in bacteriophage λ. *Proc. Natl. Acad. Sci.* **77:**1773–1777.

Vogt, V.M. and R. Eisenman. 1973. Identification of a large polypeptide precursor of avian oncornavirus proteins. *Proc. Natl. Acad. Sci.* **70:**1734–1738.

Vogt, V.M., R. Eisenman, and H. Diggelmann. 1975. Generation of avian myeloblastosis virus structural proteins by proteolytic cleavage of a precursor polypeptide. *J. Mol. Biol.* **96:**471–493.

Vogt, V.M., W. Wight, and R. Eisenman. 1979. *In vitro* cleavage of avian retrovirus *gag* proteins by viral protease p15. *Virology* **98:**154–167.

Von der Helm, K. 1977. Cleavage of Rous sarcoma viral polyprotein precursor into internal structural proteins *in vitro* by viral protein p15. *Proc. Natl. Acad. Sci.* **74:**911–915.

Von der Helm, K. and P.H. Duesberg. 1975. Translation of Rous sarcoma virus RNA in cell-free systems from ascites Krebs II cells. *Proc. Natl. Acad. Sci.* **72:**614–618.

Wang, L.-H. and P.H. Duesberg. 1973. DNA polymerase of murine sarcoma-leukemia virus: Lack of detectable RNase H and low activity with viral RNA and natural DNA templates. *J. Virol.* **12:**1512–1521.

Wang, L.-H., P.H. Duesberg, T. Robins, H. Yokota, and P.K. Vogt. 1977. The terminal oligonucleotides of avian tumor virus RNAs are genetically linked. *Virology* **82:**472–492.

Waters, L.C., B.C. Mullin, E.G. Bailiff, and R.A. Popp. 1975a. tRNA's associated with the 70S RNA of avian myeloblastosis virus. *J. Virol.* **16:**1608–1614.

Waters, L.C., B.C. Mullin, T. Ho, and W.-K. Yang. 1975b. Ability of tryptophan tRNA to hybridize with 35S RNA of avian myeloblastosis virus and to prime reverse transcription *in vitro. Proc. Natl. Acad. Sci.* **72:**2155.

Watson, K.F., P.L. Schendel, M.J. Rosok, and L.R. Ramsey. 1979. Model RNA-directed DNA synthesis by avian myeloblastosis virus DNA polymerase and its associated RNase H. *Biochemistry* **18:**3210–3219.

Weinberg, R.A. 1977. Structure of the intermediates leading to the integrated provirus. *Biochim. Biophys. Acta* **473:**39–55.

———. 1980. Integrated genomes of animal viruses. *Annu. Rev. Biochem.* **49:**197–226.

Weiss, R.A. 1971. Cell transformation induced by Rous sarcoma virus: Analysis of density dependence. *Virology* **46:**209–220.

Weiss, S.R., H.E. Varmus, and J.M. Bishop. 1977. The size and genetic composition of virus-specific RNAs in the cytoplasm of cells producing avian sarcoma-leukemia viruses. *Cell* **12:**983–992.

———. 1981. Cell-free translation of purified avian sarcoma virus *src* mRNA. *J. Virol.* **110:**476–478.

Weiss, S.R., P.B. Hackett, H. Oppermann, A. Ullrich, L. Levintow, and J.M. Bishop. 1978. Cell-free translation of avian sarcoma virus RNA: Suppression of the *gag* termination codon does not augment synthesis of the joint *gag/pol* product. *Cell* **15:**607–614.

Weissmann, C., M.A. Billeter, H.M. Goodman, J. Hindley, and H. Weber. 1973. Structure and function of phage RNA. *Annu. Rev. Biochem.* **42:**303–328.

Weller, S.K., A.E. Joy, and H.M. Temin. 1980. Correlation between cell killing and massive second-round superinfection by members of some subgroups of avian leukosis virus. *J. Virol.* **33:**494–506.

Wells, R.D., R.M. Flugel, J.E. Larson, P.F. Schendel, and R.W. Sweet. 1972. Comparison of some reactions catalyzed by deoxyribonucleic acid polymerase from avian myeloblastosis virus, *Escherichia coli,* and *Micrococcus luteus. Biochemistry* **11:**621–629.

Weymouth, L.A. and L.A. Loeb. 1978. Mutagenesis during *in vitro* DNA synthesis. *Proc. Natl. Acad. Sci.* **75:**1924–1928.

Willingham, M.C., G. Jay, and I. Pastan. 1979. Localization of the ASV *src* gene product to the plasma membrane of transformed cells by electron microscopic immunocytochemistry. *Cell* **18:**125–134.

Wist, E. and H. Prydz. 1979. The effect of aphidicolin on DNA synthesis in isolated HeLa cell nuclei. *Nucleic Acids Res.* **6:**1583–1590.

Witte, O.N. and D. Baltimore. 1978. Relationship of retrovirus polyprotein cleavages to virion maturation studied with temperature-sensitive murine leukemia virus mutants. *J. Virol.* **26:**750–761.

Yamamoto, T., B. de Crombrugghe, and I. Pastan. 1980a. Identification of a functional promoter in the long terminal repeat of Rous sarcoma virus. *Cell* **22:**787–797.

Yamamoto, T., G. Jay, and I. Pastan. 1980b. Unusual features in the nucleotide sequence of a cDNA clone derived from the common region of avian sarcoma virus messenger RNA. *Proc. Natl. Acad. Sci.* **77:**176–180.

Yang, W.K., D.M. Yang, and J.O. Kiggans, Jr. 1980a. Covalently closed circular DNAs of murine type C retroviruses: Depressed formation in cells treated with cycloheximide early after infection. *J. Virol.* **36:**181–188.

Yang, W.K., J.O. Kiggans, D.-M. Yang, C.-Y. Ou, R.W. Tennant, A. Brown, and R.H. Bassin. 1980b. Synthesis and circularization of N- and B-tropic retroviral DNA in *Fv-1* permissive and restrictive mouse cells. *Proc. Natl. Acad. Sci.* **77:**2994–2998.

Yang, Y.H.J., J.S. Rhim, S. Rasheed, V. Klement, and P. Roy-Burman. 1979. Reversion of Kirsten sarcoma virus transformed human cells: Elimination of the sarcoma virus nucleotide sequences. *J. Gen. Virol.* **43:**447–451.

Yaniv, A., T. Ohno, D. Kacian, D. Colcher, S. Witkin, J. Schlom, and S. Spiegelman. 1974. Serological analysis of reverse transcriptase of the Mason-Pfizer monkey virus. *Virology* **59:**335–338.

Yoshida, M. and K. Toyoshima. 1980. *In vitro* translation of avian erythroblastosis virus RNA: Identification of two major polypeptides. *Virology* **100:**484–487.

Yoshikura, H. 1970a. Radiological studies on the chronological relation between murine sarcoma virus infection and cell cycle. *J. Gen. Virol.* **8:**113–120.

———. 1970b. Dependence of murine sarcoma virus infection on the cell cycle. *J. Gen. Virol.* **6:**183–185.

Yoshikura, H., Y. Naito, and K. Moriwaki. 1979. Unstable resistance of G mouse fibroblasts to ecotropic murine leukemia virus infection. *J. Virol.* **29:**1078–1086.

Yoshimura, F.K. and R.A. Weinberg. 1979. Restriction endonuclease cleavage of linear and closed circular murine leukemia viral DNAs: Discovery of a smaller circular form. *Cell* **16:**323–332.

Young, H.A., T.Y. Shih, E.M. Scolnick, and W.P. Parks. 1977. Steroid induction of mouse mammary tumor virus: Effect upon synthesis and degradation of viral RNA. *J. Virol.* **21:**139–146.

Youvan, D.C. and J.E. Hearst. 1979. Reverse transcriptase pauses at N^2-methylguanine during *in vitro* transcription of *Escherichia coli* 16S ribosomal RNA. *Proc. Natl. Acad. Sci.* **76:**3751–3754.

Zamecnik, P.C. and M.L. Stephenson. 1978. Inhibition of Rous sarcoma virus replication and cell transformation by a specific oligodeoxynucleotide. *Proc. Natl. Acad. Sci.* **75:**280–284.

Ziff, E.B. and R.M. Evans. 1978. Coincidence of the promoter and capped 5′ terminus of RNA from the adenovirus 2 major late transcription unit. *Cell* **15:**1463–1475.

6

Protein Biosynthesis and Assembly

I. INTRODUCTION

To understand the transmission of viruses, a knowledge of the events that enable the viral genome to replicate, produce structural components, and become packaged into virions is required. The organization of retroviral genomes and the mechanisms involved in their replication are discussed in the preceding two chapters. Here, we describe how the genome-encoded instructions are processed by the cell to allow the accumulation of virus-specific products and how these products become associated to produce new viral particles.

Before proceeding to a discussion of the biosynthesis of retroviral proteins, we will compare retroviruses with other virus groups in a general way and discuss techniques used to study the mature viral proteins and their precursors. Following this, the characteristics shared among the different retrovirus subfamilies will be summarized. Finally, the composition and structures of virion components and the mechanisms involved in generating mature virions will be described separately and in considerable detail for some of the major retrovirus groups.

A. Comparative Strategies for Viral Protein Synthesis

Viruses use a variety of stratagems to process their genetic information into specialized enzyme activities or new structural components. This section contrasts the mechanisms used by several virus groups and compares them with those used by retroviruses.

An important feature of eukaryotic cells, relevant to the strategy of viral gene expression, is the apparent inability of eukaryotic translation systems to use more than one initiation site per mRNA molecule. Thus, unlike prokaryotic systems, eukaryotic cells synthesize only one type of polypeptide chain per mRNA species, and alternative initiation codons or polycistronic mRNA molecules are not observed. It has been proposed that this specificity is due to the ability of eukaryotic ribosomes to bind only to 5′-terminal regions of RNA molecules and subsequently to initiate synthesis at the first available AUG codon (Kozak 1978, 1980). Different groups of animal viruses use distinct strategies to direct the synthesis of more than one polypeptide chain by a single genome, including segmented genomes, synthesis of subgenomic mRNA molecules, and posttranslational cleavage of large polyprotein precursors. A second important feature of eukaryotic translation is the manner in which newly synthesized polypeptides are partitioned into intracellular proteins and cell-surface (or excreted) glycoproteins. In general, eukaryotic proteins destined for the cytoplasm are synthesized on free polysomes, whereas glycoproteins are synthesized as transmembrane proteins on polysomes associated with the rough endoplasmic reticulum. Initiation of the transmembrane processing appears to require a specific signal peptide, usually at the amino terminus of the nascent chain and composed of hydrophobic amino acids. Next, the signal peptide is cleaved from the nascent polypeptide; however, a second hydrophobic sequence (often present at the carboxyl terminus of the polypeptide) allows retention of the polypeptide in the membrane and its transport to the plasma membrane. The primary addition of sugar residues is coupled with this process of transmembrane synthesis. Thus, enveloped viruses (such as retroviruses) that mature by budding must have a fundamental difference in protein synthesis and virion assembly from those viruses that self-assemble in the cell cytoplasm and are then released by cell lysis. On the other hand, viruses that bud from the cell rely on host functions for the synthesis and transport of glycoproteins and must have appropriate signals to use these cellular systems. Some examples of the different strategies used by various groups of animal viruses follow.

Several groups of negative-strand RNA viruses (e.g., orthomyxoviruses and bunyaviruses) and all double-stranded RNA viruses (e.g., rotaviruses) have genomes consisting of up to ten discrete and unique segments of RNA. Although the overall mechanism of replication varies, each segment of RNA directs the synthesis of an mRNA species for a different viral structural protein or enzyme. Thus, each segment of RNA is a distinct gene, and there are about as many protein products as segments of the genome; relatively few additional proteins are generated by RNA processing or cleavage of polyproteins. This strategy has four effects: (1) It provides a relatively simple mechanism for separating the syntheses of internal and surface proteins. (2) It permits regulation of the relative amounts of the various proteins synthesized, for example, by varying the affinity of the various mRNA molecules for ribosomes. (3) It provides a mechanism for genetic interaction between related viruses by reassortment of subunits in progeny virions. (4) It presumably must invoke some mechanisms to ensure that a reasonable proportion of the progeny virions receive a full complement of segments.

A totally different mechanism involves the use of subgenomic-size mRNA molecules to encode viral proteins. DNA-containing viruses generally use cellular systems, at least in part, for the synthesis and processing of distinct mRNA species for different proteins. As with the segmented RNA viruses, this strategy permits regulation of the relative amount of synthesis of the various proteins and the timing of such synthesis, in this case by regulating the relative rates of synthesis of the various mRNA molecules as well as their individual translational efficiencies. Furthermore, many DNA viruses take advantage of the cellular RNA-splicing systems to synthesize different mRNA species that contain regions in common by varying the splice points in a common precursor. In this way, for example, the late mRNAs of adenovirus, which encode completely different proteins, are synthesized from a single promoter, contain common 5′ untranslated sequences, and can be coordinately regulated. Similarly, variations in splicing points within the early region of papovaviral DNA lead to mRNAs encoding proteins that share a common amino acid sequence at the amino terminus and yet differ at the carboxyl terminus.

With the exception of retroviruses, the cellular mRNA synthetic machinery is not used by RNA viruses. However, several groups of negative-strand RNA viruses, such as rhabdoviruses and paramyxoviruses, produce subgenomic mRNA species for the synthesis of distinct proteins, but these are copied from the genomic RNA by a virion enzyme immediately after infection. Because the mRNA synthesis is sequential from one end of the genome and splicing does not occur, there is less opportunity for regulation and repeated use of the same region of the genome than with DNA viruses. A different sort of subgenomic mRNA synthesis occurs with the togaviruses, which have a positive-sense RNA genome containing two coding regions; the 5′ region encodes proteins necessary for RNA replication and is translated early after infection, whereas the 3′ portion of the genome encodes capsid proteins and is not translated from the infecting genome, apparently because the internal initiation site cannot be used. Late in infection, a subgenomic-size positive-strand RNA species is synthesized in large amounts. This RNA then serves as messenger for the capsid proteins. Thus, in a fairly simple way, regulation of both the relative amounts and the time of appearance of various virus-encoded polypeptides is achieved.

Synthesis of viral structural proteins via a polyprotein precursor is another regulatory mechanism. The most extreme case is found in picornaviruses, in which the positive-sense genome is an mRNA with a single initiation site encoding a single large polyprotein. This polyprotein is cleaved by proteases, possibly one of cellular origin and some derived from the polyprotein itself, to generate at least eight final products, including both capsid and RNA-polymerase (replicase) components. Such a strategy allows the coordinated synthesis of proteins (such as capsid proteins) that are used in equimolar amounts, and cleavage can be coordinated with maturation to simplify the process of assembly. But, by the same token, what would appear to be highly excessive amounts of other proteins, like the replicase, must also be synthesized. Furthermore, temporal control of protein synthesis is not readily achieved.

The togaviruses exhibit two interesting variations in polyprotein strategy. The first is the use of a subgenomic mRNA for the capsid polyprotein discussed above. The second is the synthesis of both the core-shell protein and two surface glycoproteins from the same mRNA species. The problem of requiring both free and membrane-bound polysomes is overcome by sequential synthesis. The amino terminus of the structural polyprotein contains the capsid protein and is synthesized on free polysomes. Afterward, the nascent polypeptide is cleaved, releasing the capsid protein and exposing a signal peptide. The free polysomes can now associate with membranes, and the presence of the signal peptide allows synthesis to continue in a transmembrane fashion to produce the viral glycoproteins (Rothman and Lenard 1977).

Retroviruses display characteristics in the synthesis and control of viral proteins in common with both the RNA and DNA viruses. This is perhaps not surprising, as retroviruses contain a positive-sense single-stranded RNA genome, but they synthesize their gene products from a double-stranded DNA provirus integrated within the chromosomal DNA of the host cell. Retroviral protein synthesis involves the production of polyprotein precursors similar to those of the picornaviruses and togaviruses. As the genomic RNA is positive-sense, it can also be used to synthesize viral products in cell-free protein-synthesizing systems. Retroviruses synthesize all the products of the internal core structure as a polyprotein precursor. This allows all the components of a complex structure to achieve a three-dimensional configuration that facilitates assembly, and the precursors are subsequently cleaved with proteases to activate their specialized functions. As with DNA viruses, however, there is alternative use of splicing positions in the genome to generate different mRNA species. As maturation of retroviruses is accomplished by budding from the host-cell membrane, they are required to synthesize specific glycoproteins. Thus, the glycoproteins are also synthesized as a precursor polyprotein, but a separate spliced mRNA is produced to allow the independent synthesis of this precursor as a transmembrane protein. One interesting feature of the retrovirus group is that virus replication occurs without a concomitant inhibition of host-cell protein synthesis. In this sense, retroviruses are well-adapted parasites and utilize several of the host-cell functions (DNA-dependent RNA polymerase, RNA splicing and processing mechanisms, and the host-cell protein-synthesizing apparatus) without placing undue stress on the host-cell functions. For the investigator, however, the continuation of host-cell protein synthesis has made the study of retroviral protein synthesis more difficult.

B. Approaches to Analyzing Retroviral Protein Synthesis and Processing

Retroviral protein synthesis accounts for only about 0.5–2% of the total cellular protein production, on the same order as viral RNA synthesis. Thus, the analysis of viral protein biosynthesis necessitates the use of specific reagents to detect and isolate viral polypeptides from a profusion of host-cell proteins. Almost invariably, the most useful reagents have been antibodies prepared against disrupted viral particles or purified virion proteins or antibodies raised in animals bearing retrovirus-induced tumors.

For studies of viral protein biosynthesis, the most powerful use of such antisera has been in immunoprecipitation techniques. In this type of experiment, radioactively labeled extracts of infected cells are treated first with specific antiserum and then with either an immunoadsorbent (such as the *Staphylococcus aureus* protein A) or a second antibody directed against the first immunoglobulin. The resulting immunoprecipitate is then fractioned by SDS-polyacrylamide gel electrophoresis, which, generally speaking, separates proteins on the basis of molecular weight. After extraction from the gel, polypeptides identified in this manner can be further analyzed by peptide mapping or amino acid sequencing. When combined with different radioactive-labeling protocols and cell-fractionation procedures, the immunoprecipitation methodology has proved to be an important tool in the elucidation of virus polypeptide metabolism (see below) (for review, see Eisenman and Vogt 1978).

Cell-free translation in vitro of both virion and intracellular virus-specific RNAs has also been effectively used for identification and analysis of retroviral polypeptides. A related method is hybrid-selected translation (Ricciardi et al. 1979), which employs molecularly cloned DNA to select complementary mRNAs by hybridization, and the selected mRNAs are then released and translated in vitro. Although not yet widely used in the retrovirus system, this method may provide a means of analyzing nonstructural virus-coded proteins and *gag-onc* fusion proteins (see Chapter 9). Another recently introduced method with great promise involves electrophoretic transfer of total cellular proteins from a polyacrylamide gel to chemically activated nitrocellulose paper ("Western" blots). Virus-specific proteins are then detected by using antibody and a radioiodinated immunoadsorbent (Towbin et al. 1979). This technique is likely to prove valuable for detecting viral proteins in tissues that are difficult to grow and label in vitro.

C. Composition of Virions

A prerequisite to understanding the synthesis of the virus-specific proteins and their assembly into virions is the delineation of the number and types of structural components. Retroviruses can be concentrated and purified from the supernatant fluids of infected-cell cultures by standard virological procedures, such as velocity and equilibrium gradient centrifugation. Once separated from the culture fluids, the viral-particle preparations are suitable for a variety of analytical procedures. Virions can be disrupted with detergents, and the individual structural protein components can be separated on columns or by electrophoresis in polyacrylamide gels. Two successful column procedures involve gel filtration in the presence of the denaturing agent guanidine hydrochloride, which separates on the basis of size (Fleissner 1971; Nowinski et al. 1972), or chromatography on alkyl-agarose gels, which separates polypeptides according to their hydrophobicity (Marcus et al. 1979b). However, the most exploited procedure has been SDS-polyacrylamide gel electrophoresis, which separates polypeptides on the basis of molecular weight (Maizel et al. 1968; Laemmli 1970), although some proteins, and especially the glycoproteins, often run abnormally (Shapiro et al. 1967). The advantage of this technique is its simplicity, speed, and high resolving power.

The polypeptides separated by any of these techniques have, in the past, been given various names decided by the individual investigator. However, in 1974, a consensus was reached, and a standardized nomenclature was adopted (see August et al. 1974; Appendix A). The molecular weight in kilodaltons (10^{-3}) is prefixed by p, gp, or pp for protein, glycoprotein, and phosphoprotein, respectively (e.g., a glycoprotein with a molecular weight of 70,000 daltons would be called gp70). In a similar fashion, an identified precursor is prefixed by Pr and a polyprotein that is not known to be a precursor is designated by P. Some confusion is apparent in the literature because different electrophoresis procedures and column calibrations often result in estimates of molecular weights that may differ markedly for the same protein; however, to overcome this problem, many authors have accepted a certain molecular-weight estimate for a given protein irrespective of their own estimates (see Table 6.1).

Examination of purified virions by these techniques has led to the identification of five or six small nonglycosylated polypeptides, with molecular weights ranging from 10,000 to 30,000 daltons, and one or two larger glycoproteins. Also present in most virion preparations are a number of minor polypeptides that may be derived from cellular contaminants, as microsomes from disrupted cells band at the same density as virions. Alternatively, the proteins may be packaged, either specifically or fortuitously, during virion assembly; unfortunately, it is particularly difficult to distinguish among these possibilities. This problem also applies to the various enzymic activi-

Table 6.1 Protein composition of retroviruses based on polypeptide function

Property of proteins	Location in virion	Type of retrovirus: avian C type	murine C type	murine B type
Major hydrophobic	internal core; membrane-associated	pp19	p15	p10
Major phosphoprotein	between core and envelope; little on RNA	pp19	pp12	pp21
Most abundant; moderately hydrophobic	major structural component of core	p27	p30	p27
Highly basic	bound to RNA in core	p12	p10	p14
Reverse transcriptase	internal core	p92/p58	p70	p100
Hydrophobic (transmembrane)	envelope	gp37	p15(E)	gp36
Major glycoprotein	envelope	gp85	gp70	gp52
Protease	between core and envelope	p15	?	?

ties found associated with virion-particle preparations. These range from the ATPases, which are normally associated with plasma membranes, to enzymes involved in DNA processing, such as DNA ligases (de Thé et al. 1964; Temin and Baltimore 1972).

1. Subviral Structures

Retroviral particles can be partially disrupted, using controlled concentrations of nonionic detergents, to yield intact core structures (Coffin and Temin 1971; Davis and Rueckert 1972; Stromberg 1972; Teramoto et al. 1977). After separation by equilibrium density centrifugation, the subviral components can be analyzed by polyacrylamide gel electrophoresis and electron microscopy, which together allow an assignment of specific polypeptides to the different structural features of the virion. Other approaches have used techniques such as antibody neutralization, surface-labeling techniques, or protease treatment to define the surface components of the virion (Kennel et al. 1973; Witte et al. 1973; Hunsmann et al. 1974; Ikeda et al. 1974; Steeves et al. 1974; Rohrschneider et al. 1975; McLellan and August 1976). To complement these studies, the physical properties, and, eventually, the amino acid sequence of the purified virion proteins, can be determined directly (Oroszlan et al. 1975a) or indirectly by analysis of the nucleic acid sequence. The goals of such studies are to locate functional domains of the viral polypeptides and to construct a model for virion assembly and structure that is consistent with the biological and physical properties of the virus.

2. Isolation and Composition of Virion Cores

Mild detergent treatment of retroviruses releases core structures that band in equilibrium sucrose gradients at a density of approximately 1.24–1.26 g/ml, compared with intact virions that band at 1.16–1.18 g/ml (Coffin and Temin 1971; Davis and Rueckert 1972; Quigley et al. 1972; Bolognesi et al. 1973; Stromberg et al. 1974; Teramoto et al. 1977). The increase in density is due to the dissolution and release of the lipid-containing membrane components that remain on the top of the sucrose gradient. Identification of the cores relies primarily on negative-stain electron microscopy of the purified preparations and of the stages prior to centrifugation, in which particles are found in varying stages of disruption. Electron microscopic studies on virus and core structures using freeze-etching techniques (which are superior for preserving structural integrity) show that the murine C-type retroviral cores possess icosahedral symmetry (Nermut et al. 1972; Schafer and Bolognesi 1977). Polyacrylamide gel electrophoresis of the cores shows that they contain the most abundant nonglycosylated polypeptide found in virions (usually with a molecular weight of 24,000–30,000 daltons) and a smaller, but highly basic, polypeptide.

Further detergent treatment of the cores releases the genomic RNA associated with a highly basic polypeptide (Davis and Rueckert 1972; Bolognesi et al. 1973; Fleissner and Tress 1973) and reverse transcriptase. Internal to the virion envelope are two or three other small proteins, one of which is the major viral phosphoprotein. Some of these molecules in both murine C-type retrovirus (pp12) and avian C-type retrovirus (pp19) appear to bind specifically to the homologous virion RNA (Sen and Todaro 1977; Sen et al. 1978). However, most of the avian pp19 is located external to the core structure, is hydrophobic, and appears to exist in a multimeric form

(Montelaro et al. 1978). Thus, it is possible that a protein like pp19 may serve more than one function (see Section II.A.1.a). A very hydrophobic polypeptide is also present in murine C-type and B-type virions (Barbacid and Aaronson 1978; Cardiff et al. 1978; Marcus et al. 1978b). These hydrophobic polypeptides form the amino terminus of their respective polyprotein precursor and are believed to interact in precursor form with the internal cell membranes as a preliminary step in core assembly and budding (Bolognesi et al. 1978; Cardiff et al. 1978). Morphologically, the hydrophobic proteins may also contribute to the outer core (or inner envelope) membrane often seen in thin-section electron micrographs of budding retroviruses. The internal proteins of the virion that constitute this core structure and its outer membrane are derived from a single polyprotein precursor (discussed below), which is processed by proteases to yield the characteristic virion proteins.

3. Virion-associated RNA-dependent DNA Polymerase

The RNA-dependent DNA polymerase or reverse transcriptase of retroviruses is present in about 20–70 copies per virion, with at least one molecule presumably associated with each subunit of the virion RNA complex (Panet et al. 1975a; Krakower et al. 1977). The polymerase activity and the genomic RNA are found in close association within the core structures (Stromberg et al. 1974). The DNA polymerase is also responsible for the specific incorporation of the primer tRNA necessary for the initiation of DNA synthesis (see Chapters 4 and 5). In virions of the avian retroviruses, the majority of the DNA-polymerase activity exists as a bimolecular complex composed of the α and β subunits (Kacian et al. 1971). The $\alpha\beta$ complex is the active form of the DNA-polymerase activity and also exhibits an RNase-H activity thought to be necessary for the successful reverse transcription of the RNA genome into the double-stranded DNA form (for a complete explanation of the various enzymic activities, see Chapter 5). The murine and primate C-type retroviral polymerases occur as single polypeptide chains of about 70,000 daltons (Moelling 1974). Two sizes of polymerase molecules have been isolated from the murine mammary tumor virus (MMTV), a B-type retrovirus; however, the properties of these different molecular moieties are not yet sufficiently characterized to determine any functional significance (Dion et al. 1974b; Marcus et al. 1976).

4. The Virion Envelope

Equilibrium density centrifugation of detergent-treated virions yields the core structures as described above, but a low-density fraction remains on top of the density gradients. This fraction contains the virion lipids, glycoproteins, and often a low-molecular-weight hydrophobic polypeptide. These components are derived from the envelope of the virions (Bolognesi et al. 1972). The location of the glycoproteins to the envelope structure was convincingly confirmed by protease digestion of virions to yield "bald" particles, which by electron microscopy were shown to be virions with their lipid bilayer still intact but with all the surface proteins digested away (Rifkin and Compans 1971; Cardiff et al. 1974). Concomitant with the removal of the glycoproteins by protease digestion, there was loss of virus infectivity. In addition, antisera produced against the main glycoprotein neutralize the virus (Hunsmann et al. 1974; Rohrschneider et al. 1975); this is consistent with the exterior location of this glycoprotein and its role in host-range and interference phenomena (see Chapter 3). This major glycoprotein can also be radioactively labeled using techniques that specifically label the outer-surface proteins of the virion, such as lactoperoxidase or chloramine-T-catalyzed iodination (Kennel et al. 1973; Witte et al. 1973; Teramoto et al. 1974).

Although all retroviruses possess at least one major glycoprotein, some diversity exists in the composition of the virion envelope components (see Table 6.1). Avian C-type retroviruses and murine B-type retroviruses also possess a readily identified lower-molecular-weight glycoprotein that is more hydrophobic in nature (Marcus et al. 1978a). On the other hand, murine and primate C-type retroviruses carry a small hydrophobic nonglycosylated polypeptide instead. These smaller envelope proteins are believed to serve the same function, that of acting as anchors for the envelope components in the lipid bilayer.

D. Synthesis of the Virion Proteins

The synthesis of the proteins necessary for retrovirus replication is most easily considered as occurring in three groups that correspond to defined genetic regions. These regions are termed *gag*, which encodes the internal structural proteins of the virion; *pol*, which encodes the RNA-dependent DNA polymerase or reverse transcriptase enzyme; and *env*, which encodes the envelope components. The order of these genes for the replication-competent retroviruses that have been examined in detail is 5′-*gag-pol-env*-3′, and circumstantial evidence from many retrovirus systems would indicate that this order is invariant (see Chapter 4). Some retroviral genomes code for proteins that are not concerned with the replicative functions but determine the ability of these viruses to transform cells in vitro or induce neoplasia in vivo. Information encoding these additional genes appears to be derived by recombination of the viral genetic material with that of the host cell. The outcome of these recombinational events can be the acquisition of a new gene in addition to the replicative genes, as appears to have occurred in the replication-competent Rous sarcoma viruses (RSVs), or acquisition at the expense of the replicative genes, as appears to be the case for the murine sarcoma viruses (MSVs) and avian acute leukemia viruses. In the latter examples, the viruses are defective and unable to replicate without the aid of a replication-competent helper virus to supply the missing replicative functions. The insertion or substitution of new genetic material into the functional domains of virus replicative genes often leads to the synthesis of fusion proteins, which are composed, in part, of peptides encoded by sequences of viral origin generally, although not invariably, from *gag* and, in part, of peptides encoded by sequences derived from cellular genes. These fusion proteins can be detected with antiserum against the viral structural proteins, as they generally retain antigenic domains inherent in the viral protein sequence. In this chapter, the synthesis and processing of the replicative proteins only of competent retroviruses are discussed; the products and properties of the viruses that synthesize additional or fusion proteins are discussed in more detail in Chapter 9.

1. Synthesis of the gag*-gene Products*

All retroviruses synthesize their major internal structural proteins as a polyprotein precursor of about 70,000 to 80,000 daltons (see Fig. 6.1); for example, the avian C-type retroviruses synthesize a 76,000-dalton *gag* precursor ($Pr76^{gag}$). After synthesis, the *gag*-gene precursor polyproteins are often phosphorylated and usually associated with cell membranes, two processes that are probably part of the maturation pathway, although the molecular significance of these events is unknown. The *gag* precursor is further processed by proteases that cleave the molecule to yield the characteristic internal

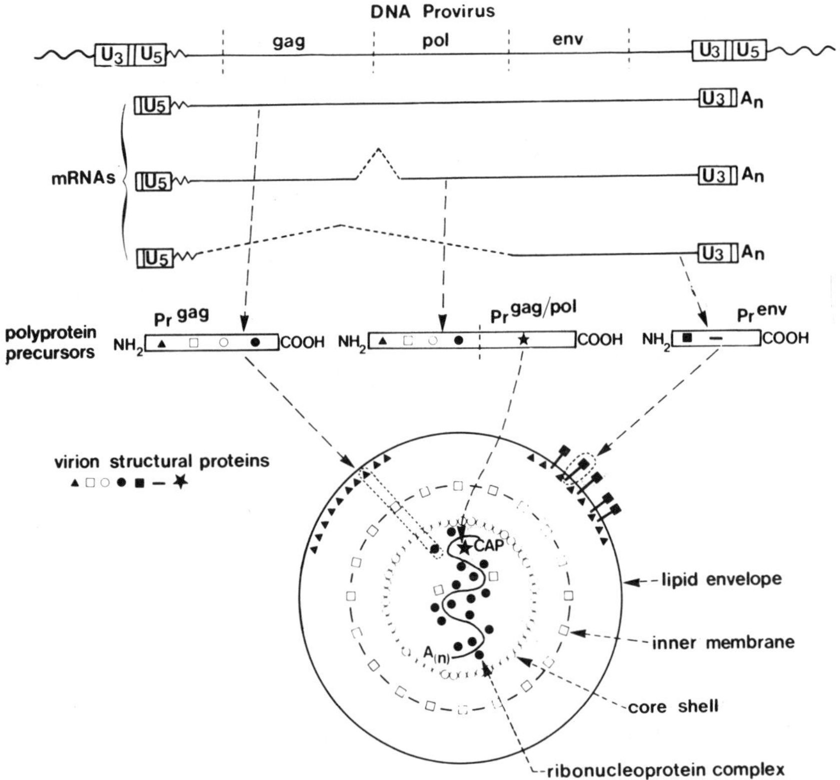

Figure 6.1 Schematic representation of retroviral protein biosynthesis from an integrated provirus. The mRNA molecules for the three structural genes are indicated, showing the leader sequence composed of R-U_5 and some adjacent sequences (shown by zigzag lines). The dashed lines in the mRNA molecules indicate the regions spliced out to create a subgenomic-size mRNA molecule. In some cases, the *pol* mRNA is thought to contain a splice near the *gag-pol* junction (see text). The arrangement of the structural proteins within the precursor polyproteins and in the virion is indicated schematically.

virion proteins. When viral particles are harvested from virus-producing cells at short intervals (2–5 min), a proportion contains uncleaved precursors, which suggests that the cleavage events occur late in the maturation pathway. The origin of these proteases is not entirely clear as yet, although candidate proteases have been isolated from virions of avian and murine retroviruses (discussed below).

Immunoprecipitation of solubilized infected-cell extracts routinely reveals a number of *gag*-related proteins of lower molecular weights than the major precursor. These proteins usually lack some tryptic peptides characteristic of the major precursor, are believed to be cleavage intermediates produced during processing, and allow the construction of precursor-processing schemes, which are described in some detail for the different viruses below.

Antisera prepared against any of the polypeptides that constitute the *gag* gene can be used to immunoprecipitate the major *gag* precursor, some of the cleavage intermediates of the precursor, and, in small amounts, a large precursor that also contains the DNA-polymerase moiety (discussed below and see Fig. 6.1). In some instances, other *gag*-related proteins, slightly larger than the major *gag* precursor, are also immunoprecipitated. For example, MMTV-infected cells synthesize an additional *gag* precursor of 110,000 daltons from which an additional virion protein (p30) not entirely encoded within *gag* is derived (see Section IV.A.1.e). A *gag*-related protein, slightly larger than the major precursor of core component, is also found in murine leukemia virus (MLV)-infected cells. This protein appears to be glycosylated and exposed on the surfaces of infected cells (see Section III.B.2).

2. Synthesis of the pol-*gene Products*

The RNA-dependent DNA polymerase is synthesized as part of a large precursor that includes the *gag* components in addition to the polymerase moiety (see Fig. 6.1). This precursor generally has a molecular weight of about 180,000 daltons and is present in virus-infected cells in 20- to 50-fold lower amounts than the major *gag*-gene precursor. As in the case of the *gag* precursor, cleavage intermediates can be found in cells, although complete cleavage of the *pol* precursor is most likely required to activate the functional enzymic activity. The final steps appear to occur after budding of the virion. Translation of virion RNA in vitro also yields this precursor in a ratio similar to that observed in vivo, although the structure of the RNA for *pol* is unknown. For reasons discussed at length in Chapter 5, it now seems likely that a splicing mechanism is used to generate a novel *pol* mRNA that lacks the *gag* termination signals. However, suppression at the *gag* termination codon by other mechanisms (Philipson et al. 1978) has not yet been rigorously excluded.

3. Synthesis of the env-*gene Products*

The components of the envelope gene are also synthesized as a single precursor, irrespective of whether the mature virion contains two glycoproteins or a glycoprotein and a smaller nonglycosylated hydrophobic polypeptide (see Fig. 6.1). The precursors are synthesized on the rough endoplasmic reticulum as transmembrane proteins, which become glycosylated prior to cleavage (with further glycosylation afterward) and eventually become situated in the plasma membrane of the host cell. The envelope components presumably act as centers for the core-protein associations or assembly. A more detailed account of the synthesis of the envelope components for the different retroviruses is given below.

E. Maturation and Morphogenesis of Retroviruses

Thin-section electron microscopy has been particularly important in formulating a conceptual model for the maturation of these viruses. In fact, it was this technique that led to the early classification of retroviruses as B-type, C-type, and later D-type on the basis of the morphology of viral particles during or after budding from the plasma membrane (for review, see Dalton 1972; de Harven 1974) (see Chapter 2). Other differences in intracytoplasmic maturation of the core structures were also noted. The B-type retroviruses demonstrate an electron-dense, eccentrically located nucleoid in thin-section electron micrographs, whereas the C-type and D-type retroviral particles exhibit an electron-dense, centrally located core structure. The core structure of the B-type and D-type particles can be found preformed in infected cells and exists as two electron-dense concentric rings with an electron-lucent center known as the intracytoplasmic A-type particle. Maturation of B-type particles occurs by budding of this intracytoplasmic A-type particle to form initially an immature B-type particle (or enveloped A-type particle), followed by the final maturation to give the classical B-type particle. Maturation of C-type retroviruses occurs at the plasma membrane where the assembly appears to take place and is observed initially as a crescent-shaped structure that eventually evolves into a fully formed core structure at the ultimate stage of budding.

II. AVIAN RETROVIRUSES

The avian sarcoma and leukemia virus family (denoted ASLV in this section) has proven to be a fruitful one for the study of the biosynthesis of viral proteins and their interactions with the host cell. ASLVs are generally produced to high titer, allowing relatively easy isolation, analysis, and preparation of serological reagents. Furthermore, the availability of numerous mutant and defective viruses, as well as partially restrictive growth conditions, enables investigations on the relationship between protein biosynthesis and the control of virus production. Information gleaned from studies of avian retroviruses has also proved to be generally applicable to other retroviruses.

A. Avian Retroviral Particles and Their Protein Constituents

As for all C-type viruses, the avian retroviral particle consists of an internal centrally located core structure surrounded by an outer membrane that is derived from the host cell during the process of virus budding. The virus-specified envelope glycoproteins are found associated with the outer surface of the membrane, whereas the internal core contains the genomic RNA as well as reverse transcriptase. The information for these structural elements is contained in the three retroviral genes concerned with virus multiplication: *gag,* encoding the major structural components of the core; *pol,* specifying reverse transcriptase; and *env,* encoding the envelope glycoproteins. The major virion structural protein precursors, intermediates, and mature virion peptides of the avian retroviruses are listed in Table 6.2. The primary translational products of all three genes are precursor polyproteins subject to posttranslational modification and processing (for review, see Eisenman and Vogt 1978). We first consider separately the virion proteins, which nearly always represent the final cleavage products of precursor polyproteins. We then review the synthesis and processing of the precursors.

1. Internal Structural gag *Proteins*

The major structural components of the virion core are four (or possibly five) nonglycosylated proteins (termed *gag* proteins), of which several thousand molecules each are present per virion (Stromberg et al. 1974). In ASLV, these proteins are p19, p12, p27, and p15.

a. p19, pp19. p19 is found in association with both viral RNA and the lipid envelope and is observed in phosphorylated (pp19) and

Table 6.2 Avian retrovirus precursor polyproteins and virion proteins

Protein	Gene	Function	Localization	Structure and properties
$Pr76^{gag}$	*gag*	precursor to virion internal structural proteins	cell cytoplasm, probably associated with inner surface of plasma membrane	phosphoprotein; NH_2-p19-p10-p27-p12-p15-COOH
$Pr66^{gag}$, $Pr60^{gag}$	*gag*	presumed intermediates in $Pr76^{gag}$ cleavage	probably associated with plasma membrane	both proteins appear to lack $p15^{gag}$; role in the processing pathway is unknown
$p27^{gag}$	*gag*	subunits of the core shell	virion core	hydrophobic; pI 7.8 (AMV)
$p19^{gag}$, $pp19^{gag}$	*gag*	may be involved in RNA processing and packaging	associated with genomic RNA in the core, also found outside core structure, possibly bound to lipid	found in phosphorylated (pp19) and nonphosphorylated (p19) forms; binds specifically to viral RNA; binds to lipid; pp19, pI 5.6 (AMV); p19, pI 6.3 (AMV)
$p15^{gag}$	*gag*	protease involved in cleavage of *gag*-protein precursors; may also cleave the β subunit of reverse transcriptase to generate α	between the virion core and the inner envelope	*gag*-specific protease; partially inhibited by thiol-specific reagents; pI 6.6 (AMV)
$p12^{gag}$	*gag*	may be involved in virion RNA packaging and folding	RNP complex within virion core	rich in arginine and lysine residues; pI 4.5 (AMV)
$p10^{gag}$	*gag*	unknown	possibly virion membrane	lacks lysine residues
$p23^{gag}$	*gag*	unknown	unknown	contains p19 plus a segment of of $Pr76^{gag}$ lying between p19 and p27

$Pr180^{gag-pol}$	*pol*	precursor to reverse transcriptase	cell cytoplasm, probably associated with the plasma membrane	phosphoprotein
$Pr130^{gag-pol}$	*pol*	probably an intermediate in $Pr180^{gag-pol}$ processing	probably associated with plasma membrane	contains reverse transcriptase and at least a portion of $p15^{gag}$
$\alpha\beta$ Subunits	*pol*	transcription of genomic RNA	virion core	RNA- and DNA-dependent polymerase and hybrid-specific RNase-H activities; β subunit is phosphorylated; $\beta = 92{,}000$ daltons; $\alpha = 58{,}000$ daltons
$p32^{pol}$	*pol*	unknown	virion core	endonuclease
$P63^{env}$	*env*	aminoterminal signal sequence allows insertion of nascent polypeptide into endoplasmic reticulum	probably associated as a nascent chain with the rough endoplasmic reticulum	contains 64-amino-acid long aminoterminal hydrophobic signal sequence plus the amino acid sequences of gp85 and gp37; represents primary translation product of *env*; observed only upon cell-free translation of *env* mRNA
$P57^{env}$	*env*	polypeptide backbone of *env*-precursor polyprotein	rough endoplasmic reticulum	observed in infected cells only after addition of inhibitors of glycosylation; represents $P63^{env}$ after removal of the signal sequence; nonglycosylated form of $Pr90^{env}$
$Pr90^{env}$	*env*	precursor to envelope glycoproteins gp85 and gp37	cell and virion membranes	glycosylated, but lacks terminal fucose

Table 6.2 (Continued)

VGP	*env*	host range; neutralization; interference; subgroup specificity	virion envelope	disulfide-bonded complex of gp85 and gp37
$gp85^{env}$	*env*	host range; neutralization; interference; subgroup specificity	virion envelope; knob structure directly associated with gp37	15% carbohydrate by weight; (subgroups B,C); nonglycosylated form = 35,000–37,000 daltons
$gp37^{env}$	*env*	may anchor gp85 to membrane	virion envelope; spike structure directly associated with membrane and gp85	nonglycosylated form = 21,000 daltons

nonphosphorylated forms. It is not yet clear to what extent phosphorylation influences the different binding functions of p19. Studies with MLVs have indicated that the extent of phosphorylation may be important in this regard (see Section III.A.1.c).

Initially, p19 was not detected in detergent-disrupted core preparations (Davis and Rueckert 1972; Stromberg et al. 1974), although it was later shown that a fraction of the p19 molecules is actually bound to virion RNA (Sen and Todaro 1977). The ability of p19 to bind preferentially to ASLV RNA in vitro parallels the highly specific binding of other retroviral phosphoproteins to their genomic RNAs (Sen et al. 1978). In its association with lipid, p19 is equivalent to MLV p15 and MMTV p10 and can be considered analogous to the lipid-associated matrix protein (M protein) of vesicular stomatitis virus (VSV) and other negative-strand viruses (Pepinsky and Vogt 1979). It has been suggested that p19 is physically associated in some way with the envelope glycoprotein gp37, which is believed to be an integral membrane protein (Schlesinger 1976; Montelaro et al. 1978). It is not known how large a fraction of the population of virion p19 molecules is actually involved in binding functions or whether single molecules of p19 engage simultaneously in both lipid binding and RNA binding. The dual properties of p19 make it an attractive candidate as a mediator of RNA packaging. In addition, a model has been advanced suggesting that p19, by virtue of its ability to bind to double-stranded regions of RNA, regulates the splicing, and therefore the production, of viral mRNAs (Leis et al. 1978). A number of viruses generated by recombination with endogenous viruses have been isolated that appear to contain deletions in p19 (Robinson et al. 1979; Shaikh et al. 1979). Although otherwise phenotypically normal, at least one of these recombinants has an altered ratio of intracellular subgenomic to genomic length mRNA, consistent with the idea that p19 may play a role in viral mRNA metabolism (Leis et al. 1981).

b. p12. p12 is also found in association with viral RNA. Unlike p19, which binds to RNA at a limited number of sites, p12 is the major protein constituent of the ribonucleoprotein (RNP) complex isolated from disrupted virions (Davis and Rueckert 1972; Bolognesi et al. 1973; Fleissner and Tress 1973). In addition, the binding of p12 to RNA is apparently nonspecific (Leis et al. 1978; Smith and Bailey 1979) and is based on ionic interactions between the RNA and the relatively high number of arginine and lysine residues in p12 (Bolognesi et al. 1973; Smith and Bailey 1979). Each bound p12 molecule has been estimated to occupy four nucleotides (Smith and Bailey 1979). In both its properties and localization, ASLV p12 appears analogous to the MLV p10 (Fleissner and Tress 1973; Schulein et al. 1978) and MMTV p14 (Arthur et al. 1978b; Nusse et al. 1980) (see Table 6.1). Evidence has also been presented indicating that p12 is a phosphoprotein (Lai 1976), but this has not been directly confirmed (Erikson et al. 1977). A possible explanation for the discrepancy may be that a fragment of pp19 comigrating with p12 has been mistaken for the p12 phosphoprotein (Shealy et al. 1980).

c. p27. p27 is not found as part of the RNP complex, but yet it is a major component of the core structure from which the RNP is isolated (Davis and Rueckert 1972; Bolognesi et al. 1973; Stromberg et al. 1974). This result has generally been interpreted to indicate that p27 forms the core "shell" that lies beneath the lipid envelope and surrounds the RNP. In fact, a distinct structure surrounding the RNP has been observed in murine viruses by electron microscopy (Nermut et al. 1972). The observed ability of p27 to form higher-order homotypic multimers when chemically cross-linked in virions (Pepinsky et al. 1980) is at least consistent with the idea that this protein may form the subunits of the core shell.

d. p15. p15 is generally absent from core preparations and from the virion surface and is thus believed to reside between the core and the inner envelope (Bolognesi et al. 1973; Stromberg et al. 1974). Perhaps the most interesting property of p15 is its ability to cleave proteolytically the *gag* precursor polyprotein into virion proteins and intermediates (Von der Helm 1977; Dittmar and Moelling 1978; Vogt et al. 1979). Biochemical studies have shown that the protease activity is inseparable from p15 and is highly specific under physiological conditions for *gag*-related polypeptides (Dittmar and Moelling 1978; Vogt et al. 1979). One exception may be the reported ability of p15 to cleave specifically the larger subunit of reverse transcriptase (Moelling et al. 1980). Although the p15 proteolytic activity is partially inhibited by thiol-specific reagents (Dittmar and Moelling 1978; Vogt et al. 1979), an analysis of the amino acid sequence of p15 suggests that its structure is different from those of known thiol proteases (R. Sauer, pers. comm.).

p15 and p12 have been completely sequenced (Sauer et al. 1981; T. Vanaman et al., pers. comm.) (see Appendix F); however, only partial amino acid sequence data and amino acid compositions are as yet available for p19 (Palmiter et al. 1978) and p27 (Herman et al. 1975). The emerging nucleotide sequence of ASLV, however, should establish the amino acid sequences of these proteins and aid in further chemical analyses.

e. p23 and p10. Two minor nonglycosylated polypeptides, p23 and p10, are found in ASLV, and at least p23 is encoded by *gag*. Peptide mapping and serological data (Robinson et al. 1979; R. Shaikh and R. Eisenman, pers. comm.) have demonstrated that p23, a phosphoprotein (Lai 1976; Erikson et al. 1977), contains the amino terminus and major peptides of p19 plus additional amino acid sequences, presumably from the region of the *gag* precursor polyprotein lying between p19 and p27 (see Section II.C.1.a). A protein related to p23 appears to be overrepresented in virions of the *gag* precursor cleavage mutant *ts* LA334 (Hunter et al. 1976; Rohrschneider et al. 1976) and in recombinant viruses containing deletions in p19 (Shaikh et al. 1979). At present, it is uncertain whether p23 plays a role in virion structure and function or whether it is simply a cleavage intermediate adventitiously packaged during budding.

The p10 polypeptide is present in variable, usually low, amounts in ASLV virions; its detection is complicated by the fact that it comigrates with the lower-molecular-weight *gag* proteins (Shealy et al. 1980). It can, however, be detected as the smallest protein in gel filtration of disrupted virions (Vogt et al. 1975). On the basis of surface-labeling studies, p10 is believed to be situated on or within the viral envelope (Bolognesi et al. 1973). Although initial peptide-mapping data indicated that p10 was not part of the *gag* protein precursor (Vogt et al. 1975), recent nucleic acid sequence studies of *gag* (see Appendix F) suggest the presence of a polypeptide segment between p19 and p27 that, by its lack of lysine residues and its size, may be p10 (E. Hunter and D. Schwartz, pers. comm.). Partial amino acid sequence analysis of p10 has confirmed that this protein is encoded within the *gag* gene (E. Hunter and R. Pepinsky, pers. comm.). Then p23 must consist of both p19 and at least a portion of p10 peptides. The possible surface localization of p10 would also make it the only *gag*-encoded protein to be found outside the viral envelope.

2. Reverse Transcriptase

In comparison with the *gag* proteins, several thousand molecules of which are present per virion, reverse transcriptase is a rather minor component with less than 100 molecules being present in viral particles (Panet et al. 1975a).

In ASLV virions, reverse transcriptase is generally recovered as a two-subunit complex: the β subunit with a molecular weight of 92,000, and the α subunit with a molecular weight of 58,000 (Kacian et al. 1971; Copeland et al. 1980). The $\alpha\beta$ complex as well as α alone and a β dimer (β_2) have been isolated and all possess both the RNA-dependent and DNA-dependent polymerase and the processive RNA-DNA hybrid-specific ribonuclease (RNase-H) activities (Grandgenett et al. 1973; Verma 1975a; Hizi and Joklik 1977a; Hizi et al. 1977; for review, see Verma 1977; Gerard and Grandgenett 1980). The enzymic functions of reverse transcriptase and their role in the virus replicative cycle are described in detail in Chapter 5.

Peptide-mapping and in vitro proteolysis studies have demonstrated convincingly that the α subunit is derived by proteolytic cleavage of the β subunit in the virion (Gibson and Verma 1974; Moelling 1975; Rho et al. 1975; Lai and Verma 1978). Another polypeptide, also encoded by *pol,* has been isolated from avian retroviral particles: a 32,000-dalton protein (p32) possessing Mn^{++}-dependent DNA endonuclease activity (Grandgenett et al. 1978). Since the p32 endonuclease activity has also been shown to be associated with the $\alpha\beta$ polymerase (Golomb and Grandgenett 1979; Samuel et al. 1979) and since p32 shares both antigenic determinants and peptides with β but not with α (Schiff and Grandgenett 1978), it seems likely that p32 is generated from β during its processing to α. Treatment of purified $\alpha\beta$ with chymotrypsin also produces the p32 endonuclease (Grandgenett et al. 1980). A smaller chymotrypsin-generated fragment with RNase-H activity has also been identified, but this peptide is contained in both α and β subunits and is thus distinct from p32 (Lai and Verma 1978). Several laboratories using different approaches have demonstrated that it is the carboxyterminal region of β that is removed to generate p32 and thus that the amino terminus constitutes α (Rettenmier et al. 1979b; Copeland et al. 1980; Eisenman et al. 1980a). A plausible scheme for the production of the reverse transcriptase complex in virions would be $\beta_2 \rightarrow \alpha\beta + \text{p32}$. The idea that the β_2 complex is a direct precursor to $\alpha\beta$ is speculative, as β_2 has been observed only in virus released from duck cells (Hizi and Joklik 1977a); thus, β_2 either is unique to this system or is a labile intermediate generally present but detected only in this special case. These cleavage events leading to the formation of reverse transcriptase appear to occur within the viral particle (Moelling 1975; Eisenman et al. 1980a), presumably during or immediately following virus budding. Results to be discussed below indicate that they represent the last in a series of cleavages of larger intracellular precursor polyproteins.

The reverse-transcriptase-related polypeptides (i.e., $\alpha\beta$ and p32) are present within the viral core structure (Stromberg et al. 1974; Grandgenett et al. 1978), and the α and β subunits copurify with the RNP complex (Stromberg et al. 1974). Present evidence suggests that reverse transcriptase is associated with virion genomic RNA by means of its specific binding to the $tRNA^{Trp}$ primer (Panet et al. 1975b). As described in Chapter 4, the primer RNA molecule is a cellular tRNA that is itself base-paired to a region located close to the 5′ terminus of the genomic RNA. The specific association between primer tRNA and reverse transcriptase in the virion raises the question of whether one of these elements determines the packaging of the other into viral particles. Two sets of experiments have shed light on this possibility. First, studies with murine retroviruses have demonstrated that packaging of primer tRNA and reverse transcriptase into the virion occurs in the absence of genomic RNA (Levin and Seidman 1979). Second, two avian retroviral mutants that produce viral particles devoid of reverse transcriptase fail to package the tRNA primer (Sawyer and Hanafusa 1979; Peters and Hu 1980). Thus, it would appear that it is reverse transcriptase that selects the primer tRNA for packaging, and not vice versa.

3. Envelope Proteins

The virion membrane that surrounds the core appears to be acquired from the host cell during the process of virus budding. Studies on the overall phospholipid content of the ASLV membrane indicate a broad compositional similarity between the viral membrane and the host-cell membrane from which the virus was released. The ratios of some components are, however, significantly different, suggesting the possibility that budding may occur in some specialized region of the membrane (Quigley et al. 1971).

Electron microscopy of avian retroviruses long ago revealed the presence of spikes, or knobs connected to the virion by spikes, on the virion surface (Bernhard et al. 1958; Bolognesi et al. 1972, 1978). Treatment of intact virions with protease leads to removal of these surface projections and loss of infectivity. Polypeptide analysis demonstrates a concomitant disappearance of only the two viral glycoproteins, gp85 and gp37 (Rifkin and Compans 1971). Peptide-mapping studies have shown these to be two distinct proteins (Mosser et al. 1977; Klemenz and Diggelmann 1978). The knoblike structure observed in the electron microscope is probably composed primarily of gp85, whereas the spike structure is composed of gp37 (Bolognesi et al. 1972; Bolognesi 1974). In viral particles, single molecules of gp85 and gp37 are linked by disulfide bonds in a dimer structure (termed VGP), and larger noncovalently linked aggregates have also been observed (Duesberg et al. 1970; Leamnson and Halpern 1976). Treatment of virions with reducing agents results in release of only gp85, whereas gp37 remains virus-associated, suggesting that the latter is membrane-associated and functions to anchor gp85 at the virion surface (Pauli et al. 1978; H. Diggelmann, pers. comm.).

Analysis of the carbohydrate content of gp85 has demonstrated significant variation among virus strains (Krantz et al. 1976) and this could be responsible for the unique adsorption properties of subgroup-A viruses (see Chapter 3). However, the amount of carbohydrate, as deduced from recent experiments with tunicamycin, differs by no more than 25–30% in subgroup A and B viruses (E. Hunter, pers. comm.). Minor variations in sugar chain length have also been detected when virus of the same subgroup is propagated in untransformed versus transformed cells (Lai and Duesberg 1972). These differences are probably the result of alterations in cellular carbohydrate metabolism that accompany transformation (see Chapter 3).

The oligosaccharide chains on gp85 appear to be linked to asparagine residues via mannose-rich cores. Chains of both the complex acidic type (containing terminal sialic acid and fucose) and the mannose-rich neutral type have been detected in a ratio of approximately 3:1 (Krantz et al. 1976; Hunt et al. 1979). Exhaustive Pronase digestion of gp85 leads to release of a collection of glycopeptides with a very broad size distribution, as determined by gel filtration (Sefton 1976). This heterogeneity appears to be due to the presence of both classes of oligosaccharide chains mentioned above, as well as to differences in the numbers of mannose units in the oligomannosyl cores (Hunt et al. 1979). Estimates have been made of the number of carbohydrate attachment sites (two to four) on gp85 (Galehouse and

Duesberg 1976), but these have not taken into account the extensive oligosaccharide heterogeneity (Hunt et al. 1979). Experiments using tunicamycin in conjunction with nucleotide sequence data indicate that gp85 of a subgroup-C virus contains about 16 carbohydrate chains, comprising about 60% of the molecular mass of gp85 (E. Hunter and D. Schwartz, pers. comm.). The high carbohydrate content of gp85 and gp37 makes accurate determination of their polypeptide chain length by electrophoresis or gel filtration extremely difficult. Recently, however, partial amino acid sequencing of the envelope glycoproteins, coupled with nucleotide sequencing of the retroviral genome, has led to estimates of 21,000 daltons for gp37 and about 36,000 daltons for gp85 (E. Hunter and D. Schwartz, pers. comm.).

As discussed in detail in Chapter 3, the envelope glycoproteins are responsible for the host-range, neutralization, interference, and subgroup specificities of retroviruses. Genetic studies with mutants containing deletions in *env* have led to the conclusion that the role of the envelope glycoproteins in the virus replication cycle is limited to mediating the adsorption and penetration of virus to the susceptible host cell (Weiss 1969; Kawai and Hanafusa 1973; Ogura and Friis 1975; Vogt 1977).

B. Immunological and Biochemical Polymorphism of Avian Retroviral Proteins

All avian viral proteins exhibit some degree of polymorphism. Variations are often detected when analogous gene products of different ASLV strains are examined by techniques such as oligonucleotide mapping, peptide mapping, radioimmunoassay, and gel electrophoresis. This should not obscure the fact that the vast majority of amino acid sequences of analogous viral proteins are highly related. For example, antisera against the *gag* proteins display broad reactivity among the different virus strains and they are thus considered to be group-specific (previously called *gs*). However, more detailed study revealed amino acid sequence and size differences, as well as antigenic determinants for *gag* proteins that were present only in certain viruses (Bolognesi et al. 1975a; Stephenson et al. 1975b; Hayman and Vogt 1976; Rettenmier and Hanafusa 1977; Shaikh et al. 1978, 1979). The presence of both unique and shared antigenic determinants has been demonstrated for p19, p15, p12, reverse transcriptase, the envelope glycoproteins, and pp60^{src}.

The envelope glycoproteins, in particular gp85, are the targets of virus-type-specific neutralizing antibodies produced during virus infection of animals. Antibodies produced against purified gp85 react with both type-specific and group-specific antigenic determinants on the molecule (Rohrschneider et al. 1975). By analogy with the murine retrovirus system, it would appear that the carbohydrate moiety does not play a major role in determining type-specific antigenic properties (Bolognesi et al. 1975b). In some cases, carbohydrate configuration may determine a more broadly reactive antigenic specificity (Van Eldik et al. 1978), which appears to be shared with a normal chicken-cell glycoprotein (Collins et al. 1978). Recently, experiments with MLV suggest that type specificity may arise from polypeptide conformational differences, whereas group-specific antibodies recognize amino acid sequences (Versteegen and Oroszlan 1980).

Among the *gag* proteins, polymorphism has been demonstrated for p27, p19, and p15 when exogenous and endogenous retroviruses have been compared (Rettenmier and Hanafusa 1977; Shaikh et al. 1978, 1979). The p27 proteins of all endogenous viruses migrate more slowly in SDS-polyacrylamide gel electrophoresis than do the analogous proteins of exogenous strains. There are some data to indicate that the size difference is due to additional amino acid sequences in the carboxyterminal region of the protein (Bhown et al. 1980).

Immunological studies have demonstrated that the reverse transcriptases from the different ASLV strains are highly related. However, type-specific antigenic determinants have been defined. Also, genus-specific differences between chicken and pheasant viruses (which are unrelated to ASLV) were detected (Bauer and Temin 1980a). In addition, the reverse transcriptases of ASLV and avian reticuloendotheliosis viruses (REVs) do not cross-react in radioimmunoassays (Bauer and Temin 1980a) (see Section V.A).

Viral particles apparently unrelated to ASLV have been detected in the allantoic fluid of embryonated chicken, quail, and goose eggs (Bauer and Hofschneider 1976). The reverse transcriptases from such particles appear biochemically and immunologically distinct from endogenous and exogenous ASLVs (Bauer et al. 1977; Bauer and Temin 1979). At present, it is not clear whether these "viruses" interact with or are in some manner related to ASLV.

C. Biosynthesis and Processing of Structural Proteins

During the late stage of retrovirus infection of permissive cells, the integrated DNA provirus serves as the template for the transcription of a series of mRNAs that encode the structural proteins of the viral particle (see Chapter 5). These mRNAs arise as the result of several processing reactions (splicing, as well as poly[A] and cap addition) performed on a primary genome-length (or possibly larger) transcript. Aside from those processing events that may be essential for RNA transport, the processing of retroviral RNAs probably serves to allow the distinction between genomic RNA and mRNAs during packaging, provides for the proper compartmentalization of viral gene products, regulates the quantities and possibly the functions of viral polypeptides, and permits translation of internal cistrons. The primary translational products of the viral mRNAs appear, in turn, to be directly involved in the mechanics of viral-particle formation, whereas, as discussed in the previous sections, the polypeptides generated as a result of processing and modification constitute the viral particle itself.

1. The gag*-gene Proteins*

a. Organization of Pr76^{gag}. The major internal structural proteins of avian retroviruses are first synthesized as a 76,000-dalton precursor polyprotein (Pr76^{gag}) (Vogt and Eisenman 1973). Pr76^{gag} is proteolytically cleaved, via several intermediates, to generate the low-molecular-weight *gag* proteins found in viral particles (see Section II.A.1). The amino acid sequences of these proteins are linked within Pr76^{gag} in the order NH_2-p19-p10-p27-p12-p15-COOH (Vogt et al. 1975; Shealy et al. 1980; D. Schwartz et al., pers. comm.). No difference in the apparent molecular weight of Pr76^{gag} synthesized by wild-type, transformation-defective or nondefective viruses, or by different virus strains has been observed (Pawson et al. 1976). Exceptions are found in certain recombinants and endogenous viruses that produce a slightly smaller protein (Shaikh et al. 1978; K. Conklin and R. Eisenman, pers. comm.).

Recent nucleotide and amino acid sequence data indicate that almost all of Pr76^{gag} is utilized to form the *gag* proteins. A region of 64 amino acids lying between p19 and p27 has been proposed to constitute p10 (E. Hunter et al., pers. comm.). In addition, a region of 9 amino acids lies between p27 and p12 (E. Hunter and D. Schwartz, pers. comm.). The amino termini of both Pr76^{gag} and p19 are identical (Palmiter et al. 1978), and the presence of a translational termination codon (UAG) immediately following the carboxyterminal amino acid of p15 (Sauer et al., pers. comm.; D. Schwartz, pers. comm.) suggests that the carboxyl termini of Pr76^{gag} and p15 are also coincident.

Considering the properties of the *gag* proteins, Pr76^{gag} can be thought of as a polyprotein with both lipid and specific RNA-binding regions at its aminoterminal end (p19), followed by the hydrophobic core-shell region (p27), a nucleic-acid-binding region (p12), and, at its carboxyl terminus, a protease capable of specifically cutting its neighboring regions (p15). Although the significance of such a functional grouping is unclear, it is interesting to recall the schematic conformation of these peptides within the viral particle (see Fig. 6.1) and to note the striking similarity to the order of the *gag* proteins within the MLV precursor polyprotein (MLV Pr65^{gag}). In MLV Pr65^{gag}, the core-shell protein p30 is also flanked by a nucleic-acid-binding protein (p10) on its carboxyterminal side and by lipid-binding protein (p15) and specific RNA-binding protein (pp12) on its aminoterminal side (NH_2-p15-pp12-p30-p10-COOH) (see Section III.A.1.a). This parallel ordering suggests that the lipid-binding functions of MLV p15 and the RNA-binding functions of MLV pp12 are, in the avian system, performed by a single protein (p19). No equivalent to the ASLV p15 *gag*-specific protease is contained within MLV Pr65^{gag}, although a protease of 10,000 daltons with the ability to cleave MLV *gag* proteins has been detected in MLV virions (Yoshinaka and Luftig 1977a,b). It remains to be determined whether the MLV *gag* protease is actually present on the *gag* precursor but so rapidly cleaved off as to prevent its detection. In any case, the similarity in the organization of the *gag*-protein precursors of two C-type retroviruses, which are otherwise unrelated as judged by nucleic acid hybridization, host range, and serology, suggests that the order of the proteins within the precursor may be of some importance to the mechanism of particle formation (see Fig. 6.1). Alternatively, the gene order may have been conserved during evolutionary diversification of C-type viruses.

It should perhaps be stressed that none of the avian *gag* proteins have yet been demonstrated to exhibit their specific properties while they are linked in a precursor. However, the isolation of MLV Pr65^{gag} on the basis of its affinity for DNA cellulose indicates that MLV p10 may retain its nucleic-acid-binding function (Oroszlan et al. 1976). Furthermore, the MLV *gag* precursor found in viral particles can be chemically cross-linked to lipid, indicating that the p15 lipid-binding function may also be retained (Pepinsky and Vogt 1979). In addition, the *gag*-protein precursor encoded by avian REV has been found associated with an intracellular RNA complex (Wong et al. 1980), suggesting that the affinity for RNA is manifested in the precursor.

$Pr76^{gag}$ is also phosphorylated, presumably at sites within p19 and possibly p12 (Lai 1976; Erikson et al. 1977), although other phosphorylation sites and other types of modifications are not excluded. Analysis of $Pr76^{gag}$ by two-dimensional electrophoresis has revealed some charge heterogeneity (Eisenman et al. 1980c).

b. Synthesis of $Pr76^{gag}$. $Pr76^{gag}$ is synthesized from an mRNA that is apparently indistinguishable from the full-length genomic RNA of the viral particle (Hayward 1977; S. Weiss et al. 1977). In fact, cell-free translation of virion RNA yields, as the predominant product in several in vitro systems, a protein identical with $Pr76^{gag}$ in size, antigenicity, and peptide map (Von der Helm and Duesberg 1975; Pawson et al. 1976). Although subtle differences may exist between the intracellular mRNA for $Pr76^{gag}$ and the virion genomic RNA, they have not yet been detected. Aminoterminal sequencing of $Pr76^{gag}$ (Palmiter et al. 1978) and nucleotide sequencing of the viral genome demonstrate that the translation of the precursor is initiated at an AUG codon 372 nucleotides from the 5′ end of genomic RNA, a region lying 271 nucleotides from the end of the U_5 region of the long terminal repeat (LTR) (R. Swanstrom and D. Schwartz, pers. comm.) (see also Chapter 4). At least three possible translational initiation codons are present on the 5′ side of the *gag* initiation sequence, one of which is preceded by a putative 18S rRNA-binding sequence (Haseltine et al. 1977; Shine et al. 1977; Stoll et al. 1977). None of these codons is directly followed by the nucleotide sequence corresponding to $Pr76^{gag}$, nor do they appear to be utilized in translation of genomic RNA in vitro (Palmiter et al. 1978). It is possible that these regions are removed by splicing from intracellular *gag* mRNA, but their apparent lack of function in translation of genomic RNA makes the avian retroviruses another example of a eukaryotic mRNA that does not initiate translation at the AUG codon nearest to the 5′ end (Kozak 1978).

Although $Pr76^{gag}$ is synthesized predominantly late in infection, small amounts of newly synthesized precursor have been detected prior to provirus integration, as early as 3 hours after infection (Gallis et al. 1976). At present, it is unclear whether this synthesis plays a role in virus infection or represents gratuitous translation of virion RNA.

Cell-fractionation studies have revealed that high levels of both genomic-length mRNA and Pr76^{gag} are present on cytoplasmic polyribosomes (Lee et al. 1979; Eisenman et al. 1980c; Purchio et al. 1980). This is in contrast to the situation with murine retroviruses, where high levels of *gag*-related precursor have been detected on membrane-bound polyribosomes (Gielkens et al. 1976), a fact that is likely to be related to the presence of glycosylated *gag* polyproteins on the surfaces of MLV-infected cells (see Section III.B.2) (Tung et al. 1976). A recent report indicates that glycosylated *gag* polyproteins may also be expressed on avian-retrovirus-producing avian cells, although they appear in amounts presumably below the level required for detection on membrane polyribosomes (Buetti and Diggelmann 1980a).

A number of membrane-associated proteins have been shown to be synthesized on cytoplasmic polyribosomes (Lodish 1973). Pr76^{gag} may also fall into this category, as several lines of indirect evidence point to some form of association of the precursor with the plasma membrane during virus budding (see Section II.D). The manner by which Pr76^{gag} becomes associated with the membrane has not been elucidated.

c. Processing of the gag *Precursor.* When ASLV-infected chick embryo cells are labeled with a radioactive amino acid for a short period (typically 10 min or less, "pulse-label"), Pr76^{gag} can be readily observed in immunoprecipitates and constitutes about 1% of total labeled protein. When the pulse-labeled cells are allowed to continue metabolizing in nonradioactive growth medium ("chase"), the levels of radioactive Pr76^{gag} diminish and the *gag* proteins (p27, p19, p12, and p15) appear. Longer chase periods show disappearance of the *gag* proteins from the cell, concomitant with their appearance within viral particles in extracellular fluids (Vogt et al. 1975). Such pulse-chase experiments indicate a half-life of about 45 minutes for Pr76^{gag} and demonstrate the precursor-product relationship between it and the virion proteins. This half-life may vary depending on the cell type and the culture conditions. Less clear are the nature and role of several presumed intermediates in this process: Pr16, Pr60, Pr66, and Pr32. The first three are often observed along with Pr76^{gag} following a pulse-label and are metabolized during the chase period. Both Pr66 and Pr60 lack p15 peptides, whereas Pr16 contains them, which suggests that a fragment somewhat larger than p15 is rapidly cleaved from Pr76^{gag}, producing Pr16 and Pr66 or Pr60 (Vogt and Eisenman 1973; Vogt et al. 1975). Pr66 and Pr60 contain p19, p27, and p12 peptides and have identical methionine tryptic peptide patterns. Sequencing studies of the *gag* region, however, demonstrate that p12 and p15 are contiguous (R. Sauer, D. W. Allen, and H. D. Niall; D. Schwartz; all pers. comm.) and thus suggest that some cleavage must occur within p12 to generate Pr16. Similarly Pr32, which appears transiently during a chase period, contains p19 plus the region of 64 amino acids (p10) between p19 and p27 and possibly a fragment of p27. The presence of such truncated polyproteins would imply rampant miscleavage leading to dead-end products that may be quickly degraded. Alternatively, these products may reflect nonconservative cleavage of Pr76^{gag}, i.e., a mechanism whereby nonequimolar amounts of the core proteins are produced. In fact, the *gag* proteins have not been detected in equal amounts in purified ASLV virions (Davis and Rueckert 1972; Stromberg et al. 1974), but the differences are not significant enough to rule out conservative cleavage.

The observation that p15 possesses a proteolytic activity specific for *gag* proteins points to a key role for this protein in the processing scheme for Pr76^{gag} (Von der Helm 1977; Dittmar and Moelling 1978; Vogt et al. 1979). Analysis of several *gag*-related polyproteins that lack p15 tends to support this view. First *ev*-3 P120, a 120,000-dalton protein encoded by an endogenous retroviral genome (*ev*-3) (Eisenman et al. 1978; Astrin and Robinson 1979), consists of p19-p27-p12 and the carboxyterminal region of reverse transcriptase but lacks p15. Second, the defective leukemia viruses, such as avian erythroblastosis virus (AEV) and avian myelocytomatosis virus (MC29), produce high-molecular-weight polyproteins lacking p15 but containing aminoterminal regions of Pr76^{gag} (AEV: NH_2-p19–p10; MC29: NH_2-p19-p27-) joined to polypeptide segments encoded by the unique regions of their respective genomes (see Chapters 4 and 9) (Bister et al. 1977; Hayman et al. 1979; Rettenmier et al. 1979a; Eisenman et al. 1980b). Neither *ev*-3 P120 nor the AEV and MC29 polyproteins are cleaved intracellularly to produce viral proteins or viral particles. However, all three proteins can be cleaved in vitro upon treatment with p15 (Vogt et al. 1979). These results imply that the absence of p15 from these polyproteins contributes to their inability to be processed. In addition, the temperature-sensitive (*ts*) mutant LA334, which cleaves Pr76^{gag} aberrantly and produces abnormal virions at the nonpermissive temperature, synthesizes a *gag* precursor with an altered p15 tryptic peptide map (Rohrschneider et al. 1976), again suggesting, but not proving, that p15 plays a role in intracellular cleavage.

Analyses of the fragments generated by cleavage of Pr76^{gag} with p15 in vitro and the nucleotide sequence of *gag* indicate that major p15 cutting sites probably lie on both sides of p27 and between p12 and p15 (Vogt et al. 1979; D. Schwartz and E. Hunter, pers. comm.) (see Fig. 6.2). The amino acid sequence preceding the amino terminus and carboxyl terminus of p27, as well as the sequence preceding p12, contains two to four hydrophobic residues followed by a methionine. Such hydrophobic clusters could thus serve as p15 cleavage sites. Since p15 itself is not preceded by this putative recognition sequence, its release from Pr76^{gag} is likely to be mediated by another protease in vivo. On the other hand, p15 seems capable of cleaving p15 accurately from p12, at least in vitro (E. Hunter and R. Eisenman, pers. comm.).

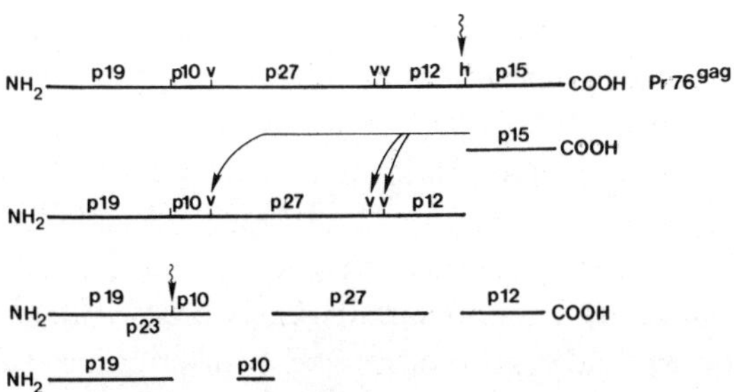

Figure 6.2 Structure and cleavage scheme for the ASLV *gag* precursor polyprotein. Processing of Pr76^{gag} commences with the removal of p15 by a putative host-cell protease that cuts Pr76^{gag} at the site marked h. The now-activated p15 protease cleaves the resulting intermediate at the three sites marked v, thus producing p12, p27, and p23. The p23 polypeptide is further processed by an unknown protease to generate p19. The segments lying between p19 and p27 (64 amino acids) and between p27 and p12 (9 amino acids) have been defined by nucleotide sequencing. This scheme was derived assuming conservative cleavage (see text). These cleavage events are intracellular, although low levels of p23 can be detected in virions.

The fact that $Pr76^{gag}$ contains a *gag*-specific protease raises the possibility that the precursor may be capable of cleaving itself and/or neighboring molecules of $Pr76^{gag}$. Autoproteolysis has in fact been observed in several other virus systems unrelated to retroviruses, including Sindbis virus (Aliperti and Schlesinger 1978), cowpea mosaic virus (Pelham 1979), and encephalomyocarditis virus (Pelham 1978). However, two lines of evidence argue against such a mechanism for avian retrovirus processing. First, in vitro translation of virion RNA yields $Pr76^{gag}$ molecules that remain stable indefinitely and are only cleaved after addition of p15 (Von der Helm 1977; R. Eisenman, pers. comm.). Second, several mammalian cell lines, transformed by RSVs, synthesize $Pr76^{gag}$ but do not cleave it to generate virion proteins or viral particles (Eisenman et al. 1975; V. Vogt and H. Oppermann, pers. comm.). With the caveat that the concentration of $Pr76^{gag}$ molecules may be low in these experiments, these data would rule out autocatalysis. Another possibility is that the p15 protease is itself generated by cleavage by a specific cell protease. Once activated in this way, p15 would then remove p12 and p27 by cutting at the putative recognition sequences mentioned above. Another protease might then separate p19 from the p10 polypeptide segment linking it to p27. Some credence is lent to this model by the fact that, in at least one of the RSV-transformed mammalian cell lines described above, $Pr76^{gag}$ is cleaved and virus is released only after fusion with permissive chick cells (Eisenman et al. 1975). This experiment is consistent with the involvement of a host-specific protease in the generation of virion proteins. Alternatively, the localization of $Pr76^{gag}$ synthesized in mammalian cells may be altered, compared with that in chicken cells, thereby rendering it less accessible to cell or other viral proteases. A proposed cleavage scheme is diagramed in Figure 6.2 and is based on predicted cleavage sites and the assumption that there is conservative cleavage. The relationship of this "idealized" pathway to all the intermediates actually observed in vivo remains to be clarified.

2. *The* pol-*gene Proteins*

a. Structure and Synthesis of $Pr180^{gag-pol}$. The primary precursor to avian retroviral reverse transcriptase is a 180,000- to 200,000-dalton polyprotein termed $Pr180^{gag-pol}$, which is a common product of the *gag* and *pol* genes. This protein can be immunoprecipitated from infected cells with antisera raised against either the *gag* proteins or reverse transcriptase. Analysis of its structure demonstrated that Pr180$^{gag-pol}$ contains polypeptide regions corresponding to both Pr76^{gag} and the β subunit of the reverse transcriptase (Oppermann et al. 1977; Hayman 1978a; Rettenmier et al. 1979b). The quantity of Pr180$^{gag-pol}$ detected in infected cells is 20-to 50-fold lower than the amount of Pr76^{gag}, consistent with the relative levels of *gag* proteins and reverse transcriptase in viral particles (Stromberg et al. 1974; Panet et al. 1975a).

The idea that Pr180$^{gag-pol}$ is a readthrough protein, produced by occasional translation past the usual *gag* termination codon at the carboxyl terminus of p15, seemed initially to be supported by cell-free translation studies. In these experiments, 39S virion genomic RNA directed the synthesis of high levels of Pr76^{gag} and low levels of Pr180$^{gag-pol}$ (Beemon and Hunter 1977; Paterson et al. 1977; Purchio et al. 1977). However, later cell-free translation experiments using yeast amber suppressor tRNA and 39S genomic RNA in an attempt to augment the frequency of readthrough into *pol* instead generated an 80,000-dalton *gag*-related protein synthesized at the expense of Pr76^{gag} with no concomitant increase in the level of Pr180$^{gag-pol}$ (Weiss et al. 1978). These studies further indicated that the 80,000-dalton protein is derived by the addition of amino acids to the carboxyl terminus of Pr76^{gag}. Thus, suppression of the UAG termination signal at the 3′ end of *gag* presumably permits translational readthrough to the next inphase terminator, but clearly not very far into *pol*. The fact that virion RNAs can normally direct the in vitro synthesis of both Pr76^{gag} and Pr180$^{gag-pol}$ therefore suggests that two populations of 39S RNA must be packaged into virions: a large population of RNA acting as message for Pr76^{gag} and a smaller population of RNA acting as message for Pr180$^{gag-pol}$ (Weiss et al. 1978).

Further light has been shed on the mechanism of Pr180$^{gag-pol}$ synthesis by nucleic acid sequencing of the *gag-pol*-junction region and amino acid sequencing of the amino terminus of reverse transcriptase. These studies have shown that the 3′ end of *gag* and the 5′ end of *pol* are separated by about 20 nucleotides and are in different translational reading frames (Copeland et al. 1980; D. Schwartz, pers. comm.). A termination codon, in phase with *gag*, has been observed about 117 nucleotides from the 3′ end of *gag*, in agreement with the in vitro translation studies described above. Moreover, putative RNA-splicing signals appear to bracket the region just preceding the carboxyl terminus of $Pr76^{gag}$ and the amino terminus of reverse transcriptase (D. Schwartz, pers. comm.). Together, these data provide strong support for the notion that separate mRNAs exist for synthesis of viral internal structural proteins. The mRNA for $Pr76^{gag}$ would possess a termination codon at the end of the *gag*-gene coding sequence. The mRNA for $Pr180^{gag\text{-}pol}$ would have this terminator removed by splicing, leading to a reading-frame shift and therefore uninterrupted translation into *pol*. The amounts of $Pr76^{gag}$ and $Pr180^{gag\text{-}pol}$ synthesized would be expected to reflect the relative abundancies of these mRNA species.

That $Pr180^{gag\text{-}pol}$ is synthesized on cytoplasmic polyribosomes can be inferred from experiments demonstrating that 39S mRNA is not detected on membrane-bound polyribosomes but is readily observed in the cytoplasmic fraction (Lee et al. 1979). Furthermore, $Pr180^{gag\text{-}pol}$ can only be detected on cytoplasmic polyribosomes (Purchio et al. 1980). Studies with MLV indicate that $Pr180^{gag\text{-}pol}$ becomes associated with cellular membranes prior to cleavage and release of mature virions (Witte and Baltimore 1978). It seems likely that the avian retrovirus polyprotein also becomes membrane-associated, although this has not been demonstrated directly.

b. Processing of Reverse Transcriptase. The fact that ASLV-infected cells synthesize a polyprotein containing both *gag*-gene and *pol*-gene products immediately raises the possibility that $Pr180^{gag\text{-}pol}$ is a common precursor to both $Pr76^{gag}$ and reverse transcriptase. However, the relatively low amounts of virion and intracellular reverse transcriptase compared with *gag* proteins would tend to argue against coordinate synthesis of these two gene products. In addition, pulse-chase experiments indicate a considerably slower turnover rate for $Pr180^{gag\text{-}pol}$ than for $Pr76^{gag}$ (half-life of 2–3 hr compared with 45 min for $Pr76^{gag}$) (Oppermann et al. 1977; Hayman 1978a; Eisenman et al. 1980a), a result incompatible with the idea that the bulk of the *gag* proteins are derived from $Pr180^{gag\text{-}pol}$. Finally, the demonstration of independent in vitro synthesis of $Pr76^{gag}$ and $Pr180^{gag\text{-}pol}$ (see above) provides strong support for the view that these proteins are not metabolically related. Thus, although $Pr180^{gag\text{-}pol}$ may be a direct precursor to reverse transcriptase, it is not the major progenitor of the *gag* proteins.

Immunoprecipitation experiments have also revealed a possible intermediate in $Pr180^{gag\text{-}pol}$ processing. This is a 130,000-dalton intracellular protein (Pr130$^{gag-pol}$) that contains tryptic peptides and antigenic determinants of reverse transcriptase and the *gag* protein p15, but not of the other *gag* proteins (Eisenman et al. 1980a). Taken together with the fact that Pr130$^{gag-pol}$ can also be immunoprecipitated with antiserum against p32 (the virion protein derived from carboxyterminal cleavage of the β-polymerase subunit), these data indicate that Pr130$^{gag-pol}$ contains the complete amino acid sequences of reverse transcriptase. Although a direct precursor-product relationship has not been demonstrated between Pr180$^{gag-pol}$ and Pr130$^{gag-pol}$, it is tempting to speculate that the cleavage event that releases p15 from Pr76^{gag} may also produce Pr130$^{gag-pol}$ from Pr180$^{gag-pol}$ (see Fig. 6.3). Pr130$^{gag-pol}$ would presumably be further processed to β by removal of the p15 *gag* segment and another region of unknown origin. The fate of the aminoterminal *gag* segment of Pr180$^{gag-pol}$ is unknown, but one possibility, especially considering the proposed membrane association of MLV reverse transcriptase precursors (Witte and Baltimore 1978), is that this fragment constitutes the recently observed *gag*-related polyprotein on the cell surface (Buetti and Diggelmann 1980a).

Proper processing of reverse-transcriptase-related polyproteins probably depends on the presence of a complete polymerase gene product. Cell lines shedding two nonconditional avian retroviral mutants (SE52d and PH9), which fail to package functional reverse transcriptase, synthesize different *gag-pol*-related proteins that are

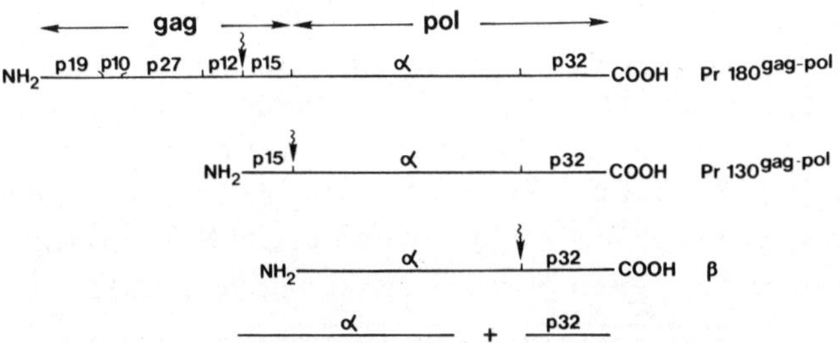

Figure 6.3 Structure and processing of the precursor to ASLV reverse transcriptase. Pr180$^{gag-pol}$, the 180,000-dalton product of the *gag* and *pol* genes, is first cleaved within the *gag* polypeptide region between p12 and p15. This cut liberates Pr130$^{gag-pol}$, which is further processed by removal of the p15 segment to generate the β subunit of reverse transcriptase. Removal of the carboxyterminal region of β results in production of the α subunit and the p32 endonuclease. Cleavage of Pr180$^{gag-pol}$ and Pr130$^{gag-pol}$ occurs within the infected cell, whereas cleavage of $\beta \rightarrow \alpha +$ p32 occurs within the virion.

deleted in the polymerase polypeptide region. These mutant proteins, which can be considered truncated forms of Pr180$^{gag\text{-}pol}$, are defective as precursors to reverse transcriptase, are not specifically cleaved, and are significantly more stable than Pr180$^{gag\text{-}pol}$ (Eisenman et al. 1980a). As both defective polyproteins apparently possess intact *gag* polypeptide regions, their inability to be processed further would argue that the mere presence of the cleavage site at p15 is not sufficient to ensure processing. The polymerase sequences may therefore be required to attain the proper conformation or cellular localization for cleavage.

Cleavage of Pr180$^{gag\text{-}pol}$ and removal of p15 from Pr130$^{gag\text{-}pol}$ apparently occur within the infected cell, rather than in viral particles, as newly budded virions contain neither of these proteins. Such virions possess a population of β subunits, a portion of which are converted to α subunits, and presumably the p32 endonuclease upon further incubation (Hayman 1978a; Schiff and Grandgenett 1978; Eisenman et al. 1980a).

As discussed in a previous section, the cleavage of β in the virion occurs by removal of a carboxyterminal segment of about 32,000 daltons, thus producing p32 and the α subunit. Mature reverse transcriptase subunits have not been detected in infected cells.

A processing scheme consistent with the available evidence is diagramed in Figure 6.3. The production of reverse transcriptase can be thought of as a two-stage process. In the first stage, the intracellular precursors Pr180$^{gag\text{-}pol}$ and Pr130$^{gag\text{-}pol}$ are cleaved by successive removal of their *gag* regions. The cleavage of Pr130$^{gag\text{-}pol}$ probably occurs at the time of, and may even be activated by, virus budding. The second stage, occurring during and immediately after the budding process, involves the cleavage of β. As p15 is capable of mediating the in vitro cleavage of $\beta \rightarrow \alpha$ (Moelling et al. 1980), the presence of p15 in Pr130$^{gag\text{-}pol}$ and its presumed release during budding may set in motion the final processing steps in reverse transcriptase maturation.

At least one other polypeptide modification occurs during processing. The phosphorylation of Pr180$^{gag\text{-}pol}$ probably occurs only within the *gag* region of the polyprotein, since Pr130$^{gag\text{-}pol}$ contains the same polymerase sequences but is not phosphorylated (Eisenman et al. 1980a). At a later stage, however, the β subunit is phosphorylated at its carboxyl terminus, since its subsequent cleavage results in the appearance of the p32 phosphoprotein (D. Grandgenett, pers. comm.) and the nonphosphorylated α subunit (Hizi and Joklik 1977b; Schiff and Grandgenett 1978). No definite role has been assigned to these differential phosphorylations, although it is plausible that they may regulate nucleic acid binding and/or polypeptide cleavage.

3. The env-*gene Proteins*

The glycosylated envelope proteins of retroviruses are synthesized from a subgenomic-size mRNA, at a different subcellular location, and are subject to a different set of modifications than the translational products of *gag* and *pol.* These differences must largely be due to the facts that they are glycoproteins and that their ultimate localization is on the outer surface of the virion envelope. As we shall see, the biosynthesis and processing of retroviral envelope glycoproteins have many features in common with the production of cellular transmembrane proteins, secreted proteins, or other viral envelope proteins (Blobel and Dobberstein 1975; Rothman and Lenard 1977; Wirth et al. 1977; Wickner 1979). First of all, unlike the *gag* and *gag-pol* mRNAs, the *env* mRNA appears to be membrane-linked, as judged by experiments localizing both RSV 28S virus-specific mRNA and glycoprotein precursor on membrane-bound polyribosomes (Lee et al. 1979; Purchio et al. 1980). The 28S mRNA has been shown to be a subgenomic-size RSV RNA consisting of a region, derived from the 5′ end of genomic 39S RNA, spliced onto the *env-src*-U_3 (or *env*-U_3 for the 21S mRNA of ALV) genetic regions (Hayward 1977; Mellon and Duesberg 1977; S. Weiss et al. 1977). RNA of this size isolated from infected cells, virions, or fragmented 39S genomes directs the in vitro synthesis of a polypeptide containing antigenic determinants of gp85 (Pawson et al. 1977, 1980; Purchio et al. 1977). Moreover, microinjection of this subgenomic RNA fraction, derived from ALV virions, into cells shedding glycoprotein-less virus (e.g., BH-RSV[−]; see Chapter 7) results in envelope complementation of the defective virus (Stacey et al. 1977). Thus, the finding that this subgenomic virus-specific mRNA size class is present on membrane-bound polyribosomes suggests that the envelope glycoproteins are initially synthesized on membranes.

Cell-free protein synthesis and glycosylation-inhibition studies have also provided insight into the nature of the primary *env*-gene translational product. When ASLV-infected cells are treated with tunicamycin or 2-deoxyglucose, inhibitors of initial glycosylation events, a nonglycosylated polypeptide of approximately 57,000 daltons ($P57^{env}$) can be immunoprecipitated with monospecific antiserum against the envelope glycoproteins (Diggelmann 1979; Stohrer and Hunter 1979). $P57^{env}$ possesses tryptic peptides of both gp85 and gp37, implying that it is the primary nonglycosylated *env*-protein precursor. However, when the size of this protein was compared directly with that of the protein synthesized in cell-free translation of 28S mRNA, it was found to be approximately 6000 daltons smaller than the in vitro product. In agreement with this difference, DNA sequencing of the *env*-gene region predicts a segment of 64 amino acids rich in hydrophobic residues, preceding the start of the mature gp85 amino acid sequence (E. Hunter and D. Schwartz, pers. comm.). These data provide evidence for the presence of a classical "membrane signal sequence" on nascent chains of the *env* translational product (Milstein et al. 1972; Blobel and Dobberstein 1975). Of particular interest here is the unusual length of the extension on the primary *env* product, which is about twice the size of signal sequences previously observed. Some form of transmembrane signal sequence, perhaps similar to that found at the carboxyterminal region of the immunoglobulin μ chain (Rogers et al. 1980), may also exist to anchor gp37 in the viral membrane.

Examination of the nucleotide sequence of RSV (Appendix E) and determination of the splice points used to produce *env* mRNA suggest some unusual aspects to the *env* signal peptide. First, the nucleotide sequence reveals a substantial overlap (about 130 nucleotides) of the 3′ terminus of *pol* and the 5′ terminus of *env*, with the two genes in different reading frames (D. Schwartz et al., pers. comm.). Second, the splice donor point resides inside the *gag* gene, approximately six codons from the 5′ end (P. Hackett et al.; D. Schwartz et al., both pers. comm.), and the splice acceptor point appears to lie eight codons from what had seemed to be the 5′ end of *env* in the genomic sequence (D. Schwartz et al., pers. comm.). Thus, the signal peptide of the *env* precursor is probably a hybrid, encoded partially in *gag* and mainly in *env*, the latter sequence overlapping with *pol*. Confirmation of these predictions will be important to an understanding of how the nascent protein associates with membranes.

The putative *env* signal sequence is probably cleaved rapidly from the nascent polypeptide chain, since it is absent from the nonglycosylated $P57^{env}$ polypeptide synthesized in vivo. In fact, the nascent polypeptide is probably glycosylated during its passage across the endoplasmic reticulum, since P57^{env} itself is detected only in ASLV-infected cells treated with glycosylation inhibitors (Diggelmann 1979; Stohrer and Hunter 1979). In pulse-labeled untreated cells, the major *env*-related protein is a 92,000-dalton glycoprotein (gPr92^{env}) containing sequences of both gp85 and gp37 in the order NH_2-gp85-gp37-COOH (England et al. 1977; Moelling and Hayami 1977; Buchhagen and Hanafusa 1978; Hayman 1978b; Klemenz and Diggelmann 1978). The inhibition of glycosylation observed in the presence of tunicamycin indicates that addition of the oligomannosyl cores to the polypeptide chains occurs via a lipid-linked dolichol intermediate (Takatsuki and Tamura 1971; for review, see Lennarz 1975). Although the enzymic machinery involved in carbohydrate chain addition to retrovirus and other small envelope glycoproteins is probably directed by the amino acid sequence of the viral polypeptide, the glycosylating enzymes themselves are likely to be host-cell-specific, considering the limited coding capacity of these viruses (Sefton 1976).

Pulse-chase experiments show gPr92^{env} to be slowly metabolized to generate gp85 and gp37 (England et al. 1977; Moelling and Hayami 1977). Because gPr92^{env} itself is deficient in fucose compared with gp85 (England et al. 1977), cleavage of the precursor may be accompanied by a final stage of glycosylation. The other observed modification, disulfide-bond formation between gp85 and gp37 (Leamnson and Halpern 1976), is also likely to occur at this stage, but whether it precedes or follows cleavage is not known. A proposed cleavage scheme is depicted in Figure 6.4.

The cleavage protease(s) involved in gPr92^{env} processing has not been identified. The inability of p15^{gag} to cut gPr92^{env} in vitro (Moelling et al. 1980), as well as the observation that the *gag*-protein-deficient mutant SE33 and the endogenous provirus *ev*-6, which lacks *gag* sequences, process the envelope precursor (Linial et al. 1980), argues against involvement of *gag*-gene products.

The site and timing of final cleavage are somewhat in dispute. Using subcellular fractionation techniques, cleavage of gPr92^{env} apparently occurs in the endoplasmic reticulum, followed by transport of the cleavage products to the plasma membrane (Hayman 1978b) where assembly of disulfide-linked gp85 and gp37 into virions occurs (Leamnson and Halpern 1976). However, rapid cleavage of gPr92^{env} has been observed in newly budded virions (Klemenz and Diggelmann 1979). Although it is difficult to reconcile these two

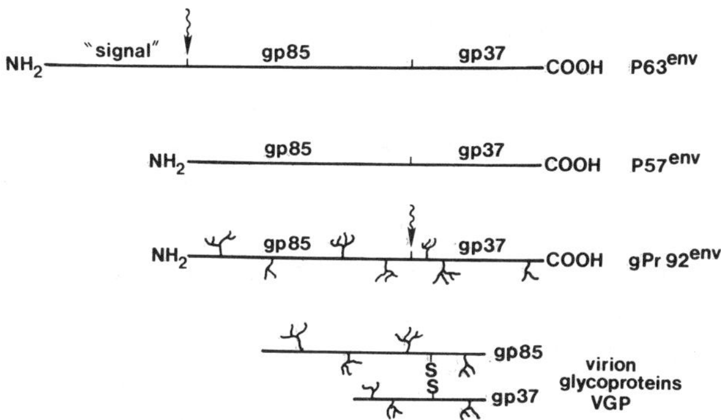

Figure 6.4 Maturation of ASLV envelope glycoproteins. The polypeptide designated P63^{env} is believed to be that synthesized by cell-free translation of *env* mRNA. Its in vivo counterpart is probably cleaved as a nascent chain after insertion into the endoplasmic reticulum. Cleavage at the site indicated by the arrow would remove the 64-amino-acid hydrophobic "signal" sequence. P57^{env} is the proposed structure of a protein observed in vivo after treatment of infected cells with inhibitors of glycosylation. Although the signal peptide is believed to have been cleaved from P57^{env}, suggesting membrane insertion, further processing does not appear to occur. In pulse-labeled ASLV-infected cells, gPr92^{env} is readily detected and is presumed to be derived from P63^{env} after membrane insertion, removal of the signal sequence, and glycosylation. Cleavage, disulfide-bond formation, and further glycosylation of gPr92^{env} generate the viral glycoproteins (VGP) (see text for details).

views, recent experiments with a *gag*-deficient mutant (SE33), which synthesizes and cleaves gPr92^{env} to functional products in the absence of particle production, would argue that virion formation is at least not a prerequisite to cleavage (Linial et al. 1980). By analogy with MLVs, we might indeed expect to find a large pool of mature glycoproteins on the cell surface (Witte et al. 1977). With another nonconditional mutant (SE521), gPr92^{env} is synthesized and is detected on the cell surface but is not further processed. The otherwise normal noninfectious particles released from these cells possess neither mature glycoproteins nor precursor (Linial et al. 1980). Although the detailed nature of the lesions in these two mutants remains unknown, these experiments provide further support for the idea, initially derived from studies with envelope deletion mutants, that particle formation and glycoprotein assembly can be uncoupled events. Furthermore, there appears to be cleavage and functional assembly of endogenous glycoproteins in the absence of C-type virion budding (Love and Weiss 1974; Bosch et al. 1978).

D. Assembly of Viral Proteins into Virions

As should be clear from the preceding sections, quite a wealth of information has been accumulated over the last few years concerning the nature and processing of the primary translational products of the genes controlling avian retrovirus multiplication. In contrast, almost nothing is known about the mechanics of particle formation. Several general themes have evolved, however, that will probably guide future experimental approaches in this area. One of these is the key role that *gag*-protein precursors and their proper cleavage products play in the genesis of a physical viral particle. Experiments in both the avian and murine retrovirus systems indicate that viral particles (albeit noninfectious ones) can be generated in the absence of envelope glycoproteins (Weiss 1969; Scheele and Hanafusa 1971; Kawai and Hanafusa 1973; Linial et al. 1980; Ramsay and Hayman 1980), reverse transcriptase (Hanafusa et al. 1972; Eisenman et al. 1980a; Ramsay and Hayman 1980), or genomic RNA (Levin et al. 1974; Linial et al. 1978). On the other hand, no physical particles are ever produced when avian virus *gag*-related polyproteins are either not synthesized or not cleaved (Eisenman et al. 1975, 1978; Bister et al. 1977; Hayman et al. 1979). Thus, $Pr76^{gag}$ can perhaps be thought of as a "particle-making machine." It should be stressed, however, that the production of infectious particles must ultimately depend on the synthesis and processing of *pol*- and *env*-, as well as of *gag*-gene products.

Although the evidence points to *gag* proteins as the crucial elements in assembly, there is still no clear idea of the mechanism by which they are assembled to form particles. In the avian system, it appears that cleavage of *gag, pol,* and *env* polyproteins immediately precedes or accompanies particle shedding. One can then speculate that processing in some manner activates virion morphogenesis. This picture may be even more complicated for the mammalian viruses, where significant levels of *gag* precursors have been detected in viral particles (Jamjoom et al. 1975). It has been demonstrated that the extracellular maturation of the core structure of murine retroviruses, as observed in the electron microscope, may be related to cleavage of the particle-associated precursor (Yoshinaka and Luftig 1977a; Pinter and de Harven 1980).

If processing activates virion morphogenesis, then what activates processing? The availability of cleavage-initiating proteases is one likely possibility. The physical association of *gag* polyproteins within the cell membrane is another. At present there is little direct evidence for association of *gag*-polyprotein cleavage with the cell membrane. Indirect evidence includes the often-visualized process of core formation just under the membrane (Sarkar et al. 1972) and the report that cleavage of ASLV $Pr76^{gag}$ in crude cell extracts is inhibited by agents that affect membrane-protein association (Vogt et al. 1975). In addition, an inhibitor of lipid biosynthesis prevents $Pr76^{gag}$ cleavage and infectious virus release from treated cells (Goldfine et al. 1978). A model has been presented that posits that *gag* and *gag-pol* polyproteins coalesce under the plasma membrane and interact at their amino termini with a transmembrane segment of the envelope-glycoprotein complex, and at their carboxyl termini with genomic RNA (Bolognesi et al. 1978). The evidence that particles can form in the absence of *env*-gene products indicates that the interaction of *gag* proteins with envelope glycoproteins, though it may occur, is not essential for virion formation. A similar situation pertains for other enveloped viruses such as VSV (Schnitzer et al. 1979). Thus, there may be other markers in the plasma membrane to direct *gag* proteins to the proper sites of assembly. In addition, with both specific viral RNA-binding and lipid-binding functions located at or proximal to the amino termini of *gag*-protein precursors, the precursors must assume a rather complex conformation in their proposed membrane association.

The notion that *gag* precursors may be organized under the plasma membrane has received some support from protein-protein cross-linking experiments. These studies show the formation of only homotypic multimeric complexes between *gag* proteins when intact ASLV virions are treated with chemical cross-linking reagents, consistent with the idea that the virion proteins are organized in concentric shells (Pepinsky et al. 1980). Such shells could perhaps most easily be derived from cleavage of parallel arrays of membrane-stabilized *gag* precursors.

A related and, in one sense, more challenging problem in retrovirus assembly is the manner by which virus-specific genomic RNA is preferentially packaged into virions. Out of the vast background of cellular structural RNAs, tRNAs, and cellular and viral mRNAs, the viral-particle-making apparatus must select and incorporate its own genome. This selection is certainly not absolute, since virions have been found to contain not only host proteins and enzymes, but also rRNA, tRNA, and subgenomic viral mRNAs. However, the RNA content of wild-type virus is predominantly genomic.

One candidate for a specific selecting molecule is reverse transcriptase, which has already been implicated as a mediator of primer tRNA packaging (Levin and Seidman 1979; Sawyer and Hanafusa 1979; Peters and Hu 1980). However, several *pol* mutants whose particles fail to incorporate reverse transcriptase nonetheless package genomic RNA; thus, it does not appear that polymerase is essential for RNA selection.

A more likely candidate than reverse transcriptase is p19 whose specific RNA-binding properties may play a role. This protein has already been implicated in the control of viral mRNA processing (Leis et al. 1981). Since unprocessed genomic RNA should contain more p19-binding sites than viral or cellular mRNA, selection may proceed on the basis of a critical number of p19 molecules bound to RNA. To carry this speculation further, a change in *gag*-precursor conformation in the membrane might accompany both the optimal binding of p19 and the massive nonspecific binding of p12. Such a conformational change could trigger cleavage, core formation, and budding. However, since particle formation occurs in the absence of genomic RNA, cleavage can proceed in any event, possibly because of nonspecific RNA binding by p12 and p19. Indeed both the packaging mutant SE21Q1b and MLV shed from actinomycin-D-treated cells incorporate cellular RNAs (Gallis et al. 1979; Levin and Seidman 1979). In the case of the mutant SE21Q1b (Linial et al. 1978), cellular mRNAs appear to be packaged on a random basis in preference to genomic RNA (Gallis et al. 1979), although it has been shown that specific VSV mRNAs can be selectively packaged in coinfected cells (Yakobson and Weiss 1981). The packaging of cellular RNAs into virions, especially those containing reverse transcriptase, may itself be an event of biological significance. The acquisition of new oncogenes to generate defective and nondefective transforming retroviruses may well occur by recombination between copackaged genomic and cellular RNAs (see Chapters 7 and 9). Thus, the specificity of packaging may have profound consequences for virus evolution.

III. MURINE C-TYPE RETROVIRUSES

A. Murine C-type Retroviral Particles and Their Protein Constituents

MLVs are enveloped particles with a nucleoprotein core. The viral envelope consists of a lipid bilayer with protruding knobs. An inner coat (or matrix) lies under the envelope and surrounds the core. The core structure consists of an icosahedral protein shell surrounding the genomic RNA that is complexed with protein (Nermut et al. 1972; for review, see Schafer and Bolognesi 1977). The viral core also contains the virus-coded reverse transcriptase (Bolognesi et al. 1973; Lange et al. 1973). Table 6.3 contains a list of MLV-encoded structural and nonstructural proteins that will be described in the following sections.

1. Internal Structural gag *Proteins*

The internal structural proteins are products of the viral *gag* gene and consist of four components: the major capsid polypeptide of 30,000 daltons (p30), a hydrophobic protein of 15,000 daltons (p15), an acidic phosphoprotein of 12,000 daltons (pp12), and a basic protein of 10,000 daltons (p10). The name *gag* was given to these proteins because the prototype protein of this class (p30) was found to bear the major antigenic determinants for group-specific antigenicity in early studies (Gregoriades and Old 1969; Schafer et al. 1969; Oroszlan et al. 1971b). It should be noted, however, that most of the *gag* proteins also carry type-specific and/or interspecies-specific determinants to greater or lesser degrees.

a. Map Order within the gag *Gene.* The physical order of *gag* proteins within the *gag* gene is NH_2-p15-pp12-p30-p10-COOH. The experiments leading to this conclusion utilized the fact that the individual *gag* proteins are derived by proteolytic cleavage of the precursor polyprotein, $Pr65^{gag}$. Barbacid et al. (1976a) studied cells transformed with different isolates of MSV. As MSV genomes contain varying amounts of the *gag* gene (see Chapters 4 and 7) depending on strain, more or less of the carboxyterminal portions of the *gag* gene have been deleted. Using radioimmunoassays for each of the *gag* proteins to analyze the *gag*-protein content of these cells, p10 could be assigned as the carboxyterminal protein, with p30 adjacent to it. Analysis of intermediate cleavage products of $Pr65^{gag}$ indicated that pp12 is also adjacent to p30, and, from this, the order of all four proteins in the *gag* gene was deduced. In cells infected with temperature-sensitive mutants of Rauscher MLV (Ra-MLV), which show impaired processing of $Pr65^{gag}$ (Reynolds and Stephenson 1977), intermediate cleavage products accumulate at the nonpermissive temperature, and a radioimmunological analysis of these intermediates yielded the same map order. A different approach involved

Table 6.3 MLV precursor polyproteins and virion proteins

Protein	Gene	Function	Localization	Structure and properties
$gP95^{gag}$	*gag*	may be precursor to $gP85^{gag}$	cell-surface membrane	glycosylated; contains sequences of $Pr65^{gag}$ and some additional aminoterminal sequences; contains GCSA antigenic determinant
$gP85^{gag}$	*gag*	unknown	cell-surface membrane	glycosylated; may lack part of p10; contains GCSA antigenic determinant
$gPr80^{gag}$	*gag*	precursor to glycosylated *gag* cell-surface proteins	rough endoplasmic reticulum	contains additional aminoterminal sequences not found in $Pr65^{gag}$; protein core = 75,000 daltons
$P75^{gag}$	*gag*	peptide core of $gPr80^{gag}$		apoprotein core of $gPr80^{gag}$; only detected after glycosidase digestion or in presence of inhibitors or glycosylation
$gP55^{gag}$	*gag*	possible cleavage product of $gP95^{gag}$	extracellular soluble protein	glycosyated
$gP45^{gag}$	*gag*	possible cleavage product of $gP95^{gag}$	extracellular soluble protein	glycosylated
$Pr65^{gag}$	*gag*	precursor to internal virion structural proteins	cytoplasm initially, later associated with membranes	only some molecules phosphorylated; NH_2-p15-pp12-p30-p10-COOH

$Pr55^{gag}$	*gag*	possible cleavage product of $Pr65^{gag}$	unknown	lacks p10 peptides
$Pr40^{gag}$	*gag*	intermediate cleavage product of $Pr65^{gag}$	cells and immature virions	contains p30 and p10 peptides
$Pr25^{gag}$	*gag*	processing intermediate	? immature virions	contains p15 and pp12 peptides; phosphorylated
$p30^{gag}$	*gag*	subunits of the core shell	virion core	neutral (pI 7.6); moderately hydrophobic
$p15^{gag}$	*gag*	may align $Pr65^{gag}$ during morphogenesis	probably resides between membrane and core or in capsid; interacts with viral membrane	very hydrophobic; pI 7.5; proline-rich; lacks methionine; contains FMR subgroup antigenic determinant
$pp12^{gag}$	*gag*	RNA binding could serve regulatory function	unknown, but may lie under viral membrane	acidic (pI 4.7); phosphorylated; minor population bound to viral RNA in type-specific manner
$p10^{gag}$	*gag*	binds to RNA	bound to RNA in RNP complex	very basic (pI 10.5)
$gPr180^{gag-pol}$	*pol*	unknown	? rough endoplasmic reticulum	fusion product of $gPr80^{gag}$ and *pol*
$Pr180^{gag-pol}$	*pol*	precursor to reverse transcriptase	cell cytoplasm and immature virions	
$Pr150^{pol}$	*pol*	possible processing intermediate	? immature virions	lacks *gag* peptides
$Pr140^{pol}$	*pol*	possible processing intermediate	? immature virions	lacks *gag* peptides
$p80^{pol}$	*pol*	transcription of genomic RNA	virion core	RNA- and DNA-dependent polymerase and hybrid-specific RNase-H activities

Table 6.3 (Continued)

$Pr80^{env}$, $Pr90^{env}$	*env*	precursor to envelope glycoproteins gp70 and p15(E)	cell and virion membranes	glycosylated; protein core = 62,000–70,000 daltons; presumed signal peptide of 10,000 daltons; NH_2-gp70-p15E-COOH (Ra-MLV has gPr90, Mo-MLV has gPr80)
$gp70^{env}$	*env*	host range; neutralization; interference; subgroup specificity	virion envelope and cell membrane; knob structure	30% carbohydrate by weight; protein core = 40,000 daltons; heterogeneous charge (pI 4.5–6.2)
$gp45^{env}$	*env*	possible degradation product of gp70		
$p15(E)^{env}$	*env*	anchors gp70 to membrane	virion envelope and cell membrane; spike structure directly associated with membrane	nonglycosylated; very hydrophobic (pI 4.4–4.6)
$p12(E)^{env}$	*env*	unknown	virion envelope only	represents aminoterminal portion of p15(E)
p24	?	proteolytic cleavage of $Pr65^{gag}$	low amounts in virions	not known whether host-coded or virus-coded

translation of Ra-MLV virion RNA in a cell-free protein-synthesizing system (Murphy and Arlinghaus 1978); the major translational product was $Pr65^{gag}$ with a variety of premature termination products (see Section III.C.1.b). Tryptic peptide analysis of these premature termination products, which lack various amounts of the carboxyl terminus of $Pr65^{gag}$, again confirmed the map order.

b. p15. p15 is the most hydrophobic of the internal structural proteins (Barbacid and Aaronson 1978) and has an approximately neutral charge. It contains approximately 45% nonpolar amino acids, lacks methionine, and is particularly rich in proline (Oroszlan et al. 1978).

The extremely hydrophobic nature of p15 suggests that it may be a constituent of the viral membrane; several other properties of p15 support this idea. First, purified p15 can associate with phospholipid vesicles (Barbacid and Aaronson 1978). Second, purification of viral membranes results in recovery of 40% of the total virion p15 (Van de Ven et al. 1978b). Third, p15 is the only internal structural protein that can be cross-linked to lipid by dimethylsuperimidate (Pepinsky and Vogt 1979). Furthermore, p15 becomes labeled after a lactoperoxidase-catalyzed reaction treatment of intact virions (Barbacid and Aaronson 1978). However, incubation of intact particles with anti-p15 serum does not lead to neutralization or to virolysis (Barbacid and Aaronson 1978). Because of these findings, the exact location of p15 in the viral particle is not yet clear. The association with the viral membrane suggests that it is the matrixlike viral protein that comprises the inner coat under the viral membrane (Pepinsky and Vogt 1979). However, purified viral cores still contain some p15 (Bolognesi et al. 1973). This has led to the proposal that p15 is actually a component of the viral capsid, which also interacts with the viral membrane (Bolognesi et al. 1978). Therefore, the hydrophobicity of p15 might be responsible for aligning $Pr65^{gag}$ in the membrane during morphogenesis (see Fig. 6.1).

Type-specific and group-specific antigenic determinants of p15 are readily demonstrated (Strand et al. 1974b; Barbacid and Aaronson 1978). On the other hand, there is little evidence for interspecies-specific antigenicity. It has also been suggested that p15 may carry the antigenic determinants that define the Friend-Moloney-Rauscher (FMR) subgroup of MLV (Strand et al. 1974b; Strand and August 1977) (see Chapter 3).

c. pp12. pp12 is an acidic phosphoprotein (pI 4.7) of 12,000 daltons. It is the only phosphoprotein in MLV virions. The phosphorylation is at serine residues, and the extent of phosphorylation per pp12 molecule is variable (Pal and Roy-Burman 1975; Pal et al. 1975). The amino acid composition indicates that the protein contains a large proportion (41%) of nonpolar residues (Oroszlan et al. 1978), but the addition of phosphates to the protein greatly alters its hydrophobicity. In fact, pp12 is one of the least hydrophobic proteins of the viral particle (Marcus et al. 1978b).

Sen et al. (1976) reported the interesting observation that pp12 interacts with virion 38S RNA in a species-specific manner; i.e., MLV pp12 will not bind to heterologous retroviral RNAs, and the homologous binding reaction cannot be competed out by heterologous pp12 molecules. It should be noted that the stoichiometry of binding indicates that only a minor fraction of the pp12 molecules in the virion is bound to RNA (about 15 molecules per 70S RNA complex). The binding of pp12 to viral RNA is influenced by the degree of pp12 phosphorylation; those pp12 molecules that bind to viral RNA are less highly phosphorylated. It has been suggested that this differential binding phenomenon might represent some sort of regulatory mechanism (Sen et al. 1977).

The location of the majority of pp12 molecules within the viral particle is unknown, as purified viral cores appear to lack pp12 completely (Bolognesi et al. 1973); presumably, the small amount of pp12 bound to viral RNA is below the level of detection. This led to the proposal that pp12 constitutes the viral inner coat (Bolognesi et al. 1978), but there is as yet no strong evidence for this supposition.

The major antigenicity of pp12 is type-specific, although some group-specific and interspecies-specific determinants can be detected (Stephenson et al. 1974). Type-specific radioimmunoassays for *gag*-gene products frequently employ this protein.

d. p30. p30 is the major component of the icosahedral shell of the viral core. It is a neutral protein and has been partially sequenced (Oroszlan et al. 1978; S. Oroszlan, T. Copeland and I. Henderson, pers. comm.) (see Appendix F). The protein is moderately hydrophobic (Marcus et al. 1978b; Swanson et al. 1978) and, as might be expected of a capsid protein, can self-associate in solution (Burnette et al. 1976).

The antigens of p30 are predominantly group-specific and provide the major antigenic determinants of MLV particles (Gregoriades and Old 1969; Schafer et al. 1969; Stephenson et al. 1974; Strand and August 1974). Radioimmunoassays utilizing this protein are the most common assays for MLV *gag* protein.

Variations in p30 have been implicated in the *Fv-1* gene restriction of MLV (see Chapters 3 and 4). NB-tropic MLV, derived by forced passage of B-tropic virus in N-type (*Fv-1*^{nn}) cells, contains p30 protein of altered electrophoretic mobility (Hopkins et al. 1977; Tennant et al. 1979). The correlation of p30 protein sequence with NB-tropism has been confirmed by two-dimensional tryptic peptide mapping (Gautsch et al. 1978a).

e. p10. This protein is a highly basic protein (pI 10.5) (Fleissner and Tress 1973; Schulein et al. 1978) with a high concentration (40%) of polar amino acids (Oroszlan et al. 1978) and is not phosphorylated. The p10 of Ra-MLV has been completely sequenced (S. Oroszlan, T. Copeland, and I. Henderson, pers. comm.) (see Appendix F) and the data suggest an actual molecular weight of 6000 daltons.

In the viral particle, p10 is located within the RNP complex, bound to viral RNA. Purification of the complex yields only RNA and p10 (Bolognesi et al. 1973). The p10 protein can be purified on the basis of its affinity for single-stranded or double-stranded nucleic acid (Davis et al. 1976), and, in viral particles, approximately 140 molecules of p10 are bound per 38S RNA molecule (Schulein et al. 1978). This protein therefore associates with the 70S viral RNA to form the RNP complex within the capsid (Nermut et al. 1972; Fleissner and Tress 1973; Bolognesi et al. 1978).

The major antigenic determinants of p10 are group-specific, with fairly strong interspecies-specific determinants and weak type-specific determinants (Barbacid et al. 1976b; Schulein et al. 1978).

2. *Reverse Transcriptase*

Reverse transcriptase is the product of the *pol* gene. There are approximately 40 molecules of reverse transcriptase per particle in Ra-MLV virions (Krakower et al. 1977). The protein has been purified from several different strains of MLV and characterized both physically and enzymically (for review, see Verma 1977). MLV reverse transcriptase is a single polypeptide of 70,000 to 80,000 daltons, as determined by SDS-polyacrylamide gel electrophoresis

(Moelling 1974; Verma 1975b; Modak and Marcus 1977). Glycerol gradient centrifugation gives a sedimentation value of approximately 4.5S for the enzymic activity, which is consistent with the results of gel analysis (Wang and Duesberg 1973; Moelling 1974; Gerard and Grandgenett 1975; Verma 1975b; Modak and Marcus 1977). This indicates that the active form of purified MLV reverse transcriptase is a monomer, in contrast to the $\alpha\beta$ dimer of avian retroviruses. However, it is still possible that the native MLV enzyme within the virion is actually a dimer, but that it is readily dissociated during purification procedures.

MLV reverse transcriptase shares antigenic determinants with some other mammalian retroviral reverse transcriptase, since antiserum raised against a heterologous viral enzyme can partially inhibit MLV enzyme activity (Parks et al. 1972; Sherr et al. 1975). Radioimmunoassays using reverse transcriptase reveal approximately equal levels of group-specific and type-specific determinants (Krakower et al. 1977). For a detailed discussion of the various enzymic properties of MLV reverse transcriptase, see Chapter 5.

3. *Envelope Proteins*

The viral envelope proteins are products of the *env* gene and consist of two principal components: a glycoprotein of approximately 70,000 daltons (gp70) (Nowinski et al. 1972; Kennel et al. 1973; Strand and August 1973; Witte et al. 1973) and a nonglycosylated protein of 15,000 daltons (p15[E]) (Ikeda et al. 1975). In addition, a smaller protein of 12,000 daltons (p12[E]), which is related to p15(E), is present in minor amounts (van Zaane et al. 1976; Karshin et al. 1977). A glycoprotein of 45,000 daltons (gp45) is also present in variable amounts and may actually represent a degradation product of gp70 (Elder et al. 1977a; Krantz et al. 1977; Henderson et al. 1978).

a. gp70. gp70, the major envelope protein, is responsible for several biological properties of the virus. First, as this protein is the major surface component of the virus, it is the principal determinant against which neutralizing antibodies are elicited (Kennel et al. 1973; Hunsmann et al. 1974; Ikeda et al. 1974; Steeves et al. 1974). The antigenicity of gp70 is not determined solely by the carbohydrate moieties, since enzymic removal of a majority of the carbohydrate does not abolish antigenicity (Bolognesi et al. 1975b). gp70 molecules carry antigenic determinants that are MLV group-specific (Kennel et al. 1973; Strand and August 1974), type-specific for certain MLV strains (Strand and August 1974; Hino et al. 1976), and also interspecies-specific in being shared with other mammalian C-type viruses (Strand and August 1973).

The adsorption of viral particles to cells is a second important biological property attributable to gp70. This adsorption takes place by an interaction of cell-surface receptors with gp70 molecules on the virion surface, followed by uptake of the particle into the cell. Receptor recognition can be used to define host range and interference groups: (1) ecotropic viruses, which infect cells of murine origin; (2) xenotropic viruses, which infect cells of many nonmurine species; (3) amphotropic viruses, which infect both mouse cells and cells of other species; and (4) dualtropic viruses (e.g., MCF [mink cell focus-forming] viruses), which have the host range of amphotropic viruses but are recombinants between ecotropic and xenotropic viruses with which they share neutralization properties (see Chapters 2 and 3). The biological interference patterns of MLVs are directly correlated with the ability of the viral gp70 to bind to the cell (DeLarco and Todaro 1976). Recently, a candidate protein for a surface receptor of gp70 has been described (Landen and Fox 1980).

gp70 is approximately 30% carbohydrate by weight (Marquardt et al. 1977). The polypeptide core of gp70 is approximately 40,000 daltons, as inferred from the fact that the polypeptide core of the *env*-protein precursor ($Pr80^{env}$) is about 62,000 daltons for Moloney MLV (Mo-MLV) (Edwards and Fan 1979; Witte and Wirth 1979) (see Section III.C.3). $Pr80^{env}$ contains the polypeptide sequences for gp70 and p15(E). Nucleic acid sequencing data indicate that the actual molecular weight of p15(E) is 22,000 daltons (Sutcliffe et al. 1980a). The core of gp70 presumably accounts for the majority of the other sequences in $Pr80^{env}$.

The oligosaccharide residues on gp70 are terminal sialic acid residues, which account for the heterogeneous charge characteristics (pI 4.5–6.2) (Witte et al. 1977). There are at least two oligosaccharide side chains in Mo-MLV gp70, as determined from the number of intermediate cleavage products generated by endoglycosidase-H digestion of $Pr80^{env}$ (Witte and Wirth 1979). More detailed analyses show that all of the carbohydrate side chains of gp70 are *N*-

asparagine-linked oligosaccharides; several dualtropic MLVs contain both complex and high-mannose oligosaccharides. Ecotropic MLV isolates additionally contain a unique complex oligosaccharide (Kemp et al. 1979, 1980), and endogenous ecotropic AKR-MLV appears to contain only complex oligosaccharides (Rosner et al. 1980a). The differences in glycosylation patterns are virus-specified, most likely due to the presence or absence of virus-coded putative glycosylation signals (Donis-Keller et al. 1980).

Structural comparisons of gp70 molecules from different MLV strains have been performed by iodination of purified gp70 followed by two-dimensional tryptic peptide analysis (Elder et al. 1977a). Molecules of gp70 from different exogenous ecotropic MLV strains are very diverse, whereas endogenous ecotropic viruses are more closely related as a group. Xenotropic virus gp70 molecules fall into two groups: one group has a unique pattern and the other group resembles amphotropic virus gp70. Thus, relatedness of gp70 proteins, as measured by peptide mapping at least, is not accurately correlated with that determined by biological interference groups. It should be noted, however, that the peptide maps of gp70 proteins labeled in vitro are influenced by a variety of factors, including primary peptide sequence, extent of glycosylation, tertiary structure, and the availability of amino acid residues for iodination.

Dualtropic MCF viruses are recombinant within the gp70 moiety of the *env* gene, with peptide sequences derived from both ecotropic and xenotropic parents (Elder et al. 1977b). More recent studies on a Rauscher MCF virus, using monoclonal antibodies (Niman and Elder 1980), showed that the aminoterminal portion of the MCF gp70 was derived from the ecotropic parent and part or all of the carboxyterminal portion was derived from a xenotropic parent.

b. p15(E) and p12(E). The other major protein component of the MLV envelope is p15(E), a virus-coded protein with a molecular weight of 15,000 daltons, as determined by conventional measurements (Ikeda et al. 1975). This protein is not glycosylated and has a relatively narrow isoelectric focusing range (pI 4.4–4.6) (Witte et al. 1977). It is the most hydrophobic MLV virion protein (Marcus et al. 1978b), and this characteristic is reflected in its tight association with the viral membrane.

The relationship between p12(E) and p15(E) has recently been determined by comparative amino acid sequencing (S. Oroszlan, pers. comm.) (see Appendix C); they share amino termini but differ at their carboxyl termini. Thus, p12(E) is derived from p15(E) by cleavage of carboxyterminal peptides (see Section III.C.3.b).

Recently, a third product of the *env* gene has been postulated, the R or rightmost gene product. This was predicted from the nucleic acid sequence of the 3′ region of the Mo-MLV *env* gene, showing an open reading frame for polypeptides that was interpreted to be in excess (by 10,000 daltons) of that required for p15(E) (Sutcliffe et al. 1980a). Antiserum raised against a chemically synthesized oligopeptide from the carboxyl terminus of the postulated R peptide precipitates $Pr80^{env}$ but not p12(E) (Sutcliffe et al. 1980b). However, more recent amino acid sequence data of the amino terminus and carboxyl terminus of p12(E) indicate that almost the entire 3′ open reading frame is required to code for p12(E) (S. Oroszlan, pers. comm.). Therefore, R is best considered to be that portion of the carboxyl terminus of p15(E) (approximately 16 amino acids) that is cleaved off during processing to p12(E) (S. Oroszlan and R. Lerner, pers. comm.) (see also Chapter 4 and Appendix C).

c. Arrangement of Proteins in the Membrane. Both gp70 and p15(E) are exposed on the external surface of the viral particle, as each is sensitive to digestion of intact viral particles with protease (Witte et al. 1977; Montelaro et al. 1978). gp70 comprises the virus knobs and can be iodinated (Kennel et al. 1973; Witte et al. 1973; McLellan and August 1976). The p15(E) moiety is more closely associated with the membrane than is gp70, because surface labeling of intact virions does not label p15(E) (Schneider and Hunsmann 1978). Additionally, monoclonal antibodies against p15(E) mediate virus lysis, whereas monoclonal antibodies to gp70 do not (Oroszlan and Nowinski 1980).

In the viral membrane, a minor fraction of p15(E) and gp70 molecules are found associated in a disulfide-linked complex (Leamnson et al. 1977; Witte et al. 1977; Montelaro et al. 1978; Pinter et al. 1978). In contrast, most of the avian retrovirus gp85 is disulfide-linked to gp37 (see Section II.A.3). The commonly held view is that p15(E) helps to anchor gp70 in the membrane by covalent disulfide bonds as well as by weaker noncovalent bonds. The weaker bonds may explain why most of the gp70 molecules from viral particles of certain MLV strains are lost during preparative procedures such as centrifugation (Witter et al. 1973).

B. Virus-coded Proteins That Do Not Appear in Viral Particles

Whereas all three of the MLV genes code for proteins that are constituents of the virion, not all virus-coded proteins are eventually incorporated into viral particles. Excess amounts of virion proteins such as gp70 may be synthesized, and some never enter virions. Also, gp70 and/or p30 is produced in some normal virus-negative mouse tissues (see Chapter 10). Furthermore, MLV-infected cells produce a glycosylated *gag* polyprotein that appears at the cell surface but does not enter virions.

1. gp70

gp70, the MLV envelope glycoprotein, is also present at the cell surface in regions not associated with maturation of viral particles, as measured by immunoelectron microscopy (Aoki et al. 1972). The cell-surface gp70 molecules contain fewer terminal sialic acid residues than those incorporated into virions produced by the same cell (Buetti and Diggelmann 1980b); this property could mediate a differential assembling process. Also, gp70 is expressed in tissues of mice that do not express other viral proteins (Strand et al. 1974a, 1977; Del Villano et al. 1975; McClintock et al. 1977). Endogenous gp70 is found in epithelial and lymphoid tissues and in particularly large amounts in tissues of the male genital tract and in seminal fluid (Lerner et al. 1976). Furthermore, gp70 contains the G_{IX} antigen detected in mice, an antigen whose immunogenicity apparently resides in the presence or absence of a single glycosylation site (Tung et al. 1975; Donis-Keller et al. 1980; Rosner et al. 1980b) (see also Chapters 2 and 4). Thus, gp70 appears to be expressed during normal mouse development, and it has been suggested that it might play some physiological role in differentiation (Lerner et al. 1976).

2. Glycosylated Cell-surface gag *Polyproteins*

The normally internal virion *gag* proteins are also present as glycosylated polyprotein forms at the cell surface. This was first observed in leukemic cells from AKR-strain mice (Tung et al. 1976), but it is now apparent that this protein is a universal feature of MLV-infected cells. Glycosylated *gag* polyprotein has also been identified in erythrocytes infected with the Friend strain of MLV (Fr-MLV) (Evans et al. 1977) and in fibroblasts productively infected with Mo-MLV (Edwards and Fan 1979; Buetti and Diggelmann 1980b), Ra-MLV

(Schultz et al. 1979), and AKR MLV (Y. C. Lin, S. Edwards, and H. Fan, pers. comm.). The surface location is evident from accessibility to lactoperoxidase iodination (Tung et al. 1976; Ledbetter et al. 1977; Buetti and Diggelmann 1980b), and glycosylation is demonstrated by metabolic labeling with radioactive sugars or binding to lectin columns (Tung et al. 1976; Evans et al. 1977; Ledbetter et al. 1977; Edwards and Fan 1979; Schultz et al. 1979). The cell-surface *gag* polyprotein exists as two molecular-weight species of 95,000 and 85,000 daltons, gP95^{gag} and gP85^{gag} (the designation gP is an extension of the standard nomenclature conventions for retroviral proteins and indicates a glycosylated polyprotein). Kinetic experiments indicate that gP95^{gag} may be the precursor to gP85^{gag} (Ledbetter et al. 1978). Also, gP95^{gag} may be cleaved into two fragments of 55,000 and 40,000 daltons and released from the cell surface (Edwards and Fan 1979; Ledbetter 1979). In fact, at steady state, these two extracellular cleavage fragments represent the majority of the glycosylated *gag* polyproteins produced by cells infected with some virus strains.

Antisera directed against any of the four *gag* proteins will immunoprecipitate gP95^{gag} (Ledbetter et al. 1977; Tung et al. 1977), which originally suggested that it might represent a glycosylated form of Pr65^{gag}, the precursor of the internal structural proteins. It was also noted that antisera to three of the *gag* proteins, but not to p10, immunoprecipitated gP85^{gag}; this suggested that gP85^{gag} might be derived from gP95^{gag} by a cleavage that removes the p10 (carboxy-terminal) portion of the *gag* polyprotein. However, tryptic peptide analysis indicated that gP85^{gag} actually contains at least some peptide sequences of p10 (Ledbetter et al. 1978). More recent experiments indicate that conversion of gP95^{gag} to gP85^{gag} may indeed involve loss of some p10 peptides (Tung and Fleissner 1980). It is unclear whether the conversion involves removal of peptides only, removal of sugars, or a conformational change.

The glycosylated *gag* polyprotein differs from Pr65^{gag} in two ways: it contains sugar residues and it contains additional peptide sequences at the amino terminus. This polyprotein is synthesized independently of Pr65^{gag} from a precursor polyprotein of 80,000 daltons, gPr80^{gag} (see Section III.C.1.c).

Glycosylated *gag* polyproteins carry the antigenic determinants of the Gross cell-surface antigen (GCSA). GCSA antigen was originally defined as an antigen on leukemic cells in AKR mice (Old et al.

1965); appearance of this antigen was correlated with the onset of leukemia. GCSA antigen is present on leukemic lymphocytes, but is not present in virus released from the cells (Aoki et al. 1972). The appearance of glycosylated *gag* polyprotein on AKR mouse lymphocytes coincides with GCSA appearance, and experiments with appropriate typing sera established that $gP95^{gag}$ and $gP85^{gag}$ carry the GCSA determinant (Ledbetter and Nowinski 1977; Snyder et al. 1977). AKR tumor cells are not the only cells that carry GCSA antigen. All cells, fibroblasts as well as lymphocytes, that produce ecotropic or dualtropic MLV are GCSA-positive, whereas cells producing xenotropic virus are GCSA-negative (O'Donnell and Stockert 1976; O'Donnell et al. 1980). The high level of GCSA on preleukemic AKR mouse lymphocytes is now believed to result from amplification of viral expression due to superinfection of the cells with dualtropic MCF virus (Kawashima et al. 1976; O'Donnell et al. 1980). It should also be emphasized, however, that GCSA-negative cells infected with xenotropic MLV do produce glycosylated cell-surface *gag* polyproteins (S. Edwards and H. Fan, pers. comm.). Thus, GCSA can be considered a type-specific or subgroup-specific determinant of cell-surface *gag* polyprotein.

Glycosylated *gag* polyprotein is present in virtually all MLV-infected cells and exhibits an affinity for extracellular matrices (S. Edwards and H. Fan, pers. comm.). The ubiquity suggests that it might play a role in the virus life cycle. Analogous proteins are also detected as minor products in cells infected by avian C-type retroviruses (Buetti and Diggelmann 1980a). Recently, several independent isolates of Mo-MLV-infected cells deficient in surface *gag* polyprotein have been isolated; most but not all are deficient in the production of viral-particles (Edwards and Fan 1981; Fitting et al. 1981). This correlation suggests that glycosylated *gag* polyprotein might be involved in virus maturation.

C. Biosynthesis and Processing of MLV-specific Proteins

1. The gag-*gene Proteins*

a. The Primary Translation Products. When MLV-infected cells are labeled with radioactive amino acids for short periods and immunoprecipitated with anti-*gag* serum, three *gag*-related polyproteins are detected. These polyproteins are 65,000, 80,000, and 180,000 daltons in size and are called $Pr65^{gag}$, $gPr80^{gag}$, and $Pr180^{gag\text{-}pol}$, respectively. $Pr65^{gag}$ and $gPr80^{gag}$ are synthesized in approximately equal amounts, whereas $Pr180^{gag\text{-}pol}$ is synthesized in 10- to 20-fold lower amounts (Jamjoom et al. 1977). All three polyproteins are detected after extremely short labels, indicating that they are independent translation products, although in early reports it was suggested that $Pr65^{gag}$ was derived from $gPr80^{gag}$ by cleavage (Arcement et al. 1977; Murphy et al. 1979). Evidence for the independent synthesis of $Pr65^{gag}$ and $gPr80^{gag}$ is discussed in the following sections. It is now clear that these three polyproteins are further modified and processed independently into three different sets of products. $Pr65^{gag}$ is analogous to avian retrovirus $Pr76^{gag}$ and is cleaved to give the internal structural *gag* proteins of the viral particle. $gPr80^{gag}$ is the precursor to the glycosylated *gag* polyprotein found at the cell surface and is itself a glycoprotein. $Pr180^{gag\text{-}pol}$ is the precursor to reverse transcriptase.

b. The $Pr65^{gag}$ Pathway. $Pr65^{gag}$ was the first *gag* polyprotein identified in MLV-infected cells (Jamjoom et al. 1975, 1977; Stephenson et al. 1975a; van Zaane et al. 1975, 1976; Shapiro et al. 1976). Immunoprecipitation with antisera specific for different *gag* proteins and peptide mapping show that it contains the peptide sequences of all four *gag* proteins. Two lines of evidence indicate that $Pr65^{gag}$ is the metabolic precursor to the *gag* proteins of the virion. First, kinetic pulse-chase experiments show the loss of radioactivity from $Pr65^{gag}$ into the mature *gag* proteins (Arcement et al. 1977; Evans et al. 1977; Ledbetter et al. 1978). The second line of evidence involves the study of temperature-sensitive MLV mutants. One class of mutants (typified by Ra-MLV *ts*25 and *ts*26) is blocked at an early stage of viral morphogenesis, and cells infected with these mutants accumulate $Pr65^{gag}$ instead of the mature *gag* proteins at the nonpermissive temperature (Stephenson et al. 1975a; Van de Ven et al. 1978a). Another class of mutants (e.g., Ra-MLV *ts*24 and Mo-MLV *ts*3) is blocked late during morphogenesis, and infected cells accumulate incompletely budded particles at the nonpermissive temperature (Wong and McCarter 1974; Wong and MacLeod 1975; Yeger et al. 1976). Upon shift to permissive temperature, particles are released that contain $Pr65^{gag}$ instead of the *gag* proteins, although continued incubation results in cleavage and processing to the mature *gag* proteins (Witte and Baltimore 1978; Lu et al. 1979).

The cleavage pathway of Pr65^{gag} has been investigated by pulse-chase experiments. A major *gag* polyprotein of intermediate size (55,000 daltons, Pr55^{gag}), lacking the peptides of the carboxy-terminal *gag* protein, p10, has been observed (Arcement et al. 1977; Ledbetter et al. 1978). This led to the suggestion that the first cleavage of Pr65^{gag} removes p10. However, other experiments indicate that another cleavage scheme may be more important. An intermediate polyprotein of 40,000 daltons has been identified that contains the sequences of p30 and p10 (Ledbetter 1979; Naso et al. 1979) and this intermediate is present in immature viral particles (Yoshinaka and Luftig 1977c). This suggests that cleavage between pp12 and p30 may occur, at least occasionally, before cleavage between p30 and p10. Furthermore, phosphate residues present in pp12 are already present in Pr65^{gag}, and the major phosphorylated intermediate in Pr65^{gag} cleavage is a phosphoprotein of 25,000 daltons, which contains p15 and pp12 (Naso et al. 1979). This provides evidence for a cleavage pathway in which the initial cleavage is between pp12 and p39, rather than one in which the initial cleavage is between p30 and p10 (the latter would have yielded a phosphorylated Pr55^{gag}). It is, in fact, suggested that Pr55^{gag} may be an artifactual product that is not further processed and raises a general note of caution for interpretation of cleavage-pathway studies.

The cleavage of Pr65^{gag} to the mature *gag* proteins is largely conservative. The combined molecular weights of the individual *gag* proteins account for essentially all of Pr65^{gag}. Also, there is no evidence for major polypeptides between the individual *gag* proteins, which are removed during processing. This has now been confirmed by sequencing of *gag* and *gag* proteins (see below). Recently, two forms of p10, differing by removal of four amino acids from the carboxyl terminus, have been identified in infected cells (L. Henderson et al., pers. comm.). A schematic cleavage pattern for this pathway is shown in Figure 6.5.

Oroszlan et al. (1978) have determined the aminoterminal and carboxyterminal peptide sequences of the individual *gag* proteins from several MLV strains (with the exception of the amino terminus of p15, which is modified). With the assumption that the cleavages of Pr65^{gag} are conservative, they postulated specific sequences for the cleavage sites between the different *gag* proteins. Two of the cleavage sites have a unique specificity, in which cleavage occurs between an aromatic amino acid and proline; a protease to perform this

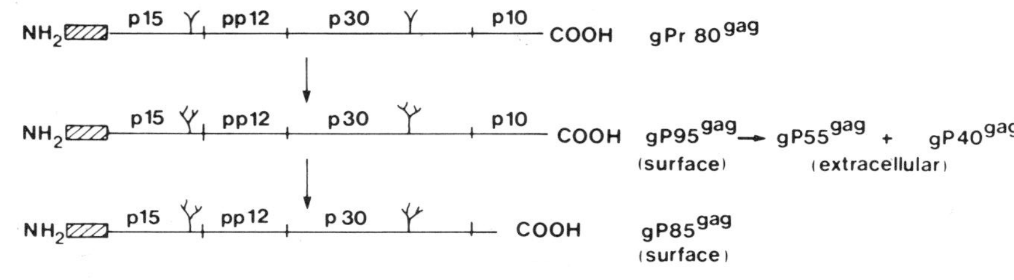

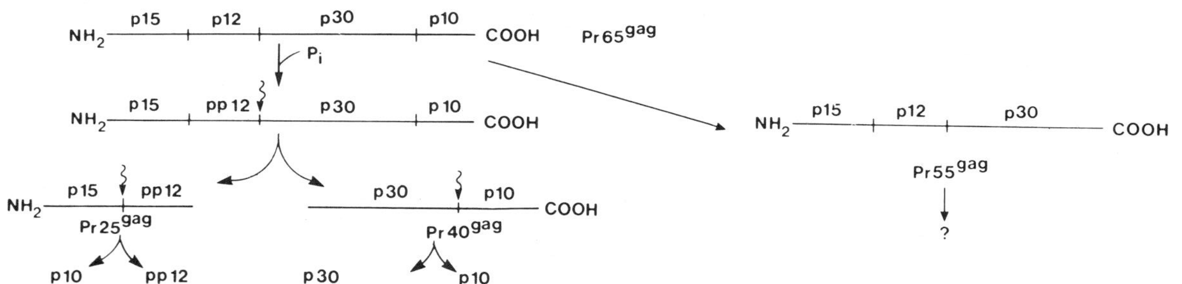

Figure 6.5 Pathways of MLV *gag*-polyprotein synthesis and processing. The two metabolic pathways of glycosylated and nonglycosylated MLV *gag* polyproteins are shown. Initiation of translation from two sites in the *gag* gene results in synthesis of the two primary translation products, $Pr65^{gag}$ and $gPr80^{gag}$. The sequences of these two molecules are probably identical except for the extra peptides, at or near the amino terminus, in $gPr80^{gag}$ denoted by the hatched box. The location of the two carbohydrate side chains is shown by the treelike structures. Modification of $gPr80^{gag}$ to $gP95^{gag}$ by further addition of oligosaccharides and its cleavage and release from the cell are discussed in the text. Phosphorylation and cleavage of $Pr65^{gag}$ to the mature internal structural proteins of the virion are also shown.

cleavage might be virus-specified. Another cleavage site (between p30 and p10) has a specificity that would be recognized by chymotryptic proteases, suggesting that this cleavage might be mediated by a cellular protease. The involvement of two different proteases in cleavage of $Pr65^{gag}$ is consistent with conclusions about avian retrovirus $Pr76^{gag}$ cleavage (see Section II.C.1) and might explain the two conflicting cleavage pathways discussed above. The proposed cleavage sites have been confirmed by nucleotide sequencing of the *gag* gene of Mo-MLV (see Appendix F).

A protease activity that can cleave $Pr65^{gag}$ has been identified and partially purified from Ra-MLV particles (Yoshinaka and Luftig 1977b). The protease cleaves $Pr65^{gag}$ in vitro into the same intermediate and final products observed in vivo. However, in contrast to avian retroviral p15 protease, the MLV protease is present in low amounts in virions and is not identifiable as a distinct product of the *gag* gene. The protease has an approximate molecular weight of 24,000 daltons (Yoshinaka and Luftig 1980), but it is as yet unclear if it is virus- or host-encoded.

c. The $gPr80^{gag}$ *Pathway.* $gPr80^{gag}$ is processed to produce the glycosylated cell-surface *gag* polyproteins. Tryptic peptide and serological analyses show that $gPr80^{gag}$ contains essentially all of the peptides present in $Pr65^{gag}$ (Arcement et al. 1976; Kerr et al. 1976). Some of the additional mass in $gPr80^{gag}$ is contributed by sugar residues. Glycosylation of $gPr80^{gag}$ was first observed by its labeling with radioactive sugar precursors (Edwards and Fan 1979). Digestion of $gPr80^{gag}$ with endoglycosidase H or labeling of cells treated with the glycosylation inhibitor tunicamycin results in a 75,000-dalton nonglycosylated core polypeptide, $P75^{gag}$ (Edwards and Fan 1979; Schultz et al. 1979). This finding indicates that $gPr80^{gag}$ contains additional peptides not found in $Pr65^{gag}$. For Mo-MLV, $gPr80^{gag}$ contains 4000 daltons of additional protein (Edwards and Fan 1980).

The locations of the additional peptides and the sugar residues in $gPr80^{gag}$ are in the aminoterminal half of the molecule (Schultz and Oroszlan 1978). This was determined from formic acid cleavage analysis of $gPr80^{gag}$ and $Pr65^{gag}$, which yielded two fragments. Immunoprecipitation with anti-p10 serum (specific for the carboxyl terminus of the *gag* gene) yields fragments of the same size from the two polyproteins. On the other hand, immunoprecipitation with anti-p15 serum (reacting with the aminoterminal peptides) gives fragments of different molecular weights, thus accounting for the disparity in mass observed between gPr80^{gag} and Pr65^{gag}. Recently, it has been determined that the additional peptide in gPr80^{gag} is at or near (within 6000 daltons) the amino terminus (Edwards and Fan 1980; Schultz et al. 1981; C. Saris, H. van Eenbergen, R. Liskamp, and H. Bloemers, pers. comm.). The location of the carbohydrate in gPr80^{gag} is in a region shared with Pr65^{gag} (Edwards and Fan 1980). In Ra-MLV and Mo-MLV gPr80^{gag}, two carbohydrate chains are present, one in the p15 region and one in the p30 region (Schultz et al. 1981; C. Saris et al., pers. comm.). Core oligosaccharides are gen amino terminus suggests that they may function as signal peptides tion (Sefton 1976); this appears to be the case for gPr80^{gag}. The sequence relationships of Pr65^{gag} and gPr80^{gag} are indicated in Figure 6.5.

The presence of a short sequence of hydrophobic amino acid residues at the amino terminus of glycoproteins may be responsible for the binding of the polyribosomes synthesizing these proteins to the rough endoplasmic reticulum, as well as the subsequent glycosylation and transport to the cell surface (Blobel and Dobberstein 1975). The location of the additional peptides in gPr80^{gag} at the amino terminus suggests that they may function as signal peptides for glycosylation and transport.

gPr80^{gag} is further modified by additional glycosylation. The sugar residues on gPr80^{gag} are of the mannose-rich core type, since they can be removed by digestion with endoglycosidase H (Edwards and Fan 1979). After synthesis, complex oligosaccharides are added to the carbohydrate side chains, with an increase in apparent molecular weight to 95,000 (Evans et al. 1977; Ledbetter et al. 1978; Edwards and Fan 1979; Schultz et al. 1979). This additional glycosylation presumably occurs during transport through the Golgi apparatus to the cell surface. The fully glycosylated 95,000-dalton form (gP95^{gag}) is described in Section III.B.2. gP95^{gag} has varying stability, depending on the strain of virus studied. It is processed to cell-surface gP85^{gag} (Ledbetter et al. 1977; Tung et al. 1977) or released from the cell as cleavage products of 55,000 and 40,000 daltons (Edwards and Fan 1979; Ledbetter 1979).

d. Independent Synthesis of Pr65^{gag} and gPr80^{gag}. Most evidence indicates that Pr65^{gag} and gPr80^{gag} are synthesized independently

(Evans et al. 1977; Edwards and Fan 1979; Ledbetter 1979), although it has also been proposed that these two polyproteins could result from rapid alternate cleavages and modifications of a single primary translation product (Schultz et al. 1979). Very short pulse labels (as short as 1 min) show labeling in both Pr65^{gag} and gPr80^{gag} (Evans et al. 1977; Edwards and Fan 1979); thus, there is no support for a precursor-product relationship between the two. In addition, the ratio of Pr65^{gag} and gPr80^{gag} synthesized can be altered by changing the growth state of the cell; resting cells produce relatively more gPr80^{gag} than Pr65^{gag} (Evans et al. 1977).

Cell-free translation experiments also support the notion of independent synthesis. When MLV virion 38S RNA is used as a template for protein synthesis, *gag*-related polyproteins indistinguishable from Pr65^{gag} and P75^{gag} (the nonglycosylated core of gPr80^{gag}) are synthesized as major products (Kerr et al. 1976; Philipson et al. 1978; Edwards and Fan 1979; Murphy et al. 1979). In particular, when isotopically labeled fMet tRNA is added to the translation mixture to label initiation sites, both Pr65^{gag} and P75^{gag} are labeled (Edwards and Fan 1979). Since the difference between these two proteins is at or near the amino terminus, two different initiation sites in MLV RNA must give rise to the two polyproteins.

The different types of chemical modifications on Pr65^{gag} and gPr80^{gag} also support the belief that these two polyproteins are synthesized and processed along independent pathways. As described above, Pr65^{gag} is phosphorylated and gPr80^{gag} is not (Witte and Baltimore 1978; Naso et al. 1979; Schultz et al. 1979). On the other hand, gPr80^{gag} is glycosylated and Pr65^{gag} is not. If one initial translation product (presumably nonglycosylated P75^{gag}) gives rise to both Pr65^{gag} and gPr80^{gag}, then cleavage of peptides and addition of phosphate and sugar residues would have to occur such that glycosylated Pr65^{gag} and phosphorylated gPr80^{gag} do not result. Longer periods of sugar and phosphate labeling also confirm that Pr65^{gag} and gPr80^{gag} are processed to different final products (Evans et al. 1977; Ledbetter 1979; Naso et al. 1979; Schultz et al. 1979).

e. mRNAs Coding for gag *Polyproteins.* In the infected cell, virus-specific, genome-size 38S mRNA codes for the *gag* polyproteins (see Chapter 5). Immunoprecipitation of polyribosomes with monospecific anti-p30 serum enriches for 38S MLV-specific mRNA (Mueller-Lantzsch and Fan 1976). Also, cell-free translation of size-selected mRNA shows that translation activity for $Pr65^{gag}$ and $gPr80^{gag}$ occurs in the 38S RNA size class (van Zaane et al. 1977; Murphy et al. 1979).

Although no differences in size of the mRNA activities coding for $Pr65^{gag}$ and $gPr80^{gag}$ have been detected, it is possible that different 38S mRNA molecules code for these two polyproteins. As discussed above, $Pr65^{gag}$ and $gPr80^{gag}$ are synthesized independently and most likely from different initiation sites on the 38S mRNA species. The simultaneous utilization of two initiation sites on the same mRNA molecule is without precedent for eukaryotic mRNA. An alternate possibility is that two 38S mRNA molecules may differ from each other by only a small splice(s). Recent nucleic acid sequence data from the 5′ portion of the Mo-MLV genome indicate that splicing does occur to produce the 38S mRNA for $gPr80^{gag}$. The AUG codon that initiates $Pr65^{gag}$ has been identified by combining DNA sequence and protein sequence data (C. van Beveren et al., pers. comm.). Three additional AUG codons in genomic RNA are on the 5′ side of the $Pr65^{gag}$ AUG, and one of these must be the initiation codon for $gPr80^{gag}$. However, all three of these AUGs are in reading frames other than the reading frame for $Pr65^{gag}$, and they are all shortly followed by termination codons in the same frame (W.N. Burnette et al., pers. comm.; see also Appendix E).

Virus-specific 38S mRNA is present in both free and membrane-bound polyribosomes (Fan and Baltimore 1973; Gielkens et al. 1974). A possible explanation is that free polyribosome-associated 38S mRNA codes for $Pr65^{gag}$, whereas membrane-bound 38S mRNA codes for $gPr80^{gag}$. Essentially all cellular glycoproteins that are to be exported are synthesized on membrane-bound polyribosomes, so one would expect $gPr80^{gag}$ synthesis to occur on membrane-bound polyribosomes. Kinetic studies of $Pr65^{gag}$ indicate that it is first present in cells as a soluble protein and later associates with membrane structures (presumably via the hydrophobic p15 portion) (Witte and Baltimore 1978). Thus, $Pr65^{gag}$ synthesis would likely occur on free polyribosomes.

2. *The* pol-*gene Proteins*

a. The Primary Translation Product. $Pr180^{gag\text{-}pol}$ is the initial translation product of the *pol* gene, and it also contains *gag*-gene determinants. Two lines of evidence show that $Pr180^{gag\text{-}pol}$ is the metabolic precursor to reverse transcriptase. First, in MLV-infected cells labeled for a short time, Pr180$^{gag-pol}$ is the only polyprotein that is immunoprecipitable with anti-reverse-transcriptase serum (Arcement et al. 1976; Ledbetter et al. 1978). Second, immature viral particles newly released from cells contain Pr180$^{gag-pol}$ rather than the mature 80,000-dalton MLV reverse transcriptase (Witte and Baltimore 1978).

Peptide-mapping and immunoprecipitation experiments indicate that Pr180$^{gag-pol}$ contains most, if not all, of the peptide sequences of Pr65^{gag} (Kerr et al. 1976; Ledbetter et al. 1978; Murphy et al. 1979). Thus, the portion of the molecule that is uniquely *pol*-encoded is 100,000 to 120,000 daltons. It should be noted that the mature form of MLV reverse transcriptase is 70,000 to 80,000 daltons; so extra peptide sequences (30,000–40,000 daltons), which are not *gag*-related and do not appear in mature reverse transcriptase, are present in Pr180$^{gag-pol}$. It is unclear whether or not these sequences are required for biological activity, but it is interesting that MLV reverse transcriptase shows several enzymic properties that more closely resemble the α subunit of avian retroviral reverse transcriptase, rather than the $\alpha\beta$ dimer form (Verma 1977) (see also Section II.A.2). The additional sequences in Pr180$^{gag-pol}$ could provide activities analogous to the β subunit.

b. The Cleavage Pathway. Cleavage of Pr180$^{gag-pol}$ to the mature 80,000-dalton reverse transcriptase occurs through two intermediates of approximately 150,000 daltons and 140,000 daltons (Arcement et al. 1976; Ledbetter et al. 1978; Witte and Baltimore 1978). These cleavage products lack the *gag* sequences (Ledbetter et al. 1978), but little is known about the localization of the mature reverse transcriptase sequences within these intermediate cleavage products or how cleavage is mediated.

Cleavage of Pr180$^{gag-pol}$ is necessary for activation of reverse transcriptase enzymic activity. Immature viral particles that contain Pr180$^{gag-pol}$ have no reverse transcriptase activity, but, upon incubation of the viral particles, Pr180$^{gag-pol}$ is cleaved and enzymic function appears (Witte and Baltimore 1978; Lu et al. 1979). It has been proposed that this might be important in preventing unpackaged reverse transcriptase from making DNA transcripts of cytoplasmic RNA in the infected cell (Witte and Baltimore 1978).

c. mRNA Coding for Pr180$^{gag-pol}$. *Pr180*$^{gag-pol}$ is also synthesized from 38S mRNA (Murphy et al. 1979), although it is unclear whether the 38S Pr180$^{gag-pol}$-specific mRNA is identical to the 38S virus-specific mRNA coding for *gag*-gene products or whether it differs by a small splice(s) (see Section III.C.1.e).

Translation of MLV virion 38S RNA in cell-free systems also leads to synthesis of Pr180$^{gag-pol}$ (Kerr et al. 1976; Murphy et al. 1978; Philipson et al. 1978). Although the ratio of Pr180$^{gag-pol}$ to Pr65^{gag} or P75^{gag} synthesis is low, Philipson et al. (1978) reported that translation of Mo-MLV 38S virion RNA in the presence of yeast amber suppressor tRNA resulted in increased synthesis of Pr180$^{gag-pol}$ at the expense of P75^{gag}. They proposed that partial suppression of the amber termination signal at the end of the *gag* gene is responsible for Pr180$^{gag-pol}$ synthesis. A more attractive hypothesis now is that splicing removes the termination codon(s) at the end of the *gag* gene, resulting in an mRNA for Pr180$^{gag-pol}$. Splicing at the *gag-pol* junction must occur in the case of the mRNA for avian retrovirus Pr180$^{gag-pol}$, because the coding sequence for *pol* apparently begins in a reading frame different from that of *gag* (see Section II.C.2.b and Chapter 5).

d. Glycosylated Pr180$^{gag-pol}$. A glycosylated form of Pr180$^{gag-pol}$ has also been detected (C. Saris et al.; S. Edwards and H. Fan; both pers. comm.). This glycosylated form appears to be a fusion product of the glycosylated gPr80^{gag} protein with *pol* sequences. It has amino-terminal sequences similar to those of gPr80^{gag}, whereas nonglycosylated Pr180$^{gag-pol}$ has aminoterminal sequences similar to those of Pr65^{gag}. Only one form of Pr180$^{gag-pol}$ (presumably the nonglycosylated form) is observed in immature viral particles (Witte and Baltimore 1978). No biological role for the glycosylated Pr180$^{gag-pol}$ has been identified, and this polyprotein may simply arise from the signals or structures in mRNA giving rise to gPr80^{gag}.

3. The env-*gene Proteins*

a. The Primary Translation Product. The initial translation product of the *env* gene is a polyprotein of 80,000 to 90,000 daltons, which contains the peptide sequences of gp70 and p15(E) (Famulari et al. 1976; Naso et al. 1976; Shapiro et al. 1976; van Zaane et al. 1976; Karshin et al. 1977; Sutcliffe et al. 1980b). This polyprotein, referred to as Pr90^{env} or Pr80^{env} (depending on virus strain), is glycosylated, although it contains only mannose-rich core oligosaccharides (Witte and Wirth 1979).

The order of gp70 and p15(E) within the *env* gene is NH_2-gp70-p15(E)-COOH, as determined by pactamycin mapping (Karshin et al. 1977). The amino acid sequences of the amino termini of Pr90^{env} and gp70 are also the same, in agreement with the pactamycin data (S. Oroszlan et al., pers. comm.). This order was also recently confirmed by direct nucleic acid sequencing of a recombinant DNA clone containing the 3′ portion of the Mo-MLV genome (Sutcliffe et al. 1980a).

The size of the *env* precursor polyprotein observed in MLV-infected cells varies with different strains of MLV. For Ra-MLV, the precursor polyprotein is 90,000 daltons (Pr90^{env}), whereas for Mo-MLV, the precursor is 80,000 daltons (Pr80^{env}) (Witte and Wirth 1979). Nevertheless, the sizes of the gp70 and p15(E) proteins from the two strains do not differ appreciably. The difference in Pr80^{env} and Pr90^{env} is also reflected in the polypeptide cores (70,000 daltons for Ra-MLV and 62,000 daltons for Mo-MLV) (Edwards and Fan 1979; Witte and Wirth 1979). However, if cellular mRNA or virion RNA from the two virus strains are translated in cell-free systems, then *env* polyproteins of more similar sizes are observed (approximately 70,000 daltons in both cases) (Gielkens et al. 1976; Philipson et al. 1978; Murphy et al. 1979). This suggests that rapid posttranslational cleavage may remove approximately 10,000 daltons of protein from the initial *env* translation product for Mo-MLV, but not for Ra-MLV. The removed protein might be a signal peptide from the amino terminus of the *env* polyprotein, as observed in the avian system (see Section II.C.3). Alternatively, the carboxyterminal sequences might be removed.

b. Modification and Cleavage of Pr90^{env}. During processing of Pr90^{env}, carbohydrate addition and proteolytic cleavage take place. The oligosaccharides present on Pr90^{env} are of the *N*-asparagine-linked, mannose-rich core variety, since they can be removed by digestion with endoglycosidase H (Witte and Wirth 1979) and are presumably added concomitantly with synthesis (Sefton 1977). The nonglycosylated core of Pr90^{env} is not observed in MLV-infected cells. After translation, the mannose-rich oligosaccharides are modified, and terminal oligosaccharides are added; terminal sugars (such as fucose) can be detected in the mature gp70 but not in Pr90^{env} (Arcement et al. 1976). Terminal sialic acid residues are also added to the sugar side chains (Witte et al. 1977), although the amount may vary (Buetti and Diggelmann 1980b). All of the glycosylation in Pr90^{env} is within the gp70 domain.

Proteolytic cleavage of Pr90^{env} first separates gp70 and p15(E). No intermediates in this cleavage have been detected, suggesting either that the cleavage of Pr90^{env} to gp70 and p15(E) conserves all protein sequences or that cleavages occur quite rapidly. In the case of Mo-MLV Pr80^{env}, it is possible for a single conservative cleavage to result in gp70 and p15(E). However, for Ra-MLV Pr90^{env}, the additional peptides must also be removed, but no intermediate cleavage products have been detected (Witte and Baltimore 1978). Subsequent to the first cleavage, some of p15(E) molecules are then cleaved to p12(E) (Van de Ven et al. 1978a,b; Sutcliffe et al. 1980b; H. Bloemers and E. Fleissner, pers. comm.).

Oligosaccharide modification and cleavage of Pr90^{env} appear to be temporally linked (Witte and Wirth 1979). All of the sugar residues in Pr90^{env} are endoglycosidase-H-sensitive, indicating that the terminal modifications do not take place prior to proteolytic cleavage. On the other hand, newly synthesized gp70 is resistant to endoglycosidase H, indicating that the sugar residues in Pr90^{env} have been modified by the time of cleavage.

c. mRNA Coding for Pr90^{env}. Pr90^{env} is coded by a subgenomic mRNA of 20S–24S (van Zaane et al. 1977; Fan and Verma 1978; Murphy et al. 1979) (see also Chapter 5). This subgenomic mRNA is a spliced molecule containing nucleotides from the 5′ terminus of 38S RNA transposed to the 5′ end of the *env* coding region (Fan and Verma 1978; Rothenberg et al. 1978). A summary of synthesis and processing of Pr90^{env} is shown in Figure 6.6.

4. Polyprotein Processing and Virion Morphogenesis

Although most studies on processing of precursor polyproteins have involved infected-cell extracts, it is important to remember that cleavage and processing of *gag* and *pol* products are temporally and physically linked with the formation of viral particles, as indicated by two lines of evidence. First, preparations of Ra-MLV cores that are enriched for the immature form (as judged by electron microscopy) also contain high levels of Pr65^{gag}, whereas preparations con-

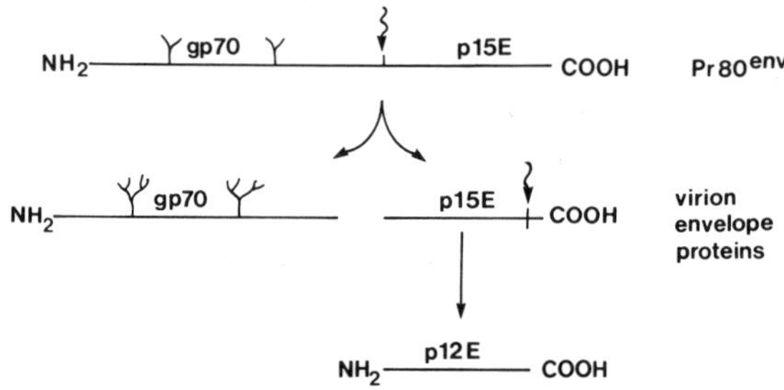

Figure 6.6 Synthesis and processing of MLV *env*-gene products. Synthesis of $Pr80^{env}$ (for Mo-MLV) or $Pr90^{env}$ (for Ra-MLV) results from translation of a subgenomic spliced 24S mRNA. Core mannose-rich oligosaccharides are present in the gp70 domain and are indicated by treelike structures. Cleavage and concomitant oligosaccharide addition results in fully modified gp70 and p15(E). Some of the p15(E) molecules are subsequently processed to p12(E).

taining mature cores contain the individual *gag* proteins instead (Yoshinaka and Luftig 1977a; Luftig and Yoshinaka 1978). Second, the experiments with temperature-sensitive mutants show that processing of $Pr65^{gag}$ and $Pr180^{gag\text{-}pol}$ does not occur until viral particles are released from the cell (see Chapter 7). Thus, cleavage of these precursors polyproteins actually occurs in budding particles, rather than in the cytoplasm. It is likely that the physical configurations of $Pr65^{gag}$ and $Pr180^{gag\text{-}pol}$ in the viral core are important requirements for the cleavage events to take place. Activation of putative virus-coded proteolytic factors might also require an appropriate conformation of the core structure.

In contrast to $Pr65^{gag}$ and $Pr180^{gag\text{-}pol}$, $Pr90^{env}$ can be at least partially processed independent of virus budding. This is suggested by the fact that gp70 molecules are present on the cell surface in regions that do not contain budding viral particles. Also, some cells, which do not produce virus particles, express endogenous MLV gp70 at the cell surface (see Section III.B.1). However, recent results indicate that cleavage of p15(E) to p12(E) may only occur in virions (Van de Ven et al. 1978a,b; H. Bloemers and E. Fleissner, pers. comm.).

IV. MURINE B-TYPE RETROVIRUSES

MMTV represents the prototype of the B-type retroviruses. The structural proteins of MMTV and their biosynthesis have been extensively studied.

A. Murine B-type Retroviruses and Their Protein Constituents

Polyacrylamide gel electrophoresis of purified MMTV consistently results in the separation and detection of seven virion-associated polypeptides (Nowinski et al. 1971b; Dickson and Skehel 1974; Teramoto et al. 1974; Sarkar and Dion 1975; Yagi and Compans 1977). Depending on the purity and source of the virion preparation, other minor proteins can often be observed; these are thought to represent contaminating cellular proteins. The estimated size of the virion-specific polypeptides often varies quite considerably for a single protein. This variation derives from the behavior of the virion proteins under the different conditions of analysis and the often inherent uncertainty of the precise molecular weights of the standard proteins used to calibrate the different analytical systems. To avoid confusion, the nomenclature used in the following discussion is presented in Table 6.4, along with previously used molecular-weight estimates from several laboratories. The proteins that comprise the MMTV virion are dealt with as the products of the three viral genes that give rise to them, namely, *gag*, the internal structural proteins; *pol*, the RNA-dependent DNA polymerase; and *env*, the envelope components. The possibility that a recently discovered open reading frame may be used to synthesize additional MMTV-specific protein(s) is considered in Chapters 4, 5, and 8.

1. Internal Structural gag *Proteins*

Thin-section electron microscopy shows the internal structure of MMTV to be composed of an eccentrically located electron-dense core, or nucleoid, surrounded by a fine inner membrane (Bernhard 1958; Dmochowski 1960; Calafat and Hageman 1969; Kramarsky et al. 1970; Sarkar et al. 1971; Dalton 1972) (see Chapter 2). The internal core structure can be released from intact virion preparations by treatment with nonionic detergents (e.g., Triton X-100, Nonidet P40, or Sterox-SL) to remove the external envelope. Subviral particles can be separated on sucrose density gradients and analyzed for structural and enzymic components (Calafat and Hageman 1969; Sarkar et al. 1971; Teramoto et al. 1977). The virion cores band in sucrose gradients at an equilibrium density of 1.24–1.26 g/ml; this is due primarily to the loss of the low-density lipid envelope of the virion. The isolated cores contain the genomic RNA, reverse transcriptase activity, and a subset of the virion polypeptides (Feldman et al. 1973; Teramoto et al. 1977). SDS-polyacrylamide

Table 6.4 Polypeptide composition of MMTV

Text nomenclature	Virion protein[a] (%)	Alternative nomenclatures[b] *A*	*B*	*C*	*D*	*E*	*F*
gp52	27	gp49	gp52	gp55	gp49	gp47	gp52
gp36	20	gp37.5/33.5	gp36	gp34	gp34	gp34	gp37/33
p30	7	p29	p30	—	p28	—	—
p27	20	p24	p28	p28	p24	p27	p24
pp21	8	p17	p22	p23	p21	p23	p17
p14	7	p13.5	p14	p18	p14	p16	p13
p10	8	p8	p10	p12	p10	p12	p8

[a]Data from Dickson and Skehel (1974).

[b]Data from the following references: A = Dickson and Skehel (1974); B = Teramoto et al. (1974); C = Sarkar and Dion (1975); D = Nusse et al. (1978); E = Sarkar et al. (1978); F = Yagi and Compans (1977).

gel electrophoresis analysis of cores shows three major polypeptides of 30,000 daltons (p30), 27,000 daltons (p27), and 14,000 daltons (p14), respectively (Teramoto et al. 1977). The p30 polypeptide is a minor component of the total virion proteins and therefore its prominence, compared with p27, in the core preparations is difficult to explain.

a. p27, pp27. The most abundant polypeptide in both virus and core preparations is p27, and for this reason, p27 is postulated to be the major structural protein of the virion core. The polypeptide has an isoelectric point of 6.5 to 6.8 (Nusse et al. 1980) and displays strong hydrophobic characteristics (Marcus et al. 1978b), two properties that are well suited for a core structural protein. p27 can also be labeled in cells using ^{32}P, demonstrating that this polypeptide is phosphorylated, although it is not the major phosphoprotein found in virion particles (Nusse et al. 1978; Sarkar et al. 1978). When injected into rabbits, this protein is strongly immunogenic and, coupled with its abundance in virions, has been exploited as the basis for several radioimmunoassays used for the detection of virus (Hendrick et al. 1978; Teramoto and Schlom 1978).

b. pp21. The major virion phosphoprotein is pp21 (Nusse et al. 1978; Sarkar et al. 1978). This polypeptide is a minor component of virions (see Table 6.4) and is not found in core preparations, although small amounts of this polypeptide could easily go undetected. The precise location of pp21 in the virion particle is not known; however, by analogy to other retroviruses, the major portion of this protein would be located between the core and the envelope components. Thus, structurally, pp21 could contribute to the inner membrane surrounding the core, and this function would be consistent with the property of this protein to exist in multimeric form in the virion (Dion et al. 1979). However, this polypeptide is the least hydrophobic (Marcus et al. 1979b) and therefore would seem to be unlikely to serve such a membrane function. A small amount of the major phosphoprotein of the avian and murine C-type retroviruses (see Sections II.A.1.a and III.A.1.c) is found specifically associated with the genomic RNA and, perhaps by analogy to these C-type retroviruses, a similar undefined function may exist for pp21 in MMTV virions.

c. p14. The core structures also contain the polypeptide p14, a highly basic protein possessing the capacity to bind to single-stranded DNA (Arthur et al. 1978b; Nusse et al. 1980). Similar, small, highly basic proteins are also found in avian and murine C-type retroviruses bound to the genomic RNA and can, in fact, be isolated in the form of a RNP complex (see Sections II.A.1.b and III.A.1.e). Thus, the basic nature of p14 and its location in the core suggest that the polypeptide may function in packaging of the genomic RNA or may affect expression of the genome during infection.

d. p10. Up to 10% of the protein in virions and bald particles (see Section IV.A.3) comprises the small hydrophobic polypeptide, p10 (see Table 6.4). Isolated cores contain a greatly diminished quantity of p10 and therefore this small polypeptide is also thought to be located external to the core structure and may be directly associated with the virion envelope (Cardiff et al. 1978; Marcus et al. 1978b). Indirect evidence for a close membrane association of p10 comes from the results of Massey and Schochetman (1979), who found that MMTV-producing cells, made semipermeable with EDTA, could be specifically lysed with anti-p10 serum. Furthermore, both p10 and the suspected transmembrane glycoprotein, gp36, can be tagged with isotopically labeled palmitic acid, a fatty acid often attached to membrane proteins (R. Nusse, pers. comm.). This hydrophobic polypeptide is synthesized at the aminoterminal end of the major internal protein precursor (see Section IV.D.1). The properties and location of p10 on the precursor suggest that it may function in interactions between the *gag* precursor and the cell membrane to facilitate assembly of the core components. It may also contribute to the association of the core with the glycoprotein envelope during budding (Cardiff et al. 1978; Dickson and Atterwill 1979).

e. p30 and p8. Analysis of MMTV virions shows the presence of two other minor components: p30, already mentioned above, and p8, a polypeptide not included formally as a *gag* polypeptide because of some uncertainty about its origin (Gautsch et al. 1978b; Dickson and Atterwill 1979; Nusse et al. 1980). p30 is related to p14 by amino acid sequence and has been postulated to be an intermediate in the processing of a *gag* precursor to yield p14 (Gautsch et al. 1978b). Further, there are unique peptides in p30 that have not been detected in the other *gag* proteins (Dickson and Atterwill 1979), nor are they found in the *gag* precursor $Pr77^{gag}$ (see Section IV.D.1). However, these peptides are present in the minor polyprotein Pr110^{gag}, suggesting that p30 might be a functionally distinct moiety from p14, although both proteins are related by a common sequence.

The p8 polypeptide is detected in virion preparations as an arginine-rich and lysine-rich, but methionine-deficient, protein of unknown function. Peptide-mapping data remain ambiguous but indicate that it may form part of the Pr77^{gag} and perhaps be analogous to the avian polypeptide p10 (see Section II.A.1.e).

2. *Reverse Transcriptase*

The reverse transcriptase is a very minor component of the virions by mass and, as such, is not easily detected by radioisotope labeling or protein staining of separated virion proteins. However, its presence is easily detected by virtue of its enzymic activity in purified virion and core preparations. The requirements for optimal enzymic activity include a divalent cation, a sulfhydryl reagent, and, like all DNA polymerases, a template and a primer (see Chapter 5) (Dickson 1973; Feldman et al. 1973; Dion et al. 1974a). A comparison of the divalent cation preference shows that magnesium is much preferred over manganese (Dickson 1973; Howk et al. 1973; Dion et al. 1974a). Consequently, with no biological assay available for MMTV, the use of the magnesium preference in a reverse transcriptase assay has been successfully utilized as an assay with some specificity to distinguish MMTV from the murine C-type retroviruses that preferentially use manganese (Dion et al. 1974a). The reverse transcriptase of MMTV has been partially purified from virions and intracytoplasmic A-type particles; the latter structures represent the intracellular form of the preformed MMTV core structure (see Section IV.C). The enzyme is reported to sediment as a protein of approximately 100,000 daltons; however, there remains some discrepancy about the structure. Dion et al. (1974b) found a single polypeptide of approximately 100,000 daltons, whereas Marcus et al. (1976) and Kohno and Ishihama (1979) found a two-subunit enzyme with molecular weights of 85,000 and 50,000 daltons, and 94,000 and 42,000 daltons, respectively. Since other retroviruses display both one- and two-subunit structures for their reverse transcriptases, further work will be required to resolve this discrepancy. Additionally, RNase-H activity is associated with MMTV polymerase (Dion et al. 1977).

3. Envelope Proteins

MMTV contains two major glycoprotein species, gp52 and gp36 (Dickson and Skehel 1974; Teramoto et al. 1974; Sarkar and Dion 1975). The carbohydrate content of these two proteins was initially demonstrated by specific chemical staining of the proteins in polyacrylamide gels with the periodic acid-Schiff reagent and by the ability of these two proteins to incorporate labeled sugars. Virus isolated from mouse milk often contains other glycoproteins associated with virion preparations; however, these do not appear to be virus encoded.

Like other retroviruses, MMTV matures by budding from the surface membrane of its host cell (Bernhard 1958). The area of cell surface at which budding is taking place is specifically modified by the accumulation of viral glycoproteins in the host-cell membrane. In thin-section electron microscopy, glycoprotein spikes are seen on the cell surface at the site of budding virions and on mature virions (Bernhard 1958; Calafat and Hageman 1969). The identity of the spikes as the virus-specific glycoproteins can be directly demonstrated by immunoelectron microscopy using ferritin-tagged antivirus serum (Tanaka and Moore 1967). Biochemically, the identity of the spikes with the virion glycoproteins has been demonstrated using several techniques. The spikes can be digested from the surface of the virion using proteases, giving rise to bald (spikeless) particles (Cardiff et al. 1974). Analysis of these bald particles by SDS-polyacrylamide gel electrophoresis demonstrates that they no longer contain gp52 or gp36 but do contain the nonglycosylated polypeptides of MMTV. The major glycoprotein, gp52, can also be specifically stripped from the virion membrane by treatment of intact viral particles with 0.05 N HCl, resulting in similar bald particles (Sarkar et al. 1976).

The surface location of at least a proportion of these glycoproteins can be demonstrated by surface-labeling techniques, such as lactoperoxidase-catalyzed iodination, which labels gp52 specifically (Witte et al. 1973; Parks et al. 1974b), and the galactose oxidase [^{3}H]potassium borohydride oxidation-reduction system, which labels both virion glycoproteins (Sheffield and Daly 1976).

A more detailed examination of gp36 shows it to migrate often as a doublet in SDS-polyacrylamide gels, with peak molecular-weight values of about 37,000 and 33,000 daltons (see Table 6.4). Tryptic peptide analysis of the two peaks shows a similar content of methionine-containing peptides (Dickson et al. 1976). Carbohydrate composition estimates for the two separable species of gp36 demonstrated 11% and 19% sugar content, respectively (Yagi et al. 1978). A lower estimate of molecular weight with the species containing more carbohydrate is probably due to the abnormal way in which glycoproteins migrate in SDS-polyacrylamide gels. The gp52 is estimated to contain minimally 9.3% carbohydrate (Yagi et al. 1978). Both glycoproteins contain mannose, fucose, galactose, *N*-acetylglucosamine, and sialic acid (Yagi et al. 1978; Dickson and Atterwill 1980). Techniques that separate proteins by charge, such as isoelectric focusing, show a far greater heterogeneity of the virion glycoproteins than SDS-polyacrylamide gel electrophoresis alone, demonstrating a series of five to six identifiable species for each glycoprotein (Nusse et al. 1980). Treatment of the glycoproteins with neuramindase prior to analysis reduces this heterogeneity, making the more neutral spots predominant. These results indicate that the microheterogeneity is, in part, the result of differing degrees of sialylation of the carbohydrate moieties, sialic acid being the most common terminal sugar of carbohydrate structures (Schloemer et al. 1976).

Membrane-component structures can be prepared from virions using nonionic detergents and organic solvents, resulting in the isolation of both gp52 and gp36. Negative-stain electron microscopy of this material shows a natural association of the glycoprotein to form rosettelike patterns, which suggest that there is some form of specific interaction (Sarkar et al. 1976). The use of chemical cross-linking reagents confirms these ideas and demonstrates the formation of homodimers and heterodimers of gp52 and gp36 (Dion et al. 1979; Racevskis and Sarkar 1980). Trimers composed of three gp52 molecules and oligomers composed of three gp52 and three gp36 molecules have also been detected and suggest an oligomeric structure for the prominent MMTV spikes seen in negative-stain electron microscopy.

B. Immunological and Biochemical Polymorphism of MMTV Proteins

The development of radioimmunoassays for most of the MMTV structural proteins (Cardiff 1973; Parks et al. 1974b; Verstraeten et al. 1975; Hendrick et al. 1978; Teramoto and Schlom 1978, 1979; Arthur and Fine 1979; Marcus et al. 1979a; Arthur et al. 1981) and the application of these assays, using different sources of MMTV, have established that these viruses exist as a multigene family. This finding is consistent with the results of the molecular analysis of the MMTV proviruses present in most strains, which also demonstrate a family of different, but related, proviral elements (see Chapter 10). Early studies using immunodiffusion demonstrated the major cross-reactivities of the viral structural proteins of different MMTV strains (Blair 1970, 1971; Daams et al. 1973), but occasionally after extensive adsorptions of antisera, differences were observed. The group-specific cross-reactivities were also confirmed using radioimmunoassays; however, judicious use of antisera and the development of heterologous radioimmunoassays demonstrated extensive polymorphism of the gp52 molecules (Teramoto et al. 1977; Arthur et al. 1978a, 1981) and limited polymorphism associated with gp36 and p27 (Teramoto and Schlom 1978; Arthur et al. 1981). Tryptic peptide mapping confirmed the immunological differences between the different gp52 and p27 polypeptides but did not show differences between the gp36 molecules from different strains (Gautsch et al. 1978b). This latter glycoprotein is thought to be the integral membrane protein of the envelope-glycoprotein complex and therefore might be expected to be more highly conserved structurally than the other glycoprotein. In strains of mice that contain more than one type of MMTV, polymorphism of the gp52 moiety has led to the detection of both antigen and antibody coexisting in mouse sera (Arthur and Fine 1978; Arthur et al. 1978a; Michalides et al. 1979); it is speculated that the antigen may derive from one strain of MMTV and that the type-specific antibody is reactive against a second strain of MMTV. Type-specific monoclonal antibodies for the MMTV proteins can also be specifically produced by hybridoma cell lines and should prove useful in classifying the various subgroups in the MMTV family (Massey et al. 1980).

C. Intracytoplasmic A-type Particles

Thin-section electron microscopy of tumors producing MMTV show three types of particles (see Chapter 2). In the cell cytoplasm, often associated with membranes, is the intracytoplasmic A-type particle that morphologically appears as two concentric rings of electron-dense material approximately 70 nm in diameter. These structures bud from the plasma membrane to form initially immature B-type particles that resemble enveloped A-type particles and eventually mature infectious B-type particles (Bernhard 1958). The mature B-type particle is characterized by a condensed electron-dense nucleoid located eccentrically in the virion and surrounded by a fine membrane.

A comparison of isolated A-type-particle proteins and MMTV proteins using antisera against either particle shows extensive cross-reactivity of the A-type-particle proteins with p27, p14, and p10 of MMTV (Tanaka et al. 1972; Sarkar and Dion 1975; Smith and Lee 1975; Tanaka 1977; Arthur et al. 1978b; Cardiff et al. 1978; Smith 1978). However, biochemical analysis has revealed very little similarity in size between the A-type-particle polypeptides and the structural proteins of MMTV (Tanaka 1977; Smith 1978). Careful isolation of A-type particles in the presence of protease inhibitors results in a particle population that is composed predominantly of a single polypeptide of about 70,000 daltons (Tanaka 1977). It is now thought that the A-type particle represents a performed MMTV core structure in which the proteins are still in their precursor form and the proteolytic processing occurs after the formation of this core structure (see Section IV.D.1).

D. Biosynthesis and Processing of MMTV Structural Proteins

Immunoprecipitation of radioactively labeled MMTV-infected cells with anti-MMTV sera results in the isolation of several virus-specific proteins. Separation of these proteins on SDS-polyacrylamide gels reveals a distribution of polypeptides quite distinct from that revealed by a similar analysis of the virion proteins. Similar experiments performed with other retrovirus systems have shown that the structural proteins and the reverse transcriptase are synthesized as precursor polyproteins, which require extensive processing by specific proteases to yield the functional virion polypeptides; MMTV is no exception to this finding. Basically, the primary translation products of the *gag, pol,* and *env* genes are expressed in the form of polyprotein precursors; a summary of these proteins is presented in Table 6.5.

Table 6.5 Murine B-type retrovirus precursor polyproteins and virion proteins

Protein	Gene	Function	Localization	Structure and properties
$Pr110^{gag}$	*gag*	may be extended form of $Pr77^{gag}$	cell cytoplasm	contains $p30^{gag}$ peptides in addition to those of $Pr77^{gag}$
$Pr77^{gag}$	*gag*	precursor to virion internal structural proteins	cell cytoplasm; rough endoplasmic reticulum; probably associated with inner surface of plasma membrane	phosphoprotein; NH_2-p10-pp21-p27-p14-COOH
$Pr34^{gag}$	*gag*	processing intermediate	found in newly budded virions and in association with plasma membrane	contains p27 and p14 peptides
$p27^{gag}$, $pp27^{gag}$	*gag*	major component of core shell	virion core	hydrophobic; phosphorylated and nonphosphorylated forms; pI 6.5–6.8
$pp21^{gag}$	*gag*	possible structural role	between core and envelope	phosphorylated
$p14^{gag}$	*gag*	may aid in packaging of RNA	RNP complex with RNA	basic protein; binds to single-stranded DNA
$p10^{gag}$	*gag*	important in aggregation and assembly of $Pr77^{gag}$	associated with virion envelope	hydrophobic
$p30^{gag}$	*gag*	unknown	minor virion component	related in amino acid sequence to p14
p8	*gag?*	unknown	minor virion component	basic protein; rich in arginine and lysine residues

$Pr160^{gag-pol}$	*pol*	presumed precursor to reverse transcriptase	cell cytoplasm, probably associated with the plasma membrane	
$Pr130^{gag-pol}$	*pol*	probably an intermediate in $Pr160^{gag-pol}$ processing	probably associated with plasma membrane	
$p100^{pol}$	*pol*	transcription of genomic RNA	virion core	RNA- and DNA-dependent polymerase and hybrid-specific RNase-H activities; conflicting reports of dimer enzymic forms
$P69^{env}$	*env*		observed in vitro only	primary translation product in vitro; presumably contains aminoterminal 9000-dalton signal sequence
$P60^{env}$	*env*		rough endoplasmic reticulum	nonglycosylated form of $Pr73^{env}$ produced only in presence of inhibitors of glycosylation
$gPr73^{env}$	*env*	precursor to envelope glycoproteins gp52 and gp36	cell cytoplasm in association with rough endoplasmic reticulum	glycosylated; NH_2-gp52-gp36-COOH
$gp52^{env}$	*env*	host range; neutralization	virion envelope; knob structure directly associated with gp36	10% carbohydrate by weight
$gp36^{env}$	*env*	may anchor gp52 to membrane	virion envelope; spike structure directly associated with membrane and gp52	10–20% carbohydrate by weight; very hydrophobic; transmembrane

1. The gag-*gene Proteins*

Immunoprecipitation of labeled cells with an anti-*gag* serum, notably anti-p27 serum, results in the detection of several proteins ranging in molecular weight from 34,000 to 160,000 daltons (Dickson and Atterwill 1978; Nusse et al. 1978; Racevskis and Sarkar 1978; Schochetman et al. 1978; Anderson et al. 1979). Using monospecific antisera to the individual *gag* proteins and peptide-mapping techniques, the major *gag* precursor, $Pr77^{gag}$, was identified on SDS-polyacrylamide gels as a doublet of 75,000 daltons and 77,000 daltons. The doublet nature of the precursor is due to a portion of the precursor population at any one time being phosphorylated, a step thought to be obligatory for further processing of the precursor (Nusse et al. 1979). The phosphorylation site appears to be conserved during processing, as all the phosphopeptides of the precursor can be found in the mature virion phosphoproteins. $Pr77^{gag}$ is the major translation product in cell-free protein-synthesizing systems primed with full-length genomic RNA and therefore is believed to be the primary *gag*-related translation product in vivo (Dahl and Dickson 1979; Nusse et al. 1979; Sen et al. 1979). A series of polypeptides with molecular weights lower than that of the $Pr77^{gag}$ are also detected in virus-infected cells and probably represent cleavage intermediates of proteolytic processing (Dickson and Atterwill 1978; Racevskis and Sarkar 1978). Immunoprecipitation with specific antisera and peptide mapping of these putative intermediates have proved useful in determining the order of the virion proteins in $Pr77^{gag}$ as NH_2-p10-pp21-p27-p14-COOH (Dickson and Atterwill 1979; Massey and Schochetman 1979). This order was confirmed by pactamycin-mapping experiments (Dickson and Atterwill 1980; Sen et al. 1980b). A scheme showing the tentative intermediates in a cleavage pathway is presented in Figure 6.7. A minor small polypeptide, p8, is also detected in virions and may form part of the $Pr77^{gag}$ precursor (see Section IV.A.1.e). The most prominent intermediate found in cells after extended chase periods has a molecular weight of 34,000 daltons and contains all the peptides of the two most predominant core polypeptides, p27 and p14. $Pr34^{gag}$ is the only intermediate that shows an increase in label with increasing times of the chase. Furthermore, virions harvested at 5-minute intervals following a pulse with [^{35}S]methionine show $Pr34^{gag}$ as a major virion structural component, which diminishes upon incubation of virions

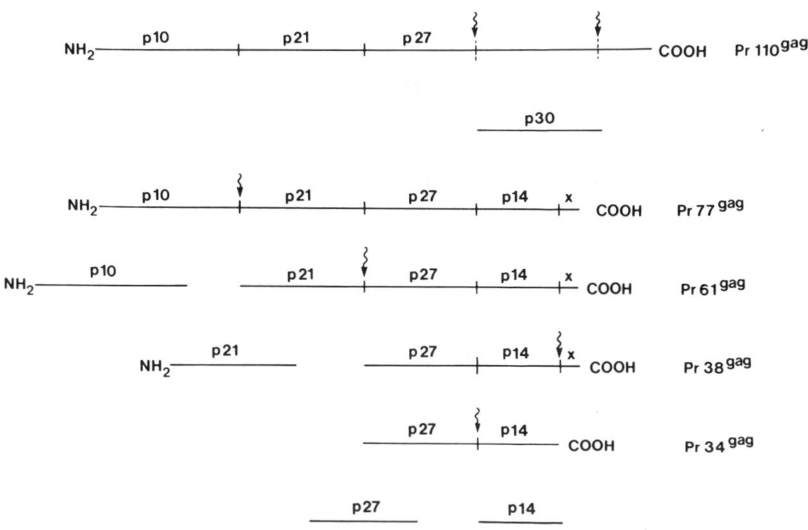

Figure 6.7 Structure and processing of the precursor to MMTV internal structural *gag* proteins. Processing of $Pr77^{gag}$ commences with the sequential removal of p10 and p21, giving rise to identifiable intermediate products, Pr61 and Pr38. Cleavage of Pr38 yields p27 and p14 and a small peptide denoted X (which could be the minor virion component p8). Cleavage of Pr34 to yield p27 and p14 apparently occurs predominantly in the virion. A second major polyprotein precursor, $Pr110^{gag}$, has been identified and contains the peptides for a minor virion protein, p30, which is not found in $Pr77^{gag}$; the location and function of p30 is not known. No virus-encoded proteases have been identified to facilitate this cleavage scheme. The above scheme was derived assuming conservative cleavage (see text). Most of these cleavage events are intracellular.

at 37°C (Dickson and Atterwill 1978). Thus, the virtual absence of p27 in infected cells and the finding of $Pr34^{gag}$ in rapidly harvested virions strongly suggest that virions bud with $Pr34^{gag}$ as the major core component. Virions harvested over longer periods contain less than 5% of their p27-related material in the form of $Pr34^{gag}$, and consequently, the proteolytic cleavage that occurs to release p27 and p14 from $Pr34^{gag}$ probably occurs after budding and may be the biochemical basis for the post-budding maturation.

A protease responsible for the specific cleavage of $Pr77^{gag}$ appears to be present in MMTV virion preparations. The protease demonstrates a marked specificity for the precursor $Pr77^{gag}$, since the analogous avian ($Pr76^{gag}$) and murine ($Pr65^{gag}$) precursors are not effectively processed (Sen et al. 1980a). Further characterization of this protease is required to determine whether it represents one of the already established virion proteins.

Two other *gag*-related proteins, Pr110^{gag} and Pr160$^{gag\text{-}pol}$, are detected by immunoprecipitation of infected cells and by cell-free translation of virion genomic RNA (Dickson and Atterwill 1978, 1979; Racevskis and Sarkar 1978; Anderson et al. 1979; Massey and Schochetman 1979). The larger of these two proteins is, by analogy to the avian and murine C-type retroviruses, the polymerase precursor (see Section IV.D.2). Pr110^{gag} contains all the peptide sequences found in Pr77^{gag} (Anderson et al. 1979; Dickson and Atterwill 1979). Some of the additional sequences found in Pr110^{gag}, but not in Pr77^{gag}, are present in the minor virion protein p30 (see Section IV.A.1.e and Fig. 6.7). p30 contains the peptides that comprise p14 and some of the unique peptides that are found only in Pr110^{gag}. Since p14 represents the carboxyl terminus of Pr77^{gag}, it has been postulated that the Pr110^{gag} is an extended form of Pr77^{gag}. The mechanism by which such an extension occurs is obscure, although suppression or deletion of a termination codon by RNA splicing are feasible possibilities.

2. The pol*-gene Proteins*

The putative primary translation product of the MMTV *pol* gene is Pr160$^{gag\text{-}pol}$. This *gag*-related polyprotein is designated as the precursor to polymerase by analogy to the processing of a similar product found in cells infected by avian and murine C-type retroviruses (see Sections II.C.2 and III.C.2). Peptide mapping indicates that Pr160$^{gag\text{-}pol}$ contains peptides found in Pr77^{gag} and Pr110^{gag}, as well as some additional peptides (Anderson et al. 1979; Dickson and Atterwill 1979). The polyprotein can be synthesized in cell-free translation systems and therefore is likely to be a primary translation product (Dahl and Dickson 1979; Sen et al. 1979). A possible intermediate of 130,000 daltons has been reported (Massey and Schochetman 1979).

3. The env*-gene Proteins*

The product of the *env* gene is a polyprotein precursor, gPr73^{env}, of 73,000 daltons, which is proteolytically cleaved to yield the virion proteins gp52 and gp36 (see Fig. 6.8) (Dickson et al. 1976; Nusse et al. 1978; Racevskis and sarkar 1978; Schochetman et al. 1978; Anderson et al. 1979). This precursor is synthesized from an mRNA

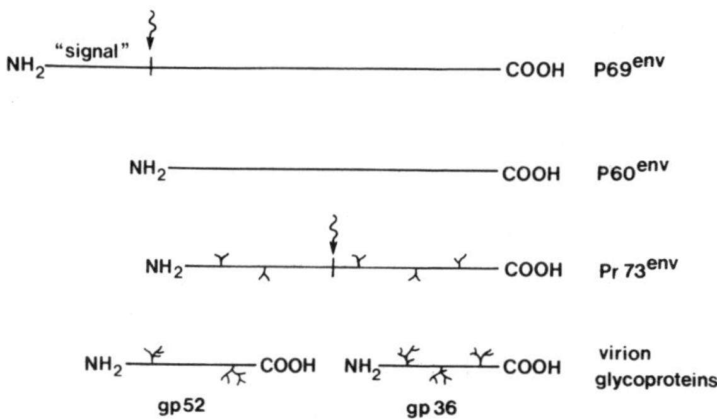

Figure 6.8 Processing and maturation of MMTV envelope glycoproteins. The polypeptide designated P69^{env} is synthesized in cell-free translation of *env* mRNA. Its in vivo counterpart is probably cleaved as a nascent chain after insertion into the endoplasmic reticulum. Cleavage at the site indicated by the arrow would remove the 9000 daltons of hydrophobic "signal" sequence. P60^{env} is the proposed structure of a protein observed in vivo after treatment of infected cells with inhibitors of glycosylation. Although the signal peptide is believed to have been cleaved from P69^{env}, suggesting membrane insertion, further processing does not appear to occur. In pulse-labeled MMTV-infected cells, gPr73^{env} is readily detected and is presumed to be derived from P69^{env} after membrane insertion, removal of the signal sequence, and glycosylation. Cleavage, disulfide-bond formation, and further glycosylation of gPr73^{env} generate the viral glycoproteins, gp52 and gp36.

(Schochetman and Schlom 1976) of subgenomic size (24S), which is derived by splicing a 5′ leader sequence to the 3′ half of the genomic RNA (Groner et al. 1979; Robertson and Varmus 1979; Sen et al. 1979; Chapter 5).

In common with other glycoproteins (Katz et al. 1977; Rothman and Lenard 1977; Rothman et al. 1978), gPr73^{env} is glycosylate during synthesis. Its synthesis as a transmembrane protein also requires the presence of a signal sequence that is proteolytically cleaved from the glycoprotein before synthesis is complete. The size of the apoprotein (i.e., without signal sequence and without carbohydrates; see Fig. 6.8) can be estimated by (1) synthesis of the precursor in cells treated with the drug tunicamycin, which inhibits glycosylation (Leavitt et al. 1977), or (2) removal of the sugar side chains with the enzyme *N*-acetyl-β-glucosaminidase H (Endo H), which cleaves unmodified primary core oligosaccharides linked to asparagine residues, leaving a single glucosamine residue on the polypeptide chain (Tarentino and Maley 1974). Both methods yield an apoprotein of 60,000 daltons (Dickson and Atterwill 1980). Lower concentrations of tunicamycin and shorter digestion times with Endo H result in incomplete inhibition or digestion. Under these suboptimal conditions, five partially glycosylated forms of the precursor can be resolved (evenly distributed in the molecular-weight range of 60,000–73,000 daltons), suggesting that the precursor receives five mannose-rich, asparagine-linked oligosaccharides during synthesis. The primary translation product in vitro of the *env* gene appears to be a polypeptide of 69,000 daltons (Dickson and Peters 1981; D. Robertson and J. Dudley, pers. comm.), indicating the existence of a 9000-dalton leader polypeptide, containing the signal sequence that would be cleaved off during synthesis in vivo (see Fig. 6.8).

Sugar labeling of the precursor shows the presence of mannose and glucosamine, but little fucose or galactose, consistent with the notion that $gPr73^{env}$ contains high-mannose-containing oligosaccharides only (Dickson and Atterwill 1980). Although the majority of the *env* precursor lacks fucose and galactose, a small proportion of the population contains these sugars and may migrate at a slightly greater molecular weight (Anderson et al. 1979; Dickson and Atterwill 1980). The order of the glycoproteins in the precursor has been determined as NH_2-gp52-gp36-COOH by hypertonic-shock-arrested initiation of protein synthesis in conjunction with pulse labeling (Schochetman and Schlom 1976; Schochetman et al. 1977a) and confirmed by pactamycin mapping (Dickson and Atterwill 1980; Sen et al. 1980b).

V. OTHER RETROVIRUS SYSTEMS

The preceding three sections have presented detailed analyses of the structures, functions, and biosynthetic pathways for the virion proteins of the avian C-type and the murine B-type and C-type virus groups. An attempt has been made to emphasize the analogies and disparities among these groups to illustrate the variety of mechanisms involved in the processing of polyprotein precursors to mature virion structural proteins. With retrovirus systems other than those just described, the biosynthetic mechanisms have not yet been examined in such depth, although similar types of analyses have been used, for example, to determine the molecular weights, chemical properties, and ordering of the protein components within genes. The presently available evidence indicates that the C-type viruses isolated from other species and the primate D-type viruses exhibit the same basic genomic organization with corresponding functional properties and utilize mechanisms for viral protein synthesis similar to those described above. Analogies can also be made for the non-structural virus-coded proteins, in particular the putative *onc* genes, which are discussed in Chapter 9. Therefore, for simplicity, but with the attempt to provide suitable references for additional reading, this information is summarized briefly in the next few pages. These virus groups have been chosen to emphasize that retroviruses isolated from a single species may be totally unrelated to one another, whereas others isolated from species that are evolutionarily only very distantly related may show very striking homologies. The viruses that fall into this latter group generally show a high degree of homology when assessed by nucleic acid hybridization studies and serological analyses, and this unexpected relatedness has led to theoretical discussions on the possibilities of trans-species transmission of retroviruses during the course of evolution (see Chapter 10). Finally, a summary table has been constructed to include reports on the protein components of retroviruses, some of which have not as yet been fully characterized (see Table 6.6). A caveat is issued here to remind the reader that many of these studies are based on detection of proteins from cell extracts or tissue-culture supernatants, observed in gels without the sensitivity and specificity provided by immunoprecipitation with anti-virus sera. Therefore, a number of the proteins observed and classified as virus-specific may represent cell or serum components.

A. Avian Reticuloendotheliosis Virus Group

At the present time, there are five antigenically related members in the REV group: the replication-defective REV strain T (REV-T) and its associated helper virus (REAV) from turkeys, duck spleen necrosis virus (SNV), duck infectious anemia virus, and chick syncytial virus. The isolation, genome structure, and pathogenicity of these viruses are described elsewhere (see Chapters 2, 4, and 8). However, despite the isolation of some of them from gallinaceous birds, the REV group does not share any genetic or immunological relationship with the avian sarcoma and leukemia C-type viruses described in Section II, although numerous antigenic and functional analogies with mammalian C-type viruses are discerned (see below).

Table 6.6 Structural virion proteins

Host species	Isolate designation	Molecular weight (kilodaltons) ($\times 10^{-3}$)[a] Internal proteins	Envelope proteins	Reverse transcriptase	Early references
Viper	VRV	p24, p18, p13, p12	?	p109	Twardzik et al (1974); Menko et al. (1976); Clark et al. (1979)
Snake	CSRV	p24, p16, p13, p12	gp72	?	Clark et al. (1979)
Birds	ALV, ASV	pp19-p27-p12-p15 (Pr76)	gp85-gp37 (gPr92)	p92 = p58-p32 (Pr180)	see text
	REAV, SNV	p29, p15, p13 (Pr63)	gp73, gp22 (Pr80)	p68 or p84 (Pr180)	see text
Mouse C type	MLV	p15-pp12-p30-p10 (Pr65)	gp70-p15(E) (Pr90)	p80 (Pr180)	see text
Mouse B type	MMTV	p10-pp21-p27-p14 (Pr77)	gp52-gp36 (Pr90)	p100 (Pr160)	see text
Rat	—	p30, p15, pp12, p10	gp70	?	Parks et al. (1974a); Pal et al. (1975)
Hamster	HLV	p37 (or p27), p23, p14	?	p68, p53	Oroszlan et al. (1971b); Charman et al. (1974); Verma et al. (1974)
Guinea pig	—	p24, p18, p16	gp70, gp36	?	Murray and Nayak (1974)
Mink	MiLV	p30, p15, pp12, p10	gp70	?	Sherr et al. (1978)

Cat	FeLV	p15-pp12-p26-p10 (Pr65)	gp70, p15(E) (gPr90)	p70	see text
	RD114	p12-pp15-p28-p10 (Pr68)	gp73	p70	see text
Pig	PK15	p30	?	p70	Todaro et al. (1974a)
Sheep	visna	p30, p16, p14	gp135 or gp70	p68	see text
Cow	BaLV	p24, p15, p12, p10 (Pr65)	gp51, gp31 (gPr85)	p70	Ferrer (1972); Onuma et al. (1976); Kaaden et al. (1977); Burny et al. (1978); Gupta and Ferrer (1978)
Deer	—	p30	?	?	Tronick et al. (1977)
Horse	EIAV	p28, p13, p11, p9	gp90, gp45	p70	Charman et al. (1976); Cheevers et al. (1978); Ishizaki et al. (1978); Parekh et al. (1980)
Primate C type	SSAV, GALV	p15-pp12-p27-p10	gp70, p15(E)	p70	see text
	BaEV	p12-pp15-p28-p10 (Pr68)	gp73	p70	see text
	MAC-1	p12-pp15-p26-p10	gp60	?	see text
	MMC-1	p12-pp15-p26-p10	gp70	?	see text
	OMC-1	p11-pp15-p29-p10	gp70	?	see text

Table 6.6 (Continued)

Primate D type	MPMV	p12-pp14-p27-p10 (Pr78)	gp68, gp20 (gPr86)	p80 (Pr180)	see text
	SMRV	p16-pp12-p35-p9 (Pr72)	gp75	p80	see text

[a]Proteins within a column are listed in order of decreasing molecular weight, except where connected by hyphens. The hyphens designate the known order of the proteins from the aminoterminal end to the carboxyterminal end within the polyprotein precursor molecule. The precursor proteins are indicated within parentheses.

Structural protein analysis has been reported for the prototype member, REAV, and for SNV. For the data presented below, we shall not distinguish these two viruses, designating them both as REV. With the exception of the major core protein, p29, the virion polypeptides of REV have not been well characterized. At least two low-molecular-weight nonglycosylated proteins, p13 and p15, are also present in purified virions, although their functional role in virus architecture is unknown (Maldonado and Bose 1975, 1976; Mosser et al. 1975). The envelope is composed of two glycosylated proteins, gp71/73 and gp22. None of these polypeptides comigrate on SDS-polyacrylamide gels with those of other avian retroviruses (Halpern et al. 1973; Maldonado and Bose 1973; Mosser et al. 1975). Not only is the major core protein p29 antigenically distinct from the ALV core protein p27 (Maldonado and Bose 1971, 1976; Moelling et al. 1975), but it is markedly different in composition and sequence; however, it is related to the MLV core protein p30, as determined by radioimmunological and sequence analysis (Hunter et al. 1978; Barbacid et al. 1979; Charman et al. 1979). REV p29 exhibits approximately 40% homology with MLV and feline leukemia virus (FeLV) p30 molecules (Hunter et al. 1978) and greater than 50% homology with the major core protein of the endogenous retroviruses of macaques (Oroszlan and Gilden 1980) (discussed in Section V.C.2.b).

REV reverse transcriptase is unrelated to other avian retroviral enzymes (Mizutani and Temin 1973, 1974, 1975; Kieras and Faras 1975; Moelling et al. 1975; Waite and Allen 1975) but is antigenically cross-reactive with those of mammalian retroviruses (Bauer and Temin 1980b). Moreover, REV reverse transcriptase has a divalent-cation requirement for manganese, as do the enzymes associated with most C-type mammalian retroviruses (Kang 1975; Moelling et al. 1975; Waite and Allen 1975). The enzyme is reported to be a single polypeptide with a molecular weight of 68,000 (Mizutani and Temin 1975) or 84,000 daltons (Moelling et al. 1975); this discrepancy has not yet been resolved. RNase-H activity, again distinct from that of ASLV, is also detected in purified REV enzyme (Mizutani and Temin 1975); the RNase-H and reverse transcriptase activities cannot be physically separated and therefore appear to be associated with the same polypeptide. A third enzymic activity associated with REV particles is an RNA-directed RNA polymerase, which, however, can be physically separated from the reverse transcriptase (Mizutani and Temin 1976). It has been postulated that this enzyme could be involved in the synthesis of RNA primers, although the association of a primer $tRNA^{Pro}$ with the genomic RNA (Peters and Glover 1980) would obviate the need for a virion-associated, RNA-directed RNA polymerase. A similar enzymic activity has not been described in other retrovirus systems and, therefore, this may represent adventitious packaging of a cellular enzyme.

The nature of the virus-specific polypeptides synthesized in REV-infected cells has not been extensively investigated. Spleen cells transformed by REV-T contain three polypeptides that can be precipitated from the cells with antiserum prepared against REAV (Hoelzer et al. 1980). These polypeptides have molecular weights of 180,000, 80,000, and 63,000 daltons. Antiserum against p29 precipitates the 63,000-dalton protein; therefore, this may be the *gag* precursor (Wong et al. 1980). By analogy to other retroviruses, the 180,000-dalton protein probably represents the *gag-pol* precursor. The 80,000-dalton protein is not immunoprecipitated by anti-p29 serum and is presumed to be the *env* precursor, although further evidence is required to prove this.

B. Feline Retroviruses

The feline retroviruses isolated from the domestic cat (*Felis cattus*) are all C-type particles and fall into two distinct unrelated groups: (1) the replication-competent FeLVs and the replication-defective feline sarcoma viruses (FeSV), which are transmitted horizontally and induce a variety of diseases, both oncogenic and nononcogenic (see Chapters 2 and 8), and (2) the RD114/CCC group representing the endogenous virus isolates, none of which show any pathogenic potential.

The lack of relatedness between the two groups was dramatically observed with the initial isolation of RD114 (McAllister et al. 1972). This isolate was obtained from a human tumor that had been injected into a fetal cat, and the recovered virus was originally thought to be of human origin because there was no cross-reaction with the known FeLV isolates with regard to protein or nucleic acid sequences. However, hybridization of RD114 nucleic acid to normal cat tissues soon belied this assumption and proved that it represented an endogenous cat virus that had replicated in the human cells

(Baluda and Roy-Burman 1973; Fujinaga et al. 1973; Gillespie et al. 1973; Neiman 1973; Okabe et al. 1973; Ruprecht et al. 1973). Isolation of viruses related to RD114 from cultured cat cells confirmed this finding (Livingston and Todaro 1973; Sarma et al. 1973). Further comparative characterization emphasized the dissimilarity between RD114 and FeLV and also pointed out the extremely high degree of relatedness between RD114 and the baboon endogenous viruses (BaEV) (see Sections V.B.2 and V.C.2.a and Chapter 2). In fact, the RD114 and BaEV isolates form a group that shows little homology with any other retroviruses, with the possible exception of the deer C-type retrovirus (Aaronson et al. 1976), lacking the interspecies reactivities shared by the other mammalian retroviruses.

1. FeLV and FeSV

Structural and polypeptide composition analysis of FeLV has shown great similarity to the murine C-type retroviruses by both physicochemical and immunological criteria. The polypeptides of the virion core have molecular weights equivalent to those of the corresponding MLV proteins (Schafer et al. 1971; Oroszlan et al. 1973; Velicer and Graves 1974; Okasinski and Velicer 1976; Khan and Stephenson 1977) (see Table 6.6). The major internal *gag* protein has a molecular weight of about 26,000 daltons and a neutral isoelectric point (pI 7.4–8.3) (Oroszlan et al. 1973; Khan and Stephenson 1977). p26 contains the interspecies antigenic determinants shared by all mammalian C-type retroviruses, although it is more highly related to the rodent group than to primates (Geering et al. 1968; Oroszlan et al. 1971a; Sarma et al. 1971; Parks and Scolnick 1972). This relatedness is further demonstrated from partial amino acid sequencing (Oroszlan et al. 1971a).

The immunological similarity of FeLV proteins to those of MLV extends to the other three internal structural *gag* polypeptides (p10, pp12, and p15), and they can be precipitated with antisera to the equivalent MLV proteins (Khan and Stephenson 1977). The isoelectric points of the small internal polypeptides are once again almost identical with the MLV counterparts, showing biochemical and biophysical relatedness as well. The polypeptide p15 is neutral (pI 7.5), pp12 is acidic (pI 5.4), and p10 is basic (pI 9.1).

The core polypeptide products of the *gag* gene are synthesized as a polyprotein precursor of 65,000 daltons ($Pr65^{gag}$). This precursor has an extremely short half-life, as it is detected only after a 2.5-minute pulse in the presence of the proline analog, L-azetidine-2-carboxylic acid. The first cleavage product is a slightly more stable intermediate of 60,000 daltons and lacks one of the small polypeptides (Okasinski and Velicer 1976, 1977). The order of the proteins within the precursor has been studied by two groups, who arrived at conflicting results. On one hand, Okasinski and Velicer (1977) determined the order as NH_2-pp12-p15-p10-p26-COOH, using the pactamycin-mapping procedure. On the other hand, Khan and Stephenson (1977) suggested the order to be NH_2-p15-pp12-p26-p10-COOH by analogy to MLV. The second order is probably correct, on the basis of our knowledge of the physical properties of the peptides.

A glycosylated *gag* protein of 40,000 daltons has been detected in the culture fluids of FeLV-infected cells. It was shown to be related to the *gag*-gene precursor by immunoprecipitation and tryptic peptide mapping (Neil et al. 1980). The synthesis of glycosylated *gag* cell-surface proteins has been described for both murine and avian C-type retroviruses (see Sections II.C.1.a and III.B.2). It is not yet known whether the FeLV glycosylated *gag* protein is normally found as a membrane protein of infected cells.

The reverse transcriptase molecule of FeLV is a monomeric molecule of 70,000 daltons (Rho and Gallo 1979). Presumably, the molecule exhibits RNA-dependent and DNA-dependent DNA polymerase reactions and RNase-H activity. By analogy to the other retroviruses, the enzyme is synthesized from a large polyprotein molecule containing both *gag*-gene and *pol*-gene sequences. Antigenically, FeLV reverse transcriptase is cross-reactive with the C-type rodent enzymes, illustrating shared interspecies determinants, although type-specific antigens are also detected (Scolnick et al. 1972a; Rho and Gallo 1979). Infected nonviremic cats often have high levels of antibody to FeLV reverse transcriptase (Jacquemin et al. 1978). Interestingly, an IgG fraction found on leukemic human cells also cross-reacts with this molecule (Rho and Gallo 1979), although the significance of this finding is obscure.

Natural isolates of FeLV often contain mixtures of two, or occasionally three, FeLV serotypes (designated subgroups A, B, and C) (see Chapters 2, 3, and 8). The subgroup differences are a function of the envelope glycoproteins and are reflected in host-range, neutralization, and interference phenomena (Sarma and Log 1971, 1973).

The *env*-gene products of FeLV are structurally analogous to those of MLV. The major envelope moiety is a glycoprotein of

70,000 daltons, gp70 (Velicer and Graves 1974; Pinter and Fleissner 1979). The majority of gp70 molecules are linked by disulfide bonds to the second component of the virion envelope, a 15,000-dalton nonglycosylated polypeptide, p15(E), to form a glycoprotein complex of 90,000 daltons (gp90) (Pinter and Fleissner 1979). These proteins are probably synthesized as a 90,000-dalton glycosylated precursor, $Pr90^{env}$.

2. RD114/CCC Group

The RD114/CCC group of viruses is distantly related to FeLV, MLV, and other rodent C-type retroviruses, as measured by interspecies radioimmunoassay, but is closely related to BaEV (Todaro et al. 1974a; Barbacid et al. 1977). The relationship between RD114/CCC and BaEV is evident from comparative studies examining the immunological, biochemical, and the physical properties of the major structural proteins of the viruses. These numerous homologies between the RD114/CCC and BaEV isolates suggest a common origin for these viruses (see Chapter 2).

The *gag* proteins are presumably processed from a 68,000-dalton precursor (Sacks et al. 1978). The major internal structural protein of RD114 has an estimated molecular weight of 33,500 daltons as determined from SDS-polyacrylamide gel electrophoresis (Oroszlan et al. 1972) and of 27,000 daltons as determined by gel filtration on agarose in the presence of 6 M guanidine hydrochloride (Stephenson et al. 1977). The purified polypeptide is neutral or slightly basic with isoelectric point estimates of 8.0 and 9.1, respectively (Oroszlan et al. 1972; Stephenson et al. 1977). Antigenically, the p27 shows a strong cross-reactivity with the p30 of BaEV (Hellman et al. 1974; Sherr and Todaro 1974; Sherr et al. 1974; Stephenson et al. 1976a) and weakly reactive interspecies determinants, using radioimmunoassays with other mammalian C-type retroviruses (Oroszlan et al. 1972; Stephenson and Aaronson 1973; Sherr and Todaro 1974; Barbacid et al. 1980b). The primary amino acid sequence of the aminoterminal portion of p27 shows significant homology with other mammalian C-type viruses, which could account for the interspecies antigenic cross-reactivity (Oroszlan et al. 1973) (see Appendix F).

The RD114 viruses also contain three other major internal polypeptides with sizes and physical properties similar to those of other retroviruses (see Table 6.6). The smallest of these polypeptides, p10, is the most basic protein with an isoelectric point of 11.2 (Stephenson et al. 1977). By analogy to other retroviruses, this protein is probably associated with the genomic RNA and should demonstrate single-stranded nucleic-acid-binding activity (see Table 6.1). RD114 p10 shows strong antigenic cross-reactivity with the BaEV p10 and weaker interspecies reactivity with the basic polypeptides from other mammalian C-type retroviruses (Barbacid et al. 1977). Similar types of antigenically cross-reactive determinants are detected when comparing the most hydrophobic protein of RD114 and BaEV, p12; in each case, the proteins exhibit a near neutral isoelectric point (pI 8.0 for RD114) (Stephenson et al. 1977). This protein corresponds in physical properties to the p15 proteins of MLV and FeLV.

The major phosphoprotein is a molecule of 15,000 daltons (Pal and Roy-Burman 1975; Pal et al. 1975) and specifically binds to the genomic RNAs of RD114 and BaEV (Sen and Todaro 1977; Sen et al. 1978). The binding of pp15 to BaEV RNA suggests that the protein-RNA recognition sites are highly conserved, adding strength to the proposal that both virus groups derive from a common evolutionary origin. This finding also suggests that RD114 pp15 is functionally homologous to the major phosphoproteins of other mammalian retroviruses. However, in the case of RD114 and BaEV, the phosphate is linked to the polypeptide on threonine residues, rather than a serine, as is the case for the rodent and FeLV C-type retroviruses (Pal et al. 1975). The significance of this difference, if any, is not known. Immunologically, the pp15 demonstrates strong type-specific antigenic determinants that allow the RD114/CCC viruses to be distinguished easily from BaEV. The type-specific antigenicity exhibited by these molecules is also a characteristic of the rodent C-type viral phosphoproteins (see Section III.A.1.c). The similar physical characteristics and interspecies cross-reactivity of three of the RD114/CCC polypeptides with those of MLV led Barbacid et al. (1977) and Stephenson et al. (1977) to postulate the order of these polypeptides within the putative *gag* precursor as NH_2-p12-pp15-p27-p10-COOH.

The reverse transcriptase of RD114 is immunologically related to that of BaEV, as might be expected (Sherr et al. 1974). Thus, antisera prepared against the RD114 enzyme inhibits its own activity and partially inhibits (66%) that of BaEV, and vice versa (Sherr et al. 1974, 1975). Similar enzyme inhibition experiments using antisera to the reverse transcriptase of other C-type viruses detect no other antigenic cross-reactivity. The reverse transcriptase enzyme of BaEV is a single polypeptide of 70,000 daltons, similar to that of MLV, and therefore the same is probably true for the RD114/CCC enzyme (Sherr et al. 1974).

The envelope proteins of RD114 virus have not been extensively studied, although they are presumably similar to those of other C-type retroviruses. A comparative examination of the host ranges of BaEV and RD114 again reflects the remarkable homology between these endogenous viruses of primate and feline origin (see Chapter 2) and suggests that close sequence homology between the envelope components might be expected.

C. Primate Retroviruses

On the basis of patterns of viral morphogenesis, primate viruses fall into two major groups: those in which the viral capsid is assembled during budding from the cell plasma membrane (C-type) and those in which the capsid is preassembled within the cytoplasm (D-type). Each group can be subdivided further on the basis of transmission (endogenous vs exogenous), species of origin, and, finally, uniqueness of the viral genetic material. The diverse origins are reflected in the structural polypeptides of the members of this group; in many instances, both the size and immunological reactivitics of a protein will distinguish it from functionally similar ones of viruses from another species. Less molecular information is available about the structure and biosynthesis of primate retroviral polypeptides than for the avian and murine retroviruses, although it is clear that the structural polypeptides are translated from intracellular mRNA as high-molecular-weight precursor proteins that are cleaved proteolytically into the individual functional units. Furthermore, the positions of polypeptides with specific functions have been highly conserved on the precursor proteins of the *gag* and *env* genes. Thus, the membrane-associated hydrophobic *gag*-gene product is invariably located at the amino terminus of the *gag*-precursor protein. Adjacent to this is a phosphorylated protein with RNA-binding properties, followed by the major structural polypeptide, and at the carboxyl terminus is a highly basic small nucleic-acid-binding protein.

Immunological approaches have been used extensively to probe the interrelationships of the functionally similar proteins of different primate viruses. The competitive radioimmunoassay is particularly powerful and can identify even relatively minor common antigenic determinants. Indeed, as discussed in Chapter 2, some of these studies have provided intriguing insights into the relationships of primate retroviruses to each other and to other retroviruses.

1. Exogenous C-type Viruses (SSAV and GALV)

The prototype virus of the group was isolated from a New World woolly monkey with multiple fibrosarcomas (Theilen et al. 1971; Wolfe et al. 1971) and is, in fact, a mixture of a replication-defective transforming simian sarcoma virus (SSV) and its associated helper virus (SSAV). The sarcoma virus component appears to be completely defective with regard to structural polypeptide synthesis, as SSV-transformed marmoset cell lines do not synthesize virus or any detectable viral proteins (Bergholz et al. 1977). On the other hand, SSAV replicates efficiently in a wide range of cell cultures and is very closely related to a group of viruses (GALV) isolated from gibbon apes.

The structural polypeptides of the SSAV/GALV group are summarized in Table 6.6. The four *gag* polypeptides have molecular weights and functions similar to those of the murine C-type retroviruses, consistent with the likely origin of the SSAV/GALV group (see Chapter 2). The major *gag*-gene polypeptide has a molecular weight of 29,000 to 30,000 daltons (Hoekstra and Deinhardt 1973/1974; Gilden et al. 1974b; Oroszlan et al. 1975a,b); tryptic peptide analyses of this polypeptide from SSAV and GALV show no differences, and the aminoterminal amino acid sequences for these same proteins are identical for at least the first 28 residues (Oroszlan et al. 1975b, 1977). In common with most other mammalian virus p30 proteins, the amino acid sequence initiates with proline-leucine-arginine and is remarkably homologous to the sequences of both MLV and FeLV. By most immunological approaches, including competition radioimmunoassays, the p30s of SSAV and GALV are essentially indistinguishable, although, by using a quantitative microcomplement fixation test and highly type-specific guinea pig sera, Gilden et al. (1974a) were able to differentiate SSAV and GALV. Nevertheless, they estimated from their results that the two polypeptides were 96–98% homologous.

The acidic phosphorylated protein, pp12, binds with high specificity to its homologous 70S and 35S virion RNAs. The precise specificity of binding allows identification of members of the SSAV/GALV group (Sen and Todaro 1976) and may reflect the highly type-specific antigenic character of this polypeptide (Tronick et al. 1974b, 1975; Stephenson et al. 1977). The other two *gag*-gene products, p15 and p10, share biochemical and antigenic properties with the murine retroviruses; p15 is a neutral (pI 6.1–6.8) hydrophobic molecule and p10 is a basic hydrophilic polypeptide. Both have interspecies antigenic determinants in common with the analogous polypeptides of mammalian viruses (Stephenson et al. 1977).

The reverse transcriptase activities of SSAV and GALV are associated with molecules of about 70,000 and 68,000 daltons, respectively (Abrell and Gallo 1973; Sarin and Gallo 1976), which are highly related to one another by immunological criteria (Kawakami et al. 1972; Scolnick et al. 1972b). SSAV/GALV reverse transcriptase shows essentially no homology with those of other primate retroviruses; however, some antigenic cross-reactivity is observed with the polymerases of the murine retroviruses, particularly the isolate from *Mus caroli*, and the endogenous virus of pigs (see Chapter 2).

The glycoprotein complex of SSAV/GALV is composed of a major glycosylated polypeptide, gp70, and a small nonglycosylated polypeptide, p15(E). By analogy to the other retroviruses, it is probable that gp70 is held into the viral membrane by disulfide linkages to the transmembrane hydrophobic p15(E). Under certain growth conditions, gp70 can be released into the growth medium in the absence of p15(E), and further proteolytic degradation of this soluble form can give rise to a smaller product, gp45 (Thiel et al. 1978). Despite the facts that complete cross-interference is observed between members of the SSAV/GALV group and that antiserum raised against one virus can neutralize the other isolates with similar titers (Kawakami and Buckley 1974; Lieber et al. 1975; Todaro et al. 1975), antigenic differences have been observed in competition radioimmunoassays.

2. Endogenous C-type Viruses

The genetically transmitted C-type primate retroviruses can be divided into three unrelated classes: those from baboons (collectively termed BaEV), those from macaques, and those from the owl monkey. Although the first two species are of Old World origin, they have presumably acquired their viruses from different sources (see Chapter 2).

a. Baboon Endogenous Viruses. Immological and nucleic acid hybridization experiments show that this group of primate viruses is highly related to the RD114/CCC endogenous cat viruses (discussed in Section V.B). This is also reflected in the polypeptides of the two virus groups.

The major *gag* polyprotein of BaEV corresponds to approximately 30% of the total virion protein and has a molecular weight in polyacrylamide gels of 28,000 to 33,000 daltons (Sherr and Todaro 1974; Stephenson et al. 1977; Bryant et al. 1978). It can be distinguished from that of the RD114/CCC viruses by its lower isoelectric point (pI 7.0 vs pI 8.0–8.8 for RD114) (Sherr and Todaro 1974; Stephenson et al. 1977). Even so, the aminoterminal amino acid sequences of BaEV and RD114 p30 proteins are identical. The sequence is similar to that of other mammalian retroviruses, but a gap has to be inserted in order to maintain alignment with murine and feline retroviruses (Oroszlan et al. 1975a,b).

The major phosphoprotein has a molecular weight of 16,000 daltons (Pal and Roy-Burman 1975), with an acidic isoelectric point (pI 4.7–5.9) (Stephenson et al. 1976a, 1977; Barbacid et al. 1977). Furthermore, Sen et al. (1978) have shown that pp16 is an RNA-binding protein that binds equally well to BaEV RNA and RD114 viral RNA (about six to eight sites per RNA subunit); no binding is observed to MLV RNA or RSV RNA. In competition binding assays, RD114 and BaEV pp16 compete equally well, indicating remarkable conservation of RNA sequence and protein conformation. It is interesting that similar studies with the primate exogenous viruses, SSAV/GALV, which share 50–75% overall nucleic acid homology, allow a clear differentiation of members within the group, yet the RNA sequence homology of BaEV and RD114 is only 20–30%. Its antigenic determinants are predominantly type-specific, allowing differentiation not only between BaEV and RD114, but also between endogenous viruses from different species of baboon (Stephenson et al. 1976a; Barbacid et al. 1977)

BaEV p12 displays hydrophobic characteristics and a neutral isoelectric point (pI 7.1–7.5) similar to those of MLV and FeLV p15 (Stephenson et al. 1976a, 1977; Barbacid et al. 1977). Indeed, it is this protein that carries interspecies antigenic determinants cross-reactive with MLV p15. The smallest *gag* polypeptide, p10, is highly basic and presumably is associated with the RNP complex within the virion; it carries interspecies antigenic determinants that cross-react with MLV p10 (Barbacid et al. 1977).

The reverse transcriptase is a polypeptide of 68,000 to 70,000 daltons with a divalent-cation preference for manganese, characteristic of other mammalian C-type retroviruses. Immunologically, the enzymes of BaEV and RD114 are closely related but distinguishable. Neither enzyme is inhibited, however, by antiserum to the reverse transcriptases of MLV, FeLV, or SSAV (Scolnick et al. 1972b; Hellman et al. 1974; Sherr et al. 1974; Todaro et al. 1974b; Sarin et al. 1977; Bryant et al. 1978).

The major *env*-gene product is a glycosylated polypeptide, gp70 (Stephenson et al. 1976b; Bryant et al. 1978; Devare et al. 1978a). It is not yet clear whether a second *env* polypeptide, equivalent to p15(E) of MLV, is present on virions, but this is most likely.

b. Macaque Endogenous Viruses. Two viruses, MAC-1 and MMC-1, have been isolated from the stumptail monkey (*Macaca arctoides*) and rhesus monkey (*Macaca mulatta*), respectively. Nucleic acid and immunological studies indicate that these are very closely related viruses, although differing in host-range properties (Bryant et al. 1978; Todaro et al. 1978a; Rabin et al. 1979).

The major structural polypeptide has a molecular weight of 26,000 daltons and is distinct, molecularly and immunologically, from other primate retroviruses. Tryptic peptide analysis of MAC-1 p26 shows that this protein is unrelated to the major core proteins of endogenous viruses from the baboon and owl monkey (Bryant et al. 1978). The aminoterminal amino acid sequence of MAC-1 p26 is also distinct from those of other endogenous primate viruses but is identical with that of MMC-1 and resembles that of the SSAV/GALV group. Unexpectedly, there is remarkable similarity (50% homology) to the avian REV p27 sequence with which it aligns, with no insertions or deletions for 15 of the first 28 residues (S. Oroszlan et al., pers. comm.). The major phosphoprotein is a polypeptide of 15,000 daltons, and the two other nonglycosylated *gag* proteins have molecular weights of 12,000 and 10,000 daltons.

Little is known about the products of the *pol* and *env* genes of the macaque viruses. The reverse transcriptase shows a divalent-cation preference for manganese and is not inhibited by antisera to various primate and mammalian viruses (Bryant et al. 1978; Todaro et al. 1978a). The major glycoproteins of MAC-1 and MMC-1 may differ in size (see Table 6.6); according to Bryant et al. (1978), there is a major glycosylated protein of 60,000 daltons in MAC-1. Whether this represents a degradation product similar to the gp45 of SSAV is not clear. The different host ranges displayed by the two isolates suggest that type-specific antigenic determinants are present on the glycoproteins (Todaro et al. 1978a; Rabin et al. 1979).

c. Owl Monkey Endogenous Virus. The first endogenous C-type virus of a New World monkey, termed OMC-1, was isolated from an owl monkey (*Aotus trivirgatus*) (Todaro et al. 1978c). The polypeptide profile of this virus resembles those of the baboon and macaque viruses, although tryptic peptide analyses show that the major polypeptide, p29, of OMC-1 is distinct from other primate retroviral proteins, and it is unreactive in the assays commonly used to detect interspecies antigenic determinants (Todaro et al. 1978c; Barbacid et al. 1980a).

3. D-type Primate Retroviruses

D-type retroviruses have now been isolated from at least three primate species. The prototype virus of this group, Mason-Pfizer monkey virus (MPMV) is a horizontally transmitted retrovirus that grows in its species of origin and in other primate cells (Chopra and Mason 1970; Jensen et al. 1970; Chopra et al. 1971) (see Chapter 2). A virus morphologically indistinguishable and antigenically related to MPMV has been isolated from a second Old World monkey, the spectacled langur (*Presbytis obscurus*) (Todaro et al. 1978b). The langur virus, designated PO-1-Lu, is endogenous in its species of origin and possesses a xenotropic host range (Benveniste and Todaro 1977; Todaro et al. 1978b) (see Chapter 2). Another D-type retrovirus was isolated from tissues of a New World squirrel monkey (*Saimiri sciureus*) (Heberling et al. 1977; Smith et al. 1977). Although structurally and antigenically distinct from the langur virus, the squirrel monkey retrovirus (SMRV) is also endogenous in its species of origin and xenotropic in its host range (Colcher et al. 1977b; Hino et al. 1977; Schochetman and Fine 1978).

On the basis of their morphogenesis, D-type viruses more closely resemble the murine B-type viruses in that intracytoplasmic A-type particles and preformed core structures are observed in infected cells. The mature virions, however, more closely resemble other primate C-type viruses to a degree, although discernible differences can be detected (Fine and Schochetman 1978; Schlom 1980) (see Chapter 2). The structural characteristics described below show that, although the D-type viruses are distinct from the primate C-type viruses, they presumably have diverged from an ancestor common to both groups.

a. MPMV and PO-1-Lu. The *gag* polypeptides of MPMV/PO-1-Lu are summarized in Table 6.6. Both viruses contain a major structural polypeptide of approximately 27,000 daltons that is unrelated to the major polypeptide of other primate retroviruses in both tryptic peptide analyses and aminoterminal amino acid sequence; the first three amino acids are proline-valine-threonine, rather than proline-leucine-arginine (Nowinski et al. 1971a; Tronick et al. 1974a; Schochetman et al. 1975; Bryant et al. 1978; Colcher et al. 1978; Charman et al. 1979). In homologous competition radioimmunoassays, the langur virus and MPMV p27 proteins are indistinguishable (Bryant et al. 1978; Colcher et al. 1978; Todaro et al. 1978b) and do not cross-react with any B-type or C-type viruses of mammalian or avian origin (Tronick et al. 1974a; Yeh et al. 1975; Schochetman et al. 1976). However, antigenic relatedness to SMRV (see Section V.C.3.b) (Devare et al. 1978b) and, perhaps surprisingly, to the viper C-type retrovirus (Andersen et al. 1979) has been detected.

The major phosphorylated polypeptide pp14, of the MPMV/ langur viruses presumably plays a functional role similar to that of MLV p12 (Bryant et al. 1978). Two other small nonglycosylated polypeptides, p12 and p10, can also be identified in virions.

MPMV *gag*-gene products are synthesized as a precursor polyprotein of 78,000 daltons that is subsequently cleaved to the individual polyproteins (Bradac and Hunter 1980). Two other *gag*-related products (180,000 and 94,000 daltons) can be detected; the former is probably the polyprotein precursor to the viral reverse transcriptase (J. Bradac and E. Hunter, pers. comm.) and the latter polypeptide may be analogous to the 110,000-dalton, *gag*-related protein found in MMTV-infected cells (see Section IV.D). Whether virus-coded or cellular enzymes are responsible for proteolytic cleavage of the $Pr78^{gag}$ to the structural polypeptides is not yet known.

The reverse transcriptase of MPMV/langur viruses is a polypeptide of 80,000 to 85,000 daltons (Marcus et al. 1978a; Todaro et al. 1978b). Both the virion-associated and purified enzymes have a divalent-cation preference for magnesium, similar to that of MMTV.

The major *env*-gene product of the MPMV/langur virus is a glycosylated polypeptide of about 70,000 daltons. A second glycoprotein, gp20, is also present in MPMV (Schochetman et al. 1975), which distinguishes this virus from mammalian C-type retroviruses. It is not clear at present whether a similar polypeptide is present in the langur virus. Type-, group-, and broadly reactive interspecies-specific antigenic determinants are present.

The glycoproteins of MPMV are synthesized as an 86,000-dalton precursor polypeptide that is subsequently processed to the individual polypeptides. This precursor is heavily glycosylated; in the presence of inhibitors of glycosylation, a carbohydrate-free polypeptide of 54,000 daltons is observed (Bradac and Hunter 1980). In this respect, the MPMV *env* precursor resembles that of the avian viruses, rather than the less heavily glycosylated protein of MMTV or MLV (Diggelmann 1979; Stohrer and Hunter 1979; Witte and Wirth 1979; Dickson and Atterwill 1980). In the presence of such inhibitors, noninfectious MPMV particles, lacking *env* proteins, are synthesized; thus, glycosylated envelope proteins are not required for virus assembly (Chatterjee et al. 1980).

b. Squirrel Monkey Retroviruses. Although clearly a D-type virus on the basis of morphogenesis, the squirrel monkey retroviruses, SMRV and M534, are unrelated to the MPMV/langur viruses, as determined by nucleic acid hybridization (Colcher et al. 1977b; Hino et al. 1977; Bryant et al. 1978). The structural proteins of SMRV are also quite distinct from those of the other two D-type viruses (see Table 6.6). The major structural polypeptide, p35, is significantly larger than that of any other primate retrovirus (Colcher et al. 1977a; Hino et al. 1977; Schochetman et al. 1977b) and is related antigenically to MPMV (Devare et al. 1978b). The major phosphorylated polypeptide in SMRV virions, pp12, is an acidic protein (pI 4.5), although the p35 and p16 proteins may also be phosphorylated to a minor extent (Bryant et al. 1978; Devare and Stephenson 1979). The p16 polypeptide resembles MLV p15 in its hydrophobic character and its tendency to aggregate in the absence of detergent, whereas a small basic polypeptide, p9, is associated with the RNP complex (Devare and Stephenson 1979; Uckert et al. 1980).

Using nonconditional mutants of SMRV (see Chapter 7), Devare and Stephenson (1979) have identified a 72,000-dalton *gag* precursor and several intermediate processing products from which they predicted a polypeptide order of NH_2-p16-pp12-p35-p9-COOH. This is consistent with the conserved arrangement of *gag*-gene products discussed earlier.

The reverse transcriptase of SMRV is similar in size and divalent-cation requirements to that of MPMV (Marcus et al. 1978a), but it can be distinguished from the latter enzyme by its preference for manganese as a divalent cation in the presence of high salt (Colcher et al. 1977b).

The major glycosylated protein of SMRV is 75,000 daltons and, like that of the MPMV/langur group, it contains type-, group-, and interspecies-specific determinants. Little is known, however, of the biosynthesis of this virion component.

D. Lentiviruses

The Lentivirinae or slow viruses comprise a unique subfamily of Retroviridae, as determined from patterns of disease production and also from the distinctive differences in nucleic acid sequence, peptide composition, and antigenicity. The subfamily consists of one isolate from goats (caprine encephalitis arthritis virus) and several isolates from sheep, including visna, maedi, progressive pneumonia virus, and zwoegerziekte virus (see Chapter 2). However, all biological and biochemical analyses performed to date indicate that these individually named viruses may actually represent highly related variants of a single prototype, the most important distinction residing in the pathological syndromes they induce (see Chapter 8).

The major virion polypeptides are gp135, p30, p16, and p14 (Mountcastle et al. 1972; Haase and Baringer 1974; Lin and Thormar 1974; Lin 1977). The gp135 apparently comprises the virion spikes and is known to elicit type-specific neutralizing antibodies (Mountcastle et al. 1972; Lin and Thormar 1979; Scott et al. 1979). There is one report of a glycopeptide of 70,000 daltons (Bruns and Frenzel 1979). Therefore, these data may suggest either that the envelope glycoprotein is more heavily glycosylated than that of other retroviruses or that there may be two smaller glycoproteins, which, however, are very resistant to the standard denaturation techniques used to separate the envelope components of other retroviruses.

The major virion protein, p30, is localized to the viral core and bears the major antigenic determinants shared by the group (Lin 1977; M. Weiss et al. 1977; Stowring et al. 1979). The smallest peptide, p14, is also located within the core. Reverse transcriptase activity is associated with a dimer composed of 68,000-dalton subunits (Lin and Thormar 1970, 1972; Stone et al. 1971; Lin et al. 1973; Haase et al. 1974; Lin and Papini 1978).

The type-specific and group-specific antigenic determinants of lentiviruses are not shared by other retroviruses, even those that exhibit similar biological functions, e.g., those associated with slow infections (equine infectious anemia virus), those that produce cell fusion (bovine syncytial virus), and those that induce cytopathic effects in vitro (REVs) (Stowring et al. 1979). Thus, the lentiviruses remain a unique class of retrovirus, sharing only the common morphological, biophysical, and functional organization without homology at the levels of nucleic acid or protein sequence.

VI. CONCLUDING REMARKS

This discourse on the nature of the structural virion proteins and their biosynthetic pathways has pointed out the overall kinship of the retroviruses. The virus groups covered in detail were chosen not only because they represent the best characterized systems, but also because they emphasize new concepts or different mechanisms. It would be too easy, and definitively inaccurate, to generalize from studies on only one virus system; there are points on which the retroviruses exhibit remarkable disparity. At this stage, it is perhaps worthwhile to recapitulate the salient features, with an emphasis on the analogies or lack thereof.

To start with the invariable mechanistic similarities, it can be concluded that each of the three viral structural genes is translated into a polyprotein precursor that requires modification and cleavage to produce the mature protein forms. This mode of synthesis and processing allows orientation of the proteins in a conformation that presumably is important in facilitating the self-assembly of viral particles. To some degree, as discussed in the Introduction (see Fig. 6.1 and Table 6.1), the order of the proteins within the gene, and consequently within the primary translational product, generally reflects the chemical nature of the protein (e.g., hydrophobicity, phosphorylation, and glycosylation), although some differences in biological function are noted. The spatial configuration of the proteins in virions, along with their order within the precursor molecules, is probably an important correlate, as it seems that a significant amount of cleavage of the precursor polyprotein occurs postbudding in extracellular virions. On one hand, this could provide an efficient means for ensuring that a major proportion of the virus-specific proteins becomes incorporated into viral particles, rather than associating with cellular proteins for which they might, individually, have some affinity. On the other hand, maintaining the product of *pol* in precursor form precludes its enzymic activity and thus impedes reverse transcription of cellular and viral mRNA molecules.

Another general feature is that both the *gag* gene and the *pol* gene are translated from mRNA molecules of genomic size. However, translation of the "downstream" *pol*-gene protein does not occur from the *gag* mRNA species, presumably because of a termination codon signal at the 3′ end (carboxyl terminus) of the *gag* gene. It is probable that the *pol* mRNA is generated by a small splice which removes the *gag*-gene termination codon (Chapter 5).

Also invariable is the synthesis of *env*-gene proteins from a subgenomic-size spliced mRNA. Like *gag* and *gag-pol* mRNAs, the *env* mRNA contains sequences derived from the 5′end of proviral DNA, the so-called leader sequence, which is composed of R-U_5-PB and at least part of the adjacent L region (Chapters 4 and 5). The primary *env* translational product is always found as a glycosylated molecule (except in the presence of inhibitors of glycosylation), which indicates that the precursor is glycosylated (at least in part) concomitant with the synthesis of the nascent peptide chain. Further glycosylation modifications occur later. The retroviruses encode one or two identifiable envelope proteins. It is possible that all retroviral *env* genes encode two separate proteins and that the smaller one has not been identified, in some cases, because of some biochemical attribute; for example, the protein could lack methionine residues and would thus not be detected in systems wherein radioactive methionine has been used to label virus-specific proteins. A second possibility, that the two *env* proteins may be joined together by strong bonds that are difficult to disrupt, is suggested in the case of visna virus, where only a single, very large glycoprotein is detected. In situations where two *env* proteins are identified, one or both of these may be glycosylated. For example, all avian retroviruses and the B-type MMTV have two glycosylated *env* proteins, whereas there is only one in the C-type murine retroviruses.

Studies of avian retroviruses have led to three distinct features that cannot be generalized to other retroviruses. First, there is the finding of more than one protein form associated with the mature *pol*-gene products. All other retroviruses studied in detail have RNA-dependent DNA polymerase, DNA-dependent DNA polymerase, and RNase-H activities associated with a protein monomer. Although visna virus apparently contains a dimer, it is not known whether the individual subunits are identical, nor is it known which of the various enzymic activities are associated with each subunit. In the case of the avian viruses, these two enzymic activities are associated with a dimeric protein, the $\alpha\beta$ complex, although the three major enzymatic activities are present in an isolated α subunit. As has been discussed, the β subunit can be found as a dimer, and apparently cleavage of one subunit gives rise to the α subunit plus the p32 protein with endonucleolytic activity.

A second feature noted from avian virus studies is the presence of a protease (p15) as an integral part of the *gag* gene. Once cleaved from its inactive form in the precursor, presumably by a host-encoded protease, the viral protease functions to cleave the remaining *gag*-gene products. Although proteases have recently been identified in both B-type and C-type murine retroviruses, there are not sufficient data to conclude whether these are virus-coded or host-coded.

The third feature so far unique to avian retroviruses is the dual binding functions of the p19 *gag* protein. Although all retroviruses examined so far have *gag* proteins that show binding to RNA and to lipid, these properties are usually associated with different proteins. In the case of the ASLV group, these two binding activities are associated with a single protein. The biological significance of this finding is as yet unknown.

One of the areas to which the murine C-type retroviruses have contributed is in understanding the independent pathways involved for synthesis of glycosylated and nonglycosylated *gag*-gene products. The former are found associated with the plasma membrane of the cell, whereas the latter are incorporated into the virion structure. Presumably, the additional aminoterminal sequences in the precursor to the glycosylated forms contain signals for glycosylation sites and hence permit transport to the plasma membrane, but the role of the glycosylated *gag* surface proteins is as yet unknown. A very interesting feature of this system is that a single eukaryotic gene sequence is translated from two separate initiation codons. Furthermore, there is now evidence for similar glycosylated *gag* cell-surface products in cells infected by avian and feline retroviruses and, therefore, this may be a phenomenon common to retroviruses.

Murine C-type retroviruses have provided information in an additional area. This subject, covered in detail in Chapter 7, involves the use of conditional (temperature-sensitive) mutants to study details of the maturation of infectious particles. Several mutants exhibiting defective cleavage of the *gag* precursor produce morphologically aberrant particles that accumulate at the cell membrane under nonpermissive conditions. Shift to permissive temperature generally restores normal cleavage, and infectious particle production ensues. Thus, such mutants indicate a temporal dependency of budding on precursor cleavage.

Morphogenesis is a process about which little is known at a biochemical level. In this regard, studies on the B-type MMTV should shed some light. For example, information is now accumulating on the structure and biosynthesis of the related intracytoplasmic A-type particle. Whether such particles are merely aberrant forms or whether they represent true precursors to the preformed core structures observed in the MMTV system is yet to be determined.

The challenging questions in the next few years will most likely involve the evolutionary relationships of the structural gene sequences, hitherto undetected functional properties, comparative studies on the biosynthetic and maturation pathways that lead to such morphologically distinct forms as B-, C-, and D-type particles, and the interactions between virus and host synthetic machineries.

REFERENCES

Aaronson, S.A., S.R. Tronick, and J.R. Stephenson. 1976. Endogenous type C RNA virus of *Odocoileus hemionus*, a mammalian species of New World origin. *Cell* **9:**489–494.

Abrell, J.W. and R.C. Gallo. 1973. Purification, characterization, and comparison of the DNA polymerases from two primate RNA tumor viruses. *J. Virol.* **12:**431–439.

Aliperti, G. and M.J. Schlesinger. 1978. Evidence for an autoprotease activity of Sindbis virus capsid protein. *Virology* **90:**366–369.

Andersen, P.R., M. Barbacid, S.R. Tronick, H.F. Clark, and S.A. Aaronson. 1979.

Evolutionary relatedness of viper and primate endogenous retroviruses. *Science* **204:** 318–321.

Anderson, S.J., R.B. Naso, J. Davis and J.M. Bowen. 1979. Polyprotein precursors to mouse mammary tumor virus proteins. *J. Virol.* **32:**507–516.

Aoki, T., R.B. Herberman, P.A. Johnson, M. Liu, and M.M. Sturm. 1972. Wild-type Gross leukemia virus: Classification of soluble antigens (GSA). *J. Virol.* **10:**1208–1219.

Arcement L.J., W.I. Karshin, R.B. Naso, and R.B. Arlinghaus. 1977. "gag" polyprotein precursors of Rauscher murine leukemia virus. *Virology* **81:**284–297.

Arcement, L.J., W.I. Karshin, R.B. Naso, G. Jamjoom, and R.B. Arlinghaus. 1976. Biosynthesis of Rauscher leukemia viral proteins: Presence of p30 and envelope p15 sequences in precursor polypeptides. *Virology* **69:**763–774.

Arthur, L.O. and D.L. Fine. 1978. Naturally occurring humoral immunity to murine mammary tumor virus (MuMTV) and MuMTV gp52 in mice with low mammary tumor incidence. *Int. J. Cancer* **22:**734–740.

———. 1979. Immunological characterization of mouse mammary tumor virus p10 and its presence in mammary tumors and sera of tumor-bearing mice. *J. Virol.* **30:**148–156.

Arthur, L.O., B.W. Altrock, and G. Schochetman. 1981. Type-specific determinants on proteins of an endogenous C3H mouse mammary tumor virus (MMTV) distinguish this virus from highly oncogenic exogenous MMTVs. *Virology* **110:**270–280.

Arthur, L.O., R.F. Bauer, L.S. Orme, and D.L. Fine. 1978a. Coexistence of the mouse mammary tumor virus (MMTV) major glycoprotein and natural antibodies to MMTV in sera of mammary tumor-bearing mice. *Virology* **87:**266–275.

Arthur, L.O., C.W. Long, G.H. Smith, and D.L. Fine. 1978b. Immunological characterization of the low-molecular-weight DNA binding protein of mouse mammary tumor virus. *Int. J. Cancer* **22:**433–440.

Astrin, S.M. and H.L. Robinson. 1979. *Gs*, an allele of chickens for endogenous avian leukosis viral antigens, segregates with *ev 3*, a genetic locus that contains structural genes for virus. *J. Virol.* **31:**420–425.

August, J.T., D.P. Bolognesi, E. Fleissner, R.V. Gilden, and R.C. Nowinski. 1974. A proposed nomenclature for the virion proteins of oncogenic RNA viruses. *Virology* **60:**595–601.

Baluda, M.A. and P. Roy-Burman. 1973. Partial characterization of RD114 virus by DNA-RNA hybridization studies. *Nat. New Biol.* **244:**59–62.

Barbacid, M. and S.A. Aaronson. 1978. Membrane properties of the *gag* gene-coded p15 protein of mouse type-C RNA tumor viruses. *J. Biol. Chem.* **253:**1408–1414.

Barbacid, M., M.D. Daniel, and S.A. Aaronson. 1980a. Immunological relationships of OMC-1, an endogenous virus of owl monkeys, with mammalian and avian type C viruses. *J. Virol.* **33:**561–566.

Barbacid, M., E. Hunter, and S.A. Aaronson. 1979. Avian reticuloendotheliosis viruses: Evolutionary linkage with mammalian type C retroviruses. *J. Virol.* **30:**508–514.

Barbacid, M., L.K. Long, and S.A. Aaronson. 1980b. Major structural proteins of type B, type C, and type D oncoviruses share interspecies antigenic determinants. *Proc. Natl. Acad. Sci.* **77:**72–76.

Barbacid, M., J.R. Stephenson, and S.A. Aaronson. 1976a. *gag* gene of mammalian type-C RNA tumour viruses. *Nature* **262:**554–559.

———. 1977. Evolutionary relationships between *gag* gene-coded proteins of murine and primate endogenous type C RNA viruses. *Cell* **10:**641–648.

———. 1976b. Structural polypeptides of mammalian type C RNA viruses. Isolation and immunologic characterization of a low molecular weight polypeptide, p10. *J. Biol. Chem.* **251:**4859–4866.

Bauer, G. and P.H. Hofschneider. 1976. An RNA-dependent DNA polymerase, different from the known viral reverse transcriptases, in the chicken system. *Proc. Natl. Acad. Sci.* **73:**3025–3029.

Bauer, G. and H.M. Temin. 1979. RNA-directed DNA polymerase from particles released from normal goose cells. *J. Virol.* **29:**1006–1013.

———. 1980a. Radioimmunological comparison of the DNA polymerases of avian retroviruses. *J. Virol.* **33:**1046–1057.

———. 1980b. Specific antigenic relationships between the RNA-dependent DNA polymerases of avian reticuloendotheliosis viruses and mammalian type C retroviruses. *J. Virol.* **34:**168–177.

Bauer, G., G. Jilek, and P.H. Hofschneider. 1977. Purification and further characterization of an RNA-dependent DNA polymerase from the allantoic fluid of leukosis-virus-free chicken eggs. *Eur. J. Biochem.* **79:**345–354.

Beemon, K. and T. Hunter. 1977. *In vitro* translation yields a possible Rous sarcoma virus *src* gene product. *Proc. Natl. Acad. Sci.* **74:**3302–3306.

Benveniste, R.E. and G.J. Todaro. 1977. Evolution of primate oncornaviruses: An endogenous virus from langurs (*Presbytis* spp.) with related virogene sequences in other Old World monkeys. *Proc. Natl. Acad. Sci.* **74:**4557–4561.

Bergholz, C.M., L.G. Wolfe, and F. Deinhardt. 1977. Establishment of simian sarcoma virus, type 1 (SSV-1)-transformed non-producer marmoset cell lines. *Int. J. Cancer* **20:**104–111.

Bernhard, W. 1958. Electron microscopy of tumor cells and tumor viruses: A review. *Cancer Res.* **18:**491–509.

Bernhard, W., R.A. Bonar, D. Beard, and J.W. Beard. 1958. Ultrastructure of viruses of myeloblastosis and erythroblastosis isolated from plasma of leukemic chickens. *Proc. Soc. Exp. Biol. Med.* **97:**48–52.

Bhown, A.S., J.C. Bennett, and E. Hunter. 1980. Alignment of the peptides derived from acid-catalyzed cleavage of an aspartylprolyl bond in the major internal structural polypeptide of avian retroviruses. *J. Biol. Chem.* **255:**6962–6965.

Bister, K., M.J. Hayman, and P.K. Vogt. 1977. Defectiveness of avian myelocytomatosis virus MC29: Isolation of long-term nonproducer cultures and analysis of virus-specific polypeptide synthesis. *Virology* **82:**431–448.

Blair, P.B. 1970. Immunology of the mouse mammary tumor virus: Comparison of the antigenicity of mammary tumor virus obtained from several strains of mice. *Cancer Res.* **30:**625–631.

———. 1971. Strain specificity in mouse mammary tumor virus virion antigens. *Cancer Res.* **31:**1473–1477.

Blobel, G. and B. Dobberstein. 1975. Transfer of proteins across membranes. I. Presence of proteolytically processed and unprocessed nascent immunoglobulin light chains on membrane-bound ribosomes of murine myeloma. *J. Cell Biol.* **67:**835–851.

Bolognesi, D.P. 1974. Structural components of RNA tumor viruses. *Adv. Virus Res.* **19:**315–359.

Bolognesi, D.P., R. Luftig, and J.H. Shaper. 1973. Localization of RNA tumor virus polypeptides. I. Isolation of further virus substructures. *Virology* **56:**549–564.

Bolognesi, D.P., H. Bauer, H. Gelderblom, and G. Huper. 1972. Polypeptides of avian RNA tumor viruses. IV. Components of the viral envelope. *Virology* **47:**551–566.

Bolognesi, D.P., R.C. Montelaro, H. Frank, and W. Schafer. 1978. Assembly of type C oncornaviruses: A model. *Science* **199:**183–186.

Bolognesi, D.P., R. Ishizaki, G. Huper, T.C. Vanaman, and R.E. Smith. 1975a. Immunological properties of avian oncornavirus polypeptides. *Virology* **64:**349–357.

Bolognesi, D.P., J.J. Collins, J.P. Leis, V. Moennig, W. Schafer, and P.H. Atkinson. 1975b. Role of carbohydrate in determining the immunochemical properties of the major glycoprotein (gp71) of Friend murine leukemia virus. *J. Virol.* **16:**1453–1463.

Bosch, V., R. Kurth, and J.E. Smart. 1978. The detection of glycoproteins immunologically related to RSV gp85 in uninfected avian cells and in sera from uninfected birds. *Virology* **86:**226–240.

Bradac, J.A. and E. Hunter. 1980. Protein synthesis in Mason-Pfizer monkey virus-infected cells. *Proc. Annu. Mtg. Amer. Soc. Microbiol.* p. 245. (Abstr.).

Bruns, M. and B. Frenzel. 1979. Isolation of a glycoprotein and two structural proteins of maedi-visna virus. *Virology* **97:** 207–211.

Bryant, M.L., C.J. Sherr, A. Sen, and G.J. Todaro. 1978. Molecular diversity among five different endogenous primate retroviruses. *J. Virol.* **28:** 300–313.

Buchhagen, D.L. and H. Hanafusa. 1978. Intracellular precursors to the major glycoprotein of avian oncoviruses in chicken embryo fibroblasts. *J. Virol.* **25:** 845–851.

Buetti, E. and H. Diggelmann. 1980a. Avian oncovirus proteins expressed on the surface of infected cells. *Virology* **102:** 251–261.

———. 1980b. Murine leukemia virus proteins expressed on the surface of infected cells in culture. *J. Virol.* **33:** 936–944.

Burnette, W.N., L.A. Holladay, and W.M. Mitchell. 1976. Physical and chemical properties of Moloney murine leukemia virus p30 protein: A major core structural component exhibiting high helicity and self-association. *J. Mol. Biol.* **107:** 131–143.

Burny, A., F. Bex, C. Bruck, Y. Cleuter, D. Dekegel, J. Ghysdael, R. Kettmann, M. Leclercq, M. Mammerickx, and M. Portetelle. 1978. Biochemical studies on enzootic and sporadic types of bovine leucosis. In *Antiviral mechanisms in the control of neoplasia* (ed. P. Chandra), pp. 83–99. Plenum Press, New York.

Calafat, J. and P. Hageman. 1969. The structure of the mammary tumor virus. *Virology* **38:** 364–368.

Cardiff, R.D. 1973. Quantitation of mouse mammary tumor virus (MTV) virions by radioimmunoassay. *J. Immunol.* **111:** 1722–1729.

Cardiff, R.D., M.J. Puentes, Y.A. Teramoto, and J.K. Lund. 1974. Structure of the mouse mammary tumor virus: Characterization of bald particles. *J. Virol.* **14:** 1293–1303.

Cardiff, R.D., M.J. Puentes, L.J.T. Young, G.H. Smith, Y.A. Teramoto, B.W. Altrock, and T.S. Pratt. 1978. Serological and biochemical characterization of the mouse mammary tumor virus with localization of p10. *Virology* **85:** 157–167.

Charman, H.P., R.V. Gilden, and S. Oroszlan. 1979. Reticuloendotheliosis virus: Detection of immunological relationship to mammalian type C retroviruses. *J. Virol.* **29:** 1221–1225.

Charman, H.P., N. Kim, and R.V. Gilden. 1974. Radioimmunoassay for the major structural protein of hamster type C viruses. *J. Virol.* **14:** 910–917.

Charman, H.P., S. Bladen, R.V. Gilden, and L. Coggins. 1976. Equine infectious anemia virus: Evidence favoring classification as a retrovirus. *J. Virol.* **19:** 1073–1079.

Chatterjee, S., J. Bradac, and E. Hunter. 1980. Effect of tunicamycin on the cell fusion induced by Mason-Pfizer monkey virus. *Proc. Annu. Mtg. Amer. Soc. Microbiol.* p. 269. (Abstr.).

Cheevers, W.P., C.M. Ackley, and T.B. Crawford. 1978. Structural proteins of equine infectious anemia virus. *J. Virol.* **28:** 997–1001.

Chopra, H.C. and M.M. Mason. 1970. A new virus in a spontaneous mammary tumor of a rhesus monkey. *Cancer Res.* **30:** 2081–2086.

Chopra, H.C., I. Zelljadt, E.M. Jensen, M.M. Mason, and N.J. Woodside. 1971. Infectivity of cell cultures by a virus isolated from a mammary carcinoma of a rhesus monkey. *J. Natl. Cancer Inst.* **46:** 127–137.

Clark, H.F., P.R. Andersen, and P.D. Lunger. 1979. Propagation and characterization of a C-type virus from a rhabdomyosarcoma of a corn snake. *J. Gen. Virol.* **43:** 673–683.

Coffin, J.M. and H.M. Temin. 1971. Comparison of Rous sarcoma virus-specific deoxyribonucleic acid polymerases in virions of Rous sarcoma virus and in Rous sarcoma virus-infected chicken cells. *J. Virol.* **7:** 625–634.

Colcher, D., Y.A. Teramoto, and J. Schlom. 1977a. Interspecies radioimmunoassay for the major structural proteins of primate type-D retroviruses. *Proc. Natl. Acad. Sci.* **74:** 5739–5743.

———. 1978. Immunological and structural relationships between langur virus and other primate type-D retroviruses. *Virology* **88:** 384–388.

Colcher, D., R.L. Heberling, S.S. Kalter, and J. Schlom. 1977b. Squirrel monkey retrovirus: An endogenous virus of a New World primate. *J. Virol.* **23:** 294–301.

Collins, J.J., R.C. Montelaro, T.P. Denny, R. Ishizaki, A.J. Langlois, and D.P. Bolognesi. 1978. Normal chicken cells (chf⁻) express a surface antigen which cross-reacts with determinants of the major envelope glycoprotein (gp85) of avian myeloblastosis virus. *Virology* **86:** 205–216.

Copeland, T.D., D.P. Grandgenett, and S. Oroszlan. 1980. Amino acid sequence analysis of reverse transcriptase subunits from avian myeloblastosis virus. *J. Virol.* **36:** 115–119.

Daams, J.H., P. Hageman, J. Calafat, and P. Bentvelzen. 1973. Antigenic structure of murine mammary tumor viruses. *Eur. J. Cancer* **9:** 567–572.

Dahl, H.-H.M. and C. Dickson. 1979. Cell-free synthesis of mouse mammary tumor virus Pr77 from virion and intracellular mRNA. *J. Virol.* **29:** 1131–1141.

Dalton, A.J. 1972. Further analysis of the detailed structure of type B and C particles. *J. Natl. Cancer Inst.* **48:** 1095–1099.

Davis, J., M. Scherer, W.P. Tsai, and C. Long. 1976. Low-molecular-weight Rauscher leukemia virus protein with preferential binding for single-stranded RNA and DNA. *J. Virol.* **18:** 709–718.

Davis, N.L. and R.R. Rueckert. 1972. Properties of a ribonucleoprotein particle isolated from Nonidet P-40-treated Rous sarcoma virus. *J. Virol.* **10:** 1010–1020.

de Harven, E. 1974. Remarks on the ultrastructure of type A, B, and C virus particles. *Adv. Virus Res.* **19:** 221–264.

DeLarco, J. and G.J. Todaro. 1976. Membrane receptors for murine leukemia viruses: Characterization using the purified viral envelope glycoprotein, gp71. *Cell* **8:** 365–371.

Del Villano, B.C., B. Nave, B.P. Croker, R.A. Lerner, and F.J. Dixon. 1975. The oncornavirus glycoprotein gp69/71: A constituent of the surface of normal and malignant thymocytes. *J. Exp. Med.* **141:** 172–187.

de Thé, G., C. Becker, and J.W. Beard. 1964. Virus of avian myeloblastosis (BAI strain A). XXV. Ultracytochemical study of virus and myeloblast phosphatase activity. *J. Natl. Cancer Inst.* **32:** 201–235.

Devare, S.G. and J.R. Stephenson. 1979. Primate retroviruses: Intracistronic mapping of type D viral *gag* gene by use of nonconditional replication mutants. *J. Virol.* **29:** 1035–1043.

Devare, S.G., R.E. Hanson, Jr., and J.R. Stephenson. 1978a. Primate retroviruses: Envelope glycoproteins of endogenous type C and type D viruses possess common interspecies antigenic determinants. *J. Virol.* **26:** 316–324.

Devare, S.G., L.O. Arthur, D.L. Fine, and J.R. Stephenson. 1978b. Primate retroviruses: Immunological cross-reactivity between major structural proteins of New and Old World primate virus isolates. *J. Virol.* **25:** 797–805.

Dickson, C. 1973. Mouse mammary tumour virus RNA-dependent DNA polymerase: Requirements and products. *J. Gen. Virol.* **20:** 243–247.

Dickson, C. and M. Atterwill. 1978. Polyproteins related to the major core protein of mouse mammary tumor virus. *J. Virol.* **26:** 660–672.

———. 1979. Composition, arrangement and cleavage of the mouse mammary tumor virus polyprotein precursor $Pr77^{gag}$ and $p110^{gag}$. *Cell* **17:** 1003–1012.

———. 1980. Structure and processing of the mouse mammary tumor virus glycoprotein precursor $Pr73^{env}$. *J. Virol.* **35:** 349–361.

Dickson, C. and G. Peters. 1981. Protein-coding potential of mouse mammary tumor virus genome RNA as examined by in vitro translation. *J. Virol.* **37:** 36–47.

Dickson, C. and J.J. Skehel. 1974. The polypeptide composition of mouse mammary tumor virus. *Virology* **58:** 387–395.

Dickson, C., J.P. Puma, and S. Nandi. 1976. Identification of a precursor protein to the major glycoproteins of mouse mammary tumor virus. *J. Virol.* **17:** 275–282.

Diggelmann, H. 1979. Biosynthesis of an unglycosylated envelope glycoprotein of Rous sarcoma virus in the presence of tunicamycin. *J. Virol.* **30:** 799–804.

Dion, A.S., A.A. Pomenti, and D.C. Farwell. 1979. Vicinal relationships between the major structural proteins of murine mammary tumor virus. *Virology* **96:** 249–257.

Dion, A.S., A.B. Vaidya, and G.S. Fout. 1974a. Cation preferences for poly(rC).oligo(dG)-directed DNA synthesis by RNA tumor viruses and human milk particulates. *Cancer Res.* **34:** 3509–3515.

Dion, A.S., C.J. Williams, and D.H. Moore. 1977. RNase H and RNA-directed DNA polymerase: Associated enzymatic activities of murine mammary tumor virus. *J. Virol.* **22:** 187–193.

Dion, A.S., A.B. Vaidya, G.S. Fout, and D.H. Moore. 1974b. Isolation and characterization of RNA-directed DNA polymerase from a B-type RNA tumor virus. *J. Virol.* **14:** 40–46.

Dittmar, K.J. and K. Moelling. 1978. Biochemical properties of p15-associated protease in an avian RNA tumor virus. *J. Virol.* **28:** 106–118.

Dmochowski, L. 1960. Viruses and tumors in the light of electron microscope studies: A review. *Cancer Res.* **20:** 977–1015.

Donis-Keller, H., J. Rommelaere, R.W. Ellis, and N. Hopkins. 1980. Nucleotide sequences associated with differences in electrophoretic mobility of envelope glycoprotein gp70 and with GIΩ antigen phenotype of certain murine leukemia viruses. *Proc. Natl. Acad. Sci.* **77:** 1642–1645.

Duesberg, P.H., G.S. Martin, and P.K. Vogt. 1970. Glycoprotein components of avian and murine RNA tumor viruses. *Virology* **41:** 631–646.

Edwards, S.A. and H. Fan. 1979. *gag*-related polyproteins of Moloney murine leukemia virus: Evidence for independent synthesis of glycosylated and unglycosylated forms. *J. Virol.* **30:** 551–563.

———. 1980. Sequence relationship of glycosylated and unglycosylated *gag* polyproteins of Moloney murine leukemia virus. *J. Virol.* **35:** 41–51.

———. 1981. Immunoselection and characterization of Moloney murine leukemia virus-infected cell lines deficient in surface *gag* antigen expression. *Virology* (in press).

Eisenman, R.N. and V.M. Vogt. 1978. The biosynthesis of oncovirus proteins. *Biochim. Biophys. Acta* **473:** 187–239.

Eisenman, R.N., W.S. Mason, and M. Linial. 1980a. Synthesis and processing of polymerase proteins of wild-type and mutant avian retroviruses. *J. Virol.* **36:** 62–78.

Eisenman, R., R. Shaikh, and W.S. Mason. 1978. Identification of an avian oncovirus polyprotein in uninfected chick cells. *Cell* **14:** 89–104.

Eisenman, R., V.M. Vogt, and H. Diggelmann. 1975. Synthesis of avian RNA tumor virus structural proteins. *Cold Spring Harbor Symp. Quant. Biol.* **39:** 1067–1075.

Eisenman, R.N., M. Linial, M. Groudine, R. Shaikh, S. Brown, and P.E. Neiman. 1980b. Recombination in the avian oncoviruses as a model for the generation of defective transforming viruses. *Cold Spring Harbor Symp. Quant. Biol.* **44:** 1235–1247.

Eisenman, R., W.N. Burnette, F. Zucco, H. Diggelmann, P. Heater, P. Tsichlis, and J. Coffin. 1980c. Synthesis and processing of the internal structural proteins of retroviruses: Site of synthesis, evidence for multiply charged species, and analysis of a mutant defective in processing. In *Biosynthesis, modification and processing of cellular and viral polyproteins* (ed. G. Koch and D. Richter). Academic Press. New York. (In press).

Elder, J.H., F.C. Jensen, M.L. Bryant, and R.A. Lerner. 1977a. Polymorphism of the major envelope glycoprotein (gp70) of murine C-type viruses: Virion associated and differentiation antigens encoded by a multi-gene family. *Nature* **267:** 23–28.

Elder, J.H., J.W. Gautsch, F.C. Jensen, R.A. Lerner, J.W. Hartley, and W.P. Rowe. 1977b. Biochemical evidence that MCF murine leukemia viruses are envelope (*env*) gene recombinants. *Proc. Natl. Acad. Sci.* **74:** 4676–4680.

England, J.M., D.P. Bolognesi, B. Dietzschold, and M.S. Halpern. 1977. Evidence that a precursor glycoprotein is cleaved to yield the major glycoprotein of avian tumor virus. *J. Virol.* **21:**810–814.

Erikson, E., J.S. Brugge, and R.L. Erikson. 1977. Phosphorylated and nonphosphorylated forms of avian sarcoma virus polypeptide p19. *Virology* **80:**177–185.

Evans, L.H., S. Dresler, and D. Kabat. 1977. Synthesis and glycosylation of polyprotein precursors to the internal core proteins of Friend murine leukemia virus. *J. Virol.* **24:**865–874.

Famulari, N.G., D.L. Buchhagen, H.-D. Klenk, and E. Fleissner. 1976. Presence of murine leukemia virus envelope proteins gp70 and p15(E) in a common polyprotein of infected cells. *J. Virol.* **20:**501–508.

Fan, H. and D. Baltimore. 1973. RNA metabolism of murine leukemia virus: Detection of virus-specific RNA sequences in infected and uninfected cells and identification of virus-specific messenger RNA. *J. Mol. Biol.* **80:**93–117.

Fan, H. and I.M. Verma. 1978. Size analysis and relationship of murine leukemia virus-specific mRNA's: Evidence for transposition of sequences during synthesis and processing of subgenomic mRNA. *J. Virol.* **26:**468–478.

Feldman, S.P., J. Schlom, and S. Spiegelman. 1973. Further evidence for oncornaviruses in human milk: The production of cores. *Proc. Natl. Acad. Sci.* **70:**1976–1980.

Ferrer, J.F. 1972. Antigenic comparison of bovine type C virus with murine and feline leukemia viruses. *Cancer Res.* **32:**1871–1877.

Fine, D. and G. Schochetman. 1978. Type D primate retroviruses: A review. *Cancer Res.* **38:**3123–3139.

Fitting, T., M. Ruta, and D. Kabat. 1981. Mutant cells which abnormally process plasma membrane glycopoteins encoded by murine leukemia virus. *Cell* (in press).

Fleissner, E., 1971. Chromatographic separation and antigenic analysis of proteins of the oncornaviruses. I. Avian leukemia-sarcoma viruses. *J. Virol.* **8:**778–785.

Fleissner, E. and E. Tress. 1973. Isolation of a ribonucleoprotein structure from oncornaviruses. *J. Virol.* **12:**1612–1615.

Fujinaga, K., A. Rankin, H. Yamazaki, K. Sekikawa, J. Bragdon, and M. Green. 1973. RD-114 virus: Analysis of viral gene sequences in feline and human cells by DNA-DNA reassociation kinetics and RNA-DNA hybridization. *Virology* **56:**484–495.

Galehouse, D.M. and P.H. Duesberg. 1976. Differences in the glycoproteins of avian tumor virus recombinants: Evidence for intragenic crossing over. In *Animal virology* (ed. D. Baltimore et al.), vol. 4, pp. 227–236. Academic Press, New York.

Gallis B.M., R.N. Eisenman, and H. Diggelmann. 1976. Synthesis of the precursor to avian RNA tumor virus internal structural proteins early after infection. *Virology* **74:**302–313.

Gallis, B., M. Linial, and R. Eisenman. 1979. An avian oncovirus mutant deficient in genomic RNA: Characterization of the packaged RNA as cellular messenger RNA. *Virology* **94:**146–161.

Gautsch, J.W., J.H. Elder, J. Schindler, F.C. Jensen, and R.A. Lerner. 1978a. Structural markers on core protein p30 of murine leukemia virus: Functional correlation with *Fv-1* tropism. *Proc. Natl. Acad. Sci.* **75:**4170–4174.

Gautsch, J.W., R. Lerner, D. Howard, Y.A. Teramoto, and J. Schlom. 1978b. Strain-specific markers for the major structural proteins of highly oncogenic murine mammary tumor viruses by tryptic peptide analyses. *J. Virol.* **27:**688–699.

Geering, G., W.D. Hardy, Jr., L.J. Old, E. de Harven, and R.S. Brodey. 1968. Shared group-specific antigen of murine and feline leukemia virus. *Virology* **36:**678–680.

Gerard, G.F. and D.P. Grandgenett. 1975. Purification and characterization of the DNA polymerase and RNase H activities in Moloney murine sarcoma-leukemia virus. *J. Virol.* **15:**785–797.

———. 1980. Retrovirus reverse transcriptase. In *Molecular biology of RNA tumor viruses* (ed. J.R. Stephenson), pp. 345–394. Academic Press, New York.

Gibson, W. and I.M. Verma. 1974. Studies on the reverse transcriptase of RNA tumor viruses. Structural relatedness of two subunits of avian RNA tumor viruses. *Proc. Natl. Acad. Sci.* **71:**4991–4994.

Gielkens, A.L.J., M.H.L. Salden, and H. Bloemendal. 1974. Virus-specific messenger RNA on free and membrane-bound polyribosomes from cells infected with Rauscher leukemia virus. *Proc. Natl. Acad. Sci.* **71:**1093–1097.

Gielkens, A.L.J., D. Van Zaane, H.P.J. Bloemers, and H. Bloemendal. 1976. Synthesis of Rauscher murine leukemia virus-specific polypeptides *in vitro. Proc. Natl. Acad. Sci.* **73:**356–360.

Gilden, R.V., K. Frank, M. Hanson, S. Bladen, R. Toni, and S. Oroszlan. 1974a. Similarity between gibbon ape and woolly monkey type C virus internal antigens by quantitative micro-complement fixation. *Intervirology* **2:**360–365.

Gilden, R.V., R. Toni, M. Hanson, D. Bova, H.P. Charman, and S. Oroszlan. 1974b. Immunochemical studies of the major internal polypeptide of woolly monkey and gibbon ape type C viruses. *J. Immunol.* **112:**1250–1254.

Gillespie, D., S. Gillespie, R.C. Gallo, J.L. East, and L. Dmochowski. 1973. Genetic origin of RD114 and other RNA tumour viruses assayed by molecular hybridization. *Nat. New Biol.* **244:**51–54.

Goldfine, H., J.B. Harley, and J.A. Wyke. 1978. Effects of inhibitors of lipid synthesis on the replication of Rous sarcoma virus. A specific effect of cerulenin on the processing of major non-glycosylated viral structural proteins. *Biochim. Biophys. Acta* **512:**229–240.

Golomb, M. and D.P. Grandgenett. 1979. Endonuclease activity of purified RNA-directed DNA polymerase from avian myeloblastosis virus. *J. Biol. Chem.* **254:**1606–1613.

Grandgenett, D.P., G.F. Gerard, and M. Green. 1973. A single subunit from avian myeloblastosis virus with both RNA-directed DNA polymerase and ribonuclease H activity. *Proc. Natl. Acad. Sci.* **70:**230–234.

Grandgenett, D.P., M. Golomb, and A.C. Vora. 1980. Activation of an Mg^{2+}-dependent DNA endonuclease of avian myeloblastosis virus $\alpha\beta$ DNA polymerase by *in vitro* proteolytic cleavage. *J. Virol.* **33:**264–271.

Grandgenett, D.P., A.C. Vora and R.D. Schiff. 1978. A 32,000-dalton nucleic acid-binding protein from avian, retrovirus cores possesses DNA endonuclease activity. *Virology* **89:**119–132.

Gregoriades, A. and L.J. Old. 1969. Isolation and some characteristics of a group-specific antigen of the murine leukemia viruses. *Virology* **37:**189–202.

Groner, B., N.E. Hynes, and H. Diggelmann. 1979. Identification of mouse mammary tumor virus-specific mRNA. *J. Virol.* **30:**417–420.

Gupta, P., and J.F. Ferrer. 1978. Detection of a precursor of bovine leukemia structural proteins in purified virions. *Ann. Rech. Vet.* **9:**619–626.

Hasse, A.T. and J.R. Baringer. 1974. The structural polypeptides of RNA slow viruses. *Virology* **57:**238–250.

Haase, A.T., A.C. Garapin, A.J. Faras, H.E. Varmus, and J.M. Bishop. 1974. Characterization of the nucleic acid product of the visna virus RNA dependent DNA polymerase. *Virology* **57:**251–258.

Halpern, M.S., E. Wade, E. Rucker, K.L. Baxter-Gabbard, A.S. Levine, and R.R. Friis. 1973. A study of the relationship of reticuloendotheliosis virus to the avian leukosis-sarcoma complex of viruses. *Virology* **53:**287–299.

Hanafusa, H., D. Baltimore, D. Smoler, K.F. Watson, A. Yaniv, and S. Spiegelman. 1972. Absence of polymerase protein in virions of alpha-type Rous sarcoma virus. *Science* **177:**1188–1191.

Haseltine, W.A., A.M. Maxam, and W. Gilbert. 1977. Rous sarcoma virus genome is terminally redundant: The 5′ sequence. *Proc. Natl. Acad. Sci.* **74:**989–993.

Hayman, N.J. 1978a. Viral polyproteins in chick embryo fibroblasts infected with avian leukosis viruses. *Virology* **85:**241–252.

———. 1978b. Synthesis and processing of avian sarcoma virus glycoproteins. *Virology* **85:**475–486.

Hayman, M.J. and P.K. Vogt. 1976. Subgroup-specific antigenic determinants of avian RNA tumor virus structural proteins: Analysis of virus recombinants. *Virology* **73:**372–380.

Hayman, M.J., B. Royer-Pokora, and T. Graf. 1979. Defectiveness of avian erythroblastosis virus: Synthesis of a 75K *gag*-related protein. *Virology* **92:**31–45.

Hayward, W.S. 1977. Size and genetic content of viral RNAs in avian oncovirus-infected cells. *J. Virol.* **24:**47–63.

Heberling, R.L., S.T. Barker, S.S. Kalter, G.C. Smith, and R.J. Helmke. 1977. Oncornavirus: Isolation from a squirrel monkey (*Saimiri sciureus*) lung culture. *Science* **195:** 289–291.

Hellman, A., P.T. Peebles, J.E. Strickland, A.K. Fowler, S.S. Kalter, S. Oroszlan, and R.V. Gilden. 1974. Baboon virus isolate M-7 with properties similar to feline virus RD-114. *J. Virol.* **14:**133–138.

Henderson, L.E., T.D. Copeland, G.W. Smythers, H. Marquardt, and S. Oroszlan. 1978. Amino-terminal amino acid sequence and carboxyl-terminal analysis of Rauscher murine leukemia virus glycoproteins. *Virology* **85:**319–322.

Hendrick, J.-C., C. Francois, C.M. Calberg-Bacq, C. Colin, P. Franchimont, L. Gosselin, S. Kozma, and P.M. Osterrieth. 1978. Radioimmunoassay for protein p28 of murine mammary tumor virus in organs and serum of mice and search for related antigens in human sera and breast cancer extracts. *Cancer Res.* **38:**1826–1831.

Herman, A.C., R.W. Green, D.P. Bolognesi, and T.C. Vanaman. 1975. Comparative chemical properties of avian oncornavirus polypeptides. *Virology* **64:**339–348.

Hino, S., J.R. Stephenson, and S.A. Aaronson. 1976. Radioimmunoassays for the 70,000-molecular-weight glycoproteins of endogenous mouse type C viruses: Viral antigen expression in normal mouse tissues and sera. *J. Virol.* **18:**933–941.

Hino, S., S.R. Tronick, R.L. Heberling, S.S. Kalter, A. Hellman, and S.A. Aaronson. 1977. Endogenous New World primate retrovirus: Interspecies antigenic determinants shared with the major structural protein of type-D RNA viruses of Old World monkeys. *Proc. Natl. Acad. Sci.* **74:**5734–5738.

Hizi, A. and W.K. Joklik. 1977a. RNA-dependent DNA polymerase of avian sarcoma virus B77. I. Isolation and partial characterization of the α, β_2 and $\alpha\beta$ forms of the enzyme. *J. Biol. Chem.* **252:**2281–2289.

———. 1977b. The β subunit of the DNA polymerase of avian sarcoma virus strain B77 is a phosphoprotein. *Virology* **78:**571–575.

Hizi, A., J.P. Leis, and W.K. Joklik. 1977. RNA-dependent DNA polymerase of avian sarcoma virus B77. II. Comparison of the catalytic properties of the α, β_2, and $\alpha\beta$ enzyme forms. *J. Biol. Chem.* **252:**2290–2295.

Hoekstra, J. and F. Deinhardt. 1973/1974. Simian sarcoma and feline leukemia virus antigens: Isolation of species- and interspecies-specific proteins. *Intervirology* **2:**222–230.

Hoelzer, J.D., R.B. Lewis, C.R. Wasmuth, and H.R. Bose, Jr. 1980. Hematopoietic cell transformation by reticuloendotheliosis virus: Characterization of the genetic defect. *Virology* **100:**462–474.

Hopkins, N., J. Schindler, and R. Hynes. 1977. Six NB-tropic murine leukemia viruses derived from a B-tropic virus of BALB/c have altered p30. *J. Virol.* **21:**309–318.

Howk, R.S., L.A. Rye, L.A. Killeen, E.M. Scolnick, and W.P. Parks. 1973. Characterization and separation of viral DNA polymerase in mouse milk. *Proc. Natl. Acad. Sci.* **70:**2117–2121.

Hunsmann, G., V. Moennig, L. Pister, E. Seifert, and W. Schafer. 1974. Properties of mouse leukemia viruses. VIII. The major viral glycoprotein of Friend leukemia virus. Seroimmunological, interfering and hemagglutinating capacities. *Virology* **62:**307–318.

Hunt, L.A., S.E. Wright, J.R. Etchison, and D.F. Summers. 1979. Oligosaccharide chains of avian RNA tumor virus glycoproteins contain heterogeneous oligomannosyl cores. *J. Virol.* **29:**336–343.

Hunter, E., A.S. Bhown, and J.C. Bennett. 1978. Amino-terminal amino acid sequence of the major structural polypeptides of avian retroviruses: Sequence homology between reticuloendotheliosis virus p30 and p30s of mammalian retroviruses. *Proc. Natl. Acad. Sci.* **75:**2708–2712.

Hunter, E., M.J. Hayman, R.W. Rongey, and P.K. Vogt. 1976. An avian sarcoma virus mutant that is temperature sensitive for virion assembly. *Virology* **69:**35–49.

Ikeda, H., W. Hardy, Jr., E. Tress, and E. Fleissner. 1975. Chromatographic separation and antigenic analysis of proteins of the oncornaviruses. V. Identification of a new murine viral protein, p15(E). *J. Virol.* **16:**53–61.

Ikeda, H., T. Pincus, T. Yoshiki, M. Strand, J.T. August, E.A. Boyse, and R.C. Mellors. 1974. Biological expression of antigenic determinants of murine leukemia virus proteins gp69/71 and p30. *J. Virol.* **14:**1274–1280.

Ishizaki, R., R.W. Green, and D.P. Bolognesi. 1978. The structural polypeptides of equine infectious anemia virus. *Intervirology* **9:**286–294.

Jacquemin, P.C., C. Saxinger, and R.C. Gallo. 1978. Surface antibodies of human myelogenous leukaemia leukocytes reactive with specific type-C viral reverse transcriptases. *Nature* **276:**230–236.

Jamjoom, G.A., R.B. Naso, and R.B. Arlinghaus. 1977. Further characterization of intracellular precursor polyproteins of Rauscher leukemia virus. *Virology* **78:**11–34.

Jamjoom, G., W.L. Karshin, R.B. Naso., L.J. Arcement, and R.B. Arlinghaus. 1975. Proteins of Rauscher murine leukemia virus: Resolution of a 70,000 dalton, nonglycosylated polypeptide containing p30 peptide sequences. *Virology* **68:**135–145.

Jensen, E.M., I. Zelljadt, H.C. Chopra, and M.M. Mason. 1970. Isolation and propagation of a virus from a spontaneous mammary carcinoma of a rhesus monkey. *Cancer Res.* **30:**2388–2393.

Kaaden, O.R., B. Frenzel, B. Dietzschold, F. Weiland, and M. Mussgay. 1977. Isolation of a p15 polypeptide from bovine leukemia virus and detection of specific antibodies in leukemic cattle. *Virology* **77:**501–509.

Kacian, D.L., K.F. Watson, A. Burny, and S. Spiegelman. 1971. Purification of the DNA polymerase of avian myeloblastosis virus. *Biochim. Biophys. Acta* **246:**365–383.

Kang, C.-Y. 1975. Characterization of endogenous RNA-directed DNA polymerase activity of reticuloendotheliosis viruses. *J. Virol.* **16:**880–886.

Karshin, W.L., L.J. Arcement, R.B. Naso, and R.B. Arlinghaus. 1977. Common precursor for Rauscher leukemia virus gp69/71, p15(E), and p12(E). *J. Virol.* **23:**787–798.

Katz, F.N., J.E. Rothman, V.R. Lingappa, G. Blobel, and H.F. Lodish. 1977. Membrane assembly *in vitro*: Synthesis, glycosylation, and asymmetric insertion of a transmembrane protein. *Proc. Natl. Acad. Sci.* **74:**3278–3282.

Kawai, S. and H. Hanafusa. 1973. Isolation of defective mutant of avian sarcoma virus. *Proc. Natl. Acad. Sci.* **70:**3493–3497.

Kawakami, T.G. and P.M. Buckley. 1974. Antigenic studies on gibbon type-C viruses. *Transplant. Proc.* **6:**193–196.

Kawakami, T.G., S.D. Huff, P.M. Buckley, D.L. Dungworth, S.P. Snyder, and R.V. Gilden. 1972. C-type virus associated with gibbon lymphosarcoma. *Nat. New Biol.* **235:**170–171.

Kawashima, K., H. Ikeda, E. Stockert, T. Takahashi, and L.J. Old. 1976. Age-related changes in cell surface antigens of preleukemic AKR thymocytes. *J. Exp. Med.* **144:**193–208.

Kemp, M.C., S. Basak, and R.W. Compans. 1979. Glycopeptides of murine leukemia viruses. I. Comparison of two ecotropic viruses. *J. Virol.* **31:**1–7.

Kemp, M.C., N.G. Famulari, P.V. O'Donnell, and R.W. Compans. 1980. Glycopeptides of murine leukemia viruses. II. Comparison of xenotropic and dual-tropic viruses. *J. Virol.* **34:**154–161.

Kennel, S.J., B.C. Del Villano, R.L. Levy, and R.A. Lerner. 1973. Properties of an oncornavirus glycoprotein: Evidence for its presence on the surface of virions and infected cells. *Virology* **55:**464–475.

Kerr, I.M., U. Olshevsky, H.F. Lodish, and D. Baltimore. 1976. Translation of murine leukemia virus RNA in cell-free systems from animal cells. *J. Virol.* **18:**627–635.

Khan, A.S. and J.R. Stephenson. 1977. Feline leukemia virus: Biochemical and immunological characterization of *gag* gene-coded structural proteins. *J. Virol.* **23:**599–607.

Kieras, R.M. and A.J. Faras. 1975. DNA polymerase of reticuloendotheliosis virus: Inability to detect endogenous RNA-directed DNA synthesis. *Virology* **65:**514–523.

Klemenz, R. and H. Diggelmann. 1978. The generation of the two envelope glycoproteins of Rous sarcoma virus from a common precursor polypeptide. *Virology* **85:**63–74.

———. 1979. Extracellular cleavage of the glycoprotein precursor of Rous sarcoma virus. *J. Virol.* **29:**285–292.

Kohno, M. and A. Ishihama. 1979. Purification and properties of RNA-dependent DNA polymerase from cytoplasmic A-type particles of murine mammary tumor virus. *Eur. J. Biochem.* **97:**257–266.

Kozak, M. 1978. How do eucaryotic ribosomes select initiation regions in messenger RNA? *Cell* **15:**1109–1123.

———. 1980. Evaluation of the "scanning model" for initiation of protein synthesis in eucaryotes. *Cell* **22:**7–8.

Krakower, J.M., M. Barbacid, and S.A. Aaronson. 1977. Radioimmunoassay for mammalian type C viral reverse transcriptase. *J. Virol.* **22:**331–339.

Kramarsky, B., E.Y. Lasfargues, and D.H. Moore. 1970. Ultrastructural and quantitative studies of mammary tumor virus production in cultured mouse mammary tumor cells. *Cancer Res.* **30:**1102–1108.

Krantz, M.J., Y.C. Lee, and P.P. Hung. 1976. Characterization and comparison of the major glycoprotein from three strains of Rous sarcoma virus. *Arch. Biochem. Biophys.* **174:**66–73.

Krantz, M.J., M. Strand, and J.T. August. 1977. Biochemical and immunological characterization of the major envelope glycoprotein gp69/71 and degradation fragments from Rauscher leukemia virus. *J. Virol.* **22:**804–815.

Laemmli, U.K. 1970. Cleavage of structural proteins during the assembly of the head of bacteriophage T4. *Nature* **227:**680–685.

Lai, M.C. 1976. Phosphoproteins of Rous sarcoma viruses. *Virology* **74:**287–301.

Lai, M.M.C. and P.H. Duesberg. 1972. Differences between the envelope glycoproteins and glycopeptides of avian tumor viruses released from transformed and from nontransformed cells. *Virology* **50:**359–372.

Lai, M.-H.T. and I.M. Verma. 1978. Reverse transcriptase of RNA tumor viruses. V. In vitro proteolysis of reverse transcriptase from avian myeloblastosis virus and isolation of a polypeptide manifesting only RNase H activity. *J. Virol.* **25:**652–663.

Landen, B. and C.F. Fox. 1980. Isolation of BPgp70, a fibroblast receptor for the envelope antigen of Rauscher murine leukemia virus. *Proc. Natl. Acad. Sci.* **77:**4988–4992.

Lange, J., H. Frank, G. Hunsmann, V. Moennig, R. Wollmann, and W. Schafer. 1973. Properties of mouse leukemia viruses. VI. The core of Friend virus; isolation and constituents. *Virology* **53:**457–462.

Leamnson, R.N. and M.S. Halpern. 1976. Subunit structure of the glycoprotein complex of avian tumor virus. *J. Virol.* **18:**956–968.

Leamnson, R.N., M.H.M. Shander, and M.S. Halpern. 1977. A structural protein complex in Moloney leukemia virus. *Virology* **76:**437–439.

Leavitt, R., S. Schlesinger, and S. Kornfield. 1977. Tunicamycin inhibits glycosylation and multiplication of Sindbis and vesicular stomatitis viruses. *J. Virol.* **21:**375–385.

Ledbetter, J.A. 1979. Two-dimensional analysis of murine leukemia virus *gag*-gene polyproteins. *Virology* **95:**85–98.

Ledbetter, J. and R.C. Nowinski. 1977. Identification of the Gross cell surface antigen associated with murine leukemia virus-infected cells. *J. Virol.* **23:** 315–322.

Ledbetter, J., R.C. Nowinski, and S. Emery. 1977. Viral proteins expressed on the surface of murine leukemia cells. *J. Virol.* **22:** 65–73.

Ledbetter, J.A., R.C. Nowinski, and R.N. Eisenman. 1978. Biosynthesis and metabolism of viral proteins expressed on the surface of murine leukemia virus-infected cells. *Virology* **91:** 116–129.

Lee, J.S., H.E. Varmus, and J.M. Bishop. 1979. Virus-specific messenger RNAs in permissive cells infected by avian sarcoma virus. *J. Biol. Chem.* **254:** 8015–8022.

Leis, J.P., J. McGinnis, and R.W. Green. 1978. Rous sarcoma virus p19 binds to specific double-stranded regions of viral RNA: Effect of p19 on cleavage of viral RNA by RNase III. *Virology* **84:** 87–98.

Leis, J.P., P. Scheible, and R.E. Smith. 1981. Correlation of RNA binding affinity of avian oncornavirus p19 proteins with the extent of processing of virus genome RNA in cells. *J. Virol.* (in press).

Lennarz, N.J. 1975. Lipid linked sugars in glycoprotein synthesis. *Science* **188:** 986–991.

Lerner, R.A., C.B. Wilson, B.C. Del Villano, P.J. McConahey, and F.J. Dixon. 1976. Endogenous oncornaviral gene expression in adult and fetal mice: Quantitative, histologic, and physiologic studies of the major viral glycoprotein, gp70. *J. Exp. Med.* **143:** 151–166.

Levin, J.G. and J.G. Seidman. 1979. Selective packaging of host tRNA's by murine leukemia virus particles does not require genomic RNA. *J. Virol.* **29:** 328–335.

Levin, J.G., P.M. Grimley, J.M. Ramseur, and I.K. Berezesky. 1974. Deficiency of 60 to 70S RNA in murine leukemia virus particles assembled in cells treated with actinomycin D. *J. Virol.* **14:** 152–161.

Lieber, M.M., C.J. Sherr, G.J. Todaro, R.E. Benveniste, R. Callahan, and H.G. Coon. 1975. Isolation from the Asian mouse *Mus caroli* of an endogenous type C virus related to infectious primate type C viruses. *Proc. Natl. Acad. Sci.* **72:** 2315–2319.

Lin, F.H. 1977. Polyacrylamide gel electrophoresis of visna virus polypeptides isolated by agarose gel chromatography. *J. Virol.* **25:** 207–214.

Lin, F.H. and M. Papini. 1978. Evidence for two forms of RNA-dependent DNA polymerase in visna virus. *Biochim. Biophys. Acta* **561:** 383–395.

Lin, F.H. and H. Thormar. 1970. Ribonucleic acid-dependent deoxyribonucleic acid polymerase in visna virus. *J. Virol.* **6:** 702–704.

———. 1972. Properties of maedi nucleic acid and the presence of ribonucleic acid- and deoxyribonucleic acid-dependent deoxyribonucleic acid polymerase in the virions. *J. Virol.* **10:** 228–233.

———. 1974. Substructures and polypeptides of visna virus. *J. Virol.* **14:** 782–790.

———. 1979. Precipitation of visna viral proteins by immune sera of rabbits and sheep. *J. Virol.* **29:** 536–539.

Lin, F.H., M. Genovese, and H. Thormar. 1973. Multiple activities of DNA polymerase from visna virus. *Prep. Biochem.* **3:** 525–539.

Linial, M., E. Medeiros, and W.S. Hayward. 1978. An avian oncovirus mutant (SE21Q1b) deficient in genomic RNA: Biological and biochemical characterization. *Cell* **15:** 1371–1381.

Linial, M., J. Fenno, W.N. Burnette, and L. Rohrschneider. 1980. Synthesis and processing of viral glycoproteins in two nonconditional mutants of Rous sarcoma virus. *J. Virol.* **36:** 280–290.

Livingston, D.M. and G.J. Todaro. 1973. Endogenous type C virus from a cat cell clone with properties distinct from previously described feline type C virus. *Virology* **53:** 142–151.

Lodish, H.F. 1973. Biosynthesis of reticulocyte membrane proteins by membrane-free polyribosomes. *Proc. Natl. Acad. Sci.* **70:** 1526–1530.

Love, D.N. and R.A. Weiss. 1974. Pseudotypes of vesicular stomatitis virus determined by exogenous and endogenous avian RNA tumor viruses. *Virology* **57:**271–278.

Lu, A.H., M.M. Soong, and P.K.Y. Wong. 1979. Maturation of Moloney murine leukemia virus. *Virology* **93:**269–274.

Luftig, R.B. and Y. Yoshinaka. 1978. Rauscher leukemia virus populations enriched for "immature" virions contain increased amounts of P70, the *gag* gene product. *J. Virol.* **25:**416–421.

Maizel, J.V., Jr., D.O. White, and M.D. Scharff. 1968. The polypeptides of adenovirus. I. Evidence for multiple protein components in the virion and a comparison of types 2, 7A, and 12. *Virology* **36:**115–125.

Maldonado, R.L. and H.R. Bose, Jr. 1971. Separation of reticuloendotheliosis virus from the avian tumor viruses. *J. Virol.* **8:**813–815.

———. 1973. Relationship of reticuloendotheliosis virus to the avian tumor viruses: Nucleic acid and polypeptide composition. *J. Virol.* **11:**741–747.

———. 1975. Polypeptide and RNA composition of the reticuloendotheliosis viruses. *Intervirology* **5:**194–204.

———. 1976. Group-specific antigen shared by the members of the reticuloendotheliosis virus complex. *J. Virol.* **17:**983–990.

Marcus, S.L., R. Kopelman, and N.H. Sarkar. 1979a. Simultaneous purification of murine mammary tumor virus structural proteins: Analysis of antigenic reactivities of native gp34 by radioimmunocompetition assays. *J. Virol.* **31:**341–349.

Marcus, S.L., N.H. Sarkar, and M.J. Modak. 1976. Purification and properties of murine mammary tumor virus DNA polymerase. *Virology* **71:**242–254.

———. 1978a. Template-specific requirements for DNA synthesis by the Mason-Pfizer monkey virus DNA polymerase: Unique aspects. *Biochim. Biophys. Acta* **519:**317–330.

Marcus, S.L., S.W. Smith, J. Racevskis, and N.H. Sarkar. 1978b. The relative hydrophobicity of oncornaviral structural proteins. *Virology* **86:**398–412.

———. 1979b. Purification of murine oncornaviral phosphoproteins using alkyl-agarose derivatives. *J. Biol. Chem.* **254:**4809–4813.

Marquardt, H., R.V. Gilden, and S. Oroszlan. 1977. Envelope glycoproteins of Rauscher murine leukemia virus: Isolation and chemical characterization. *Biochemistry* **16:**710–717.

Massey, R.J. and G. Schochetman. 1979. Gene order of mouse mammary tumor virus precursor polyproteins and their interaction leading to the formation of a virus. *Virology* **99:**358–371.

Massey, R.J., L.O. Arthur, R.C. Nowinski, and G. Schochetman. 1980. Monoclonal antibodies identify individual determinants on mouse mammary tumor virus glycoprotein gp52 with group, class, or type specificity. *J. Virol.* **34:**635–643.

McAllister, R.M., M. Nicolson, M.B. Gardner, R.W. Rongey, S. Rasheed, P.S. Sarma, R.J. Huebner, M. Hatanaka, S. Oroszlan, R.V. Gilden, A. Kabigting, and L. Vernon. 1972. C-type virus released from cultured human rhabdomyosarcoma cells. *Nat. New Biol.* **235:**3–6.

McClintock, P.R., J.N. Ihle, and D.R. Joseph. 1977. Expression of AKR murine leukemia virus gp71-like and BALB(X) gp71-like antigens in normal mouse tissues in the absence of overt virus expression. *J. Exp. Med.* **146:**422–434.

McLellan, W.L. and J.T. August. 1976. Analysis of the envelope of Rauscher murine oncornavirus: In vitro labeling of glycopeptides. *J. Virol.* **20:**627–636.

Mellon, P. and P.H. Duesberg. 1977. Subgenomic, cellular Rous sarcoma virus RNAs contain oligonucleotides from the 3′ half and the 5′ terminus of virion RNA. *Nature* **270:**631–634.

Menko, A.S., F. Sokol, H.F. Clark, and K.B. Tan. 1976. Structural and enzymatic characterization of viper C-type virus. *Arch. Virol.* **50:**125–135.

Michalides, R., E. Wagenaar, and R. Nusse. 1979. Autogenous antibodies against the murine mammary tumor virus in strains of mice with low incidences of mammary tumors. *J. Natl. Cancer Inst.* **62:**935–941.

Milstein, C., G.G. Brownlee, T.M. Harrison, and M.B. Mathews. 1972. A possible precursor of immunoglobulin light chains. *Nat. New Biol.* **239:**117–120.

Mizutani, S. and H.M. Temin. 1973. Lack of serological relationship among DNA polymerases of avian leukosis-sarcoma viruses, reticuloendotheliosis viruses, and chicken cells. *J. Virol.* **12:**440–448.

———. 1974. Specific serological relationships among partially purified DNA polymerases of avian leukosis-sarcoma viruses, reticuloendotheliosis viruses, and avian cells. *J. Virol.* **13:**1020–1029.

———. 1975. Purification and properties of spleen necrosis virus DNA polymerase. *J. Virol.* **16:**797–806.

———. 1976. RNA polymerase activity in purified virions of avian reticuloendotheliosis viruses. *J. Virol.* **19:**610–619.

Modak, M.J. and S.L. Marcus. 1977. Purification and properties of Rauscher leukemia virus DNA polymerase and selective inhibition of mammalian viral reverse transcriptase by inorganic phosphate. *J. Biol. Chem.* **252:**11–19.

Moelling, K. 1974. Characterization of reverse transcriptase and RNase H from Friend-murine leukemia virus. *Virology* **62:**46–59.

———. 1975. Reverse transcriptase and RNase H: Present in a murine virus and in both subunits of an avian virus. *Cold Spring Harbor Symp. Quant. Biol.* **39:**969–973.

Moelling, K. and M. Hayami. 1977. Analysis of precursors to the envelope glycoproteins of avian RNA tumor viruses in chicken and quail cells. *J. Virol.* **22:**598–607.

Moelling, K., A. Scott, K.E.J. Dittmar, and M. Owada. 1980. Effect of p15-associated protease from an avian RNA tumor virus on avian virus-specific polyprotein precursors. *J. Virol.* **33:**680–688.

Moelling, K., H. Gelderblom, G. Pauli, R.R. Friis, and H. Bauer. 1975. A comparative study of the avian reticuloendotheliosis virus: Relationship to murine leukemia virus and viruses of the avian sarcoma-leukosis complex. *Virology* **65:**546–557.

Montelaro, R.C., S.J. Sullivan, and D.P. Bolognesi. 1978. An analysis of type-C retrovirus polypeptides and their associations in the virion. *Virology* **84:**19–31.

Mosser, A.G., R.C. Montelaro, and R.R. Rueckert. 1975. Polypeptide composition of spleen necrosis virus, a reticuloendotheliosis virus. *J. Virol.* **15:**1088–1095.

———. 1977. Proteins of Rous-associated virus type 61: Polypeptide stoichiometry and evidence that glycoprotein gp35 is not a cleavage product of gp85. *J. Virol.* **23:**10–19.

Mountcastle, W.E., D.H. Harter, and P.W. Choppin. 1972. The proteins of visna virus. *Virology* **47:**542–545.

Mueller-Lantzsch, N. and H. Fan. 1976. Monospecific immunoprecipitation of murine leukemia virus polyribosomes: Identification of p30 protein-specific messenger RNA. *Cell* **9:**579–588.

Murphy, E.C., Jr. and R.B. Arlinghaus. 1978. Tryptic peptide analyses of polypeptides generated by premature termination of cell-free protein synthesis allow a determination of the Rauscher leukemia virus *gag* gene order. *J. Virol.* **28:**929–935.

Murphy, E.C., Jr., D. Campos, III, and R.B. Arlinghaus. 1979. Cell-free synthesis of Rauscher murine leukemia virus "gag" and "env" gene products from separate cellular mRNA species. *Virology* **93:**293–302.

Murphy, E.C., Jr., J.J. Kopchick, K.F. Watson, and R.B. Arlinghause. 1978. Cell-free synthesis of a precursor polyprotein containing both *gag* and *pol* gene products by Rauscher murine leukemia virus 35S RNA. *Cell* **13:**359–369.

Murray, P.R. and D.P. Nayak. 1974. Characterization of bromodeoxyuridine-induced endogenous guinea pig virus. *J. Virol.* **14:**679–688.

Naso, R.B., W.L. Karshin, Y.H. Wu, and R.B. Arlinghaus. 1979. Characterization of 40,000-

and 25,000-dalton intermediate precursors to Rauscher murine leukemia virus *gag* gene products. *J. Virol.* **32:** 187–198.

Naso, R.B., L.J. Arcement, W.L. Karshin, G.A. Jamjoom, and R.B. Arlinghaus. 1976. A fucose-deficient glycoprotein precursor to Rauscher leukemia virus gp69/71. *Proc. Natl. Acad. Sci.* **73:** 2326–2330.

Neil, J.C., J.E. Smart, M.J. Hayman, and O. Jarrett. 1980. Polypeptides of feline leukemia virus: A glycosylated *gag*-related protein is released into culture fluids. *Virology* **105:** 250–253.

Neiman, P.E. 1973. Measurement of RD114 virus nucleotide sequences in feline cellular DNA. *Nat. New Biol.* **244:** 62–64.

Nermut, M.V., H. Frank, and W. Schafer. 1972. Properties of mouse leukemia viruses. III. Electron microscopic appearance as revealed after conventional preparation techniques as well as freeze-drying and freeze-etching. *Virology* **49:** 345–358.

Niman, H.L. and J.H. Elder. 1980. Molecular dissection of Rauscher virus gp70 by using monoclonal antibodies: Localization of acquired sequences of related envelope gene recombinants. *Proc. Natl. Acad. Sci.* **77:** 4524–4528.

Nowinski, R.C., E. Edynak, and N.H. Sarkar. 1971a. Serological and structural properties of Mason-Pfizer monkey virus isolated from the mammary tumor of a rhesus monkey. *Proc. Natl. Acad. Sci.* **68:** 1608–1612.

Nowinski, R.C., E. Fleissner, N.H. Sarkar, and T. Aoki. 1972. Chromatographic separation and antigenic analysis of proteins of the oncornaviruses. II. Mammalian leukemia-sarcoma viruses. *J. Virol.* **9:** 359–366.

Nowinski, R.C., N.H. Sarkar, L.J. Old, D.H. Moore, D.I. Scheer, and J. Hilgers. 1971b. Characteristics of the structural components of the mouse mammary tumor virus. II. Viral proteins and antigens. *Virology* **46:** 21–38.

Nusse, R., H. Janssen, L. deVries, and R. Michalides. 1980. Analysis of secondary modifications of mouse mammary tumor virus proteins by two-dimensional gel electrophoresis. *J. Virol.* **35:** 340–348.

Nusse, R., F.A.M. Asselbergs, M.H.L. Salden, R.J.A.M. Michalides, and H. Bloemendal. 1978. Translation of mouse mammary tumor virus RNA: Precursor polypeptides are phosphorylated during processing. *Virology* **91:** 106–115.

Nusse, R., L. van der Ploeg, L. van Duijn, R. Michalides, and J. Hilgers. 1979. Impaired maturation of mouse mammary tumor virus precursor polypeptides in lymphoid leukemia cells, producing intracytoplasmic A particles and no extracellular B-type virions. *J. Virol.* **32:** 251–258.

O'Donnell, P.V. and E. Stockert. 1976. Induction of G_{IX} antigen and Gross cell surface antigen after infection by ecotropic and xenotropic murine leukemia viruses in vitro. *J. Virol.* **20:** 545–554.

O'Donnell, P.V., E. Stockert, Y. Obata, A.B. DeLeo, and L.J. Old. 1980. Murine-leukemia-virus-related cell-surface antigens as serological markers of AKR ecotropic, xenotropic and dualtropic viruses. *Cold Spring Harbor Symp. Quant. Biol.* **44:** 1255–1264.

Ogura, H. and R. Friis. 1975. Further evidence for the existence of a viral envelope protein defect in the Bryan high-titer strain of Rous sarcoma virus. *J. Virol.* **16:** 443–446.

Okabe, H., R.V. Gilden, and M. Hatanaka. 1973. Extensive homology of RD114 virus DNA with RNA of feline cell origin. *Nat. New Biol.* **244:** 54–56.

Okasinski, G.F. and L.F. Velicer. 1976. Analysis of intracellular feline leukemia virus proteins. II. Identification of a 60,000-dalton precursor of feline leukemia virus p30. *J. Virol.* **20:** 96–106.

———. 1977. Analysis of intracellular feline leukemia virus proteins. II. Generation of feline leukemia virus structural proteins from precursor polypeptides. *J. Virol.* **22:** 74–85.

Old, L.J., E.A. Boyse, and E. Stockert. 1965. The G (Gross) leukemia antigen. *Cancer Res.* **25:** 813–819.

Onuma, M., C. Olson, and D.M. Driscoll. 1976. Properties of two isolated antigens associated with bovine leukemia virus infection. *J. Natl. Cancer Inst.* **57:** 571–578.

Oppermann, H., J.M. Bishop, H.E. Varmus, and L. Levintow. 1977. A joint product of the genes *gag* and *pol* of avian sarcoma virus: A possible precursor of reverse transcriptase. *Cell* **12:** 993–1005.

Oroszlan, S. and R.V. Gilden. 1980. Primary structure analysis of retrovirus proteins. In *Molecular biology of RNA tumor viruses* (ed. J.R. Stephenson), pp. 299–344. Academic Press, New York.

Oroszlan, S. and R.C. Nowinski. 1980. Lysis of retroviruses with monoclonal antibodies against viral envelope proteins. *Virology* **101:** 296–299.

Oroszlan, S., R.J. Huebner, and R.V. Gilden. 1971a. Species-specific and interspecies antigenic determinants associated with the structural proteins of feline C-type virus. *Proc. Natl. Acad. Sci.* **68:** 901–904.

Oroszlan, S., C.W. Long, and R.V. Gilden. 1976. Isolation of a murine type-C virus p30 precursor protein by DNA-cellulose chromatography. *Virology* **72:** 523–526.

Oroszlan, S., M. Summers, and R.V. Gilden. 1975b. Amino-terminal sequence of baboon type C virus p30. *Virology* **64:** 581–583.

Oroszlan, S., T. Copeland, M.R. Summers, and R.V. Gilden. 1973. Feline leukemia and RD-114 virus group-specific proteins: Comparison of amino terminal sequence. *Science* **181:** 454–456.

Oroszlan, S., C. Foreman, G. Kelloff, and R.V. Gilden. 1971b. The group-specific antigen and other structural proteins of hamster and mouse C-type viruses. *Virology* **43:** 665–674.

Oroszlan, S., T. Copeland, G. Smythers, M.R. Summers, and R.V. Gilden. 1977. Comparative primary structure analysis of the p30 protein of woolly monkey and gibbon type C viruses. *Virology* **77:** 413–417.

Oroszlan, S., T. Copeland, M.R. Summers, G. Smythers, and R.V. Gilden. 1975b. Amino acid sequence homology of mammalian type C RNA virus major internal proteins. *J. Biol. Chem.* **250:** 6232–6239.

Oroszlan, S., D. Bova, M.H.M. White, R. Toni, C. Foreman, and R.V. Gilden. 1972. Purification and immunological characterization of the major internal protein of the RD-114 virus. *Proc. Natl. Acad. Sci.* **69:** 1211–1215.

Oroszlan, S., L.E. Henderson, J.R. Stephenson, T.D. Copeland, C.W. Long, J.N. Ihle, and R.V. Gilden. 1978. Amino- and carboxyl-terminal amino acid sequences of proteins coded by *gag* gene of murine leukemia virus. *Proc. Natl. Acad. Sci.* **75:** 1404–1408.

Pal, B.K. and P. Roy-Burman. 1975. Phosphoproteins: Structural components of oncornaviruses. *J. Virol.* **15:** 540–549.

Pal, B.K., R.M. McAllister, M.B. Gardner, and P. Roy-Burman. 1975. Comparative studies on the structural phosphoproteins of mammalian type C Viruses. *J. Virol.* **16:** 123–131.

Palmiter, R.D., J. Gagnon, V.M. Vogt, S. Ripley, and R.N. Eisenman. 1978. The NH_2-terminal sequence of the avian oncovirus *gag* precursor polyprotein ($Pr76^{gag}$). *Virology* **91:** 423–433.

Panet, A., D. Baltimore, and H. Hanafusa. 1975a. Quantitation of avian RNA tumor virus reverse transcriptase by radioimmunoassay. *J. Virol.* **16:** 146–152.

Panet A., W.A. Haseltine, D. Baltimore, G. Peters, F. Harada, and J.E. Dahlberg. 1975b. Specific binding of tryptophan transfer RNA to avian myeloblastosis virus RNA-dependent DNA polymerase (reverse transcriptase). *Proc. Natl. Acad. Sci.* **72:** 2535–2539.

Parekh, B., C.J. Issel, and R.C. Montelaro. 1980. Equine infectious anemia virus, a putative lentivirus, contains polypeptides analogous to prototype-C oncornaviruses. *Virology* **107:** 520–525.

Parks W.P. and E.M. Scolnick. 1972. Radioimmunoassay of mammalian type-C viral proteins: Interspecies antigenic reactivities of the major internal polypeptide. *Proc. Natl. Acad. Sci.* **69:** 1766–1770.

Parks, W.P., E.M. Scolnick, M.C. Noon, and C.J. Watson. 1974a. Immunological cross-reactions between two low-molecular-weight polypeptides from a murine type C virus. *J. Virol.* **14:**430–433.

Parks, W.P., R.S. Howk, E.M. Scolnick, S. Oroszlan, and R.V. Gilden. 1974b. Immunochemical characterization of two major polypeptides from murine mammary tumor virus. *J. Virol.* **13:**1200–1210.

Parks, W.P., E.M. Scolnick, J. Ross, G.J. Todaro, and S.A. Aaronson. 1972. Immunological relationships of reverse transcriptases from ribonucleic acid tumor viruses. *J. Virol.* **9:**110–115.

Paterson, B.M., D.J. Marciani, and T.S. Papas. 1977. Cell-free synthesis of the precursor polypeptide for avian myeloblastosis virus DNA polymerase. *Proc. Natl. Acad. Sci.* **74:**4951–4954.

Pauli, G., W. Rohde, and E. Harms. 1978. The structure of the Rous sarcoma virus glycoprotein complex. *Arch. Virol.* **58:**61–64.

Pawson, T., R. Harvey, and A.E. Smith. 1977. The size of Rous sarcoma virus mRNAs active in cell-free translation. *Nature* **268:**416–420.

Pawson, T., G.S. Martin, and A.E. Smith. 1976. Cell-free translation of virion RNA from nondefective and transformation-defective Rous sarcoma viruses. *J. Virol.* **19:**950–967.

Pawson, T., P. Mellon, P.H. Duesberg, and G.S. Martin. 1980. *env* gene of Rous sarcoma virus: Identification of the gene product by cell-free translation. *J. Virol.* **33:**993–1003.

Pelham, H.R.B. 1978. Translation of encephalomyocarditis virus RNA *in vitro* yields an active proteolytic processing enzyme. *Eur. J. Biochem.* **85:**457–462.

———. 1979. Synthesis and proteolytic processing of cowpea mosaic virus proteins in reticulocyte lysates. *Virology* **96:**463–477.

Pepinsky, R.B. and V.M. Vogt. 1979. Identification of retrovirus matrix proteins by lipid-protein cross-linking. *J. Mol. Biol.* **131:**819–837.

Pepinsky, R.B., D. Cappiello, C. Wilkowski, and V.M. Vogt. 1980. Chemical cross-linking of proteins in avian sarcoma and leukemia viruses. *Virology* **102:**205–210.

Peters, G.G. and C. Glover. 1980. Low-molecular-weight RNAs and initiation of RNA-directed DNA synthesis in avian reticuloendotheliosis virus. *J. Virol.* **33:**708–716.

Peters, G.G. and J. Hu. 1980. Reverse transcriptase as the major determinant for selective packaging of tRNA's into avian sarcoma virus particles. *J. Virol.* **36:**692–700.

Philipson, L., P. Andersson, U. Olshevsky, R. Weinberg, D. Baltimore, and R. Gesteland. 1978. Translation of MuLV and MSV RNAs in nuclease-treated reticulocyte extracts: Enhancement of the gal-pol polypeptide with yeast suppressor tRNA. *Cell* **13:**189–199.

Pinter, A. and E. de Harven. 1980. Protein composition of a defective murine sarcoma virus particle possessing the enveloped type-A morphology. *Virology* **99:**103–110.

Pinter, A. and E. Fleissner. 1979. Structural proteins of retroviruses: Characterization of oligomeric complexes of murine and feline leukemia virus envelope and core components formed upon cross-linking. *J. Virol.* **30:**157–165.

Pinter, A., J. Lieman-Hurwitz, and E. Fleissner. 1978. The nature of the association between the murine leukemia virus envelope proteins. *Virology* **91:**345–351.

Purchio, A.F., E. Erikson, and R.L. Erikson. 1977. Translation of 35S and of subgenomic regions of avian sarcoma virus RNA. *Proc. Natl. Acad. Sci.* **74:**4661–4665.

Purchio, A.F., S. Jovanovich, and R.L. Erikson. 1980. Sites of synthesis of viral proteins in avian sarcoma virus-infected chicken cells. *J. Virol.* **35:**629–636.

Quigley, J.P., D.B. Rifkin, and R.W. Compans. 1972. Isolation and characterization of ribonucleoprotein substructures from Rous sarcoma virus. *Virology* **50:**65–75.

Quigley, J.P., D.B. Rifkin, and E. Reich. 1971. Phospholipid composition of Rous sarcoma virus, host cell membranes and other enveloped RNA viruses. *Virology* **46:**106–116.

Rabin, H., C.V. Benton, M.A. Tainsky, N.R. Rice, and R.V. Gilden. 1979. Isolation and characterization of an endogenous type C virus of rhesus monkeys. *Science* **204:**841–842.

Racevskis, J. and N.H. Sarkar. 1978. Synthesis and processing of precursor polypeptides to murine mammary tumor virus structural proteins. *J. Virol.* **25:** 374–383.

———. 1980. Murine mammary tumor virus structural protein interactions: Formation of oligomeric complexes with cleavable cross-linking agents. *J. Virol.* **35:** 937–948.

Ramsay, G. and M.J. Hayman. 1980. Analysis of cells transformed by defective leukemia virus OK10: Production of noninfectious particles and synthesis of $Pr76^{gag}$ and an additional 200,000-dalton protein. *Virology* **106:** 71–81.

Rettenmier, C.W. and H. Hanafusa. 1977. Structural protein markers in the avian oncoviruses. *J. Virol.* **24:** 850–864.

Rettenmier, C.W., S.M. Anderson, M.W. Riemen, and H. Hanafusa. 1979a. *gag*-related polypeptides encoded by replication-defective avian oncoviruses. *J. Virol.* **32:** 749–761.

Rettenmier, C.W., R.E. Karess, S.M. Anderson, and H. Hanafusa. 1979b. Tryptic peptide analysis of avian oncovirus *gag* and *pol* gene products. *J. Virol.* **32:** 102–113.

Reynolds, R.K. and J.R. Stephenson. 1977. Intracistronic mapping of the murine type C viral *gag* gene by use of conditional lethal replication mutants. *Virology* **81:** 328–340.

Rho, H.M. and R.C. Gallo. 1979. Characterization of reverse transcriptase from feline leukemia virus by radioimmunoassay. *Virology* **99:** 192–196.

Rho, H.M., D.P. Grandgenett, and M. Green. 1975. Sequence relatedness between the subunits of avian myeloblastosis virus reverse transcriptase. *J. Biol. Chem.* **250:** 5278–5280.

Ricciardi, R.P., J.S. Miller, and B.E. Roberts. 1979. Purification and mapping of specific mRNAs by hybridization-selection and cell-free translation. *Proc. Natl. Acad. Sci.* **76:** 4927–4931.

Rifkin, D.B. and R.W. Compans. 1971. Identification of the spike proteins of Rous sarcoma virus. *Virology* **46:** 485–489.

Robertson, D.L. and H.E. Varmus. 1979. Structural analysis of the intracellular RNAs of murine mammary tumor virus. *J. Virol.* **30:** 576–589.

Robinson, H.L., R. Eisenman, A. Senior, and S. Ripley. 1979. Low frequency production of recombinant subgroup E avian leukosis viruses by uninfected $V\text{-}15_B$ chicken cells. *Virology* **99:** 21–30.

Rogers, J., P. Early, C. Carter, K. Calame, M. Bond, L. Hood, and R. Wall. 1980. Two mRNAs with different 3′ ends encode membrane-bound and secreted forms of immunoglobulin μ chain. *Cell* **20:** 303–312.

Rohrschneider, L., H. Bauer, and D.P. Bolognesi. 1975. Group-specific antigenic determinants of the large envelope glycoprotein of avian oncornaviruses. *Virology* **67:** 234–241.

Rohrschneider, J.M., H. Diggelmann, H. Ogura, R.R. Friis, and H. Bauer. 1976. Defective cleavage of a precursor polypeptide in a temperature-sensitive mutant of avian sarcoma virus. *Virology* **75:** 177–187.

Rosner, M.R., L.S. Grinna, and P.W. Robbins. 1980a. Differences in glycosylation patterns of closely related murine leukemia viruses. *Proc. Natl. Acad. Sci.* **77:** 67–71.

Rosner, M.R., J.-S., Tung, N. Hopkins, and P.W. Robbins. 1980b. Relationship of G_{IX} antigen expression to the glycosylation of murine leukemia virus glycoprotein. *Proc. Natl. Acad. Sci.* **77:** 6420–6424.

Rothenberg, E., D.J. Donoghue, and D. Baltimore. 1978. Analysis of a 5′ leader sequence on murine leukemia virus 21S RNA: Heteroduplex mapping with long reverse transcriptase products. *Cell* **13:** 435–451.

Rothman, J.E. and J. Lenard. 1977. Membrane asymmetry. *Science* **195:** 743–753.

Rothman, J.E., F.N. Katz, and H.F. Lodish. 1978. Glycosylation of a membrane protein is restricted to the growing polypeptide chain but is not necessary for insertion as a transmembrane protein. *Cell* **15:** 1447–1454.

Ruprecht, R.M., N.C. Goodman, and S. Speigelman. 1973. Determination of natural host taxonomy of RNA tumor viruses by molecular hybridization: Application to RD-114, a candidate human virus. *Proc. Natl. Acad. Sci.* **70:** 1437–1441.

Sacks, T.L., S.G. Devare, G.R. Blennerhassett, and J.R. Stephenson. 1978. Non-conditional replication mutants of type C and type D retroviruses defective in *gag* gene-coded polyprotein post-translational processing. *Virology* **91:**352–363.

Samuel, K.P., T.S. Papas, and J.G. Chirikjian. 1979. DNA endonucleases associated with the avian myeloblastosis virus DNA polymerase. *Proc. Natl. Acad. Sci.* **76:**2659–2663.

Sarin, P.S. and R.C. Gallo. 1976. Purification and characterization of gibbon ape leukemia virus DNA polymerase. *Biochim. Biophys. Acta* **454:**212–221.

Sarin, P.S., B. Friedman, and R.C. Gallo. 1977. Purification and characterization of baboon endogenous virus DNA polymerase. *Biochim. Biophys. Acta* **479:**198–206.

Sarkar, N.H. and A.S. Dion. 1975. Polypeptides of the mouse mammary tumor virus. I. Characterization of two group-specific antigens. *Virology* **64:**471–491.

Sarkar, N.H., D.H. Moore, and R.C. Nowinski. 1972. Symmetry of the nucleocapsid of the oncornaviruses. In *RNA viruses and host genome in oncogenesis* (ed. P. Emmelot and P. Bentvelzen), pp.71–79. North-Holland, Amsterdam.

Sarkar, N.H., R.C. Nowinski, and D.H. Moore. 1971. Characteristics of the structural components of the mouse mammary tumor virus. I. Morphological and biochemical studies. *Virology* **46:**1–20.

Sarkar, N.H., N.E. Taraschi, A.A. Pomenti, and A.S. Dion. 1976. Polypeptides of the mouse mammary tumor virus. II. Identification of two major glycoproteins with the viral structure. *Virology* **69:**677–690.

Sarkar, N.H., E.S. Whittington, J. Racevskis, and S.L. Marcus. 1978. Phosphoproteins of the murine mammary tumor virus. *Virology* **91:**407–422.

Sarma, P.S. and T. Log. 1971. Viral interference in feline leukemia-sarcoma complex. *Virology* **44:**352–358.

———. 1973. Subgroup classification of feline leukemia and sarcoma viruses by viral interference and neutralization tests. *Virology* **54:**160–169.

Sarma, P.S., J. Tseng, Y.K. Lee, and R.V. Gilden. 1973. Virus similar to RD114 virus in cat cells. *Nat. New Biol.* **244:**56–59.

Sarma, P.S., R.J. Huebner, H.C. Turner, R.V. Gilden, and T.-S. Log. 1971. Feline leukaemia viral antigens and antisera to the group specific antigens of the murine leukaemia viruses. *Nat. New Biol.* **230:**50–52.

Sawyer, R.C. and H. Hanafusa. 1979. Comparison of the small RNAs of polymerase-deficient and polymerase-positive Rous sarcoma virus and another species of avian retrovirus. *J. Virol.* **29:**863–871.

Schafer, W. and D.P. Bolognesi. 1977. Mammalian C-type oncornaviruses: Relationships between viral structural and cell-surface antigens and their possible significance in immunological defense mechanisms. *Contemp. Top. Immunobiol.* **6:**127–167.

Schafer, W., F.A. Anderer, H. Bauer, and L. Pister. 1969. Studies on mouse leukemia viruses. I. Isolation and characterization of a group-specific antigen. *Virology* **38:**387–394.

Schafer, W., J. Lange, D.P. Bolognesi, F. de Noronha, J.E. Post, and C.G. Rickard. 1971. Isolation and characterization of two group-specific antigens from feline leukemia virus. *Virology* **44:**73–82.

Scheele, C.M. and H. Hanafusa. 1971. Proteins of helper-dependent RSV. *Virology* **45:**401–410.

Schiff, R.D. and D.P. Grandgenett. 1978. Virus-coded origin of a 32,000-dalton protein from avian retrovirus cores: Structural relatedness of p32 and the β polypeptide of the avian retrovirus DNA polymerase. *J. Virol.* **28:**279–291.

Schlesinger, M.J. 1976. Formation of an infectious virus-antibody complex with Rous sarcoma virus and antibodies directed against the major virus glycoprotein. *J. Virol.* **17:**1063–1067.

Schloemer, R.H., J. Schlom, G. Schochetman, P. Kimball, and R.R. Wagner. 1976. Sialylation of glycoproteins of murine mammary tumor virus, murine leukemia virus, and Mason-Pfizer monkey virus. *J. Virol.* **18:**804–808.

Schlom, J. 1980. Type B and type D retroviruses. In *Molecular biology of RNA tumor viruses* (ed. J.R. Stephenson), pp. 447–484. Academic Press, New York.

Schneider, J. and G. Hunsmann. 1978. Surface expression of murine leukemia virus structural polypeptides on host cells and the virion. *Int. J. Cancer* **22:**204–213.

Schnitzer, T.J., C. Dickson, and R.A. Weiss. 1979. Morphological and biochemical characterization of viral particles produced by the *tsO45* mutant of vesicular stomatitis virus at restrictive temperature. *J. Virol.* **29:**185–195.

Schochetman, G. and D.L. Fine. 1978. Natural distribution of squirrel monkey retrovirus proviral sequences in primate DNAs. *J. Gen. Virol.* **40:**257–260.

Schochetman, G. and J. Schlom. 1976. Independent polypeptide chain initiation sites for the synthesis of different classes of proteins for an RNA tumor virus: Mouse mammary tumor virus. *Virology* **73:**431–441.

Schochetman, G., M. Boehm-Truitt, and J. Schlom. 1976. Antigenic analysis of the major structural protein of the Mason-Pfizer monkey virus. *J. Immunol.* **117:**168–173.

Schochetman, G., K. Kortright, and J. Schlom. 1975. Mason-Pfizer monkey virus: Analysis and localization of virion proteins and glycoproteins. *J. Virol.* **16:**1208–1219.

Schochetman, G., S. Oroszlan, L. Arthur, and D. Fine. 1977a. Gene order of the mouse mammary tumor virus glycoproteins. *Virology* **83:**72–83.

Schochetman, G., D. Fine, L. Arthur, R. Gilden, and R. Heberling. 1977b. Characterization of a retravirus isolated from squirrel monkeys. *J. Virol.* **23:**384–393.

Schochetman, G., C.W. Long, S. Oroszlan, L. Arthur, and D.L. Fine. 1978. Isolation of separate precursor polypeptides for the mouse mammary tumor virus glycoproteins and nonglycoproteins. *Virology* **85:**168–174.

Schulein, M., W.N. Burnette, and J.T. August. 1978. Stoichiometry and specificity of binding of Rauscher oncovirus 10,000-dalton (p10) structural protein to nucleic acids. *J. Virol.* **26:**54–60.

Schultz, A.M. and S. Oroszlan. 1978. Murine leukemia virus *gag* polyproteins: The peptide chain unique to Pr80 is located at the amino terminus. *Virology* **91:**481–486.

Schultz, A.M., E.H. Rabin, and S. Oroszlan. 1979. Post-translational modification of Rauscher leukemia virus precursor polyproteins encoded by the *gag* gene. *J. Virol.* **30:**255–266.

Schultz, A.M., S.M. Lockhart, E.M. Rabin and S.O. Oroszlan. 1981. Structure of glycosylated and unglycosylated *gag* polyproteins of Rauscher murine leukemia virus: Carbohydrate attachment sites. *J. Virol.* **38:**581–592.

Scolnick, E.M., W.P. Parks, and D.M. Livingston. 1972a. Radioimmunoassay of mammalian C-type proteins. I. Species specific reactions of murine and feline viruses. *J. Immunol.* **109:**570–577.

Scolnick, E.M., W.P. Parks, G.J. Todaro, and S.A. Aaronson. 1972b. Immunological characterization of primate C-type virus reverse transcriptases. *Nat. New Biol.* **235:**35–40.

Scott, J.V., L. Stowring, A.T. Haase, O. Narayan, and R. Vigne. 1979. Antigenic variation in visna virus. *Cell* **18:**321–327.

Sefton, B.M. 1976. Virus-dependent glycosylation. *J. Virol.* **17:**85–93.

———. 1977. Immediate glycosylation of Sindbis virus membrane proteins. *Cell* **10:**659–668.

Sen, A. and G.J. Todaro. 1976. Specificity of in vitro binding of primate type C viral RNA and the homologous viral p12 core protein. *Science* **193:**326–328.

———. 1977. The genome-associated, specific RNA binding proteins of avian and mammalian type C viruses. *Cell* **10:**91–99.

Sen, A., C.J. Sherr, and G.J. Todaro. 1976. Specific binding of the type C viral core protein p12 with purified viral RNA. *Cell* **7:**21–32.

———. 1977. Phosphorylation of murine type C viral p12 proteins regulates their extent of binding to the homologous RNA. *Cell* **10:**489–496.

———. 1978. Endogenous feline (RD-114) and baboon type C viruses have related specific RNA-binding proteins and genome binding sites. *Virology* **84:**99–107.

Sen, G.C., H.C. Haspel, and N.H. Sarkar. 1980a. Presence of a proteolytic activity in murine mammary tumor virus. *J. Biol. Chem.* **255:** 7098–7101.

Sen, G.C., W. Zablocki, and N.H. Sarkar. 1980b. Gene order of murine mammary tumor virus *gag* proteins and *env* proteins. *Virology* **106:** 152–154.

Sen, G.C., S.W. Smith, S.L. Marcus, and N.H. Sarkar. 1979. Identification of the messenger RNAs coding for the *gag* and *env* gene products of the murine mammary tumor virus. *Proc. Natl. Acad. Sci.* **76:** 1736–1740.

Shaikh, R., M. Linial, J. Coffin, and R. Eisenman. 1978. Recombinant avian oncoviruses. I. Alterations in the precursor to the internal structural proteins. *Virology* **87:** 326–338.

Shaikh, R., M. Linial, S. Brown, A. Sen, and R. Eisenman. 1979. Recombinant avian oncoviruses. II. Alterations in the *gag* proteins and evidence for intragenic recombination. *Virology* **92:** 463–481.

Shapiro, A.L., E. Vinuela, and J.V. Maizel, Jr. 1967. Molecular weight estimation of polypeptide chains by electrophoresis in SDS-polyacrylamide gels. *Biochem. Biophys. Res. Commun.* **28:** 815–820.

Shapiro, S.Z., M. Strand, and J.T. August. *1976.* High molecular weight precursor polypeptides to structural proteins of Rauscher murine leukemia virus. *J. Mol. Biol.* **107:** 459–477.

Shealy, D.J., A.G. Mosser, and R.R. Rueckert. 1980. Novel p19-related protein in Rous-associated virus type 61: Implications for avian *gag* gene order. *J. Virol.* **34:** 431–437.

Sheffield, J.B. and T.M. Daly. 1976. Extrinsic labeling of MuMTV with a galactose oxidase-tritiated borohydride method. *Virology* **70:** 247–250.

Sherr, C.J. and G.J. Todaro. 1974. Radioimmunoassay of the major group specific protein of endogenous baboon type C viruses: Relation to the RD-114/CCC group and detection of antigen in normal baboon tissues. *Virology* **61:** 168–181.

Sherr, C.J., R.E. Benveniste, and G.J. Todaro. 1978. Endogenous mink (*Mustela vison*) type C virus isolated from sarcoma virus-transformed mink cells. *J. Virol.* **25:** 738–749.

Sherr, C.J., L.A. Fedele, R.E. Benveniste, and G.J. Todaro. 1975. Interspecies antigenic determinants of the reverse transcriptases and p30 proteins of mammalian type C viruses. *J. Virol.* **15:** 1440–1448.

Sherr, C.J., M.M. Lieber, R.E. Benveniste, and G.J. Todaro. 1974. Endogenous baboon type C virus (M7): Biochemical and immunologic characterization. *Virology* **58:** 492–503.

Shine, J., A.P. Czernilofsky, R. Friedrich, J.M. Bishop, and H.M. Goodman. 1977. Nucleotide sequence at the 5′ terminus of the avian sarcoma virus genome. *Proc. Natl. Acad. Sci.* **74:** 1473–1477.

Smith, B.J. and J.M. Bailey. 1979. The binding of an avian myeloblastosis virus basic 12,000 dalton protein to nucleic acids. *Nucleic Acids Res.* **7:** 2055–2072.

Smith, G.C., R.L. Heberling, R.J. Helmke, S.T. Barker, and S.S. Kalter. 1977. Oncornavirus-like particles in squirrel monkey (*Saimiri sciureus*) placenta and placenta culture. *J. Natl. Cancer Inst.* **59:** 975–979.

Smith, G.H. 1978. Evidence for a precursor-product relationship between intracytoplasmic A particles and murine mammary tumour virus cores. *J. Gen Virol.* **41:** 193–200.

Smith, G.H. and B.K. Lee. 1975. Mouse mammary tumor virus polypeptide precursors in intracytoplasmic A particles. *J. Natl. Cancer Inst.* **55:** 493–496.

Snyder H.W., Jr., E. Stockert, and E. Fleissner. 1977. Characterization of molecular species carrying Gross cell surface antigen. *J. Virol.* **23:** 302–314.

Stacey, D.W., V.G. Allfrey, and H. Hanafusa. 1977. Microinjection analysis of envelope-glycoprotein messenger activities of avian leukosis virus RNAs. *Proc. Natl. Acad. Sci.* **74:** 1614–1618.

Steeves, R.A., M. Strand, and J.T. August. 1974. Structural proteins of mammalian oncogenic RNA viruses: Murine leukemia virus neutralization by antisera prepared against purified envelope glycoprotein. *J. Virol.* **14:** 187–189.

Stephenson, J.R. and S.A. Aaronson. 1973. Expression of endogenous RNA C-type virus group-specific antigens in mammalian cells. *J. Virol.* **12:**564–569.

Stephenson, J.R., R.K. Reynolds, and S.A. Aaronson. 1976a. Comparisons of the immunological properties of two structural polypeptides of type C RNA viruses endogenous to Old World monkeys. *J. Virol.* **17:**374–384.

Stephenson, J.R., S.R. Tronick, and S.A. Aaronson. 1974. Analysis of type specific antigenic determinants of two structural polypeptides of mouse RNA C-type viruses. *Virology* **58:**1–8.

———. 1975a. Murine leukemia virus mutants with temperature-sensitive defects in precursor polypeptide cleavage. *Cell* **6:**543–548.

Stephenson, J.R., S. Hino, E.W. Garrett, and S.A. Aaronson. 1976b. Immunological cross reactivity of Mason-Pfizer monkey virus with type C RNA viruses endogenous to primates. *Nature* **261:**609–611.

Stephenson, J.R., R.K. Reynolds, S.G. Devare, and F.H. Reynolds. 1977. Biochemical and immunological properties of *gag* gene-coded structural proteins of endogenous type C RNA tumor viruses of diverse mammalian species. *J. Biol. Chem.* **252:**7818–7825.

Stephenson, J.R., E.J. Smith, L.B. Crittenden, and S.A. Aaronson. 1975b. Analysis of antigenic determinants of structural polypeptides of avian type C tumor viruses. *J. Virol.* **16:**27–33.

Stohrer, R. and E. Hunter. 1979. Inhibition of Rous sarcoma virus replication by 2-deoxyglucose and tunicamycin: Identification of an unglycosylated *env* gene product. *J. Virol.* **32:**412–419.

Stoll, E., M.A. Billeter, A. Palmenberg, and C. Weissmann. 1977. Avian myeloblastosis virus RNA is terminally redundant: Implications for the mechanism of retrovirus replication. *Cell* **12:**57–72.

Stone, L.B., E. Scolnick, K.K. Takemoto, and S.A. Aaronson. 1971. Visna virus: A slow virus with an RNA dependent DNA polymerase. *Nature* **229:**257–258.

Stowring, L., A.T. Haase, and H.P. Charman. 1979. Serological definition of the lentivirus group of retroviruses. *J. Virol.* **29:**523–528.

Strand, M. and J.T. August. 1973. Structural proteins of oncogenic ribonucleic acid viruses. *Interspec* II, a new interspecies antigen. *J. Biol. Chem.* **248:**5627–5633.

———. 1974. Structural proteins of mammalian oncogenic RNA viruses: Multiple antigenic determinants of the major internal protein and envelope glycoprotein. *J. Virol.* **13:**171–180.

———. 1977. Purification and analysis of a Gross murine oncornavirus protein with a molecular weight of about 12,000 specific for the Gross virus subgroup. *Virology* **79:**129–143.

Strand, M., J.T. August, and R. Jaenisch. 1977. Oncornavirus gene expression during embryonal development of the mouse. *Virology* **76:**886–890.

Strand, M., F. Lilly, and J.T. August. 1974a. Host control of endogenous murine leukemia virus expression: Concentrations of viral proteins in high and low leukemia mouse strains. *Proc. Natl. Acad. Sci.* **71:**3682–3686.

Strand, M., R. Wilsnack, and J.T. August. 1974b. Structural proteins of mammalian oncogenic RNA viruses: Immunological characterization of the p15 polypeptide of Rauscher murine virus. *J. Virol.* **14:**1575–1583.

Stromberg, K. 1972. Surface-active agents for isolation of the core component of avian myeloblastosis virus. *J. Virol.* **9:**684–697.

Stromberg, K., N.E. Hurley, N.L. Davis, R.R. Rueckert, and E. Fleissner. 1974. Structural studies of avian myeloblastosis virus: Comparison of polypeptides in virion and core component by dodecyl sulfate-polyacrylamide gel electrophoresis. *J. Virol.* **13:**513–528.

Sutcliffe, J.G., T.M. Shinnick, I.M. Verma, and R.A. Lerner. 1980a. Nucleotide sequence of Moloney leukemia virus: 3′ end reveals details of replication, analogy to bacterial transposons, and an unexpected gene. *Proc. Natl. Acad. Sci.* **77:**3302–3306.

Sutcliffe, J.G., T.M. Shinnick, N. Green, F.-T. Liu, H.L. Niman, and R.A. Lerner. 1980b. Chemical synthesis of a polypeptide predicted from nucleotide sequence allows detection of a new retroviral gene product. *Nature* **287:**801–805.

Swanson, S.K., E. Sulkowski, and K.F. Manly. 1978. Hydrophobic binding site(s) on Moloney-murine leukemia virus p30. *Virology* **85:**211–221.

Takatsuki, A. and G. Tamura. 1971. Effect of tunicamycin on the synthesis of macromolecules in cultures of chick embryo fibroblasts infected with Newcastle disease virus. *J. Antibiot.* **24:**785–794.

Tanaka, H. 1977. Precursor-product relationship between nonglycosylated polypeptides of A and B particles of mouse mammary tumor virus. *Virology* **76:**835–850.

Tanaka, H. and D.H. Moore. 1967. Electron microscopic localization of viral antigens in mouse mammary tumors by ferritin-labeled antibody. I. The homologous systems. *Virology* **33:**197–214.

Tanaka, H., A. Tamura, and D. Tsujimura. 1972. Properties of the intracytoplasmic A particles purified from mouse tumors. *Virology* **49:**61–78.

Tarentino, A.L. and F. Maley. 1974. Purification and properties of an endo-β-*N*-acetylglucosaminidase from *Streptomyces griseus. J. Biol. Chem.* **249:**811–817.

Temin, H.M. and D. Baltimore. 1972. RNA-directed DNA synthesis and RNA tumor viruses. *Adv. Virus Res.* **17:**129–186.

Tennant, R.W., J.A. Otten, A. Brown, W.K. Yang, and S.J. Kennel. 1979. Characterization of Fv-1 host range strains of murine retroviruses by titration and p30 protein characteristics. *Virology* **99:**349–357.

Teramoto, Y.A. and J. Schlom. 1978. Radioimmunoassays that demonstrate type-specific and group-specific antigenic reactivities for the major internal structural protein of murine mammary tumor viruses. *Cancer Res.* **38:**1990–1995.

———. 1979. Radioimmunoassays for the 36,000-dalton glycoprotein of murine mammary tumor viruses demonstrate type, group, and interspecies determinants. *J. Virol.* **31:**334–340.

Teramoto, Y.A., R.D. Cardiff, and J.K. Lund. 1977. The structure of the mouse mammary tumor virus: Isolation and characterization of the core. *Virology* **77:**135–148.

Teramoto, Y.A., M.J. Puentes, L.J.T. Young, and R.D. Cardiff. 1974. Structure of the mouse mammary tumor virus: Polypeptides and glycoproteins. *J. Virol.* **13:**411–418.

Theilen, G.H., D. Gould, M. Fowler, and D.L. Dungworth. 1971. C-type virus in tumor tissue of a woolly monkey (*Lagothrix spp.*) with fibrosarcoma. *J. Natl. Cancer Inst.* **47:**881–889.

Thiel, H.-J., H. Beug, T. Graf, H. Schwarz, W. Schafer, C. Bergholz, and F. Deinhardt. 1978. Studies of simian sarcoma and simian sarcoma-associated virus. II. Isolation of the major viral glycoprotein, properties of this component and its specific antiserum. *Viriology* **90:**360–365.

Todaro, G.J., R.E. Benveniste, M.M. Lieber, and C.J. Sherr. 1974a. Characterization of a type C virus released from the porcine cell line PK(15). *Virology* **58:**65–74.

Todaro, G.J., R.E. Benveniste, S.A. Sherwin, and C.J. Sherr. 1978a. MAC-1, a new genetically transmitted type C virus of primates: "Low frequency" activation from stumptail monkey cell cultures. *Cell* **13:**775–782.

Todaro, G.J., C.J. Sherr, R.E. Benveniste, M.M. Lieber, and J.L. Melnick. 1974b. Type C viruses of baboons: Isolation from normal cell cultures. *Cell* **2:**55–61.

Todaro, G.J., R.E. Benveniste, C.J. Sherr, J. Schlom, G. Schidlovsky, and J.R. Stephenson. 1978b. Isolation and characterization of a new type D retrovirus from the Asian primate, *Presbytis obscurus* (spectacled langur). *Virology* **84:**189–194.

Todaro, G.J., M.M. Leiber, R.E. Benveniste, C.J. Sherr, C.J. Gibbs, Jr., and D.C. Gajdusek. 1975. Infectious primate type C viruses: Three isolates belonging to a new subgroup from the brains of normal gibbons. *Virology* **67:**335–343.

Todaro, G.J., C.J. Sherr, A. Sen, N. King, M.D. Daniel, and B. Fleckenstein. 1978c.

Endogenous New World primate type C viruses isolated from owl monkey (*Aotus trivirgatus*) kidney cell line. *Proc. Natl. Acad. Sci.* **75:** 1004–1008.

Towbin, H., T. Staehelin, and J. Gordon. 1979. Electrophoretic transfer of proteins from polyacrylamide gels to nitrocellulose sheets: Procedure and some applications. *Proc. Natl. Acad. Sci.* **76:** 4350–4354.

Tronick, S.R., J.R. Stephenson, and S.A. Aaronson. 1974a. Immunological properties of two polypeptides of Mason-Pfizer monkey virus. *J. Virol.* **14:** 125–132.

———. 1974b. Comparative immunological studies of RNA C-type viruses: Radioimmunoassay for a low molecular weight polypeptide of woolly monkey leukemia virus. *Virology* **57:** 347–356.

Tronick, S.R., M.M. Golub, J.R. Stephenson, and S.A. Aaronson. 1977. Distribution and expression in mammals of genes related to an endogenous type C RNA virus of *Odocoileus hemionus*. *J. Virol.* **23:** 1–9.

Tronick, S.R., J.R. Stephenson, S.A. Aaronson, and T.G. Kawakami. 1975. Antigenic characterization of type C RNA virus isolates of gibbon apes. *J. Virol.* **15:** 115–120.

Tung, J.-S. and E. Fleissner. 1980. Amplified *env* and *gag* products on AKR cells. Origin from different murine leukemia virus genomes. *J. Exp. Med.* **151:** 975–979.

Tung, J.-S., A. Pinter, and E. Fleissner. 1977. Two species of type C viral core polyprotein on AKR mouse leukemia cells. *J. Virol.* **23:** 430–435.

Tung, J.-S., T. Yoshiki, and E. Fleissner. 1976. A core polyprotein of murine leukemia virus on the surface of mouse leukemia cells. *Cell* **9:** 573–578.

Tung, J.-S., E.S. Vitetta, E. Fleissner, and E.A. Boyse. 1975. Biochemical evidence linking the G_{IX} thymocyte surface antigen to the gp69/71 envelope glycoprotein of murine leukemia virus. *J. Exp. Med.* **141:** 198–205.

Twardzik, D.R., T.S. Papas, and F.H. Portugal. 1974. DNA polymerase in virions of a reptilian type C virus. *J. Virol.* **13:** 166–170.

Uckert, W., V. Wunderlich, E. Bender, G. Sydow, and D. Bierwolf. 1980. The protein pattern of PMF virus, a type D retrovirus from malignant permanent human cell lines. *Arch. Virol.* **64:** 155–166.

Van de Ven, W.J.M., D. van Zaane, C. Onnekink, and H.P.J. Bloemers. 1978a. Impaired processing of precursor polypeptides of temperature-sensitive mutants of Rauscher murine leukemia virus. *J. Virol.* **25:** 553–561.

Van de Ven, W.J.M., A.J.M. Vermorken, C. Onnekink, H.P.J. Bloemers, and H. Bloemendal. 1978b. Structural studies on Rauscher murine leukemia virus: Isolation and characterization of viral envelopes. *J. Virol.* **27:** 595–603.

Van Eldik, L.J., J.C. Paulson, R.W. Green, and R.E. Smith. 1978. The influence of carbohydrate on the antigenicity of the envelope glycoprotein of avian myeloblastosis virus and B77 avian sarcoma virus. *Virology* **86:** 193–204.

van Zaane, D., M.J.A. Dekker-Michielsen, and H.P.J. Bloemers. 1976. Virus-specific precursor polypeptides in cells infected with Rauscher leukemia virus: Synthesis, identification, and processing. *Virology* **75:** 113–129.

van Zaane, D., A.L.J. Gielkens, M.J.A. Dekker-Michielsen, and H.P.J. Bloemers. 1975. Virus-specific precursor polypeptides in cells infected with Rauscher leukemia virus. *Virology* **67:** 544–552.

van Zaane, D., A.L.J. Gielkens, W.G. Hesselink, and H.P.J. Bloemers. 1977. Identification of Rauscher murine leukemia virus-specific mRNAs for the synthesis of *gag*- and *env*-gene products. *Proc. Natl. Acad. Sci.* **74:** 1855–1859.

Velicer, L.F. and D.C. Graves. 1974. Properties of feline leukemia virus. II. In vitro labeling of the polypeptides. *J. Virol.* **14:** 700–703.

Verma, I.M. 1975a. Studies on reverse transcriptase of RNA tumor viruses. I. Localization of thermolabile DNA polymerase and RNase H activities on one polypeptide. *J. Virol.* **15:** 121–126.

———. 1975b. Studies on reverse transcriptase of RNA tumor viruses. III. Properties of purified Moloney murine leukemia virus DNA polymerase and associated RNase H. *J. Virol.* **15:** 843–854.

———. 1977. The reverse transcriptase. *Biochim. Biophys. Acta* **473:** 1–38.

Verma, I.M., N.L. Meuth, H. Fan, and D. Baltimore. 1974. Hamster leukemia virus DNA polymerase: Unique structure and lack of demonstrable endogenous activity. *J. Virol.* **13:** 1075–1082.

Versteegen, R.J. and S. Oroszlan. 1980. Effect of chemical modification and fragmentation on antigenic determinants of internal protein p30 and surface glycoprotein gp70 of type C retroviruses. *J. Virol.* **33:** 983–992.

Verstraeten, A.A., R. van Nie, H.G. Kwa, and P.C. Hageman. 1975. Quantative estimation of mouse mammary tumor virus (MTV) antigens by radioimmunoassay. *Int. J. Cancer* **15:** 270–281.

Vogt, P.K. 1977. Genetics of RNA tumor viruses. In *Comprehensive virology* (ed. H. Fraenkel-Conrat and R. Wagner), vol. 9, pp.341–455. Plenum Press, New York.

Vogt, V.M. and R. Eisenman. 1973. Identification of a large polypeptide precursor of avian oncornavirus proteins. *Proc. Natl. Acad. Sci.* **70:** 1734–1738.

Vogt, V.M., R. Eisenman, and H. Diggelmann. 1975. Generation of avian myeloblastosis virus structural proteins by proteolytic cleavage of a precursor polypeptide. *J. Mol. Biol.* **96:** 471–493.

Vogt, V.M., W. Wight, and R. Eisenman. 1979. *In vitro* cleavage of avian retrovirus *gag* proteins by viral protease p15. *Virology* **98:** 154–167.

Von der Helm, K. 1977. Cleavage of Rous sarcoma viral polyprotein precursor into internal structural proteins *in vitro* involves viral protein p15. *Proc. Natl. Acad. Sci.* **74:** 911–915.

Von der Helm, K. and P.H. Duesberg. 1975. Translation of Rous sarcoma virus RNA in a cell-free system from ascites Krebs II cells. *Proc. Natl. Acad. Sci.* **72:** 614–618.

Waite, M.R.F. and P.T. Allen. 1975. RNA-directed DNA polymerase activity of reticuloendotheliosis virus: Characterization of the endogenous and exogenous reactions. *J. Virol.* **16:** 872–879.

Wang. L.-H. and P.H. Duesberg. 1973. DNA polymerase of murine sarcoma-leukemia virus: Lack of detectable RNase H and low activity with viral RNA and natural DNA templates. *J. Virol.* **12:** 1512–1521.

Weiss, M.J., E.P. Zeelon, R.W. Sweet, D.H. Harter, and S. Spiegelman. 1977. Immunological cross-reactions of the major internal protein component from "slow" viruses of sheep. *Virology* **76:** 851–854.

Weiss, R.A. 1969. Interference and neutralization studies with Bryan strain Rous sarcoma virus synthesized in the absence of helper virus. *J. Gen. Virol.* **5:** 529–539.

Weiss, S.R., H.E. Varmus, and J.M. Bishop. 1977. The size and genetic composition of virus-specific RNAs in the cytoplasm of cells producing avian sarcoma-leukemia viruses. *Cell* **12:** 983–992.

Weiss, S.R., P.B. Hackett, H. Oppermann, A. Ullrich, L. Levintow, and J.M. Bishop. 1978. Cell-free translation of avian sarcoma virus RNA: Suppression of the *gag* termination codon does not augment synthesis of the joint *gag/pol* product. *Cell* **15:** 607–614.

Wickner, W. 1979. The assembly of proteins into biological membranes: The membrane trigger hypothesis. *Annu. Rev. Biochem.* **48:** 23–45.

Wirth, D.F., F. Katz, B. Small, and H.F. Lodish. 1977. How a single Sinbis vius mRNA directs the synthesis of one soluble protein and two integral membrane proteins. *Cell* **10:** 253–263.

Witte, O.N. and D. Baltimore. 1978. Relationship of retrovirus polyprotein cleavages to virion maturation studied with temperature-sensitive murine leukemia virus mutants. *J. Virol.* **26:** 750–761.

Witte, O.N. and D.F. Wirth. 1979. Structure of the murine leukemia virus envelope glycoprotein precursor. *J. Virol.* **29:** 735–743.

Witte, O.N., A. Tsukamoto-Adey, and I.L. Weissman. 1977. Cellular maturation of oncornavirus glycoproteins: Topological arrangement of precursor and product forms in cellular membranes. *Virology* **76:** 539–553.

Witte, O.N., I.L. Weissman, and H.S. Kaplan. 1973. Structural characteristics of some murine RNA tumor viruses studied by lactoperoxidase iodination. *Proc. Natl. Acad. Sci.* **70:** 36–40.

Witter, R., H. Frank, V. Moennig, G. Hunsmann, J. Lange, and W. Schafer. 1973. Properties of mouse leukemia viruses. IV. Hemagglutination assay and characterization of hemagglutinating surface components. *Virology* **54:** 330–345.

Wolfe, L.G., F. Deinhardt, G.H. Theilen, H. Rabin, T. Kawakami, and L.K. Bustad. 1971. Induction of tumors in marmoset monkeys by simian sarcoma virus, type 1 (*Lagothrix*): A preliminary report. *J. Natl. Cancer Inst.* **47:** 1115–1120.

Wong, P.K.Y. and R. MacLeod. 1975. Studies on the budding process of a temperature-sensitive mutant of murine leukemia virus with a scanning electron microscope. *J. Virol.* **16:** 434–442.

Wong, P.K.H. and J.A. McCarter. 1974. Studies of two temperature-sensitive mutants of Moloney murine leukemia virus. *Virology* **58:** 396–408.

Wong, T.C., R.B. Lewis, H.R. Bose, Jr., and C.Y. Kang. 1980. Assembly of avian reticuloendotheliosis virus: Association of the core precursor polypeptide with the intracellular ribonucleoprotein complex. *J. Virol.* **34:** 484–489.

Yagi, M.J. and R.W. Compans. 1977. Structural components of mouse mammary tumor virus. I. Polypeptides of the virion. *Virology* **76:** 751–766.

Yagi, M.J., M. Tomana, R.E. Stutzman, B.H. Robertson, and R.W. Compans. 1978. Structural components of mouse mammary tumor virus. III. Composition and tryptic peptides of virion polypeptides. *Virology* **91:** 291–304.

Yakobson, E. and R.A. Weiss. 1981. Mutant retrovirus particles package vesicular stomatitis virus mRNA during mixed infection. *Virology* **108:** 183–187.

Yeger, H., V.I. Kalnins, and J.R. Stephenson. 1976. Electron microscopy of mammalian type-C RNA viruses: Use of conditional lethal mutants in studies of virion maturation and assembly. *Virology* **74:** 459–469.

Yeh, J., M. Ahmed, J. Lyles, D. Larson, and S.A. Mayyasi. 1975. Competition radioimmunoassay for Mason-Pfizer monkey virus: Comparison with recent isolates. *Int. J. Cancer* **15:** 632–639.

Yoshinaka, Y. and R.B. Luftig. 1977a. Murine leukemia virus morphogenesis: Cleavage of P70 *in vitro* can be accompanied by a shift from a concentrically coiled internal strand ("immature") to a collapsed ("mature") form of the virus core. *Proc. Natl. Acad. Sci.* **74:** 3446–3450.

———. 1977b. Properties of a P70 proteolytic factor of murine leukemia viruses. *Cell* **12:** 709–719.

———. 1977c. Characterization of Rauscher leukemia virus (RLV) P40-42, an intermediate cleavage product of the group specific antigen (*gag*) precursor polyprotein, P65-70. *Biochem. Biophys. Res. Commun.* **79:** 319–325.

———. 1980. Physiochemical characterization and specificity of the murine leukaemia virus $Pr65^{gag}$ proteolytic factor. *J. Gen. Virol.* **48:** 329–340.

7

Genetics of Retroviruses

I. INTRODUCTION

In the nine years since the first edition of this book (Tooze 1973), many advances have been made in our understanding of the structure and function of the genomes of the RNA tumor viruses. Much of the progress has been aided by the isolation and subsequent characterization of viral mutants, both conditional and nonconditional. When the earlier edition was written, attempts were being made to classify viral mutants into groups on the basis of their biological behavior in temperature-shift experiments as well as their effect on replication and/or transformation. The major gene products, which have been subsequently identified, mapped, and characterized, were unknown. And yet many of the mutants isolated prior to 1973 are still being used to obtain a more detailed understanding of the viral genome.

This chapter includes descriptions of the early results with mutants (mainly of avian Rous sarcoma virus [RSV]) in light of what is currently known. The characteristics of spontaneous and induced mutants and variants of nondefective (*nd*) and defective RNA tumor viruses are presented, as well as the usefulness of such mutants in the elucidation of our current understanding of the viral genome and its functions. Finally, viral phenotypic and genotypic interactions are described, including the high-frequency recombination unique to the retroviruses.

Most of the information on the coding capacity of the genomes of RNA tumor viruses, as well as detailed analysis of the various gene products, has come from the study of the nondefective transforming avian sarcoma virus, RSV. RSV has been most useful because it is competent for both virus replication and transformation of fibroblasts in culture, leading to a simple in vitro assay with single-hit kinetics. Much of the discussion in this chapter centers around RSV, although isolation and characterization of mutants of nondefective murine leukemia viruses (MLV) is well under way. Work is just beginning on the genetics of the defective murine sarcoma viruses (MSV) and the acute leukemia viruses, such as Abelson murine leukemia virus (Ab-MLV), avian myelocytomatosis (MC29) virus, and avian erythroblastosis virus (AEV). Excellent review articles giving many details of viral mutants and genetics are available (Vogt 1977; Friis 1978; Wang 1978; Hunter 1980).

II. STRUCTURE AND FUNCTION OF THE VIRAL GENOME

A. Definition of the Genome and the Genetic Maps

A detailed discussion of the retroviral genome is found in Chapter 4; however, it is worth recapitulating the salient features before we consider the results of genetic analysis in the remainder of this chapter.

The genomes of the RNA tumor viruses are diploid. In the case of prototype RSV, the genome is a 70S RNA molecule that dissociates upon heating to yield two identical 35S–39S single-stranded RNAs with a molecular size of about 9–10 kb. The viral subunits are not permuted; thus, the same fixed gene order is found on each subunit (Wang and Duesberg 1974; Coffin and Billeter 1976; Wang et al. 1976c). A genome of this size could code for about 3.3×10^5 daltons of protein in a single reading frame. Protein products of four coding domains of RSV (Fig. 7.1) have been identified; the genes coding for these were termed *gag, pol, env,* and *onc* by Baltimore (1975). Since that time, *onc* has been replaced by *src* for the RSV transforming gene (Wang et al. 1976a), and *onc* has been used as a more general term for viral genes that may be responsible for the induction of neoplastic disease and for cell transformation in culture but might or might not be related to the *src* gene of RSV. It should be pointed out that the genes of retroviruses are unusual in many respects. For instance, the primary translation product of *pol* may be a polyprotein containing *gag* sequences as well. These features are discussed in detail in Chapters 4 and 6. The known molecular weights of these four gene products total about 2.9×10^5, making it unlikely that other gene products will be found, although one or two small proteins synthesized in the same reading frame, or proteins synthesized in other reading frames, cannot yet be excluded. The *gag* gene is known to encode the internal structural proteins of the virus (in the case of RSV, p27, p19, p15, p10, and p12); *pol,* the reverse transcriptase; *env,* the viral glycoproteins; and *src,* the transforming protein. Evidence for the virus-coded specificity of at least three of the gene products has been provided by mutants (see Sections V.A.1 and V.B and Chapter 6). In addition to the four regions encoding viral products, two other regions of the RSV genome have been described: (1) a stretch of 370 bases near the 5′ end, which is not known to encode any protein and has been termed the leader sequence, as this

Rous Sarcoma Virus

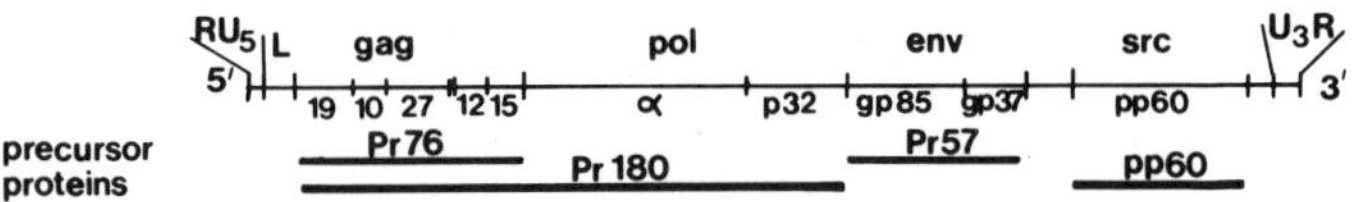

Avian Leukosis Virus

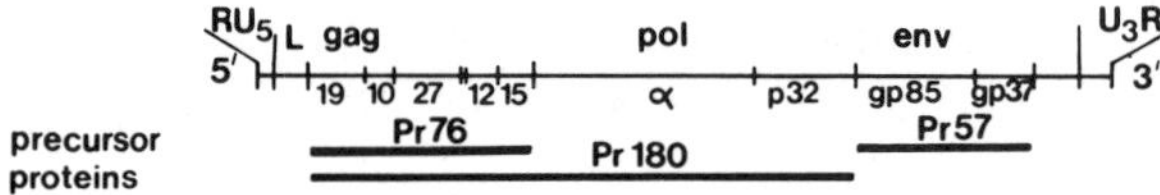

Murine Leukemia Virus

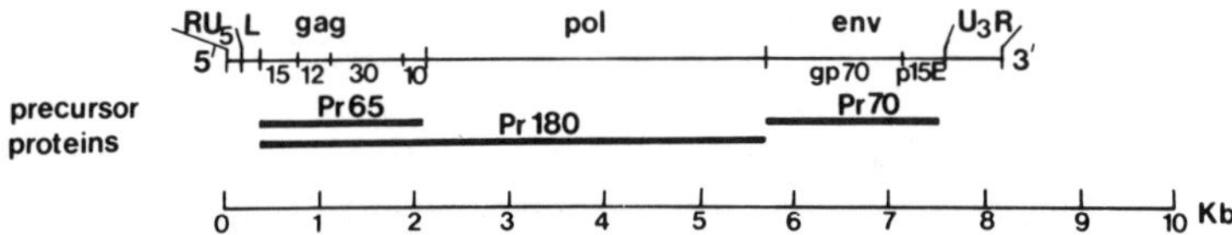

Figure 7.1 Genomic coding regions and gene products. The genomic structures of the following replication-competent viruses are depicted: Rous sarcoma virus (RSV), avian leukosis virus (ALV), and murine leukemia virus (MLV). The three structural genes for each (*gag, pol,* and *env*) and the *src* gene of RSV are shown, subdivided according to the known gene products. Also noted are the polyprotein precursors for each gene. The terminal regions (U_3, R, U_5, and L) are discussed in detail in Chapter 4. Genomic structures for the replication-defective viruses are also presented in Chapter 4.

information appears on both genomic and subgenomic mRNAs; and (2) a region of about 500 bases near the 3′ end of the genome. This last region is not known to encode any protein, although there is much speculation that at least some part of it might be involved in regulation of virus replication and/or leukemogenesis (see Section V.C.2 and Chapter 4).

Early attempts to order the viral genes were genetic (Mason et al. 1974; Friis et al. 1975; Hunter and Vogt 1976), and some evidence for gene linkage was obtained. Current consideration of the properties of recombination (see Section VI.B) in the avian RNA tumor viruses makes it difficult to understand how linkage patterns were obtained, or how these studies yielded what proved to be the correct gene order. The earliest studies utilized the presence of the *src* gene in RSV, and its absence in avian leukosis virus (ALV), and the subgroup variations in the *env* gene (see Chapter 3) as selected markers. Temperature-sensitive (*ts*) mutants in other genes, such as *gag* and *pol*, were then mapped by their recombination frequencies relative to *env* and *src*. As discussed in detail in Chapter 4, biochemical and physical analyses of mutants and recombinants have been much more fruitful for mapping the genome. The sum of a myriad of experiments has yielded the gene order depicted in Figure 7.1. The four known genes are ordered 5′-*gag-pol-env-src*-3′ on both the genomic RNA and integrated proviral DNA. Three of the genes, *gag, pol,* and *env,* encode precursors and polyproteins that are processed; the current order of the proteins is listed under each gene from the amino terminus to the carboxyl terminus (see also Chapters 4 and 6). There has been some uncertainty in the order of the *gag* proteins with regard to the positions of p12 and p27. Several groups ordered them NH_2-p12-p27-COOH using peptide analysis of partial cleavage products (Reynolds et al. 1977; Rettenmier et al. 1979b; V. Vogt et al. 1979), but the correct order from sequencing data is NH_2-p27-p12-COOH (D. Schwartz and W. Gilbert, pers. comm.; see also Chapter 6 and Appendix E). The order of polymerase subunits has been obtained by using deletion mutants in the *pol* gene (see Section V.B.2.a) (Eisenman et al. 1980c). The envelope-gene glycoproteins have been ordered by tryptic peptide mapping (Klemenz and Diggelmann 1978; Shealy and Rueckert 1978).

B. Analysis of Viral Mutants—An Historical Perspective

The classical approach to the genetic analysis of viruses is to isolate mutants that can be characterized both physiologically and genetically. Such mutants fall into two classes: (1) conditional mutants, in which the gene containing the mutation continues to function under permissive conditions but fails to function under nonpermissive situations, and (2) nonconditional mutants, which are altered or inactive under all conditions. Mutated avian and murine RNA tumor viruses of both classes have been identified, and a systematic nomenclature (used in this chapter) of the mutant avian viruses has been proposed (Vogt et al. 1974). In the case of mammalian viruses, no standard nomenclature has yet been adopted. Some of the abbreviations used most frequently in this chapter are listed in Table 7.1.

The conditional mutants of RNA tumor viruses isolated to date

Table 7.1. Commonly used abbreviations for different virus strains and variants

Abbreviation	Strain/variant
AcLV	acute defective leukemia virus
AEV	avian erythroblastosis virus
MC29	avian myelocytomatosis virus
AMV	avian myeloblastosis virus
ALV	avian leukemia virus
ASV	avian sarcoma virus
rASV	recovered avian sarcoma virus
FeSV	feline sarcoma virus
LLV	lymphoid leukemia virus
MLV	murine leukemia virus
Ra-MLV	Rauscher strain of MLV
Mo-MLV	Moloney strain of MLV
Ab-MLV	Abelson strain of MLV
MSV	murine sarcoma virus
Ha-MSV	Harvey strain of MSV
Ki-MSV	Kirsten strain of MSV
Mo-MSV	Moloney strain of MSV
RAV	Rous-associated virus
RSV	Rous sarcoma virus
BH-RSV(−), RSV(−)	Bryan high-titer strain of RSV
B77-RSV	Bratislava strain of RSV
PR-RSV	Prague strain of RSV
SR-RSV	Schmidt-Ruppin strain of RSV
nd (*wt*)	nondefective (wild type)
rd	replication defective
td	transformation defective
ts	temperature sensitive

In the text, *ts* is used as an adjective or as a superscript to designate a conditional mutant (e.g., *ts src* or src^{ts}). Similarly, nonconditional mutants are designated by the adjective *td* or by the superscript minus sign (e.g., *td src* or src^{-}). The wild-type gene is designated either by a plus sign or by the superscript *wt* (e.g., src^{wt} or src^{+}).

are all temperature-sensitive. The functions of genes carrying *ts* mutations may be identified by complementation tests, and their mode of action can be determined by studying the physiological consequences of shifts between permissive and nonpermissive temperatures. On the other hand, nonconditional mutants, which carry defects in essential genes, can only be propagated by coinfection with helper viruses or by multiplication of cells containing the mutant provirus. As temperature-shift experiments are inapplicable, their use in studying virus physiology is restricted. However, nonconditional mutants, particularly those which involve deletions or major alterations of genetic information, are far more stable than *ts* mutants, and this is an advantage in fine genetic analysis. They have proved very useful in mapping the genome by physical methods (see Chapter 4). Such mutants are also invaluable in identifying the biochemical function of a gene, since there is no background due to leakiness as in the case of *ts* mutants. Nonconditional mutants of transforming viruses can easily be maintained as proviruses in transformed cell lines. In addition, MLV mutants can be maintained as infected cell lines.

The first RNA tumor virus *ts* mutants were isolated by Toyoshima and Vogt (1969) and by Martin (1970); both groups used *nd* RSV as the parental virus. Subsequently, many laboratories have isolated *ts* mutants of RSV. In the early 1970s, *ts* mutants were also isolated from MLV (Stephenson et al. 1972; Wong et al. 1973) and MSV (Scolnick et al. 1972), viruses for which convenient in vitro biological assays are available. This section is limited to the early work done to classify the *ts* mutants of *nd* RSV; other mutants will be discussed in later sections of this chapter.

In general, *ts* mutants of RNA tumor viruses have permissive temperatures of 31–32° C (mammalian viruses) and 35–37° C (avian viruses) and nonpermissive temperatures of 37–40° C and 40–42° C, respectively. RSV *ts* mutants were originally characterized by studying the temperature sensitivity of two simple parameters in tissue culture: fibroblast transformation and production of infectious virus. These tests defined three physiological classes of mutants: fibroblast transformation-defective (*td;* class T), replication-defective (*rd;* class R), and those with a coordinate defect in both transformation and virus production (class C). Screening for *ts* mutants is still based on the ability either to transform or to replicate at one temperature, but not at the other. For instance, T-or C-class mutants are able to induce transformation as measured by focus formation at permissive temperatures, but not at nonpermissive temperatures. R-class mutants, on the other hand, induce foci at both temperatures, but particles produced under nonpermissive conditions are not competent to transform or replicate at the permissive temperature in the next round of infection (see Table 7.3).

These three classes were further subdivided by studying the effect of shifting infected cultures from permissive to nonpermissive temperature, and vice versa, at various times after infection (Friis et al. 1971; Wyke and Linial 1973). Such temperature-shift experiments showed that some functions ("early" functions) were absolutely necessary only during the first 24 hours or so of infection if subsequent replication and/or transformation were to occur. In contrast, other functions ("late" functions) played no role in the initiation of infection, but their activity was continuously required thereafter for virus replication or cell transformation to be maintained.

Wyke and Linial (1973) described six classes of T and C *ts* mutants on the basis of temperature-shift studies. This classification into T1, T2, and C1–C4 is no longer considered very useful, as several categories consisted of mutants now known to contain multiple mutations in several genes (for review, see Wyke 1974). No R-class mutants were studied in this work. For the purpose of this discussion, we confine our classification of *ts* mutants to T and R classes. Certain mutants of the polymerase gene, encoding a temperature-sensitive enzyme (Linial and Mason 1973), are unable either to transform or to replicate and are truly coordinate (C) mutants; however, the failure to transform is not a consequence of a dysfunctional *src* gene but an effect of the inability to synthesize viral DNA. Therefore, such mutants will be considered as replicative mutants. The term coordinate mutant served a function historically, but, since all the coordinate mutations either are in *pol* or have been shown to be multiple mutations, the term will not be used here. It should be noted that the classification of mutants into T, R, and C groups by the simple criteria outlined here is not very useful when applied to mutants of any other retrovirus. For example, MLV does not possess any gene for fibroblast transformation, and therefore, by definition, all mutants must belong to class R. Conversely, MSV is not competent for replication, and therefore one could not readily detect defects in any replicative functions the virus might possess.

Although the physiological approach taken by Martin (1970), Friis et al. (1971), and Wyke and Linial (1973) was useful in the initial characterization of mutants, subsequent virus isolation and identification has focused on correlation of biochemical properties with biological parameters. Temperature-shift experiments for focus formation or agar colony formation will continue to be useful in initially defining whether a *ts* mutation is required for initation only, for maintenance of the transformed phenotype, or for virus replication. However, the current emphasis is on isolation of nonconditional mutants, which are much easier to map biochemically, although they are, of course, not amenable to physiological manipulations.

III. SPONTANEOUS MUTANTS AND VARIANTS OF RNA TUMOR VIRUSES

A. Naturally Occurring Viruses

As mentioned previously, most laboratory strains of RSV are nondefective and can replicate in and transform fibroblasts in tissue culture after solitary infection. Commonly used strains of *nd* RSV are Prague (PR), Schmidt-Ruppin (SR), and Bratislava (B77). These viruses are unique, since no other species have yielded retroviruses competent for both replication and in vitro cell transformation. Furthermore, no strains of *nd* avian sarcoma virus (ASV) have been isolated recently, and it is unclear whether the three aforementioned *nd* strains all arose from the original Rous tumor isolate (Rous 1911) after passage or as independent isolates in different laboratories (see Chapter 8). The *nd* RSVs may represent an unwitting laboratory selection. In any event, *nd* RSV has been an extremely popular and useful laboratory tool, despite the fact that its importance as a cause of disease in the field is rather limited. A fourth strain of RSV, the Bryan high-titer strain (BH), is known to be replication-defective, containing a large deletion in the *env* gene. This virus and other defective transforming viruses are discussed below.

The most commonly occurring avian oncoviruses are ALVs, also called lymphoid leukosis viruses (LLV) or Rous-associated viruses (RAV). These viruses are not defective for replication but lack all or part of the *src* gene and do not transform fibroblasts in culture. They may, however, cause neoplasms in birds (see Chapter 8). In the laboratory, transformation-defective variants of RSV can be isolated from virus stocks, either spontaneously or after mutagenesis, and these closely resemble field isolates of ALV. All these viruses can function as helper viruses for replication-defective viruses by supplying *gag, pol,* and *env* functions. In addition, many independent isolates of acute defective leukemia viruses have been obtained (see Chapters 2, 4, and 8). These viruses generally have the property of transforming fibroblasts as well as specific hematopoietic target cells in vitro. They are all defective for replication and lack all or part of the *gag, pol,* and *env* genes. Examples are MC29, Mill Hill virus (MH2), and AEV. Other naturally defective viruses have been described that are defective both for replication in and for transformation of fibroblasts in vitro, although they do transform other target tissues; an example is avian myeloblastosis virus (AMV). All the naturally occurring defective avian viruses appear to contain deletions in their genomes when compared with *nd* RSV. It appears that a portion of the viral genome has been replaced by cellular genetic material, some or all of which may represent *onc* sequences.

Among the mammalian RNA tumor viruses, there are no examples of a single retrovirus that is competent for both replication and transformation. The MLVs, like the ALVs, are replication-competent but do not transform fibroblasts. Mutants in the MLV replicative genes have been isolated and characterized (Section V.B); they are easier to obtain than ALV mutants because there is a convenient in vitro plaque assay for some MLV strains (Rowe et al. 1970), as well as focus assays based on the ability of MLV to induce transformed foci on certain morphologically flat cells (Hackett and Sylvester 1972) or on flat clones of MSV-transformed cells (S^+L^-, Bassin et al. 1970, 1971b; 15F, McCarter 1977). MSVs are all defective for replication but competent for fibroblast transformation. The most commonly studied MSV strains are Moloney (Mo-MSV), Harvey (Ha-MSV) and Kirsten (Ki-MSV). Coinfection with a competent MLV (or other compatible retrovirus helper) is required for MSV to replicate and spread by reinfection; but, at high virus dilution, a single MSV pseudotype particle can infect and transform a cell, and cell clones produced in this way are free of helper virus. By analyzing both the expression of viral genes in such cells and the genetic constitution of virus rescued by superinfection with helper, the replicative defects of MSV have now been characterized. The genomes of these viruses are discussed in some detail in Chapter 4. In summary, the Ha-MSV, Ki-MSV, and Mo-MSV strains are viruses that transform cells but lack *gag, env,* and *pol* functions because of genomic deletions. Therefore, these viruses are more defective than the prototype defective BH-RSV(−), which lacks only the *env* gene. Some MSV strains are less defective; certain Mo-MSV strains seem to possess the entire *gag* gene (Aaronson et al. 1972; Fischinger et al. 1972a), and some Ki-MSV strains encode the *env*-gene product (Bilello et al. 1974).

B. Replication-defective RSV

Two types of viruses with deleted genomes have been isolated from stocks of RSV. These were the first well-characterized RSV variants, and analysis of their genomes led to the first glimmer of understanding of the organization of the *nd* RSV genome. These two variants are the *rd* BH-RSV, also referred to as BH-RSV(−) or RSV(−), and a whole series of *td* mutants of RSV, which have been isolated in many laboratories and are found normally in stocks of all strains of RSV. The use of these mutants in mapping viral genes is discussed in Chapter 4; what follows here is a brief description of the isolation and biological characterization of these viruses.

The existence of the envelope-defective BH-RSV(−) strain has been known for two decades (Hanafusa et al. 1963,1964 Temin 1963). Stocks of BH-RSV(−) and helper virus can infect cells, but, at high virus dilution, individual clones of transformed cells do not produce infectious virus. Subsequent work has shown that the BH-RSV(−) particles lack the two major virion glycoproteins, gp85 and gp37 (Scheele and Hanafusa 1971). These particles therefore have no subgroup specificity. The BH-RSV(−) defect can be compensated by phenotypic mixing with the envelope glycoproteins of other viruses, both retroviruses and other animal viruses, a phenomenon described in Section VI.A. BH-RSV(−) can also be introduced into cells by fusion, using inactivated Sendai virus or polyethylene glycol (Weiss 1969; T. Hanafusa et al. 1970b; Rohde et al. 1978). The transformed cultures again produce noninfectious particles. This result illustrates that the envelope glycoproteins are necessary only for early stages of infection (absorption and/or penetration) and not for subsequent replication or virion assembly. BH-RSV(−) was used to show that certain chicken cells were producing endogenous viral glycoprotein and the cells were termed chick helper factor positive or chf$^+$ (Weiss 1969; H. Hanafusa et al. 1970) (see Chapter 3).

One problem in using BH-RSV(−) in mapping experiments is that the origin of this variant is unknown and therefore the parental virus is unavailable for comparison. This problem was circumvented by the use of an *rd* mutant isolated from SR-RSV-A (Kawai and Hanafusa 1973) called *rd* NY8 SR-RSV or, more simply, NY8. NY8 has the same biological properties as BH-RSV(−); neither reverts to *nd* virus and both contain large deletions in the RNA genome (Duesberg et al. 1975). NY8 has been used to map the location of the *env* gene, using a variety of physical and biochemical methods, discussed in detail in Chapter 4.

C. Transformation-defective RSV

The second type of spontaneously occurring variants of RSV is the *td* virus. These viruses are fully competent for replication in tissue culture and in birds. Variants of this type were originally called RAV (Rubin and Vogt 1962) and arise spontaneously in stocks of *nd* RSV (Dougherty and Rasmussen 1964; Hanafusa and Hanafusa 1966; Duff and Vogt 1969; Vogt 1971a; Martin and Duesberg 1972). The frequency of *td* viruses, even in cloned sarcoma virus stocks, is high, varying from 4% to 17% in different RSV strains (Vogt 1971a). The *td* viruses possess the same envelope properties as the sarcoma virus stocks from which they arise, and their incidence is the same in stocks of sarcoma virus grown in cells expressing endogenous virus functions as it is in stocks propagated in cells in which endogenous virus is not expressed (Vogt 1971a). Their origin, therefore, probably does not normally involve recombination between the genomes of sarcoma viruses and those of endogenous viruses. The majority of *td* viruses have genomic deletions. Originally, *td* viruses appeared to have rather uniformly sized deletions in their genomes, measuring about 10–15% of the RSV genome (Duesberg and Vogt 1973; Neiman et al. 1974; Bernstein et al. 1976). More recently, a variety of *td* mutants have been obtained that contain only partial deletions in *src;* these are discussed in Section V.A.1. Just as NY8 was invaluable in localizing the *env* gene and defining the *env*-gene product, *td* mutants have helped to locate the *src* gene and to identify the transforming protein it encodes, $pp60^{src}$ (Brugge and Erikson 1977; Purchio et al. 1978) (see Chapters 4 and 9).

td mutants derived in tissue culture are indistinguishable biologically from field isolates of avian LLV. Unlike RSV, they fail to induce sarcomas in birds, but they do induce bursal lymphomas after long latent periods (Biggs et al. 1973; Purchase et al. 1977). Again, as in the case of NY8, the advantage of using *td* derivatives of cloned *nd* RSV, rather than the field-isolated LLVs or the RAVs (which were isolated from mixed stocks of RSV), is that the parental virus is available for comparison.

IV. MUTAGENESIS AND SELECTION OF MUTANTS

A variety of physical and chemical agents have been utilized to obtain types of mutants that were not found to arise spontaneously from stocks of *nd* viruses. Both nonconditional mutants and mutants sensitive to elevated temperature (*ts* mutants) have been obtained, and it might be possible to isolate other types of conditional mutants, such as pH-sensitive viruses. However, with two exceptions, a spontaneous cold-sensitive mutant of Mo-MSV (Somers and Kit 1973) and a mutant of RSV cold-sensitive for some *src* properties and heat-sensitive for others (Weber and Friis 1979), none have been described. Almost all of the *ts* mutants have been isolated after mutagenesis, and many of the nonconditional mutants have arisen spontaneously in virus stocks and have been identified by random picking of clones. A concise discussion of mutagenesis and selection of RSV mutants is available (Wyke 1976).

Both nonconditional and *ts* mutants proved very useful in delineating gene functions. The *ts* mutants are often reversible, and the mode of action of the mutated gene product can be determined by studying the physiological and/or biochemical consequences of shifts between permissive and nonpermissive temperatures. It is easy to propagate *ts* mutants (although frequent recloning is necessary to maintain good stocks with tight temperature restrictions), and they can be used in complementation and recombination tests for genetic analysis. The major disadvantage of *ts* mutants is their leakiness, which often makes genetic and/or biochemical analysis difficult. This is especially true for mutants in RSV replicative functions. In addition, since probably only single-base changes are responsible for the mutation, they are not useful for mapping studies by heteroduplex or oligonucleotide-mapping analysis (see Chapter 4).

Nonconditional mutants generally contain deletions, insertions, or substitutions in their genomes and are therefore very stable. However, in the case of replicative mutants, if one desires to move the mutant genome into another cell type, it must first be rescued with a replication-competent virus, and the subsequent steps of end point dilution to remove the helper, cloning of infected cells, and retesting for the mutant phenotype can be laborious. Nonconditional mutants are nevertheless extremely useful for mapping studies (see Chapter 4) (Wang 1978) and in complementation tests with different nonconditional mutants or with *ts* mutants. Finally, a great advantage of nonconditional mutants is that they can be isolated with mutations in noncoding regions of the genome, whereas *ts* mutants would only be evident in regions coding for viral protein. To date, only one RSV mutant containing a deletion in a region of the genome outside of the four viral genes has been isolated and characterized (Linial et al. 1978a; Shank and Linial 1980) (see Section V.C.1). Current techniques of restriction mapping allow detailed analysis of the provirus of nonconditional mutants, even if they are so defective that no genomic RNA and/or viral particles are produced.

The most commonly used mutagens are listed in Table 7.2. A more detailed summary may be found in the review by Friis (1978). Mutagens such as 5-azacytidine, which is incorporated into virion RNA, and those such as 5-bromodeoxyuridine (BrdU), which interact with proviral DNA, have been used very effectively. In most cases, mutant isolation is accomplished after mutagenesis by screening large numbers of clones. Several "selective" procedures have been developed. For instance, Wyke (1973a) described a negative-selection technique for obtaining *ts* transformation mutants with the lesion in maintenance of transformation. Transformed and normal cells are put into methylcellulose under conditions in which only transformed cells can divide. The cultures are then treated with BrdU and blue light to kill only those cells that are dividing. In reconstruction experiments, this enriched the survival of normal cells 20-fold over transformed cells. When this technique was used at the nonpermissive temperature to enrich for *ts* mutants of RSV, it resulted in only a 2.5-fold enrichment for *ts* mutants over random picking. Wyke (1973a) also described a second procedure to enrich for early mutants that might be mutated in a function required for the establishment, but not maintenance, of transformation. Cells are infected with virus at the permissive temperature and shifted to the nonpermissive temperature after 1 day. Later, small foci are picked, with the idea that they had resulted from cell proliferation rather than virus replication, and spread. A classic *ts* polymerase mutant, LA335, was isolated in this way. Using MLV, Wong et al. (1973) devised a selective procedure to isolate spontaneous *ts* mutants, based on the observation that certain MSV nonproducer clones (S^+L^-) round up and become less adherent after infection with MLV (Bassin et al. 1971a). A selective procedure similar to that described

Table 7.2 Some mutagens used for isolation of temperature-sensitive mutants

Mutagen	Virus	Initial isolation
5-Azacytidine	B77-RSV	Toyoshima and Vogt (1969)
	Ki-MSV	Scolnick et al. (1972)
	Pr-RSV-A,C	Wyke (1973a)
	PR-RSV-C	Linial and Mason (1973)
	PR-RSV-A	Friis and Hunter (1973)
	PR-RSV-D	Calothy and Pessac (1976)
	PR-RSV-C	Mason and Yeater (1977)
	AEV	Graf et al. (1978)
	PR-RSV-A,C	Mason et al. (1979a)
5-Bromodeoxyuridine	BH-RSV(−)	Bader and Brown (1971)
	Ki-MSV	Scolnick et al. (1972)
	Ki-MLV	Stephenson et al. (1972)
	Ra-MLV	Stephenson and Aaronson (1973)
	BH-RSV(−)	Balduzzi (1976)
	PR-RSV-A	Becker et al. (1977)
	PR-RSV-C	Alevy and Vogt (1978)
5-Fluorouracil	SR-RSV-B	Kawai and Hanafusa (1971)
	SR-RSV-D	Biquard and Vigier (1972)
	PR-RSV-C	Alevy and Vogt (1978)
Nitrosoguanidine	SR-RSV-A	Martin (1970)
	SR-RSV-A	Kawai et al. (1972)
	Ki-MLV	Stephenson et al. (1972)
	Ra-MLV	Stephenson and Aaronson (1973)
Ultraviolet light	PR-RSV-C	Wyke and Linial (1973)
None (selected)	Mo-MLV	Wong et al. (1973)

by Wyke (1973a) has also been used to select nonconditional mutants of Ki-MSV and Mo-MSV as nontransformed cell revertants, using cytosine arabinoside to kill selectively the transformed cells in the population (Greenberger and Aaronson 1974; Blair et al. 1979).

RSV *ts* mutants have been isolated in all the replicative functions, as well as in the transforming gene. Different screening procedures have been used depending on whether the goal was a replicative mutant or a maintenance-of-transformation mutant. For the latter, mutagenized virus is screened for focus formation (most commonly) or agar colony formation at permissive and nonpermissive temperatures. This simple procedure also works for early mutants in which the mutant function is required for initiation of focus formation or replication, such as *ts* polymerase mutants. However, for late-replication mutants, in which the defect may be in the synthesis, but not in the functioning, of the mutant protein at 41°C, another approach is taken. Clones are screened at both temperatures by picking foci and testing the progeny virus for the ability to initiate new transforming events at both temperatures. A simplified scheme for the type of screening necessary for the identification of three distinct *ts* mutant types is presented in Table 7.3. Temperature-shift experiments for focus formation are also quite revealing. For instance, *ts* transformation mutants show complete reversibility of transformation no matter when the temperature is shifted up or down, but pol^{ts} (initiation of infection) mutants are fixed early after infection so that a shift-up at late times does not prevent focus formation and a shift-down does not initiate it (Friis et al. 1971; Linial and Mason 1973; Wyke and Linial 1973; for review, see Wyke 1975).

One point that must be emphasized is that many of the *ts* mutants isolated by mutagenesis and described as having complex biological phenotypes have turned out to contain multiple mutations. Using the nomenclature of Vogt et al. (1974), these have been designated with a number followed by the letter m. For instance, LA334m and LA338m (Toyoshima and Vogt 1969; Wyke and Linial 1973) were found to contain two and three mutations, respectively. Using selective recombination with wild-type viruses, Owada and Toyoshima (1973) and Hunter and Vogt (1976) were able to obtain *ts* virus clones containing only one of the mutations. Mutants containing both conditional and nonconditional defects can also be obtained. Transformation-defective derivatives of *ts* RSV have been isolated, such as *td ts* LA337, which retains the *ts* polymerase mutation of the parental *ts* LA337 (Mason et al. 1979a).

Whereas most *ts* mutants have generally been isolated after mutagenesis, most of the nonconditional avian RNA tumor virus mutants have arisen spontaneously in cloned stocks. However, γ-irradiation or UV-irradiation have been used to produce *rd* and *td* variants (Golde 1970; Kawai and Yamamoto 1970), although neither procedure resulted in the establishment of long-term mutant cultures. UV-irradiation was used by Martin et al. (1979) to obtain noncondi-

Table 7.3 Screening for three types of *ts* RSV mutants

Mutant phenotype	Mutant example	Lesion	Foci produced at		Viral particles produced at		Ability of particles produced at 41° C to transform at 35° C
			35° C	41° C	35° C	41° C	
Maintenance of transformation	LA24 (Wyke 1973a)	*src*	+	–	+	+	+
Iniation of replication and transformation	LA337 (Linial and Mason 1973)	*pol*	+	–	+	–	n.a.
Late replication	LA672 (Friis and Hunter 1973)	*pol*	+	+	+	+	–

n.a. indicates not applicable.

tional *rd* PR-RSV clones and by Yoshida and colleagues (Yoshida and Ikawa 1977; Yoshida et al. 1979) to obtain *td* deletion mutants that retain part of the *src* gene. However, it is unclear whether these mutants preexisted in the stocks or were induced by the UV treatment.

Since *td* mutants can replicate normally, there is no problem in maintaining cultures of these variants as virus stocks. However, the nonconditional *rd* RSV mutants are most conveniently maintained as proviruses in transformed cell clones. As transformed chicken cells cannot be cultured indefinitely, the nonconditional mutants have been maintained as transformed turkey cells (Murphy 1977), rat cells (Quade 1979; Steimer and Boettiger 1979), or, most commonly, quail cells (Friis et al. 1975; Murphy 1977; Linial et al. 1978a,b, 1980; Martin et al. 1979; Mason et al. 1979b). MLV *rd* mutants present no problem for propagation as the uninfected mouse or rat cells used to propagate the viruses, such as NIH-3T3 or NRK, are established cell lines (Shields et al. 1978). Since nontransformed avian cells cannot be maintained indefinitely (a few long-term cultures such as the pheasant cells described by Linial [1976] become resistant to infection at high passage) and no selection exists for ALV-infected cells, no conditional *rd* mutants of ALV have been described, although it might be possible to isolate ALV *ts* mutants using the plaque assay described by Graf (1972).

There is another category of virus variants that, although not mutants per se, will be discussed in this chapter (see Sections V.B, V.C, and VI.B) and in more detail in Chapters 4 and 10. These are the viral recombinants between parental viruses with different biological or biochemical properties that can be detected or selected in the progeny. In the case of avian viruses, these include recombinants between endogenous and exogenous viruses (Weiss et al. 1973; Hayward and Hanafusa 1975; Linial and Neiman 1976; Shaikh et al. 1978, 1979; Robinson et al. 1979; Tsichlis and Coffin 1980) or recombinants between two viruses with different biological properties in vivo (E. Schmidt et al., pers. comm.). Another type of virus variant exhibits variation in host range; such variants may represent recombinants with endogenous cellular information within the *env* gene or spontaneous mutants in *env* (Shoyab et al. 1975; Zarling et al. 1977; Tsichlis et al. 1980). Recombinants between MLVs are numerous, as are host-range variants; these are discussed in Chapters 4, 8 and 10.

V. USE OF MUTANTS IN DELINEATING VIRAL GENE FUNCTION

In the last 10 years, many avian retrovirus mutants have been isolated and characterized, as well as a smaller number of murine virus mutants. Initially, a large effort was directed toward a physiological description of the mutants. As our knowledge of the molecular biology of RNA tumor virus infection progressed, the mutants became more and more useful as tools to determine whether proteins were virus-coded, as well as to demonstrate the biological consequence of biochemical changes. Thus, mutants in the transforming (*src*) gene of RSV were used to identify the elusive transforming protein (see Chapter 9). Details of the replicative cycle have been provided by mutant analysis as well. In this section, we provide a review of the use of mutants in developing our understanding of virus transformation and replication. The mutants will be considered in three main groups: (1) those in regions affecting transforming functions (both *src* and other *onc* genes), (2) those in the replicative genes, and (3) those in regions not as yet known to code for any viral proteins. (Tables 7.4a–l, 7.5a,b, and 7.6a,b, which can be found as an appendix to this chapter, list all the retroviral mutants [avian, murine, and mammalian, respectively] that have been isolated and at least partially characterized as of January 1981.)

A. Transforming Genes

Chapter 9 includes a discussion of the biochemistry of *onc*-gene products, such as $pp60^{src}$ (the product of the *src* gene of RSV), as well as facts and speculation about the origin of viral transforming genes. The purpose of this section is to present information on the wide variety of *ts* mutants and nonconditional *td* mutants, in particular those derived from *nd* RSV and from MSV. Prototype mutants of this sort, isolated from RSV, were used to show that a transforming protein was encoded by the RSV genome and was required for virus-induced transformation of fibroblasts in vitro, as well as for sarcoma formation in birds. A large number of morphological and biochemical cellular changes have been associated with the *src* gene (see Chapters 3 and 9). Now that the *src*-gene product has been identified, interest has shifted to partial *td* mutants that retain part of the *src*-gene function. These mutants are of use in determining which of the measurable changes in transformation can be related to the primary action of pp60^{src} and in dissecting the pleiotropic effects of this protein. Mutants in transforming genes of other viruses are also beginning to have a similar input and are described below.

Although the RSV *src* gene is by far the best characterized of the transforming genes, other avian RNA tumor viruses have sequences unrelated to *src* that are presumably responsible for transforming fibroblasts and other target cells in vivo and in vitro (Sheiness et al. 1978; Stehelin and Graf 1978; Roussel et al. 1979). In addition, there are mammalian transforming viruses that have no sequence homology to the transforming gene of MSV but can transform fibroblasts and other cell types. These viruses have been called acute leukemia viruses (AcLV), defective leukemia viruses (DLV), or defective transforming viruses (DTV). The biology and biochemistry of these viruses are discussed in Chapters 4, 8, and 9. All of these viruses have genomes that contain 5′ and 3′ ends in common with nondefective viruses and a large insert thought to contain the transforming gene(s) (*onc*). A set of specific names for the various sequences has been proposed (see Appendix A and Chapters 4 and 9). Most of the AcLVs encode polyproteins containing some viral *gag* peptides linked to nonviral peptides, thereby permitting precipitation by antiserum to the viral structural proteins. The polyproteins vary in size, depending on the particular virus, and contain varying amounts of *gag* peptides as well as non-*gag* peptides.

1. src

The first *ts src* mutants were isolated by Martin (1970). These mutants, and all the *ts src* mutants that have been subsequently isolated, replicate normally at both restrictive and permissive temperatures (unless they contain multiple mutations) but do not transform infected cells at the nonpermissive temperature. Generally, the criterion of transformation used for isolation is the ability to induce foci of transformed cells under a hard agar overlay. The temperature sensitivity is completely reversible; shortly after cells are shifted from 41°C to 35°C, transformed cells appear, but their appearance is blocked by protein-synthesis inhibitors. Conversely, upon shift from 35°C to 41°C, there is a rapid morphological reversion to a normal phenotype. A *ts* change in cell morphology is usually accompanied by temperature sensitivity of several behavioral characteristics of transformed cells, e.g., altered-cell interactions typified by growth to a higher saturation density (density independence), and growth when suspended in semisolid media (agar colony formation) (Martin 1970; Friis et al. 1971; Kawai and Hanafusa 1971; Wyke and Linial 1973). However, there are exceptions to this pattern of morphological changes. For instance, Wyke and Linial (1973) reported that cells infected with 2 of 13 mutants for the maintenance of transformation (LA25 and LA28) did not form agar colonies or foci at 41°C but did grow to a higher saturation density at this temperature. More recently, mutants GI251–253 (Becker et al. 1977; Weber and Friis 1979) have been shown to induce agar colony formation and grow to high density at 41°C without forming foci. Conversely, CU11-infected cells (Anderson et al. 1980) do not form foci at either permissive or nonpermissive temperatures, but they are temperature-sensitive for growth in agar and density-independent growth. In addition, GI251 (Weber and Friis 1979) is heat-sensitive for many biochemical parameters such as 2-deoxyglucose uptake but cold-sensitive for cell growth. Thus, many mutants show some dissociation of the biochemical and morphological parameters of transformation discussed in Chapter 3.

The relationship of parameters of transformation measured in vitro to tumorigenicity in vivo is somewhat unclear. Several groups (Kawai and Hanafusa 1971; Toyoshima et al. 1973; Becker et al. 1977) found that *ts src* mutants produced a lower incidence of sarcomas in chickens when inoculated into the wing web (the body temperature of the chicken is 41°C, which is a nonpermissive temperature for the mutants); here, tumor formation could be due to leakiness or back mutations. The results of Toyoshima et al. (1973) were particularly dramatic in that they attempted to control the wing-web temperature artificially and could show a direct correlation between temperature and tumorigenicity. However, Purchase et al. (1977) found that there was no difference in tumor formation between wild-type virus and *ts* mutants when inoculated intra-abdominally, a site that should be less subject to temperature variation than the wing web. Poste and Flood (1979) did an extensive study on "tumorigenicity" of *ts* mutants as measured by migration across the chick chorioallantoic membrane (CAM). They found that ten lines of rat NRK cells transformed by ten different *ts src* mutants produced tumors at both temperatures as efficiently as cells transformed by wild-type virus. Because rat cells do not produce infectious RSV, virus spread and replication are not complicating factors in these experiments, although experiments with infected chicken cells were also carried out. Furthermore, virus rescued from the CAM was still temperature-sensitive in vitro. In contrast, a chemically transformed rat cell line mutant, which was temperature-sensitive for the transformed phenotype, produced tumors only at the permissive temperature. These results could be interpreted to mean that the *ts* phenotype does not extend to tumorigenicity or, alternatively, that the CAM is a permissive environment in which *src* defects can be complemented by endogenous factors to allow tumor formation. It would be of interest to look at the level and activity of the endogenous cellular *src*-related (*c-src*) protein in the CAM, since this protein has many of the same properties as $pp60^{src}$ (see Chapter 9). Complementation between *ts src* mutants and chemicals to overcome, at least in part, the *ts* phenotype in vitro has been reported by Bissell et al. (1979). They found that addition of the phorbol ester TPA to *ts src*-mutant-infected cultures at 41°C produced changes in cell morphology and biochemical properties more characteristic of transformed cells. Because of the complexity of virus activation in vivo and conflicting reports in the literature, it is currently difficult to equate the thermolability of the *src*-gene product of *ts* mutants in vitro and in vivo.

ts src mutants have been studied also for their interactions with target cells other than fibroblasts in vitro. Wild-type RSV transforms myoblasts, chondroblasts, and neural and pigmented retinal epithelial cells. Myoblasts infected with RSV form myotubes that eventually vacuolate and degenerate, leaving cultures of replicating transformed cells. Myoblasts infected with the *ts src* mutant LA24 become transformed at 35°C, but at 41°C cell fusion and myotube formation proceed normally. Cells infected with *ts src* mutants at 35°C rapidly differentiate when shifted to 41°C, suggesting that the differentiation program is blocked only transiently by expression of the *src*-gene product. However, if these cells are shifted down to 35°C, the myotubes rapidly degenerate and die (Fiszman and Fuchs 1975; Holtzer et al. 1975). This suggests that expression of the transforming gene product in postmitotic differentiated cells can be a lethal event. A similar picture is seen with chick embryo retinal epithelial melanocytes infected with *ts src* mutants (Boettiger et al. 1977); again a shift from 35°C to 41°C causes transformed cells to differentiate (as measured by melanin synthesis), but a shift from

41°C to 35°C causes the differentiated cells to degenerate rapidly. A different result is seen with chondroblasts transformed by *ts* LA24; in this case, the phenotype is completely reversible in either direction (Pacifici et al. 1977). The differentiated cell marker, sulfated proteoglycan, ceases to be synthesized at 35°C even if infection is initiated at 41°C, but the cells do not die after shift-down.

An interesting result has been reported by Calothy and colleagues (Calothy and Pessac 1976; Calothy et al. 1978, 1980). Neuroretinal (NR) cells from chick embryos infected with wild-type RSV become morphologically transformed and are stimulated to proliferate more rapidly than uninfected NR cells. PA2, a *ts src* mutant, induces greatly enhanced rates of NR-cell proliferation at both temperatures, although morphological transformation is not seen at 41°C. Several *td* mutants, PA101–104, have been isolated that do not transform fibroblasts or NR cells but cause enhanced proliferation of NR cells. Other *td* RSV mutants do not induce proliferation, suggesting that PA101–104 are *td* mutants that have dissociated transforming and proliferative functions. The mitogenic effect of PA101–104 is temperature-sensitive; they induce NR-cell proliferation at 37°C but not at 41.5°C. Other *td* viruses with partially expressed transforming functions are discussed below.

A second type of *ts* transformation mutant has been reported. In addition to a defect in the maintenance of transformation, these mutants (LA30m, LA338m, LA343m, and MI100m) were originally thought to have mutations in a function required for initiation of transformation but not for replication (Wyke and Linial 1973; Bookout and Sigel 1975; Hunter and Vogt 1976). The direct evidence for such a virus function has not been forthcoming, and it now seems most likely that these contain multiple mutations (in *src* and a replicative gene) that are leakier for replication than for transformation. More recent work has shown that LA338m is defective in *pol,* as well as in *src,* because it is deficient in proviral DNA synthesis; however, the polymerase is only slightly thermolabile in vitro (Verma et al. 1976; Moelling and Friis 1979). Hunter (1980) reported that LA338m may be temperature-sensitive in *env* as well, making it a triple mutant. LA30m appears to have mutations in *src* and *env,* because the early temperature-sensitive defect is no longer observed once viral particles have penetrated the cell, and the virions are heat labile unless they exist as pseudotypes (Tato et al. 1978). LA343m and MI100m have not been characterized further but probably contain multiple mutations as well. LA343m, in particular, has the same phenotype as LA338m (Wyke and Linial 1973).

A large number of nonconditional transformation mutants (*td*) have been isolated. These mutants may have large or small deletions in *src* or, in some cases, point mutations. *td* mutants appear with fairly high frequency in stocks of wild-type RSV and have been isolated in many laboratories. The *td* mutants in which most or all of *src* has been deleted do not recombine with *ts src* mutants to produce wild-type virus (Bernstein et al. 1976). Of special interest are deletion mutants that have not deleted the entire *src* gene, originally called long *td* (*ltd*) or partial *td* (*ptd*) mutants (Kawai et al. 1977; Lai et al 1977; Yoshida and Ikawa 1977; Yoshida et al. 1979; Fincham et al. 1980). Although the term *ptd* originally described mutants with partial deletions of *src* genetic information but no detectable *src* function, it has also been applied to mutants with a partial functional expression of *src;* to avoid such confusion, this term will not be used hereafter in this chapter. *td* viruses may exhibit dissociation of parameters of the transformed phenotype. For example, *td* TY9-infected cells do not form foci, although agar colony formation occurs after the cells have been passaged several times (Yoshida and Ikawa 1977). Another unusual mutant of RSV, CU2, forms minicolonies in soft agar and induces an unusual "blebby" morphology, whereas CU12 induces fusiform morphology and large colonies in soft agar (Anderson et al. 1980). *td* mutants with partial deletions have been used in recombination experiments with cellular *src*-related sequences (*c-src*) to form new sarcomagenic viruses in vivo (recovered ASV or rASV) (Hanafusa et al. 1977; Vigne et al. 1979). This is discussed in more detail in Section VI.B.7 (see also Chapters 4 and 9). Fincham et al. (1980) have isolated 11 *td* viruses with various deletions from PR-RSV-A and have done a genetic analysis of the ability of these viruses to recombine with *ts src* mutants (see below).

Varmus and colleagues (Oppermann et al. 1981; Varmus et al. 1981) have described mutants in the *src* gene obtained by selecting revertants of a transformed rat line, B31, containing a single copy of B77-RSV-C proviral DNA. Although several revertants lost the RSV provirus, the majority had acquired mutations in the *src* gene. Three classes of *src* mutants were detected biochemically: class-I mutants encode *src* proteins of normal size with little or no protein kinase activity; class-II mutants encode smaller proteins related to $pp60^{src}$ that lack protein kinase activity; and class-III mutants encode no detectable $pp60^{src}$-related proteins. One mutant, SF/LO104, displays a cell-dependent phenotype after rescue; it induces fusiform transformation in chicken cells in which a high level of $pp60^{src}$-associated protein kinase activity is detected. However, the *src* product in the original revertant line exhibits very little protein kinase activity and the rescued virus does not transform rat cells. No deletions could be detected in any of the 30 mutants by restriction enzyme digestion of the proviral DNAs. Some of the truncated proteins encoded by class-II mutants represent the amino terminus of $pp60^{src}$ and may result from nonsense mutations.

Current biochemical data suggest that there is only one RSV transforming gene and one gene product, $pp60^{src}$ (see Chapter 9). However, the genetic data suggest that there is heterogeneity among *td* phenotypes (Calothy et al. 1978; Weber and Friis 1979). This could be explained either by a multifunctional gene product and/or by different amounts of leakiness for different *src*-gene functions. For instance, if $pp60^{src}$ acts upon more than one target, mutations could differentially affect action on those targets. Weber and Friis (1979) examined *ts* GI251, which shows only some parameters of transformation at 42°C; they found that the phenotype is probably not caused by leakiness and concluded that there is more than one primary target for $pp60^{src}$.

Genetic evidence also supports the concept of a single transforming gene product. Two early studies (Kawai et al. 1972; Wyke 1973b) showed that simultaneous infection by two different *ts src* mutants could result in transformation at the nonpermissive temperature. This phenomenon was originally thought to be genetic complementation; however, it was later named cooperative transformation when it became clear that recombination of the two *ts* mutants to produce wild-type virus was involved (Wyke et al. 1975; Balduzzi 1976). This conclusion was reached because it was found that reinfection was necessary in order to produce transformation, whereas true complementation should occur within a single cell, and no clear evidence for true phenotypic complementation has been presented. Cooperative transformation experiments have shown that induction of transformation at 41°C by mixed infection permits categorization of *ts src* mutants into at least four groups (Wyke 1973b). The four groups correlated, in part, with the diversity of phenotypes found for these mutants (Wyke and Linial 1973). One interesting result of Wyke's study (1973b) was that PR-RSV mutants would not reproducibly transform cooperatively with *ts src* mutants of SR-RSV or B77-RSV to the same extent as with other PR-RSV mutants. Balduzzi (1976) performed similar coinfection experiments with mutants of BH-RSV(−) and PR-RSV and found that a few of the BH-RSV(−) mutants did recombine with PR-RSV mutants, although at an efficiency much lower than that at which PR-RSV mutants recombined with each other. More recently, recombinants between the two *ts src* mutants, NY68 SR-RSV-A and LA24 PR-RSV-C, have been observed with high efficiency, some of which appear to have hybrid $pp60^{src}$ molecules (M. Linial, pers. comm.). Since the *src* proteins of SR-RSV and PR-RSV appear very similar by tryptic peptide mapping (Sefton et al. 1978), it is not clear why cooperative transformation between PR-RSV and SR-RSV was not seen originally. It is also still unclear why *ts src* mutants should fall into cooperative-transformation groups at all, since recombination among the avian tumor viruses appears to occur with high frequency throughout the genome (see Section VI.B.1). One possibility is the existence of "hot spots" for recombination.

In contrast to the results of Bernstein et al. (1976), who showed that a *td* mutant with a complete deletion of *src* could not recombine with *ts src* mutants, Kawai et al. (1977) observed recombination between a *td* mutant (with a partial *src* deletion) and *ts src* NY68. Fincham et al. (1980) have isolated 11 *td* mutants of PR-RSV-A and have used these in recombination experiments with *ts src* mutants in mapping studies. Deletions in the *src* gene allow physical mapping of the missing sequence by restriction enzyme analysis and Southern transfer (see Chapter 4). These workers used four *ts src* mutants of Wyke's different cooperative-transformation groups that had tentatively been ordered within the *src* gene in recombination experiments by Balduzzi et al. (1978). Several of the *td* mutants contained no detectable deletions by restriction enzyme analysis, whereas three had large deletions (of 1.0 kb, 1.5 kb, and 1.6 kb) in the *src* gene, as compared with 1.7–2.0 kb for standard *td* mutants. The stable *td* mutants with no visible deletion (indicating either a point mutation or a very small deletion) recombine with all the tested *ts* mutants. Those with observable deletions recombined with some, but not all, of the *ts* mutants. All the *td* mutants recombine with LA29, in which the lesion appears to map close to the 3′ end of the *src* gene (Balduzzi et al. 1978). Although Lai et al. (1977) suggested that all partial *td* mutants tend to retain the 5′ end of *src* (on the basis of heteroduplex mapping), H. Hanafusa et al. (1980) have found *td* viruses lacking the 5′ end of *src* but retaining the 3′ end of *src* (see Chapter 4). Finer restriction mapping of the mutant *src* genes should localize the deletions with more precision.

As mentioned briefly above, partial *td* mutants can recombine with *c-src* sequences in vivo to produce wild-type ASV, called rASV (Hanafusa et al. 1977). This phenomenon is discussed in more detail in Section VI.B.7 (also see Chapters 4 and 9). An interesting set of rASV variants was obtained after injection of birds with *td* NY109m (Kawai et al. 1977), which was shown to be missing an oligonucleotide in the *env* region as well as most of the *src* region. The missing *env*-region oligonucleotide is not necessary for replication as *td* NY109m is replication-competent (H. Hanafusa et al. 1980). rASV particles isolated after injection of *td* NY109m into chickens are defective and of three types: *env*$^-$ or *pol*$^-$*env*$^-$ or *gag*$^-$*pol*$^-$*env*$^-$. The recombination model proposed by these authors suggests that these *rd* rASVs are generated because of homologous sequences at the *env-src* junction (utilized for formation of other rASVs) and the *pol-env* junction, which are used in recombination to generate *env*$^-$ rASV. However, this cannot explain the formation of all the mutant rASV phenotypes. Recently, it has been found that there are homologous sequences at either side of *src* that might allow specific deletion of the *src* gene (Czernilofsky et al. 1980; Yamamoto et al. 1980).

Variants of RSV with abnormal *src* genes but wild-type phenotypes have been described. Quail cells harboring the provirus of PH1 are transformed and synthesize wild-type virions (Mason et al. 1979b). The provirus of PH1 contains an insertion of about 250 bases in the *src* region, enough to encode an additional 80 amino acids of protein. But the pp60^{src} synthesized by PH1 is normal (W. Mason, pers. comm.); therefore, the insertion must not be in the coding region of the gene. In addition, both *src* and *env-src* mRNAs contain the insertion (G. Mark and J. Taylor, pers. comm.). Oppermann et al. (1981) and Varmus et al. (1981) have described another virus variant of B77-RSV with a *src*-gene insert. A flat revertant of B77-RSV-transformed Rat-1 cells (line B31), called OOO (rescued virus called SF/LO208), was shown to encode a 45,000-dalton *src*-related protein lacking peptides at the amino terminus of pp60^{src}. A back mutant, SF/LO2082-1, was isolated that encodes a 68,000-

dalton protein with kinase activity that contains extra amino acids near the amino terminus. The provirus of the back mutant contains an insert of about 200 bp at or near the 5′ end of the *src* gene.

Two groups have described experiments in which the presence of the *src* gene in certain strains of RSV appears to retard or prevent virus replication. Neiman et al. (1978) reported that, in MSB-1 cells (a line of chicken lymphoid cells derived from tumors induced by Marek's disease herpesvirus), replication of *td* RSV proceeded normally, whereas replication of some wild-type RSV strains was restricted. Infection with either *td* RSV or RSV leads to synthesis of unintegrated viral DNA copies, but, in the case of restricted strains of RSV, this DNA does not become integrated and disappears 2 days after infection. Therefore, the presence of some *src*-gene sequences may prevent integration and stable infection. Shimakage et al. (1979) found that wild-type B77-RSV-C replication in duck embryo fibroblasts was retarded compared with replication in chick embryo fibroblasts. However, a *td* mutant appeared during duck-cell propagation that replicated similarly in duck and chick cells. No further molecular analysis was done, but again *src* sequences seem to inhibit replication. It is not known in either case how *src* interferes with replication.

2. fps

Fujinami sarcoma virus (FuSV) is an example of a replication-defective oncogenic avian retrovirus whose pathogenic spectrum, like that of RSV, is limited to the induction of sarcomas (Fujinami and Inamoto 1914). Its 4.5-kb genomic RNA encodes a 140,000-dalton polyprotein (P140) that contains *gag,* but neither *pol* nor *env* sequences (T. Hanafusa et al. 1980; Lee et al. 1980) (see Chapter 4). P140 from transformed cells is highly phosphorylated and has an associated protein kinase activity (Bister et al. 1980). The cell-derived inserted sequences, which are unrelated to those of RSV *src,* have been designated *fps.* Pawson et al. (1980) have recently reported a strain of FuSV that induces temperature-sensitive transformation of fibroblasts. They show that the phosphorylation of P140 and its associated kinase activity are reduced at the nonpermissive temperature.

PRCII is another replication-defective ASV (Carr and Campbell 1958) and shows a high degree of homology to the *fps*-specific sequences of FuSV (Shibuya et al. 1980). The PRCII genome encodes a 105,000-dalton polyprotein, which, like the products of *src* and of FSV *fps,* is a phosphoprotein with protein kinase activity (Breitman et al. 1981; Neil et al. 1981a,b). Three conditional mutants have been isolated following mutagenesis (Hirano and Vogt 1981). Two of these, *ts* LA42 and *ts* LA47, exhibit temperature-sensitive transformation of fibroblasts with no other apparent defect in any other genes they may contain or in the replicative genes of the accompanying helper virus. On the other hand, the third mutant, *ts* LA46, in addition to exhibiting the temperature-sensitive transformation of fibroblasts, shows a replication defect in that there is decreased particle production at the nonpermissive temperature and the virions are thermolabile. Thus, the helper virus presumably contains a *ts* defect as well.

3. ras

Two well-known strains of MSV were derived after the passage of MLV through rats. These strains, called Ha-MSV (Harvey 1964) and Ki-MSV (Kirsten and Mayer 1967), contain rat-cell-derived sequences that have been termed *ras.*

The first mammalian sarcoma virus mutants isolated were derived from Ki-MSV (Scolnick et al. 1972, 1975; Carchman et al. 1974). These isolates (*ts*1, *ts*2, *ts*3, and *ts*6) were obtained as nonproducer cell lines following mutagenesis of Ki-MSV(MLV) mixtures. They are temperature-sensitive for the maintenance of transformation but exhibit only a slow reversibility between transformed phenotype and normal phenotype upon temperature shift. All the mutants can be rescued by superinfection with MLV. Rescued virus is able to transform cells, producing clones that are also temperature-sensitive. Interestingly, cells infected with *ts*2 and *ts*6 exhibit a transformed phenotype at the nonpermissive temperature when superinfected with helper virus (Scolnick et al. 1975), a phenomenon not seen with RSV *ts src* mutants. A similar apparent dependence of the *ts* phenotype on the presence or absence of replication-competent helper virus has been reported for Mo-MSV *ts* mutants (Blair et al. 1979), but the mechanism and significance of this phenomenon are unknown.

Further analysis of these conditional Ki-MSV mutants was difficult until the recent identification of a 21,000-dalton phosphoprotein (p21) in nonproducer cells transformed by both Ki-MSV and Ha-MSV (Shih et al. 1979a,b). The p21 of both Ha-MSV and Ki-MSV can be immunoprecipitated from transformed cells by antisera obtained from rats bearing tumors from MSV-transformed syngeneic cells. The same protein can be immunoprecipitated from translation products synthesized in vitro from virion RNA (Shih et al. 1979a; Shih and Scolnick 1980). Anti-p21 serum was used in the biochemical analysis of one mutant of Ki-MSV called *ts*371, which was isolated as a nonproducer focus of NRK cells. *ts*371-infected cells show temperature sensitivity for transformation in both focus and agar colony assays (Shih et al. 1979b). Cells coinfected with *ts*371 and wild-type Mo-MLV show a reversible shift from transformed morphology to a near normal morphology after being shifted from permissive temperature to nonpermissive temperature (see Fig. 7.2). The amount of p21 that can be immunoprecipitated from extracts of cells infected with *ts*371 is markedly decreased by heating the extracts to 36° C for 5 minutes, whereas the precipitability of p21 from extracts of cells infected with wild-type virus is unaffected. Mixing experiments suggest that there is no heat-activated component in the mutant cells capable of blocking precipitation. p21 synthesized by *ts*371 exhibits other altered properties as well. Wild-type p21 is phosphorylated at both 34° C and 39° C in vivo; however, when *ts*371 cells are labeled with ^{32}P, p21 cannot be detected in immunoprecipitates from cells grown at either temperature, suggesting that the *ts*371 p21 is not phosphorylated. Furthermore, sera raised against either Ha-MSV or Ki-MSV tumors exhibit differential abilities to precipitate p21 from *ts*371-transformed cells at 34° C or 39° C. Ki-MSV antiserum precipitates p21 at both temperatures, whereas Ha-MSV antiserum precipitates much less p21 from cells grown at 39° C. A phenotypically wild-type revertant has been shown to regain the precipitation and phosphorylation characteristics of wild-type Ki-MSV (Shih et al. 1979b). Which, if any, of the altered properties of *ts*371 p21 are directly related to the expression of temperature-sensitive transformation remains to be determined.

Ki-MSV-transformed cells have been reported to express a 35,000-dalton polypeptide that copurifies with lactate dehydrogenase activity and has been called LDH_K (Anderson et al. 1979). Studies of *ts*371-infected cells indicate that the protein, which appears to consist of four 35,000-dalton subunits and one 22,000-dalton subunit, has thermolabile enzymic activity both in vivo and in vitro, although the difference in activity is not large (about twofold at 42° C) (G.

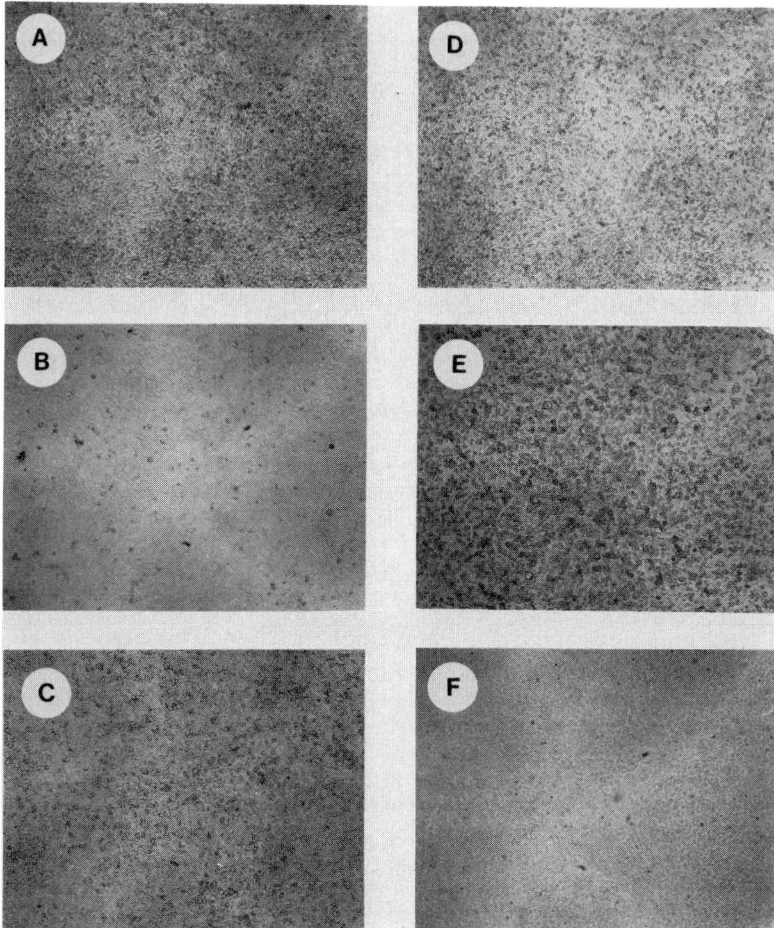

Figure 7.2 Morphological changes associated with transformation of mouse cells by wild-type Ki-MSV or a mutant temperature-sensitive for transformation (*ts*371 Ki-MSV) at permissive and nonpermissive temperatures. In all cases, the helper virus is wild-type Mo-MLV. Infected cells were grown for approximately 7 days at 34° C, reseeded into fresh dishes, and grown for 48 hr at either 34° C or 39.5° C before photographing. The *ts*371 Ki-MSV-infected cells grown at 39.5° C were subcultured again at 34° C for 60 hr to show the effects of a temperature shift-down. (*A*) *ts*371 Ki-MSV(Mo-MLV) at 34° C; (*B*) *ts*371 Ki-MSV(Mo-MLV), 34° C → 39.5° C; (*C*) *ts*371 Ki-MSV(Mo-MLV), 34° C → 39.5° C → 34° C; (*D*) wild-type Ki-MSV(Mo-MLV) at 34° C; (*E*) wild-type Ki-MSV(Mo-MLV), 34° C → 39.5° C; (*F*) Mo-MLV alone at 34° C. (Reprinted, with permission, from Shih et al. 1979b.)

Anderson et al., pers. comm.). It is not known whether any of the LDH_K subunit peptides share any homology with the p21 protein described by Shih et al. (1979a).

Nonconditional mutants of Ki-MSV were first described by Greenberger and colleagues (Greenberger and Aaronson 1974; Greenberger et al. 1974) following mutagenesis of nonproducer transformed BALB/3T3 mouse cells and selection for morphological revertants. The revertants fall into two classes (Bensinger et al. 1977): class I consists of cell clones that appear to have lost the viral genome, and class II consists of clones that appear to contain an altered virus genome that can be rescued. Cells infected with the virus rescued from class-II cells do not become transformed. However, if class-II clones spontaneously transform, wild-type transforming virus can be rescued. The properties of these class-II Ki-MSV revertants resemble closely revertants of feline sarcoma virus (FeSV)-transformed cells (Donner et al. 1980) (see Section V.A.4) and revertants of B77-RSV-transformed rat cells, described above (Oppermann et al. 1981; Varmus et al. 1981). The revertants that contain a viral genome are readily retransformed by wild-type Ki-MSV, but there is no evidence of complementation or recombination between mutant and wild-type genomes (Greenberger et al. 1974; Bensinger et al. 1977). Clearly, an immunological analysis of these revertant cell lines with anti-p21 sera, as well as a detailed characterization of the mutant viral genomes, would be extremely interesting.

4. mos

Mo-MSV and its naturally occurring genetic variants are among the most extensively characterized of the mammalian defective C-type viruses. Mo-MSV was initially derived following passage of Mo-MLV in BALB/c mice (Moloney 1966) from which a number of different strains have been isolated. These strains share the common feature of inducing transformation of fibroblasts in vitro but differ in the nature and extent of the sequences they share with helper MLV (Hu et al. 1977; Canaani et al. 1979; Donoghue et al. 1979; Vande Woude et al. 1979, 1980). They also differ in the size of the cell-derived insert, called *mos*, they contain (Canaani et al. 1979; Vande Woude et al. 1979, 1980) (see Chapter 4) and in the amount and size of the MLV *gag*-containing polypeptides they express (Robey et al. 1977; Stephenson et al. 1978). These naturally occurring variants have demonstrated clearly that expression of *gag*-, *pol*-, and *env*-gene products is not required for fibroblast transformation by MSV (Robey et al. 1977). In addition, not all of the *mos* sequences carried by certain strains, such as HT-1 (Huebner et al. 1966) or 124 (Ball et al. 1973), are required for the expression of the transforming function of these viruses (Canaani et al. 1979; Vande Woude et al. 1979, 1980). The sequence diversity seen among the MSV variants could be caused by multiple recombination events between the Mo-MLV and *c-mos* sequences that occurred during the original mouse passage. However, it seems more likely that the genetic diversity has arisen as a result of deletions and genetic rearrangements acquired during the course of virus propagation in tumors and in tissue culture. Deletions have been shown to occur readily in vitro in both MLV and MSV genomes (Shields et al. 1978; Canaani and Aaronson 1980). The problem in sorting out the evolution of MSV strains is that parental viruses are not available for comparison. Strain HT-1 may represent a virus closest to the original recombination event. This idea is based on the large size of its *mos* insert and the amount of MLV information it contains (Vande Woude et al. 1979, 1980). Interestingly, HT-1 expresses no detectable MLV-related polypeptides (Robey et al. 1977), although it appears to contain all the *gag* coding sequences present in the m1 MSV strain, which does express a *gag*-gene product (Vande Woude et al. 1979). The reason for this is not known.

td deletions of *mos* sequences have not been isolated, although some of the revertants of Mo-MSV-transformed mink and mouse cells described by Fischinger et al. (1972b) may represent nonconditional transformation-defective genomes similar to those described for Ki-MSV (Greenberger et al. 1974; see also below). However, a large number of spontaneous deletion variants of the 124 strain of MSV have been described (Canaani and Aaronson 1980). These variants arose during multiple cycles of virus growth, in a manner reminiscent of the generation of *td* variants of RSV. In the case of MSV, transformation functions are retained while *gag* coding sequences are deleted. In one well-characterized virus (clone 14), 45% of the parental 124 genome was deleted, resulting in a viral genome of 3.5–3.9 kb. Clone 14 is nevertheless fully capable of transformation and can be efficiently rescued by MLV upon superinfection (Canaani et al. 1979). Indeed, the deleted genomes appear to have a replicative advantage and grow to a higher titer in the presence of helper than does the parental MSV (Canaani and Aaronson 1980).

Conditionally defective transformation mutants of Mo-MSV have been difficult to isolate and maintain. Attempts to define the lesion in the few *ts* Mo-MSV mutants that do exist have been hampered by the fact that no gene product of *mos* has been identified. No antitumor serum has been found that detects expression of a transformation-specific protein, as has been found in the case of RSV, Ki-MSV, and Ha-MSV. Nevertheless, a number of Mo-MSV mutants that are defective in either establishment or maintenance of transformation have been described, and their properties are consistent in most cases with defects in *mos.*

The first conditionally defective mutant of Mo-MSV transformation was MSV-1b, described by Somers and Kit (1973). This mutant is unique among retroviruses in that it is cold-sensitive for transformation. Cells infected with MSV-1b express a transformed phenotype at 39°C and a normal phenotype at 33°C. A number of different phenotypic characteristics of the transformed state exhibit this temperature dependence (May et al. 1973; Steiner et al. 1974). The reacquisition of the transformed phenotype following a shift to the permissive temperature is blocked by inhibitors of protein synthesis, but not by inhibitors of RNA or DNA synthesis (Somers et al. 1973). K. Somers (pers. comm.) has also isolated three *ts* Mo-MSV mutants that express the transformed phenotype at 33°C and a normal phenotype at 39°C, but these have not been characterized further.

Nine Mo-MSV mutants were isolated following UV-light mutagenesis of a virus stock derived from a subclone of strain 124 that contained a large excess of MSV particles over helper virus. The nine isolates, designated *ts*101–*ts*106 and *ts*108–*ts*110, have been cloned as rat nonproducer transformed cells at 34°C. Selection for these mutants consisted of multiple cycles of growth in methylcellulose in the presence of cytosine arabinoside at 39°C (the nonpermissive temperature) to eliminate cells expressing the transformed phenotype (Blair et al. 1979). All nine isolates exhibit a temperature-dependent expression of the transformed phenotype as measured by several parameters, but it is unclear whether they all contain different mutations. The *ts*110 mutant has been characterized in some detail. Pseudotype particles, produced after MLV superinfection of *ts*110-infected nonproducer cells, contain a low-molecular-weight protein with actin-binding kinase activity that exhibits an increased sensitivity to temperature inactivation compared with that of parental virus (Sen et al. 1979b). The presence of this kinase activity is characteristic of MSV pseudotype preparations, and it has been suggested that this may represent a virus-coded enzyme (Sen and Todaro 1979). The apparent thermolability of this kinase activity in *ts*110 suggests that, like the avian *src* product pp60^{src}, this could represent a product of at least part of the *mos* sequence, but no direct proof exists.

Analysis of the *gag*-related products present in *ts*110-transformed NRK cells has revealed some interesting temperature-dependent properties. At the permissive temperature, two polypeptides, P58 and P85, can be precipitated with anti-MLV *gag* serum (Horn et al. 1980; Wood et al. 1980). Analyses by immunoprecipitation and peptide mapping indicate that P58 and P85 contain peptides of three of the MLV *gag*-gene-encoded proteins, p15, p12, and p30, but no sequences related to the fourth *gag*-gene protein, p10 (the carboxy-terminal protein of *gag*). P85 appears to contain all of P58, plus an additional 27,000 daltons of protein of unknown origin. *ts*110-infected NRK cells grown at the nonpermissive temperature contain P58, but no P85, indicating that the expression of P85 is a characteristic of the transformed state. In vitro translation studies indicate that both P58 and P85 can be synthesized from RNA isolated from *ts*110 virions following rescue with helper virus (J. Horn et al., pers. comm.). Recent studies with inhibitors of RNA synthesis indicate that the reappearance of P85 following a shift from the nonpermissive temperature to the permissive temperature is blocked by actinomycin D (J. Horn et al., in prep.). It has been suggested that the additional peptide sequences present in P85 could represent *mos*-encoded information (Wood et al. 1980), but this remains to be established directly.

Another Mo-MSV *ts* mutant, designated CP27 (Forchhammer and Turnock 1978) has been characterized for its in vivo effects (Klarlund and Forchhammer 1980). Nonproducer cells infected with CP27 or wild-type MSV were inoculated into nude mice (which are more sensitive than hairy mice to ambient temperature) subsequently incubated at either 28°C or 39°C. CP27-infected cells induced tumors only at 28°C, whereas wild-type-transformed cells were tumorigenic at both temperatures. When animals bearing tumors induced by CP27 at 28°C were shifted to 36°C, the tumors regressed. Some secondary tumor growth appeared after regression, but this appeared to represent host-cell modification, rather than

CP27 reversion, because cells recovered from these tumors induced tumor formation at the permissive temperature only and the virus recovered retains temperature sensitivity for focus formation (Karlund and Forchhammer 1980). Further studies employing this technique of in vivo temperature sensitivity of oncogenesis should prove exciting.

5. fes

The techniques of genetic analysis have only recently been applied to the FeSV and feline leukemia virus (FeLV) systems, but the first results indicate that these viruses are amenable to such studies and mutants of FeSV with interesting properties have already been obtained. Although three strains of FeSV have been isolated from cat tumors (see Chapters 2 and 8), thus far mutants of only the Snyder-Theilen (ST) strain (Snyder and Theilen 1969) have been reported. The only known product of the ST-FeSV genome is a phosphoprotein of about 80,000 daltons, called $pp80^{fes}$ or $P80^{fes}$, consisting of *gag* polypeptides (related to those produced by the helper FeLV) linked to a protein sequence encoded totally, or in part, by the cell-derived *fes* sequences (Porzig et al. 1979; Barbacid et al. 1980; Ruscetti et al. 1980; Van de Ven et al. 1980b,c). This protein is phosphorylated and apparently contains an associated phosphokinase activity (Van de Ven et al. 1980a).

Two nonconditional mutants of ST-FeSV were isolated following infection and single-cell cloning of mink cells (Donner et al. 1980). Cells infected by these two mutants (designated B2 and B7) exhibit flat, nontransformed morphology and spontaneously convert at a low frequency to the transformed phenotype. B2- and B7-infected cells express normal levels of FeSV viral RNA and $P80^{fes}$. The FeSV genomes can be rescued by helper virus and transmitted to mink cells, again inducing FeSV gene products in the absence of morphological transformation. This indicates that B2 and B7 are transformation-defective viral mutants (Donner et al. 1980). Consistent with this, the DNA of cells infected with these *td* mutants is unable to induce transformation of recipient cells in transfection assays (L. Turek et al., pers. comm.). Recent evidence indicates that the P80 of these mutants is defective in the associated kinase activity found in wild-type P80 (Van de Ven et al. 1980a). Mink cells infected with B7 FeSV express little or no FOCMA-S, which is an antigen detected on the surfaces of FeSV-transformed rat and mink cells, that cross-reacts with the FOCMA-L antigen detected on the surface of transformed cat lymphoid cells (Sher et al. 1980) (see Chapter 8). Spontaneous retransformants of B7, however, exhibit normal levels of immunofluorescence after probing with anti-FOCMA-S sera, suggesting that expression of FOCMA-S determinants correlates with the transformed phoneotype (Sher et al. 1980).

A second type of FeSV variant has been isolated in which the defect can less clearly be defined as viral (L. Turek et al., pers. comm.). NRK rat cell clone A3 exhibits a flat morphology but contains a single integrated copy of a normal ST-FeSV provirus. This clone spontaneously segregates transformed variants at a frequency of about 3×10^{-7} per cell generation, consistent with the hypothesis of a somatic-cell mutation. NRK-A3 cells contain neither detectable FeSV-specific viral RNA nor $P80^{fes}$, although treatment with iododeoxyuridine results in the induction of detectable levels of FeLV-related p15 antigen. However, DNA from NRK-A3 cells superinfected with FeLV is only fivefold less efficient at inducing transformation in transfection assays than cellular DNA derived from NRK cells transformed by wild-type FeSV. This would indicate that the block to FeSV expression in NRK-A3 cells either is cellular in nature (and unlinked to the FeSV genome) or represents a lesion in the virus that is readily rectified during the transfection or rescue process.

6. erb, myc, *and* myb

The two best-studied avian AcLVs are AEV (insert called *erb*), which encodes a 75,000-dalton polyprotein (P75) (Hayman et al. 1979), and MC29 (insert called *myc*), which encodes a 110,000-dalton polyprotein (P110) (Bister et al. 1977). The non-*gag* peptides of AEV P75 and MC29 P110 are unrelated (Rettenmier et al. 1979a; Eisenman et al. 1980b; Kitchener and Hayman 1980). In addition to the *gag*-related polyproteins, there are reports of a gag-unrelated protein found by translation in vitro of AEV RNA that might also be a candidate for a transforming protein. This non-*gag* protein is translated from subgenomic 20S RNA and has a size of 40,000-46,000 daltons (P40); it contains no *gag*-related tryptic peptides (Lai et al. 1980; Pawson and Martin 1980; Yoshida and Toyoshima 1980). In addition, the peptide maps of P75 and P40 are distinct, suggesting different coding regions (Lai et al. 1980). An antiserum specific for the non-*gag* portion of the AEV polyprotein P75 has been described (Beug et al. 1981). This serum precipitates P75 via the *erb* determinants of this molecule but does not precipitate P40.

A key question concerning the AcLVs is the nature of the transforming protein(s). AEV and MC29 both transform fibroblasts, as well as specific hematopoietic cells (erythrocyte precursors in the case of AEV and macrophage lineage cells in the case of MC29) but contain different unique sequences (see Chapters 4 and 9). Therefore, it is possible that each encodes a fibroblast-transforming protein and a second hematopoietic-cell-transforming protein, or that one transforming protein is responsible for the specific spectrum of transformation. It is known that the specificity of hematopoietic-cell transformation is not merely a function of infection. Graf et al. (1980) have shown that AEV can replicate and synthesize P75 in macrophage precursor cells, which it does not transform in vivo, and, conversely, that MC29 can replicate and synthesize P110 in erythroid cells. However, the erythroid cells used in these experiments were already transformed by AEV, so it is not possible to determine whether MC29 could transform such cells in vitro. This suggests that the transforming target for the *onc* products is cell-lineage-specific. It should be pointed out that, although AEV-transformed fibroblasts resemble RSV-transformed fibroblasts in both biological and biochemical properties (Quade 1979), MC29-transformed fibroblasts are quite different. They have, for instance, the unique property of an accelerated growth rate (Royer-Pokora et al. 1978) (see Chapters 8 and 9).

As in the case of *src,* transformation mutants of the AcLVs would be of great help in elucidating the functions of the various viral sequences. Graf and his colleagues have isolated two mutants of AEV defective in transformation and are beginning to characterize these viruses. Erythroid cells transformed by wild-type AEV fail to synthesize globin, the criterion used for screening clones for viral mutants. One *ts* mutant of AEV, *ts*34, was originally reported to be temperature-sensitive for transformation of erythroblasts but not of fibroblasts (Graf et al. 1978). The defective product in *ts*34 is required for maintenance of erythroid transformation, since after a shift to nonpermissive temperature, erythroid cells infected with *ts*34 start synthesizing globin and an erthrocyte-specific cell-surface glycoprotein (K. Savin and H. Beug, pers. comm.). In addition, leukemogenicity of the mutant is reduced. One conclusion from this work is that transformation of erythroid cells by AEV results in a block of differentiated cell functions and that this block depends on a virus-coded protein. The dissociation of thermolability of erythroid transformation and fibroblast transformation is not complete, as later studies have shown that many parameters of transformation are temperature-sensitive in *ts*34-infected fibroblasts (Beug and Graf 1980). For instance, neither focus formation nor agar colony formation is temperature-sensitive, although sarcomagenicity, hexose uptake, and induction of plasminogen activator are temperature-sensitive. Therefore, *ts*34 behaves like a partial transforming virus in fibroblasts at 41°C. This result makes it unclear as to whether a single mutant product in *ts*34 is responsible for the defects in both erythroid transformation and fibroblast transformation, with transformation of fibroblasts being leakier, or whether there are two mutations.

The second AEV mutant, *td*359, is nonconditionally defective for erythroid-cell transformation but is fully able to transform fibroblasts (Royer-Pokora et al. 1979). *td*359 does not induce erythroblastosis in vivo, although one of ten chicks developed a sarcoma at the site of injection, and *td*359-transformed fibroblasts are tumorigenic in vivo. Initial biochemical studies (Beug et al. 1980a,b) showed that *td*359 has a small deletion in the *gag* containing P75 polyprotein, lacking 3 of 53 peptides found in the wild-type virus. The deletion is in the non-*gag* part of P75. There is no detectable change in P40 in this mutant, consistent with P75 being required for erythroblast transformation.

Three clones of MC29, a myelocytomatosis virus, have been isolated that encode smaller P110-related proteins (P90, P95, and P100) (Beug et al. 1980b; Ramsay et al. 1980). These variants were obtained by recloning the virus from a line of MC29-transformed quail fibroblasts, and they have a 100-fold reduced ability to transform macrophagelike cells and thus may represent *td* MC29 variants. The characterization of such variants is preliminary but potentially quite exciting.

A mutant of AMV has recently been isolated. This mutant (FL 907/7) replicates to equal titer at 35°C and 41°C but transforms yolk sac and bone marrow cells about tenfold more efficiently at 35°C than at 41°C (C. Moscovici and M. Moscovici, pers. comm.). Thus, the lesion may be in the AMV *onc* or *myb* gene.

7. abl

Ab-MLV is a replication-defective, rapidly transforming retrovirus that was derived, presumably by recombination, after passage of Mo-MLV in a steroid-treated BALB/c mouse (Abelson and Rabstein 1970) (see also Chapter 8). Like a number of avian (MC29, AEV) and mammalian (FeSV) viruses, its genome encodes a polyprotein consisting of *gag*-protein sequences derived from the helper virus, linked to peptides encoded by the cell-derived insert, *abl* (see Chapters 4 and 9). Ab-MLV transforms lymphoid cells and fibroblasts in vitro (Sklar et al. 1974; Rosenberg et al. 1975; Scher and Siegler 1975), but in vivo it transforms only lymphoid cells, inducing a rapid pre-B-cell lymphoma (Abelson and Rabstein 1970; Boss et al. 1979; Rosenberg and Baltimore 1980). This specificity contrasts to those of AEV and MC29, which can induce sarcomas and carcinomas, as well as leukemias, in vivo. The prototype strain, derived from NIH-3T3-transformed fibroblasts designated ANN-1 (Scher and Siegler 1975), encodes a 120,000-dalton polyprotein (P120) that contains MLV p15, pp12, and p30 determinants (Reynolds et al. 1978; Witte et al. 1978; Van de Ven et al. 1979). P120 contains a protein kinase activity that autophosphorylates one or more tyrosine residues (Reynolds et al. 1980; Van de Ven et al. 1980a; Witte et al. 1980a).

A number of variants and mutants of Ab-MLV have been recently isolated. Analysis of these isolates indicates that P120 and its kinase activity are directly involved in the transforming function of Ab-MLV. Sacks et al. (1979) have described the isolation of two types of *td* Ab-MLV-infected cell lines. Class I consists of four clones that were selected as spontaneous revertants of an Ab-MLV mink-cell clone. These clones (class I) express no detectable *gag* determinants. They become retransformed upon superinfection with helper virus and then release low levels of Ab-MLV capable of transforming mink or rat cells. These variants probably result from epigenetic events affecting regulation of proviral expression and are similar to ST-FeSV revertants described by Porzig et al. (1979) or to RSV revertants described by Deng et al. (1974, 1977). Class II consists of 20 clones of nontransformed mink cells isolated after Ab-MLV infection. These clones contain different levels of pp12, correlating with the degree of transformation as measured by morphology or growth in soft agar. Several of these class-II mink-cell clones, as well as other Ab-MLV isolates derived in rat cells (Reynolds et al. 1980), produce a P120 product that is deficient in its associated kinase activity in vitro and contains altered phosphorylation patterns. Several of the rat cell mutants are nontumorigenic in syngeneic rats. Both class-I and class-II mutants show levels of binding of epidermal growth factor similar to the levels in normal cells, in contrast to the reduced levels found in cells transformed by wild-type Ab-MLV (Blomberg et al. 1980).

Rosenberg and colleagues (Rosenberg and Witte 1980; Rosenberg et al. 1980) have isolated variants of Ab-MLV that encode polyproteins of different sizes. The P160-producing strain is apparently naturally occurring (or perhaps represents the initial isolate) and, like the P120 strain, transforms both lymphoid and fibroblastic cells in vitro. The strains that encode smaller proteins (P90 and P100) are deficient in their ability to transform lymphoid cells in vitro or to induce Abelson disease in vivo. The P90 and P100 proteins are less stable than P120 or P160 and, interestingly, have reduced kinase activity. However, both P90 and P100 can be efficiently phosphorylated in the presence of active wild-type P120 kinase. It appears that the difference between P120 and the smaller proteins resides in the *abl*-specific portion of the polyprotein and that P90 and P100 are probably premature termination products from a genome of normal size (O. Witte, pers. comm.) (see Chapter 4).

Witte et al. (1980b) have described a second type of mutant of Ab-MLV. The mutant *td* Ab-MLV-P92 encodes a 92,000-dalton protein (P92) and has in its genome a deletion of about 600 bp, which has been mapped in the *abl* region. Whereas P90 and P100 are less efficient in transformation of lymphoid cells but can transform fibroblasts, the P92 encoded by the *td* mutant is deficient in transformation of both fibroblasts and lymphoid cells. Although wild-type transformation is not observed, infected cells form microcolonies in soft agar after long periods of incubation. The P92 protein, unlike that of P90 and P100, has no detectable kinase activity in vitro, but it can be phosphorylated by wild-type P120. P90 and P100, which do contain residual kinase activity, can transform fibroblasts. Since P92, P90, and P100 defects occur in the same portion of the Ab-MLV polyprotein, the available data suggest that, although kinase activity is needed for transformation of both cell types, lymphoid-cell transformation is more sensitive to loss of enzymic activity than is fibroblast transformation (O. Witte, pers. comm.). Therefore, one gene product may be responsible for transformation of two cell types in the Ab-MLV system.

In summary, the genetic studies of the acute leukemia viruses are providing information on the transforming genes of these viruses, but additional mutants will be invaluable in defining the virus-coded nature of the various proteins associated with these viruses, as well as their roles in oncogenesis. There are no reports of avian AcLV mutants with defects in fibroblast transformation. It is too early to judge whether this is indicative of an important feature of avian AcLV transformation, such as a tight coupling of infection of fibroblasts and their ultimate transformation. The results with Ab-MLV show that it is possible to isolate a *td* variant that does not transform fibroblasts and that both hematopoietic-cell transformation and fibroblast transformation presumably may occur via the same gene product. The success of mutant isolation has and will depend on an ability to grow and assay the hematopoietic target cells. This is well under way for the erythroid target of AEV and the pre-B-cell target of Ab-MLV (see Chapter 8). For the viruses that transform avian myeloid cells, such as MC29 or AMV, work is just commencing (Gazzolo et al. 1979).

B. Replicative Genes

By far the greatest number of conditional and nonconditional RSV mutants are of the *src* mutation class. This may possibly be a function of the assays used to screen for mutants and/or the general leakiness of mutations in replicative functions and/or complementation or recombination with endogenous viral or cellular products. Alternatively, *src* mutants may be easier to detect because of a greater sensitivity of the transformed phenotype to small decreases in $pp60^{src}$, than of the replicative phenotypes to decreases in their gene products. Nonetheless, the isolation of complex RSV mutants containing lesions in replicative functions actually preceded the isolation of Martin's *ts src* mutants by a year (Toyoshima and Vogt 1969). These mutants, LA334m and LA336m, contained mutations in both replicative and transforming functions. The first temperature-sensitive replication mutants to be well-characterized biochemically were those with polymerase lesions, and such mutants conclusively proved the virus-encoded nature of this enzyme in avian viruses (Linial and Mason 1973; Mason et al. 1974; Verma et al. 1974) and in murine viruses (Stephenson and Aaronson 1973; Tronick et al. 1975). Several nonconditional *pol* mutants have been isolated and characterized as well (Hanafusa and Hanafusa 1971; Linial et al. 1978a; Gerwin et al. 1979; Eisenman et al. 1980a). Of the three replicative genes, *pol* has been the one in which most mutants of avian viruses have been isolated. Only one well-characterized avian *ts gag* mutant exists, and it is a derivative of LA334m (Hunter and Vogt 1976); however, there are many murine *ts* and nonconditional *gag* mutants (Stephenson and Aaronson 1973; Wong et al. 1973; Shields et al. 1978). A handful of conditional and nonconditional RSV *env* mutants have been described that differ from BH-RSV(−).

1. gag

a. Avian Retroviruses. Although much is known about the synthesis, processing, and functions of the *gag*-gene proteins (see Chapter 6), very little information has been contributed by avian *gag*-gene mutants. For the purpose of this discussion, we briefly review *gag*-gene synthesis in avian oncoviruses. The *gag* gene is located near the 5′ end of the viral RNA (Fig. 7.1). The RSV gene encodes a polyprotein, $Pr76^{gag}$, which is processed intracellularly into five internal structural proteins. At the amino terminus of *gag* is located p19, which specifically interacts with the virion RNA. p15, at the carboxyl terminus of the *gag* gene, is a protease that is cleaved from the precursor, presumably by a host-cell enzyme, and, in turn, processes the other proteins. The other structural proteins are p27, the major core capsid protein, and p12, a protein that binds nonspecifically to the genomic RNA. In addition, sequencing data suggests that a fifth protein, p10, is present in $Pr76^{gag}$ (see Chapter 6 and Appendix F).

LA334m (Toyoshima and Vogt 1969) was shown to be a mutant with multiple lesions (Friis et al. 1971; Owada and Toyoshima 1973), one of which resides in *gag* (Blair et al. 1976). By crossing LA334m with PR-RSV-B, Hunter and Vogt (1976) were able to produce a recombinant that lacked the transforming mutation but retained the replicative defect. This recombinant (LA3342) was then analyzed biochemically (Hunter et al. 1976). Similar studies were also performed on LA334m itself (Friis et al. 1976; Rohrschneider et al. 1976). The major conclusion from these studies was that the defect was in virus maturation, probably due to a defective core protein. Atypical viral structures were seen budding from cells, and new intermediate $Pr76^{gag}$ cleavage products were noted; in addition, cleavage of the precursor was slower at the nonpermissive temperature. Rohrschneider et al. (1976) performed tryptic peptide analysis of LA334m proteins and found an altered p15 peptide. Since p15 has been shown to be the viral protease responsible for maturation of the other *gag* proteins (Von der Helm 1977), this alteration in p15 is consistent with the phenotype. However, leakiness of LA334m makes it difficult to obtain a completely clear picture.

Mason et al. (1979a) have described three additional temperature-sensitive replication mutants that appear to have lesions in *gag,* since they produce reduced quantities (five- to tenfold lower) of virions at 41°C with infectivity reduced 5- to 1000-fold. PH954 seems to be deficient in p27. Processing of $Pr76^{gag}$ appears slower in cells infected with PH954 and the other two mutants, PH943m and LA669, than in wild-type infections at 41°C. These mutants appear to have normal *env*-gene function. No further information on the *gag*-gene lesions is available, but PH943m is probably mutant in *gag* and *src.*

Several nonconditional mutants of *gag* have been isolated, but none of these have been very useful in elucidating the function of the various *gag* component proteins. P. Vogt et al. (1979) have described a mutant of SR-RSV-A (LA7365) that does not synthesize infectious progeny, although it has functional *env* and *src* genes. Since LA7365 has a significant rate of reversion to wild type, it probably contains a point mutation. No complementation is seen between LA7365 and the *ts gag* mutant LA3342. $Pr76^{gag}$ is not cleaved in LA7365-infected cells and therefore this mutant could have a defect either in $Pr76^{gag}$ at a key cleavage site or in p15 itself. It is suggested that LA7365 may additionally contain a second defect in *pol,* but this does not fit with its high reversion rate. A second nonconditional mutant called BO10m (Eisenman et al. 1980c) is highly defective, containing a large deletion in *pol* and *env* and a small deletion in *gag*. The virus does not encode the three major structural precursors: $gPr92^{env}$, $Pr180^{gag\text{-}pol}$, or $Pr76^{gag}$. A *gag*-related protein (P63) is synthesized but not cleaved. This protein contains the peptides of p19, p12, and p15, but not p27. P63 is cleaved poorly by p15 in vitro, but some p15 is released. Therefore, it appears that a deletion in the p27 portion of the *gag* gene may change the conformation of the precursor protein so that in vivo a host-cell protease cannot cleave p15 from the precursor; alternately, the deletion could be in the p15 cleavage site. However, since exogenously added p15 can cleave P63 to a degree, the second interpretation is less likely.

Nonconditional avian viral mutants have been isolated that synthesize small *gag*-related proteins of about 30,000 daltons, but no $Pr76^{gag}$. PH7 and PH14 each show deletions of about 90 bases in *gag* (W. Mason et al., pers. comm.), and SE33, with no detectable deletion, also produces a 30,000-dalton protein (Linial et al. 1980). The SE33 P30 protein contains determinants of p19 but not of p27 (as measured by immunoprecipitation). None of these mutants make viral particles and each is $pol^{-}env^{+}src^{+}$. The pol^{-} phenotype in these mutants can be explained if polymerase is generated from a *gag-pol* readthrough product that is not synthesized in the mutants because of a new termination signal in *gag*.

None of the RSV mutants isolated to date provide information on the role of the viral structural proteins in replication, with the possible exception of p15. Temperature-sensitive or nonconditional mutants that affect only one *gag* protein would be most useful in answering key questions about the roles of p27, p19, and p12 in virus maturation and infection. For instance, RSV p19 binds specifically to certain sites of its viral RNA (Sen and Todaro 1977; Leis et al. 1978), and it would be of great interest to investigate the effect of a p19 mutation on infectivity.

Variants of RSV have been described that are not defective per se but encode altered viral structural proteins (Shaikh et al. 1978, 1979). Recombinant viruses selected for markers in *env* and *src* or *env* and *pol* were analyzed for *gag*-gene precursors and products. It was found that many recombinants synthesize a Pr76 molecule with a greater electrophoretic mobility than that of wild-type, called ΔPr76. Recombinants from a cross between an exogenous virus and an endogenous virus (which differ in p19 tryptic peptides) encode ΔPr76 and also often encode new forms of p19, termed p19α and p19β, with apparent molecular weights of 20,000 and 15,000, respectively. Both forms of p19 are phosphorylated and contain specific p19 peptides characteristic of both parental viruses, as well as new peptides, indicating that they are recombinant proteins. p19α and p19β do not seem to affect the stability or specific infectivity of the virions and viral RNA. There is some evidence (J. Leis, pers. comm.) that p19α and p19β do not bind as tightly to viral RNA as nonrecombinant p19. It has also been demonstrated (Rettenmier and Hanafusa 1977; Shaikh et al. 1979) that the mobility of p27 proteins from an endogenous virus such as RAV-0 and exogenous RSV differ; that of endogenous virus (termed $p27_0$) is slightly slower. These results indicate that the *gag*-gene proteins can withstand some diversity in size and structure without altering their function. It is surprising that mutants have not been isolated in which *gag* changes lead to nonfunctional, but processed, structural proteins.

b. Mammalian Retroviruses. The *gag* gene of MLV also encodes a polyprotein, $Pr65^{gag}$. Four *gag* proteins (p15, pp12, p30, and p10 from amino terminus to carboxyl terminus; see below and Fig. 7.1) are processed from this precursor. A large number of both conditional and nonconditional mutants of MLV exhibit defective processing of the *gag* precursor polypeptides. Of 12 *ts* Rauscher MLV (Ra-MLV) mutants, seven (*ts*20, *ts*21, *ts*23, *ts*24, *ts*25, *ts*26, and *ts*27) express *gag* antigenic determinants at the nonpermissive temperature, in the absence of particle production (Stephenson and Aaronson 1973; Stephenson et al. 1974a). Ra-MLV *ts*25 and *ts*26 accumulate the nonglycosylated $Pr65^{gag}$ precursor (Stephenson et al. 1975). Van de Ven et al. (1978) reported that *ts*26 was slightly leaky and thus accumulated small amounts of cleaved p30. Both Ra-MLV *ts*24 (Stephenson and Aaronson 1973) and the Mo-MLV mutant *ts*3 (Wong and McCarter 1973) accumulate $Pr65^{gag}$ and the polymerase precursor $Pr180^{gag\text{-}pol}$ at the cell membrane under nonpermissive conditions (Witte and Baltimore 1978), but the exact nature of the lesion(s) is unknown. Genetic analysis of Ra-MLV *ts*25 indicates that the *ts* lesion segregates with the 3′end of the *gag* region, perhaps within the sequences encoding p10 (Aaronson and Barbacid 1980). Ra-MLV *ts*17 appears to be defective in an early function when infection is initiated at the nonpermissive temperature (Stephenson and Aaronson 1973) and accumulates uncleaved $Pr65^{gag}$ when the infection is initiated at the permissive temperature and the cells are then shifted to the nonpermissive temperature (Van de Ven et al. 1978). The relationship of the *gag*-gene lesion to the early defect is unknown.

Ra-MLV *ts*29-infected cells (Stephenson and Aaronson 1973) accumulate partially cleaved *gag* intermediates. One intermediate contains pp12, p30, and p10 antigenic determinants, and a smaller one contains p15 and pp12 determinants. A third small fragment contains pp12 and p30 determinants. Thus, this mutant made it possible to deduce that the order of the *gag* proteins on the Ra-MLV precursor is NH_2-p15-pp12-p30-p10-COOH (Reynolds and Stephenson 1977).

It has been suggested that the defects in *ts*25, *ts*26, and *ts*29 Ra-

MLV lead to precursors with altered structures that prevent normal *gag*-gene-product cleavage, rather than to defects in a virion-coded cleavage enzyme. This conclusion was reached because no complementation for Ra-MLV production was observed at the nonpermissive temperature in cells doubly infected with the *ts* mutants and a wild-type xenotropic MLV (Reynolds and Stephenson 1977). The picture is clouded, however, by the fact that both *ts*29 and *ts*26 appear to contain multiple mutations. *ts*29 contains a defect in *pol* (Tronick et al. 1975), and *ts*26 is defective in the processing of *env* precursors (Ruta et al. 1979). No attempt has yet been made to manipulate these mutants genetically, as in the case of the RSV multiple mutants; so no direct evidence exists for multiple mutations. The possibility that the *gag* cleavage defect in *ts*26 is due to a pleiotropic effect of an *env*-gene lesion has been suggested (Ruta et al. 1979). Several recently isolated *ts* Mo-MLV mutants contain defects in the *pol* gene that lead to the accumulation of unprocessed *gag* precursors (P. Traktman and D. Baltimore, pers. comm.). This suggests that a mammalian equivalent of the avian virus p15 protease may be present in the $Pr180^{gag\text{-}pol}$ precursor and that lesions within this structure may have a pleiotropic effect on both cleavage and polymerase function.

A number of nonconditional MLV mutants that affect *gag* synthesis or *gag* processing have been isolated either by cloning chronically infected cells (Besmer et al. 1979) or by cloning single cells immediately after MLV infection (Shields et al. 1978). In the latter case, 10 out of 31 clones derived from an infection with a cloned Mo-MLV stock appeared to contain nonconditionally defective MLV genomes. Several of the defective clones were analyzed phenotypically. M11 produces a replicating virus that induces no XC plaques, and M10 induces small XC plaques only. These are similar in their properties to variants with normal *gag* synthesis and processing patterns that had been previously reported (Hopkins and Jolicoeur 1975; Rapp and Nowinski 1976; Rein et al. 1978). Two other clones, M13 and M6, produce defective particles that lack both polymerase activity and intracellular $Pr180^{gag\text{-}pol}$. The particles released by these clones contain $Pr65^{gag}$ as a major component, suggesting that these viruses are defective in some function necessary for normal *gag* processing. Pulse-chase experiments with M13-infected cells and particles support this hypothesis. These two variants differ, however, in that M13-infected cells contain a relatively high level of the *env* precursor, gPr80^{env} (equal to or greater than wild-type levels), whereas M6-infected cells express a much lower level. The sensitivity to superinfection with either MLV pseudotypes of vesicular stomatitis virus (VSV) or MLV itself seems to parallel the gPr80^{env} levels, cells infected with M6 being about 20- to 50-fold more sensitive to superinfection than those with M13 (Shields et al. 1978). The obviously pleiotropic nature of the defect seen in these variants raises questions about the number and nature of the lesions involved. It is possible that a single defect at the level of RNA splicing, for example, could account for all of the proposed variations; alternatively, the possibility that a component of Pr180$^{gag\text{-}pol}$ is involved in processing of the other viral structural proteins, as suggested above, must also be considered.

A fifth variant, M23 (Shields et al. 1978), appears to have arisen as the result of a 1000–1500-base deletion. Infected cells release low levels of particles containing RNA slightly smaller than 70S; upon denaturation, the RNA yields clearly smaller subunits. M23-infected cells contain unprocessed Pr65^{gag} but no detectable Pr180$^{gag\text{-}pol}$ or gPr80^{env}. M23-infected cells are completely susceptible to MLV superinfection and, as with M6, would probably be superinfected with wild-type MLV under mass culture conditions. The exact location of the deletion in M23 is unknown, and the determination of this, as well as the effect of the deletion on the generation of subgenomic *env* message, would be of great interest. These mutants indicate that, as in the avian system, murine retroviral particles lacking polymerase or lacking both polymerase and glycoprotein can be assembled. However, since M23 (which produces low levels of particles) lacks glycoprotein, it has been suggested that the production of glycoprotein may increase the efficiency of particle budding (Hanafusa et al. 1972; Kawai and Hanafusa 1973; Eisenman et al. 1980a; Linial et al. 1980). This is consistent with the behavior of Ra-MLV *ts*26, where a block in gp70 production results in a decrease in particle production at the nonpermissive temperature (Ruta et al. 1979).

Shields et al. (1978) also described mutants of Mo-MLV in nonproducer rat NRK cells, called NX-1 through NX-4. Recent data (Yoshimura and Yamamura 1981) show that these mutants synthesize Pr65^{gag} and gPr80^{env}, but only NX-1 makes Pr180$^{gag\text{-}pol}$. However, processing of the virion *gag* proteins by the mutants is defective. XC-negative, polymerase-negative virions are produced that contain viral RNA, Pr65^{gag}, and/or Pr40^{gag}, but little or no mature *gag*-gene proteins. Only NX-4 has a detectable proviral deletion, lacking 1.7 kb in the *pol* region. The RNA packaged by the mutants is 38S, except in the case of NX-4, which packages 33S RNA. These results indicate that RNA can be packaged and exported from the cell in the absence of mature *gag* proteins, but such virions are noninfectious.

Another type of nonconditionally defective Mo-MLV has been isolated by Besmer et al. (1979) from BALB/c mouse JLS-V11 cells. These cells, designated V11-NP, contain an MLV provirus with a deletion of about 1000 nucleotides. They produce no detectable Pr180$^{gag\text{-}pol}$ or Pr65^{gag}, but a 45,000-dalton *gag* product is detectable. gPr80^{env} production and processing are normal in these cells. The cells are resistant to superinfection and contain an apparently normal gp70 on their surface. Treatment of these cells with iododeoxyuridine generates an N-tropic XC^{+} MLV, which is probably a recombinant between an endogenous BALB/c N-tropic provirus and the large-XC-plaque morphology marker of the mutant Mo-MLV.

The ease of isolation of nonconditional variants reported by Shields et al. (1978) and Besmer et al. (1979) indicates that at least some isolates of MLV are highly mutable. Because similar mutants were isolated in both mouse and rat cells, it would be of interest to determine whether this high rate of spontaneous mutation is a common characteristic of all mammalian C-type viruses in different cell types.

A number of nonconditional mutants have been isolated from other mammalian retroviruses, but they have been only partially characterized. By selecting for cell clones that express viral antigens but fail to release infectious virus, a number of apparently nonconditional defective mutants of RD114 (cat endogenous virus), M7 (baboon endogenous virus), and D-type squirrel monkey retrovirus (SMRV) have been isolated. All of these mutants appear to be defective in the processing of *gag*-gene polyproteins (Sacks et al. 1978). Although the susceptibility of these clones to superinfection and their similarity to certain conditional MLV mutants favor the assumption that they represent viral mutants, this has not been conclusively demonstrated. Two of these mutants, SMRV 103-10 and

SMRV 86-9, have been useful in establishing the order of proteins in the *gag* gene of SMRV as NH_2-p16-pp12-p35-p9-COOH (Devare and Stephenson 1979).

2. pol

a. Avian Retroviruses. The majority of the temperature-sensitive replication mutants of RSV have been assigned to the *pol*-gene class, and these mutants have made important contributions to our understanding of RNA-dependent DNA-polymerase (reverse transcriptase) structure and function (see Chapter 5). The *pol* gene is located adjacent to *gag*, and the candidate primary translational precursor protein for *pol* is a 180,000-dalton *gag-pol* protein, called $Pr180^{gag-pol}$ (Oppermann et al. 1977; Paterson et al. 1977; Purchio et al. 1977). Mature avian virus polymerase contains two subunits, α (58,000 daltons) and β (92,000 daltons). Three enzymic activities, RNA-dependent and DNA-dependent polymerases and RNase H, are associated with the α subunit, which is processed from the β subunit, and an endonuclease activity is associated with the other cleavage product of β, p32 (see Chapters 5 and 6).

The first *ts* polymerase mutants identified were LA337 and LA335 (Linial and Mason 1973; Wyke 1973a). These mutants have a coordinate *ts* defect in both replication and transformation. The *ts* function is required only during the first few hours after infection; once infection is initiated at 35° C, a shift to 41° C has no effect. Conversely, when infection is initiated at 41° C, infectivity decays rapidly (see Table 7.2). The infectivity of LA335 and LA337 virions is inactivated more rapidly at 41° C than that of wild-type virus, and the activity of the virion reverse transcriptase is temperature-sensitive. Both wild-type recombinants, obtained after coinfection with ALV, and revertants have reverse transcriptase that is no longer thermolabile (Mason et al. 1974). Verma and his colleagues purified the enzyme from mutant viruses and showed that the RNA-dependent and DNA-dependent polymerase, as well as RNase H, activities were thermolabile (Verma 1975) (see also Chapter 5) and associated with the α subunit of polymerase. In cells infected with LA335 or LA337, the synthesis of both strands of proviral DNA is reduced at the nonpermissive temperature (Verma et al. 1974, 1976; Varmus et al. 1975). These results showed conclusively that the RNA-dependent DNA polymerase of RSV is a virus-coded enzyme responsible for intracellular viral DNA synthesis.

Another mutant, LA336m (Toyoshima and Vogt 1969), contains multiple mutations. The early defect in LA336m is a thermolabile polymerase, but this was not revealed until the enzyme was purified, as virions are not heat-sensitive. Apparently, the enzyme in LA336m virions is protected from denaturation by association with the viral RNA template. All three enzymic activities in LA336m are thermolabile (Verma et al. 1976).

LA672 represents a third type of *ts* polymerase mutant with a defect late in replication (Friis and Hunter 1973). Virus produced at 35° C can transform cells at 35° C and 41° C, but viral particles produced at 41° C are noninfectious at either temperature (see Table 7.3). Within 3 hours of a shift from 35°C to 41° C, only noninfectious particles are produced. Virus produced at 35° C contains temperature-stable enzyme, but that produced at 41° C has a 20-fold reduction in polymerase activity (Friis et al. 1975). Later studies by Moelling and Friis (1979) demonstrated by radioimmunoassay and enzyme purification that LA672 particles produced at 41° C contain less than half the level of polymerase molecules, compared with that of wild-type virions, and that the protein is inactive in both the synthetic and endonucleolytic activities. Therefore, LA672 contains a mutation that affects the maturation of polymerase.

Moelling and Friis (1979) reexamined LA338m (see Sections V.A.1 and V.B.3), which contains a *src* mutation as well as a replication defect. They found that the polymerase activity in LA338m is slightly thermolabile and loses activity on synthetic template: primers more rapidly than on endogenous viral RNA. In addition, the early mutation described for LA343m may also be in the *pol* gene (Panet et al. 1978), since less polymerase is incorporated into the virions produced at 41° C; however, this assignment is very tentative and awaits further study.

A large number of additional *ts pol* mutants have been isolated that resemble LA335, LA337, and LA672. Alevy and Vogt (1978) isolated 27 replication mutants of PR-RSV-C (LA351–377), all of which appear to be early coordinate mutants with thermolabile polymerase, like LA335 and LA337, but which have leakier properties. None of these mutants map at the same site as LA337, because they recombine with LA337 to yield wild-type virus. Mason et al. (1979a) isolated six additional *pol* mutants, four of which are like LA337 (PH543, PH553, PH568, and PH620). The mutations of three of these viruses map at sites distinct from that of LA337, but

PH543 does not recombine with LA337 (LA335 and LA337 apparently map at the same site). Two other *pol* mutants with late replicative defects include PH912 and PH1045. Like LA672, they can replicate at both temperatures, but virus produced at 41°C is noninfectious. In addition, PH1045 virions harvested at 35°C are heat-sensitive, as is the polymerase activity; so there could be two mutations or a single mutation affecting both thermostability and maturation.

Studies to distinguish the defective functions in the various polymerase mutants are in their infancy, but some interesting results have been obtained. The Mn^{++}-dependent DNA endonuclease activity associated with $\alpha\beta$ polymerase (Golomb and Grandgenett 1979) was examined in four *ts pol* mutants with similar biological phenotypes: LA335, LA337, PH553, and PH568 (Golomb et al. 1981). It was found that the endonuclease activities of LA335 and LA337 were more thermolabile than that of wild type, whereas the activities in PH553 and PH568 were as stable as that of wild type. This correlates well with the fact that LA335 and LA337 appear to map at the same site, whereas PH553 and PH568 contain a different mutation. These results also show that the Mn^{++}-dependent endonuclease activity is a virus-coded function, but they do not identify a function for the endonuclease in the virus life cycle. It should be pointed out that all *ts pol* mutants that have been tested for RNase-H activity are temperature-sensitive for both RNase-H activity and polymerase activity and that no mutants have been isolated that are temperature-sensitive for RNase-H activity alone. In addition, no *ts pol* mutants in DNA endonuclease activity alone have been isolated.

A number of nonconditional mutants of *pol* have also been isolated from RSV. The first polymerase-defective deletion mutants, described by Hanafusa and coworkers, were found in stocks of envelope-defective BH-RSV(−) and NY8. These were named α mutants (Hanafusa and Hanafusa 1968; Hanafusa et al. 1970; Kawai and Hanafusa 1973). RSV(−)α and NY8α virions contain no polymerase activity and, in the case of RSV(−)α, the virion contains no cross-reactive protein (Hanafusa and Hanafusa 1971; Hanafusa et al. 1972; Kawai and Hanafusa 1973; Panet et al. 1975). Murphy (1977) obtained a $pol^{-}env^{+}$ clone of BH-RSV(−)-transformed turkey cells, called α48T, which separated the two mutations. (Although the mechanism by which subgroup-A specificity has been acquired by this virus has not been fully examined, it is possible that recombination may have occurred during one of the many passages as a pseudotype with helper virus.) The genome of NY8α is only slightly smaller than that of NY8, suggesting a small *pol* deletion (Wang 1978). The absence of polymerase in α virions did not present conclusive evidence that the enzyme was virus-coded. Other explanations for the lack of polymerase were entirely plausible, such as a defect in virus packaging or in a cellular enzyme required for infectivity.

Other nonconditional polymerase mutants have been described that synthesize nonfunctional polyproteins containing polymerase peptides. SE52d was isolated as a polymerase-defective mutant from a cross of PR-RSV-C and RAV-0 (Linial et al. 1978b). It was originally thought to contain a deletion in the polymerase gene, but subsequent experiments revealed that the apparent deletion may be due to substitution of endogenous quail cell information. A probe made to the specific sequences of SE52d virion RNA hybridized to a specific restriction fragment in uninfected quail cells. The fragment was quail-specific, because these sequences were not detected in chicken, pheasant or other avian DNAs (Eisenman et al. 1980b; P. Neiman and M. Linial, pers. comm.). Antisera to *gag* or *pol* precipitate a 125,000-dalton protein from SE52d-transformed cells. This protein (P125) contains *gag* peptides but no detectable polymerase peptides. The origin of the non-*gag* portion of SE52d P125 is an unresolved question, but the immunoprecipitation data suggest that at least a small part comes from *pol*.

Another nonconditional polymerase mutant, PH9, has a deletion of 0.62 kb near the 3′ end of the *pol* gene. Instead of $\mathrm{Pr180}^{gag\text{-}pol}$, a protein of 140,000 daltons (P140) is synthesized that contains *gag* and *pol* peptides and probably terminates near the deletion boundary (Mason et al. 1979b; Eisenman et al. 1980a). This mutant has proved useful in determining the order of the α and β subunits in the polymerase gene (Fig. 7.1). Grandgenett and his coworkers have shown that a 32,000-dalton protein (p32) with endonucleolytic activity is contained within the β, but not the α, subunit and is derived by cleavage from $\beta : \beta \rightarrow \alpha + \mathrm{p32}$ (Grandgenett et al. 1978, 1980; Schiff and Grandgenett 1978). Eisenman et al. (1980a) were able to show that anti-p32 serum did not precipitate the PH9 P140 protein synthesized from the 5′ end of *pol*. The simplest interpretation of these results is that α and β share aminoterminal sequences and that p32 is cleaved from the carboxyl terminus of *pol* (Fig. 7.1). This model has been confirmed by protein sequencing, which shows that the α- and β-polymerase subunits do indeed contain the same aminoterminal amino acids (Copeland et al. 1980).

Several other nonconditional mutants in *pol* have been partially characterized (W. Mason, pers. comm.). PH16m has a 0.75-kb deletion in *pol* extending into *env* and produces no detectable *pol*- or *env*-gene products. PH17m encodes a protein smaller than Pr180$^{gag-pol}$ of about 170,000 daltons. Neither PH16m nor PH17m complements *env* mutants, such as BH-RSV(−), nor do they synthesize any *env*-related protein. No deletion has been found in the PH17m provirus.

b. Mammalian Retroviruses. The *pol* gene of murine viruses encodes a single polypeptide of 80,000 daltons, which is the active form of reverse transcriptase. The enzyme is processed from a 180,000-dalton precursor containing *gag* and *pol* information (Pr180$^{gag-pol}$; see Fig. 7.1 and Chapter 6). Genetic evidence that this is virus-coded was based on Ra-MLV *ts*29, which was shown to encode a thermolabile reverse transcriptase (Tronick et al. 1975). Further analysis of *ts*29 demonstrated that both reverse transcriptase and RNase-H activity copurify as a single peptide and that both activities are two- to threefold more thermolabile than the activities derived from wild-type Ra-MLV. A revertant capable of growing at the nonpermissive temperature was also shown to contain polymerase and RNase-H activities with normal heat stability (Lai et al. 1978).

Analysis of two mutants, Ra-MLV *ts*24 (Stephenson and Aaronson 1973) and Mo-MLV *ts*3 (Wong et al. 1973), indicates that the reverse transcriptase is enzymically inactive in its Pr180$^{gag-pol}$ precursor form and is activated only after cleavage to p80. At the nonpermissive temperature, these mutants fail to cleave Pr180$^{gag-pol}$. Cleavage apparently occurs after virion release, as polymerase activity is found only in virions released after shifting to the permissive temperature cells infected by these mutants (Witte and Baltimore 1978). These experiments lend credence to the idea that Pr180$^{gag-pol}$ is the actual precursor that is cleaved to mature polymerase. A *ts* mutant that does not cleave polymerase precursors has not been found in the avian retrovirus system.

A nonconditional mutant of MLV has also been isolated in which the defect appears to be within the polymerase or its precursor (Gerwin et al. 1979). A clone derived from a cell originally infected with this variant (clone 23) does not contain any detectable intracellular $Pr180^{gag-pol}$ but does contain 114,000-dalton and 117,000-dalton peptides precipitable by anti-*pol* sera. The small amount of active polymerase that can be recovered from the noninfectious virions produced by this cell line appears smaller in glycerol gradients than that of wild-type virus. How these peptides relate to normal polymerase is not yet known.

In addition, several nonconditional variants that release defective particles and are defective in the production of $Pr180^{gag-pol}$ have been described by Shields et al. (1978) and are discussed more fully in the section on MLV *gag* mutants (see Section V.B.1.b).

One mutant of a D-type retrovirus has been isolated that may have a defect in polymerase. This mutant of Mason-Pfizer monkey virus (MPMV) is called rd 1 (S. Chatterjee and E. Hunter, pers. comm.). Cells infected with this mutant contain normal $Pr78^{gag}$ and $gPr86^{env}$ precursors but apparently make no *gag-pol* precursor.

3. env

a. Avian Retroviruses. The viral-envelope gene of ALV and ASV encodes two viral glycoproteins, gp85 and gp37, which are synthesized as a single precursor molecule. The precursor, $gPr92^{env}$, is cleaved by an unknown enzyme into the mature products. The nonglycosylated form of $gPr92^{env}$ has a molecular weight of 57,000 to 62,000, depending on the virus strain (see Chapter 6). gp85 and gp37 are required only for virus adsorption and/or penetration (Weiss 1969; T. Hanafusa et al. 1970b); once an envelope-defective virion enters the cell, it is replicated normally, producing new virions lacking glycoproteins. The prototype env^- mutant BH-RSV(−) is described in Section III.B. Several other RSV *env* deletion mutants have been isolated, as well as four *ts* mutants. Some are recombinants with viral or endogenous cellular sequences. Such viruses exhibit altered or extended host ranges or different biological properties. Some of these are considered in this section, although, in a few cases, it is unclear as to whether the altered sequences are within the *env* gene or outside the gene near the 3′ end of the RNA.

LA30m and LA338m (Wyke 1973a) have mutations in the *env* gene in addition to other lesions. Tato et al. (1978) showed that the early defect in LA30m renders the virions heat-labile and that the early lesion is temperature-sensitive only before penetration. A biochemical analysis of LA30m has not been reported. However, coinfection with LA30m and an ALV of different host range leads to production of transforming virus that is more stable than that produced in a single infection by LA30m. In addition, virus from mixed infection can show the LA30m host range. Therefore, the particles are phenotypically mixed. LA338m, which was described above (Sections V.A.1 and V.B.2.a) as having mutations in *pol* and *src,* also has an *env* mutation (Hunter 1980). LA338m particles produced at 41°C have reduced amounts of gp85 and gp37 but do contain $gPr92^{env}$. After long chases, labeled precursor associated with virions is cleaved, but the products are not found in virions. Glycoprotein, apparently the size of gp85, is found in the medium (J. Hardwick and E. Hunter, pers. comm.). Thus, this mutant appears to have a defect in *env* that prevents normal processing.

A third *ts env* mutant, PH734, has been reported by Mason and Yeater (1977). This virus contains a mutation only in *env* and is a late-replication mutant. Virions produced at 41°C are deficient in gp85 and gp37. If PH734-infected cells are superinfected at 41°C with an ALV of a different subgroup, the particles produced do not have the PH734 subgroup specificity. Furthermore, PH734 cannot complement BH-RSV(−) at the nonpermissive temperature. These results indicate that PH734 virions lack subgroup determinants at 41°C. Glycoprotein appears to accumulate in PH734-infected cells at 41°C; however, it is unknown whether the accumulated glycoprotein is mature gp85 or the precursor $gPr92^{env}$. If the latter were the case, these mutants might be defective in cleavage. The fourth *ts env* mutant PH668 (Mason et al. 1979a) is similar to PH734 but has not been further characterized. Clearly, additional biochemical analysis of these mutants is required to define the steps that are affected in glycoprotein synthesis or processing.

As described earlier in this chapter, BH-RSV(−) was the first defective variant of RSV reported. The virus was shown by Scheele and Hanafusa (1971) to lack the major viral glycoproteins. In 1973, Kawai and Hanafusa described NY8, a derivative of SR-RSV-A, that has a phenotype similar to that of BH-RSV(−) and also lacks glycoproteins. The RNA of NY8 is 21% smaller than that of the parental virus. It is assumed that the entire envelope region is deleted, and this has been used as the physical definition of the *env* region (Duesberg et al. 1975). Several other nonconditional *env* mutants with different phenotypes have been isolated. PH10 (Mason et al. 1979b) bears a deletion of about 130 bases in *env*. The deletion is near the 3′ end of the *env* gene so that only the gp37 region might be affected. Virions produced by PH10 cells are noninfectious. However, after superinfection with ALV, transforming virus is produced with the PH10 host range, suggesting that the deletion is not involved in subgroup specificity. Intracellularly, PH10 directs the synthesis of a protein slightly smaller than the normal glucosamine- and mannose-containing precursor, but virions contain no glycoprotein (W. Mason and M. Linial, pers. comm.). The inactive precursor must contain the specificity for host range and is presumably cleaved and incorporated into virions upon superinfection. A mutant with a similar phenotype has also been described by Steimer and Boettiger (1979). PN3/2 cells were derived by infection of rat embryo cells by SR-RSV-D. Virus rescued from PN3/2 cells is *env*$^-$ but exhibits the host-range specificity of SR-RSV-D upon rescue by fusion with chicken cells infected with ALV of different subgroups. Glycoprotein synthesized intracellularly in PN3/2-infected nonproducer chicken cells is not incorporated into virions (Steimer and Boettiger 1980).

SE521 is another type of nonconditional *env* mutant (Linial et al. 1980). The provirus exhibits no detectable deletion; however, the virus behaves like a deletion mutant, since no revertants are produced. A gPr92^{env} molecule with apparently normal glycosylation is synthesized, and the nonglycosylated form of gp85, P57^{env}, is the same size as that of the parental wild type. However, the glycoprotein precursor in this mutant is not cleaved to mature glycoprotein or to any aberrant products and appears to remain associated with the cell surface. This suggests that transport of precursor to the cell surface precedes the additional steps (e.g., cleavage and/or further glycosylation) necessary to produce mature glycoproteins. The mutation is not cellular because superinfecting viruses replicate normally. The uncleaved gPr92^{env} is able to induce subgroup-specific virus interference (see Chapter 3), since superinfecting viruses of the same, but not of different, subgroups are prevented from superinfection. SE521 differs from LA338m in that uncleaved gPr92^{env} is packaged at the nonpermissive temperature into LA338m virions (J. Hardwick and E. Hunter, pers. comm.).

Linial et al. (1980) also described experiments on glycoprotein processing, utilizing a nonconditional mutant in the *gag* gene, SE33. This mutant makes no mature *gag* or *pol* proteins and no particles, but gPr92^{env} is synthesized. Moreover, the precursor is cleaved to mature glycoprotein faster than in cells infected with wild-type virus, suggesting that particle production is not required for cleavage. The glycoprotein that is synthesized is found on the cell surface. PH7 and PH14 (W. Mason, pers. comm.) have phenotypes similar to that of SE33 (e.g., particle$^-$*env*$^+$), but have not been analyzed in detail.

The *env* gene is responsible for the host range (see Chapter 3) and thus defines a genetic marker in avian viruses. Mutations within the host-range-determining (or subgroup-specific) sequences of *env* could alter the host range without producing replication-defective virus. Such mutations are extremely rare. However, *env* changes in avian virus recombinants have been described by Tsichlis et al. (1980); two recombinants between either subgroups B and E (NTRE-4) or subgroups D and E (SR-DE-1) were obtained that exhibit dual host range, in that they can infect T/BD and C/E cells with equal efficiency. A single subgroup-E-associated oligonucleotide was identified in the *env* region of each virus. A third variant, BO1, was described as a mutant in *env* with B and E dual host range. The authors suggested that these viruses interact with subgroup-B receptors on chicken cells and subgroup-E receptors on turkey cells. It is not known whether these viruses can use the subgroup-E-specific receptor coded by the *tv-e* locus in chicken cells. More recent work indicates that BO1 might be a recombinant with the endogenous chicken virus locus *ev*-1 (K. Conklin and J. Coffin, pers. comm.). Recombination with endogenous viral sequences could be a mechanism for generation of these rare variants.

b. Mammalian Retroviruses. The *env* gene of the MLVs encodes 80,000-dalton or 90,000-dalton precursor peptides (for Moloney or Rauscher viruses, respectively) which are processed into gp70 (the major viral-envelope glycoprotein) and the nonglycosylated p15(E) (see Figure 7.1 and Chapter 6). The murine, and other mammalian, sarcoma viruses are naturally occurring *env*$^-$ deletion/substitution mutants and lack most or all of the helper-virus *env*-gene sequences, as is the case for BH-RSV(−). There are also a large number of naturally occurring *env* variants (ecotropic and xenotropic MLVs), as well as apparent *env*-gene recombinants (HIX and MCF viruses) (see Chapters 4 and 10).

Only one MLV *ts* mutant has been described that appears to contain a lesion affecting *env*-gene expression. Cells infected with the Ra-MLV mutant *ts*26, initially described as being defective in *gag* precursor cleavage (see Section V.B.1.b) (Stephenson et al. 1975), were subsequently shown by Ruta et al. (1979) to accumulate the glycoprotein precursor, gPr90^{env}, rapidly upon shift from permissive to nonpermissive growth conditions. Upon such shift, formation of gp70 and p15(E) ceases, the cell surface becomes depleted of gp70 antigens, and the cells release defective virions that lack gp70 and p15(E). The rate of Pr65^{gag} processing also is reduced but not blocked, and the noninfectious particles contain p30 with altered charge properties, as well as a lower relative level of reverse transcriptase activity. Whether these multiple effects represent multiple lesions or simply pleiotropic effects of a single lesion remains unresolved, although further genetic analysis should clarify this question.

Two nonconditional Mo-MLV mutants described by Shields et al. (1978) express altered levels of gPr80^{env} intracellularly. M23-infected cells lack detectable gPr80^{env} and are completely susceptible to superinfection, whereas M6-infected cells produce low levels of gPr80^{env} and are moderately susceptible to MLV superinfection. These two mutants are discussed more fully in Section V.B.1.b.

In addition, Vaidya et al. (1980) have recently described a mutant of mouse mammary tumor virus (MMTV) that appears to be defective in the *env* gene. The absence of *env* proteins in virions and the presence of *env* precursor and cleaved *env* products in the supernates suggest a resemblance to the *env* lesion described for the avian retrovirus mutant *ts* LA338m described above (see Section V.B.3.a.).

4. Virus Assembly and Maturation

The availability of several mutants of both Mo-MLV (*ts*3) and Ra-MLV (*ts*24, *ts*25, and *ts*29), which are blocked late in the virus life cycle, has allowed a dramatic visualization of the process of virus maturation and assembly. By combining transmission and scanning electron microscopy with biochemical analysis, and by utilizing temperature shifts that result in the highly synchronized assembly and release of viral particles, it has been possible to observe visually the stages of virus budding, release, and subsequent maturation (Wong and MacLeod 1975; Yeger et al. 1976, 1978; Yuen and Wong 1977; Witte and Baltimore 1978; Yeger and Kalnins 1978; Lu et al. 1979). These studies indicate that processing of Pr180$^{gag\text{-}pol}$ and most, if not all, of the Pr65^{gag} occurs after virus release (see also Chapter 6).

Assembly of MLV particles at the cell surface can occur at 0° C (Demsey et al. 1979), but particle release is blocked, suggesting that release may involve an energy-dependent step. Conversion of free virus from an immature to a mature C-type structure requires up to 3 hours at 37° C in cell-free medium (Yuen and Wong 1977; Lu et al. 1979), but some viral particles never undergo maturation. Data obtained using purified immature particles suggest that these particles are deficient in virion-associated protease (Yoshinaka et al. 1980) (see Chapter 6). The nature of this protease is unknown because, as yet, no murine virus analog of the avian virus p15 protease has been definitively identified.

C. Other Regions of the Viral Genome

1. 5′ Region Involved in Packaging

A unique nonconditional mutant of RSV has been described by Linial et al. (1978b). The mutant, SE21Q1b, which is maintained in a line of transformed quail cells, directs the synthesis of all the known intracellular viral mRNAs and proteins. Noninfectious particles are produced, containing normal *gag-*, *pol-*, and *env*-gene products. However, instead of packaging viral 38S genomic RNA, SE21Q1b particles package predominantly cellular RNA. The packaged RNA is primarily polyadenylated and is highly efficient as a template for translation in vitro, suggesting that it is mRNA. The proteins translated in vitro resemble qualitatively those found in quail cells (Gallis et al. 1979). It appears that cellular mRNAs are packaged randomly, including some virus-specific RNAs that represent about 0.7% of the packaged RNA (Linial et al. 1978a), or roughly the same proportion as in the total cellular RNA (see Chapter 5). This virus can be considered an RNA-packaging mutant. Recent work on packaging of VSV mRNA after superinfection of SE21Q1b cells demonstrates that there may be some specificity in RNA packaging, as SE21Q1b virions contain mRNA species for VSV M and NS gene proteins but not VSV G or N gene protein mRNAs (Yakobson and Weiss 1981).

The defect in SE21Q1b is a deletion of about 150 bases located between 300 and 600 bases from the 5′ terminus of the integrated proviral DNA (or 100–400 bases from the 5′ end of the viral RNA) (Shank and Linial 1980). The deletion does not include the 5′ end of *gag*, since the amino terminus of p19 is normal in SE21Q1b virions (R. Eisenman and M. Linial, pers. comm.). Rare wild-type recombinants with ALV no longer exhibit this deletion, suggesting that it is responsible for the phenotype (Shank and Linial 1980). However, this description may be an oversimplification because the mutation in SE21Q1b is *trans*-dominant. That is, superinfection of SE21Q1b cells by wild-type ALV or wild-type RSV results in replication of wild-type virus (at about 10% the normal titer), but the released virions contain 90% cellular RNA and 10% viral RNA (Linial et al. 1978a). A deletion alone could not account for the packaging of cellular RNA in the presence of bona fide viral genomes, and it is possible that there is a defect in a specific packaging protein as well. Therefore, either the SE21Q1b deletion that was mapped in the leader sequence (see Fig. 7.1 and Chapter 4) is actually in a protein-coding region or there is a second mutation in the genome that has not been detected.

As the deletion in SE21Q1b is not in a known coding region of the genome, it represents a type of mutation that could be detected only as a nonconditional mutant. It illustrates that there are probably regulatory sequences in RSV outside of the known coding regions and that a small sequence at the 5′ end of the genome is necessary for efficient packaging of viral genomic RNA. Since the packaging sequence deleted in the SE21Q1b mutation is normally part of the leader sequence spliced onto subgenomic mRNAs, and the mRNAs synthesized by this mutant function normally, it would appear that the entire leader region is not required for mRNA function (see Chapters 4 and 5).

2. Alterations at the 3′ End (U_3 Region)

The sequences (about 500 bases) 3′ to the *env* and *src* genes, in ALV and RSV, respectively, are unlikely to encode any viral proteins in view of the published nucleotide sequence (Czernilofsky et al. 1980) (see Appendix E). The 3′-terminal portion of this region (U_3) has been implicated in control of replication, because the sequences are duplicated at the ends of proviral DNA and contain putative regulatory signals (see Chapters 4 and 5). In addition, the sequences are well conserved in all exogenous viruses that replicate efficiently and cause disease in vivo, but differ from those at the 3′ end of endogenous viruses that replicate poorly in most cell types and are nonpathogenic in vivo (for details, see Chapters 4, 8, and 10).

It is interesting to speculate as to whether or not a specific gene exists for induction of cell proliferation of bursal lymphomas or other slowly developing tumors. Since endogenous nononcogenic avian retroviruses differ from the exogenous oncogenic avian retroviruses primarily at the 3′ end (Hayward 1977; Neiman et al. 1977; Coffin et al. 1978), one idea is that this region is involved in induction of disease. However, since these viruses also differ in efficiency of virus replication (Linial and Neiman 1976; Robinson 1976), the role of the 3′-end sequences in control of replication alone, without a specific gene product, could be responsible for the difference in tumorigenicity. Tsichlis and Coffin (1980) examined the oligonucleotide sequences in recombinants between exogenous and endogenous viruses and concluded that the U_3 region contains the major determinant responsible for growth rates in vitro. They suggest that there are two "alleles" for the U_3 region, U_3^n (endogenous) and U_3^x (exogenous). Viruses with endogenous viral *env* sequences and U_3^x regions cause lymphoid leukosis in birds (Crittenden et al. 1980; Robinson et al. 1980). One exception is a virus (NTRE-7) that is identical to nonleukemogenic RAV-0, except in the U_3 region (NTRE-7 contains at least part of U_3^x), and is apparently only weakly transforming in vivo (Coffin et al. 1980). More viruses will be needed to determine the relationship of the 3′ end of the genome to oncogenicity.

Many of the ALVs show differences in the spectrum of neoplasms induced in susceptible birds (for review, see Purchase and Burmester 1978; and Chapter 8). The major tumors induced by ALV are the slowly progressing lymphoid leukoses and the more rapidly appearing diseases, osteopetrosis and nephroblastoma. ALVs of different pathogenesis seem to differ in the sequences near the 3′ end of the genome. Neiman (1978) found that a field-isolated ALV, which predominantly causes lymphoid leukosis, and MAV-2(O), which predominantly causes osteopetrosis (Smith and Moscovici 1969), differ in sequences clustered near the 3′ end of the genome. The divergent sequences were localized closer to the 3′ end of the genome than the *env* deletion on BH-RSV(−). In further studies by Schmidt et al. (1982), shared oligonucleotides were assigned to the 3′ end of the genomes of four osteopetrosis-inducing viruses. These oligonucleotides appear to map at a location analogous to that of oligonucleotides in RSV that are not in *env* but are retained in *td* leukosis-inducing viruses (i.e., between *env* and *src* coding regions). Although viruses of several subgroups can cause osteopetrosis, the role of *env* sequences in specificity of disease cannot definitely be eliminated.

D. Large Deletion Mutants

There are several nonconditional RSV mutants with deletions spanning several genes. The existence of such variants is in itself interesting, although they cannot be used to elucidate functions of their individual deleted genes. Dierks et al. (1979) described a spontaneous variant of B77-RSV propagated in duck cells that contains two large noncontiguous deletions in the virion RNA. The major viral RNA is about 2.3 kb and contains two deletions, one in *src* and one in *pol.* This RNA encodes a 130,000-dalton protein (P130) that contains p27 and gp85 sequences and is therefore a *gag-env* fusion product. Since the deleted virus lacks *src* sequences, it has not been possible to maintain the mutant in a cell line in the absence of helper virus. Coffin and coworkers (J. Coffin, pers. comm.) obtained a similar mutant that arises after many passages of RSV in tissue culture. This virus has been termed *ld* (for long deletion) and was derived from PR-RSV-B. *ld* PR-RSV-B has two deletions: one of *src* and a second extending from some point in *gag* to near the 3′ end of *env. ld* PR-RSV-B is highly defective but can replicate more rapidly than *td* PR-RSV-B in mixed infection and is eventually found in three- to fivefold excess.

Two groups of investigators have described mutants, isolated in transformed quail cells, that have deletions of all the replicative genes but retain the *src* gene. PH2 is a spontaneous mutant of B77-RSV lacking 6 kb in its provirus. The long terminal repeats (LTRs) and *src* are retained, and PH2 synthesizes pp60^{src} (Mason et al. 1979b). BK301, BK303, and BK305 were derived after UV-irradiation of PR-RSV-A and apparently have similar deletions of 6 kb (Martin et al. 1979). These clones also synthesize pp60^{src} but no other viral gene products. In addition, Hughes et al. (1978) characterized the proviruses in 15 clones of RSV-transformed rat cells and found that seven clones contained mutant proviruses. One clone (clone 12) contained a deletion of 6 kb spanning *env, pol,* and most of *gag;* it appears similar to the deletion mutants just described. Virus could not be rescued from clone 12 by fusion with either uninfected or RAV-infected chicken cells. The existence of these mutants shows that the LTRs and the *src* gene are sufficient for the maintenance of transformation.

H. Hanafusa et al. (1980) have described deletion mutants obtained after injection of chickens with *td* NY109m RSV that lacks nucleotides in the *env* region (but is replication-competent). Defective viruses were found among the recovered sarcoma virus (see Section V.A.1). The intracellular proteins produced by these mutants have not been determined, but genomic maps of the RNA show that rASV 3812 has a deletion of all of *env* and part of *pol* and that rASV 398 has a deletion of *pol* and *env* extending into part of *gag*. It would be of interest to determine whether the latter synthesizes a *gag-src* readthrough product analogous to the *gag-env* product reported by Dierks et al. (1979).

E. Mutants with Unknown Lesions

Several RSV mutants have been reported for which no specific defect can be identified. These might prove to be very interesting, since they do not fall into any of the categories described previously and appear to synthesize normal gene products from all four RSV genes. These might be mutants in more subtle functions, such as primer tRNA binding or correct protein assembly. PH11 is a non-conditional mutant of B77-RSV-C that contains no detectable proviral deletion (Mason et al. 1979b). It produces noninfectious virus, but PH11-infected cells complement mutants in *gag, pol,* and *env* (M. Linial and W. Mason, pers. comm.). Viral particles contain polymerase activity and normal structural proteins, as well as genomic RNA. Superinfection with ALV leads to efficient rescue of focus-forming virus (Mason et al. 1979b). Interestingly, after repeated passage, PH11-infected cells contain tandem repeats of provirus or unintegrated circles (W. Mason, pers. comm.). The relationship of this to the noninfectious phenotype is unknown.

Mason et al. (1979a) described two *ts* replication mutants that cannot be assigned to *gag, pol, env,* or *src.* These mutants (PH746 and PH1369) produce particles at 41°C that contain apparently normal *gag* and *pol* proteins but have greatly reduced infectivity. In addition, infection with ALV rescues the mutant subgroup specificity with high efficiency, indicating normal envelope protein (or at least gp85). Since the virus produced at 35°C initiates a normal infection at 41°C, it is assumed that neither virions nor polymerase is heat-sensitive. Additional experiments to analyze details of the replicative cycle will be required to elucidate the defect in these mutants.

A number of mammalian virus mutants have also been described for which the nature of the lesion is not precisely defined. Some of these will probably be shown to be similar to other mutants in known genes when they are more extensively characterized, but others may represent defects in as yet undefined virus functions. Two Ra-MLV mutants, *ts*17 and *ts*19, were initially classified as having early defects (Stephenson and Aaronson 1973) but appear to have normal reverse transcriptase activity (Tronick et al. 1975); so the exact nature of the early defect is unknown. Another early mutant with an unidentified lesion is *ts*1 Mo-MLV (Wong et al. 1973; Wong and McCarter 1974). Again, a polymerase defect does not seem to be involved, and this mutant, in contrast to its wild-type parent, induces lower-limb paralysis and lower-spinal-cord necrosis when injected into some strains of mice (McCarter et al. 1977).

A mutant of Mo-MLV (*ts*7), described by Wong and Gallick (1978), produces particles that are about six times more heat labile at 39°C than at 34°C. Cells infected by this mutant show only a slight reduction in particle production at 39°C, but the majority of the particles are noninfectious because of their rapid heat inactivation. The reverse transcriptase activity in the virions is not heat-sensitive, indicating that a more subtle virion defect is involved that renders the virions heat labile.

Several nonconditional murine virus mutants have been described that show an interesting phenotype, but for which no lesion has been defined. These include the NP-N variants (Hopkins and Jolicoeur 1975), several XC^- variants of AKR virus (Rapp and Nowinski 1976), and clones 8A and AK24 (Rein et al. 1978, 1979a,b). Clone 8A was isolated after high-multiplicity infection of MSV-transformed mouse 3T3 cells with a stock of Mo-MLV. This cell clone exhibits a high level of particle production, a low level of infectious MSV production, and almost no infectious MLV production when scored in either the S^+L^- focus assay or the XC plaque assay (Rein et al. 1978). The infectivity of this defective virus can be detected by its low-level ability to complement a non-XC-plaque-forming amphotropic MLV for plaque formation (Rein and Bassin 1978). When infected by 8A virus in the absence of helper, cells initially show no alteration, but then spontaneously begin to produce normal wild-type XC^+ MLV after 6 to 8 weeks in culture (Rein et al. 1978). 8A virus was able to donate its N tropism to other viruses (Kashmiri et al. 1977). The properties of 8A-infected cells and virus are consistent with 8A being a leukemia virus analog of replication-defective MSV

(Rein et al. 1979a), although 8A virus has no pathogenic effect when injected into mice (Rein et al., 1978).

AK24 was derived from an AKR lymphoma cultured in vitro. Cells containing the AK24 genome produce no particles and release no particle-associated reverse transcriptase activity (Rein et al. 1979b). Thus, this virus is even more defective than clone 8A, but nothing further is known about the genomic lesion.

VI. VIRUS INTERACTIONS

The genetic and nongenetic interactions between RNA tumor viruses are diverse and undoubtedly play an important role in their life cycles. Both genetic and structural components of biologically different viruses are thought to appear in individual viruses after coinfection. This explains how highly defective viruses, such as the acute defective leukemia viruses, may be propagated in nature. In the laboratory, the complex interactions involved in RNA tumor virus replication have allowed the propagation of interesting mutants and recombinants. On the other hand, they have complicated the elucidation of the mechanisms of individual types of stable genetic recombination.

In this section, we describe the two types of virus interactions: phenotypic mixing of structural components and genetic recombination. In addition, the genetic exchange between retrovirus and host genetic elements is discussed in relation to the origin and diversity of RNA tumor viruses.

A. Phenotypic Mixing

When two related viruses infect the same cell, progeny may be formed that possess the genome of one parent, but the structural proteins, and hence the phenotypes, of either or both parents (for review, see Boettiger 1979). Retrovirus populations are frequently polymorphous, and phenotypic mixing is an important aspect of their propagation, especially for replication-defective retroviruses. Phenotypic mixing has also proved to be an extremely useful tool for studying virion protein functions and for altering the host range of retroviruses, e.g., for the introduction of avian retroviral genomes into mammalian cell lines (Hanafusa and Hanafusa 1966; Quade

1979). Phenotypic mixing should not be confused with genetic reassortment or recombination following mixed infection (see Section VI.B.1). In phenotypic mixing, only the structural proteins are exchanged and, hence, any change in the phenotype is not heritable.

1. Rescue of Defective Retroviruses by Phenotypic Mixing

Phenotypic mixing was first demonstrated among RNA tumor viruses in the rescue of BH-RSV(−), which lacks envelope glycoproteins, by the associated helper viruses RAV-1 and RAV-2 (Hanafusa et al. 1963, 1964). In this example of unilateral phenotypic mixing, the *env*-defective BH-RSV(−) is able to assemble envelope glycoproteins synthesized from the *env* genes of the helper virus; the envelope properties of the BH-RSV(−), reflected in its response to neutralizing antisera, host range, and interference pattern, are determined by the helper virus (see Chapter 3) (Hanafusa et al. 1964; Vogt 1964, 1965; Hanafusa 1965; Rubin 1965). Rubin (1965) coined the term pseudotype for RSV virions bearing RAV envelope glycoproteins, and this term is now generally used for virions carrying the genome of one virus and one or more of the proteins of another virus. Envelope pseudotypes have been very extensively used in studies of the biological properties of virion glycoproteins (see Chapter 3).

Phenotypic mixing also occurs with structural components other than envelope glycoproteins and is crucial for the propagation of replication-defective strains of transforming viruses. In the absence of helper virus, cells infected by replication-defective viruses produce either defective virions or no virions at all, depending on the nature of the defect. *gag* proteins and functions appear to be essential for the formation of virions, whereas those of *pol* and *env* are not. The BH-RSV(−)α variants of RSV lack both *pol*- and *env*-gene products, yet cells transformed by these defective genomes produce large numbers of noninfectious particles (Hanafusa and Hanafusa 1968, 1971). Superinfection with helper ALV rescues infectious BH-RSV(−)α as glycoprotein and polymerase pseudotypes. Thus, phenotypic mixing of *pol,* as well as *env,* products readily occurs. Almost every strain of mammalian sarcoma virus isolated to date is defective in at least one structural gene. Indeed, many strains are defective for *gag, pol,* and *env,* so that all the structural components of the sarcoma virus pseudotype particle are provided by the accompanying helper virus. Defective avian leukemia viruses, such as AMV (Moscovici and Vogt 1968), AEV (Graf et al. 1976), and MC29 (Bister et al. 1977) also need to be rescued by helper viruses for infectious propagation. These defective avian and mammalian transforming viruses represent the most extreme forms of phenotypic mixing when the genome of the defective virus is mixed with structural proteins entirely derived from the helper virus. The defective viral genomes can be reestablished in nonproducer cells by infection at multiplicities low enough to prevent infection of the same cells by helper virus.

Complementation of two defective strains of retrovirus has also been demonstrated through phenotypic mixing. Murphy (1977) showed that fusion of turkey cells carrying *env*⁻ and *pol*⁻ variants resulted in the production of competent infectious virus, although wild-type recombinants were not obtained (see Section V.B.2.a). Linial (1981) has similarly rescued MC29 for a single round of infection by fusion of MC29 nonproducer cells with quail cells carrying the RNA-packaging mutant RSV SE21Q1b (see Section V.C.1). In this case, the structural proteins of SE21Q1b are competent for the functional packaging of MC29 genomic RNA.

2. Phenotypic Mixing between Unrelated Viruses

During the last 10 years, numerous examples of phenotypic mixing between quite unrelated enveloped animal viruses have been reported (for review, see Zavada 1976; Boettiger 1979; Weiss 1980). Phenotypic mixing between avian or murine retroviruses and vesicular stomatitis virus (VSV) was first reported by Zavada (1972a,b). The phenotypically mixed virion components are restricted to the envelope antigens that are exchanged reciprocally, i.e., both VSV particles bearing retroviral antigens and retroviral particles bearing VSV glycoproteins can be detected in mixed virus stocks (Weiss et al. 1975, 1977; Livingston et al. 1976). In other virus combinations, only one type of virion may assemble envelope glycoproteins derived from the other virus; e.g., in mixed infection between RSV and Sindbis virus, pseudotypes of RSV with Sindbis envelope antigens are detectable, but Sindbis virions with RSV antigens are not detectable (Zavadova et al. 1977).

VSV pseudotypes bearing retroviral envelope antigens have been extensively used in studies of the host range of retroviruses and the role of virion glycoprotein cell-receptor interactions in the determination of host range (for review, see Chapter 3). The formation of

VSV pseudotypes has also been used to detect retroviral glycoproteins in latently infected cells such as chf$^+$ chick cells (Love and Weiss 1974), human cells expressing D-type retroviral antigens (Zavada et al. 1975; Altstein et al. 1976), or cells latently infected with lentiviruses (D. Gilden and R. Weiss, pers. comm.). Pseudotypes of VSV, bearing glycoproteins of retroviruses for which there are no efficient in vitro biological assays, have been used "by proxy" to probe the potential host range of the retrovirus and the action of neutralizing antibodies, for example, in the MMTV system (Zavada et al. 1977). Phenotypic mixing between VSV and retroviruses has also been used for rescue of defective mutants. ALV and RSV readily complement VSV mutants temperature-sensitive for glycoprotein maturation, although MLV is much less efficacious in rescue (Zavada and Rosenbergova 1972; Witte and Baltimore 1977; Weiss and Bennett 1980). Conversely, VSV acts as a helper virus in rescuing *env*-defective BH-RSV(−) but not other retroviral defects (Weiss et al. 1977).

In view of the widespread phenotypic mixing between envelope glycoproteins of retroviruses and VSV, it was expected that mixed assembly of envelope antigens would also occur between unrelated species of retroviruses themselves. Following Levy's (1975) discovery that xenotropic MLV can replicate in avian cells such as quail, the rescue of *env*-defective RSV by xenotropic MLV, as well as by a variety of other mammalian C-type viruses, e.g., FeLV, simian sarcoma-associated virus (SSAV), and gibbon ape leukemia virus (GALV), was demonstrated (Levy 1977; Weiss and Wong 1977). Similarly, rescue of BH-RSV(−) by the unrelated avian reticuloendotheliosis-associated virus (REAV) was observed (Sawyer and Hanafusa 1977; Vogt et al. 1977).

Phenotypic mixing among completely unrelated retroviruses seldom extends beyond envelope mixing. For example, *env$^-$pol$^-$* BH-RSV(−)α cannot be rescued by REAV (Sawyer and Hanafusa 1977) or by mammalian C-type viruses (Weiss and Wong 1977). However, it has long been known that the highly defective MSV strains can be rescued by a wide range of mammalian C-type retroviruses, such as SSAV, FeLV, and baboon endogenous virus (BaEV), which are only distantly related to MSV (see Chapters 2 and 3). In a more disparate case, MSV can be rescued as an envelope pseudotype of the B-type MMTV by cocultivation of MSV nonproducer cells with a cell line producing both MMTV and MLV (Schochetman et al.

1979). Whether MMTV is capable of complementing MSV defects other than *env* was not resolved in this experiment. Recently, the rescue of infectious MSV from nonproducer dog or rat cells has been demonstrated with avian REAV (R. Weiss and M. Harrison, pers. comm.); it should be recalled that REAV shows protein homology with the mammalian, but not avian, retroviruses (see Chapters 2 and 6). In this case, only the $S^{+}L^{-}$ strain of Mo-MSV was rescuable; infection by REAV of nonproducer cells carrying other MSV strains, such as Ki-MSV, Finkel-Biskis-Jinkins MSV (FBJ-MSV), or Ab-MLV genomes, did not result in the production of pseudotypes.

In contrast to phenotypic mixing between unrelated retroviruses in fully permissive replicative systems, there is little evidence that a second retrovirus can rescue virus in a cell type nonpermissive for one of the viruses. Thus, MLV will not rescue infectious RSV from rat cells (Weiss and Wong 1977), although simultaneous infection may transiently increase permissiveness of mammalian cells for RSV transformation and/or replication (Levy 1977).

3. Phenotypic Mixing between Nondefective Viruses

Mixed infection between nondefective retroviruses leads to the formation of virions with mixed components, rather than pure pseudotypes. Mixed infection of nondefective RSV and RAV of another envelope subgroup results in an extension of the RSV host range (Hanafusa and Hanafusa 1966; Vogt 1967). There is some evidence from antibody neutralization studies that particles with dual host range are formed (Vogt 1967). These studies were performed before the discovery of genetic reassortment of envelope markers (Vogt 1971b; Kawai and Hanafusa 1972); so it is possible that genetic exchange may also have occurred. However, it is now clear that virions with envelopes bearing a mosaic of glycoproteins, and hence a dual host range, are formed in mixed infections where recombination does not occur (Weiss and Bennett 1980). BH-RSV(−) particles bearing both RAV and VSV glycoproteins are produced when quail cells producing a RAV-1 pseudotype of BH-RSV(−) are superinfected with VSV, and it appears that there is no competition, but rather enhancement, of mixed assembly between the viral glycoproteins (Weiss et al. 1977). Selective neutralization by antisera to either parent restricts the host range of the pseudotypes to that specified by the other glycoprotein (Vogt 1967; Weiss and Bennett 1980). VSV particles phenotypically mixed with retroviruses also bear mosaic envelopes. In some cases, these are neutralizable with antiserum specific to either of the parental glycoprotein species (Zavada et al. 1975), but usually a nonneutralizable fraction is obtained that may appear to be a pure pseudotype. However, the combination of antiserum and complement has indicated mixed envelopes even in these pseudotypes (Weiss et al. 1975; Witte and Baltimore 1977), and a quantitative study, including the use of monoclonal antibodies, has shown that the vast majority of progeny particles resulting from mixed infection in permissive conditions for both RSV and VSV have mosaic envelopes (Weiss and Bennett 1980). It is important to realize, therefore, that the specification of a pseudotype, as carrying the genome of one virus and the envelope of another, is defined by function, rather than by structure. In its host-range and neutralization properties, a virion may behave as a pure pseudotype, yet the envelope may also contain a minor proportion of glycoproteins encoded by its own genome.

B. Genetic Recombination

1. Recombination following Mixed Infection

Genetic exchange between RNA tumor viruses was not fully recognized until about 10 years ago, largely because of the prevalence of phenotypic mixing in mixed infections, and because stable recombination between defective viruses and helper viruses had been sought but not found (Rubin 1964). Nevertheless, some evidence in avian tumor viruses for the acquisition of stable phenotypic markers from distinct genetic sources accrued during the late 1960s. Hanafusa and Hanafusa (1968) observed the frequent conversion of the $pol^- env^-$ BH-RSV(−)α strain to the pol^+ env$^-$ BH-RSV(−) variant following rescue with $pol^+ env^+$ helper viruses; because recombination was limited to *pol,* it was not fully recognized at first. The stable rescue of a new envelope marker by RSV or RAV passaged through chf$^+$ cells (Weiss 1969; H. Hanafusa et al. 1970; Weiss and Payne 1971) was also subsequently shown to result from genetic recombination (Weiss et al. 1973; Hanafusa et al. 1975).

The first formal demonstration of genetic exchange came from experiments involving mixed infections between nondefective strains of RSV and RAV (Vogt 1971b; Kawai and Hanafusa 1972), resulting in the stable recombination of the *env* gene of RAV (or *td* RSV) with the *src* gene of RSV. Because recombination occurred at high frequency (about 10% of all progeny) and the genome was known to be composed of subunits, it was at first thought that a reassortment of nonidentical subunits was occurring, as is seen with other RNA viruses with segmented genomes, such as reovirus and influenza virus. However, the discovery of heterozygous RSV particles (Weiss et al. 1973) led to the postulation of polyploid models for retroviral genomes (Vogt 1973; Weiss 1973), in which two or more allelic subunits may be assembled in one virion. It was later shown that the genome was, in fact, diploid and that intermolecular exchange was involved in recombination. This was accomplished by using the techniques of oligonucleotide fingerprinting of parental and recombinant 35S–39S genomic RNAs using parents that differed in defined oligonucleotides (Beemon et al. 1974; Joho et al. 1975). In an extensive analysis of the variables involved in recombination, Blair (1977) confirmed the earlier findings that the frequency of recombination is extremely high; 10–40% of the sarcoma virus progeny isolated from cells coinfected with RSV and *td* RSV undergo at least one recombinational event in crosses between *env* and *src*. Recombination frequencies are extremely high even in cases involving single genes, such as within the *src* gene (Wyke et al. 1975; Balduzzi et al. 1978), *env* gene (Wang et al. 1976b; Galehouse and Duesberg 1978), or *gag* gene (Linial and Brown 1979; Shaikh et al. 1979). Oligonucleotide mapping of recombinants obtained after several rounds of infection shows that nucleotides less than 1 kb apart behave as unlinked markers (Coffin 1979).

Recombination between viruses with different markers has also been well documented in the murine viruses. The *ts* mutants of both Mo-MLV and Ra-MLV recombine at high frequency (Wong and McCarter 1973; Stephenson et al. 1974a,b), and recombination experiments have been used to identify MLV genetic elements that cosegregate with certain biological properties. For instance, plaque variants of N-tropic and B-tropic Mo-MLVs were recombined, and the results indicated that there was a linkage between N tropism or B tropism and p30 (Schindler et al. 1977). Recombination experiments also demonstrated a linkage between the viral gp70 and the G_{IX} antigenic type expressed on the surfaces of infected cells (O'Donnell and Stockert 1976). Furthermore, although large-plaque versus small-plaque morphology could not be specifically linked to any viral gene, the evidence suggested that the determinants might map near gp70. Since recombination occurs with such high frequency, linkage probably really means identity of the biological marker and the protein marker.

2. Recombination between Exogenous and Endogenous Virus Markers

Exogenous viruses can also undergo recombination with endogenous viral genomes (see Chapter 10). For example, infection of chicken cells with RAV-2 or RSV leads to recovery among the progeny of a virus, RAV-60, which possesses the host range of the chicken endogenous virus RAV-0 (env^{E}), but differs from RAV-0 in its ability to replicate in quail cells (T. Hanafusa et al. 1970a; Weiss and Payne 1971; Hanafusa et al. 1975). The genetic compositions of Hanafusa's RAV-60 isolates appear to be intermediate between those of RAV-2 and RAV-0, as judged by nucleic acid hybridization (Hayward and Hanafusa 1975). RAV-60 viruses are presumably recombinants between a leukosis virus and viral genes (particularly env^{E}) endogenous to most normal chickens. This conclusion is supported by fingerprint analysis of RAV-60 RNAs (Robinson et al. 1980; J. Coffin, pers. comm.). The various genetic loci that encode viral structural genes (the *ev* loci) are described in detail in Chapter 10.

Nondefective RSV can also recombine with chicken endogenous virus, yielding transforming virus with an endogenous (subgroup-E) viral-envelope marker (Weiss et al. 1973). Recombination with the endogenous env^{E} gene is dependent on its expression in the cell. Whereas 2–5% of RSV progeny carried the env^{E} gene after passage through chf^{+} cells, no detectable recombinants (< 0.001%) were found in chf^{-} cells. In a more recent study, Eisenman et al. (1980b) have estimated that 0.1–0.5% of virions released after RSV infection of chf^{+} cells are recombinant for the endogenous envelope gene.

Recombination between endogenous and exogenous mammalian viruses has been demonstrated both in tissue culture (Stephenson et al. 1974b) and in leukemic mice (Barbacid et al. 1978). Recently, a tissue-culture system has been described that has allowed the more reproducible generation of such recombinants (Aaronson and Barbacid 1980). Recombinants between the endogenous xenotropic BALB virus 2 and the NB-tropic Ra-MLV *ts*25 mutant were isolated following cocultivation of the two viruses in wild-mouse embryo cells. Recombinants were characterized immunologically and for the expression of various biological parameters, including host range and N/B ecotropism; the former is a property of *env* determinants, and the latter is governed at an intracellular level and is attributed to the *gag* gene (see Chapters 3 and 4). Multiple crossover events were found to have occurred within each isolated recombinant. Analysis of the tropism of the ecotropic recombinants showed that NB tropism segregated with p30 of Ra-MLV, whereas those recombinants that contained the BALB-virus-2 p30 were N-tropic. The conclusion that xenotropic virus p30 specifies N tropism is consistent with the theory that these viruses arise as a result of recombination with an endogenous N-tropic MLV (Barbacid et al. 1978).

3. Heterozygous Virions

Just as virions may carry structural components from two different parents, single particles can also carry nonidentical 35S–39S RNA subunits. Such heterozygous genomes have been detected genetically (Weiss et al. 1973; Wyke et al. 1975) but not physically. Heterozygotes would appear to be a consequence of the diploid nature of the RNA tumor virus genome and may be an obligatory intermediate in stable genetic recombination.

Weiss et al. (1973) first detected heterozygotes in experiments between endogenous glycoproteins (env^{E}) and nondefective RSV of subgroup B or D. Using selectively resistant cells in infectious center assays, they were able to demonstrate that single particles appeared to carry genetic information for both parental envelopes. Some dual-host-range heterozygous clones exhibited this property for several infectious cycles, but eventually all proved to be unstable and segregated into either parental types or stable recombinants. Wyke et al. (1975) investigated in detail a single cross between two *ts* RSV mutants ($pol^{+}env^{C}src^{ts}$ and $pol^{ts}env^{A}src^{+}$) in which all progeny viruses could be identified in a nonselective manner. They distinguished 12 phenotypes and grouped the phenotypes according to the type of virus (parental, recombinant, or heterozygote) that would be able to produce it. Of 193 progeny virus examined, 75% fell into a parental class and the other 25% fell into a heterozygous class. No progeny were unambiguously recombinant after a single cycle of infection. Stable recombinants were obtained only after recloning stocks that were heterozygous. In these experiments, virus was filtered through

Millipore filters to try to eliminate the complicating factor of virus aggregates.

The experiments of Weiss et al. (1973) and Wyke et al. (1975) strongly suggest that recombination does not occur after one round of infection and that unstable heterozygotes are the progenitors of true recombinants. Reinfection appears to be required for the generation of stable recombinants. Further experiments by Wyke and Beamand (1979) again showed that true recombinants are rare during a single cycle of infection, whereas heterozygotes make up about 25% of the population. Recloning heterozygotes again led to recombinants. Other workers have also detected heterozygotes in recombination experiments (Balduzzi et al. [1978], in *src* × *src* crosses, and Alevy and Vogt [1978], in *pol* × *pol* crosses). In addition, experiments with MLVs have shown that heterozygotes are found during mixed infection by wild-type and *ts* MLVs (McCarter 1977).

Viral mRNA species may be encapsidated into retroviruses. Particles that are heterozygous or recombinant for the env^{E} marker are readily detected after RSV or RAV infection of cells expressing the endogenous chf mRNA in the absence of full expression of the endogenous virus RAV-0 (Weiss et al. 1973; Hayward and Hanafusa 1975). Direct evidence also exists that avian retroviruses assemble viral mRNA. Stacey (1979) demonstrated that 21S *env* mRNA could function as active mRNA and became encapsidated in viral particles following microinjection into envelope-defective BH-RSV(–)-transformed cells. The 21S *env* mRNA was found to be associated with high-molecular-weight RNA in virions. It appears that, in RAV-2 particles, about 5–10% of the virion RNA molecules are 21S *env* RNA and 90–95% are 35S genomic-size RNA, whereas, in the cell, the molar ratio of the two RNAs is about 1:1 (W. Hayward, pers. comm.). Other workers have found lower efficiencies of packaging of mRNAs in other strains of avian oncoviruses (J. Bishop and H. Varmus, pers. comm.). Therefore, viral mRNA appears to be packaged, but at a lower frequency than genomic RNA. It has not been possible to prove that genomic and messenger RNAs exist as heterodimers in virions, although the packaged mRNAs are associated with 60S–70S RNA. Stacey (1979) provided indirect evidence for synthesis of proviral DNA, which can, in turn, serve as a template for the synthesis of *env* mRNA, after infection by virions containing *env* mRNA. In confirmation of this conclusion, the truncated MMTV provirus studied by Majors and Varmus (1980, 1981) appears to be a product of synthesis from a packaged MMTV *env* mRNA, since the deletion endpoints correspond to conventional sites for splicing eukaryotic RNA (J. Majors and H. Varmus, pers. comm.).

Another type of possible heterozygote is seen in the case of the RNA-packaging mutant SE21Q1b. Superinfection of SE21Q1b cells with RAV leads to production of particles with a new size class of undenatured RNA of about 50S–60S, which could represent complexes of cellular mRNA and RAV genomic 35S RNA (Linial et al. 1978a). Friend leukemia virus, propagated in erythroid cells, has also been shown to package about 1 copy of globin mRNA per 1000 copies of viral RNA (Ikawa et al. 1974). Although the existence of viral mRNA:genomic RNA or cellular RNA:genomic RNA heterodimers has yet to be proved, they could have important implications for recombination, resulting in new types of avian and mammalian RNA tumor viruses (see Section VI.B.7).

4. Recombination following DNA Transfection

Another interesting type of recombination, shown to occur in tissue culture, is the marker rescue seen in transfection experiments with DNA fragments and mutant viruses; however, there is no evidence that such a phenomenon occurs in nature. Cooper and Castellot (1977) showed that fragments of DNA containing proviral sequences could rescue temperature-sensitive markers (*gag*^{ts} or *pol*^{ts}) if DNA and virus were added sequentially. Because infections were performed at the permissive temperature for 6 to 9 days, reinfections could certainly occur. Marker rescue was about 10^{-3} as efficient as transfection by intact RSV proviral DNA. Thermolabile polymerase markers could also be converted to wild type by cellular DNAs from a wide variety of avian species at even lower frequencies (Cooper 1978), indicating that marker rescue could also occur with cellular genetic information. In an examination of the mechanism of transfection, Cooper and Okenquist (1978) found that, in chick embryo cells, recombination may follow the formation of heterozygous particles. Similarly, the encapsidation of viral mRNA into virions (Stacey 1979) described above could lead to recombination.

Recombinant DNA technology allows the formation of recombinants in vitro. For example, it has been used to join cellular *c-mos* sequences to MLV LTRs (Blair et al. 1980; Oskarsson et al. 1980) (see Chapter 4). The recombinant DNA molecules were transfected into cells and could subsequently be rescued by helper MLV. In addition, recombinant DNA technology has led to the ability to perform site-specific mutagenesis on the proviral DNA genomes of retroviruses (Wei et al. 1980), which should allow more detailed analysis of the structures and functions of *onc* sequences and other viral genes and structural elements (see Chapters 5 and 9).

5. Unique Features of Retrovirus Recombination

There are features characteristic of RNA tumor virus recombination that appear to be unique to this family of viruses. First, recombination occurs with an extremely high frequency and can be observed between any two markers. The probability of recombination at any site is about 10 to 50 times that seen in bacteriophage T4, or about 100-fold greater than that in poliovirus. This alone implies a mechanism different from those used by other DNA or RNA viruses. Linkage between adjacent markers appears similar to linkage between distal markers. In some experiments, linkage patterns could be defined and genes could be roughly mapped (Mason et al. 1974; Friis et al. 1975; Hunter and Vogt 1976; Balduzzi et al. 1978), whereas in others, where all the progeny were examined (Wyke et al. 1975; Linial and Brown 1979; Wyke and Beamand 1979; Tsichlis and Coffin 1980), no linkage order could be established. This is discussed further below.

Second, recombination between unselected markers is very frequent, and multiple recombination events occur with very high frequency (Joho et al. 1975; Wang et al. 1976c; Shaikh et al. 1979). In one recombinant studied in detail by Shaikh et al. (1979), eight crossovers were detectable phenotypically, without the use of techniques (such as oligonucleotide mapping) that detect recombinational events not necessarily associated with phenotype. It must be pointed out that it is difficult to prove that isolated recombinants have arisen from a single round of recombination. Even if they have been isolated from a single infectious cycle, it is not known what constitutes a round of recombination, and one cannot assume that there is only one round of recombination per infectious cycle.

Several other unique features of avian RNA tumor virus recombination have been described. However, these are not as critical in considering models of recombination, either because alternative explanations are plausible or because conflicting data have been obtained. The first is that recombinants tend to have terminal oligonucleotides from one of the two parents, thereby causing the termini to appear genetically linked (Wang et al. 1977; Joho et al. 1978). This could, however, be a function of further replication of the virus after recombination, rather than recombination itself; as pointed out by Coffin (1979), identical termini are very likely to result from the mechanism for synthesis of DNA copies of the termini by reverse transcriptase (see Chapter 5). A second feature is nonreciprocal recombination. Kawai and Hanafusa (1976) found that in a cross between NY8 (*env*$^-$) and *ts* NY68 (*src*^{ts}), a majority of recombinants carried both defects (e.g., *src*^{ts}*env*$^-$), whereas wild-type recombinants were almost undetectable. NY8α (*pol*$^-$*env*$^-$) crossed with *ts* NY68 yielded a majority of recombinant progeny with triple defects. However, this result has not been obtained in other experiments. For instance, Wyke and Beamand (1979) found that in following the progeny from individual crosses between two *ts* mutants, certain markers predominated, making it appear as if recombination is not reciprocal, as described by Kawai and Hanafusa (1976). However, when the recombinants from the same cross were examined in a mass population, the levels of all recombinant combinations were fairly equal. Hunter (1980) has reported that *ts* NY68 (*src*^{ts}) crossed with *ts* LA335 (*pol*^{ts}) does generate wild-type recombinants. Furthermore, in a cross involving two nonoverlapping deletions, Martin et al. (1980) found that nondefective viruses could be generated at a very low frequency in crosses between heterologous strains (PR-RSV-derived *gag*$^-$*pol*$^-$*env*$^-$ BK303 and SR-RSV-derived *td* NY106). Balduzzi et al. (1980) found that after superinfection of BH-RSV(−) (*env*$^-$ *src*$^+$) chronically infected chicken cells by *ts src* mutants of PR-RSV-A (LA29) or SR-RSV-A (BK1), they could find few, if any, recombinants. Of 225 clones examined, only three were wild type (which could represent revertants) and ten were double mutants, representing a frequency of recombination of less than 6%. Thus, in these heterologous crosses (between different RSV strains), the rate of recombination was found to be low, in contrast to results of others with crosses between homologous strains. The implications of this finding are unclear, since, in earlier studies, Balduzzi (1976) found a higher rate of recombination between *ts src* mutants of PR-RSV and BH-RSV(−).

Another feature of recombination that was an enigma for a long time is that recombination between deletion mutants was rare or nonexistent. The *env*-defective strains, BH-RSV(−) or NY8, would not recombine with *td* RSV to yield wild-type virus (Kawai et al. 1972; Kawai and Hanafusa 1973; Weiss et al. 1973). However, this can now be explained by overlapping deletions. In fact, deletion mutants do recombine with *ts* mutants, and, more importantly (as mentioned above), nonoverlapping deletion mutants recombine to yield wild-type virus.

Most of the evidence available indicates that recombinants do not arise from a single cycle of infection but that heterozygotes are obligate intermediates, as shown in Figure 7.3 (Weiss et al. 1973; Wyke et al. 1975; Wyke and Beamand 1979). However, Alevy and Vogt (1978) found that infection by two *ts* polymerase mutants could yield wild-type virus in the first 24 hours after infection. This is unlikely to be enough time for two rounds of infection, although this possibility was not rigorously excluded. The RNA-packaging mutant SE21Q1b described above does not package its own genome with any specificity. When cells shedding this virus are superinfected with ALV, recombinants arise very rarely (less than 10^{-6}) (Linial et al. 1978a; Shank and Linial 1980). This result is certainly supportive of recombinational models requiring copackaging of RNAs into heterozygous particles for high-frequency recombination (Vogt 1973; Weiss 1973). Another result favoring a role for heterozygotes is the finding (M. Pettigrew, pers. comm.) that recombinants could be generated as early as 3 hours after fusion of cells infected with two different *ts* mutants.

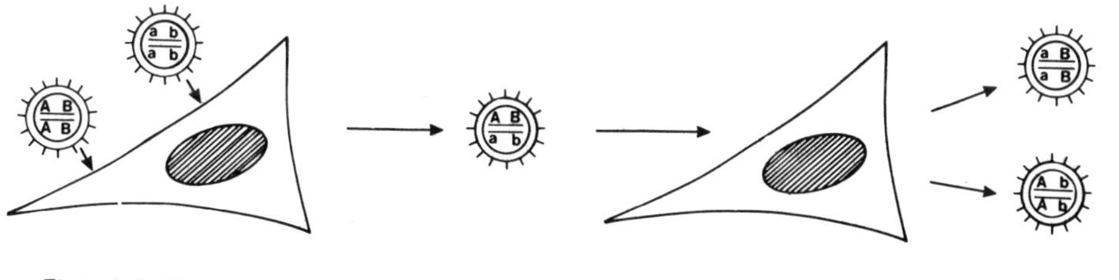

Figure 7.3 Formation of heterozygous particles as a mechanism for recombination. During the first infection, involving two different viruses, progeny particles may contain heterodimeric genomic RNA containing one subunit of each parental virus. During the second infection, these heterozygous viruses undergo recombination (by any of the possible mechanisms described in the text) and may generate reciprocal or nonreciprocal recombinant progeny.

6. *Mechanisms of Recombination*

Several mechanisms of recombination have been proposed (for reviews, see Hunter 1978; Coffin 1979). Because RNA tumor virus recombination occurs much more frequently than that of other viruses, and because reverse transcription is a unique feature of the RNA tumor virus life cycle, it is thought likely that the mechanism of recombination is inherent in this unique aspect of the retrovirus life cycle. However, there is no evidence to rule out recombination between RNA molecules, although recombination among other RNA viruses is rare, and where it does occur (e.g., with picornaviruses), it is of much lower frequency. Furthermore, unlike retroviruses, picornaviruses synthesize abundant double-stranded RNA as a replication intermediate, and picornavirus recombination might involve this RNA. Similarly, although recombination between integrated genomes is theoretically possible, eukaryotic-cell mitotic recombination occurs at extremely low frequency, if at all (Rosenstraus and Chasin 1978), and stable integration of tandem proviruses does not seem to occur (see Chapter 5). Recombination between two circular viral DNA molecules would present a situation similar to that observed with the DNA tumor viruses (polyoma virus and SV40), which has been shown to be very infrequent (Ishikawa and di Mayorca 1971; Dubbs et al. 1974).

When transformed clones are selected after infection with BH-RSV(−) and helper virus at high dilution, they produce no infectious virus (Vogt 1977). In addition, the data of Weiss et al. (1973) suggest that producer clones are found with two-hit kinetics. These results imply that if heterozygotes containing BH-RSV(−) RNA and RAV RNA in a single 70S complex are present in the virus stocks, then only one of the viral genomes, recombinant or otherwise, can become stably integrated. Although direct evidence for heterozygotes and their obligatory roles in recombination is not available, the models of recombination that have been proposed take this reasoning into account and do not include recombination occurring between two integrated viral genomes.

Three models of recombination that have been proposed and considered seriously meet many of the restrictions placed upon model building by the currently available genetic and biochemical information. These are (1) formation of oligomeric closed circular DNA intermediates from which new monomeric circles are formed by crossing-over (Blair et al. 1976; Stoll et al. 1977); (2) recombination between single-stranded DNA fragments (probably of plus polarity) and double-stranded viral DNA (either closed circular or linear forms) leading to partially heterozygous molecules ("strand-invasion" model, as described for bacteriophage ΦX174 recombination [Hunter 1978]); and (3) "copy choice" by polymerase during reverse transcription of heterozygotic RNA dimers (Vogt 1973; Weiss 1973; Coffin 1979).

The evidence for the first model is the weakest, although it cannot be ruled out. Although oligomeric circles (dimers and trimers) have been detected in cells (Goubin and Hill 1979; Kung et al. 1980), they are of low abundance and have not been analyzed for recombinant molecules after dual infection. However, in the case of SV40, Wake and Wilson (1980) found that artificially constructed circular oligomers generated genetic recombinants about 500 times more frequently than mixtures of circular monomers. In addition, the ends of retroviral recombinants generally are derived from the same parent (Wang et al. 1977; Joho et al. 1978), a finding that does not fit with the predictions of this model. This could be the result of virus replication; i.e., the initially formed recombinants could contain different ends, but by the time these recombinants can be analyzed, replication would generate identical termini.

A corollary of the second model, that of the single-strand invasion, is that recombinational repair of large deletions either would not occur or would be very rare. Martin et al. (1980) have shown that two viruses with very little homology do recombine to yield wild-type virus (BK303 lacks *gag, pol,* and *env* and *td* NY106 lacks *src,* and thus they share homologies mainly in the 300 bases of the LTR and perhaps in the *env-src* intercistronic region and the L region between the LTR and *gag*). However, as the frequency of recombinant formation between BK303 and *td* NY106 is very low (about 10^{-5}), these results do not unequivocally rule out this model. For instance, rare recombination between deletion mutants could occur by a secondary mechanism. Another argument against this model is that only avian retroviruses appear to make highly fragmented plus-strand DNA copies (Gilboa et al. 1979; Chen and Temin 1980; Kung et al. 1981).

The copy-choice mechanism makes specific predictions as well. Since two dissimilar RNA subunits would yield only one double-stranded DNA molecule with identical sequences in both strands, no partial heterozygotes should ever be isolated. This prediction needs to be carefully examined. Moreover, since the copy-choice model predicts that "jumps" from strand to strand by reverse transcriptase would be initiated by a break in the RNA strand being copied at the time, two corollaries should be true: (1) virus that is harvested at very short intervals from mixedly infected cells and has a high specific infectivity (Smith 1974) should recombine at much lower frequency than virus harvested at 24-hour intervals (which has a much lower specific infectivity), assuming that loss of specific infectivity is related to breaks in the genome; (2) UV-irradiation or other treatments that cause single-strand breaks should increase recombinational frequencies. However, in one cross (*ts* LA24 × *ts* LA31), it was found that UV-irradiation did not increase the recombinational frequency of about 3% (M. Pettigrew, pers. comm.). The presence of heterozygotes that are apparently stable for several rounds of recombination (Weiss et al. 1973; Wyke et al. 1975) also argues against this model. To sum up, we do not know the molecular basis of recombination.

7. Recombination between Viral and Cellular Genetic Information

The fascinating aspect of recombination to the devotee of retroviruses is that it occurs not only between viral sequences (whether exogenous or endogenous), but also between viral and normal cellular sequences that appear to be the progenitors of the viral transforming genes. Recombination can also account for the diversity of this virus family, and examples of rapid virus variation can easily be seen in vitro and in vivo. Several examples of such recombination are mentioned below.

At the outset, it should be recalled that every exogenously initiated virus replication cycle is a recombinational event per se, involving not only the insertion of viral DNA into chromosomes, but also the generation of repeated sequences in the flanking cellular DNA. This phenomenon is discussed in detail in Chapter 5.

As described in greater detail in Chapter 9, cellular sequences that have been called *sarc,* or more recently *c-src,* are highly homologous to the *src* sequences of RSV (Stehelin et al. 1976). A similar situation exists with the *onc* genes of many other viruses (see Chapter 9). Thus, most MSV strains do not appear to be naturally occurring viruses but were isolated following experimental passage of MLV through animals. Two model systems have been described for the generation of transforming viruses in tissue culture: (1) Rapp and Todaro (1978a,b, 1980) described the isolation of viruses causing leukemias, sarcomas, or carcinomas following induction with halogenated pyrimidines of either normal C3H/10T½ cells (for isolation of leukemia viruses) or chemically transformed cells of the same type (for isolation of leukemia, sarcoma, and carcinoma viruses). At least two viruses isolated in this manner appear to specify phosphoproteins that differ from the well-characterized laboratory strains (Sen et al. 1979a). (2) Rasheed et al. (1978) have isolated a fibroblast-transforming rat sarcoma virus from rat embryo cell cultures by cocultivating, with chemically transformed rat cell lines, a nontransformed rat cell line that spontaneously releases rat ecotropic leukemia virus. This recovered transforming virus appears to encode a 29,000-dalton protein that shares homology with the p21 of Ki-MSV (Young et al. 1979). Both the animal and tissue-culture models suggest that recombinations between cellular and viral sequences are rare events that depend on specific conditions and factors yet to be identified and understood. The tissue-culture model systems should be extremely useful in determining the mechanism of this complex event.

Another example of virus-cell recombination has been demonstrated by several groups (Hanafusa et al. 1977; Vigne et al. 1979; Wang et al. 1979) who have shown that inoculation of birds with *td* mutants of RSV, which retain part of *src,* led to the recovery of new sarcoma viruses with at least partial cellular *c-src* sequences. rASV are not defective, except in the cases mentioned in Section V.A.1, where partial *td* viruses with other mutations were used to generate recombinants (H. Hanafusa et al. 1980). The origins of sarcoma viruses are discussed in greater detail elsewhere in this volume (see Chapter 9).

In most cases, when a replication-competent leukemia virus recombines with cellular sequences to produce a virus containing an *onc* gene, some of the replicative functions of the parental leukemia virus are lost. This is the case with all the replication-defective transforming viruses that presumably have arisen as recombinants between lymphoid leukemia viruses and cellular sequences. Some evidence exists for the generation of these defective viruses by recombination of the helper virus with which they are isolated and endogenous information (Rettenmier et al. 1979a; Eisenman et al. 1980b); however, how and where this might have occurred is not known.

Since replication-defective viruses can only be propagated in vitro and in vivo by phenotypic mixing with replication-competent helper viruses, they may be constantly undergoing subtle changes in their genomes through recombination with new helper viruses. For example, Duesberg et al. (1979) reported that, using one MC29 nonproducer cell line, stocks of MC29 rescued by different helpers contained different oligonucleotides near the 5′ end related to the specific helper virus used for rescue. In the converse of this experiment, Tsichlis and Coffin (1979) showed that helper virus could acquire MC29-specific oligonucleotides near the 5′ and 3′ ends after rescue.

It is attractive to postulate that low-frequency recombination between cellular sequences and viral sequences involves heterozygotes (Weiss 1973), although the evidence for this is lacking. Infecting retroviruses could, on rare occasions, package cellular sequences and initiate new infections, and recombination could occur during or after reverse transcription of the cellular sequences. Some nucleic acid homology between virus and cell might be required to form a heterozygous complex in the virion (Fig. 7.4) and for recombination to occur. In the case of recombination between *td* viruses retaining part of *src* and *c-src* sequences, recombination may result from homology in the *src* region ("legitimate" recombination), generating viruses that retain the entire *td* parental viral genome. Recombination between *c-src* and a helper-virus genome could be envisioned as occurring during reverse transcription by a copy-choice mechanism (Fig. 7.4A), when the enzyme would copy *c-src* RNA. An alternative model (Fig. 7.4B) utilizes a break-and-join mechanism, which would be possible if the 5′ end of *c-src* has sequence homology with RSV, perhaps at a noncoding region at the *env-src* junction. In this case, recombination could occur after DNA copies of both the *td* genome and *c-src* are transcribed. H. Hanafusa et al. (1980) have postulated such regions of homology to explain the types of defective rASVs, lacking some *env*-region oligonucleotides, which arise after infection in vivo with *td* NY109m.

In the case of recombination of virus and *c-onc* leading to the generation of transforming viruses, the actual parental viruses are unknown. Recombination could be a complex event, with the generation of many intermediate viruses, ultimately leading to the tumorigenic strains studied in the laboratory. It is not clear whether a limited number of classes of replication-defective transforming vir-

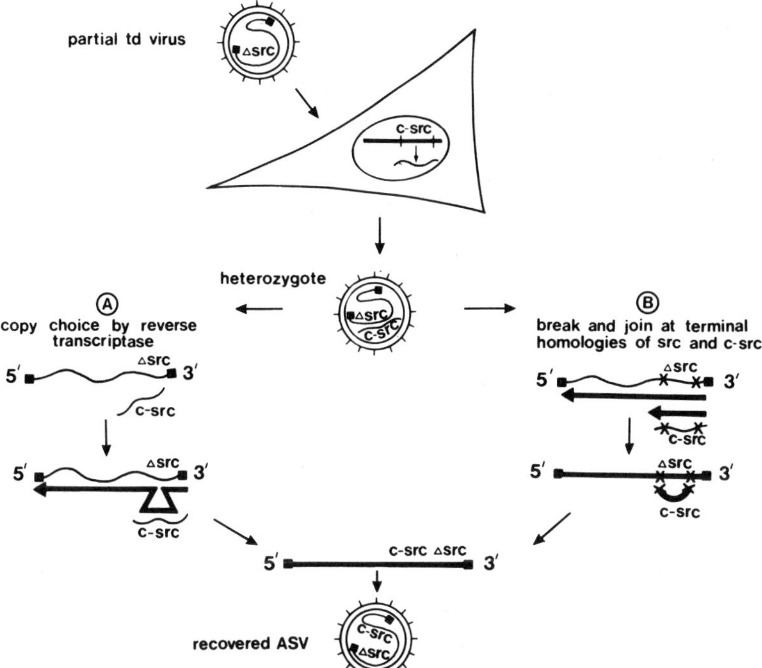

Figure 7.4 Formation of recovered avian sarcoma virus (rASV) following inoculation of chickens in vivo with a transformation-defective leukosis virus having a deletion of part of the *src* gene. (〜) RNA; (—) DNA; (■) noncoding terminal regions; (x) presumably homologous regions in the viral *src* gene and the cellular *c-src* sequences, which could facilitate "legitimate" recombination. Heavy lines with arrowheads represent potential DNA transcripts generated by reverse transcriptase activity. Two possible mechanisms, both involving the formation of heterozygous virions, are discussed further in the text and are indicated by two separate pathways: copy choice by reverse transcriptase (*A*) and break and join at terminal homologies (*B*).

uses have been isolated because only certain cellular sequences have homology with oncoviral genomes, which in turn allows recombination, or because only a few cellular sequences confer a selectable transforming phenotype on the virus, or for both reasons. Homology between *c-onc* and a specific region of the parental progenitor virus does not seem likely, since the known acute leukemia viruses have genomes containing deletions of different viral sequences; therefore, homologies would have to exist in many places on the parental viral genome or in the terminal-repeat regions. If homology between viral and cellular sequences is not necessary for recombination, then stocks of viruses should contain particles with any cellular sequence. However, as these particles would most likely be replication-defective and there would be difficulties in selecting for them, they would not be identified.

Another possibility is that integration of helper-virus DNA near a *c-onc* sequence could play a role in the genesis of transforming viruses. This idea has gained credibility in light of recent evidence that ALV DNA integrates near *c-myc* during bursal lymphomagenesis (Hayward et al. 1981; see Chapters 8 and 9). Since the ALV proviruses contain extensive deletions (Payne et al. 1981), it is possible that deletion of the 3′ LTR in a provirus situated on the 5′ side of *c-onc* could produce a "readthrough" transcript containing viral sequences linked to *c-onc* sequences. Such RNAs would be more abundant than normal *c-onc* RNA and would contain viral sequences that promote packaging (see Sec. V.C.1.). Packaging of such hybrid RNAs followed by illegitimate recombination with helper RNA during or after reverse transcription could then produce recombinants with the observed 3′ termini. Goldfarb and Weinberg (1981a,b) have shown that infectious Ha-MSV could be recovered after MLV superinfection of cells transformed by Ha-MSV DNA lacking the 3′ LTR. However, reports of the isolation of transforming viruses from ALV bursal lymphomas, where ALV is integrated next to *c-myc*, have not been forthcoming.

How recombination could occur in the absence of sequence homology (illegitimate recombination) and why recombination is almost always accompanied by deletion of viral replicative gene sequences are not presently known. Speculation and model construction await more detailed knowledge of the structure of cellular *onc* genes and their relationship to the viruses that have acquired them.

VII. APPENDIX

Tables of Avian, Murine and Other Mammalian Retroviral Mutants

The tables in this appendix were compiled as a guide to the retrovirus mutants and, in some cases, variants that have been isolated and at least partially characterized. Obviously, numerous other mutants have been reported in the literature, but the lack of genetic or biochemical data precluded listing them here. At present, considerably more information is known about the genetic defects in the avian retroviral mutants than about those in the mammalian retroviral mutants. Therefore, Table 7.4, which deals with avian viruses, has been subdivided according to specific genes as well as on the basis of conditional and nonconditional mutant categories. The viruses are generally ordered by the date of isolation. Mutants containing identifiable multiple mutations are cross-referenced in the appropriate sections of the table.

The murine retroviral mutants (Table 7.5) are separated into conditional and nonconditional classes. Within these classifications, the viruses are ordered with regard to virus strain, leukemia or sarcoma virus, and C-type or B-type particle.

The remaining mammalian retroviruses (Table 7.6) are segregated on the basis of conditional or nonconditional status.

Table 7.4 Avian retroviral mutants

Mutant(s)	Parental virus(es)	Mutant gene(s)	Major phenotype	Isolation reference	Other references	Other comments
			(a) *ts src* or *ts onc*			
ts LA334m	B77-RSV-C	*src* *gag*	*ts* maintenance of transformation and late defect, possibly p15	Toyoshima and Vogt (1969)	Friis et al. (1971); Rohrschneider et al. (1976)	originally called *ts*75
ts LA336m	B77-RSV-C	*src* *pol*	*ts* maintenance of transformation, *ts pol,* virions not thermolabile	Toyoshima and Vogt (1969)	Verma et al. (1976)	originally called *ts*149
ts BK1–6	SR-RSV-A	*src*	*ts* maintenance of transformation	Martin (1970)		first *ts* mutants in *src* alone
ts PA19	SR-RSV-D	*src*	*ts* maintenance of transformation	Biquard and Vigier (1970)	Biquard and Vigier (1972)	originally called FU–19
ts BE1m	BH-RSV(−)	*src* *env*	*ts* maintenance of transformation	Bader and Brown (1971)	Bader (1972)	originally called Ta; nonconditional for *env* like BH-RSV(−) parent
ts NY68	SR-RSV-A	*src*	*ts* maintenance of transformation	Kawai and Hanafusa (1971)	Kawai and Hanafusa (1972)	supports plaques of ALV
ts NY10 *ts* NY19	SR-RSV-A	*src*	*ts* maintenance of transformation	Kawai et al. (1972)		

ts LA334 A-1 *ts* LA334 A-2	*ts* LA334m B77-RSV-C × RAV-1	*src*	*ts* maintenance of transformation	Owada and Toyoshima (1973)		no longer have *gag* replication defect of *ts* LA334m parent
ts OS260 *ts* OS122 *ts* OS538	B77-RSV-C SR-RSV-D SR-RSV-A	*src*	*ts* maintenance of transformation	Toyoshima et al. (1973)		
ts LA22–29, *ts* LA31–35	PR-RSV-A	*src*	*ts* maintenance of transformation	Wyke (1973a)	Wyke and Linial (1973)	LA25 and LA28 induce overgrowth at 41°C and allow ALV plaque formation
ts LA30m	PR-RSV-A	*src* *env*	*ts* maintenance of transformation and *ts env*	Wyke (1973a)	Wyke and Linial (1973); Tato et al. (1978)	
ts LA338m	PR-RSV-C	*src* *pol* *env*	*ts* maintenance of transformation; thermolabile *pol;* reduced glycoproteins at 41°C	Wyke (1973a)	Wyke and Linial (1973); Hunter and Vogt (1976); Verma et al. (1976) Moelling and Friis (1979); Hunter (1980)	enzyme protected by virion RNA but not by synthetic template primer; virion contains uncleaved $gPr92^{env}$ at 41°C
ts LA343m	PR-RSV-C	*src* *pol*? other?	*ts* maintenance of transformation and replication defect	Wyke and Linial (1973)	Panet et al. (1978)	replication defect may be in *pol* but not completely clear

Table 7.4 (Continued)

Mutant(s)	Parental virus(es)	Mutant gene(s)	Major phenotype	Isolation reference	Other references	Other comments
ts MI100m	SR-RSV-B	*src* other?	*ts* maintenance of transformation and replication defect	Bookout and Sigel (1975)		
ts RO1m, RO19m, etc.	BH-RSV(−)	*src* *env*	*ts* maintenance of transformation; nonconditional for *env*	Balduzzi (1976)		
ts PA2	SR-RSV-D	*src*	*ts* maintenance of transformation	Calothy and Pessac (1976)		induces proliferation of neuroretinal cells at both temperatures
*ts*68/*env*$^-$	*ts* NY68 SR-RSV-A × NY8 SR-RSV-A	*src* *env*	*ts* maintenance of transformation; nonconditional for *env*	Kawai and Hanafusa (1976)		
*ts*68 α/*env*$^-$	*ts* NY68 SR-RSV-A × NY8	*src* *env* *pol*	*ts* maintenance of transformation; nonconditional replication defect	Kawai and Hanafusa (1976)		nonconditional for *env* and *pol*

ts GI201–205	PR-RSV-A	*src*	*ts* maintenance of transformation	Becker et al. (1977)	Weber and Friis (1979)	
ts GI251–253	PR-RSV-A	*src*	*ts* maintenance of transformation (partial)	Becker et al. (1977)	Weber and Friis (1979)	density independent and agar colonies at 41° C; GI251 cold-sensitive for growth but heat-sensitive for 2-deoxyglucose uptake
ts PH943m	PR-RSV-B	*src* *gag*	*ts* maintenance of transformation and replication defect; reduced particle production at 41° C	Mason et al. (1979a)		
ts CU11	SR-RSV-A	*src*	*ts* maintenance of transformation (partial)	Anderson et al. (1980)	Anderson et al. (1981)	decreased kinase activity and no foci at 36° C or 41° C; *ts* for anchorage dependence, *ts* for fibronectin
ts PA1, 5, 15	SR-RSV-D	*src*	*ts* maintenance of transformation	Gionti et al. (1980)		
ts PA2, 3, 7, 8, 11, 13, 14	SR-RSV-A	*src*	*ts* maintenance of transformation	Gionti et al. (1980)		PA13 forms agar colonies at 41° C

Table 7.4 (Continued)

Mutant(s)	Parental virus(es)	Mutant gene(s)	Major phenotype	Isolation reference	Other references	Other comments
ts ST529	SR-RSV-A	*src*	*ts* maintenance of transformation	Fujita et al. (1981)		fusiform foci at 35° C, no disruption of actin cables, no parameters of transformation at 41°C
*ts*34	AEV (strain ESR)	*erb*	*ts* for erythroblast transformation and some parameters of fibroblast transformation	Beug and Graf (1980); Graf et al. (1978)		
	FuSV	*fps*	*ts* maintenance of transformation	Pawson et al. (1980)		phosphorylation of $P140^{fps}$ and protein kinase activity are reduced at 41.5° C
ts LA42 *ts* LA47	PRCII	*fps*	*ts* maintenance of transformation	Hirano and Vogt (1981)		
ts LA46	PRCII	*fsp* other?	*ts* maintenance of transformation and replication defect	Hirano and Vogt (1981)		other lesion could be in helper virus; particles thermolabile; decreased particle production
ts FL 907/7	AMV	*myb*	*ts* maintenance of macrophage transformation	C Moscovici and M. Moscovici (pers. comm.)		

(b) *ts gag*

ts LA334m	B77-RSV-C	*gag* *src*	*ts* maintenance of transformation and late defect, possibly p15	Toyoshima and Vogt (1969)	Friis et al. (1971); Rohrschneider et al. (1976)	originally called *ts* 75; atypical budding particles; unusual $Pr76^{gag}$ cleavage intermediates
ts LA3342	*ts* LA334m B77-RSV-C	*gag*	derivative of LA334m with *gag* mutation only	Hunter and Vogt (1976)	Hunter et al. (1976)	
ts LA669	PR-RSV-A	*gag*	replication mutant; reduced particle production at 41°C	Mason et al. (1979a)		slower $Pr76^{gag}$ processing
ts PH954	PR-RSV-A	*gag*	replication mutant; reduced particle production at 41°C	Mason et al. (1979a)		slower $Pr76^{gag}$ processing; deficient in p27
ts PH943m	PR-RSV-A	*gag* *src*	*ts* maintenance of transformation and replication mutant with reduced p27 at 41°C	Mason et al. (1979a)		slower $Pr76^{gag}$ processing

Table 7.4 (Continued)

Mutant(s)	Parental virus(es)	Mutant gene(s)	Major phenotype	Isolation reference	Other references	Other comments
			(c) *ts pol*			
ts LA336m	B77-RSV-C	*pol* *src*	*ts* maintenance of transformation; *ts pol,* but virions not thermolabile	Toyoshima and Vogt (1969)	Verma et al. (1976)	first *ts pol* mutant; originally called *ts*149
ts LA335	PR-RSV-C	*pol*	early coordinate defect; thermolabile polymerase	Wyke (1973a)	Linial and Mason (1973)	
ts LA338m	PR-RSV-C	*pol* *env* *src*	*ts* maintenance of transformation; *pol* slightly thermolabile	Wyke (1973a)	Wyke and Linial (1973); Hunter and Vogt (1976); Verma et al. (1976); Moelling and Friis (1979); Hunter (1980)	reduced glycoproteins at 41°C, although virions contain uncleaved $gPr92^{env}$; enzyme protected by virion RNA but not by synthetic template primer
ts LA337	PR-RSV-C	*pol*	early coordinate defect; thermolabile polymerase	Linial and Mason (1973)	Verma et al. (1976)	
ts LA672	PR-RSV-A	*pol*	late replication defect; virions produced at	Friis and Hunter (1973)		

			41°C are defective in polymerase activity			
ts LA351–377	PR-RSV-C	*pol*	early coordinate defect; thermolabile polymerase	Alevy and Vogt (1978)		
ts PH563, 568, and 620	PR-RSV-C	*pol*	early coordinate defect; thermolabile polymerase	Mason et al. (1979a)		
ts NY21	SR-RSV-A	*pol*		Sawyer et al. (1979)		
			(d) *ts env*			
ts LA30m	PR-RSV-A	*env* *src*	*ts* maintenance of transformation and *ts env*	Wyke (1973a)	Tato et al. (1978)	
ts LA338m	PR-RSV-C	*env* *pol* *src*	*ts* maintenance of transformation, thermolabile *pol;* virions at 41°C contain $gPr92^{env}$ instead of mature glycoproteins	Wyke and Linial (1973)	Wyke and Linial (1973); Hunter and Vogt (1976); Verma et al. (1976); Moelling and Friis (1979); Hunter (1980)	enzyme protected by virion RNA but not by synthetic template primer
PH734	PR-RSV-C	*env*	lacks gp85 and gp37 at 41°C	Mason and Yeater (1977)		virions lack host-range determinants
ts PH668	PR-RSV-C	*env*	similar to PH734	Mason et al. (1979a)		

Table 7.4 (Continued)

Mutant(s)	Parental virus(es)	Mutant gene(s)	Major phenotype	Isolation reference	Other references	Other comments
			(e) *ts* in another part of genome			
ts PH746 *ts* PH1369	PR-RSV-C	?	replication mutants; noninfectious virus produced at 41°C	Mason et al. (1979a)		*gag, pol,* and *env* seem normal at 41°C
			(f) Nonconditional in *src* or *onc*			
td NY101 *td* NY105 *td* NY107 *td* NY108	SR-RSV-A	*src*	recombine with endogenous *c-src* to yield rASV	Kawai et al. (1977)	H. Hanafusa et al. (1980)	
td NY109m	SR-RSV-A	*src* *env*	recombines with endogenous *c-src* to yield rASV	Kawai et al. (1977)	H. Hanafusa et al. (1980)	generated rASV, are env^-, $pol^- env^-$, or $gag^- pol^- env^-$; *env* mutation does not affect phenotype but may facilitate loss during recombination
*ptd*3 *ptd*14	SR-RSV-D	*src*	recombine with endogenous *c-src* to yield rASV	Lai et al. (1977)	Vigne et al. (1979)	75% deletion in *src*; possibly insertion in *src*
td TY9	PR-RSV-C	*src*	no focus formation; induces density	Yoshida and Ikawa (1977)		

			independence; slowly developing agar colonies			
td PA101	SR-RSV-D	*src*	does not transform fibroblasts or neuroretinal cells; *ts* for proliferation of neuroretinal cells	Calothy et al. (1978)	Calothy et al. (1980)	*ts* for mitogenic effect; may have *env* defect
PH1	B77-RSV-C	*src*	wild-type virus; cells transformed	Mason et al. (1979b)		0.25-kb insertion in *src* region; normal-sized *src* protein
td CU2	SR-RSV-A	*src*	minicolonies in soft agar with "blebby" morphology	Anderson et al. (1980)	Anderson et al. (1981)	decreased kinase activity; no increase in hexose transport; no decrease in adhesiveness
td CU12	SR-RSV-A	*src*	large agar colonies; fusiform morpology	Anderson et al. (1980)	Anderson et al. (1981)	no decrease in adhesiveness
td PA102–104	SR-RSV-A	*src*	similar to *td* PA101	Calothy et al. (1980)		
td LO5611 *td* LO5621	PR-RSV-A	*src*		Fincham et al. (1980)		no detectable deletions by restriction mapping
td LO2622	PR-RSV-A	*src*		Fincham et al. (1980)		deletion of 1.6 kb in *src*
td LO0041	PR-RSV-A	*src*		Fincham et al. (1980)		deletion of 1.5 kb in *src*

Table 7.4 (Continued)

Mutant(s)	Parental virus(es)	Mutant gene(s)	Major phenotype	Isolation reference	Other references	Other comments
td LO00431	PR-RSV-A	*src*		Fincham et al. (1980)		deletion of 1.0 kb in *src*
td SF/LO104	B77-RSV-C	*src*	transformed chick cells fusiform; does not transform rat cells	Varmus et al. (1981)	Oppermann et al. (1981)	revertant of B31 Fischer rat cells transformed by B77-RSV; originally called mutant L
td SF/LO101, 102, 103, 105, and 15 others	B77-RSV-C	*src*	$pp60^{src}$ has little or no kinase activity	Varmus et al. (1981)	Oppermann et al. (1981)	normal provirus B31 revertant class I
td SF/LO201, 202, 205–208	B77-RSV-C	*src*	smaller *src* proteins	Varmus et al. (1981)	Oppermann et al. (1981)	normal provirus B31 revertant class II
td SF/LO301 *td* SF/LO302	B77-RSV-C	*src*	no detectable $pp60^{src}$	Varmus et al. (1981)	Oppermann et al. (1981)	normal provirus B31 revertant class III
*td*359	AEV (strain ESR)	*erb*	*td* for erythroblast transformation but not for fibroblasts	Royer-Pokora et al. (1979)	Beug et al. (1980a)	small deletion in *erb* portion of P75
td LO1599 *td* LO1600 *td* LO1601	MC29	*myc*	*td* for myeloid cell transformation but not for fibroblasts	Ramsay et al. (1980)	Beug et al. (1980b)	transformation of myeloid cells reduced about 100-fold

(g) Nonconditional in *gag*						
PN3/1	SR-RSV-D	*gag*	*gag*$^-$*pol*$^+$, migration of precursors Pr76^{gag} and Pr180$^{gag-pol}$ more rapid in gels	Steimer and Boettiger (1979)	Steimer and Boettiger (1980)	
LA7365	SR-RSV-A	*gag* *pol*	Pr76^{gag} not cleaved	P. Vogt et al. (1979)		
BO10m	PR-RSV-B × RAV-0	*gag* *env* *pol*	P63^{gag} synthesized but not cleaved; lacks part of p27; no *env* or *pol* precursors	Eisenman et al. (1980c)		probably small deletion in *gag*, large deletions in *pol* and *env*
SE33	*ts* LA335 PR-RSV-C × RAV-0	*gag* *pol*	no particles; P30^{gag} contains p19 but not p27 antigens; no polymerase activity; normal gPr92^{env}	Linial et al. (1980)		*pol*$^-$ phenotype possibly due to *gag* defect (could still have cryptic *ts pol* lesion of *ts* LA335 parent); no detectable deletion
PH7 PH14	PR-RSV-A	*gag*	no particles, P30^{gag} protein produced	W. Mason (pers. comm.)		90-base deletion in *gag*; *pol*$^-$ phenotype possibly due to *gag* defect
(h) Nonconditional in *pol*						
RSV(−)α	BH-RSV(−)	*pol* *env*	no glycoproteins or polymerase activity	Hanafusa and Hanafusa (1968)	Hanafusa and Hanafusa (1971)	spontaneous mutant

Table 7.4 (Continued)

Mutant(s)	Parental virus(es)	Mutant gene(s)	Major phenotype	Isolation reference	Other references	Other comments
NY8α	NY8 SR-RSV-A	*pol* *env*	no glycoproteins or polymerase activity	Kawai and Hanafusa (1973)		
*ts*68α/*env*	*ts*NY68 SR-RSV-A × NY8 SR-RSV-A	*src* *env* *pol*	*ts* maintenance of transformation; nonconditional replication defects	Kawai and Hanafusa (1976)		nonconditional for *env* and *pol*
α48T	BH-RSV(−)	*pol*	no polymerase activity	Murphy (1977)		recombinant between BH-RSV(−) and ?; subgroup-A *env*
α40T	BH-RSV(−)	*pol* *env*	no glycoproteins or polymerase activity	Murphy (1977)		same phenotype as RSV(−)α
SE52d	PR-RSV-C × RAV-0	*pol*	makes $P125^{gag-pol}$; no functional *pol*	Linial et al. (1978b)	Eisenman et al. (1980a)	substitution of quail-cell information for part of *pol* gene; subgroup-C *env*
PH9	PR-RSV-A	*pol*	makes $P140^{gag-pol}$; no functional *pol*	Mason et al. (1979b)	Eisenman et al. (1980a)	0.62-kb deletion in *pol* near 3′ end
BO10m	PR-RSV-B × RAV-0	*pol* *env* *gag*	$P63^{gag}$ synthesized but not cleaved; lacks part of p27; no *env* or *pol* precursors	Eisenman et al. (1980c)		probably small deletion in *gag*; large deletion in *pol* and *env*

PH16m	PR-RSV-A	*pol* *env*	no *pol*- or *env*-gene products	W. Mason (pers. comm.)		0.75-kb deletion in *pol* extending into *env*
PH17m	PR-RSV-A	*pol* *env*	makes P170$^{gag\text{-}pol}$; no *env*-gene products	W. Mason (pers. comm.)		no detectable deletion
			(i) Nonconditional in *env*			
RSV(−)= BH-RSV(−)	?	*env*	no glycoproteins	Hanafusa et al. (1963); Temin (1963)	Scheele and Hanafusa (1971)	large deletion in *env*
RSV(−)α	BH-RSV(−)	*env* *pol*	no glycoproteins or polymerase activity	Hanafusa and Hanafusa (1968)	Hanafusa and Hanafusa (1971)	spontaneous mutant
ts BE1m	BH-RSV(−)	*env* *src*	no glycoproteins; *ts* for maintenance of transformation	Bader and Brown (1971)	Bader (1972)	originally called Ta
NY8	SR-RSV-A	*env*	no glycoproteins	Kawai and Hanafusa (1973)	Duesberg et al. (1975)	21% of genome deleted in *env*
NY8α	NY8 SR-RSV-A	*env* *pol*	no glycoproteins or polymerase activity	Kawai and Hanafusa (1973)		
ts RO1m, 19m, etc.	BH-RSV(−)	*env* *src*	*ts* for maintenance of transformation; no glycoproteins	Balduzzi (1976)		nonconditional for *env*, like BH-RSV(−) parent

Table 7.4 (Continued)

Mutant(s)	Parental virus(es)	Mutant gene(s)	Major phenotype	Isolation reference	Other references	Other comments
*ts*68/*env*$^-$	*ts*NY68 SR-RSV-A × NY8 SR-RSV-A	*src* *env*	*ts* maintenance of transformation; no glycoproteins	Kawai and Hanafusa (1976)		nonconditional for *env*
*ts*68α/*env*$^-$	*ts* NY68 SR-RSV-A × NY8 SR-RSV-A	*src* *env* *pol*	*ts* maintenance of transformation; nonconditional replication defects	Kawai and Hanafusa (1976)		nonconditional for *env* and *pol*
td NY109m	SR-RSV-A	*env* *src*	recombines with endogenous *c-src* to yield rASV	Kawai et al. (1977)	H. Hanafusa et al. (1980)	generated rASVs are *env*$^-$, *pol*$^-$, or *gag*$^-$*pol*$^-$*env*$^-$; *env* mutation does not affect phenotype but may facilitate loss of *env*, *pol*, and/or *gag* during recombination
α40T	BH-RSV(−)	*env* *pol*	no glycoproteins or polymerase activity	Murphy (1977)		same phenotype as RSV(−)α
PH10	B77-RSV-C	*env*	noninfectious virions; no glycoproteins	Mason et al. (1979b)		0.13-kb deletion in 3′ part of *env* (?gp37); retains subgroup specificity

PH18	PR-RSV-A	*env*	no glycoproteins in virions	Mason et al. (1979b)		
PN3/2	SR-RSV-D	*env*	*env*-gene defect but contains sub-group-specific determinants	Steimer and Boettiger (1979)	Steimer and Boettiger (1980)	rat-cell clone
SE521	PR-RSV-E	*env*	makes $gPr92^{env}$, which is not cleaved	Linial et al. (1980)		no detectable deletion; $gPr92^{env}$ associated with cell surface
NTRE-4	*td* PR-RSV-B × RAV-0	*env*	dual host range; infects, but does not transform, C/E chick and T/B turkey cells	Tsichlis et al. (1980)		
SR-DE-1	SR-RSV-D × chf^{+}	*env*	dual host range; transforms C/E chick and T/BD turkey cells	Tsichlis et al. (1980)		
BO1	PR-RSV-B	*env*	dual host range; transforms C/E chick and T/BD turkey cells	Tsichlis et al. (1980)	K. Conklin (pers. comm.)	may be recombinant with endogenous virus *ev-1* locus
BO10m	PR-RSV-B × RAV-0	*env* *pol* *gag*	$P63^{gag}$ synthesized but not cleaved; lacks part of p27; no *env* or *pol* precursors	Eisenman et al. (1980c)		probably small deletion in *gag;* large deletion in *pol* and *env*

Table 7.4 (Continued)

Mutant(s)	Parental virus(es)	Mutant gene(s)	Major phenotype	Isolation reference	Other references	Other comments
PH16m	PR-RSV-A	*env* *pol*	no *pol*- or *env*-gene products	W. Mason (pers. comm.)		0.75-kb deletion in *pol* extending into *env;*
PH17m	PR-RSV-A	*env* *pol*	no *env*-gene products; makes $P170^{gag-pol}$	W. Mason (pers. comm.)		no detectable deletion
			(j) Nonconditional in leader region			
SE21Q1b	PR-RSV-E	5′ end (leader)	RNA-packaging mutant; particles lack genome	Linial et al. (1978a)	Shank and Linial (1980)	150-bp deletion in 5′ end of proviral DNA preceding *gag* gene
			(k) Nonconditional large deletions			
NRK clone 12	SR-RSV-D	*gag* *pol* *env*		Hughes et al. (1978)		nonrescuable genome
BK301 BK303 UV-BK305	PR-RSV-A	*gag* *pol* *env*	src^{+}, makes $pp60^{src+}$	Martin et al. (1979)		6-kb deletion in *gag*, *pol*, and *env*; UV-induced mutant BK303 contains some *env* sequences but makes no *env* proteins

PH2	B77-RSV-C	*gag* *pol* *env*	*src*$^+$, makes pp60^{src}	Mason et al. (1979b)	6-kb deletion in *gag*, *pol*, and *env*; spontaneous mutant
BO10m	PR-RSV-B × RAV-0	*gag* *pol* *env*	P63^{gag} synthesized but not cleaved; lacks part of p27; no *env* or *pol* precursors	Eisenman et al. (1980c)	probably small deletion in *gag*; large deletions in *pol* and env
rASV 3812	*td* NY109m SR-RSV-A × *c-src*	*pol* *env*		H. Hanafusa et al. (1980)	
rASV 398	*td* NY109m SR-RSV-A × *c-src*	*gag* *pol* *env*		H. Hanafusa et al. (1980)	
ld PR-RSV-B	PR-RSV-B	*gag* *pol* *env* *src*	defective; replicates more rapidly than *td* helper	J. Coffin (pers. comm.)	retains 3′- and 5′-terminal regions and 3′ end of *env*; genome is about 4 kb
			(l) Nonconditional in unknown region		
PH11	B77-RSV-C	?	*gag*$^+$*pol*$^+$*env*$^+$*src*$^+$ RNA$^+$ noninfectious virions	Mason et al. (1979b)	no detectable deletion in genome; superinfection with ALV recovers infectious transforming virus

Table 7.5 Murine retrovirus mutants

Mutant(s)	Parental virus(es)	Mutant gene(s)	Major phenotype	Isolation reference	Other references	Other comments
			(a) Conditional			
*ts*3, *ts*7	Ki—MLV	?	no particles at 39° C	Stephenson et al. (1972)	Stephenson and Aaronson (1973)	first mammalian C-type mutants
*ts*6, *ts*9	Ki-MLV	?	defective particles produced	Stephenson et al. (1972)		
K23	Ki-MLV	*env* *gag*?	uncleaved $Pr65^{gag}$ and $Pr180^{gag-pol}$ at 39° C; no particles at 39° C; no $gPr80^{env}$ at 34° C or 39° C	A. Horwich et al. (pers. comm.)		nonconditional for *env; ts* for particle production; no *env* 21S mRNA
*ts*17	Ra-MLV	*gag*?	preintegration defect; $Pr65^{gag}$ not processed	Stephenson and Aaronson (1973)	Yeger et al. (1976); Van de Ven et al. (1978)	*pol* apparently normal; may be multiple mutant
*ts*18–20 *ts*23	Ra-MLV	?	preintegration defect; defective *gag* at 39° C	Stephenson and Aaronson (1973)		
*ts*24	Ra-MLV	*gag*?	partial $Pr65^{gag}$ cleavage; $Pr180^{gag-pol}$ not cleaved	Stephenson and Aaronson (1973)	Reynolds and Stephenson (1977)	

*ts*25	Ra-MLV	*gag*?	uncleaved $Pr65^{gag}$	Stephenson and Aaronson (1973)	Van de Ven et al. (1978); Ruta et al. (1979); Aaronson and Barbacid (1980)	budding particles assemble at surface after shift-down; lesion appears to be in 3′ end of *gag* (?p10)
*ts*26	Ra-MLV	*gag*? *env*	uncleaved $Pr65^{gag}$; releases particles without gp70 on upshift	Stephenson and Aaronson (1973)	Van de Ven et al.; (1978); Ruta et al. (1979)	defective *env* processing
*ts*27	Ra-MLV	?	defective particles produced at 39°C	Stephenson and Aaronson (1973)		
*ts*28	Ra-MLV	?	defective particles produced at 39°C	Stephenson and Aaronson (1973)	Yeger et al. (1976); Van de Ven et al. (1978)	particles are distorted; normal $Pr65^{gag}$ cleavage at 39°C
*ts*29	Ra-MLV	*pol* *gag*	thermolabile polymerase; uncleaved $Pr65^{gag}$ at 39°C	Stephenson and Aaronson (1973)	Tronick et al. (1975); Yeger et al. (1976)	probably multiple mutant; maturation defect; partially cleaved *gag* intermediates
*ts*1	Mo-MLV	?	early defect	Wong et al. (1973)	McCarter et al. (1977)	causes paralysis in mice
*ts*3	Mo-MLV	*gag*?	particles accumulate at cell surface in late budding stage	Wong and McCarter (1973)	Yuen and Wong (1977); Witte and Baltimore (1978)	accumulates uncleaved *gag* and *gag-pol* precursors in the cell membrane at 39°C

Table 7.5 (Continued)

Mutant(s)	Parental virus(es)	Mutant gene(s)	Major phenotype	Isolation reference	Other references	Other comments
*ts*7	Mo-MLV	?	thermolabile particles	Wong et al. (1977)		normal polymerase
*ts*1 *ts*3	Ki-MSV	*ras*?	*ts* for maintenance of transformation	Scolnick et al. (1972)		first isolates of mammalian sarcoma viral mutants
*ts*2	Ki-MSV	*ras*?	*ts* for maintenance of transformation	Scolnick et al. (1972)		helper-infected cells are wild type
*ts*6	Ki-MSV	*ras*?	similar to *ts*2	Carchman et al. (1974)	Scolnick et al. (1975)	cellular cAMP levels parallel *ts* morphology changes
*ts*371	Ki-MSV	*ras*	*ts* for transformation	Shih et al. (1979b)	G. Anderson et al. (pers. comm.)	thermolabile MSV-specific $P21^{ras}$; thermolabile LDH_K
MSV-1b	Mo-MSV	*mos*?	cold-sensitive for maintenance of transformation	Somers and Kit (1973)		
3 Isolates	Mo-MSV	*mos*?	*ts* for focus formation in helper-dependent assay	Yuasa and Shimojo (1977)		maintenance of transformation is not *ts*
CP27	Mo-MSV	*mos*?	*ts* for maintenance of transformation	Forchhammer and Turnock (1978)	Klarlund and Forchhammer (1980)	tumorigenicity of transformed cells is *ts* in nude mice
*ts*110	Mo-MSV	*mos*?	*ts* for maintenance of transformation	Blair et al. (1979)	Sen et al. (1979b); Wood et al. (1980)	*ts* for production of $P85^{gag}$; rescued pseudotypes con-

						tain *ts* low-molecular-weight protein kinase activity
*ts*101–109	Mo-MSV	*mos*?	similar to *ts*110	Blair et al. (1979)		
ts 124/2 *ts* 143/1	MPSV	?	*ts* for maintenance of fibroblast transformation, *ts* for focus formation, defective for hematopoietic cell transformation	Ostertag et al. (1981)		$Pr65^{gag}$ of *ts* 124/2 is not affected
			(b) Nonconditional			
NP-N 2 Isolates	BALB/c-N	?	no XC plaques	Hopkins and Jolicoeur (1975)		converts to XC^+ large plaques on passage of infected cells
SP-N	BALB/c-N	?	minute XC plaques	Hopkins and Jolicoeur (1975)		spreads slowly within culture
C3H	C3H-MLV	?	no XC plaques	Rapp and Nowinski (1976)		induced from C3H/10T½ cells; converts to XC^+ large plaques
8A	Mo-MLV	?	poor replication; cells release high levels of reverse transcriptase	Rein et al. (1978)	Rein et al. (1979a)	converts to XC^+ after long passage of infected cells; replication defect is relative, not absolute

Table 7.5 (Continued)

Mutant(s)	Parental virus(es)	Mutant gene(s)	Major phenotype	Isolation reference	Other references	Other comments
M6	Mo-MLV	?	no $Pr180^{gag-pol}$; low $gPr80^{env}$; particles lack *pol*	Shields et al. (1978)		70S RNA is apparently normal
M10	Mo-MLV	?	small XC plaques	Shields et al. (1978)		like SP-N
M11	Mo-MLV	?	no XC plaques	Shields et al. (1978)		converts to XC^{+} on passage
M13	Mo-MLV	*pol*? other	no $Pr180^{gag-pol}$; high $gPr80^{env}$; particles lack *pol*	Shields et al. (1978)		70S RNA is apparently normal
M23	Mo-MLV	*env*? other	no $Pr180^{gag-pol}$; no $gPr80^{env}$; few particles released	Shields et al. (1978)		23% (1.0–1.5 kb) deletion in RNA; $Pr65^{gag}$ not cleaved
NX-1	Mo-MLV	*gag*?	$Pr65^{gag}$ slightly smaller; normal *pol* and *env*	Shields et al. (1978)	Yoshimura and Yamamura (1981)	NRK clone
NX-2	Mo-MLV	*pol*?	no $Pr180^{gag-pol}$; normal *gag* and *env*	Shields et al. (1978)	Yoshimura and Yamamura (1981)	NRK clone
NX-3	Mo-MLV	*pol*?	normal *gag* and *env*	Shields et al. (1978)	Yoshimura and Yamamura (1981)	NRK clone
NX-4	Mo-MLV	*pol*	$Pr180^{gag-pol}$ smaller; normal *gag* and *env*	Shields et al. (1978)	Yoshimura and Yamamura (1981)	NRK clone has 1.7-kb deletion in *pol*

V11-NP	Mo-MLV	*gag*? *pol*?	no particles released; no $Pr180^{gag-pol}$ or $Pr65^{gag}$; makes $gPr80^{env}$ and $P45^{gag}$	Besmer et al. (1979)		proviral deletion of 1.0 kb; cells make gp70 and are resistant to superinfection
4 Isolates	Ra-MLV	?	low levels of *gag* products; one has uncleaved $Pr65^{gag}$	Sacks et al. (1978)		produce low levels of gp70; resistant to Ra-MLV superinfection
K23	Ki-MLV	*env* *gag*?	uncleaved $Pr65^{gag}$ and $Pr180^{gag-pol}$ at 39°C; no particles at 39°C; no $gPr80^{env}$ at 34°C or 39°C	A. Horwich et al. (pers. comm.)		*ts* for particle production; nonconditional for *env;* no *env* 21S mRNA
AK24	AKR-MLV	?	poor replication; cells release high levels of reverse transcriptase	Nowinski et al. (1977)	Rein et al. (1979b)	probably derived from ecotropic MLV
7C	Fr-MLV	*gag*?	noninfectious particles	Collins and Chesebro (1981)		clone of Friend erythroleukemia cells; particles contain uncleaved $Pr65^{gag}$ and decreased amounts of gp70; *pol* is 70,000 daltons

Table 7.5 (Continued)

Mutant(s)	Parental virus(es)	Mutant gene(s)	Major phenotype	Isolation reference	Other references	Other comments
4 Isolates	Ab-MLV	*gag*?	nontransformed revertants of mink cell clones; no *gag* proteins	Sacks et al. (1979)		retransform upon helper-virus superinfection; rescuable transforming virus
20 Isolates	Ab-MLV	?	nontransformed; $p15^{+}$, $pp12^{+}$	Sacks et al. (1979)		not rescuable; several show reduced kinase activity
Ab-MLV-P100	Ab-MLV	*abl*?	produces variant $P100^{abl}$; reduced kinase activity	Rosenberg and Witte (1980)	Rosenberg et al. (1980)	transforms fibroblasts but not lymphoid cells
Ab-MLV-P90	Ab-MLV	*abl*?	produces variant $P90^{abl}$; reduced kinase activity	Rosenberg and Witte (1980)	Rosenberg et al. (1980)	transforms fibroblasts but not lymphoid cells
Ab-MLV-P92	Ab-MLV	*abl*	produces variant $P92^{abl}$ protein; no kinase activity; no transformation, but microcolonies in soft agar	Witte et al. (1980b)		600-bp deletion in *abl* does not transform fibroblasts or lymphoid cells
NRK6, NRK7, NRK8	Ki-MSV	*gag*	env^{+} cells; no particles produced	Bilello et al. (1974)	Bilello et al. (1977)	rat-cell clones; resistant to superinfection with ecotropic MLV; rescuable with xenotropic

						MLV, SSAV, or endogenous rat virus; no detectable p30
R20 and 7 others	Ki-MSV	?	phenotypically flat cells; low frequency of retransformation	Greenberger and Aaronson (1974)	Greenberger et al. (1974)	helper-virus infection rescues transforming virus at low frequency
R30, R54, R70	Ki-MSV	?	similar to R20	Greenberger and Aaronson (1974)	Bensinger et al. (1977)	
MLA	MMTV (B type)	*env*	particles contain little gp52 or gp36	Vaidya et al. (1980)		$gPr73^{env}$ cleaved in supernatant but not found in virions

Table 7.6 Other mammalian retrovirus mutants

Mutant(s)	Parental virus	Mutant gene(s)	Major phenotype	Isolation reference	Other references	Other comments
(a) Conditional						
103–10, 86–9, and 7 others	SMRV (D type)	*gag*	defective for replication; accumulation of $Pr63^{gag}$ and partially cleaved intermediates	Sacks et al. (1978)	Devare and Stephenson (1979)	
(b) Nonconditional						
RD-49	RD114	*gag*? *env*?	replication defective; uncleaved $Pr65^{gag}$, little gp70	Sacks et al. (1978)		four additional nonproducer clones contain both *gag* and *env* proteins

RD-54	RD114	*gag*? *env*?	replication defective; expresses *gag* but little *env*	Sacks et al. (1978)		
3 Isolates	M7-baboon	?	replication defective; reduced *gag* and gp70 levels	Sacks et al. (1978)		
B2, B7	ST-FeSV	?	flat subclones express viral RNA and phosphorylated $P80^{fes}$	Donner et al. (1980)		helper superinfection rescues high level of infectious FeSV capable of low efficiency transformation only
rd1	MPMV (D type)	*pol*?	normal $Pr78^{gag}$ and $gPr86^{env}$, no $Pr180^{gag-pol}$	S. Chatterjee and and E. Hunter (pers. comm.)		

REFERENCES

Aaronson, S.A. and M. Barbacid. 1980. Viral genes involved in leukemogenesis. I. Generation of recombinants between oncogenic and nononcogenic mouse type-C viruses in tissue culture. *J. Exp. Med.* **151:** 467–480.

Aaronson, S.A., R.H. Bassin, and C.Weaver. 1972. Comparison of murine sarcoma viruses in nonproducer and $S^{+}L^{-}$-transformed cells. *J. Virol.* **9:** 701–704.

Abelson, H.T. and L.S. Rabstein. 1970. Influence of prednisolone on Moloney leukemogenic virus in BALB/c mice. *Cancer Res.* **30:** 2208–2212.

Alevy, M.C. and P.K. Vogt. 1978. *Ts pol* mutants of avian sarcoma viruses: Mapping and demonstration of single cycle recombinants. *Virology* **87:** 21–33.

Altstein, A.D., V.M. Zhdanov, T.N. Omelchenko, S.G. Dzagurov, G.G. Miller, and J. Zavada. 1976. Phenotypic mixing of vesicular stomatitis virus and D-type oncornavirus. *Int. J. Cancer* **17:** 780–784.

Anderson, D.D., D.W. Salter, L.R. Rohrschneider, and M.J. Weber. 1980. Genetic and biochemical approaches to analyzing transformation by Rous sarcoma virus. *Cold Spring Harbor Symp. Quant. Biol.* **44:** 1031–1041.

Anderson, D.D. R.P. Beckmann, E.H. Harms, K. Nakamura, and M.J. Weber. 1981. Biological properties of "partial" transformation mutants of Rous sarcoma virus and characterization of their $pp60^{src}$ kinase. *J. Virol.* **37:** 445–458.

Anderson G.R., K.R. Marotti, and P.A. Whitaker-Dowling. 1979. A candidate rat-specific gene product of the Kirsten murine sarcoma virus. *Virology* **99:** 31–48.

Bader, J.P. 1972. Temperature-dependent transformation of cells infected with a mutant of Bryan Rous sarcoma virus. *J. Virol.* **10:** 267–276.

Bader, J.P. and N.R. Brown. 1971. Induction of mutations in an RNA tumour virus by an analogue of a DNA precursor. *Nat. New Biol.* **234:** 11–12.

Balduzzi, P.C. 1976. Cooperative transformation studies with temperature-sensitive mutants of Rous sarcoma virus. *J. Virol.* **18:** 332–343.

Balduzzi, P., J.R. Christensen, and M.F.D. Notter. 1980. Studies on recombination in heterologous crosses of Rous sarcoma virus. *J. Gen. Virol.* **50:** 173–178.

Balduzzi, P.C., J.A. Beamand, J.R. Christensen, Y.M. Pearson, and J.A. Wyke. 1978. Provisional mapping of transformation defective temperature sensitive mutants of Rous sarcoma virus. In *Avian RNA tumor viruses* (ed. S. Barlati and C. de Giuli-Morghen), pp. 112–121. Piccin, Padua.

Ball, J.K., J.A. McCarter, and S.M. Sunderland. 1973. Evidence for helper independent murine sarcoma virus. I. Segregation of replication-defective and transformation-defective viruses. *Virology* **56:** 268–284.

Baltimore, D. 1975. Tumor viruses: 1974. *Cold Spring Harbor Symp. Quant. Biol.* **39:** 1187–1200.

Barbacid, M., A.V. Lauver, and S.G. Devare. 1980. Biochemical and immunological characterization of polyproteins coded for by the McDonough, Gardner-Arnstein, and Snyder-Theilen strains of feline sarcoma virus. *J. Virol.* **33:** 196–207.

Barbacid, M., K.C. Robbins, S. Hino, and S.A. Aaronson. 1978. Genetic recombination between mouse type C RNA viruses: A mechanism for endogenous viral gene amplification in mammalian cells. *Proc. Natl. Acad. Sci.* **75:** 923–927.

Bassin, R.H., N. Tuttle, and P.J. Fischinger. 1970. Isolation of murine sarcoma virus-transformed cells which are negative for leukemia virus from agar suspension cultures. *Int. J. Cancer* **6:** 95–107.

———. 1971a. Rapid cell culture assay technique for murine leukaemia viruses. *Nature* **229:** 564–566.

Bassin R.H., L.A. Phillips, M.J. Kramer, D.K. Haapala, P.T. Peebles, S. Nomura, and P.J.

Fischinger. 1971b. Transformation of mouse 3T3 cells by murine sarcoma virus: Release of virus-like particles in the absence of replicating murine leukemia helper virus. *Proc. Natl. Acad. Sci.* **68:** 1520–1524.

Becker, D., R. Kurth, D. Critchley, R. Friis, and H. Bauer. 1977. Distinguishable transformation-defective phenotypes among temperature-sensitive mutants of Rous sarcoma virus. *J. Virol.* **21:** 1042–1055.

Beemon, K., P. Duesberg, and P. Vogt. 1974. Evidence for crossing-over between avian tumor viruses based on analysis of viral RNAs. *Proc. Natl. Acad. Sci.* **71:** 4254–4258.

Bensinger, W.I., K.C. Robbins, J.S. Greenberger, and S.A. Aaronson. 1977. Different mechanisms for morphologic reversion of a clonal population of murine sarcoma virus-transformed nonproducer cells. *Virology* **77:** 750–761.

Bernstein, A., R. MacCormick, and G.S. Martin. 1976. Transformation-defective mutants of avian sarcoma viruses: The genetic relationship between conditional and nonconditional mutants. *Virology* **70:** 206–209.

Besmer, P., H. Fan, M. Paskind, and D. Baltimore. 1979. Isolation and characterization of a mouse cell line containing a defective Moloney murine leukemia virus genome. *J. Virol.* **29:** 1023–1034.

Beug, H. and T. Graf. 1980. Transformation parameters of chicken embryo fibroblasts infected with the *ts*34 mutant of avian erythroblastosis virus. *Virology* **100:** 348-356.

Beug, H., T. Graf, and M.J. Hayman. 1981. Production and characterization of antisera specific for the *erb*-portion of p75, of the presumptive transforming protein of avian erythroblastosis virus, p75 AEV. *Virology* **111:** 201–210.

Beug, H., G. Kitchener, G. Doederlein, T. Graf, and M.J. Hayman. 1980a. Mutant of avian erythroblastosis virus defective for erythroblast transformation: Deletion in the *erb* portion of p75 suggests function of the protein in leukemogenesis. *Proc. Natl. Acad. Sci.* **77:** 6683–6686.

Beug, H., G. Ramsay, S. Saule, D. Stehelin, M.J. Hayman, and T. Graf. 1980b. Transformation defective mutants of AEV and MC29 avian leukemia viruses synthesize smaller *gag*-related proteins. In *Animal virus genetics* (ed. B.N. Fields et al.), pp. 551–567. Academic Press, New York.

Biggs, P.M., B.S. Milne, T. Graf, and H. Bauer. 1973. Oncogenicity of non-transforming mutants of avian sarcoma viruses. *J. Gen. Virol.* **18:** 399–403.

Bilello, J.A., M. Strand, and J.T. August. 1974. Murine sarcoma virus gene expression: Transformants which express viral envelope glycoprotein in the absence of the major internal protein and infectious particles. *Proc. Natl. Acad. Sci.* **71:** 3234–3238.

———. 1977. Expression of viral envelope glycoprotein and transformation genes in cells transformed by a defective Kirsten murine sarcoma virus. *Virology* **77:** 233–244.

Biquard, J.-M. and P. Vigier. 1970. Isolement et etude d'un mutant conditionnel du virus de Rous a capacite transformante thermosensible. *C. R. Acad. Sci. Ser. D.* **271:** 2430–2433.

———. 1972. Characteristics of a conditional mutant of Rous sarcoma virus defective in ability to transform cells at high temperature. *Virology* **47:** 444–455.

Bissell, M.J., C. Hatie, and M. Calvin. 1979. Is the product of the *src* gene a promoter? *Proc. Natl. Acad. Sci.* **76:** 348–352.

Bister, K., M.J. Hayman, and P.K. Vogt. 1977. Defectiveness of avian myelocytomatosis virus MC29: Isolation of long-term nonproducer cultures and analysis of virus-specific polypeptide synthesis. *Virology* **82:** 431–448.

Bister, K., W.-H. Lee, and P.H. Duesberg. 1980. Phosphorylation of the nonstructural proteins encoded by three avian acute leukemia viruses and by avian Fujinami sarcoma virus. *J. Virol.* **36:** 617–621.

Blair, D.G. 1977. Genetic recombination between avian leukosis and sarcoma viruses. Experimental variables and the frequencies of recombination. *Virology* **77:** 534–544.

Blair, D.G., M.A. Hull, and E.A. Finch. 1979. The isolation and preliminary characterization of temperature-sensitive transformation mutants of Moloney sarcoma virus. *Virology* **95:** 303–316.

Blair, D.G., W.S. Mason, E. Hunter, and P.K. Vogt. 1976. Temperature-sensitive mutants of avian sarcoma viruses: Genetic recombination between multiple or coordinate mutants and avian leukosis viruses. *Virology* **75:** 48–59.

Blair, D.G., W.L. McClements, M.K. Oskarsson, P.J. Fischinger, and G.F. Vande Woude. 1980. Biological activity of cloned Moloney sarcoma virus DNA: Terminally redundant sequences may enhance transformation efficiency. *Proc. Natl. Acad. Sci.* **77:** 3504–3508.

Blomberg, J., F.H. Reynolds, Jr., W.J.M. Van de Ven, and J.R. Stephenson. 1980. Abelson murine leukaemia virus transformation involves loss of epidermal growth factor-binding sites. *Nature* **286:** 504–507.

Boettiger, D. 1979. Animal virus pseudotypes. *Prog. Med. Virol.* **25:**37–68.

Boettiger, D., K. Roby, J. Brumbaugh, J. Biehl, and H. Holtzer. 1977. Transformation of chicken embryo retinal melanoblasts by a temperature-sensitive mutant of Rous sarcoma virus. *Cell* **11:** 881–890.

Bookout, J.B. and M.M. Sigel. 1975. Characterization of a conditional mutant of Rous sarcoma virus with alterations in early and late functions of cell transformation. *Virology* **67:** 474–486.

Boss, M., M. Greaves, and N. Teich. 1979. Abelson virus transformed haematopoietic cell lines with pre-B-cell characteristics. *Nature* **278:** 551–553.

Breitman, M.L., J.C. Neil, C. Moscovici, and P.K. Vogt. 1981. The pathogenicity and defectiveness of PRCII: A new type of avian sarcoma virus. *Virology* **108:** 1–12.

Brugge, J.S. and R.L. Erikson. 1977. Identification of a transformation-specific antigen induced by an avian sarcoma virus. *Nature* **269:** 346–348.

Calothy, G. and B. Pessac. 1976. Growth stimulation of chick embryo neuroretinal cells infected with Rous sarcoma virus: Relationship to viral replication and morphological transformation. *Virology* **71:** 336–345.

Calothy, G., F. Poirier, G. Dambrine, and B. Pessac. 1978. A transformation defective mutant of Rous sarcoma virus inducing chick embryo neuroretinal cell proliferation. *Virology* **89:** 75–84.

Calothy, G., F. Poirier, G. Dambrine, P. Mignatti, P. Combes, and B. Pessac. 1980. Expression of viral oncogenes in differentiating chick embryo neuroretinal cells infected with avian tumor viruses. *Cold Spring Harbor Symp. Quant. Biol.* **44:** 983–990.

Canaani, E. and S.A. Aaronson. 1980. Isolation and characterization of naturally occurring deletion mutants of Moloney murine sarcoma virus. *Virology* **105:** 456–466.

Canaani, E., K.C. Robbins, and S.A. Aaronson. 1979. The transforming gene of Moloney murine sarcoma virus. *Nature* **282:** 378–383.

Carchman, R.A., G.S. Johnson, I. Pastan, and E.M. Scolnick. 1974. Studies on the levels of cyclic AMP in cells transformed by wild-type and temperature-sensitive Kirsten sarcoma virus. *Cell* **1:** 59–64.

Carr, J.G. and J.G. Campbell. 1958. Three new virus-induced fowl sarcomata. *Br. J. Cancer* **12:** 631–635.

Chen, I.S.Y. and H.M. Temin. 1980. Ribonucleotides in unintegrated linear spleen necrosis virus DNA. *J. Virol.* **33:** 1058–1073.

Coffin, J.M. 1979. Structure, replication, and recombination of retrovirus genomes: Some unifying hypotheses. *J. Gen. Virol.* **42:** 1–26.

Coffin, J.M. and M.A. Billeter. 1976. A physical map of the Rous sarcoma virus genome. *J. Mol. Biol.* **100:** 293–318.

Coffin, J.M., M. Champion, and F. Chabot. 1978. Nucleotide sequence relationships between the genomes of an endogenous and an exogenous avian tumor virus. *J. Virol.* **28:** 972–991.

Coffin, J.M., P.N. Tsichlis, and H.L. Robinson. 1980. Genetics of leukemogenesis by avian leukosis viruses. In *Modern trends in human leukemia IV* (ed. R. Neth et al.). Springer-Verlag, Berlin. (In press.)

Collins, J.K. and B. Chesebro. 1981. Replication-defective Friend murine leukemia virus particles containing uncleaved *gag* polyproteins and decreased levels of envelope glycoprotein. *J. Virol.* **37:** 161–170.

Cooper, G.M. 1978. Marker rescue of endogenous cellular genetic information related to the avian leukosis virus gene encoding RNA-directed DNA polymerase. *J. Virol.* **25:** 788–796.

Cooper, G.M. and S.B. Castellot. 1977. Assay of noninfectious fragments of DNA of avian leukosis virus-infected cells by marker rescue. *J. Virol.* **22:** 300–307.

Cooper, G.M. and S. Okenquist. 1978. Mechanism of transfection of chicken embryo fibroblasts by Rous sarcoma virus DNA. *J. Virol.* **28:** 45–52.

Copeland, T.D., D.P. Grandgenett, and S. Oroszlan. 1980. Amino acid sequence analysis of reverse transcriptase from avian myeloblastosis virus. *J. Virol.* **36:** 115–119.

Crittenden, L.B., W.S. Hayward, H. Hanafusa, and A.M. Fadly. 1980. Induction of neoplasms by subgroup E recombinants of exogenous and endogenous avian retroviruses (Rous-associated virus type 60). *J. Virol.* **33:** 915–919.

Czernilofsky, A.P., A.D. Levinson, H.E. Varmus, J.M. Bishop, E. Tischer, and H.M. Goodman. 1980. Nucleotide sequence of an avian virus oncogene (*src*) and proposed amino acid sequence for gene product. *Nature* **287:** 198–203.

Demsey, A., D. Kawka, S. Galuska, and C.W. Stackpole. 1979. Assembly of a temperature-sensitive mutant of Rauscher murine leukemia virus at the cell surface induced by low temperature and by ligands. *Virology* **95:** 235–240.

Deng, C.-T., D. Boettiger, I. Macpherson, and H.E. Varmus. 1974. The persistence and expression of virus-specific DNA in revertants of Rous sarcoma virus-transformed BHK-21 cells. *Virology* **62:** 512–521.

Deng, C.-T., D. Stehelin, J.M. Bishop, and H.E. Varmus. 1977. Characteristics of virus-specific RNA in avian sarcoma virus-transformed BHK-21 cells and revertants. *Virology* **76:** 313–330.

Devare, S.G. and J.R. Stephenson. 1979. Primate retroviruses: Intracistronic mapping of type D viral *gag* gene by use of nonconditional replication mutants. *J. Virol.* **29:** 1035–1043.

Dierks, P.M., P.E. Highfield, and J.T. Parsons. 1979. Deletion mutant of the Bratislava-77 strain of Rous sarcoma virus containing a fusion of the group-specific antigen and envelope genes. *J. Virol.* **32:** 567–582.

Donner, L., L.P. Turek, S.K. Ruscetti, L.A. Fedele, and C.J. Sherr. 1980. Transformation-defective mutants of feline sarcoma virus which express a product of the viral *src* gene. *J. Virol.* **35:** 129–140.

Donoghue, D.J., P.A. Sharp, and R.A. Weinberg. 1979. Comparative study of different isolates of murine sarcoma virus. *J. Virol.* **32:** 1015–1027.

Dougherty, R.M. and R. Rasmussen. 1964. Properties of a strain of Rous sarcoma virus that infects mammals. *Natl. Cancer. Inst. Monogr.* **17:** 337–350.

Dubbs, D.R., M. Rachmeler, and S. Kit. 1974. Recombination between temperature-sensitive mutants of simian virus 40. *Virology* **57:** 161–174.

Duesberg, P.H. and P.K. Vogt. 1973. Gel electrophoresis of avian leukosis and sarcoma viral RNA in formamide: Comparison with other viral and cellular RNA species. *J. Virol.* **12:** 594–599.

Duesberg, P.H., K. Bister, and C. Moscovici. 1979. Avian acute leukemia virus MC29: Conserved and variable RNA sequences and recombination with helper virus. *Virology* **99:** 121–134.

Duesberg, P.H., S. Kawai, L.-H. Wang, P.K. Vogt, H.M. Murphy, and H. Hanafusa. 1975.

RNA of replication-defective strains of Rous sarcoma virus. *Proc. Natl. Acad. Sci.* **72:** 1569–1573.

Duff, R.G. and P.K. Vogt. 1969. Characteristics of two new avian tumor virus subgroups. *Virology* **39:** 18–30.

Eisenman, R.N., W.S. Mason, and M. Linial. 1980a. Synthesis and processing of polymerase proteins of wild-type and mutant avian retroviruses. *J. Virol.* **36:** 62–78.

Eisenman, R.N., M. Linial, M. Groudine, R. Shaikh, S. Brown, and P.E. Neiman. 1980b. Recombination in the avian oncoviruses as a model for the generation of defective transforming viruses. *Cold Spring Harbor Symp. Quant. Biol.* **44:** 1235–1247.

Eisenman, R., W.N. Burnette, F. Zucco, H. Diggelmann, P. Heater, P. Tsichlis, and J. Coffin. 1980c. Synthesis and processing of the internal structural proteins of retroviruses: Site of synthesis, evidence for multiply charged species and analysis of a mutant defective in processing. In *Biosynthesis, modification and processing of cellular and viral polyproteins* (ed. G. Koch and D. Richter) pp. 233–247. Academic Press, New York. (In press.)

Fincham, V.J., P.E. Neiman, and J.A. Wyke. 1980. Novel nonconditional mutants in the *src* gene of Rous sarcoma virus: Isolation and preliminary characterization. *Virology* **103:** 99–111.

Fischinger, P.J., W. Schäfer, and E. Seifert. 1972a. Detection of some murine leukemia virus antigens in virus particles derived from 3T3 cells transformed only by murine sarcoma virus. *Virology* **47:** 229–235.

Fischinger, P.J., S. Nomura, P.T. Peebles, D.K. Haapala, and R.H. Bassin. 1972b. Reversion of murine sarcoma virus transformed mouse cells: Variants without a rescuable sarcoma virus. *Science* **176:** 1033–1035.

Fiszman, M.Y. and P. Fuchs. 1975. Temperature-sensitive expression of differentiation in transformed myoblasts. *Nature* **254:** 429–431.

Forchhammer, J. and G. Turnock. 1978. Glycoproteins from murine C-type virus are more acidic in virus derived from transformed cells than from nontransformed cells. *Virology* **88:** 177–182.

Friis, R.R. 1978. Temperature-sensitive mutants of avian RNA tumor viruses: A review. *Curr. Top. Microbiol. Immunol.* **79:** 261–293.

Friis, R.R. and E. Hunter. 1973. A temperature-sensitive mutant of Rous sarcoma virus that is defective for replication. *Virology* **53:** 479–483.

Friis, R.R., K. Toyoshima, and P.K. Vogt. 1971. Conditional lethal mutants of avian sarcoma viruses. I. Physiology of *ts* 75 and *ts* 149. *Virology* **43:** 375–389.

Friis, R.R., W.S. Mason, Y.C. Chen, and M.S. Halpern. 1975. A replication defective mutant of Rous sarcoma virus which fails to make a functional reverse transcriptase. *Virology* **64:** 49–62.

Friis, R.R., H. Ogura, H. Gelderblom, and M.S. Halpern. 1976. The defective maturation of viral progeny with a temperature-sensitive mutant of avian sarcoma virus. *Virology* **73:** 259–272.

Fujinami, A. and K. Inamoto. 1914. Ueber Geschwulste bei japanischen Haushuhnern insbesondere uber einen transplantablen Tumor. *Z. Krebsforsch.* **14:** 94–119.

Fujita, D.J., C.B. Boschek, A. Ziemiecki, and R.R. Friis. 1981. An avian sarcoma virus mutant which produces an aberrant transformation affecting cell morphology. *Virology* **111:** 223–238.

Galehouse, D.M. and P.H. Duesberg. 1978. Glycoproteins of avian tumor virus recombinants: Evidence for intragenic crossing-over. *J. Virol.* **25:** 86–96.

Gallis, B., M. Linial, and R. Eisenman. 1979. An avian oncovirus mutant deficient in genomic RNA: Characterization of the packaged RNA as cellular messenger RNA. *Virology* **94:** 146–161.

Gazzolo, L., C. Moscovici, M.G. Moscovici, and J. Samarut. 1979. Response of hemopoietic cells to avian acute leukemia viruses: Effects on the differentiation of the target cells. *Cell* **16:** 627–638.

Gerwin, B.I., A. Rein, J.G. Levin, R.H. Bassin, B.M. Benjers, S.V.S. Kashmiri, D. Hopkins, and B.J. O'Neill. 1979. Mutant of B-tropic murine leukemia virus synthesizing an altered polymerase molecule. *J. Virol.* **31:** 741–751.

Gilboa, E., S.W. Mitra, S. Goff, and D. Baltimore. 1979. A detailed model of reverse transcription and tests of crucial aspects. *Cell* **18:** 93–100.

Gionti, E., C. Kryceve-Martinerie, M.C. Aupoix, and G. Calothy. 1980. Phenotypic heterogeneity among temperature-sensitive mutants of Rous sarcoma virus. Studies with inhibitors of protein synthesis. *Virology* **100:** 219–228.

Golde, A. 1970. Radio-induced mutants of the Schmidt-Ruppin strain of Rous sarcoma virus. *Virology* **40:** 1022–1029.

Goldfarb, M. and R.A. Weinberg. 1981a. Structure of the provirus within NIH 3T3 cells transfected with Harvey sarcoma virus DNA. *J. Virol.* **38:** 125–135.

———. 1981b. Generation of novel, biologically active Harvey sarcoma virus via apparent illegitimate recombination. *J. Virol.* **38:** 136–150.

Golomb, M. and D.P. Grandgenett. 1979. Endonuclease activity of purified RNA-directed DNA polymerase from avian myeloblastosis virus. *J. Biol. Chem* **254:** 1606–1613.

Golomb, M., D.P. Grandgenett, and W.S. Mason. 1981. Virus-coded DNA endonuclease from avian retrovirus. *J. Virol.* **38:** 548–555.

Goubin, G. and M. Hill. 1979. Monomer and multimer convalently closed circular forms of Rous sarcoma virus DNA. *J. Virol.* **29:** 799–804.

Graf, T. 1972. A plaque assay for avian RNA tumor viruses. *Virology* **50:** 567–578.

Graf, T., N. Ade, and H. Beug. 1978. Temperature-sensitive mutant of avian erythroblastosis virus suggests a block of differentiation as mechanism of leukaemogenesis. *Nature* **275:** 496–501.

Graf, T., H. Beug, and M.J. Hayman. 1980. Target cell specificity of defective avian leukemia viruses: Hematopoietic target cells for a given virus type can be infected but not transformed by strains of a different type. *Proc. Natl. Acad. Sci.* **77:** 389–393.

Graf, T., B. Royer-Pokora, G.E. Schubert, and H. Beug. 1976. Evidence for the multiple oncogenic potential of cloned leukemia virus: *in vitro* and *in vivo* studies with avian erythroblastosis virus. *Virology* **71:** 423–433.

Grandgenett, D.P., M. Golomb, and A.C. Vora. 1980. Activation of an Mg^{+2} -dependent DNA endonuclease of avian myeloblastosis virus $\alpha\beta$ DNA polymerase by in vitro proteolytic cleavage. *J. Virol.* **33:** 264–271.

Grandgenett, D.P., A.C. Vora, and R.D. Schiff. 1978. A 32,000-dalton nucleic acid-binding protein from avian retrovirus cores possesses DNA endonuclease activity. *Virology* **89:** 119–132.

Greenberger, J.S. and S.A. Aaronson. 1974. Morphologic revertants of murine sarcoma virus transformed nonproducer BALB/3T3: Selective techniques for isolation and biologic properties *in vitro* and *in vivo*. *Virology* **57:** 339–346.

Greenberger, J.S., G.R. Anderson, and S.A. Aaronson. 1974. Transformation-defective virus mutants in a class of morphologic revertants of sarcoma virus transformed nonproducer cells. *Cell* **2:** 279–286.

Hackett, A.J. and S.S. Sylvester. 1972. Cell line derived from Balb/3T3 that is transformed by murine leukaemia virus: a focus assay for leukaemia virus. *Nat. New Biol.* **239:** 164–166.

Hanafusa, H. 1965. Analysis of the defectiveness of Rous sarcoma virus. III. Determining influence of a new helper virus on the host range and susceptibility to interference of RSV. *Virology* **25:** 248–255.

Hanafusa, H. and T. Hanafusa. 1966. Determining factor in the capacity of Rous sarcoma virus to induce tumors in mammals. *Proc. Natl. Acad. Sci.* **55:** 532–538.

———. 1968. Further studies on RSV production from transformed cells. *Virology* **34:**630–636.

———. 1971. Noninfectious RSV deficient in DNA polymerase. *Virology* **43:**313–316.

Hanafusa, H., T. Hanafusa, and H. Rubin. 1963. The defectiveness of Rous sarcoma virus. *Proc. Natl. Acad. Sci.* **49:**572–580.

———. 1964. Analysis of the defectiveness of Rous sarcoma virus. II. Specification of RSV antigenicity by helper virus. *Proc. Natl. Acad. Sci.* **51:**41–48.

Hanafusa, H., T. Miyamoto, and T. Hanafusa. 1970. A cell-associated factor essential for formation of an infectious form of Rous sarcoma virus. *Proc. Natl. Acad. Sci.* **66:**314–321.

Hanafusa, H., C.C. Halpern, D.L. Buchhagen, and S. Kawai. 1977. Recovery of avian sarcoma virus for tumors induced by transformation-defective mutants. *J. Exp. Med.* **146:**1735–1747.

Hanafusa, H., W.S. Hayward, J.H. Chen, and T. Hanafusa. 1975. Control of expression of tumor virus genes in uninfected chicken cells. *Cold Spring Harbor Symp. Quant. Biol.* **39:**1139–1144.

Hanafusa, H., D. Baltimore, D. Smoler, K.F. Watson, A. Yaniv, and S. Spiegelman. 1972. Absence of polymerase protein in virions of alpha-type Rous sarcoma virus. *Science* **177:**1188–1191.

Hanafusa, H., L.-H. Wang, T. Hanafusa, S.M. Anderson, R.E. Karess, and W.S. Hayward. 1980. The nature and origin of the transforming gene of avian sarcoma viruses. In *Animal virus genetics* (ed. B.N. Fields et al.), pp.483–497. Academic Press, New York.

Hanafusa, T., H. Hanafusa, and T. Miyamoto. 1970a. Recovery of a new virus from apparently normal chick cells by infection with avian tumor viruses. *Proc. Natl. Acad. Sci.* **67:**1797–1803.

Hanafusa, T., T. Miyamoto, and H. Hanafusa. 1970b. A type of chicken embryo cell that fails to support formation of infectious RSV. *Virology* **40:**55–64.

Hanafusa, T., L.-H. Wang, S.M. Anderson, R.E. Karess, W.S. Hayward, and H. Hanafusa. 1980. Characterization of the transforming gene of Fujinami sarcoma virus. *Proc. Natl. Acad. Sci.* **77:**3009–3013.

Harvey, J.J. 1964. An unidentified virus which causes the rapid production of tumours in mice. *Nature* **204:**1104–1105.

Hayman, M.J., B. Royer-Pokora, and T. Graf. 1979. Defectiveness of avian erythroblastosis virus: Synthesis of a 75K *gag*-related protein. *Virology* **92:**31–45.

Hayward, W.S. 1977. Size and genetic content of viral RNAs in avian oncovirus-infected cells. *J. Virol.* **24:**47–63.

Hayward, W.S. and H. Hanafusa. 1975. Recombination between endogenous and exogenous RNA tumor virus genes as analyzed by nucleic acid hybridization. *J. Virol.* **15:**1367–1377.

Hayward, W.S., B.G. Neel, and S.M. Astrin. 1981. Activation of a cellular *onc* gene by promoter insertion ALV-induced lymphoid leukosis. *Nature* **290:**475–480.

Hirano, A. and P.K. Vogt. 1981. Avian sarcoma virus PRCII: Conditional mutants temperature sensitive in the maintenance of fibroblast transformation. *Virology* **109:** 193–197.

Holtzer, H., J. Biehl, G. Yeoh, R. Meganathan, and A. Kaji. 1975. Effect of oncogenic virus on muscle differentiation. *Proc. Natl. Acad. Sci.* **72:**4051–4055.

Hopkins, N. and P. Jolicoeur. 1975. Variants of N-tropic leukemia virus derived from BALB/c mice. *J. Virol.* **16:**991–999.

Horn, J.P., T.G. Wood, D.G. Blair, and R.B. Arlinghaus. 1980. Partial characterization of a Moloney murine sarcoma virus 85,000-dalton polypeptide whose expression correlates with the transformed phenotype in cells infected with a temperature-sensitive mutant virus. *Virology* **105:**516–525.

Hu, S., N. Davidson, and I.M. Verma. 1977. A heteroduplex study of the sequence relationships between the RNAs of M-MSV and M-MLV. *Cell* **10:** 469–477.

Huebner, R.J., J.W. Hartley, W.P. Rowe, W.T. Lane, and W.I. Capps. 1966. Rescue of the defective genome of Moloney sarcoma virus from a noninfectious hamster tumor and the production of pseudotype sarcoma viruses with various murine leukemia viruses. *Proc. Natl. Acad. Sci.* **56:** 1164–1169.

Hughes, S.H., P.R. Shank, D.H. Spector, H.-J. Kung, J.M. Bishop, H.E. Varmus, P.K. Vogt, and M.L. Breitman. 1978. Proviruses of avian sarcoma virus are terminally redundant, co-extensive with unintegrated linear DNA and integrated at many sites. *Cell* **15:** 1397–1410.

Hunter, E. 1978. The mechanism for genetic recombination in the avian retroviruses. *Curr. Top. Microbiol. Immunol.* **79:** 295–309.

———. 1980. Avian oncoviruses: Genetics. In *Viral oncology* (ed. G. Klein), pp.1–38. Raven Press, New York.

Hunter, E. and P.K. Vogt. 1976. Temperature-sensitive mutants of avian sarcoma viruses. Genetic recombination with wild type sarcoma virus and physiological analysis of multiple mutants. *Virology* **69:** 23–34.

Hunter, E., M.J. Hayman, R.W. Rongey, and P.K. Vogt. 1976. An avian sarcoma virus mutant that is temperature sensitive for virion assembly. *Virology* **69:** 35–49.

Ikawa, Y., J. Ross, and P. Leder. 1974. An association between globin messenger RNA and 60S RNA derived from Friend leukemia virus. *Proc. Natl. Acad. Sci.* **71:** 1154–1158.

Ishikawa, A. and G. di Mayorca. 1971. Recombination between two temperature-sensitive mutants of polyoma virus. In *The biology of oncogenic viruses* (ed. L.G. Silvestri), pp.294–299. North-Holland, Amsterdam.

Joho, R.H., M.A. Billeter, and C. Weissmann. 1975. Mapping of biological functions of RNA of avian tumor viruses: Location of regions required for transformation and determination of host range. *Proc. Natl. Acad. Sci.* **72:** 4772–4776.

———. 1978. Concordance of the RNA termini of recombinants from crosses between avian retroviruses with different termini. *Virology* **85:** 364–377.

Kashmiri, S.V.S., A. Rein, R.H. Bassin, B.I. Gerwin, and S. Gisselbrecht. 1977. Donation of N- or B-tropic phenotype to NB-tropic murine leukemia virus during mixed infections. *J. Virol.* **22:** 626–633.

Kawai, S. and H. Hanafusa. 1971. The effects of reciprocal changes in temperature on the transformed state of cells infected with a Rous sarcoma virus mutant. *Virology* **46:** 470–479.

———. 1972. Genetic recombination with avian tumor virus. *Virology* **49:** 37–44.

———. 1973. Isolation of defective mutant of avian sarcoma virus. *Proc. Natl. Acad. Sci.* **70:** 3493–3497.

———. 1976. Recombination between a temperature-sensitive mutant and a deletion mutant of Rous sarcoma virus. *J. Virol.* **19:** 389–397.

Kawai, S. and T. Yamamoto. 1970. Isolation of different kinds of non-virus producing chick cells transformed by Schmidt-Ruppin strain (Subgroup A) of Rous sarcoma virus. *Jpn. J. Exp. Med.* **40:** 243–256.

Kawai, S., P.H. Duesberg, and H. Hanafusa. 1977. Transformation-defective mutants of Rous sarcoma virus with *src* gene deletions of varying length. *J. Virol.* **24:** 910–914.

Kawai, S., C.E. Metroka, and H. Hanafusa. 1972. Complementation of functions required for cell transformation by double infection with RSV mutants. *Virology* **49:** 302–304.

Kirsten, W.H. and L.A. Mayer. 1967. Morphologic responses to a murine erythroblastosis virus. *J. Natl. Cancer. Inst.* **39:** 311–335.

Kitchener, G. and M.J. Hayman. 1980. Comparative tryptic peptide mapping studies suggest a role in cell transformation for the *gag*-related protein of avian erythroblastosis virus and avian myelocytomatosis virus strains CMII and MC29. *Proc. Natl. Acad. Sci.* **77:** 1637–1641.

Klarlund, J.K. and J. Forchhammer. 1980. Temperature-sensitive tumorigenicity of cells transformed by a mutant of Moloney sarcoma virus. *Proc. Natl. Acad. Sci.* **77:** 1501–1505.

Klemenz, R. and H. Diggelmann. 1978. The generation of the two envelope glycoproteins of Rous sarcoma virus from a common precursor polypeptide. *Virology* **85:** 63–74.

Kung, H.-J., P.R. Shank, J.M. Bishop, and H.E. Varmus. 1980. Identification and characterization of dimeric and trimeric circular forms of avian sarcoma virus-specific DNA. *Virology* **103:** 425–433.

Kung, H.-J., Y.K. Fung, J.E. Majors, J.M. Bishop, and H.E. Varmus. 1981. Synthesis of plus strands of retroviral DNA in cells infected with avian sarcoma virus and mouse mammary tumor virus. *J. Virol.* **37:** 127–138.

Lai, M.-H.T., I.M. Verma, S.R. Tronick, and S.A. Aaronson. 1978. Mammalian retrovirus-associated RNase H is virus coded. *J. Virol.* **27:** 823–825.

Lai, M.M.C., S.S.F. Hu, and P.K. Vogt. 1977. Occurrence of partial deletion and substitution of the *src* gene in the RNA genome of avian sarcoma virus. *Proc. Natl. Acad. Sci.* **74:** 4781–4785.

Lai, M.M.C., J.C. Neil, and P.K. Vogt. 1980. Cell-free translation of avian erythroblastosis virus RNA yields two specific and distinct proteins with molecular weights of 75,000 and 40,000. *Virology* **100:** 475–483.

Lee, W.-H., K. Bister, A. Pawson, T. Robins, C. Moscovici, and P.H. Duesberg. 1980. Fujinami sarcoma virus: An avian RNA tumor virus with a unique transforming gene. *Proc. Natl. Acad. Sci.* **77:** 2018–2022.

Leis, J.P., M. McGinnis, and R.W. Green. 1978. Rous sarcoma virus p19 binds to specific double-stranded regions of viral RNA: Effect of p19 on cleavage of viral RNA by RNase III. *Virology* **84:** 87–98.

Levy, J.A. 1975. Host range of murine xenotropic virus: Replication in avian cells. *Nature* **253:** 140–142.

———. 1977. Murine xenotropic type C viruses. III. Phenotypic mixing with avian leukosis and sarcoma viruses. *Virology* **77:** 811–825.

Linial, M. 1976. A line of ring-necked pheasant cells susceptible to infection by avian oncornaviruses. *Virology* **73:** 548–552.

———. 1981. Transfer of defective avian tumor virus genomes by a Rous sarcoma virus RNA packaging mutant. *J. Virol.* **38:** 380–382.

Linial, M. and S. Brown. 1979. High frequency recombination within the *gag* gene of Rous sarcoma virus. *J. Virol.* **31:** 257–260.

Linial, M. and W.S. Mason. 1973. Characterization of two conditional early mutants of Rous sarcoma virus. *Virology* **53:** 258–273.

Linial, M. and P.E. Neiman. 1976. Infection of chick cells by subgroup E viruses. *Virology* **73:** 508–520.

Linial, M., S. Brown, and P. Neiman. 1978a. A nonconditional mutant of Rous sarcoma virus containing defective polymerase. *Virology* **87:** 130–141.

Linial, M., E. Medeiros, and W.S. Hayward. 1978b. An avian oncovirus mutant (SE21Q1b) deficient in genomic RNA: Biological and biochemical characterization. *Cell* **15:** 1371–1381.

Linial, M., J. Fenno, W.N. Burnette, and L. Rohrschneider. 1980. Synthesis and processing of viral glycoproteins in two nonconditional mutants of Rous sarcoma virus. *J. Virol.* **36:** 280–290.

Livingston, D.M., T. Howard, and C. Spence. 1976. Identification of infectious virions which are vesicular stomatitis virus pseudotypes of murine type C virus. *Virology* **70:** 432–439.

Love, D.N. and R.A. Weiss. 1974. Pseudotypes of vesicular stomatitis virus determined by exogenous and endogenous avian RNA tumor viruses. *Virology* **57:**271–278.

Lu, A.H., M.M. Soong, and P.K.Y. Wong. 1979. Maturation of Moloney murine leukemia virus. *Virology* **93:**269–274.

Majors, J.E. and H.E. Varmus. 1980. Learning about the replication of retroviruses from a single cloned provirus of mouse mammary tumor virus. In *Animal virus genetics* (ed. B.N. Fields et al.), pp.241–253. Academic Press, New York.

———. 1981. Nucleotide sequences at host-proviral junctions for mouse mammary tumour virus. *Nature* **289:**253–258.

Martin, G.S. 1970. Rous sarcoma virus: A function required for the maintenance of the transformed state. *Nature* **227:**1021–1023.

Martin, G.S. and P.H. Duesberg. 1972. The *a* subunit in the RNA of transforming avian tumor viruses. I. Occurence in different virus strains. II. Spontaneous loss resulting in nontransforming variants. *Virology* **47:**494–497.

Martin, G.S., W.-H. Lee, and P.H. Duesberg. 1980. Generation of nondefective Rous sarcoma virus by asymmetric recombination between deletion mutants. *J. Virol.* **36:**591–594.

Martin, G.S., K. Radke, S. Hughes, N. Quintrell, J.M. Bishop, and H.E. Varmus. 1979. Mutants of Rous sarcoma virus with extensive deletions of the viral genome. *Virology* **96:**530–546.

Mason, W.S. and C. Yeater. 1977. A mutant of Rous sarcoma virus with a conditional defect in the determinant(s) of viral host range. *Virology* **77:**443–456.

Mason, W.S., R.R. Friis, M. Linial, and P.K. Vogt. 1974. Determination of the defective function in two mutants of Rous sarcoma virus. *Virology* **61:**559–574.

Mason, W.S., C. Yeater, J.V. Bosch, J.A. Wyke, and R.R. Friis. 1979a. Fourteen temperature-sensitive replication mutants of Rous sarcoma virus. *Virology* **99:** 226–240.

Mason, W.S., T.W. Hsu, C. Yeater, J.L. Sabran, G.E. Mark, A. Kaji, and J.M. Taylor. 1979b. Avian sarcoma virus-transformed quail clones defective in the production of focus-forming virus. *J. Virol.* **30:**132–140.

May, J.T., K.D. Somers, and S.D. Kit. 1973. Temperature-dependent alterations in 2-deoxyglucose uptake in rat cells transformed by a cold-sensitive murine sarcoma virus mutant. *Int. J. Cancer* **11:**377–384.

McCarter, J.A. 1977. Genetic studies of the ploidy of Moloney murine leukemia virus. *J. Virol.* **22:**9–15.

McCarter, J.A., J.K. Ball, and J.V. Frei. 1977. Lower limb paralysis induced in mice by a temperature-sensitive mutant of Moloney leukemia virus. *J. Natl. Cancer Inst.* **59:**179–183.

Moelling, K. and R.R. Friis. 1979. Two avian sarcoma virus mutants with defects in the DNA polymerase-RNase H complex. *J. Virol.* **32:**370–378.

Moloney, J.B. 1966. A virus-induced rhabdomyosarcoma of mice. *Natl. Cancer Inst. Monogr.* **22:**139–142.

Moscovici, C. and P.K. Vogt. 1968. Effect of genetic cellular resistance on cell transformation and virus replication in chicken hematopoietic cell cultures infected with avian myeloblastosis virus (BAI-A). *Virology* **35:**487–497.

Murphy, H.M. 1977. A new replication-defective variant of the Bryan high-titer strain Rous sarcoma virus. *Virology* **77:**705–721.

Neil, J.C., M.L. Breitman, and P.K. Vogt. 1981a. Characterization of a 105,000 molecular weight *gag*-related phosphoprotein from cells transformed by the defective avian sarcoma virus PRCII. *Virology* **108:**98–110.

Neil, J.C., J. Ghysdael, and P.K. Vogt. 1981b. Tyrosine-specific protein kinase activity associated with p105 of avian sarcoma virus PRCII. *Virology* **109:**223–228.

Neiman, P.E. 1978. Mapping by competitive hybridization of sequences which differ between endogenous and exogenous chicken leukosis viruses. *Virology* **85:**9–16.

Neiman, P., C. McMillin-Helsel, and G.M. Cooper. 1978. Specific restriction of avian sarcoma viruses by a line of transformed lymphoid cells. *Virology* **89:**360–371.

Neiman, P.E., S. Das, D. MacDonnell, and C. McMillin-Helsel. 1977. Organization of shared and unshared sequences in the genomes of chicken endogenous and sarcoma viruses. *Cell* **11:**321–329.

Neiman P.E., S.E. Wright, C. McMillin, and D. MacDonnell. 1974. Nucleotide sequence relationships of avian RNA tumor viruses: Measurement of the deletion in a transformation-defective mutant of Rous sarcoma virus. *J. Virol.* **13:**837–846.

Nowinski, R.C., E.F. Hays, T. Doyle, S. Linkhart, E. Medeiros, and R. Pickering. 1977. Oncornaviruses produced by murine leukemia cells in culture. *Virology* **81:**363–370.

O'Donnell, P.V. and E. Stockert. 1976. Induction of G_{IX} antigen and Gross cell surface antigen after infection by ecotropic and xenotropic murine leukemia viruses in vitro. *J. Virol.* **20:**545–554.

Oppermann, H., A.D. Levinson, and H.E. Varmus. 1981. The structure and protein kinase activity of proteins encoded by nonconditional mutants and back mutants in the *src* gene of avian sarcoma virus. *Virology* **108:**47–70.

Oppermann, H., J.M. Bishop, H.E. Varmus, and L. Levintow. 1977. A joint product of the genes *gag* and *pol* of avian sarcoma virus: A possible precursor of reverse transcriptase. *Cell* **12:**993–1005.

Oskarsson, M., W.L. McClements, D.G. Blair, J.V. Maizel, and G.F. Vande Woude. 1980. Properties of a normal mouse cell DNA sequence (sarc) homologous to the src sequence of Moloney sarcoma virus. *Science* **207:**1222–1224.

Ostertag, W. et al. 1981. In *Expression of differentiated functions in cancer cells* (ed. P.P. Revoltella), pp. 000–000. Raven Press, New York.

Owada, M. and K. Toyoshima. 1973. Analysis on the reproducing and cell-transforming capacities of a temperature sensitive mutant (*ts* 334) of avian sarcoma virus B77. *Virology* **54:**170–178.

Pacifici, M., D. Boettiger, K. Roby, and H. Holtzer. 1977. Transformation of chondroblasts by Rous sarcoma virus and synthesis of the sulfated proteoglycan matrix. *Cell* **11:**891–899.

Panet, A., D. Baltimore, and T. Hanafusa. 1975. Quantitation of avian RNA tumor virus reverse transcriptase by radioimmunoassay. *J. Virol.* **16:**146–152.

Panet, A., G. Weil, and R.R. Friis. 1978. Binding of tryptophanyl-tRNA to the reverse transcriptase of replication-defective avian sarcoma viruses. *J. Virol.* **28:**434–443.

Paterson, B.M., D.J. Marciani, and T.S. Papas. 1977. Cell-free synthesis of the precursor polypeptide for avian myeloblastosis virus DNA polymerase. *Proc. Natl. Acad. Sci.* **74:**4951–4954.

Pawson, T. and G.S. Martin. 1980. Cell-free translation of avian erythroblastosis virus RNA. *J. Virol* **34:**280–284.

Pawson, T., J. Guyden, T.-H. Kung, K. Radke, T. Gilmore, and G.S. Martin. 1980. A strain of Fujinami sarcoma virus which is temperature-sensitive in protein phosphorylation and cellular transformation. *Cell* **22:**767–775.

Payne, G.S., S.A. Courtneidge, L.B. Crittenden, A.M. Fadly, J.M. Bishop, and H.E. Varmus. 1981. Analysis of avian leukosis virus DNA and RNA in bursal tumors: Viral gene expression is not required for maintenance of the tumor state. *Cell* **23:**311–322.

Porzig, K.J., M. Barbacid, and S.A. Aaronson. 1979. Biological properties and translational products of three independent isolates of feline sarcoma virus. *Virology* **92:** 91–107.

Poste, G. and M.K. Flood. 1979. Cells transformed by temperature-sensitive mutants of avian sarcoma virus cause tumors in vivo at permissive and nonpermissive temperatures. *Cell* **17:**789–800.

Purchase, H.G. and B.R. Burmester. 1978. Leukosis/sarcoma group. In *Diseases of poultry,* 7th edition (ed. M.F. Hofstad et al.), pp.418–468. Iowa State University Press, Ames.

Purchase, H., W. Okazaki, P. Vogt, H. Hanafusa, B. Burmester, and L. Crittenden. 1977. Oncogenicity of avian leukosis viruses of different subgroups and of mutants of sarcoma viruses. *Infect. Immun.* **15:** 423–428.

Purchio, A.F., E. Erikson, and R.L. Erikson. 1977. Translation of 35S and of subgenomic regions of avian sarcoma virus RNA. *Proc. Natl. Acad. Sci.* **74:** 4661–4665.

Purchio, A.F., E. Erikson, J.S. Brugge, and R.L. Erikson. 1978. Identification of a polypeptide encoded by the avian sarcoma virus *src* gene. *Proc. Natl. Acad. Sci.* **75:** 1567–1571.

Quade, K. 1979. Transformation of mammalian cells by avian myelocytomatosis virus and avian erythroblastosis virus. *Virology* **98:** 461–465.

Ramsay, G., T. Graf, and M.J. Hayman. 1980. Mutants of avian myelocytomatosis virus with smaller *gag* gene-related proteins have an altered transforming ability. *Nature* **288:** 170–172.

Rapp, U.R. and R.C. Nowinski. 1976. Endogenous ecotropic mouse type C viruses deficient in replication and production of XC plaques. *J. Virol.* **18:** 411–417.

Rapp, U.R. and G.J. Todaro. 1978a. Generation of oncogenic type C viruses: Rapidly leukemogenic viruses derived from C3H mouse cells *in vivo* and *in vitro*. *Proc. Natl. Acad. Sci.* **75:** 2468–2472.

———. 1978b. Generation of new mouse sarcoma viruses in cell culture. *Science* **201:** 821–824.

———. 1980. Generation of oncogenic mouse type C viruses: *in vitro* selection of carcinoma-inducing variants. *Proc. Natl. Acad. Sci.* **77:** 624–628.

Rasheed, S., M.B. Gardner, and R.J. Huebner. 1978. *In vitro* isolation of stable rat sarcoma viruses. *Proc. Natl. Acad. Sci.* **75:** 2972–2976.

Rein, A. and R.H. Bassin. 1978. Replication-defective ecotropic murine leukemia viruses: Detection and quantitation of infectivity using helper-dependent XC plaque formation. *J. Virol.* **28:** 656–660.

Rein, A., B.M. Benjers, B.I. Gerwin, R.H. Bassin, and D.R. Slocum. 1979a. Rescue and transmission of a replication-defective variant of Moloney murine leukemia virus. *J. Virol.* **29:** 494–500.

Rein, A., B.I. Gerwin, R.H. Bassin, L. Schwarm, and G. Schidlovsky. 1978. A replication-defective variant of Moloney murine leukemia virus. I. Biological characterization. *J. Virol.* **25:** 146–156.

Rein, A., E. Athan, B.M. Benjers, R.H. Bassin, B.I. Gerwin, and D.R. Slocum. 1979b. Isolation of a replication-defective murine leukaemia virus from cultured AKR leukaemia cells. *Nature* **282:** 753–754.

Rettenmier, C.W. and H. Hanafusa. 1977. Structural protein markers in the avian oncoviruses. *J. Virol.* **24:** 850–864.

Rettenmier, C.W., S.M. Anderson, M.W. Riemen, and H. Hanafusa. 1979a. *gag*-related polypeptides encoded by replication-defective avian oncoviruses. *J. Virol.* **32:** 749–761.

Rettenmier, C.W., R.E. Karess, S.M. Anderson, and H. Hanafusa. 1979b. Tryptic peptide analysis of avian oncovirus *gag* and *pol* gene products. *J. Virol.* **32:** 102–113.

Reynolds, F.H., Jr., W.J.M. Van de Ven, and J.R. Stephenson. 1980. Abelson murine leukemia virus transformation-defective mutants with impaired P120-associated protein kinase activity. *J. Virol.* **36:** 374–386.

Reynolds, F.H., Jr., C.A. Hanson, S.A. Aaronson, and J.R. Stephenson. 1977. Type C viral *gag* gene expression in chicken embryo fibroblasts and avian sarcoma virus-transformed mammalian cells. *J. Virol.* **23:** 74–79.

Reynolds, F.H., Jr., T.L. Sacks, D.N. Deobagkar, and J.R. Stephenson. 1978. Cells non-productively transformed by Abelson murine leukemia virus express a high molecular weight polyprotein containing structural and nonstructural components. *Proc. Natl. Acad. Sci.* **75:** 3974–3978.

Reynolds, R.K. and J.R. Stephenson. 1977. Intracistronic mapping of the murine type C viral *gag* gene by use of conditional lethal replication mutants. *Virology* **81:** 328–340.

Robey, W.G., M.K. Oskarsson, G.F. Vande Woude, R.B. Naso, R.B. Arlinghaus, D.K. Haapala, and P.J. Fischinger. 1977. Cells transformed by certain strains of Moloney sarcoma virus contain murine p60. *Cell* **10:** 79–89.

Robinson, H.L. 1976. Intracellular restriction on the growth of induced subgroup E avian type C viruses in chicken cells. *J. Virol.* **18:** 856–866.

Robinson, H.L., R. Eisenman, A. Senior, and S. Ripley. 1979. Low frequency production of recombinant subgroup E avian leukosis viruses by uninfected V-15_B chicken cells. *Virology* **99:** 21–30.

Robinson, H.L., M.N. Pearson, D.W. DeSimone, P.N. Tsichlis, and J.M. Coffin. 1980. Subgroup-E avian-leukosis-virus-associated disease in chickens. *Cold Spring Harbor Symp. Quant. Biol.* **44:** 1133–1142.

Rohde, W., G. Pauli, J. Henning, and R.R. Friis. 1978. Polyethylene glycol-mediated infection with avian sarcoma viruses. *Arch. Virol.* **58:** 55–59.

Rohrschneider, J.M., H. Diggelmann, H. Ogura, R.R. Friis, and H. Bauer. 1976. Defective cleavage of a precursor polypeptide in a temperature-sensitive mutant of avian sarcoma virus. *Virology* **75:** 177–187.

Rosenberg, N. and D. Baltimore. 1980. Abelson virus. In *Viral oncology* (ed. G. Klein), pp.187–203. Raven Press, New York.

Rosenberg, N. and O.N. Witte. 1980. Abelson murine leukemia virus mutants with alterations in the virus-specific P120 molecule. *J. Virol.* **33:** 340–348.

Rosenberg, N., D. Baltimore, and C.D. Scher. 1975. *In vitro* transformation of lymphoid cells by Abelson murine leukemia virus. *Proc. Natl. Acad. Sci.* **72:** 1932–1936.

Rosenberg, N.E., D.R. Clark, and O.N. Witte. 1980. Abelson murine leukemia virus mutants deficient in kinase activity and lymphoid cell transformation. *J. Virol.* **36:** 766–774.

Rosenstraus, M.J. and L.A. Chasin. 1978. Separation of linked markers in Chinese hamster cell hybrids: Mitotic recombination is not involved. *Genetics* **90:** 735–760.

Rous, P. 1911. A sarcoma of the fowl transmissible by an agent separable from the tumor cells. *J. Exp. Med.* **13:** 397–411.

Roussel, M., S. Saule, C. Lagrou, C. Rommens, H. Beug, T. Graf, and D. Stehelin. 1979. Three new types of viral oncogene of cellular origin specific for haematopoietic cell transformation. *Nature* **281:** 452–455.

Rowe, W.P., W.E. Pugh, and J.W. Hartley. 1970. Plaque assay techniques for murine leukemia viruses. *Virology* **42:** 1136–1139.

Royer-Pokora, B., S. Grieser, H. Beug, and T. Graf. 1979. Mutant avian erythroblastosis virus with restricted target cell specificity. *Nature* **282:** 750–752.

Royer-Pokora, B., H. Beug, M. Claviez, H.-J. Winkhardt, R.R. Friis, and T. Graf. 1978. Transformation parameters in chicken fibroblasts transformed by AEV and MC29 avian leukemia viruses. *Cell* **13:** 751–760.

Rubin, H. 1964. Virus defectiveness and cell transformation in the Rous sarcoma. *J. Cell. Comp. Physiol.* **64** (suppl. 1): 173–180.

———. 1965. Genetic control of cellular susceptibility to pseudotypes of Rous sarcoma virus. *Virology* **26:** 270–276.

Rubin, H. and P.K. Vogt. 1962. An avian leukosis virus associated with stocks of Rous sarcoma virus. *Virology* **17:** 184–194.

Ruscetti, S.K., L.P. Turek, and C.J. Sherr. 1980. Three independent isolates of feline sarcoma virus code for three distinct gag-x polyproteins. *J. Virol.* **35:** 259–264.

Ruta, M., M.J. Murray, M.C. Webb, and D. Kabat. 1979. A murine leukemia virus mutant with a temperature-sensitive defect in membrane glycoprotein synthesis. *Cell* **16:** 77–88.

Sacks, T.L., E.J. Hershey, and J.R. Stephenson. 1979. Abelson murine leukemia virus-infected cell lines defective in transformation. *Virology* **97:**231–240.

Sacks, T.L., S.G. Devare, G.R. Blennerhassett, and J.R. Stephenson. 1978. Nonconditional replication mutants of type C and type D retroviruses defective in *gag* gene-coded polyprotein post-translational processing. *Virology* **91:**352–363.

Sawyer, R.C. and H. Hanafusa. 1977. Formation of reticuloendotheliosis virus pseudotypes of Rous sarcoma virus. *J. Virol.* **22:**634–639.

Sawyer, R.C., C.W. Rettenmier, and H. Hanafusa. 1979. Formation of Rous associated virus-60: Origin of the polymerase gene. *J. Virol.* **29:**856–862.

Scheele, C.M. and H. Hanafusa. 1971. Proteins of helper-dependent RSV. *Virology* **45:**401–410.

Scher, C.D. and R. Siegler. 1975. Direct transformation of 3T3 cells by Abelson murine leukaemia virus. *Nature* **253:**729–731.

Schiff, R.D. and D.P. Grandgenett. 1978. Virus-coded origin of a 32,000-dalton protein from avian retrovirus cores: Structural relatedness of p32 and the β polypeptide of the avian retrovirus DNA polymerase. *J. Virol.* **28:**279–291.

Schindler, J., R. Hynes, and N. Hopkins. 1977. Evidence for recombination between N- and B-tropic murine leukemia viruses: Analysis of three virion proteins by sodium dodecyl sulfate-polyacrylamide gel electrophoresis. *J. Virol.* **23:**700–707.

Schmidt, E.V., J.D. Keene, M. Linial, and R.E. Smith. 1982. Association of 3′ terminal RNA sequences with avian leukosis viruses causing a high incidence of osteoporosis. *Virology* **116:**163–180.

Schochetman, G., C. Long, and R. Massey. 1979. Generation of a mouse mammary tumor virus (MMTV) pseudotype of Kirsten sarcoma virus and restriction of MMTV *gag* expression in heterologous infected cells. *Virology* **97:**342–353.

Scolnick, E.M., R.J. Goldberg, and W.P. Parks. 1975. A biochemical and genetic analysis of mammalian RNA-containing sarcoma viruses. *Cold Spring Harbor Symp. Quant. Biol.* **39:**885–895.

Scolnick, E.M., J.R. Stephenson, and S.A. Aaronson. 1972. Isolation of temperature-sensitive mutants of murine sarcoma virus. *J. Virol.* **10:**653–657.

Sefton, B.M., K. Beemon, and T. Hunter. 1978. Comparison of the expression of the *src* gene of Rous sarcoma virus in vitro and in vivo. *J. Virol.* **28:**957–971.

Sen, A. and G.J. Todaro. 1977. The genome-associated, specific RNA binding proteins of avian and mammalian type C viruses. *Cell* **10:**91–99.

———. 1979. A murine sarcoma virus-associated protein kinase: Interaction with actin and microtubular protein. *Cell* **17:**347–356.

Sen, A., D.O. Halverson, U.R. Rapp, and G.J. Todaro. 1979a. Sarcoma virus-specific phosphoproteins are packaged in "rescued" type C virions. *Virology* **92:**245–251.

Sen, A., G.J. Todaro, D.G. Blair, and W.G. Robey. 1979b. Thermolabile protein kinase molecules in a temperature-sensitive murine sarcoma virus pseudotype. *Proc. Natl. Acad. Sci.* **76:**3617–3621.

Shaikh, R., M. Linial, J. Coffin, and R. Eisenman. 1978. Recombinant avian oncoviruses. I. Alterations in the precursor to the internal structural proteins. *Virology* **87:**326–338.

Shaikh, R., M. Linial, S. Brown, A. Sen, and R. Eisenman. 1979. Recombinant avian oncoviruses. II. Alterations in the *gag* proteins and evidence for intragenic recombination. *Virology* **92:**463–481.

Shank, P.R. and M. Linial. 1980. Avian oncornavirus mutant (SE21Q1b) deficient in genomic RNA: Characterization of a deletion in the provirus. *J. Virol.* **36:**450–456.

Shealy, D.J. and R.R. Rueckert. 1978. Proteins of Rous-associated virus 61, an avian retrovirus: Common precursor for glycoproteins gp85 and gp35 and use of pactamycin to map translational order of proteins in the *gag, pol,* and *env* genes. *J. Virol.* **26:**380–388.

Sheiness, D., L. Fanshier, and J.M. Bishop. 1978. Identification of nucleotide sequences which may encode the oncogenic capacity of avian retrovirus MC29. *J. Virol.* **28:** 600–610.

Sher, C.J., L. Donner, L.A. Fedele, L. Turek, J. Even, and S.K. Ruscetti. 1980. Molecular structure and products of feline sarcoma and leukemia viruses: Relationship to FOCMA expression. In *Feline leukemia virus* (ed. W.D. Hardy, Jr. et al.), pp.293–307. Elsevier/ North Holland, New York.

Shibuya, M., T. Hanafusa, H. Hanafusa, and J.R. Stephenson. 1980. Homology exists among the transforming sequences of avian and feline sarcoma viruses. *Proc. Natl. Acad. Sci.* **77:** 6536–6540.

Shields, A., O.N. Witte, E. Rothenberg, and D. Baltimore. 1978. High frequency of aberrant expression of Moloney murine leukemia virus in clonal infections. *Cell* **14:** 601–609.

Shih, T.Y. and E.M. Scolnick. 1980. Molecular biology of mammalian sarcoma viruses. In *Viral oncology* (ed. G. Klein), pp.135–160. Raven Press, New York.

Shih, T.Y., M.O. Weeks, H.A. Young, and E.M. Scolnick. 1979a. Identification of a sarcoma virus-coded phosphoprotein in nonproducer cells transformed by Kirsten or Harvey murine sarcoma virus. *Virology* **96:** 64–79.

———. 1979b. p21 of Kirsten murine sarcoma virus is thermolabile in a viral mutant temperature sensitive for the maintenance of transformaton. *J. Virol.* **31:** 546–556.

Shimakage, M.I., T. Kamahora, A. Hakura, and K. Toyoshima. 1979. Selective replication of transformation-defective avian sarcoma virus mutants in duck embryo fibroblasts. *J. Gen. Virol.* **45:** 99–105.

Shoyab, M., P.D. Markham, and M.A. Baluda. 1975. Host induced alteration of avian sarcoma virus B-77 genome. *Proc. Natl. Acad. Sci* **72:** 1031–1035.

Sklar, M.D., B.J. White, and W.P. Rowe. 1974. Initiation of oncogenic transformation of mouse lymphocytes *in vitro* by Abelson leukemia virus. *Proc. Natl. Acad. Sci.* **71:** 4077–4081.

Smith, R.E. 1974. High specific infectivity avian RNA tumor viruses. *Virology* **60:** 543–547.

Smith, R.E. and C. Moscovici. 1969. The oncogenic effects of nontransforming viruses from avian myeloblastosis virus. *Cancer Res.* **29:** 1356–1366.

Snyder, S.P. and G.H. Theilen. 1969. Transmissible feline fibrosarcoma. *Nature* **221:** 1074–1075.

Somers, K. and S. Kit. 1973. Temperature-dependent expression of transformation by a cold-sensitive mutant of murine sarcoma virus. *Proc. Natl. Acad. Sci.* **70:** 2206–2210.

Somers, K.D., J.T. May, and S. Kit. 1973. Control of gene expression in rat cells transformed by a cold-sensitive murine sarcoma virus (MSV) mutant. *Intervirology* **1:** 176–184.

Stacey, D.W. 1979. Messenger activity of virion RNA for avian leukosis viral envelope glycoprotein. *J. Virol.* **29:** 949–956.

Stehelin, D. and T. Graf. 1978. Avian myelocytomatosis and erythroblastosis viruses lack the transforming gene *src* of avian sarcoma viruses. *Cell* **13:** 745–750.

Stehelin, D., H.E. Varmus, J.M. Bishop, and P.K. Vogt. 1976. DNA related to the transforming gene(s) of avian sarcoma viruses is present in normal avian DNA. *Nature* **260:** 170–173.

Steimer, K.S. and D. Boettiger. 1979. Cell fusion for genetic analysis of two nonconditional Rous sarcoma virus replication mutants. *J. Virol.* **32:** 175–186.

———. 1980. Envelope assembly mutant of Rous sarcoma virus. *J. Virol.* **36:** 883–888.

Steiner, S.M., J.L. Melnick, S. Kit, and K.D. Somers. 1974. Fucosylglycolipids in cells transformed by a temperature-sensitive mutant of murine sarcoma virus. *Nature* **248:** 682–684.

Stephenson, J.R. and S.A. Aaronson. 1973. Characterization of temperature-sensitive mutants of murine leukemia virus. *Virology* **54:** 53–59.

Stephenson, J.R., S.G. Devare, and F.H. Reynolds, Jr. 1978. Translational products of type-C RNA tumor viruses. *Adv. Cancer Res.* **27:** 1–53.

Stephenson, J.R., R.K. Reynolds, and S.A. Aaronson. 1972. Isolation of temperature-sensitive mutants of murine leukemia virus. *Virology* **48:** 749–756.

Stephenson, J.R., S.R. Tronick, and S.A. Aaronson. 1974a. Temperature-sensitive mutants of murine leukemia virus. IV. Further physiological characterization and evidence for genetic recombination. *J. Virol.* **14:** 918–923.

———. 1975. Murine leukemia virus mutants with temperature-sensitive defects in precursor polypeptide cleavage. *Cell* **6:** 543–548.

Stephenson, J.R., G.R. Anderson, S.R. Tronick, and S.A. Aaronson. 1974b. Evidence for genetic recombination between endogenous and exogenous mouse RNA type C viruses. *Cell* **2:** 87–94.

Stoll, E., M.A. Billeter, A. Palmenberg, and C. Weissmann. 1977. Avian myeloblastosis virus RNA is terminally redundant: Implications for the mechanism of retrovirus replication. *Cell* **12:** 57–72.

Tato, F., J.A. Beamand, and J.A. Wyke. 1978. A mutant of Rous sarcoma virus with a thermolabile defect in the virus envelope. *Virology* **88:** 71–81.

Temin, H.M. 1963. Separation of morphological conversion and virus production in Rous sarcoma virus infection. *Cold Spring Harbor Symp. Quant. Biol.* **27:** 407–414.

Tooze, J. 1973. *The molecular biology of tumour viruses.* Cold Spring Harbor Laboratory, Cold Spring Harbor, New York.

Toyoshima, K. and P.K. Vogt. 1969. Temperature sensitive mutants of an avian sarcoma virus. *Virology* **39:** 930–931.

Toyoshima, K., M. Owada, and Y. Kozai. 1973. Tumor producing capacity of temperature sensitive mutants of avian sarcoma viruses in chicks. *Biken J.* **16:** 103–110.

Tronick, S.R., J.R. Stephenson, I.M. Verma, and S.A. Aaronson. 1975. Thermolabile reverse transcriptase of a mammalian leukemia virus mutant temperature sensitive in its replication and sarcoma virus helper functions. *J. Virol.* **16:** 1476–1482.

Tsichlis, P.N. and J.M. Coffin. 1979. Recombination between the defective component of an acute leukemia virus and Rous associated virus 0, an endogenous virus of chickens. *Proc. Natl. Acad. Sci.* **76:** 3001–3005.

———. 1980. Recombinants between endogenous and exogenous avian tumor viruses: Role of the C region and other portions of the genome in the control of replication and transformation. *J. Virol.* **33:** 238–249.

Tsichlis, P.N., K.F. Conklin, and J.M. Coffin. 1980. Mutant and recombinant avian retroviruses with extended host range. *Proc. Natl. Acad. Sci.* **77:** 536–540.

Vaidya, A.B., C.A. Long, J.B. Sheffield, A. Tamura, and H. Tanaka. 1980. Murine mammary tumor virus deficient in the major glycoprotein: Biochemical and biological studies on virions produced by a lymphoma cell line. *Virology* **104:** 279–293.

Van de Ven, W.J.M., F.H. Reynolds, Jr., and J.R. Stephenson. 1980a. The nonstructural components of polyproteins encoded by replication-defective mammalian transforming retroviruses are phosphorylated and have associated protein kinase activity. *Virology* **101:** 185–197.

Van de Ven, W.J.M., F.H. Reynolds, Jr., R.P. Nalewaik, and J.R. Stephenson. 1979. The nonstructural component of the Abelson murine leukemia virus polyprotein P120 is encoded by newly acquired genetic sequences. *J. Virol.* **32:** 1041–1045.

———. 1980b. Characterization of a 170,000-dalton polyprotein encoded by the McDonough strain of feline sarcoma virus. *J. Virol.* **35:** 165–175.

Van de Ven, W.J.M., D. van Zaane, C. Onnekink, and H.P.J. Bloemers. 1978. Impaired processing of precursor polypeptides of temperature-sensitive mutants of Rauscher murine leukemia virus. *J. Virol.* **25:** 553–561.

Van de Ven, W.J.M., A.S. Khan, F.H. Reynolds, Jr., K.T. Mason, and J.R. Stephenson. 1980c. Translational products encoded by newly acquired sequences of independently derived feline sarcoma virus isolates are structurally related. *J. Virol.* **33:** 1034–1045.

Vande Woude, G.F., M. Oskarsson, L.W. Enquist, S. Nomura, M. Sullivan, and P.J. Fischinger. 1979. Cloning of integrated Moloney sarcoma proviral DNA sequences in bacteriophage λ. *Proc. Natl. Acad. Sci.* **76:** 4464–4468.

Vande Woude, G.F., M. Oskarsson, W.L. McClements, L.W. Enquist, D.G. Blair, P.J. Fischinger, J.V. Maizel, and M. Sullivan. 1980. Characterization of integrated Moloney sarcoma provirus and flanking host sequences cloned in bacteriophage λ. *Cold Spring Harbor Symp. Quant. Biol.* **44:** 735–745.

Varmus, H.E., N. Quintrell, and J. Wyke. 1981. Revertants of an ASV-transformed rat cell line have lost the complete provirus or sustained mutations in *src*. *Virology* **108:** 28–46.

Varmus, H.E., R.V. Guntaka, C.T. Deng, and J.M. Bishop. 1975. Synthesis, structure and function of avian sarcoma virus-specific DNA in permissive and nonpermissive cells. *Cold Spring Harbor Symp. Quant. Biol.* **39:** 987–996.

Verma, I.M. 1975. Studies on reverse transcriptase of RNA tumor viruses. I. Localization of thermolabile DNA polymerase and RNase H activities on one polypeptide. *J. Virol.* **15:** 121–126.

Verma, I.M., H.E. Varmus, and E. Hunter. 1976. Characterization of "early" temperature-sensitive mutants of avian sarcoma viruses: Biological properties, thermolability of reverse transcriptase *in vitro,* and synthesis of viral DNA in infected cells. *Virology* **74:** 16–29.

Verma, I., W.S. Mason, S.D. Drost, and D. Baltimore. 1974. DNA polymerase activity from two temperature-sensitive mutants of Rous sarcoma virus is thermolabile. *Nature* **251:** 27–31.

Vigne, R., M.L. Breitman, C. Moscovici, and P.K. Vogt. 1979. Restitution of fibroblast-transforming ability in *src* deletion mutants of avian sarcoma virus during animal passage. *Virology* **93:** 413–426.

Vogt, P.K. 1964. Fluorescence microscopic observations on the defectiveness of Rous sarcoma virus. *Natl. Cancer Inst. Monogr.* **17:** 523–541.

———. 1965. A heterogeneity of Rous sarcoma virus revealed by selectively resistant chick embryo cells. *Virology* **25:** 237–247.

———. 1967. Phenotypic mixing in the avian tumor virus group. *Virology* **32:** 708–717.

———. 1971a. Spontaneous segregation of nontransforming viruses from cloned sarcoma viruses. *Virology* **46:** 939–946.

———. 1971b. Genetically stable reassortment of markers during mixed infection with avian tumor viruses. *Virology* **46:** 947–952.

———. 1973. The genome of avian RNA tumor viruses: A discussion of four models. In *Possible episomes in eukaryotes* (ed. L.G. Silvestri), vol. 4, pp. 35–41. North-Holland, Amsterdam.

———. 1977. Genetics of RNA tumor viruses. In *Comprehensive virology* (ed. H. Fraenkel-Conrat and R.R. Wagner), vol. 9, pp.341–455. Plenum Press, New York.

Vogt, P.K., R.A. Weiss, and H. Hanafusa. 1974. Proposal for numbering mutants of avian leukosis and sarcoma viruses. *J. Virol.* **13:** 551–554.

Vogt, P.K., M. Hayman, E. Hunter, and P.H. Duesberg. 1979. A nonconditional replication-defective mutant of the Schmidt-Ruppin strain of Rous sarcoma virus. *Virology* **92:** 285–290.

Vogt, P.K., J.L. Spence, W. Okazaki, R.L. Witter, and L.B. Crittenden. 1977. Phenotypic mixing between reticuloendotheliosis virus and avian sarcoma viruses. *Virology* **80:** 127–135.

Vogt, V.M., A. Wight, and R. Eisenman. 1979. *In vitro* cleavage of avian retrovirus *gag* proteins by viral protease p15. *Virology* **98:** 154–167.

Von der Helm, K. 1977. Cleavage of Rous sarcoma viral polypeptide precursor into internal structural proteins *in vitro* involves viral protein p15. *Proc. Natl. Acad. Sci.* **74:** 911–915.

Wake, C.T. and J.H. Wilson. 1980. Defined oligomeric SV40 DNA: A sensitive probe of general recombination in somatic cells. *Cell* **21:** 141–148.

Wang, L.-H. 1978. The gene order of avian RNA tumor viruses derived from biochemical analyses of deletion mutants and viral recombinants. *Annu. Rev. Microbiol.* **32:** 561–592.

Wang, L.-H. and P. Duesberg. 1974. Properties and location of poly(A) in Rous sarcoma virus RNA. *J. Virol.* **14:** 1515–1529.

Wang, L.-H., P.H. Duesberg, S. Kawai, and H. Hanafusa. 1976a. Location of envelope-specific and sarcoma-specific oligonucleotides on RNA of Schmidt-Ruppin Rous sarcoma virus. *Proc. Natl. Acad. Sci.* **73:** 447–451.

Wang, L.-H., P.H. Duesberg, P. Mellon, and P.K. Vogt. 1976b. Distribution of envelope-specific and sarcoma-specific nucleotide sequences from different parents in the RNAs of avian tumor virus recombinants. *Proc. Natl. Acad. Sci.* **73:** 1073–1077.

Wang, L.-H., C. Moscovici, R.E. Karess, and H. Hanafusa. 1979. Analysis of the *src* gene of sarcoma viruses generated by recombination between transformation-defective mutants and quail cellular sequences. *J. Virol.* **32:** 546–556.

Wang, L.-H., P.H. Duesberg, T. Robins, H. Yokota, and P.K. Vogt. 1977. The terminal oligonucleotides of avian tumor virus RNAs are genetically linked. *Virology* **82:** 472–492.

Wang, L.-H., D. Galehouse, P. Mellon, P. Duesberg, W.S. Mason, and P.K. Vogt. 1976c. Mapping oligonucleotides of Rous sarcoma virus RNA that segregate with polymerase and group-specific antigen markers in recombinants. *Proc. Natl. Acad. Sci.* **73:** 3952–3956.

Weber, M.J. and R.R. Friis. 1979. Dissociation of transformation parameters using temperature-conditional mutants of Rous sarcoma virus. *Cell* **16:** 25–32.

Wei, C.-M., D.R. Lowy, and E.M. Scolnick. 1980. Mapping of transforming region of the Harvey murine sarcoma virus genome by using insertion-deletion mutants constructed *in vitro*. *Proc. Natl. Acad. Sci.* **77:** 4674–4678.

Weiss, R.A. 1969. The host range of Bryan strain Rous sarcoma virus synthesized in the absence of helper virus. *J. Gen. Virol.* **5:** 511–528.

———. 1973. Transmission of cellular genetic elements by RNA tumor viruses. In *Possible episomes in eukaryotes* (ed. L.G. Silvestri), vol. 4, pp.130–141. North-Holland, Amsterdam.

———. 1980. Rhabdovirus pseudotypes. In *Rhabdoviruses* (ed. D.H.L. Bishop), vol. 3, pp.51–65. CRC Press, Boca Raton.

Weiss, R.A. and P.L.P. Bennett. 1980. Assembly of membrane glycoproteins studied by phenotypic mixing between mutants of vesicular stomatitis virus and retroviruses. *Virology* **100:** 252–274.

Weiss, R.A. and L.N. Payne. 1971. The heritable nature of the factor in chicken cells which acts as a helper virus for Rous sarcoma virus. *Virology* **45:** 508–515.

Weiss, R.A. and A.L. Wong. 1977. Phenotypic mixing between avian and mammalian RNA tumor viruses. I. Envelope pseudotypes of Rous sarcoma virus. *Virology* **76:** 826– 834.

Weiss, R.A., D. Boettiger, and D.N. Love. 1975. Phenotypic mixing between vesicular stomatitis virus and avian RNA tumor viruses. *Cold Spring Harbor Symp. Quant. Biol.* **39:** 913–918.

Weiss, R.A., D. Boettiger, and H.M. Murphy. 1977. Pseudotypes of avian sarcoma viruses with the envelope properties of vesicular stomatitis virus. *Virology* **76:** 808–825.

Weiss, R.A., W.S. Mason, and P.K. Vogt. 1973. Genetic recombinants and heterozygotes derived from endogenous and exogenous avian RNA tumor viruses. *Virology* **52:** 535-552.

Witte, O.N. and D. Baltimore. 1977. Mechanism of formation of pseudotypes between vesicular stomatitis virus and murine leukemia virus. *Cell* **11:** 505–511.

———. 1978. Relationship of retrovirus polyprotein cleavages to virion maturation studied with temperature-sensitive murine leukemia virus mutants. *J. Virol* **26:** 750–761.

Witte, O.N., A. Dasgupta, and D. Baltimore. 1980a. Abelson murine leukaemia virus protein is phosphorylated *in vitro* to form phosphotyrosine. *Nature* **283:** 826–831.

Witte, O.N., S. Goff, N. Rosenberg, and D. Baltimore. 1980b. A transformation-defective mutant of Abelson murine leukemia virus lacks protein kinase activity. *Proc. Natl. Acad. Sci.* **77:** 4993–4997.

Witte, O.N., N. Rosenberg, M. Paskind, A. Shields, and D. Baltimore. 1978. Identification of an Abelson murine leukemia virus-encoded protein present in transformed fibroblast and lymphoid cells. *Proc. Natl. Acad. Sci.* **75:** 2488–2492.

Wong, P.K.Y. and G.E. Gallick. 1978. Preliminary characterization of a temperature-sensitive mutant of Moloney murine leukemia virus that produces particles at the restrictive temperature. *J. Virol.* **25:** 187–192.

Wong, P.K.Y. and R. MacLeod. 1975. Studies of the budding process of a temperature-sensitive mutant of murine leukemia virus with a scanning electron microscope. *J. Virol.* **16:** 434–442.

Wong, P.K.Y. and J.A. McCarter. 1973. Genetic studies of temperature-sensitive mutants of Moloney-murine leukemia virus. *Virology* **53:** 319–326.

———. 1974. Studies of two temperature-sensitive mutants of Moloney murine leukemia virus. *Virology* **58:** 396–408.

Wong, P.K.Y., L.J. Russ, and J.A. McCarter. 1973. Rapid, selective procedure for isolation of spontaneous temperature-sensitive mutants of Moloney leukemia virus. *Virology* **51:** 424– 431.

Wong, P.K.Y., P.H. Yuen, R. MacLeod, E.H. Chang, M.W. Myers, and R.M. Friedman. 1977. The effect of interferon on the de novo infection of Moloney murine leukemia virus. *Cell* **10:** 245–252.

Wood, T.G., J. Peltier-Horn, W.G. Robey, D.G. Blair, and R.B. Arlinghaus. 1980. Characterization of virus-specified proteins present in NRK cells infected with a temperature-sensitive transformation mutant of Moloney murine sarcoma virus. *Cold Spring Harbor Symp. Quant. Biol.* **44:** 747–754.

Wyke, J.A. 1973a. The selective isolation of temperature-sensitive mutants of Rous sarcoma virus. *Virology* **52:** 587–590.

———. 1973b. Complementation of transforming functions by temperature-sensitive mutants of avian sarcoma virus. *Virology* **54:** 28–36.

———. 1974. The genetics of C-type RNA tumor viruses. *Int. Rev. Cytol.* **38:** 67–109.

———. 1975. Temperature sensitive mutants of avian sarcoma viruses. *Biochim. Biophys. Acta* **417:** 91–121.

———. 1976. Selection, screening, and isolation of temperature-sensitive mutants of avian sarcoma viruses. *Methods Cell Biol.* **14:** 251–264.

Wyke, J.A. and J.A. Beamand. 1979. Genetic recombination in Rous sarcoma virus: The genesis of recombinants and lack of evidence for linkage between *pol, env* and *src* genes in three factor crosses. *J. Gen. Virol.* **43:** 349–364.

Wyke, J.A. and M. Linial. 1973. Temperature-sensitive avian sarcoma viruses: A physiological comparison of twenty mutants. *Virology* **53:** 152–161.

Wyke, J.A., J.G. Bell, and J.A. Beamand. 1975. Genetic recombination among temperature-sensitive mutants of Rous sarcoma virus. *Cold Spring Harbor Symp. Quant. Biol.* **39:** 897–905.

Yakobson, E. and R.A. Weiss. 1981. Mutant retrovirus particles package vesicular stomatitis virus mRNA during mixed infection. *Virology* **109:** 183–187.

Yamamoto, T., J.S. Tyagi, J.B. Fagan, G. Jay, B. deCrombrugge, and I. Pastan. 1980. Molecular mechanism for the capture and excision of the transforming gene of avian sarcoma virus as suggested by analysis of recombinant clones. *J. Virol.* **35:** 436–443.

Yeger, H., and V.I. Kalnins. 1978. Immunocytochemical localization of gp70 over virus-related submembranous densities in *ts* mutant Rauscher murine leukemia virus-infected cells at the nonpermissive temperature. *Virology* **91:** 489–492.

Yeger, H., V.I. Kalnins, and J.R. Stephenson. 1976. Electron microscopy of mammalian type-C RNA viruses: Use of conditional lethal mutants in studies of virion maturation and assembly. *Virology* **74:**459–469.

———. 1978. Type-C retrovirus maturation and assembly: Post-translational cleavage of the *gag*-gene coded precursor polypeptide occurs at the cell membrane. *Virology* **89:**34–44.

Yoshida, M. and Y. Ikawa. 1977. Induction of some transformation-related properties by a transformation-defective mutant of avian sarcoma virus. *Virology* **83:**444–448.

Yoshida, M. and K. Toyoshima. 1980. *In vitro* translation of avian erythroblastosis virus RNA: Identification of two major polypeptides. *Virology* **100:**484–487.

Yoshida, M., M. Yamashita, and A. Nomoto. 1979. Transformation-defective mutants of Rous sarcoma virus with longer sizes of genome RNA and their highly frequent occurrences. *J. Virol.* **30:**453–461.

Yoshimura, F.K. and J.M. Yamamura. 1981. Four Moloney murine leukemia virus-infected rat cell clones producing replication-defective particles: Protein and nucleic acid analysis. *J. Virol.* (in press).

Yoshinaka, Y., K. Ishigame, T. Ohno, S. Kageyama, K. Shibata, and R.B. Luftig. 1980. Preparations enriched for "immature" murine leukemia virus particles that remain in tissue culture fluids are deficient in $Pr65^{gag}$ proteolytic activity. *Virology* **100:**130–140.

Young, H.A., T.Y. Shih, E.M. Scolnick, S. Rasheed, and M.B. Gardner. 1979. Different rat-derived transforming retroviruses code for an immunologically related intracellular phosphoprotein. *Proc. Natl. Acad. Sci.* **76:**3523–3527.

Yuasa, Y. and H. Shimojo. 1977. Isolation and preliminary characterization of temperature-sensitive mutants of the murine sarcoma leukaemia virus complex. *J. Gen. Virol.* **36:**257–266.

Yuen, P.H. and P.K.Y. Wong. 1977. A morphological study on the ultrastructure and assembly of murine leukemia virus using a temperature-sensitive mutant restricted in assembly. *Virology* **80:**260–274.

Zarling, D.A., A.G. Mosser, and H.M. Temin. 1977. Spontaneous mutations affecting the host range of the B77 strain of avian sarcoma virus involve type-specific changes in the virion envelope antigen. *J. Virol.* **21:**105–112.

Zavada, J. 1972a. Pseudotypes of vesicular stomatitis virus with the coat of murine leukaemia and of avian myeloblastosis viruses. *J. Gen. Virol.* **15:**183–191.

———. 1972b. VSV pseudotype particles with the coat of avian myeloblastosis virus. *Nat. New Biol.* **240:**122–124.

———. 1976. Viral pseudotypes and phenotypic mixing. *Arch. Virol.* **50:**1–15.

Zavada, J. and M. Rosenbergova. 1972. Phenotypic mixing of vesicular stomatitis virus with fowl plague virus. *Acta Virol.* **16:**103–114.

Zavada, J., C. Dickson, and R. Weiss. 1977. Pseudotypes of vesicular stomatitis virus with envelope antigens provided by murine mammary tumor virus. *Virology* **82:**221–231.

Zavada, J., J. Bubenik, R. Widmaier, and Z. Zavadova. 1975. Phenotypically mixed vesicular stomatitis virus particles produced in human tumor cell lines. *Cold Spring Harbor Symp. Quant. Biol.* **39:**907–912.

Zavadova, Z., J. Zavada, and R. Weiss. 1977. Unilateral phenotypic mixing of envelope antigens between togaviruses and vesicular stomatitis virus or avian RNA tumour virus. *J. Gen. Virol.* **37:**557–567.

8

Pathogenesis of Retrovirus-induced Disease

I. INTRODUCTION

Retroviral infections manifest a variety of pathological syndromes. The very nature of provirus integration and persistence emphasizes the close interrelationship between virus and host that often, but by no means always, results in disease. Although neoplasia has always been foremost in investigations of pathogenesis, retroviruses also elicit several kinds of nonmalignant diseases that represent significant causes of morbidity and mortality in infected host populations.

The diseases most commonly associated with retroviruses can be divided into four groups: (1) malignant tumors; (2) proliferative diseases that, although not necessarily neoplastic, may nonetheless be fatal; (3) anemias; and (4) slow, sporadic or chronic, degenerative diseases sometimes resembling "autoimmune" disease, affecting hematopoietic, neural, and other tissues. Tumors can be further classified on the basis of the tissue or origin: (1) sarcomas, which arise from connective (mesenchymal) tissue (e.g., fibroblasts, muscle cells, and chondrocytes); (2) carcinomas, which arise from epithelial tissues (e.g., epithelia of mammary glands); and (3) leukemias and lymphomas, which involve cells of the hematopoietic system. The majority of retrovirus-induced tumors fall into this third category, and therefore one section of this chapter is devoted to a general description of the hematopoietic lineages, using the mouse as a model system. Now that the molecular genetics of retroviruses is well established, it has become increasingly important to understand the underlying cellular mechanisms involved in normal differentiation in order to elucidate the alterations that occur during the pathogenic process or neoplastic conversion. Such studies can be undertaken at two levels: the target cell and the whole animal.

In this chapter, the major types of retrovirus disease are very briefly noted, followed by a short description of normal hematopoiesis in the mouse, necessary as a prelude to discussing leukemogenesis. The pathogenesis of the main taxonomic groups of retroviruses is then surveyed. We cover the following parameters for each virus or related virus group, where applicable: (1) historical perspective; (2) pathological syndrome, including some basic histological and gross anatomical characteristics, cofactors, host genes governing susceptibility or resistance, modifying immunological responses, and transmission; (3) oncogenic mechanisms operating in vivo; and (4) transformation in vitro of fibroblasts, hematopoietic cells, or cells of other origins. Only a minimum of histology and pathology is presented here; for details, see the excellent treatise by Gross (1970). The molecular aspects of oncogenes and their gene products are the subject of Chapter 9.

II. DISEASES CAUSED BY RETROVIRUSES

A. Apathogenic Infections

Among the exogenous retroviruses, only the foamy viruses (subfamily Spumavirinae) have not been associated with disease. These viruses frequently occur in neural tissue (Hooks and Gibbs 1975) (see Chapter 2). Although infected cultures give rise to vacuolated (foamy) syncytia, infection in vivo is not known to cause overt pathological symptoms, although some immunosuppressive effects have been noted.

Among the endogenous retroviruses, on the other hand, nonpathogenicity is the rule. Only those viruses resident in inbred strains of mice specially selected for high incidence of disease have been found to have oncogenic potential, e.g., the murine leukemia virus (MLV) genomes residing at the *Akv* loci in AKR mice and the murine mammary tumor virus (MMTV) genome of GR mice. Under natural selection, the intimate persistence of endogenous retroviruses, perhaps over millions of years, has probably ensured a nonpathogenic, symbiotic relationship between virus and host. The evolution of xenotropism, whereby replication and amplification of endogenous viruses in their natural host species are restricted (see Chapters 2 and 3), may be important in preventing disease; pathogenic variants and recombinants are known to arise in mice such as AKR and C58 in which the replication of an ecotropic endogenous virus is unrestricted (Cloyd et al. 1980). However, xenotropism does not entirely explain nonpathogenicity. AKR endogenous ecotropic virus does not induce disease in mouse strains susceptible to infection, and the endogenous viruses of chickens, such as RAV-0, appear to be completely nonpathogenic in chickens permissive for their replication to reasonably high titer (Motta et al. 1975; Robinson et al. 1980, 1982; Crittenden et al. 1982). The possible pathogenicity of such viruses and of xenotropic viruses in foreign hosts susceptible to infection has not been adequately studied; however, Weiss and Frisby (1982) have presented evidence suggesting that RAV-0 may induce lymphoma and wasting disease in a related species of fowl.

Although endogenous viruses generally are not themselves pathogenic, they may play a role in protecting the host from pathogenic sequelae of exogenous virus infection. There is evidence, for instance, that those endogenous viral elements in chickens which express envelope (*env*)-related genes modify the host response to avian leukosis viruses (ALVs) in a beneficial way (Crittenden et al. 1982; Weiss and Frisby 1982).

B. Acute Neoplasms

Some C-type retroviruses cause the appearance of malignant tumors within a few days of infection. For instance, tumors induced by Rous sarcoma virus (RSV) in the wing web of a chicken may reach 10 mm in diameter within 1 week of inoculation with virus; chickens die of acute erythroblastic or myeloblastic leukemia within 2 to 3 weeks of infection by the causative viruses. Splenomegaly caused by the Friend erythroleukemia virus complex in mice is also manifest within 2 weeks of infection at high doses. The tumors that appear so early after infection are probably not clonal growths but involve transformation of many target cells. This was studied in detail for Rous sarcoma by Ponten

(1964), who, using sex chromosome markers, showed that the rapid growth of sarcomas resulted from the recruitment of newly infected and transformed cells.

Acutely oncogenic retroviruses induce specific kinds of leukemias or solid tumors in animals. Most of these viruses also transform corresponding, and sometimes inappropriate, target cells in vitro and carry specific transforming sequences called *onc* genes (Baltimore 1975). *onc* genes usually occur as inserts substituting for portions of the viral structural genes, rendering the virus defective for replication (see Chapter 4). The viral (*v-onc*) genes causing cell transformation are derived from cellular (*c-onc*) genes that apparently exert their oncogenic effect when recombined into the viral genome governed by strong promoter signals in the proviral long terminal repeat (LTR) (see Chapter 4). These *onc* genes and their products are discussed in detail in Chapter 9. Almost all of the acutely oncogenic viruses carry *onc* genes; thus, they can be considered analogous to transducing bacteriophages or as cloning vectors that reintroduce genetic sequences back into appropriate target cells. It is reasonable to suppose that these sequences, when present in the cellular genomes of normal cells, play an important role in normal differentiation or development. Thus, studies on the molecular and cell biology of transforming viruses (Chapter 9) should provide insight into the genetic basis of normal differentiation, including hematopoiesis.

Some defective, acutely oncogenic viruses carry transforming genes derived not from host genes but from viral *env* genes, e.g., the spleen focus-forming component of Friend virus. A discussion of these viruses is included in this chapter. There are also selected variants of nondefective MLVs that cause acute disease (Haas 1980; Oliff et al. 1980; Van Griensven and Vogt 1980). These viruses possibly carry recombinant genes whose products may still function as virion components while additionally exerting an oncogenic effect. This may also be true of some recombinant viruses arising during nonacute leukemogenesis (see below).

Although acutely oncogenic viruses have been studied more intensively than other retroviruses, they are found only rarely and sporadically in nature, suggesting that each isolate represents a new recombinant virus. They are not naturally transmitted from one host to another, perhaps because they are defective or because they are so rapidly pathogenic that there is strong selection against natural persistence by transmission. Nevertheless, acutely oncogenic viruses are proving to be extraordinarily powerful tools in experimental and natural carcinogenesis through studies of the functions of *v-onc* and *c-onc* genes (Chapter 9).

C. Slow Neoplasms

These are tumors induced by retroviruses that do not carry oncogenes as part of their genomes. As the tumor may be fast growing and highly malignant, the "slowness" indicates a long latent period between infection and manifestation of the disease. Tumors induced by slow retroviruses usually appear in animals that are chronically viremic, whether chickens (Rubin et al. 1962), mice (Rowe 1973), cats (Essex 1975), or gibbons (Kawakami and McDowell 1980). However, restriction enzyme analyses of host-virus integration sites, in murine thymic lymphoma (Steffen and Weinberg 1978), murine mammary carcinoma (Cohen et al. 1979), bovine leukemia (Kettmann et al. 1980), and avian bursal lymphoma (Neiman et al. 1980a), indicate that the tumors are clonal in origin. As described below for specific instances, it appears to be a general feature of the "slow" oncogenic viruses that many more potential target cells become infected with the virus than progress to form a malignant tumor. Thus, tumorigenesis is an extremely rare consequence of infection at the cellular level, although the probability that an infected animal will develop a tumor is usually quite high.

Viral oncogenesis induced by nonacute retroviruses also appears to be a multistage process, as is typical for nonviral tumors (Armitage and Doll 1961; Peto 1978; Whittemore 1978). This is clearly seen in avian and murine virus lymphomagenesis. Following infection of newly hatched chicks by ALV, large numbers of potential target cells in the bursa of Fabricius become infected. Within 1 month of infection, a preneoplastic transformation is seen in that 10–100 follicles in the bursa become filled with immature blast cells, which are called transformed follicles (Cooper et al. 1968; Neiman et al. 1980b). About 1 in 50 of the transformed follicles grow to form small nodules 5–10 mm in diameter. Most nodules do not appear until approximately 5 months after infection. During physiological regression of the bursa, disseminated disease occurs, and it is likely that the progressively growing nodules give rise to the metastases, since the pattern of viral restriction fragments is similar or identical in bursal and metastatic tumors in the same animal (Neiman et al. 1980a; Fung et al. 1981; Payne et al. 1981).

Thymic lymphomagenesis in mice also involves several stages of progression. An important step in lymphomagenesis by endogenous ecotropic viral genomes in AKR mice is the generation of variant or recombinant viruses with altered *env* genes. The altered host range of these viruses may also render them especially effective in infecting and transforming thymic lymphocytes (Hartley et al. 1977; Cloyd et al. 1980).

In murine mammary carcinogenesis, endocrine factors play an important role in addition to virus infection, but again, only a few of the millions of infected, hormone-responsive mammary cells develop into malignant clones (Cohen et al. 1979).

Recent evidence strongly suggests that specific *c-onc* host genes may play a role in oncogenesis by nonacute tumor viruses. Neel et al. (1981) and Payne et al. (1981) found that the LTR of ALVs promotes the expression of a cellular gene in avian lymphomas. In the majority of bursal lymphomas, the cellular gene is *c-myc,* the host homolog of the oncogene of the myelocytomatosis virus MC29 and related viruses (Hayward et al. 1981). The LTR is able to enhance *c-myc* expression by integration adjacent to the host gene in the infected cell. The right-hand (3′) LTR appears to be most active in promotion when the left-hand (5′) LTR is missing; therefore, in many lymphomas, it is a defective viral genome that activates the expression of the cellular gene by "downstream promotion." In some tumors, the nearby ALV LTR enhances expression of *c-myc* by mechanisms other than provision of a viral promoter (Payne et al. 1982) (see Section IV.B.3).

These findings reveal a common mechanism of oncogenesis between some acutely transforming and slowly transforming retroviruses: the ectopic expression of cellular genes. With acute viruses, the gene is transduced by the virus and has a high probability of expression under the control of the left-hand LTR of each integrated provirus. With nonacute viruses, the virus will integrate next to the specific cellular gene to augment its expression only very rarely indeed.

In avian bursal lymphomas, a second host gene has been identified through DNA transfection studies (Cooper and Neiman

1980). This gene is not linked to viral LTR sequences or to *c-myc* (Cooper and Neiman 1981), and its expression may represent a later step in oncogenesis than *c-myc* activation (see Section IV.B.3).

It is not established yet whether enhanced expression of cellular genes by viral LTRs is a widespread phenomenon in oncogenesis by nonacute retroviruses, nor is its mechanistic role in tumor induction understood. The activation of *c-myc* has also been observed in avian lymphomas induced by chick syncytial virus (CSV) (Noori-Daloii et al. 1981), a virus unrelated to ALV. Similar *c-onc* activations are being sought in tumors induced by mammalian nonacute viruses (see Section VII.G). It is possible, however, that other mechanisms of oncogenesis may be involved. For example, the LTR of MMTV is unusual in having an open-reading-frame sequence that codes for polypeptides when translated in vitro (Dickson et al. 1981) (see Chapter 4 and Section VII.G). If such polypeptides are synthesized in vivo, they might play a role in carcinogenesis.

As already mentioned, thymic lymphomagenesis by MLV involves the generation of "thymotropic" host-range variants. These variants may be required simply to deliver an LTR to the target cell where it might activate a *c-onc* gene; on the other hand, the changes within the *env* gene itself may be directly concerned with oncogenesis, as well as with infectivity for the appropriate target cell. It has been suggested by McGrath and Weissman (1979) that viral glycoproteins encoded by recombinant *env* genes recognize unique receptors on the surfaces of individual T lymphocytes. These authors postulate that the interaction with the receptor not only allows entry of the virus, but also is mitogenic. The infected lymphocyte thus synthesizes *env* glycoprotein, which acts as a autocrine mitogen, leading to the clonal proliferation of the infected cell into a tumor. In this model, the recombinant *env* gene is effectively an oncogene. The various models of oncogenesis by nonacute retroviruses are discussed in more detail in sections devoted to particular viruses.

D. Anemia, Wasting, and "Autoimmune" Disorders

Many C-type viruses cause anemias. These may be aplastic through destruction of bone-marrow stem cells, hyperplastic through a block in hematopoietic maturation (as with the anemia strain of Friend virus), or hemolytic as in several "autoimmune" syndromes associated with retroviruses. For example, feline leukemia virus (FeLV), particularly the subgroup-C serotype, induces aplastic or hemolytic anemia as frequently as it causes leukemia (Jarrett 1980).

Equine infectious anemia virus (EIAV) is a retrovirus of worldwide distribution (Henson and McGuire 1974). EIAV is currently considered to be a member of the Oncovirinae subfamily (see Chapter 2), although it is not known to be oncogenic. The only cell type in which it is known to replicate in vitro is the macrophage, causing cellular degeneration (Kobayashi and Kono 1967). Following an acute febrile illness, the chronic phase of the disease caused by EIAV involves lymphoproliferative disorders, glomerulonephritis, and hemolytic anemia. The latter symptoms are presumably a result of a secondary, humoral response to virus infection.

MLVs may exacerbate the autoimmune disease of (NZB × NZW) F_1 mice that resembles systemic lupus erythematosus (SLE) of man (Talal and Steinberg 1974) and the necrotizing arthritis and glomerulonephritis of SL/Ni mice that resembles human polyarteritis nodosa (Yoshiki et al. 1979). The pathological lesion in these conditions is the result of deposition of immune complexes in the walls of blood vessels and glomeruli. In affected mice, these complexes include antibodies to nucleic acids and to virion components (Mellors 1968; Yoshiki et al. 1974). There is no correlation, however, between development of disease and antibodies to the viral *env*-gene product gp70 (Izui et al. 1978), and in genetic crosses in which virus expression is diminished, full-blown autoimmune disease develops (Datta et al. 1978). It would appear that retroviruses are not the primary cause of these conditions in inbred mice.

There is increasing evidence, however, that retroviruses, including those classically considered as leukemia viruses, cause wasting, runting, and degenerative syndromes in several virus-host systems. Congenital transmission of FeLV frequently induces abortion or runting in the newborn. Subgroup-B and -D ALVs, which are somewhat cytopathic for fibroblasts in culture, can cause a degenerative syndrome involving bursal and thymic atrophy, liver necrosis, and wasting. Subgroup-A and -E viruses elicit similar symptoms in fowl not possessing or expressing endogenous virus genes (Robinson et al. 1980; Crittenden et al. 1982; Weiss and Frisby 1982). Osteopetrosis is another common disease associated with ALV infection (Smith and Moscovici 1969) and is discussed in detail in Section IV. Avian reticuloendotheliosis-associated virus (REAV), like the subgroup-B and -D ALVs, is cytopathic in fibroblast cultures early after infection. In vivo, spleen and liver necrosis is observed. Since these viruses are cytopathic in vitro, one may question whether the in vivo necrosis is immunologically mediated.

Visna (wasting) and maedi (shortness of breath) are neurological and pulmonary manifestations of persistent infection by the same retrovirus in sheep (Haase 1975; Petursson et al. 1979). Both forms of the disease are inflammatory, involving infiltration of lymphocytes and macrophages in the central nervous system or in the septa dividing the alveoli of the lung. Caprine arthritis-encephalitis virus causes an acute leukoencephalitis that resembles the disease produced in goats inoculated with visna virus. Persistent infection of adult goats causes a chronic arthritis in which the joints become infiltrated with lymphocytes, the synovial cells proliferate, and cartilage is broken down (Crawford et al. 1980).

It is apparent, then, that retroviruses are associated with a wide variety of disorders resembling autoimmune diseases of man. The mechanisms of pathogenesis are not well understood, although antibody complexed with viral antigens is presumably implicated in hemolytic anemia, glomerulonephritis, and arthritis. In other tissues, the virus may have a direct cytopathic effect not mediated through immune lysis.

E. Neural Diseases

The inflammatory degeneration of the central nervous system during the long course of visna virus infection (Haase 1975; Petursson et al. 1979) has already been alluded to as an autoimmune disease that probably reflects the host response to chronic virus infection. Antigenic changes in virus-envelope glycoproteins and subsequent production of matching neutralizing antibodies (see Section XIV) indicate a continuing immunological response to chronic infection by visna virus, to the detriment of the nervous system.

A different kind of neurological disorder is found in feral Californian mice infected with a congenitally transmitted C-type virus (Andrews and Gardner 1974; Gardner et al. 1980a). This virus causes lymphoma and hind-limb paralysis; the two diseases are not linked and they both occur relatively late in life. The paralysis is caused by a noninflammatory destruction of motor neurons in the spinal cord, resembling poliomyelitis. Persistent viremia is essential for the development of the disease, and passive immunization of newborn mice is highly protective (Gardner et al. 1980a). Numerous viral particles are seen in affected neural tissue, including bizarre rod-shaped virions atypical of C-type particles (Andrews and Gardner 1974). A temperature-sensitive mutant of Moloney MLV (Mo-MLV) (*ts*1) also induces neurological paralysis in mice (McCarter et al. 1977).

This brief survey of diseases associated with retroviruses emphasizes the variety of syndromes and host-virus interactions evident in persistent infections. A more detailed discussion of the pathogenesis of particular retroviruses is presented in later sections of this chapter.

III. HEMATOPOIESIS IN THE MOUSE

Because leukemia is often viewed as blocked or aberrant hematopoietic cell differentiation, an understanding of the mechanism of transformation by the leukemia viruses must begin with a discussion of current thinking about normal hematopoietic cell differentiation. The description here will be brief, as there are a number of excellent recent reviews on hematopoiesis (Metcalf 1977; Quesenberry and Levitt 1979; Till and McCulloch 1980). Although this discussion concerns hematopoiesis in the mouse specifically, similar studies have derived related schemes for hematopoietic cell differentiation in other animals.

The hematopoietic system is made up of a hierarchy of cells with different developmental, functional, and proliferative capacities (see Fig. 8.1). Throughout the life span of the individual, the hematopoietic system must be able to generate new, fully differentiated cells to replace those cells that are continually lost as the cells mature and die. In addition, the rate of production of the mature differentiated cells must be sensitive to the continuously

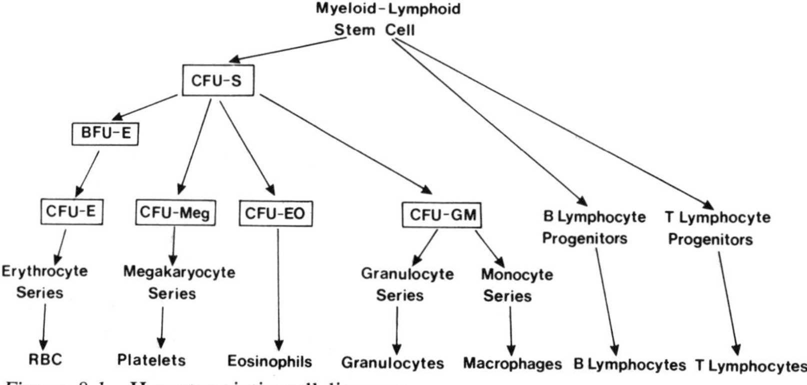

Figure 8.1 Hematopoietic cell lineages.

changing demands that occur for the specific cells under different physiological conditions.

An understanding of the cellular organization of this differentiating system has come largely from the development of functional colony assays for various hematopoietic progenitor cells. Using these colony techniques, both the relative frequency and developmental capacity of a number of such progenitor cells have been established.

The first assay system described was the spleen-colony assay (Till and McCulloch 1961). This assay detects hematopoietic cells, called the CFU-S (colony-forming units, spleen), that can form macroscopic spleen colonies 9–12 days after injection into lethally irradiated mice. There is now extensive evidence (for review, see McCulloch et al. 1965a) that this assay detects a class of cells with the expected properties of a myeloid stem cell; as commonly used, this term implies that the cells can serve as precursors to all the cells of the hematopoietic system, excluding the lymphoid series. Some of the properties of the spleen-colony assay include: (1) The number of colonies formed is linearly related to the number of cells injected (generally spleen or bone-marrow cells), and cytogenetic studies have demonstrated that each colony is derived from a single cell. (2) The spleen colonies contain cells of the erythroid, granulocytic, and megakaryocytic pathways. (3) The colonies still contain CFU-S, indicating that CFU-S have self-renewal capacity. (4) The cell-cycle status of CFU-S is sensitive to differing demands for mature cells.

It is not yet clear whether an even more primitive stem cell, capable of giving rise to both myeloid and lymphoid progeny, is also detected by the spleen-colony assay. No mature B (bone-marrow-derived) or T (thymus-derived) lymphoid cells have been conclusively detected in spleen colonies, nor is it clear whether less-differentiated lymphoid progenitor cells (pre-B or pre-T cells) are present in CFU-S-derived colonies. However, the notion that a myeloid-lymphoid pluripotent stem cell exists is suggested by the work of Abramson et al. (1977), who, using radiation-induced chromosomal markers, demonstrated the presence of mature myeloid and lymphoid cells that had clearly descended from a common stem cell in the adult mouse. Thus, there appear to be at least two distinguishable classes of hematopoietic stem cells: (1) a population of cells that is restricted to differentiate along the myeloid lineages and (2) a more primitive stem-cell population that is capable of differentiating along either the myeloid or the lymphoid system (see Fig. 8.1).

Following the development of the in vivo spleen-colony assay, additional colony assays were developed using semisolid media such as agar, methylcellulose, or plasma clots, widening the spectrum of progenitor cells that can be detected and enumerated. These in vitro colony assays also serve as useful bioassays for factors, usually glycoproteins, that appear to be necessary for the proliferation and/or differentiation of a number of normal hematopoietic progenitor cells. Characterization of these factors, and their mechanism of action, is of particular interest when considering leukemic transformation by retroviruses, because transformation by these viruses is often accompanied by the appearance of cells with a factor-independent phenotype.

Historically, the first cell-culture colony assays detected progenitor cells committed to differentiation into granulocytes and macrophages (Pluznik and Sachs 1965; Bradley and Metcalf 1966). The growth of these colony-forming cells, termed either colony-forming units in culture (CFU-C) or granulocyte-macrophage colony-forming units (CFU-GM), from normal mice is absolutely dependent on the presence of a glycoprotein called colony-stimulating factor or activity (CSF or CSA) that can be obtained and purified from conditioned medium or cell extracts from a number of different sources (Burgess et al. 1977; Stanley et al. 1978).

Clonal assays for red-cell progenitors, based on their ability to form colonies in semisolid medium, have also been described (Stephenson et al. 1971; Axelrad et al. 1972; Iscove 1978). At least two distinct classes of erythroid precursors can be detected by these assays: relatively mature precursors, referred to as CFU-E (colony-forming units, erythroid), form small colonies of 20–60 hemoglobinized cells after 48 hours in culture, whereas more primitive erythroid progenitors, referred to as BFU-E (burst-forming units, erythroid), form large colonies that do not start to become hemoglobinized until after 4–6 days in culture. The growth and differentiation of CFU-E are absolutely dependent on the presence of low doses of a normal hormone, erythropoietin, in the culture medium. In addition to requiring erythropoietin, BFU-E also require a glycoprotein factor, termed BPA (burst-promoting activity), for their proliferation and differentiation; conditioned medium obtained from lectin-stimulated mouse spleen cells is a rich source of this activity (Iscove 1978; Iscove et al. 1980).

The above-mentioned culture systems all describe colony-forming cells that appear to be committed along one of the myeloid differentiation pathways and thus are more differentiated than the pluripotent stem cell detected in the spleen-colony assay. Recently, Johnson and Metcalf (1977) have described an agar colony-forming assay that appears to detect a multipotent stem cell equivalent to CFU-S assayed in vivo. These "mixed" colony-forming cells give rise to large colonies of predominantly erythroid cells, but some also contain macrophages, neutrophils, eosinophils and megakaryocytes. In addition, these mixed colonies contain very low numbers of CFU-S (Metcalf and Johnson 1978; Humphries et al. 1979). Thus, an in vitro cell-culture assay is now available that detects a primitive stem-cell population equivalent to, or perhaps even less differentiated than, that detected by the spleen-colony assay.

Colony assays have also been developed for the two distinct populations of lymphoid cells: B cells generated mainly in the bone marrow and involved in immunoglobulin biosynthesis and T cells whose differentiation is thymus-dependent. Mature B lymphocytes can be identified by a number of B-cell-specific membrane markers, including membrane immunoglobulin, and by receptors for the Fc portion of immunoglobulins and the C3 component of complement. Mouse T cells, many of which can be identified by the presence of the antigen Thy-1 on their surfaces, interact with B cells (either positively or negatively) and are involved in cell-mediated immune responses, particularly against virus-infected cells.

Techniques for obtaining colonies of B lymphocytes in agar have been described by Metcalf et al. (1975a,b). The assay requires the presence of 2-mercaptoethanol (5×10^{-5} M), fetal calf serum, and a B-cell mitogen, such as lipopolysaccharide. Analysis of the properties of the colony-forming cell (CFU-B) suggests that it is a relatively mature B cell, rather than the less-differentiated pre-B cell (Metcalf 1977). CFU-B appear rather late in embryogenesis, they represent a very high proportion of hematopoietic cell populations, and they are found in the peripheral blood. Evidence that the assay detects B cells comes from an examination of the membrane properties of the B-lymphocyte colony cells. They express Fc receptors, membrane-bound IgM, and Ly-4.1 and Ly-4.2 antigens, but they do not have Thy-1 (Metcalf et al. 1975a).

The production of murine T-lymphocyte colonies in semisolid medium (Sredni et al. 1976; Jacobs and Miller 1979) requires the presence of either a T-cell mitogen or conditioned medium from mitogen-stimulated leukocytes. The colony cells express surface Thy-1 and a high proportion of the colonies contain cytotoxic lymphocyte precursors (Ching and Miller 1980).

Until recently, early events in hematopoietic cell differentiation have been difficult to study for two major reasons. First, studies on CFU-S or early-committed progenitor cells (either or both of which are likely target cells for transformation by the leukemia viruses discussed in this chapter) are hampered by the fact that populations that contain these cells are extremely heterogeneous, with stem cells making up a very small fraction of the total. It seems to be generally true that the less differentiated a cell is, the rarer it is. This latter conclusion arises from the fact that differentiation is usually accompanied by extensive cell proliferation. For example, the best estimates assess the frequency of CFU-S in normal bone-marrow populations at 10^{-2} to 10^{-3}. Attempts to enrich these populations for particular cell types by physical or immunological techniques have provided useful information about these cells but have not yet yielded purified populations of progenitor cells.

The second major technical problem in working with hematopoietic progenitor cells has been the inability to maintain these cells in long-term culture in vitro. Recently, however, Dexter and his colleagues have described tissue-culture procedures for the long-term (3 months or more) proliferation of certain hematopoietic progenitor cells, including CFU-S, CFU-GM, CFU-E, and BFU-E, in suspension over an adherent monolayer of cells derived from bone marrow or spleen (Dexter and Testa 1976; Dexter et al. 1977; Eliason et al. 1979). As discussed in Section VIII below, these cultures have been extremely useful for studying the effects of certain murine retroviruses, including Friend and Abelson leukemia virus complexes, in a more controlled environment than the intact animal.

From the cellular hematologists' perspective, leukemia viruses provide the opportunity to transfer, with high efficiency, genetic information into hematopoietic cells. The functional consequences of this genetic manipulation can then be analyzed by the techniques now becoming available for the characterization of hematopoietic progenitor cells. Recent studies on the origin of the transforming sequences of acute leukemia and sarcoma viruses have indicated that these sequences, in most cases, originated in normal cells and have been acquired by a recombinational event between a replication-competent retrovirus and the host genome (see Chapter 9). In addition, transformation by some of the ALVs and MLVs (discussed in Sections IV and VIII) can lead to the generation of clonal cell lines that have retained the capacity to differentiate along one or more hematopoietic cell lineages. Such cell lines provide a relatively homogeneous population of cells that are useful in the development of a molecular genetics approach to the study of both normal and leukemic hematopoietic cell differentiation. Thus, studies on these viruses should yield information not only on viral leukemogenesis, but also on the cellular and genetic events involved in a complex differentiation system.

IV. PATHOGENESIS OF AVIAN LEUKOSIS VIRUSES

Since the beginning of this century, evidence has accumulated linking viruses with a number of neoplastic or hyperplastic disorders in domestic fowl. Interest in these agents was at first meager, for clinicians and pathologists were interested primarily in man and secondarily in other mammals. Birds are clearly very different from mammals, possessing anatomical and physiological peculiarities that are dictated by their adaptation to flight and are yet strongly reminiscent of the body organization of diapsid reptiles. These differences fostered the idea that the study of avian tumors would tell us little about neoplasia in man. This prejudice was exacerbated by the fact that most virus-induced disorders in fowl involved the hematopoietic system in which the pathologists' usual criteria for distinguishing benign from malignant neoplasia and neoplasia from hyperplasia are harder to apply. It was thus suggested that many of these diseases reflected hyperplasia, chronic inflammation, or aberrant immune responses, rather than true neoplasia. These distinctions are, of course, important in terms of the basic mechanisms of cell proliferation. Although neoplasia may be responsive to external influences, its induction involves stable genetic or epigenetic alterations in the cells themselves, whereas hyperplasia is an abnormal proliferative response of normal cells to particular external stimuli.

Two unlinked developments generated widespread interest in the avian tumor viruses. First, the introduction of modern practices of intensive fowl husbandry resulted in an increased occurrence of hematopoietic neoplasms, which became a major cause of economic loss in the industry. Second, it was found that viruses were also involved in mammalian neoplasia (see Chapter 1), suggesting that the avian diseases might yet provide appropriate experimental models.

A. Early Studies on Avian Leukosis

For the first 50 years, research on these disorders was principally clinical and pathological, and from the outset, it was clear that the disease pattern was complex (for a full review of research during this period, see Gross [1970], for a review of histopathology, see Beard [1980]). In studies on induction of erythromyeloblastosis by cell-free filtrates, Ellermann and Bang (1908, 1909) distinguished "leukemic" disease, in which the peripheral blood contained large numbers of immature blood cells, from "aleukemic" disease, in which neoplastic cells infiltrated the viscera (mainly the spleen and liver) but were not present in massive numbers in the blood. These two disease patterns were clearly linked, for the same filtrate could cause either disease upon inoculation; and Ellermann and Bang coined the term leukosis to include both forms of disorder. Not only the location, but also the type of the predominant immature blood cell involved was variable. The leukosis studied by Ellermann and Bang comprised both erythroblasts (erythroid cell precursors) and myeloblasts (progenitors of granulocytes and macrophages) in variable proportions, but by serial laboratory passage, Ellermann and other workers obtained strains that produced predominantly or entirely leukosis of one or the other histological type. However, even these laboratory strains could show complex behavior, for it was later shown that, under certain conditions, some strains of erythroblastosis virus could cause sarcomas (Oberling and Guerin 1934) or renal adenocarcinomas (Carr 1956). Moreover, although the myeloblastosis and erythroblastosis strains showed differences in their patterns of disease production (e.g., the former produced disease most readily in very young chicks [Beaudreau et al. 1956], whereas older birds were more susceptible to the latter [Eckert et al. 1955a]), they were also clearly related antigenically (Eckert et al. 1955b), and some chicken strains were resistant to both viruses.

A spectrum of different disease patterns was also found in studies on the agents that caused avian lymphomatosis, a disease characterized by diffuse or nodular infiltration of internal organs with primitive lymphoid cells. Sites of infiltration showed characteristic differences, either viscera (mainly liver and spleen), nerves (notably the brachial, sciatic, and femoral), or the iris being involved in the typical forms of the disease. One form of the disease, in which visceral lymphomas are associated with neural and ocular lymphomatosis, comprises a complex called Marek's disease. The other form of visceral lymphomatosis is now more widely called lymphoid leukosis. This disease was sometimes associated with osteopetrosis, a thickening of the bones, principally in the leg, as a result of excessive osteoblast activity in the endosteum and periosteum. Sarcomas of various types, e.g., erythroblastosis, endotheliomas (hemangiomas), and nephroblastomas, were also sometimes associated with lymphoid leukosis, and even passaged strains of virus seemed capable of inducing a variety of neoplasia (Burmester et al. 1959a). As with the erythroid and myeloid leukoses, strains of chickens were discovered that showed resistance to disease.

These complex findings posed important questions (Gross 1970). Many of the diseases are caused by related viruses, but are these viruses identical? In other words, must one explain the plethora of disease manifestations in terms of different, perhaps specific, interactions between a single strain of virus and its host? Such interactions could be influenced by factors such as the route of infection, dose of infecting virus, age and physiological status of the host, strain-specific or individual genetic variations in host susceptibility, and postinfection modulation or mutation in the virus. On the other hand, are there a number of different viruses each responsible for producing a disease of distinct histological type? In this case, the variable disease patterns would be attributable to infection of individuals or flocks by varying proportions of more than one agent. These questions have been clarified, although not yet fully answered, by work over the last 20 years in which the techniques of modern virology and cell and molecular biology have been applied to these viruses (for review, see Graf and Beug 1978). At the same time, new knowledge of hematopoietic differentiation and modern hematological methods have led to a reappraisal of some of the pathological findings. With the benefit of hindsight, we now realize that many of the studies outlined above involved mixtures of viruses, but some of these agents do indeed have the potential to induce tumors of more than one type. It is also clear that, in some isolates, virus mixtures are unavoidable because many of the oncogenic viruses have replication defects and can only be propagated with the assistance of a helper virus (see Chapter 3). Moreover, we now know a great deal about the mode of transmission of these agents and the genetic basis of host resistance (see below and Chapter 3), facts that help to explain some of the variable host responses observed by earlier workers.

B. Classification and In Vivo Pathogenesis of Avian Leukoses

1. Classification

A modern classification of avian leukosis can be based logically on the nature of the causative viruses, which can be divided into three main groups. The first of these causes Marek's disease and is a horizontally transmitted herpesvirus, which, as such, is outside the scope of this work. It is dealt with in the companion volume to this book (Tooze 1980) and by Nazerian (1980). Suffice it to say that the virus replicates in feather follicle epithelium in both clinically susceptible and clinically resistant birds and is spread in contaminated dander and litter. Infection of clinically susceptible birds leads to proliferation of T lymphoblasts, infiltration of viscera and nerves (sometimes with ocular involvement), and paralysis in birds from the age of 4–6 weeks onwards. Diagnostic differentiation between the lymphomas of Marek's disease and those of retrovirus-induced lymphoid leukosis is important, because prophylactic measures can be taken against Marek's disease using vaccines that employ either natural or attenuated avirulent strains or a related turkey herpesvirus that is avirulent in chickens.

The second group contains the retroviruses with nondefective replication that typically cause lymphoid leukosis, whereas the third group is made up of replication-defective retroviruses causing a variety of leukemias and tumors of other tissues. The nondefective lymphoid leukosis viruses (LLVs) produce neoplasms with a long clinical latency, and they are not known to encode a gene product that mediates this oncogenic change. The replication-defective leukemia viruses (DLVs), on the other hand, produce disease with short latency, apparently as a result of the functioning of a viral transforming gene (see Chapters 4 and 9). It seems likely that their replication defect has been incurred because they have recombined with cellular genetic material to acquire this transforming gene (Roussel et al. 1979; Sheiness and Bishop 1979) (see Chapter 9). Their helper viruses are nondefective leukosis viruses that thus may themselves be pathogenic.

2. Transmission

The natural spread of ALVs has been studied mainly with the LLVs, which are the commonest of this group of pathogens. Since these agents are the helper for DLV, most of which lack any functional virus replicative genes (see Chapter 4), factors that influence their spread are likely also to affect the defective agents.

Unlike endogenous retroviruses (see Chapter 10), which are genetically transmitted as proviruses, ALVs are passed from bird to bird by congenital vertical transmission and by horizontal transmission (see Chapter 2 and Fig. 2.3). Horizontal infection of adult birds is usually countered by an effective development of neutralizing antibodies to envelope antigens, and the birds rarely develop leukosis (Rubin et al. 1962). However, virus may be present in ovarian follicles and oviducts (DiStefano and Dougherty

1966; Spencer et al. 1977; Payne et al. 1979), and this can lead to congenital transmission of virus via the egg, particularly in the case of the younger laying hens (Burmester et al. 1955; Burmester and Waters 1956). The chicks thus infected become viremic in embryo and are immunologically tolerant to the virus (Rubin et al. 1961, 1962). Such birds grow normally but shed virus in saliva and other secretions (Zeigel et al. 1964) and frequently develop leukosis later in life. If these virus-shedding birds are housed with susceptible virus-free chicks in the brooder, the contacts can show very heavy losses from lymphomatosis; however, if mixing occurs at a later stage, the contacts mount a protective immune response after transient viremia and the cycle can be repeated.

3. Nondefective Leukosis Viruses (Lymphoid Leukosis Viruses)

a. Lymphoid Leukosis. This is a common neoplasm in susceptible flocks and is typified by an enlarged liver and spleen, infiltrated with B lymphoblasts, and a concomitant anemia. The position of the tumor cells within the B-cell developmental pathway is defined by the presence on their surfaces of IgM, but not IgG or IgA, molecules (Cooper et al. 1974). The tumor cells originate in the bursa of Fabricius, a lymphoid organ of birds located dorsal to the proctodeum (posterior cloaca). Here, lymphoblast accumulation within the follicles is seen as early as 1 month after infection (Cooper et al. 1968; Neiman et al. 1980b). Most of these transformed follicles disappear with the natural regression of the bursa at 5–6 months of age, but a small percentage form progressively growing nodules at 3–4 months, which grow slowly for a while and then produce rapidly growing metastatic lymphomas at 6–8 months (Neiman et al. 1980b). The clinical disease can run either a brief or rather prolonged course, typified by pallor, listlessness, and diarrhea. The importance of the bursa in tumor development is demonstrated by the observation that bursectomy during the first 3 months of life prevents the development of visceral lymphomatosis (Peterson et al. 1966).

b. Osteopetrosis and Nephroblastoma. An unusual effect of bursectomy, if it is performed on hatchlings infected experimentally with LLV at 1 day of age, is an increased incidence of osteopetrosis (Peterson et al. 1966). However, osteopetrosis is also sometimes seen in the natural disease, and in experimental transmission, it can appear more rapidly than lymphoid tumors. The disease is

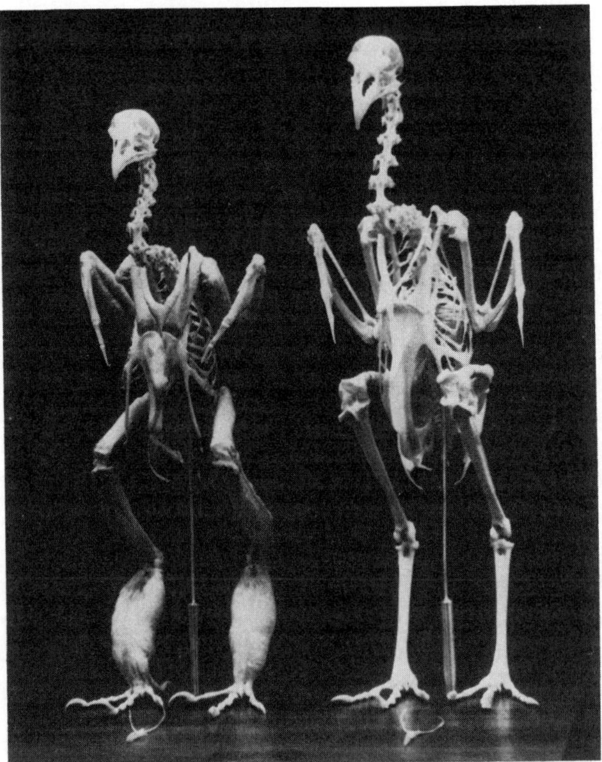

Figure 8.2 Osteopetrosis induced by MAV-2(O) in a chicken. The skeleton of an infected bird (*left*) shows massive thickening of the long bones in both fore and hind limbs; also note thickening and malformations in sternum. An uninfected bird (*right*) is shown for comparison. (Photograph courtesy of R.E. Smith).

typified by an excessive formation of hard bone, particularly in the legs (see Fig. 8.2), but there is uncertainty as to the primary lesion leading to this disorder. In mammals, osteopetrosis apparently reflects failure of bone resorption, probably resulting from a lack of the monocytes that are the precursors of osteoclasts (Marks and Walker 1976). Such a defect may contribute to some avian osteopetrosis, because the disease is often accompanied by lymphoid involution and anemia, and monocytes may thus also be suppressed (Smith and Ivanyi 1980; Schmidt et al. 1982). However, hematopoietic lesions do not always accompany osteopetrosis, and other workers suggest that virus infection primarily causes osteoblast proliferation, the reduction in osteoclast activity being secondary to a diminution of the bone-marrow space by excessive bone deposition (Boyde et al. 1978). These authors suggest that the avian disease is not comparable to that in mammals and should preferably be classified as avian osteogenic osteoblastoma.

Strains of nondefective LLV have been described that produce predominantly osteopetrosis, most notably MAV-2(O), which is a helper for avian myeloblastosis virus (AMV) strain BAI/A (Smith and Moscovici 1969; Smith et al. 1976). Unlike other helper viruses, MAV-2(O) is capable of stimulating the proliferation and cloning ability of embryonic chick bone cells (Schmidt and Smith 1981), which may indicate some target-cell specificity. Other cloned helper viruses isolated from this AMV strain cause a high incidence of renal tumors that, like osteopetrosis, arise after a short latency (Fourcade et al. 1974; Ogura et al. 1974). These kidney neoplasms were originally described as adenocarcinomas but are now usually considered to be nephroblastomas, histologically comparable to Wilms' tumor in man (see Gross 1970). It is interesting that Ogura's isolate of nephroblastoma virus causes mainly osteopetrosis when injected into birds of another flock (R. Smith, cited in Graf and Beug 1978), suggesting that host factors modify the pathogenesis of the virus (see Section IV.B.5). It is also interesting that transformation-defective (*td*) deletion mutants of some RSV strains, such as PR-RSV-B, induce osteopetrosis as their primary disease (Robinson et al. 1982), whereas others, such as *td* SR-RSV-A, induce principally lymphomas (Neel et al. 1981).

c. Anemia. Chickens developing neoplasia, particularly erythroblastosis and osteopetrosis, often show an accompanying anemia. It is conceivable that this could be explained solely as a consequence of the presence of the tumor, which either obliterates the marrow cavity (in the case of osteopetrosis) or obstructs normal erythropoiesis (in the case of erythroblastosis). However, it is clear that anemia induction is, at least in part, an inherent property of the retroviruses themselves (Graf et al. 1976a; Paterson and Smith 1978). For example, LLV helpers for the defective avian erythroblastosis virus (AEV) strains R and ES4 can induce anemia even when cloned free of AEV (Graf et al. 1976a). The viruses that induce anemia are mainly those of envelope subgroups B and D (Schmidt et al. 1982); since LLVs of subgroups B and D are also able to produce cytotoxic changes in vitro (see Section IV.C.1), it is possible that such cellular toxicity may contribute to the mechanism of anemia. Whatever the molecular basis of the disorder, it is clear that LLV can induce this nonneoplastic disease, and in this respect, they can be compared with the murine and feline leukemia viruses whose pathogenic potential also extends beyond the induction of neoplasia (see Sections VIII and X).

d. Pathogenesis. We do not understand how nondefective leukosis viruses induce these diseases, but recent investigations on genomic structure and function provide intriguing clues to possible mechanisms of pathogenesis.

First, LLV and transformation-defective derivatives of Rous sarcoma viruses all replicate efficiently in tissue culture and cause disease in birds (Biggs et al. 1973; Purchase et al. 1977). In contrast, the endogenous chicken retroviruses of envelope subgroup E (see Chapter 3) are nonpathogenic and replicate relatively poorly in most host cells. The nonpathogenicity of endogenous viruses is not dictated by their envelope subgroup because recombinant viruses, known as RAV-60, can be obtained by crosses between exogenous viruses and the endogenous virus RAV-0, and these recombinants are leukemogenic even though they have subgroup-E envelope specificity (Crittenden et al. 1980; Robinson et al. 1980). However, endogenous and exogenous viruses of chickens differ not only in the *env* gene, but also in the U_3 region at the 3′ end of the genomic RNA (see Chapter 4), and other recombinational analyses between endogenous and exogenous viruses have directly associated the structure of the U_3 region with replicative ability; recombinants that replicate well always possess the U_3 region from the exogenous parent (Tsichlis and Coffin 1980). As the promoter for viral transcription is probably situated in the U_3 portion of the genome (Chapter 5), it seems likely that differences in the replication of endogenous and exogenous viruses reflect differences in their promoter regions. It is tempting to extrapolate this reasoning to explain the differences in pathogenicity between endogenous and exogenous viruses, particularly since those leukemogenic RAV-60 isolates that have been examined all have U_3 regions derived from their exogenous parent (Crittenden et al. 1980; Robinson et al. 1980). However, a similar sort of recombinant with a lesser amount of exogenous virus information has been found to have greatly reduced pathogenicity compared with that of the exogenous parent, although it induces significantly more disease than RAV-0 (Robinson et al. 1982). According to partial nucleotide sequence determination, and oligonucleotide and restriction maps, this virus contains only noncoding regions (the U_3 region and about 200 nucleotides 5′ of U_3) from the exogenous parent (PR-RSV-B), with the remainder from RAV-0 (Tsichlis and Coffin 1980; L. Donehower and P. Tsichlis, pers. comm.). Thus, regions outside of U_3 must also have a determining effect on pathogenicity, and analysis of more recombinants of this type will be required to resolve the issue.

In a second set of studies, several groups have investigated the status of lymphoid leukosis proviruses in infected birds by restriction enzyme analyses (explained in Chapter 5). With either a field isolate of LLV (Neiman et al. 1980a) or the laboratory strains RAV-1 and RAV-2 (Fung et al. 1981; Hayward et al. 1981; Neel et al. 1981; Payne et al. 1981), it was found that provirus integration occurred at many sites in normal tissue during infection, but at only one or a few sites in the cells from each tumor, including the early bursal nodules. These data strongly indicated that the individual tumors were of monoclonal origin. Although the apparent clonality could be explained in several ways, the situation was experimentally advantageous in that it permitted a detailed analysis of proviral DNA and viral RNA in each tumor (see below). Most groups found that the same integration sites were occupied in the primary bursal tumors and in metastatic lesions in the liver and spleen (Fung et al. 1981; Hayward et al. 1981; Neel et al. 1981; Payne et al. 1981), although Neiman et al. (1980a) described one case in which the pattern of proviruses in the metastasis was more complex than in the primary tumor. Some birds carried additional tumors (hemangiomas and nephroblastomas) in which the pattern of integrated proviruses differed from that in the lymphomas from the same bird (Neiman et al. 1980b; Fung et al. 1981), suggesting that histologically different tumors in each animal arose independently.

These two lines of investigation promoted the hypothesis that an efficiently replicating LLV can cause a spreading infection in which a rare virus-cell interaction predisposes the host cell to neoplastic change. The presumably random occurrence of this event (or series of events) could explain the long and variable latency of the lymphoid leukoses compared with the rapid onset of diseases caused by the defective leukemia viruses bearing transforming genes; alternatively, the long latency could reflect a requirement for secondary events (see below). It is also possible that the long latency is related to the apparent necessity for multiple random events following the initial rare virus-cell interaction (Neiman et al. 1980a; Cooper and Neiman 1981).

Provocative insight into the nature of the virus-host interaction responsible for neoplastic conversion by LLV has come from recent studies of viral DNA and RNA in LLV-induced tumors. The several unexpected conclusions that have been drawn from these experiments can be summarized as follows: (1) Expression of viral genes is not required for maintenance of the tumor state, although all tumors retain at least a portion of an LLV provirus. (2) Most LLV-induced tumors, lymphomas and perhaps nephroblastomas, carry at least one provirus inserted in the vicinity of the cellular homolog of the putative transforming sequence of the myelocytomatosis-29 (MC29) virus (*c-myc;* see Chapters 4 and 9). (3) The insertion appears to activate the expression of the *c-myc* locus, in many cases as a consequence of provision of a viral promoter in an LTR positioned to the 5′ side of *c-myc*. The view fostered by these conclusions is that LLV, and perhaps other oncogenic viruses that lack transforming genes, can initiate an oncogenic mechanism by introducing proviral DNA (presumably as a rare event) near a cellular oncogene (*c-onc*) and thereby enhancing the expression of *c-onc*.

Several pieces of evidence led to the formulation summarized above. First, all tumors that have been examined to date contain at least a portion of one LLV provirus (Neiman et al. 1980a, 1981; Neel et al. 1981; Payne et al. 1981). Since many tumors contain only a single insertion of LLV DNA (Neel et al. 1981; Payne et al. 1981), the failure to find tumors lacking any vestige of LLV DNA argues strongly for the role of viral DNA in the maintenance, if not also the initiation, of the tumor phenotype. In contrast, there is considerable reason to believe that expression of virus-specific sequences per se is not necessary to maintain the tumor state. (The question of whether viral sequences and gene products might be involved in *initiation* of tumor growth is presently moot.) Several tumors have been found to lack infectious virus, normal species of viral mRNA, or any intact proviruses. This has been shown by tests for infectivity of tumor extracts (Payne et al. 1981), by examination of virus-specific RNA in tumors by gel electrophoresis and transfer to activated cellulose sheets for hybridization (Neel et al.

1981; Payne et al. 1981), and by mapping proviruses with restriction endonucleases (Fung et al. 1981; Neel et al. 1981; Neiman et al. 1981; Payne et al. 1981). For example, Payne et al. (1981) performed detailed mapping of the solitary proviruses in four RAV-2-induced bursal lymphomas and showed that one provirus retained little more than an LTR sequence and that each of the three others had incurred small deletions involving portions of the provirus (5′ copy of the LTR or splicing sites) believed to be important in the production of normal species of viral mRNA. Less extensive analysis of DNA from additional tumors was consistent with the occurrence of frequent deletions involving the left end of proviral DNA. It has been proposed that such deletions may have been selected for by immune responses to tumor cells that carry unaffected proviruses and express viral structural antigens. The deletions may have little to do with the mechanisms of oncogenesis, even though they illustrate that viral gene products are dispensable, at least at late stages. Alternatively, the use of the 3′ LTR as a downstream promoter might be facilitated by deletions that eliminate normal transcription of the provirus.

Mapping studies from several laboratories suggested that one (or more) of the proviruses in each tumor might be located in a single region of the host genome (Fung et al. 1981; Neel et al. 1981; Payne et al. 1981). This was an attractive idea because several of the tumors studied by Neel et al. (1981) and a few examined by Payne et al. (1981) contained RNA species detectable with cDNA specific for the U_5 region ($cDNA_{5'}$), but not with cDNA transcribed from other regions of the LLV genome. These findings conformed to prior suggestions (Tsichlis and Coffin 1980) and published evidence (Quintrell et al. 1980) that proviruses could promote the expression of cellular sequences flanking the 3′ side of the provirus. This could be explained most simply by the use of the 3′ LTR as a promoter to initiate transcription of downstream cellular DNA, but it could also reflect readthrough transcription beyond the 3′ LTR of transcripts initiated at the usual site in the 5′ LTR, with subsequent splicing to remove most of the viral sequences (see Fig. 8.3). In at least one of the tumors examined by Payne et al. (1981), the former mechanism was strongly favored by the absence of the 5′ LTR from the defective single provirus in that tumor.

Powerful light was shed on this problem by the experiments performed by Hayward et al. (1981), who chose to test hybridization

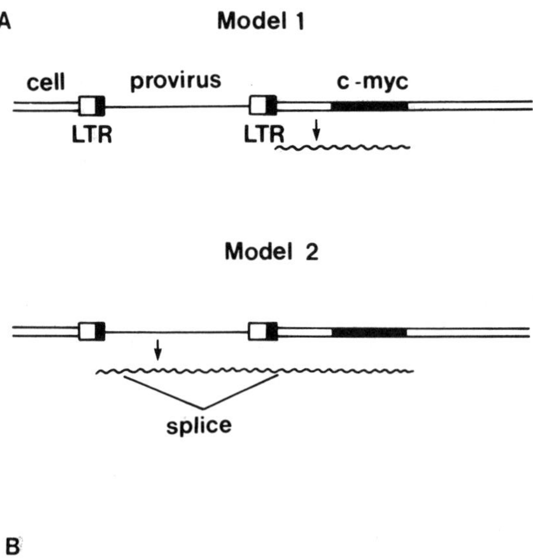

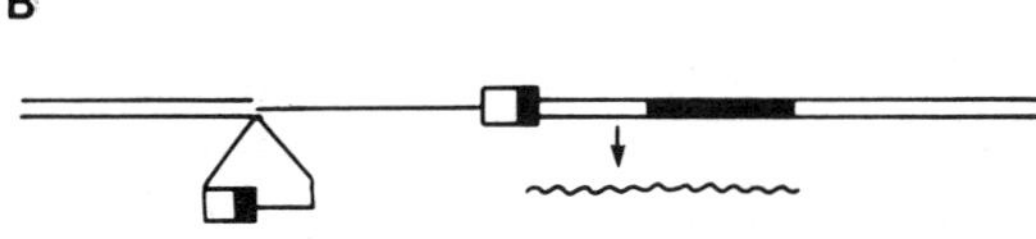

Figure 8.3 Promoter insertion model of ALV leukemogenesis. (*A*) In the first model, transcription initiates in the right LTR and proceeds directly into flanking cellular DNA. The second model postulates that transcription originates in the left LTR and reads through possible termination signals in the right LTR. The final transcript is formed by a processing event that removes most of the viral sequences. (*B*) The structure of a provirus in an ALV-induced tumor from which the left LTR and some of the viral coding sequences have been deleted. The probable origin of the RNA that anneals to $cDNA_{5'}$ only is drawn below the provirus. (Redrawn from Payne et al. 1981.)

reagents available for five unrelated avian virus oncogenes (*src, myc, myb, fps,* and *erb;* see Chapters 4 and 9) for their ability to anneal to the RNA from LLV-induced lymphomas. With few exceptions, the tumors were shown to contain relatively high concentrations of RNA complementary to cDNA representing the transformation-specific sequence (*myc*) of MC29 virus. The cellular homolog of the viral *myc* sequences, *c-myc,* is a highly conserved locus of apparently single-copy DNA, normally transcribed at low levels (about 1–5 copies/cell) into stable RNA species of 2.5 kb

(Sheiness and Bishop 1979; Roussel et al. 1979; Sheiness et al. 1980). In the tumor cells, Hayward et al. (1981) found a 50-fold elevation of the concentration of *myc*-specific RNA; this RNA varied in size from 2 kb to 4 kb from tumor to tumor, but in each case, comigrating bands were detected with cDNA for *myc* sequences and $cDNA_{5'}$, suggesting that the U_5 and *myc* sequences were covalently linked. The proposal that augmented *c-myc* expression was accompanied by insertion of an LLV provirus upstream from the *c-myc* locus was supported by the striking demonstration that restriction endonuclease digests of tumor DNA contained novel fragments annealing with both cDNA for *myc* sequences and $cDNA_{5'}$ (Hayward et al. 1981) and was confirmed by molecular cloning (W. Hayward; G. Payne; both pers. comm.). The tumor DNAs also yielded a *myc*-specific fragment identical with that present in digests of normal DNA from normal tissues; this band presumably represented the undisrupted locus from the homologous chromosome.

Several investigators have since confirmed the findings of Hayward et al. using additional tumors, including one nephroblastoma and early lymphoid nodules induced by LLV (Cooper and Neiman 1981), numerous LLV-induced bursal tumors (Fung et al. 1981; Payne et al. 1982; H. Robinson, pers. comm.) and B-cell lymphomas induced in chickens by chicken syncytial virus, a reticuloendotheliosis virus (Noori-Daloii et al. 1981) (see Section VI.D) One surprising finding has emerged from the recent studies of Payne et al. (1982): In some tumors, an LLV provirus has been found upstream from the *c-myc* locus, but in the opposite transcriptional orientation, and in at least one other tumor, an LLV provirus was located on the 3′ side of the *c-myc* locus. Nevertheless, the unexpected configurations appear to produce enhanced expression of *c-myc* (Payne et al. 1982), indicating that stimulation of *c-myc* does not depend solely on the promoter-insertion mechanism, in which a viral promoter is appropriately positioned to initiate transcription of *c-myc*.

Although these provocative studies provide evidence for a novel mode of oncogenesis, parallel experiments by Cooper and Neiman (1980, 1981) indicate that the oncogenic process may be more complex. They found that high-molecular-weight DNA from several LLV-induced bursal tumors, early nodules, and a nephroblastoma morphologically transformed NIH-3T3 cells, whereas similarly prepared DNA from normal organs of the same animals did not. High-molecular-weight DNA retrieved from the transformed NIH-3T3 cells could transfer the altered phenotype at the same high frequency to produce secondary transformants. However, tests with probes for LLV-specific sequences (including the LTR) and for *c-myc*-specific sequences indicated that the transforming DNA was unlinked to any LLV provirus and especially to that provirus inserted in the *c-myc* locus. Cooper and Neiman interpret these findings to mean that at least two classes of obligatory events are involved in tumorigenesis. One is an insertion of an LLV provirus in a position to activate expression of *c-myc,* and the other is an inheritable alteration in the host genome (due to deletion, transposition, inversion, etc.) that activates a cellular gene capable of transforming NIH-3T3 cells morphologically.

The existence of two such definable events can be considered further evidence in favor of a multistep development of lymphoid leukosis (Neiman et al. 1980b), although the second step has yet to be defined biochemically. If these diseases do indeed require events in addition to an appropriate virus-cell interaction, this may explain why LLVs induce predominantly only a limited spectrum of tumors; a weakness of models such as the promoter-insertion model is that random promotion of cell gene expression might predict the induction of a much wider spectrum of tumor types with no particular type predominating. In addition, the apparent involvement of the *c-myc* locus in B-cell leukemogenesis is surprising in view of the reported pathogenic effects of MC29 and other viruses containing *v-myc:* carcinomas, sarcomas, myelocytomas, and perhaps endotheliomas (see IV.B.4.c), but not B-cell neoplasms.

Models of viral leukemogenesis must also account for the fact that LLV can induce osteopetrosis and anemia (see above), diseases that do not show a long latency but become apparent in a majority of birds within 3 weeks. The rapid appearance of these diseases suggests that LLV may induce them by a more direct mechanism than that inducing lymphoma. Even though these viruses are known to code for virus replicative genes only, it is worth considering that they may encode functions that directly influence the infected-cell phenotype.

The striking findings with LLV-induced lymphoma have stimulated attempts to demonstrate analogous mechanisms for other virus-induced proliferative disease, with only partial success to date. Neiman et al. (1981) presented preliminary evidence for a specific LTR–cell-DNA interaction in DNA from osteopetrotic bone tissue. This study, however, involved only one bird and was complicated by large amounts of unintegrated DNAs. In studies of MMTV-induced mammary carcinoma, R. Nusse and H. Varmus (pers. comm.) have found that some 15% of independent tumors have a new MMTV provirus integrated within the same 10-kb region of the mouse-cell genome, although specific transcripts associated with these integrations have not yet been identified. It should be noted that it is possible that the LTR may exert an effect on transcription at considerable distance; if so, then direct evidence for gene activating mechanisms may be difficult to obtain in many cases.

4. Defective Leukemia Viruses

There have been many reports of virus-associated neoplasms in birds in which an incubation period of a few weeks is followed by an acute and fatal disease. As suggested in the preceding section, some of these acute diseases may be caused by LLV, but most of those studied proved to be due to defective viruses propagated by coinfection with a nondefective helper. Detailed studies on some of these defective leukemia viruses (DLVs) have divided them into three groups: the avian erythroblastosis virus (AEV)-type strains, the avian myeloblastosis virus (AMV)-type strains, and the avian myelocytomatosis virus (MC29)-type strains. These subdivisions, presumably reflecting the existence of three types of oncogenes (see Chapters 4 and 9), are based on: (1) their in vivo pathogenic spectrum and in vitro cell-transforming capacity (Table 8.1; Section IV.C.4), (2) similarities within a group in the specific genomic sequences that are absent from their helpers but are related to host-cell sequences (see Chapters 4 and 9 and Table 8.1), and (3) similarities within a group in their specific gene products, coded in part by these specific genomic sequences (see Chapters 4 and 9).

a. Avian Erythroblastosis Viruses. The original isolates of these agents were probably mixed with other viruses and produced disease after a latency of 1 month or more. With further animal passage, the latent period decreased to about 1 week, although the reason for this is not clear. Birds infected intravenously with

Table 8.1 Properties of commonly studied defective leukosis viruses

Virus strain	Country and year of isolation	Predominant neoplasms induced in chickens	Annealing of viral RNA (% S1 resistance) with			Oncogene product
			$cDNA_{erb}$	$cDNA_{myc}$	$cDNA_{myb}$	
AEV	Denmark 1931 (strain R) 1933 (strain ES4)	erythroblastosis, sarcomas	100	<3	<3	$P75^{gag\text{-}erb\text{-}A}$ $p40^{erb\text{-}B}$
AMV-BAI/A	United States 1941	myeloblastosis	<3	<3	100	$p35^{myb}$ (?)
E26	Bulgaria 1962	erythroblastosis[a]	<3	<3	68	$P150^{gag\text{-}myb}$ (?)
MC29	Bulgaria 1964	myelocytomas, hepatocarcinomas, renal carcinomas, sarcomas, mesotheliomas, endotheliomas (?)	<3	100	<3	$P110^{gag\text{-}myc}$
CMII	West Germany 1964	myelocytomas	<3	96	<3	$P90^{gag\text{-}myc}$
MH2	England 1927	hepatocarcinomas, sarcomas, renal carcinomas, endotheliomas (?), monocytic leukemia (?)	<3	66	<3	$P100^{gag\text{-}myc}$
OK10	Finland 1975	carcinomas	<3	91	<3	$P200^{gag\text{-}pol\text{-}myc}$

For further details, see Graf and Beug (1978). Data from Roussel et al. (1979); $cDNA_{erb}$, $cDNA_{myc}$, and $cDNA_{myb}$ are probes specific for the unique sequences of AEV, MC29, and AMV, respectively. (?) indicates uncertainty.

[a]This agent was originally claimed to cause erythroblastosis. In view of the finding that chicken hematopoietic cells transformed in vitro with E26 have, like AMV-BAI/A-transformed cells, the phenotype of myeloblasts (Beug et al. 1979), this claim requires reexamination.

passage-adapted strains show dramatic anemia, thrombocytopenia (a deficiency of blood platelets resulting in poor clotting), and leukemia with up to 6×10^5 erythroblasts/μl. Graf et al. (1976b) suggested that the anemia is due largely to the helper virus, which can cause this condition in solitary infection. However, the massive accumulation of erythroblasts leading to enlarged and brown-red or cherry-red liver and spleen and almost total obliteration of the bone-marrow cavity also seems likely to lead per se to anemia. Infected birds may die suddenly before these hematological changes are fully developed, but if not, the majority die only a few days after showing symptoms of progressive weakness. Long-term survivors of inoculation may later develop visceral lymphomatosis, presumably as a result of helper-virus infection (Burmester et al. 1959b).

The incidence of disease is reduced and the onset of symptoms is delayed if the virus is injected intramuscularly, and even more so if administered subcutaneously (Eckert et al. 1955a). Under these conditions, sarcomas may develop rapidly at the site of inoculation (Engelbreth-Holm and Rothe Meyer 1935; Graf et al. 1977a).

Two strains of AEV, R and ES4, are currently being studied. They are apparently indistinguishable, so they may be separate isolates of the same agent. It is worth stressing here that viruses are no respecters of frontiers, and birds are hardly less reprehensible in this respect. Even domestic fowl travel by human agency, so the fact that the isolation of agents is separated in space and time does not guarantee that they are different. One should guard against this when drawing conclusions on the basis of similarities between different isolates; unless there is other evidence suggesting that they are indeed different viruses, such conclusions may be invalid. Thus, one can infer little from the similarity of the specific regions in AEV-R and AEV-ES4. On the other hand, the extent of sequence homology between the specific regions of MC29, CMII, MH2, and OK10 (see below and Table 8.1) and the incomplete similarities in the proteins encoded by these regions (see Chapters 4 and 9) do provide prima facie evidence that these are clearly separate agents with related regions in their genomes apparently involved in the property they have in common, oncogenesis.

b. Avian Myeloblastosis Viruses. The latency, symptoms and outcome of avian myeloblastosis resemble those of erythroblastosis. The blood contains up to 2×10^6 myeloblasts/μl with associated anemia and thrombocytopenia, and the enlarged liver and spleen are more gray than in cases of erythroblastosis. Unlike erythroblastosis viruses, the myeloblastosis agents do not cause sarcomas at the site of inoculation.

c. MC29-type Viruses. This category comprises four agents whose affinities are more obvious from biochemical studies in vitro (see below) than from their behavior in vivo. The prototype, MC29, was isolated from a case of myelocytomatosis. Upon inoculation, it induces not only this disease, but also liver and kidney carcinomas, mesotheliomas, and anaplastic round- or spindle-cell "soft-tissue" sarcomas (Moscovici et al. 1978). The virus CMII is an isolate from a separate case of myelocytomatosis, and MH2 is another isolate that causes liver and kidney carcinomas and soft-tissue sarcomas. MH2 was originally thought to cause endotheliomas (Begg 1927), but it probably resembles a fourth isolate, OK10 (Oker-Blom et al. 1975, 1978), and the tumors are now considered by some to be carcinomas (Moscovici et al. 1978). The uncertainty about whether any of these agents causes endotheliomas probably reflects partly pathological fashion and partly the difficulty of demonstrating that ill-defined tumors actually arise from vascular endothelium. OK10 has not been reported to cause myelocytomas (Hortling 1978), but the RAV-3 pseudotype of MH2 does cause leukemia, probably of monocytic nature (Moscovici et al. 1978).

d. Role of the Helper Virus. The helpers for DLV are necessary for successful infection by the defective agents and can themselves be pathogenic (see Section IV.B.3). However, it is not clear whether or not the helpers contribute to the pathology of the acute disease primarily attributed to the defective viruses. Since the helpers are obligatory, this point is difficult to clarify but could be approached by (1) studying the behavior of nonproducer cells transformed by DLV (see below) both in vitro and in vivo and (2) observing whether different helpers materially alter the pathogenic behavior of a given DLV. A possible example of helper effect is the leukemia that is only induced by the RAV-3 pseudotype of MH2 (Moscovici et al. 1978). It should be noted, however, that formation of recombinants between the helper- and defective-virus genomes may complicate the interpretations of such studies.

5. Host Factors Preventing or Modifying Infection by ALVs

Naturally occurring ALVs are of envelope subgroups A or B, with subgroup A predominating. Subgroups specificity resides in the glycoprotein product of the viral *env* gene (see Chapters 4 and 6). Host susceptibility to viruses of various subgroups is governed by independent autosomal loci at which susceptibility is dominant (see Chapter 3). These loci probably encode receptors for the viral glycoproteins so that chicken strains homozygous for (recessive) alleles at any particular locus will not code for the appropriate receptor and will be resistant to infection by virus of the corresponding envelope subgroup. This mechanism is the basis of the resistance of certain chicken strains to naturally occurring avian leukosis. Genetically resistant strains form the bulk of modern commercial poultry stocks and, as a result, the incidence of lymphoid leukosis on poultry farms has been greatly reduced.

However, expression of cell receptors for viral glycoproteins is not governed entirely by the cell's genotype. Gazzolo et al. (1974, 1975), in studies on transformation of macrophages by avian sarcoma viruses, reported that macrophages are susceptible only to viruses of envelope subgroups B and C whereas fibroblasts from the same birds are additionally susceptible to subgroup-A and -D viruses. Anomalously, however, AMV can be rescued from nonproducer transformed yolk-sac cells by subgroup-D virus (Moscovici and Zanetti 1970), and both subgroup-A and -D viruses can act as helpers to enable MC29, CMII, and MH2 viruses to transform macrophages (Graf et al. 1977b; Moscovici et al. 1978). Moreover, a leukemogenic AMV exists that has subgroup-A helper only (Ishizaki et al. 1975), although this agent appears incapable of macrophage transformation in vitro. These discrepant findings have yet to be resolved, but it should be noted that the various studies cited utilized not only different transforming viruses, but also macrophages from different tissues, either yolk sac or bone marrow.

As indicated at the end of Section IV.A, dose of virus, route of inoculation, age and physiological status of the host, modulation of the virus by prior animal passage, and the types of tumor cells from which the virus is isolated all have an effect, albeit modest, on the disease pattern (for review, see Graf and Beug 1978). However, a more dramatic effect on the pathogenic spectrum can be seen when an exotic host is used in experimental infection. Thus, the E26 strain of myeloblastosis virus will cause myelocytomas in guinea fowl (Nedyalkov et al., quoted in Graf and Beug 1978) and an immature leukemia with predominantly erythroblast cells in Japanese quail (C. Moscovici et al., pers. comm.). AEV inoculation of Japanese quail produces predominantly myeloblastosis with erythroblastosis less in evidence (C. Moscovici et al., pers. comm), and yet another example is the nephroblastoma virus that produces osteopetrosis in some chicks (R. Smith, quoted in Graf and Beug 1978) (see Section IV.B.3.a). The target-cell specificity of the viruses (see below) is thus presumably different in different host strains or species, but the reason for this is unknown.

C. In Vitro Studies on Avian Leukosis

1. Nondefective Leukosis Viruses

Studies on LLV have been hampered by the lack of an in vitro system that detects neoplastic conversion of a target cell. Some workers have, however, reported minor morphological and cytopathic alterations in fibroblasts (Calnek 1964; Oker-Blom et al. 1975). Some leukosis viruses, particularly of subgroups B, D, and F, can be induced to form plaques in fibroblast cultures by careful manipulation of the medium (Dougherty and Rasmussen 1964; Graf 1972; Moscovici et al. 1976) or by preinfection of the cells at restrictive temperature with temperature-sensitive transformation mutants of RSV (Kawai and Hanafusa 1972; Wyke and Linial 1973). Plaque formation by the subgroup-A viruses MAV-1, RAV-1, and RAV-3 has also been reported, but only in certain cell types (Moscovici et al. 1976). The cytopathic effect of subgroup-B, -D, and -F leukosis viruses is associated with a transient accumulation of unintegrated linear viral DNA and seems to result from massive superinfection (Weller et al. 1980).

2. Defective Leukemia Viruses

Transformation of hematopoietic cells in vitro by AMV was first described 20 years ago (Beaudreau et al. 1960), and such transformation has since been shown to be a property of all DLVs that have been tested (see Baluda and Goetz [1961] and Moscovici et al. [1975] for AMV; Graf [1975] and Graf et al. [1976b] for AEV-R;

Langlois et al. [1969] and Graf [1973] for MC29; Graf et al. [1977b] for CMII; Moscovici et al. [1978] for MH2; and Graf et al. [1979] for OK10 and AMV-E26). Bone-marrow or yolk-sac cultures provide the source of the cells, and transformation is observed either as a loose, nonadherent focus of transformed cells above the substrate of adherent or semiadherent normal cells or as a colony of transformed cells suspended in semisolid medium, both phenomena permitting enumeration of transforming events (see Fig. 8.4).

It was also shown that MC29 (Langlois et al. 1967), AEV (Ishizaki and Shimizu 1970), MH2 (Payne and Biggs 1970; Moscovici et al. 1978), OK10 (Oker-Blom et al. 1975), and CMII (Graf et al. 1977b) could transform cultures of chick embryo fibroblasts, whereas AMV-E26 could transform quail fibroblasts (Graf et al. 1979). Although it is possible that in some studies the transformed cells were contaminants of hematopoietic origin, this

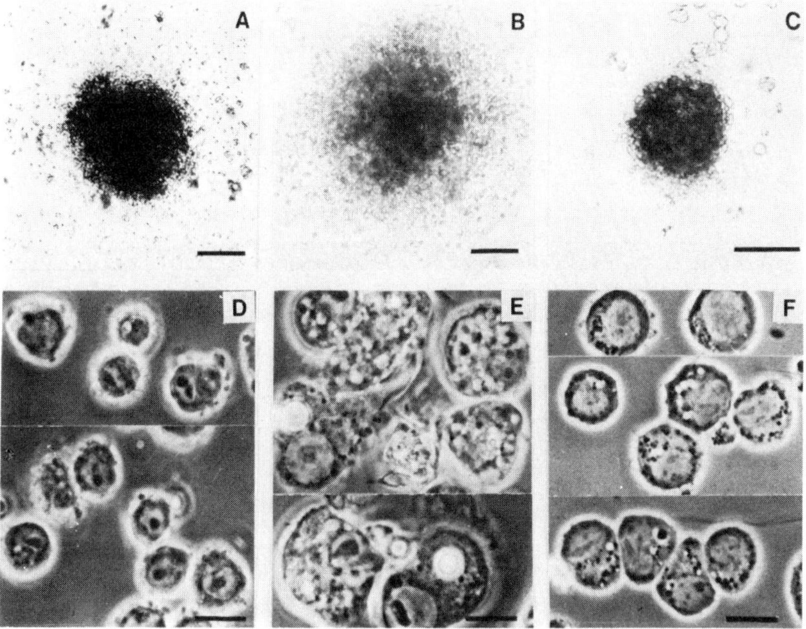

Figure 8.4 Transformation by DLV of avian bone-marrow cultures. (*A–C*) Colonies of transformed cells; (*D–F*) phase-contrast micrographs of individual cells from the colonies. Transformation by AEV (*A,D*), by AMV (*B,E*), and by MC29 (*C,F*). (Photograph courtesy of T. Graf.)

is very unlikely in three other sets of experiments. In the first, Graf and his coworkers showed that cloned lines of chick fibroblasts could be transformed by AEV, MC29, and CMII (Graf 1973; Graf et al. 1976b, 1977b; Royer-Pokora et al. 1978). In the second experiment, Quade (1979) found that AEV and MC29 can transform the rat fibroblastlike line F2408; Copeland and Cooper (1980) showed in the third experiment that DNA extracted from AEV- and MC29-transformed chick cells could transform NIH-3T3 mouse cells by transfection. It is interesting that fibroblasts transformed by various MC29-type viruses resemble one another and are distinct from those transformed by AEV or RSV (see Table 8.2) (Royer-Pokora et al. 1978). This suggests that these two types of DLVs interact in different ways with fibroblasts, a conclusion strengthened by the finding of K. Quade (pers. comm.) that distinctive phenotypes are also shown by transformed rat cells (Table 8.2).

Fibroblast transformation by MC29-type viruses and AEV probably reflects their ability to induce sarcomas in vivo. Conversely, AMV, which does not induce sarcomas, apparently cannot transform fibroblasts (Graf and Beug 1978), although the related E26 strain has been reported to transform quail fibroblasts (Graf et al. 1979). Since members of the MC29 group can also cause carcinomas (see above), it would be interesting to know if they can transform epithelial cells. There is preliminary evidence that they can, for epithelioid-transformed cells have been observed following infection of whole embryo, liver, kidney, or retinal cell cultures with MC29, CMII, and OK10 viruses (Bonar and Paulson 1974; Langlois et al. 1976; Graf and Beug 1978; Zeller et al. 1980; R. Weiss and M. Harrison, pers. comm.). However, it is not clear in these cases whether the progenitor of the epithelioid-transformed cell was itself epithelial, although this seems likely. Moreover, AMV, which is not known to induce carcinomas, might nonetheless transform cells of epithelial origin (Baluda 1963; Bonar and Paulson 1974), although here again, cellular heterogeneity makes the identity of the target for transformation uncertain. It should be noted that some helpers for AMV induce nephroblastomas and, although cloned nephroblastoma virus has so far failed to transform in vitro (Ogura et al. 1974), it may do so in concert with AMV, or if the appropriate target cell is available, and this might explain the apparent AMV-induced transformation.

Table 8.2 Comparison of selected transformation parameters induced by AEV and MC29 in chick and rat fibroblasts

Parameter	AEV		MC29		RSV	
	chick	rat	chick	rat	chick	rat
Colony formation in semisolid medium	+	+	+	+	+	+
Morphological and cell-surface alterations	+	+	+	+	+	+
Disappearance of actin/myosin cables	+	+	+	(+)	+	+
Disappearance of fibronectin	+	n.d.[a]	-	n.d.	+	n.d.
Fibrinolytic activity of cells	(+)	+	-	-	+	+
Increased hexose uptake	+	+	-	(-)	+	+
Increased growth rate	-	+	+	-	-	(+)
Sarcoma formation	+	+	–[b]	+	+	+

Data from Royer-Pokora et al. (1978) for chick cells and from K. Quade (pers. comm.) for rat cells. Results with RSV are included for comparison. Uninfected cells score as negative for all parameters listed.

[a]n.d. indicates not determined.

[b]Note that Royer-Pokora et al. (1978) were unable to induce sarcomas with MC29-transformed chick cells, whereas Moscovici et al. (1978) stated that this virus is sarcomagenic in chickens, and transformed rat cells are clearly sarcomagenic.

These in vitro transformation systems have been profoundly important catalysts in the study of DLV. Cloned transformed cells can be isolated after infection at low multiplicity and can be shown to be "nonproducers" containing only the transforming genome and no helper virus. DLV can be rescued from such cell clones with a variety of helpers, and AEV and MC29-type viruses cloned in this fashion can transform both hematopoietic and fibroblast cultures in vivo and in vitro (proving that the dual oncogenic potential is not due to virus mixtures). Moreover, the choice of helper virus has no apparent influence on the phenotype of DLV-transformed cells (Graf 1973; Graf et al. 1976b, 1977a,b). Nonproducer clones also enable analysis of DLV DNA, RNA, and proteins in the absence of helper-virus functions, and this has greatly facilitated the elucidation of the DLV genomic structures and gene products described in Chapters 4 and 9. In vitro transformation also permits one to modify the DLV genome in a controlled fashion and to monitor the effects of such manipulation on the transformed-cell phenotype. By analogy with studies on RSV, mutants so obtained should be invaluable in dissecting the mechanism of viral oncogenesis (see Chapter 7). These important aspects of the study of DLVs are discussed elsewhere in this volume, but we shall dwell here on two problems of DLV pathogenesis that have been elucidated by the study of in vitro transformation: (1) What is the phenotype of the transformed hematopoietic cell? (2) Which cell(s) in the hematopoietic lineage is the target(s) susceptible to DLV infection and subsequent transformation?

a. Phenotype of DLV-transformed Hematopoietic Cells. Beug et al. (1979) and Gazzolo et al. (1979) used a battery of tests characteristic for hematopoietic cells at various stages of the different cell lineages to identify those transformed by DLV (for a brief account of the sequence of normal hematopoiesis, see Section III). They found that DLVs induce three distinct transformation phenotypes (Table 8.3), the viruses behaving in accordance with the division of DLV into the three groups outlined above. Cells transformed by AEV are small and round, and they resemble erythroblasts, expressing heme, globin, carbonic anhydrase, and erythrocyte surface antigen, but at much lower levels than in mature erythrocytes, and possessing histone H5 at levels

Table 8.3 Differentiation parameters of bone-marrow cells transformed by defective leukosis viruses

Transforming virus	Cell morphology	Differentiation parameters: erythroid: heme[a]	globin[b]	histone H5	carbonic anhydrase	erythrocyte antigen	erythroblast antigen	"late" myeloid: Fc receptors	phagocytosis	macrophage antigen	"early" myeloid: ATPase	myeloblast antigen
AEV	10 μm, round, nonadherent	+	+	+++	+	+	+++	-	-	-	-	-
MC29	15–20 μm, polar, amoeboid;	-	-	-	-	-	-	+++	+++	+++	(+)	(+)
CMII	slightly adherent; many lamellipodia;	-	n.d.[c]	-	n.d.	-	-	+++	+++	+++	(+)	(+)
OK10	granular	-	n.d.	-	n.d.	-	-	+++	+++	+++	(+)	(+)
MH2	cytoplasm	-	n.d.	n.d.	n.d.	-	-	+++	+++	+++	(+)	(+)
AMV	10 μm, round, nonadherent	-	-	-	-	-	-	+	+	+	+++	+++
E26	eccentric nucleus; granular cytoplasm	-	-	-	-	-	-	+	+	+	+++	+++
Normal erythrocytes		+++	+++	+++	+++	+++	-	-	-	-	-	-
Normal macrophages		-	-	-	-	-	-	+++	+++	+++	-	(+)

The data, taken from Beug et al. (1979), show results for in vitro-transformed cells only. However, cells transformed in vivo by the prototype strains of AEV, MC29, and AMV were similar.

[a]Benzidine staining for hemoglobin.

[b]Radioimmunoassay for hemoglobin, probably detects only globin moiety.

[c]n.d. indicates not done.

similar to those in erythrocytes. Cells transformed by MC29-type viruses are large, amoeboid, and slightly adherent; possess Fc receptors; react with macrophage-specific sera; and exhibit phagocytosis. Cells transformed by AMV-BAI and AMV-E26 are small and nonadherent but, unlike the AEV transformants, they often contain an irregular eccentric nucleus and some cytoplasmic granulation. The AMV-type-transformed cells express macrophage-specific markers weakly and are presumed to represent more primitive myeloid cells. They occasionally convert to a more adherent morphology (Moscovici and Vogt 1968) and show a concomitant increase in macrophage characteristics (Beug et al. 1979; Boettiger and Durban 1980). Cells derived from in vivo infections with AEV, MC29, and AMV resemble their in vitro-transformed counterparts, although it should be remembered that this parallel probably cannot be extended to OK10, which is not known to produce hematopoietic neoplasms in vivo (Table 8.1).

b. Target Cells for DLV Infection and Transformation. From the results outlined in the previous section, it seems that DLV-transformed cells resemble immature members of the hematopoietic lineages. Do DLVs have a predilection for infecting cells at these intermediate stages of development and preventing their further maturation, do they infect more primitive cells and perhaps direct aberrant maturation along abortive pathways, or do they cause dedifferentiation of more mature cells (in analogous fashion to the dedifferentiation seen when RSV transforms certain cell types)? To answer this question, it is necessary to identify the target cells for transformation. This difficult task has been approached in several ways (Graf et al. 1976a, 1981; Gazzolo et al. 1979, 1980; Boettiger and Durban 1980; Durban and Boettiger 1981a,b).

Direct quantitative assays of the numbers of target cells per million for the three types of DLVs in bone marrow gave estimates of 3500 for MC29, 700 for AMV, and 50 for AEV (Graf et al. 1981). Although these are presumably minimum estimates, limited by the sensitivity of the assay, they are informative in two ways. First, they indicate that the targets for the three virus types are present in different quantities and are therefore different cells (although one could postulate that this simply reflects some difference in threshold for different viral *onc* genes or a difference in efficiency of infection). Second, these results vividly demonstrate the rarity of target cells and the attendant problems in studying them. Attempts have been made to enrich various cell compartments by (1) separating cells of different sizes on gradients, (2) separating adherent cells (predominantly macrophages) from nonadherent cells, (3) using a magnet to remove phagocytic cells (macrophages) that have ingested iron filings, and (4) immunocytolysis using antisera specific for erythroid or myeloid lineages. These experiments have confirmed that AEV and the MC29- and AMV-type viruses transform different target cells and do not transform a progenitor stem cell common to both erythroid and myeloid lineages (Graf et al. 1976a, 1981; Gazzolo et al. 1979). The failure to transform a wider range of cells is not, however, because virus infection is unsuccessful in other cells. For example, AEV will replicate in macrophages, but it will transform erythroid cells only. Conversely, MC29 can replicate in erythroid cells (at least in those transformed by AEV) but is only known to transform macrophages (Graf et al. 1980); similarly, AMV will also replicate in cell types other than the macrophage precursors that it transforms (Baluda and Goetz 1961). Thus, target cells for one type of DLV can be infected, but are not transformable, by other DLV strains.

Precise identification of the target cells is still somewhat equivocal, but the available data suggest that the target-cell phenotype in vivo is very similar to that of the equivalent DLV-transformed cell. Thus, the AEV targets are erythrocyte precursors, their rarity suggesting that they are more immature than the late (CFU-E) precursors (Graf et al. 1981). Cell-fractionation and immunocytolysis studies indicate that the targets may be the burst-forming erythroid cells (BFU-E) (Gazzolo et al. 1980). The targets for MC29 are macrophagelike, but possibly a little more primitive than the corresponding transformed cells (Graf et al. 1981). However, the MC29 targets are apparently more mature than the AMV target cells, as judged from their greater adherence and phagocytosis. Thus, it is thought that AMV usually transforms an earlier cell of the myeloid lineage (Gazzolo et al. 1979; Graf et al. 1981), although it is clear that AMV is able to transform cultures of mature differentiated macrophages in vitro (Durban and Boettiger 1981a). After AMV infection, it seems that the macrophage progenitors continue differentiation and become more adherent before exhibiting the less-adherent transformed phenotype (Boettiger and Durban 1980).

c. Mechanisms of Cell Transformation by DLV. The findings outlined above have led to the concept that transformation by different DLVs results from blocks at specific points in various hematopoietic lineages (Graf and Beug 1978). Since DLVs encode putative transforming genes related to genetic material in normal cells (see Chapters 4 and 9), it has been postulated that these viral genes mimic the effect of normal cellular genes that are specifically active at the transformation-sensitive stage of development. The viral genes may be aberrant in function or, being presumably controlled by viral promoters, they may be inappropriately expressed. Whatever the reason, they effectively seem to block further maturation of the host cell. The behavior of a temperature-sensitive mutant of AEV (see Chapter 7) supports this concept of interference with maturation; at the restrictive temperature, transformed erythroid cells proceed further along the path of erythrocyte development and synthesize hemoglobin (Graf et al. 1978; Savin and Beug 1981).

These hypotheses account for the target-cell specificity of DLV transformation, they make some experimentally testable predictions, and they suggest interesting avenues for future research: (1) If the DLV-transforming gene functions are specific to particular differentiation states, then cells at or near that stage of development should contain cellular target molecules common to both the viral oncogene product and its cellular counterpart. The target cells may even contain relatively large amounts of this normal-cell counterpart of the DLV-transforming protein; in this connection, it is significant that a probe for the AMV-specific (*myb*) sequence detects an RNA in normal chick cells that is present at about 20 copies/cell in bone marrow, but at only 1 copy/cell in embryo fibroblasts (Chen et al. 1980). (2) Differentiation is possibly regulated by a series of stage-specific gene products analogous to the cellular progenitors of DLV oncogenes. If so, then tumor viruses of different specificities may evolve by recombination between the virus and these genes. A search for novel oncogenic agents may thus extend the available range of probes capable of specifically perturbing development. (3) At a more immediately pragmatic level, DLV infection expands particular compartments of immature hematopoietic cells that are not otherwise obtainable in quantities sufficient for study. Not only is it now possible to examine these precursor cells, but, by the use of temperature-shift experiments in cultures infected with the temperature-sensitive AEV mutant, the partial maturation of large numbers of erythroid cells can also be monitored (Savin and Beug 1981). Thus, temperature-sensitive mutants of other DLVs should also prove useful in kinetic analyses of other pathways of hematopoietic maturation.

It is clearly important to characterize, in detail, the products of both the DLV oncogenes and their cellular counterparts. We have, at present, no information on the functions of these proteins (e.g., none of the *gag-onc* proteins of DLVs have been found to have protein kinase activity [Chapter 9]), but observations on virus pathogenesis suggest that their roles may be related or to some extent interchangeable. Thus, AEV and MC29 can both transform fibroblasts, although MC29-transformed chick cells show a narrower range of transformation parameters than those transformed by AEV (Royer-Pokora et al. 1978) (see Table 8.2); it is possible that fibroblast transformation is mediated by a different function, or even a different gene product, from that which mediates hematopoietic transformation (see Chapter 7). Another curious feature of virus pathology is that the tumors induced seem to depend on the host cell infected; the disparate observations on sarcoma formation by MC29 (see footnote to Table 8.2) may simply reflect the use of different chicken strains or variation in protocol. More strikingly, the observation that AEV in quail induces predominantly myeloblastosis (C. Moscovici et al., pers. comm.) suggests that the target-cell lineages for DLV oncogenesis can be altered in related species and indicates that the different DLV oncogenes may share a great deal of functional homology. A full understanding of DLV oncogenesis must explain these intricacies of virus-cell interaction.

V. PATHOGENESIS OF AVIAN SARCOMA VIRUSES

Connective tissue tumors of nonhematopoietic origin are, with exceptions (Perek 1960), less-frequent causes of morbidity and death in poultry than the leukoses. The commonest mesenchymal tumors that have probable virus etiology are fibromas, myxomas, chondromas, osteomas and the malignant counterparts (sarcomas) of these tumors, and histiocytic sarcomas (Purchase and Burmester

1978). Two groups of viruses have been implicated in the causation of these tumors: (1) the various strains of RSV, most of which are nondefective for growth and have a unique genomic structure (Chapter 4) and (2) the defective sarcoma viruses (strains Fujinami, PRCII, PRCIV, Esh, Y73, UR-1, and UR-2; see below) that have genetic structures similar to those of the DLVs (see Chapter 4 and Section IV.B.4). On the basis of pathogenicity and in vitro-transforming activities, the defective sarcoma viruses resemble RSV. This likeness is emphasized in the similar biochemical changes in cells transformed by the defective sarcoma viruses and RSV (Section V.C and Chapter 9), suggesting a common mechanism of transformation by the various avian sarcoma viruses.

A. History

The first cell-free tumor filtrates that induced a solid neoplasm were described by Rous (1911). The virus from his tumor no. 1, a spindle-cell sarcoma, has given rise to the various RSV strains. Soon afterward, Fujinami and Inamoto (1914) isolated the replication-defective Fujinami sarcoma virus (FuSV) and its associated helper virus (FAV). Recent work on FuSV has led to controversy because some stocks were found to hybridize with probes to the RSV *src* gene. However, the recently characterized Fujinami virus can apparently be traced back to the original isolate of 1914 (Hanafusa et al. 1980; Lee et al. 1980), implying that some stocks have been contaminated recently with RSV. No such doubts exist concerning the pedigree of PRCII, isolated at the Poultry Research Centre (hence PRC) in Edinburgh (Carr and Campbell 1958), or Esh sarcoma virus, isolated in Pennsylvania by Wallbank et al. (1966). PRCIV virus was isolated at the same time from the same source as PRCII; since the two viruses are closely related, it is difficult to provide convincing evidence that PRCII and PRCIV arose independently. The latest avian sarcoma viruses isolates include Y73 (Itohara et al. 1978), isolated in Yamaguchi, Japan in 1973, and the UR-1 and UR-2 viruses, isolated from tumor material provided from Cornell University in 1969 and the University of Connecticut in 1963, respectively (Balduzzi et al. 1981). All of these avian sarcoma viruses were obtained from spontaneous tumors of chickens.

B. Pathogenesis In Vivo

Data on pathogenesis come partly from observations on the sporadic mesenchymal tumors seen in the field and partly from experimental tumor induction, largely by RSV (for review, see Purchase and Burmester 1978; Beard 1980). The various laboratory strains of nondefective RSV have acquired a wide host range, including galliform and other birds and mammals, most notably rodents and lagomorphs, but also primates and others (Munroe et al. 1964; Svoboda 1964). This wide host range is accompanied by a broad pathogenic spectrum, particularly in unusual hosts and as a result of inoculation at various sites.

A sufficiently large inoculum of RSV will produce a tumor within 1 week at the site of inoculation. Metastases and/or spread of virus may result in distant tumors becoming apparent later, but the tumors may often also regress, possibly as a result of an immune response to viral or tumor antigens (Wainberg et al. 1977). The tumors comprise mainly cells of mesodermal origin, such as fibroblasts or histiocytes, surrounded by varying amounts of an appropriate collagenous, mucoid, cartilaginous, or osseous matrix. Intracerebral inoculation of birds produces tumors of the connective tissue of brain membranes (meningiomas), but inoculation at the same site in mammals can induce neural tumors, gliomas of ectodermal origin.

Studies referenced by Hanafusa et al. (1980) and Lee et al. (1980) concluded that the oncogenic spectrum of FuSV was like that of early strains of RSV, with some differences in tumor-cell morphology and in the incidence of tumor regression. Recent studies on FuSV have supported these conclusions. FuSV induces fibrosarcomas in young chickens after a short latent period (7–10 days), which occur at the site of inoculation (wing web). Attempts to induce hematopoietic tumors by intravenous inoculation produced only sarcomas close to the inoculation site (Hanafusa et al. 1980; Lee et al. 1980).

PRCII induces tumors similar to those of FuSV, described as myxofibrosarcomas by Carr and Campbell (1958). The description of the tumor cells (spindle cells) matches well with the morphology of PRCII- and FuSV-transformed cells in vitro. Recent analysis of the best-characterized stock of PRCII has shown it to be much less pathogenic than the original isolate; inoculated birds show a relatively low incidence of tumors, and the regression rate is significant. There is some reason to believe that PRCII has undergone genetic change during passage, since stocks exist that have larger genomic RNA, encode larger transformation-specific proteins, and show an oncogenic efficiency reminiscent of the original isolate (Breitman et al. 1980). However, there is not yet sufficient evidence to link unequivocally the genetic change with altered pathogenicity.

The first report of Esh sarcoma virus (ESV) described a soft myxoid tumor that was classified as a spindle-cell sarcoma (Wallbank et al. 1966). High rates of tumor induction were obtained only when the inoculum consisted of minced tumor tissue rather than cell-free filtrates. The tumors only rarely progressed and were generally small, showing no metastases (Wallbank et al. 1966). Recent work with ESV confirms these findings (Ghysdael et al. 1981).

UR-1 and UR-2 were isolated from spontaneous tumors and have been shown to induce myxosarcomas and fibrosarcomas (Balduzzi et al. 1981). The similarity of the in vivo pathogenesis and the morphology of cells transformed in vitro with the UR-1, FuSV, and PRC isolates also is emphasized by the fact that they all contain the related oncogene sequence, *fps* (Wang et al. 1981) (see below).

Y73 virus was isolated from a transplantable tumor that had been passaged many times. Like the other defective sarcoma viruses, Y73 induces exclusively sarcomas (Itohara et al. 1978).

The factors that govern the transmission of sarcoma viruses and the outcome of infection have not been studied in detail. However, since helper viruses are usually necessary for the sarcoma agents to complete their life cycles, the influences that affect the helpers (as discussed in Section IV.B.4.d) are likely also to apply to sarcoma virus infections. Bear in mind that, as with DLV, the helper may modify pathogenicity and that helper-virus proteins may also be important in eliciting the immune responses to tumors referred to above.

C. In Vitro Studies on Sarcoma Viruses

The broad oncogenic potential of RSV is reflected in its ability to transform a wide range of cell types in vitro. In addition to embryo fibroblasts, RSV will transform other mesenchymal cells, such as myoblasts (Kaighn et al. 1966; Fiszman and Fuchs 1975) and chondroblasts (Pacifici et al. 1977). It also transforms epithelial cells from chick iris (Ephrussi and Temin 1960) and retina, including both the pigmented retina (Boettiger et al. 1977) and the underlying neural retina (Pessac and Calothy 1974). In cells that express differentiation-specific markers and molecules, the general effect of RSV transformation is to disrupt such expression. Thus, retinal melanoblasts cease pigment synthesis (Boettiger et al. 1977), chondroblasts no longer synthesize appropriate proteoglycans and type-II collagen (Pacifici et al. 1977; Durban and Boettiger 1981b), and myoblasts fail to fuse into myotubes (Fiszman and Fuchs 1975; Holtzer et al. 1975) and show decreased synthesis of the muscle-specific acetylcholine receptor protein (Miskin et al. 1978).

These changes in the differentiation programs are presumably mediated at the molecular level by the action of the RSV *src* gene, whose manifestations and functions are dealt with in Chapters 7 and 9. However, it should be remembered that most studies on the action of *src* have been performed on transformed fibroblasts. There is little or no information available on the interaction of the *src*-gene product, $pp60^{src}$, with targets in cells of other types. One piece of knowledge we do have is that RSV can replicate in macrophages yet cannot transform them (Durban and Boettiger 1981b), a situation like that seen in DLV infections (Section IV.C.2). Although we do not know whether $pp60^{src}$ is synthesized in these infected macrophages, it is possible that it is, and thus, although many cells respond to this protein, the response is not universal.

All the replication-competent avian sarcoma viruses carry the *src* gene. The *env*-defective Bryan high-titer strain, BH-RSV(−), also contains *src*. However, all of the replication-defective avian sarcoma viruses contain other distinct oncogenes that so far fall into three classes: (1) *fps,* found in FuSV, PRCII, PRCIV, and UR-1, (2) *yes,* found in Y73 and ESV; and (3) *ros,* the oncogene of UR-2 (Chapter 9). No detailed studies have yet been performed on the cell targets of the defective sarcoma viruses. From their pathological propensities, we anticipate that they will share many targets with RSV.

Changes in cell phenotype that result from the expression of the RSV *src* gene have been carefully reviewed by Hanafusa (1977) and only the most elementary discussion of the transformed cell phenotype is presented here. It is possible, of course, that some changes described here for RSV will not be observed in all instances of viral transformation of fibroblasts or that there may be quantitative differences between host cells in some parameters. It is of obvious interest and importance to determine whether a given phenotypic alteration is due to a direct action of the *src*-gene product or whether it is the consequence of another event that has preceded it. Furthermore, two changes need not necessarily be causally related, but rather may be parallel expressions of two different *src*-induced events. Unfortunately, in this regard, there is little definitive information available. Merely placing one alteration in a certain time frame with respect to another may be misleading, because various changes can be detected with different levels of sensitivity, making assessment of the point at which they began difficult. Furthermore, late changes in cell culture may nevertheless be important for the ultimate formation of a tumor.

One end point of viral transformation is the morphological alteration of a cell, as observed by light microscopy. It is also the most easily recognized and is the basis for the original quantitative assays for RSV (Manaker and Groupé 1956; Temin and Rubin 1958). Morphological alteration may begin with the appearance of surface ruffles, as observed by scanning electron microscopy. Using an RSV mutant temperature-sensitive for transformation, Ambros et al. (1975) showed that, upon shift from the nonpermissive temperature to the permissive temperature, surface ruffles appear within 1 hour, marking one of the earliest events reported. This surface activity increases with time until larger blebs appear and the cell shows less adherence to the surface of the culture dish.

Concomitantly, modifications of the cytoskeletal components within the cell take place. Numerous reports have indicated that both microfilaments and microtubules undergo redistribution, although, of the two structures, microfilaments exhibit more alteration. Specifically, they appear thinner than normal and are reduced in number (Wang and Goldberg 1979). It has not been reported whether the morphological alterations at the cell surface are linked to the cytoskeletal changes, but it is obviously of interest to explore this question.

It is tempting to imagine that a change in either the cell surface or the cytoskeleton, or in a component between the two, could result in the alteration of the other. That close contact occurs between the cell surface and the cytoskeleton was shown by studies which revealed that microfilaments extend to the plasma membrane and are separated by only 8–22 nm from the external cell-surface glycoprotein, fibronectin (Singer 1979). Fibronectin, a major cell-surface component of normal fibroblasts in culture, is lost from the surfaces of RSV-transformed cells (Hynes 1974), possibly as a result of changes in a structure under the plasma membrane (Vaheri and Ruoslahti 1975). In this regard, it is interesting that in normal cells the organization and distribution of microfilaments under the plasma membrane are correlated with those of fibronectin above (Hynes and Destree 1978), as judged by immunofluorescence studies.

Many investigators have suggested that increased fluidity of transformed-cell membranes accounts for some parameters of the transformed phenotype observed. According to the fluid mosaic membrane model of Singer and Nicolson (1972), proteins in the lipid bilayer are able to move laterally; thus, increased fluidity may permit proteins, such as lectin receptors, to move readily and cluster in response to external molecules. This fluidity may be reflected in transformed cells by increased lectin agglutination, for although transformed cells have the same number of binding sites as normal cells, the clustered receptors might permit more stable cross-bridging between transformed cells. More recently, however, Ben-Zeév et al. (1979) have suggested that protein-protein interactions may play a greater role in stabilizing the plasma membrane than is the case for other cellular membranes. Thus, some caution is necessary in attempting to relate the diversity of membrane changes to increased fluidity.

Other reports also focus on another aspect of the plasma membrane, namely, the increased uptake of a number of nutrients by transformed cells as compared with the uptake by their normal counterparts. For example, an increase in hexose transport in RSV-transformed fibroblasts has been attributed to an increase of the V_{max} in the transport system. This result was interpreted to mean that there was an increase in the number of functional transportation sites within the cell (Kletzien and Perdue 1975); thus, the increase in hexose transport may be unrelated to the other cytoskeletal/plasma-membrane perturbations observed. These observations may be related to those of other investigators (Shiu et al. 1977), who showed that the levels of at least two normal membrane proteins are elevated because of glucose starvation resulting from the rapid depletion of glucose that occurs in the medium in which RSV-transformed cells are grown. Thus, the increase in the levels of these proteins may be an example of a secondary change that occurs later than other events, such as the appearance of surface ruffles. The enhanced rate of aerobic glycolysis resulting in glucose starvation is a general feature of tumor cells, including RSV-transformed fibroblasts, and appears to be closely linked to the expression of the *src* gene (R. Carroll et al. 1978). Despite considerable effort, however, the enzymic mechanisms that underlie enhanced glycolysis are still not completely understood.

Many of these observations point to important alterations at the level of the cytoskeleton and the plasma membrane as the result of *src* expression and suggest that many other properties of transformed cells may be secondary to these initial events. These alterations may also be related to the capacity of a transformed cell to grow in semisolid medium, whereas normal fibroblasts cannot. Anchorage-independent growth of this sort by RSV-transformed fibroblasts, in turn, strongly correlates with the capacity of a cell transformed in culture to produce a tumor upon injection into the appropriate host.

One dramatic biochemical event that has received considerable attention is that RSV-transformed cells excrete a proteolytic enzyme termed plasminogen activator (Unkeless et al. 1974). It has been suggested that production of such a proteolytic enzyme may facilitate metastasis of tumor cells and invasion of other sites. However, increased levels of plasminogen activator apparently cannot account for the morphological changes in RSV-transformed cells, as shown by studies which revealed that about 25% of RSV-transformed cell clones had low proteolytic activity, but nevertheless appeared transformed by the criteria of morphology and growth in soft agar (Wolf and Goldberg 1976).

Furthermore, Ash et al. (1976) showed that when cells infected with a temperature-sensitive transformation mutant of RSV were treated with inhibitors of protein synthesis at the permissive temperature, they assumed a more normal morphology with concomitant changes to a more normal arrangement of cytoskeletal components and membrane receptors. These experiments indicate that all components necessary for normal cellular architecture are present in transformed cells and that, upon inactivation or turnover of the temperature-sensitive *src*-gene product, they are reassembled without the necessity of protein synthesis. Such a result seems to eliminate protease activity, in general, as the cause of the cytoskeletal alterations and suggests that the product of *src* may be directly or indirectly involved in a readily reversible modification of component(s) involved in the maintenance of cell structure.

Although attention is now directed at the cytoplasm and, in particular, at the cytoskeletal or membrane components as primary *src*-gene targets, the results which reveal that changes in certain mRNA levels also occur in RSV-transformed cells should be considered. Transcriptional activation of cellular genes occurs in RSV-transformed cells, as judged from the presence of new mRNA transcripts and increased sensitivity of certain genes to deoxyribonuclease I, an assay for transcriptionally active chromatin (Groudine and Weintraub 1980). Other studies, showing greatly decreased levels of collagen mRNAs, also imply alterations in transcriptional controls, although other explanations are available (Adams et al. 1979). These changes may result from action on primary targets in the cytoplasm that only indirectly alter transcription but, nevertheless, may have important consequences with regard to sarcoma formation.

VI. PATHOGENESIS OF AVIAN RETICULOENDOTHELIOSIS VIRUSES

The five members of the avian reticuloendotheliosis virus (REV) group, already discussed in Chapters 2, 4, and 6, share many biological, biochemical, and pathogenic properties. By most criteria, they are unrelated to the avian sarcoma and leukemia viruses and show some similarities to the mammalian C-type viruses. The group comprises the replication-defective strain-T virus (REV-T) (Sevoian et al. 1964; Theilen et al. 1966; Witter et al. 1970; Robinson and Twiehaus 1974), its associated helper virus (REAV, also referred to as REV-A) (Hoelzer et al. 1979), duck infectious anemia virus (DIAV) (Ludford et al. 1972), Trager duck spleen necrosis virus (SNV) (Trager 1959), and chick syncytial virus (CSV) (Cook 1969).

A. Pathogenicity

The prototype REV-T was isolated from an adult turkey that died with extensive visceral reticuloendotheliosis and infiltrative nerve lesions (Robinson and Twiehaus 1974). The progression of disease in chickens is extremely rapid; the incubation period can be as short as 3 days, but death generally occurs between 7 and 10 days (Theilen et al. 1966). The mortality rate after intraperitoneal inoculation of 1-day-old chicks approaches 100% (Sevoian et al. 1964; Bose and Levine 1967). Young chicks experimentally infected with REV-T develop a severe hepatosplenomegaly with either lymphoproliferative or necrotic lesions (Sevoian et al. 1964; Theilen et al. 1966; Mussman and Twiehaus 1971; Taylor and Olson 1973). Some lesions are composed almost entirely of large undifferentiated lymphoreticular cells, whereas other lesions are composed predominantly of smaller lymphoid cells, suggestive of an immunological response to the primary lesion. Initially it was unclear whether REV-T induced a neoplastic or hyperplastic disease (Olson 1967; Mussman and Twiehaus 1971); however, REV-T induces tumors at the site of inoculation (Campbell et al. 1971; Linna et al. 1974), and transplantable tumors and transformed nonproducer cell lines have been obtained (see below), providing evidence of oncogenicity. Because REV-T is replication-defective (Hoelzer et al. 1979), infectious stocks exist as pseudotypes with a replication-competent nontransforming helper virus, generally REAV. The severe runting syndrome, anemia, peripheral nerve lesions, and paralysis that result from inoculation of chicks with low doses of REV-T (Witter et al. 1970) occur as a consequence of infection with REAV (Scofield et al. 1978; Hoelzer et al. 1979).

The nondefective REV cause a wide variety of syndromes, including visceral reticuloendotheliosis, splenomegaly, spleen necrosis, lymphoproliferative nerve lesions, lymphomas, and anemia (Trager 1959; Witter et al. 1970; Ludford et al. 1972; Purchase et al. 1973; Witter and Crittenden 1979). Generally death occurs rapidly. Some of these properties are presented in Table 8.4.

B. Role of the Helper Virus

Superinfection of REV-T-transformed nonproducer cells (see below) by the nontransforming REV results in rescue of REV-T (Hoelzer et al. 1980). REV-T pseudotypes with virion polypeptides

Table 8.4 Pathogenic properties of reticuloendotheliosis viruses

Virus	Host (age)	Anemia	Visceral lesions	Nerve lesions	Lethality
REV-T(REAV)	ducks (2 weeks)	+	-/+	+	+
	ducks (4 days)	+	+	-	+
	chicks (1 day)	+	+	+	+
	turkeys	-	+	-	+
CSV	ducks (2 weeks)	-	-/+	-	-
	chicks (1 day)	-	+	+	-/+
DIAV	ducks (2 weeks)	+	+	-	+
	chicks (1 day)		+	+	+
SNV	ducks (4 days)	+	+	-	+
	chicks (1 day)	+	+	+	+

Data from Purchase and Witter 1975.

provided by any nondefective REVs are equally efficient in transforming hematopoietic cells in vitro and inducing lethal reticuloendotheliosis in chickens. The transforming potential of REV-T is therefore independent of the helper virus.

It is generally thought that the helper viruses associated with avian acute leukemia viruses may play an important role in pathogenesis, and REAV is no exception. In addition to providing virion polypeptides for the defective REV-T, the helper viruses rapidly and severely depress the cellular immune response of the infected bird (Smith and van Eldik 1978; Rup et al. 1979, 1981). Thymus-derived T lymphocytes recognize and destroy tumor cells and therefore have been postulated to play a significant role in protection from malignant diseases (Burnet 1970). REAV, as well as the other nontransforming members of the REV group, induces or activates a suppressor-cell population in the spleens of infected chickens which, in turn, cytostatically inhibits the proliferation of T cells (Carpenter et al. 1978b; Scofield and Bose 1978; Rup et al. 1979). This manifestation appears to be a contact-mediated event involving a trypsin-sensitive protein on the surface of the suppressor cell (Carpenter et al. 1977). Although blastogenesis is blocked, cell-mediated cytotoxic function is unaltered (Carpenter et al. 1978a). The suppressor cells do not express viral antigens and therefore are presumably not activated by virus infection and replication (Carpenter et al. 1978b). The induction of the suppressor-cell population in birds infected with REAV has been shown to correlate with the level of viremia (Rup et al. 1979) and can be detected within 3 days after infection (Carpenter et al. 1978b). Although the immunosuppression induced by REAV alone is transient, of about 4 weeks duration, it is within this time period that birds coinfected by REV-T die of reticuloendotheliosis. Chickens that exhibit a suppressed proliferative response develop reticuloendotheliosis, whereas, in the absence of immunosuppression, birds fail to develop visible tumor foci or lethal reticuloendotheliosis (Rup et al. 1979). The rapid induction of the suppressor-cell population that prevents T-cell proliferation may therefore permit the unrestricted replication of REV-T-transformed lymphocytes.

Helper viruses associated with other avian acute leukemia viruses (AMV, AEV, and MC29) also cause rapid suppression of T-cell proliferation in infected birds (Smith and van Edik 1978; Rup et al. 1981). However, spleen cells from birds infected with these acute leukemia viruses fail to suppress T-cell proliferative responses in vitro of lymphocytes from uninfected chickens (Dent et al. 1968; Purchase et al. 1968; Meyers et al. 1976), suggesting that these viruses, unlike the REV group, do not induce a suppressor-cell population. Thus, the immunosuppressive activity induced by the helper viruses associated with all avian acute leukemia viruses may greatly influence the virulence of the acute defective leukemia viruses.

C. Infection In Vitro by Nondefective REV

The nondefective REV do not transform cultured cells; instead, acute infection is characterized by extensive cytopathic effects (Temin and Kassner 1974, 1975; Hoelzer et al. 1979). At this stage, large amounts of unintegrated viral DNA accumulate and multiple proviral DNA copies are detected (Battula and Temin 1978; Keshet and Temin 1979). Keshet and Temin (1979) suggest that cell death during the acute phase is a consequence of the toxic effects of the large numbers of unintegrated viral DNA copies present in many of the cells. However, UV-inactivated REV, incapable of producing viral DNA copies, also inhibits cell-protein synthesis and induces cytopathology in fibroblasts and hematopoietic cells in a dose-dependent relationship (H. Bose et al., pers.

comm.), suggesting that a virion component is most likely responsible for the development of these acute effects. Survivors of the acute phase proliferate to form chronically infected cultures in which the level of unintegrated viral DNA is decreased 50–100-fold and only one or a few copies of proviral DNA are detected in integrated form (Battula and Temin, 1977, 1978; Keshet and Temin 1979). Nothing is known about whether or not REVs cause similar cytopathic effects during the acute infectious process in vivo.

D. Transformation In Vitro by REV-T

REV-T is the only member of the REV group shown to be capable of transforming cells in vitro. There is close agreement between the dose-dependent response for transformation and for oncogenicity, as measured by (1) colony formation in soft agar with spleen cells, (2) focus formation in quail embryo fibroblasts, and (3) the development of reticuloendotheliosis in chicks following intraperitoneal injection. REV-T-transformed cells produce approximately 10^5 infectious REV-T particles and 10^7 infectious REAV particles (Hoelzer et al. 1979; Breitman et al. 1980). However, analysis of the viral RNA from some cloned populations of REV-T-transformed cells shows the presence of a considerable excess of particles containing the REV-T genome. These results indicate that the assays for REV-T in spleen cells or in fibroblasts in vitro or in infected birds are not as sensitive as the plaque assay for REAV in fibroblasts or that only a small fraction of the REV-T particles contain transformation-competent genomes.

REV-T-transformed nonproducer hematopoietic cells induce lethal reticuloendotheliosis when injected into birds matched at the histocompatibility *B* locus (Rup et al. 1979; Lewis et al. 1981). In fact, certain clones of REV-T-transformed cells are as lethal as virus-producing cells, indicating that helper-virus functions are not required for expression of tumorigenicity. Moreover, REV-T presumably recognizes and transforms the same target cell in vitro as it does in vivo.

In the last few years, several studies have been conducted to identify the lineage and maturation stage of the REV-T-transformed cell. Franklin et al. (1974), studying transformed cells from the bone marrow of infected chickens, detected a nonadherent population with lymphoblastoid morphology, and Keller et al. (1979) suggested that the cell had a B-lymphoblast phenotype. However, more recently, Beug et al. (1981) and Lewis et al. (1981) proposed that their results on cells transformed in vitro by REV-T are more consistent with a less mature lymphoid cell, perhaps a pre-B, pre-T progenitor or a pre-pre-B cell. This conclusion is based on the following findings: (1) Antigenic determinants found on mature T and B cells are generally absent from REV-T-transformed cells. (2) Surface immunoglobulins are absent. (3) Intracytoplasmic μ chains (characteristic of pre-B cells) have been found in only one of many cell lines tested. (4) The enzyme, terminal deoxynucleotidyl transferase, characteristically found in mature T cells and expressed in some very immature lymphoid cells (for review, see Bollum 1979), is detected in some, but not all, cell lines at very low concentrations. (5) Markers specific to erythroid or myelomonocytic cells are invariably absent. Although it is not entirely clear that T and B cells develop from a common stem cell (Till and McCulloch 1980), the REV-T-transformed cell has a phenotype consistent with that of an uncommitted lymphoid progenitor cell. In addition, many of the clones of REV-T-transformed cells derived in vivo or by in vitro procedures show a great deal of variability in morphology and growth properties, suggesting that REV-T may be capable of transforming more than one cell type.

E. Mechanism of Tumorigenesis

Little is known about the mechanisms by which the various members of the REV group cause the acute proliferative disease. Because REV-T is capable of transforming cells in vitro, the presence of an *onc*-gene sequence, *rel,* has been postulated (see Chapters 2 and 9).

No *onc* sequences have been described for the replication-competent viruses, although they may cause very rapid mortality. Very young chickens inoculated with CSV develop B-cell lymphomas by 17–43 weeks postinfection (Witter and Crittenden 1979); interestingly, the integration of CSV proviral DNA frequently occurs near the *c-myc* gene (Noori-Daloii et al. 1981), much in the manner of the less acute ALVs described above (Section IV.B.3).

Thus, it is possible that two unrelated virus groups cause B-cell tumors in chickens by a similar mechanism.

VII. PATHOGENESIS OF MOUSE MAMMARY TUMOR VIRUSES

A. Discovery of MMTV-induced Carcinogenesis

Reciprocal genetic crosses between mice from strains with high and low incidences of mammary carcinomas, which were performed in the early 1930s by the Staff of the Jackson Memorial Laboratory (1933) and by Korteweg (1934, 1936) in Holland, revealed that the incidence of mammary carcinomas in progeny mice was maternally determined. By appropriate fostering experiments, Bittner (1936) proved that a "maternal extrachromosomal factor" was present in the milk of A and C3H strains of mice and that it was responsible for the high incidence of mammary carcinoma in these strains. Subsequent analysis of C3H milk showed the "factor" to be a virus (for review, see Gross 1970; Hilgers and Bentvelzen 1978). This virus, and the closely related variants that have subsequently been isolated, shows the diagnostic biochemical properties that define retroviruses, although the morphology and morphogenesis of the virions differ from most other RNA tumor viruses (see Chapters 2 and 6).

B. Tumors and Preneoplastic Lesions Induced by MMTV

MMTV induces mammary adenocarcinomas that derive from the secretory epithelial cells of the mammary gland. The tumors usually retain features of glandular differentiation and often contain blood-filled cysts and areas of necrosis. The histological classification most frequently used was proposed by Dunn (1959) and covers all mammary tumors found in inbred strains of mice, including those believed to be of nonviral origin. The virus-induced tumors are most frequently adenocarcinomas of types A and B and rarely of type C. The type-A tumors are well differentiated, display small acini and tubules composed of small cuboidal cells, and occasionally show foci of secretory activity. Type-B tumors are less well differentiated but usually retain tubule type structures and are often cystic, whereas the type-C tumors are very cystic. Adenoacanthomas are also quite common among the virus-induced tumors; in these tumors, the bulk of the tumor tissue resembles adenocarcinomas of types A and B, but at least one-quarter of the tumor tissues must show epidermoid differentiation (e.g., stratified squamous epithelium). Mice carrying the milk-borne virus also exhibit preneoplastic lesions in the mammary gland, known as hyperplastic alveolar nodules (DeOme et al. 1959), in which a nodule of epithelial cells is produced by acinar hyperplasia. These lesions occur early in susceptible virus-infected mice, especially in conjunction with hormonal stimulation (e.g., pituitary isografts) and have been used as a basis for a biological assay for MMTV (Nandi 1963). Another important neoplastic structure, particularly associated with the GR strain of mice, has been termed a plaque (Foulds 1956); these structures appear as densely packed branching tubules arranged in a radial fashion and are further characterized by being dependent on the hormonal stimulation of pregnancy for growth. Thus, these structures arise during pregnancy and regress after parturition, but they eventually become independent of hormones and give rise to an autonomously growing tumor (Foulds 1956; Muhlbock 1965).

C. Transmission of MMTV

Since the discovery of MMTV and of its extrachromosomal transmission in C3H mice, several other variants of the virus have been detected in other mouse strains. Their transmission has been investigated in the natural host strain and following transfer to new host strains. These studies demonstrate that MMTV can be transmitted by two principal routes: by congenital infection of suckling mice by milk-borne virus and genetically as an endogenous provirus (see Chapter 10). In the latter instance, the endogenous proviruses of both parents can segregate during gametogenesis like any other inherited character (Cohen and Varmus 1979).

Most strains of inbred mice with a high incidence of mammary tumors (e.g., A, C3H, DBA, and RIII) harbor a highly oncogenic, milk-transmitted MMTV, and the viruses are named according to the host of origin, e.g., MMTV(C3H) or MMTV(RIII). In these mouse strains, the congenitally acquired virus replicates in the mammary glands and leads to a high concentration of virus in the milk of lactating mice. The virus can be isolated from the milk or mammary tumors and can be used to induce tumors in other strains of mice with varying degrees of success (see Section VI.D).

Most mouse strains (e.g., C3H and DBA) can be freed of the highly oncogenic milk-borne virus they naturally harbor by foster-nursing neonates on mothers of a low-incidence strain to yield strains designated, for example, as C3Hf and DBAf. These mice have a lower incidence of mammary carcinomas than the prefoster generations, but a substantial percentage still succumb to mammary carcinomas in old age (at 1–2 years). Genetic cross experiments, in conjunction with electron microscopy and immunological analysis of the mammary glands and milks, have shown that C3Hf mice retain an endogenous MMTV of low oncogenic potential which is genetically transmitted (Boot and Muhlbock 1956; Pitelka et al. 1964; Vlahakis et al. 1970; van Nie and Verstraeten 1975). Further backcross analysis has established that expression of virus in the milk appears to be regulated by a single dominant locus (*Mtv-1*), which is linked to the albino locus on chromosome 7 (van Nie and Verstraeten 1975; Verstraeten and van Nie 1978). Virus produced from the provirus present at this locus is called MMTV(C3Hf) and is apparently responsible for the induction of late mammary tumors (Cohen and Varmus 1980; Michalides et al. 1981a).

In one strain of mouse so far examined (GR strain), a very high incidence of early mammary tumors is associated with the presence of a genetically transmitted MMTV. The first indications of the genetic transmission derived from extensive breeding experiments between GR and low-incidence mouse strains (Muhlbock 1965; Bentvelzen 1968; Muhlbock and Bentvelzen 1968; Hilgers and Bentvelzen 1978). More direct support for this notion came from the embryo-transplantation experiments of Zeilmaker (1969). Fertilized GR eggs were implanted into pseudopregnant females from a strain with a low incidence of mammary carcinoma. The subsequent GR progeny had the high incidence of the disease characteristic of the GR strain. Conversely, when fertilized eggs of a low-incidence strain were transferred to GR females and the progeny mice were foster-nursed by a female of a low-incidence strain to avoid possible milk transmission by the GR mother, the offspring had a low incidence of the disease. Thus, the fertilized GR eggs were infected prior to transfer, whereas the fertilized eggs of the low-incidence strain were not infected by MMTV after implantation in the uterus of a GR female. More extensive genetic analysis of hybrid and backcross populations between GR mice and low-incidence mice led Bentvelzen to postulate that a single dominant Mendelian locus controlled the early appearance of mammary tumors in GR mice (Bentvelzen 1968, 1972; Bentvelzen and Daams 1969; Varmus et al. 1973), a view that was contested by other investigators (see Chapter 10).

The establishment of a congenic strain of GR mice with a low incidence of mammary carcinomas (van Nie and de Moes 1977), and the subsequent molecular analysis of the DNA of these mice, yielded results that strongly support the notion that a single provirus is responsible for early tumor development in the GR mouse strain. The low-incidence congenic strain of GR mouse (GR/*Mtv-2*$^-$) lacks the DNA of a single provirus, does not contain infectious virus in the milk, and rarely develops mammary carcinomas (van Nie and de Moes 1977; Michalides et al. 1978a, 1981a). Thus, the *Mtv-2* locus of the GR mouse appears to encode a provirus that is responsible for the high yield of infectious virus in the milk and the high incidence of mammary carcinomas. Furthermore, similar breeding experiments aimed at introducing the *Mtv-2* locus into a low-incidence strain succeeded in showing a coincident gain of the proviral DNA, with an increase in the incidence of mammary tumors (Michalides et al. 1981a,b). A further general discussion of *Mtv-1, Mtv-2,* and other endogenous MMTV proviruses is presented in Chapter 10.

D. Susceptibility and Resistance to Exogenous Infection and Tumor Induction

The lack of in vitro assay systems for MMTV has hindered the analysis of cell susceptibility to infection by this virus. However, many in vivo experiments have been performed where the end point has been measured by the induction of mammary tumors. Tumor incidence depends on susceptibility to virus replication as well as infection and on other nonviral factors that directly affect subsequent tumor progression; consequently, it is often difficult to ascribe observed effects to virus-cell interactions. Direct titration studies using a variety of virus isolates in different mouse strains has revealed a spectrum of susceptibility in mice; some are highly resistant, some are highly susceptible, and others can be either, depending on the virus isolate used to induce disease (Moore et al. 1970, 1974, 1979). However, genetic and hormonal factors can invariably be demonstrated to modify drastically the response of mice to virus infection. For example, C57BL and I strains of mice are resistant to mammary tumorigenesis by exogenous MMTV, but the F_1 hybrids are susceptible (Andervont 1940, 1945). If mammary-gland fragments of either parental strain are transplanted into F_1 hybrids, the fragments are then susceptible to infection and transformation, like the surrounding F_1 host tissue, which indicates that resistance was not at the level of the virus-cell interaction (Nandi et al. 1972; Nandi 1974). The influence of sex hormones is suggested by the observations that (1) the incidence of mammary carcinoma is lowest in virgin mice and highest in multiparous mice (see Gross 1970) and (2) males of high-incidence strains have a low incidence compared with that of the females, although this is increased by castration followed by administration of estrogens (Muhlbock and Boot 1959; Boot 1970). In general, administration of estrogens and progestins increases the incidence of the disease, but tumors are not always accompanied by overt expression of MMTV (Muhlbock and Boot 1959). Alleles of the *H-2* histocompatibility locus also influence susceptibility to exogenous infections (Dux 1972; Muhlbock and Dux 1974). However, the relative importance of genetic, hormonal, dietary, and other environmental factors, as well as age (Dmochowski 1953; Heston 1965; Bentvelzen 1972; Nandi and McGrath 1973; Moore et al. 1974), in determining the induction of the mammary carcinoma by MMTV is complex and remains obscure.

E. Expression of MMTV In Vivo

The presence of replicating MMTV can be detected by immunological tests, electron microscopy, and biologically by its ability to induce tumors or hyperplastic nodules in mammary glands of susceptible mice following hormone stimulation (Dmochowski 1953; DeOme et al. 1962; Nandi 1963; Moore et al. 1970).

1. Viral Particles

Mature extracellular MMTV particles have a characteristic B-type morphology and are associated with their precursors, intracytoplasmic A-type particles (see Chapters 2 and 6). Typical B-type particles (Bernhard 1958) have been seen under the electron microscope in sections of mammary gland and mammary tumor tissue, as well as in milk preparations from most high-incidence strains of mice and several low-incidence strains (Dmochowski 1953; Bernhard et al. 1956; Pitelka et al. 1964; Tanaka and Moore 1967; Calafat 1968; Dmochowski et al. 1968; Hageman et al. 1968). Occasionally, B-type particles have been seen budding from cells of the seminal vesicles, epididymis, and submaxillary gland and from cells of lung adenomas and ependymoblastomas (Smith 1966; Nandi and McGrath 1973; Rongey et al. 1975). In addition, positive bioassays for MMTV have been obtained with extracts from epididymis, testis, kidney, and salivary gland (see Parks et al. 1972; Nandi and McGrath 1973; Bentvelzen and Brinkhof 1977). The synthesis of infectious MMTV by the accessory sex organs of male mice has been well documented in GR mice (see Hilgers and Bentvelzen 1978), although no neoplasia seems to result from this expression of virus. Intracytoplasmic A-type particles have also been detected in many tissues and tumors, independent of the presence of mature B-type particles. A-type particles or the viral structural proteins have, for example, been detected in lymphomas and leukemias (Dalton et al. 1961; Granboulan and Riviere 1962; Brandes et al. 1966; Tanaka et al. 1972; Nusse et al. 1979), in Leydig cell tumors (Pourreau-Schneider et al. 1968; Nowinski et al. 1971), and in hepatomas and lung adenomas (Rongey et al. 1975). The significance of the partial virus expression is still uncertain.

2. Viral Antigens

Immunochemical tests, such as immunodiffusion, immunofluorescence, radioimmunoprecipitation, cytotoxicity, and complement-fixation assays, have been used to detect specific MMTV antigens (see Chapters 2 and 6). Viral antigens are readily detected in mammary tumors, tissues, and milk from strains of mice with a high incidence of the disease and in exogenously infected mice (Blair 1965; Charney et al. 1969; Nandi and McGrath 1973; Moore et al. 1979). In mammary tissues, the amount of detectable antigen is higher in strains with a high incidence of the disease, is greater in tumor tissues than in their normal counterparts, and increases during pregnancy (Blair 1965; Nowinski et al. 1971; Parks et al.

1972; Hilgers et al. 1973, 1975; Noon et al. 1975; Verstraeten et al. 1975). In some low-incidence strains, hormonal stimulation can specifically increase viral antigen concentration in the mammary gland, a finding that is not reflected in the subsequent tumors (Nusse et al. 1980). MMTV antigens have also been detected in several other tissues, e.g., in spleen, lymphoid organs, kidney, liver, placenta, epididymis, seminal vesicles, and male ejaculate (for reviews, see Dmochowski 1953; Bentvelzen 1972; Hageman et al. 1972; Nandi and McGrath 1973; Hilgers and Bentvelzen 1978), but the amount of antigen is usually low and varies both with the strain and the age of the individual mouse (Daams 1970; Daams et al. 1970; Hilgers et al. 1973; Gillette et al. 1974; Charyulu et al. 1979).

The presence of antigen in the kidney could result from the deposition of antigen-antibody complexes, since MMTV antigens and antibodies have been detected in mouse serum (Hilgers et al. 1973; Verstraeten et al. 1975; Ihle et al. 1976a; Arthur and Fine 1978; Michalides et al. 1979; Schochetman et al. 1979), but kidney cells in culture are also capable of supporting the replication of MMTV (Calafat et al. 1974). It is also noteworthy that cell-free extracts of liver and brain of GR mice, which show only a low level of virus-specific immunofluorescence, induce mammary carcinomas when injected into test mice (Bentvelzen and Daams 1970; Daams 1970).

3. *Virus-specific RNA*

In mouse strains with a high incidence of early mammary tumors, induced by either milk-borne or genetically transmitted MMTVs, the mammary glands and the mammary tumors express high levels of virus-specific RNA concomitant with viral protein production (Axel et al. 1972; Schlom et al. 1973; Varmus et al. 1973; C. McGrath et al. 1978; Michalides et al. 1978b). Mammary glands from certain strains (e.g., C57BL/6 or I) also exhibit moderate or even high levels of MMTV RNA, even in the absence of infection by milk-borne virus (see Chapter 10). Examination of other nontarget tissues, such as spleen, liver, and kidney, rarely shows significant levels of MMTV RNA, suggesting that exogenous infection or efficient expression of endogenous proviruses is unusual in those tissues (Schlom et al. 1973; Varmus et al. 1973). In some spontaneous tumors from virus-free animals, this RNA seems to be transcribed from regions at the 3′ half of endogenous proviruses (Dudley et al. 1978). The appearance of these transcripts may be correlated with hypomethylation in the 3′ half of endogenous proviruses (J.C. Cohen, pers. comm.). Mammary-gland tropism of milk-transmitted MMTV has been confirmed by tests for MMTV proviral DNA in livers and mammary glands of naturally infected animals; new proviruses were detected only in mammary-gland DNA (Cohen et al. 1979).

The low level of expression of endogenous MMTV DNA in the mammary glands of some mouse strains with a low incidence of mammary tumors had led several investigators to inquire whether other agents that induce mouse mammary tumors, such as hormonal stimulation, chemical carcinogens, radiation, or combinations of these treatments, exert their action by activation of endogenous proviruses. The results of these studies have not yielded clear answers. In many cases, resultant mammary tumors can be shown to produce MMTV (Timmermans et al. 1969; Schlom et al. 1973; C. McGrath et al. 1978; Svec et al. 1979), suggesting an association of virus production with tumorigenesis. On the other hand, tumors can be induced without the obvious activation of MMTV; in some other instances, viral products can be detected in the mammary glands during treatment but are not detected in the subsequent tumors (Michalides et al. 1978b, 1979; Pauley et al. 1979; Nusse et al. 1980). Thus, the role of endogenous MMTV in tumor induction by these agents is questionable.

4. Biological Activity of MMTV in the Absence of Viral Particles

Nucleated cells of the spleen, bone marrow, and blood may contain MMTV antigens and also transmit MMTV infection from one animal to another (Dux and Muhlbock 1968; Hageman et al. 1972; Nandi et al. 1974). These cells do not, however, appear to shed B-type particles readily, and their MMTV biological activity is inactivated by procedures such as mechanical disruption and doses of X-irradiation to which virions are quite stable (Hageman et al. 1972; Nandi and Helmich 1974; Nandi et al. 1974). It appears, therefore, that leukocytes may be implicated in the widespread distribution of MMTV biological activity in many organs and tissues. However, although many tissues have MMTV antigens and may even produce both A-type and B-type particles, MMTV has not been associated with tumors other than mammary carcinoma, with the possible exception of lymphoid leukemias.

F. Association of MMTV with Lymphoid Leukemias

In DBA/2 and GR mice, T-cell lymphomas occur at a low frequency, more often in male mice, and appear to be associated with the intracellular expression of MMTV products (Stuck et al. 1964; Tanaka et al. 1972; Hilgers et al. 1975; Nusse et al. 1979; Vaidya et al. 1980). In GR mice, amplification of the endogenous MMTV provirus is also a consistent feature of the leukemia cells (R. Michalides et al., pers. comm.). Thus, the expression of MMTV, which is usually restricted to the mammary glands of female mice and the gonads of male mice, is also found in some T-cell lymphomas, suggesting some form of association. In the case of CFW mice, a virus that morphologically resembles MMTV has been isolated and shown to induce a thymic lymphoma upon injection into the thymus, providing more-stringent evidence of MMTV expression being associated with this form of neoplasia in some mouse strains (G. Dekaban and J. Ball, pers. comm.). Further molecular characterization of this virus should be enlightening.

G. Mechanisms of Tumorigenesis by MMTV

Although the manner by which MMTV induces mammary carcinomas is not known, recent work suggests several features of the virus and its interaction with the host cell that are probably pertinent to the oncogenic mechanism: (1) Like other retroviruses that induce tumors after lengthy latency and fail to transform cultured cells, MMTV appears to carry genes required for replication only; i.e., there is no evidence for a viral *onc* gene derived from a cellular gene. (2) Virus-induced tumors almost always carry new proviruses and are clonal with respect to acquired proviruses. (3) It is possible that certain integration sites predispose to oncogenesis and that cellular oncogenes (either adjacent or unlinked) are activated during tumor production. Some of the findings that support these postulates are described briefly below.

MMTV induces adenocarcinomas of the mammary gland with a relatively long latency period of 4–9 months (Nandi and McGrath 1973; Hilgers and Bentvelzen 1978). The virus can infect a variety of target cells in vitro, albeit with a low efficiency, but does not appear to cause any alterations in cell morphology or in cell-growth characteristics (Lasfargues et al. 1974, 1976; Vaidya et al. 1976). Thus, in both its pathogenic properties and its behavior in vitro, MMTV closely resembles the avian and murine leukemia viruses. These viruses too are equipped with genes for replication only, and viral oncogenesis is, at least in the case of ALV (see Section IV.B.3.d), apparently dependent on the activation of cellular genes.

Genetic, biochemical, and physical mapping of the MMTV genome (see Chapter 4) demonstrates the three replicative genes common to all replication-competent retroviruses, but no substantial evidence has been obtained for a viral oncogene. Differences between endogenous and milk-borne strains, at one time considered to be a possible manifestation of a transforming gene, can probably be ascribed to minor variations in sequence distributed throughout the MMTV genome (see Chapter 10), and molecular hybridization experiments have not identified a conserved cellular gene homologous to any part of the viral genome.

An unexpectedly long open reading frame was recently discovered in the U_3 region of the MMTV LTR using in vitro translation systems (Dickson and Peters 1981; Dickson et al. 1981), and the open frame has been confirmed by nucleotide sequencing of several MMTV LTRs (Donehower et al. 1981; H. Diggelmann; J. Majors; C. Dickson; all pers. comm.) (see Chapters 4 and 5). However, there is as yet no evidence that this potential coding region is actually expressed in cells. There are conflicting data about the nature of the minor species of intracellular MMTV RNAs, but none of the species observed to date appears to be a likely candidate for expression of the family of proteins encoded in the LTR. Efforts to detect the predicted proteins in vivo have been hampered by the lack of a suitable antiserum. Hence, the role of the putative LTR-encoded proteins in oncogenesis remains an unresolved issue.

Integration of MMTV DNA into the host chromosome may be a critical event in oncogenesis. Initially, acquisition of MMTV proviruses was studied by reassociation hybridization kinetics. In general, tumors that were induced by milk-transmitted MMTV had acquired new provirus information (Michalides et al. 1976; Morris et al. 1977). Subsequently, with the use of restriction enzymes and Southern blotting, a more detailed analysis of the integration process was possible (Cohen et al. 1979; Fanning et al. 1980a; Groner and Hynes 1980; Groner et al. 1980). Milk-transmitted MMTV could be distinguished from endogenous proviruses, and restriction fragments that were specific for milk-transmitted MMTV were detected in DNA from MMTV-infected, nontumorous mammary-gland cells. These new proviral elements are integrated at numerous sites in the cell genome. The tumors that arise from infected mammary-gland cells also contain the restriction fragments specific for the milk-transmitted MMTV, but in contrast to the infected mammary-gland cells, specific host DNA–proviral DNA restriction fragments were detected in the tumor cells, indicating that the integration site is identical in at least a large number of cells within a single tumor (Cohen et al. 1979). Thus, it appears that virally induced tumors are clonal, i.e., arise from a single infected mammary-gland cell, and that proviral integration per se is not sufficient for neoplastic transformation, although the site of integration may be important. When independent tumors are compared, MMTV DNA seems to be integrated at different sites, but this pattern is complicated because most tumors contain more than one provirus in addition to the endogenous ones (Cohen et al. 1979). Recent experiments, using cloned chromosomal DNA flanking an MMTV provirus as a probe, indicate that in 5 of 35 independent tumors, MMTV DNA is integrated in the same region of the host genome (R. Nusse and H. Varmus, pers. comm.). It is as yet unknown whether this flanking sequence is relevant to the oncogenic process.

In the C3Hf and GR mouse strains, the development of mammary tumors is under the control of genes that are identical to the endogenous MMTV proviruses, *Mtv-1* and *Mtv-2,* respectively (Michalides et al. 1981a). Endogenous MMTV seems to be amplified in most of the mammary tumors in these strains, even in the absence of milk-transmitted virus (Cohen and Varmus 1980; Fanning et al. 1980b), but some tumors do not contain additional proviruses, suggesting that the expression of *Mtv-1* and *Mtv-2* per se would be sufficient for oncogenesis (Michalides et al. 1981b). In the BALB/c strain, mammary tumors also develop without reintegration of proviruses, but in this case, as in many tumors in other strains, it is not clear whether MMTV is causally related to tumorigenesis. In some tumors without proviral amplification, a relatively low level of methylation of the DNA at the 3′ half of endogenous proviruses has been observed. Hypomethylation has been correlated with gene activation in general and may, in the case of MMTV proviruses, indicate that these genes are activated during tumorigenesis (Cohen 1980).

High-molecular-weight DNA from mammary tumors is capable of transforming mouse NIH-3T3 fibroblasts in tissue culture. The sequences responsible for transformation do not seem to contain MMTV-related information. Interestingly, the transforming sequences are inactivated by the same set of restriction enzymes when DNAs from several MMTV-induced tumors and one chemically induced mouse mammary tumor, and the known mammary tumor cell, MCF7, are compared (Lane et al. 1981).

VIII. PATHOGENESIS OF MURINE SARCOMA AND ACUTE LEUKEMIA VIRUSES

The following sections encompass discussions of those murine retroviruses that rapidly induce neoplastic disease. Many of these viruses contain identified oncogene sequences presumably responsible for the ability of the virus to transform fibroblasts and/or hematopoietic cells in vitro and for the capability to induce sarcomas and leukemias. Others do not contain classic *onc*-gene sequences, defined generically as normal-cell sequences unrelated to known endogenous viral genes that are acquired in the course of generating highly oncogenic viruses; for example, in the case of the various components of the Friend virus complex, the sequences considered most important in the oncogenic process appear to derive from endogenous retroviruslike elements. In addition, following Friend virus infection in vivo, cell-free tumor extracts may contain other infectious viruses, such as the mink-cell focus-inducing (MCF) viruses (see Section IX) whose involvement in the induction of disease is not clearly understood. The functions of *onc* genes and their products are described in Chapter 9; here, we deal with the pathogenic considerations concerning the changes that occur within specific organs and cells in vivo and we describe how these are manifested in classic fibroblast transformation assays or quantitative hematopoietic colony formation in vitro.

A. Friend Leukemia Virus

1. Origin and Pathology

The original isolate of Friend virus was obtained as a cell-free extract from a Swiss mouse that had developed erythroleukemia following inoculation with Ehrlich mouse carcinoma cells (Friend 1957). The disease induced by this initial extract could subsequently be serially transmitted by injecting filtrates prepared from spleen extracts. Early description of the pathology of Friend disease (for review, see Tambourin 1978; Tambourin et al. 1979) indicated that the original isolate, when injected into susceptible adult mice, induced a thymus-independent disease characterized by rapid enlargement of the spleen (splenomegaly) (Fig. 8.5) and anemia. In addition, the peripheral blood contained numerous hyperbasophilic cells, called Friend cells, that morphologically resemble proerythroblast progenitor cells. The susceptibility to anemia in vivo caused by this original isolate, now termed FV-A, appears to be affected by factors that determine the demand for erythroid differentiation: hypoxia, bleeding, and erythropoietin (Epo) increase susceptibility, whereas repeated red-cell transfusions (which lower Epo levels in vivo) prolong the survival of FV-A-infected mice. Thus, as suggested by Tambourin et al. (1979), the enhanced erythropoiesis observed after FV-A infection remains sensitive to Epo levels.

Two groups independently obtained derivatives of the original Friend virus preparation that induced a rapid splenomegaly, characterized by polycythemia (increased levels of red blood cells in the peripheral blood), rather than anemia (Mirand et al. 1961; Sassa et al. 1968). Studies by Mirand and his colleagues (Mirand 1967; Mirand et al. 1968a) demonstrated that in mice infected with the polycythemic strain of Friend virus (FV-P), erythropoiesis proceeded in the absence of Epo. Thus, the diseases induced by FV-A and FV-P can be distinguished not only by their effects on hematocrit levels (the proportion of red cells in a volume of whole blood), but also on the basis of the responsiveness of erythroid cells to Epo in vivo. This latter point is discussed further below.

Both FV-A and FV-P stocks contain at least two viral compo-

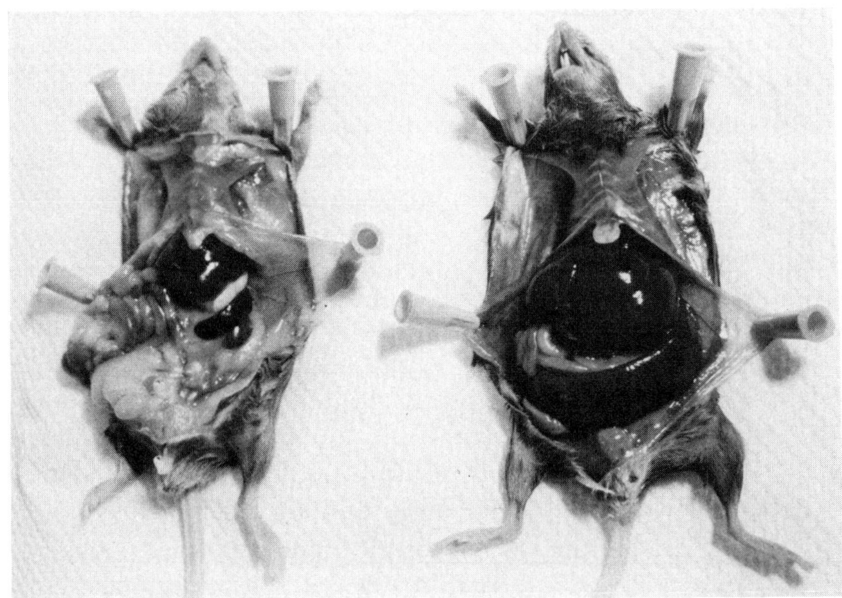

Figure 8.5 Gross pathology of FV-P-induced disease in a susceptible DBA/2 adult mouse. Compare the massive spleen and liver enlargement in the FV-P-infected animal (*right*) with the uninoculated control (*left*). (Photograph courtesy of J. Silver, National Institutes of Health.)

nents: a replication-competent helper virus (Friend murine leukemia virus [Fr-MLV]) and a replication-defective spleen focus-forming virus (SFFV). Wherever it is necessary to distinguish the origin of a particular component, a subscript (A for anemia, P for polycythemia) will be used; the reasons for these annotations will become clear in ensuing sections.

2. Cellular Aspects of Friend Disease

The erythroleukemia induced by either the anemia- or polycythemia-inducing Friend virus isolates exhibits two distinct stages: an early stage characterized by a rapid increase in the number of relatively mature erythroid progenitor cells with limited proliferative capacity and a later stage characterized by the emergence of relatively undifferentiated progenitor cells with very extensive proliferative capacity. By far the fullest characterization has been of the cellular changes that occur after infection with FV-P, although more recently, similar analyses of hematopoietic progenitors after infection with FV-A have been carried out. As discussed below, these studies support the view that this virally induced erythroleukemia has an early polyclonal "preleukemic" phase, followed by a true leukemia characterized by the appearance of immortal leukemic stem-cell clones.

a. FV-P: Early. Within days after infection of susceptible mice with FV-P, changes are observed in hematopoietic progenitor cell populations. The most dramatic alteration is the large (100-fold) increase in the number of cells from the spleen or marrow capable of forming small (32–64 cells) erythroid colonies after 2 days in plasma clots or methylcellulose in medium containing fetal calf serum without Epo (Horoszewicz et al. 1975; Liao and Axelrad 1975). The growth of these erythroid colonies is not due to trace amounts of Epo in the serum, because these colonies can also be obtained from FV-P mice under serum-free conditions (Rossi and Peschle 1980; MacDonald et al. 1981). Thus, the proliferation and differentiation of FV-P-infected erythroid progenitor cells, in parallel with the disease in vivo, appear totally independent of Epo, the hormonal regulator of normal erythropoiesis. As discussed below (Section VIII.A.3.a), these effects appear to be due to the replication-defective $SFFV_P$ component of FV-P, rather than to the helper $Fr\text{-}MLV_P$.

Within 2 to 4 weeks, infection of susceptible mice with FV-P also leads to marked increases in the number of cells capable of forming spleen colonies (CFU-S) in irradiated secondary recipients (Wendling et al. 1974). The CFU-S concentration in the spleen remains constant, but because the spleen cellularity increases approximately 20-fold after infection with FV-P, the total number of spleen CFU-S increases about 20-fold. The number of CFU-S in the peripheral blood also increases by a remarkable 500-fold 25 days postinfection, whereas very little, if any, change in either the concentration or total number of CFU-S is observed in the bone marrow. The histology and spectrum of morphologically distinct cell types observed in the spleen colonies from donor mice infected with FV-P appear to be the same as those seen with normal CFU-S (Wendling et al. 1974); however, it remains to be determined whether these spleen colony-forming cells behave as functionally normal hematopoietic stem cells.

b. FV-A: Early. Recently, it has been shown that FV-A, like FV-P, also induces an increase in the number of splenic erythroid colony-forming cells early after infection of susceptible mice (Steinheider et al. 1979; Fagg et al. 1980; MacDonald et al. 1980b). However, unlike the results described above for FV-P, no Epo-independent erythroid progenitor cells are observed after FV-A infection; these findings are consistent with the in vivo observations (see Section VIII.A.1). The early effects of FV-A on the number of erythroid progenitor cells in adult mice are attributed to the $SFFV_A$ activity present in stocks of FV-A, and not to its helper Fr-MLV_A (see Section VIII.A.3.b).

c. FV-P and FV-A: Late. Although infection of susceptible mice with either FV-A or FV-P leads to the rapid proliferation of erythroid cells in the spleen, several experiments suggest that, at least early after infection, the vast majority of these cells have only limited proliferative capacity. First, fragments of the grossly enlarged spleens of mice infected with either virus complex cannot be successfully transplanted subcutaneously to syngeneic hosts early (2 weeks) after infection. Only very late after infection (more than 3 weeks) is it possible to obtain tumor cell lines (Buffett and Furth 1959; Friend and Haddad 1960; Dawson et al. 1963). These cell lines, once established, have the well-described property that they can be induced by certain chemicals, such as dimethylsulfoxide (DMSO) (Friend et al. 1971), to undergo terminal erythroid differentiation.

Second, when the spleen cells from mice infected 1–2 weeks previously with FV-P are cloned in a semisolid medium, only small erythroid colonies are observed 2 days after plating. The cells in these small colonies have none of the expected properties of a virally transformed cell: they are relatively differentiated along the erythroid pathway and have lost any further capacity to divide.

Third, attempts to develop an in vivo assay for possible Friend-virus-induced tumor colony-forming units (TCFU) early after infection have so far failed to detect such leukemic stem cells. In these experiments, spleen cells from animals infected with Friend virus were transplanted into secondary recipients, which were then observed for tumor colony formation. However, because the donor spleen cells continuously release virus, the secondary recipients were chosen to be resistant to de novo virus infection. For this reason, in the initial attempt to develop such a TCFU assay, mice that were *Fv-1* restrictive (see Section VIII.A.6.b) for virus replication and spleen focus formation were used (Thomson and Axelrad 1968). However, later studies, using *H-2* and sex chromosome markers, demonstrated that the spleen colonies present in the secondary hosts were of host, rather than donor, origin (Steeves et al. 1978; Wendling and Tambourin 1978). Thus, transplantation of spleen cells from animals infected with Friend virus into *Fv-1* nonpermissive hosts detects infectious centers of virus production, rather than the clonal growth of donor leukemic stem cells.

These observations suggest that there are at least two distinct stages to the disease induced by either FV-A or FV-P (Levy et al. 1979; Tambourin et al. 1979): an early phase, with rapid changes in various hematopoietic progenitor cells, and a later phase, characterized by the emergence of truly malignant Friend-virus-transformed cells. The relationship between the early and late hematopoietic cell populations is unknown. It is possible that some of the early infected cells evolve or progress with time such that the probability of self-renewal, and hence extensive proliferative capacity, increases while the probability of terminal differentiation decreases. Alternatively, truly malignant Friend-virus-transformed cells may arise de novo from a population of target cells different from that affected early after infection with either FV-A or FV-P. The discrete biological roles of SFFV and Fr-MLV in the late transformation process are also unknown. The Fr-MLV may only be providing virus functions necessary for the replication of SFFV. Alternatively, because Fr-MLV$_A$ and Fr-MLV$_P$ both have erythroleukemic potential in neonates (Section VIII.A.4), these helper viruses may be more directly involved in the late transformation process.

Attempts to answer these and other questions concerning the mechanism of malignant transformation by FV-A and FV-P have been hampered by the lack of a quantitative assay for Friend-virus-transformed cells. Recently, two colony assays, one using irradiated *Sl/Sl*^{d} mice (Mager et al. 1980) (see Section VIII.A.7.b) and one in cell culture in methylcellulose, have been developed to detect a cell population with the properties expected of a Friend-virus-transformed leukemic stem cell (Mager et al. 1981a,b): (1)

The colony-forming cells only appear quite late after infection with either FV-A or FV-P, in agreement with the earlier transplantation studies. (2) Approximately 1–5% of the cells in the colonies spontaneously differentiate to produce hemoglobin. (3) Cells in the colony are productively infected. (4) FV-A-induced colonies, designated CFU-FV-A, have a high self-renewal probability, and correspondingly, a high proportion of the colonies give rise directly to permanent cell lines. (5) Cells in the primary colony can form spleen colonies in irradiated hosts and form tumors when injected subcutaneously into unirradiated hosts.

In addition to these common properties, Friend tumor colony-forming cells, and cell lines derived from them, exhibit a number of important differences (Mager et al. 1981b), some of which parallel the differences seen in the early stage of the diseases: (1) In adult DBA/2J (highly susceptible) mice, CFU-FV-P are detected as early as 3 weeks postinfection, whereas CFU-FV-A are not detected until 8 weeks. A similar difference in the kinetics of appearance of tumorigenic cells after infection with FV-A and FV-P has also been reported, using an assay that detects tumor formation in the omentum of secondary irradiated recipients (Wendling et al. 1981). (2) Tumor cells transformed by FV-A have an extensive capacity to self-renew (i.e., form secondary colonies in methylcellulose), whereas a significant proportion of the corresponding FV-P cells do not. (3) The initial CFU-FV-P colonies are diploid or pseudodiploid, whereas a high proportion of CFU-FV-A are hyperploid. (4) Cell lines derived from these tumorigenic colony-forming cells differ in their differentiating properties. Clonal cell lines from CFU-FV-A have a low level of hemoglobin-containing cells, whereas newly isolated lines from CFU-FV-P exhibit a high level (>25%) of cells with detectable hemoglobin. In addition, these lines differ in their response to chemical inducers such as Epo or DMSO. With Epo, most CFU-FV-A-derived cell lines accumulate spectrin (an erythroid-cell-specific membrane protein) and hemoglobin, whereas those derived from CFU-FV-P do not. Conversely, some of the cell lines derived from CFU-FV-P respond to low (1%) levels of DMSO, whereas the CFU-FV-A cell lines do not.

The clonal analysis of tumorigenic Friend-virus-transformed cells indicates that these leukemic colony-forming cells retain at least one attribute of normal hematopoietic cells (the property of self-renewal and terminal differentiation), but they have also acquired two attributes considered characteristic of malignant transformation: autonomous growth and a high self-renewal capacity. Both CFU-FV-A and CFU-FV-P form large colonies in cell culture in the absence of Epo or other added regulatory factors (other than those that may be present in the serum). In addition, CFU-FV-P proliferate to form macroscopic spleen colonies in genetically anemic *Sl*/*Sl*^{d} mice (Mager et al. 1980). These mice carry two mutations at the steel (*Sl*) locus, resulting in a defective cellular microenvironment that prevents spleen colony formation by normal hematopoietic cells. Thus, the final stage of Friend leukemia is characterized by the emergence of tumorigenic cells that appear to be partially or totally autonomous of both humoral and cellular factors that regulate the behavior of normal progenitor cells. As discussed below (Section VIII.A.5.b), analysis of the effects of FV-P on long-term bone-marrow cultures has led to similar conclusions (Dexter et al. 1981).

The late stages of the erythroleukemia induced by Friend virus are progressive and usually lethal; death often occurs due to rupture of the enormously enlarged spleen. There are, however, several circumstances where quite a remarkable regression of the disease and/or viremia can occur. Regression of Friend leukemia is under host genetic control (discussed more fully in Section VII.A.6). In addition, spontaneous regression of Friend disease occurs regularly with a regression strain of Friend virus (RFV) (Rich et al. 1969). The regressing property of this virus appears to be due to the helper Fr-MLV, rather than to the SFFV component of the complex (Dietz et al. 1977). Regression of RFV-induced erythroleukemia appears to have an immunological basis involving macrophage function. Macrophages and their precursors (CFU-GM) become infected with virus early after infection. However, in regressor mice, the infected progenitor cells are replaced by uninfected macrophage progenitor cells prior to regression (Marcelletti and Furmanski 1979). Furthermore, transfer of normal macrophages to leukemic mice with progressive disease causes regression (Marcelletti and Furmanski 1978).

3. Replication-defective Friend SFFVs

a. SFFV$_P$. FV-P, like other rapidly transforming mammalian viruses, is actually a complex of two viruses: SFFV$_P$, which induces macroscopic spleen foci 9 days after injection into susceptible mice (Axelrad and Steeves 1964) (Fig. 8.6), and Fr-MLV$_P$, which provides functions necessary for SFFV$_P$ replication (for review, see Steeves 1975). The spleen foci induced by FV-P are actively engaged in hemoglobin synthesis (Stephenson et al. 1972). When the concentration of helper virus is limiting (Bernstein et al. 1977) or when its replication is restricted because of host resistance genes (for review, see Steeves 1975 and Section VIII.A.6), the spleen foci titrate with multi-hit kinetics, suggesting that they arise by a process of continuous recruitment of newly infected cells rather than from clonal growth of a single transformed cell.

Early attempts to analyze the biological and molecular relationships between various Friend virus isolates were frustrated by the apparent inability to propagate SFFV in mouse fibroblasts. Eckner (1975) reported the successful growth in vitro of FV-P complex (SFFV$_P$ and Fr-MLV$_P$) in primary mouse embryo cells, and Clarke et al. (1976) isolated a nonerythroid adherent cell line from the spleen of a chronically infected mouse. Following this work, productive infection of cloned BALB/3T3 and NIH-3T3 fibroblasts with FV-P was reported (Bernstein et al. 1977; Troxler et al. 1977b). Furthermore, starting with FV-P stocks containing SFFV$_P$ in either equal or excess titer to its helper, it was possible to isolate mouse and rat fibroblast cell clones nonproductively infected with SFFV$_P$ (Bernstein et al. 1977; Troxler et al. 1977b; Dresler et al. 1979). Such clones have been useful in identifyng the translation products encoded by the SFFV$_P$ genome and also for analyzing the biological properties that can be attributed separately to SFFV and its helper.

To determine which component was responsible for the Epo-independent nature of the erythropoiesis in FV-P-infected mice, SFFV$_P$ nonproducer clones were superinfected with a variety of helper viruses, including Fr-MLV$_A$, Fr-MLV$_P$, Moloney MLV (Mo-MLV), amphotropic MLV, and Gross MLV. In each case, the disease induced by the SFFV pseudotypes was characterized by the appearance of large numbers of Epo-independent erythroid colony-forming cells (Fagg et al. 1980; MacDonald et al. 1980b). Thus, although the helper virus is necessary for the spread of the disease, the qualitative nature of the disease is specified by SFFV$_P$. More recent evidence has shown that a molecularly cloned SFFV$_P$, rescued by various helper viruses, can induce a disease very similar

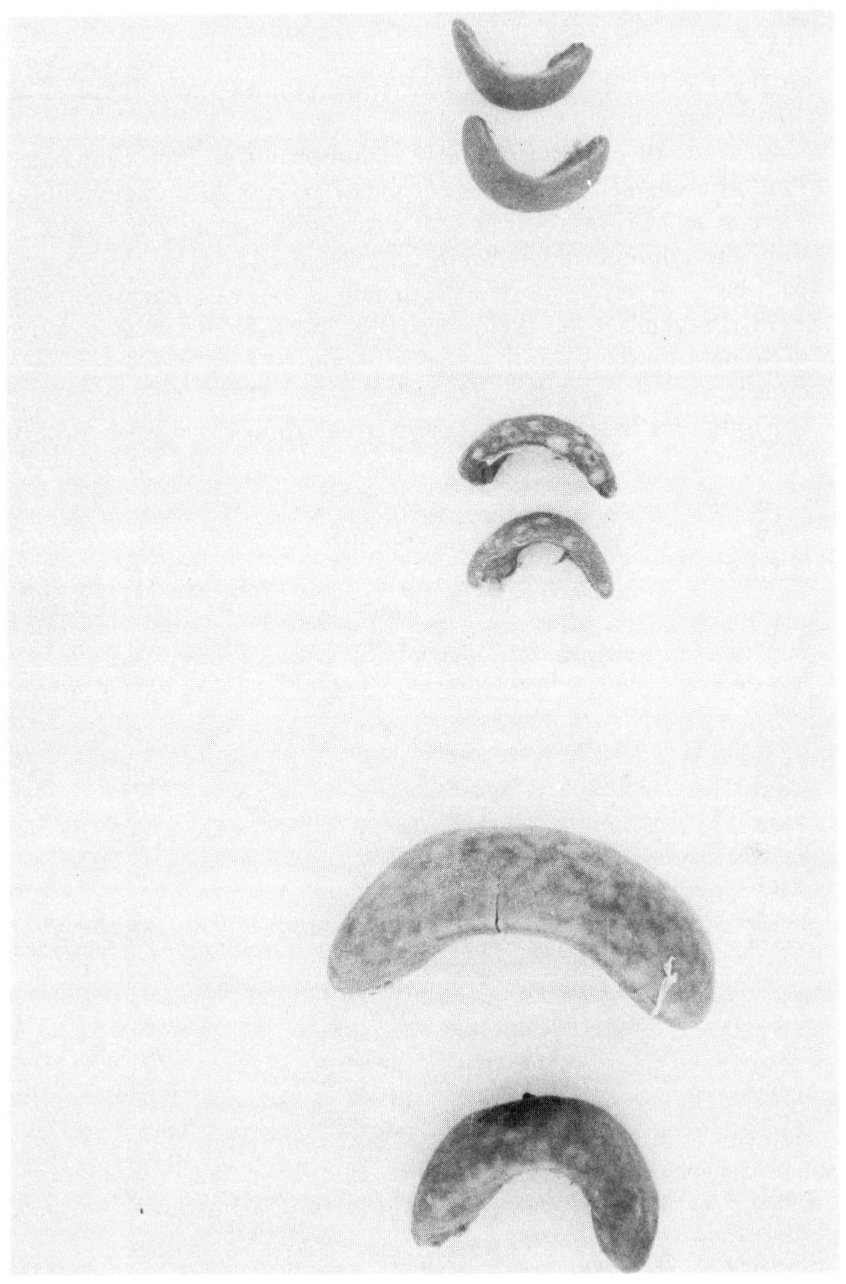

Figure 8.6 Induction of discrete spleen foci by FV-P. A control spleen is seen at the top. The macoscopically visible foci are observed with or without staining with Bouin's fixative. Microscopically, the foci are seen to contain centers of proliferating erythroid cells. (Photograph courtesy of A. Bernstein, Ontario Cancer Institute, Toronto.)

to the FV-P-induced erythroleukemia in adult mice (Oliff et al. 1980; Yamamoto et al. 1981).

Analysis of a variety of $SFFV_P$ nonproducer clones indicated that different $SFFV_P$ isolates encode or express different extents of the *gag* gene. Nonproducer cells expressing no *gag*-gene proteins, only the aminoterminal *gag*-gene protein p15, or both p15 and p12, have all been reported (Bernstein et al. 1977; Barbacid et al. 1978; Pragnell et al. 1980) (see Table 8.5). No proteins reactive with determinants of the *gag* proteins p30 or p10 have been detected.

Mouse erythroleukemic cells derived from FV-P-infected mice

Table 8.5 Biological and molecular properties of Friend erythroleukemia viruses

	Replication-competent		Replication-defective	
Property	$Fr\text{-}MLV_A$	$Fr\text{-}MLV_P$	$SFFV_A$	$SFFV_P$
Genomic size	8.2 kb	8.2 kb	5.2 kb	6.0 kb
gag-gene expression				
p15	+	+	+	– + +
p12	+	+	+	– – +
p30	+	+	+	– – –
p10	+	+	–	– – –
env-gene expression				
gp70	+	+	–	–
gp52	–	–	+	+
Age of susceptible host	newborn only	newborn only	newborn and adult	newborn and adult
Host gene control				
W	unknown	unknown	+	+
Sl	unknown	unknown	+	+
Fv-1	+	+	–	–
Fv-2	unknown	unknown	+	+
Fv-5	unknown	unknown	unknown	+
Fv-6	+	+	–	–
Latent period till spleen enlargement	4–6 weeks	4–6 weeks	1–3 weeks	1–2 weeks
Induction of spleen foci	–	–	+	+
Hematocrit	very low	very low	low or normal	very high
Increased spleen colony-forming cells	+ Epo-dependent	+ Epo-dependent	++ Epo-dependent	++ Epo-independent
Induction of erythroid bursts in vitro	–	–	+	+

(Racevskis and Koch 1977), as well as fibroblast nonproducer $SFFV_P$ clones (Dresler et al. 1979; Ruscetti et al. 1979), contain a glycoprotein of 52,000–55,000 daltons (gp52) that shares both immunological properties and tryptic peptides with the *env*-related gene product gp70 of certain mouse xenotropic and MCF leukemia viruses. As discussed in Chapter 4, it has been suggested that the xenotropic-virus-related sequences included within the $SFFV_P$ genome (Troxler et al. 1977a) and encoding the gp52 (Yoshida and Yoshikura 1980) may be directly associated with the erythroleukemic potential of $SFFV_P$ (Troxler et al. 1977a; Ruscetti et al. 1980).

b. $SFFV_A$. Although an SFFV component was detected in some stocks of FV-A (Mirand et al. 1968b), it was originally assumed to be $SFFV_P$. More recent experiments, however, indicate that the SFFV found in stocks of FV-A ($SFFV_A$) can be distinguished by both biological and molecular criteria from $SFFV_P$. Rescue of the $SFFV_A$ genome from rat nonproducer clones by different helper viruses has shown, analogous to the $SFFV_P$ experiments, that all of the different pseudotypes of $SFFV_A$ induce splenomegaly, anemia, and an increase in only Epo-dependent erythroid colony-forming cells (Troxler et al. 1980; MacDonald et al. 1980b). No Epo-independent precursors have been detected in $SFFV_A$-infected mice.

Although $SFFV_A$ and $SFFV_P$ induce distinct effects on erythroid precursors, they are subject to regulation by the same host gene loci (MacDonald et al. 1980b) (see Section VIII.A.8). Thus, these two SFFVs appear to be highly related, both historically and biologically.

Further evidence that $SFFV_A$ and $SFFV_P$ are distinct but related viruses has come from an analysis of the translational products expressed in nonproducer cells. Unlike any of the $SFFV_P$ isolates described above, $SFFV_A$ encodes the *gag*-gene proteins p15, p12, and p30 (MacDonald et al. 1980b). The $SFFV_A$ genome includes sequences highly related to specific sequences on the $SFFV_P$ genome (Troxler et al. 1980) and encodes 52,000–55,000-dalton glycoprotein that is antigenically related to the *env* gene of MCF MLV (MacDonald et al. 1980b; Troxler et al. 1980). The *env*-related glycoprotein encoded by $SFFV_A$, however, is not identical to that found in $SFFV_P$-infected cells and can be distinguished by tryptic peptide analysis (MacDonald et al. 1980b).

4. Replication-competent Fr-MLVs. In addition to the replication-defective SFFV components present in any Friend virus complex, stocks of FV-A and FV-P contain replication-competent C-type viruses, designated Fr-MLV$_A$ and Fr-MLV$_P$ (the viruses are given separate names to denote their origin, rather than to imply any biological or molecular differences between them). A replication-competent virus was first isolated free of SFFV$_P$ by passage of the FV-P complex through mice or rats resistant to SFFV$_P$ (Dawson et al. 1966; Steeves et al. 1971). The virus recovered from these animals induced lymphatic leukemia involving T cells in both mice and rats; for this reason, the replication-competent virus isolated from FV-P was originally designated Fr-LLV, for Friend lymphatic leukemia virus. More recent studies, using T-cell-depleted newborn mice, indicate that stocks of LLVs also induce erythroleukemia after a long latent period (Dawson et al. 1979). In addition, clonal isolates of replication-competent Friend leukemia virus, obtained by end-point dilution and cloning in fibroblasts in vitro (Troxler and Scolnick 1978; MacDonald et al. 1980a) or by molecular cloning in bacteriophage (Oliff et al. 1980) induce an erythroleukemia, rather than a lymphoid leukemia, in newborn mice. Injection of either Fr-MLV$_A$ (Troxler and Scolnick 1978; MacDonald et al. 1980a) or Fr-MLV$_P$ (MacDonald et al. 1980a) into newborn BALB/c or NIH-Swiss mice results in splenomegaly and profound anemia within 25 to 45 days, which is generally lethal. In addition, the disease induced by these replication-competent viruses is associated with a large increase in both the number and proportion of erythroid progenitor cells, as determined by measuring the number of spleen and marrow Epo-dependent erythroid burst-forming cells (BFU-E) (Niho et al. 1982) and the proportion of cells that stain positively for spectrin (MacDonald et al. 1980a). On the basis of these hematological parameters, the disease induced by Fr-MLV$_A$ and Fr-MLV$_P$ in neonates is similar to the Fr-SFFV$_A$-induced erythroleukemia described above. However, unlike stocks containing SFFV$_A$, which are pathogenic in both newborn and adult mice, the leukemogenic potential of Fr-MLV$_A$ and Fr-MLV$_P$ (Troxler and Scolnick 1978; MacDonald et al. 1980a) and their effects on erythroid colony-forming cells (MacDonald et al. 1980a) appear to be restricted to newborn animals. Induction of splenomegaly in newborn mice is also under host genetic control. Although it is possible to induce splenomegaly in NIH-Swiss and BALB/c mice, other mouse strains (e.g., DBA/2J) are resistant because of the *Fv-6* gene (see Section VIII.A.6.e). The basis for the age-dependent responses to Fr-MLV-induced diseases is unknown. Because the immune system of the mouse is not fully developed at birth, it is possible that newborn mice are functionally immunodeficient and hence more susceptible to viral transformation. Alternatively, the differences in susceptibility of newborn and adult mice to Fr-MLV_A and Fr-MLV_P may reflect either changes in the hematopoietic target-cell populations of mice of different ages or the ability to induce other endogenous viruses, e.g., MCF viruses (Ruscetti et al. 1981); the latter hypothesis is supported by the presence of MCF-specific *env*-gene expression in transplantable cell lines isolated from Fr-MLV-infected animals (Oliff et al. 1981).

Similar to the disease induced by FV-P and FV-A, the erythroleukemia induced by Fr-MLV in newborn mice appears to be a multistage disease. Transplantable cell lines or cells capable of forming cell lines in vitro can be detected in spleens of Fr-MLV-infected animals only late after infection (Oliff et al. 1981; Shibuya and Mak 1982).

5. *Transformation of Hematopoietic Cells In Vitro*

Analysis of the cellular and viral events that lead to erythroleukemia by Friend virus would be facilitated by the development of quantitative and reproducible assays for the transformation of hematopoietic cells in vitro. Several reports have now appeared that describe both short-term and long-term infections of hematopoietic cells by different isolates of Friend virus.

a. Short-term Cultures. Clarke et al. (1975) reported the induction of erythroid colonies without the use of erythropoietin 2 days after infection of bone-marrow cells in vitro with a preparation of FV-P. The induction of these small Epo-independent colonies appears to parallel results observed in vivo (see Section VIII.A.2). Unfortunately, activity in this in vitro assay is restricted to a preparation of FV-P harvested from the medium of the IS cell, an adherent cell line derived from the leukemic spleen of an FV-P-infected mouse (Clarke et al. 1976). Infection of bone-marrow cells in vitro with other FV-P preparations did not give rise to Epo-independent colonies (Clarke et al. 1975).

Using a similar approach, Hankins et al. (1978) have described the appearance of very large erythroid "bursts" in semisolid medium 5 days after infection of bone-marrow cells in vitro with FV-P. Biological and physical characterizations indicate that the cells which give rise to these bursts are erythroid progenitor cells that are closely related to CFU-E (see Fig. 8.1) (Kost et al. 1979). Poorly hemoglobinized erythroid bursts have also been observed 5 days postinfection with FV-A (Hankins and Troxler 1980). Rescue of SFFV nonproducer cell clones with different helper viruses suggests that it is the SFFV component, rather than the helper, that has the capability to induce bursts in vitro (Hankins and Troxler 1980).

Like the infected cells in the early stages of Friend disease (see Section VIII.A.2.a), the cells in the in vitro-induced Epo-independent colonies or bursts are not tumorigenic and have no capacity to self-renew. There have now been two reports that infection of hematopoietic cell populations in vitro with either FV-P or FV-A leads to the establishment of permanent cell lines that produce tumors in syngeneic mice after subcutaneous injection. Revoltella et al. (1979) reported the appearance of two cell lines after in vitro infection of adult DBA/2 mouse bone-marrow cells with FV-P, and Golde et al. (1979) isolated one tumorigenic cell line after infection of fetal liver cells with FV-A. In both instances, the cell lines have similar properties: They grow in suspension, they can be induced to synthesize hemoglobin after treatment with DMSO, and they have an abnormal karyotype, including the presence of metacentric chromosomes. The efficiency of these in vitro-transformation systems is very low, and any quantitation must await the development of a clonal transformation assay.

b. Long-term Cultures. More recently, long-term bone marrow cultures have been described in which hematopoietic progenitor cells, including erythroid progenitors, continue to self-renew and differentiate. Infection of these cultures with FV-P results in cellular changes that parallel the results seen after in vivo infection (Dexter et al. 1981), including the appearance of large numbers of Epo-independent CFU-E and the proliferation of large numbers of primitive erythroid cells. These cells appear to represent an intermediate state between the early and late stages of Friend leukemia: They form spleen colonies in irradiated mice and can be cloned in semisolid medium in vitro, but they depend on an adherent layer for their growth. However, this population, after passage onto a fresh adherent layer, does give rise to autonomous cell lines similar to those described by Mager et al. (1981a).

6. Host Resistance Genes

The genetic control of susceptibility to leukemia induction in mice is best illustrated by the rapidly transforming acute MLV, especially Friend erythroleukemia virus, where specific mammalian genes governing host-range restriction have been identified. Some of these viral susceptibility genes were first identified because of their effects on normal development and hematopoiesis, whereas others were identified by virtue of their effects on the growth or expression of the virus. Although the exact mechanisms of resistance mediated by these genes have not been elucidated, it seems likely that they act by influencing one or more of the steps in either virus replication or transformation. A number of such possible steps include (1) direct inhibition of SFFV replication, (2) inhibition of Fr-MLV replication, (3) reduction in the number of target cells available for viral transformation and/or replication, (4) suppression of the proliferation of infected or transformed cells; and (5) regulation of the number of target or transformed cells by host immune systems.

Early studies established that mice of various inbred strains exhibit marked heterogeneity of susceptibility to Friend virus infection, suggesting that multiple genetic loci are involved (Fieldsteel et al. 1961; Odaka and Yamamoto 1962; Axelrad 1966). To facilitate further investigation, many groups have constructed mouse strains differing only at single gene loci (congenic pairs). To date, several well-defined genetic loci have been identified that affect susceptibility to the polycythemia strain of Friend virus complex. Although most of these studies were carried out with FV-P, studies using FV-A (MacDonald et al. 1980b) indicate that these genes are also involved in the control of both strains of viruses. A list of these loci and their possible modes of action are presented in Table 8.6.

a. Fv-2. The genetic basis of susceptibility to erythroleukemia induction by Friend virus was first established through studies by Odaka and Yamamoto (1962). These authors presented evidence that RF and C57BL/6 strains of mice differed markedly in their susceptibility to FV-P and that susceptibility behaved as a single

Table 8.6 Host genes controlling susceptibility to Friend erythroleukemia viruses

Gene locus	Chromosome	Mechanism of resistance	Degree of resistance
Fv-1	4	helper-virus replication inhibited	10–100-fold
Fv-2	9	SFFV replication inhibited; spleen foci inhibited	10–1000-fold complete
Fv-4	not known	replication of helper virus?	100–1000-fold
Fv-6	not known	replication/generation of MCF virus?	complete
Rfv-3	not known	control of anti-viral antibody production	200-fold
Sl	10	inhibition of transformed cell growth in *Sl*-defective microenvironment?	100-fold
W	5	target cell defect?	100-fold
f	13	not known	not known
H-2	17	immunological? replication of SFFV?	incomplete

genetic determinant with the susceptibility allele being dominant over the resistance allele. This gene, located on chromosome 9, was subsequently established as being the *Fv-2* gene (Lilly 1970; Odaka 1970). Mice that are susceptible to erythroleukemia induction by Friend virus complex are $Fv\text{-}2^{ss}$, and mice resistant to Friend virus are $Fv\text{-}2^{rr}$. Mice heterozygous at this locus ($Fv\text{-}2^{rs}$) show intermediate susceptibility to FV-P. Most inbred mouse strains are $Fv\text{-}2^{ss}$; only the C57BL/6 series, including C57L, C58, and B10 mice, carry the $Fv\text{-}2^{r}$ allele. The degree of susceptibility of these inbred strains to Friend virus infection also varies, indicating a multiple-gene phenomenon. Dissection of these multiple-gene effects has been greatly facilitated by the construction of mouse strains congenic at defined loci. For studies of the *Fv-2* locus, three pairs of congenic mice and a pair of partially congenic mice have been constructed. Axelrad and coworkers have introduced the $Fv\text{-}2^{s}$ allele of SIM mice into the C57BL/6 ($Fv\text{-}2^{rr}$) background, producing the B6.S ($Fv\text{-}2^{ss}$) strain (Axelrad and Van der Gaag 1969; Axelrad et al. 1972). Odaka (1970) similarly constructed a $Fv\text{-}2^{ss}$ strain on a C57BL/6 ($Fv\text{-}2^{rr}$) background and also introduced the $Fv\text{-}2^{r}$ allele from C57BL/6 into the DDD mouse, producing the DDD.Fv-2^{r} strain. A strain of mice (D2.Fv-2) partially congenic at the *Fv-2* locus, developed from DBA/2 × C57BL crosses, carries the $Fv\text{-}2^{r}$ allele (Lilly 1970).

The *Fv-2* locus controls both leukemic transformation by Friend virus and replication of the $SFFV_P$ component itself (Dawson et al. 1966; Steeves et al. 1971). Because SFFV presumably replicates better in vivo in rapidly proliferating transformed cells than in normal hematopoietic cells, it is not evident whether the *Fv-2* locus acts by inhibiting replication of SFFV directly or by affecting the target cells for transformation by Friend virus. Alternatively, because SFFV is replication-defective, the *Fv-2* locus might control the replication of the helper virus in hemapoietic cells and might thereby only indirectly control the replication of SFFV in vivo. This latter possibility is suggested by recent experiments indicating that $SFFV_P$ can replicate in vitro in fibroblasts (Evans et al. 1980) and in bone-marrow cultures (Yoosook et al. 1980) derived from *Fv-2*^{rr} mice. Therefore, the *Fv-2*^{r} phenotype, at least as it pertains to virus replication, may only be expressed in vivo and perhaps only in hematopoietic cells.

Passage of FV-P through C57BL mice selects for virus stocks that can now replicate and induce spleen foci in *Fv-2*^{rr} mice (Steeves et al. 1970) (see Chapter 2 for comments on the BSB virus complex). Biological cloning of the SFFV and helper components of this host-range variant complex has been accomplished and indicates that nonproducer cells containing the replication-defective genome do not express $SFFV_P$ gp52, although two *env*-related proteins (a 50,000-dalton nonglycosylated protein and a 43,000-dalton glycoprotein) have been identified (Teich and Rowe 1982). Further studies should aid in determining whether it is the replication-defective or replication-competent viruses in the FV-P complex that are controlled by *Fv-2*.

More direct evidence that the action of the *Fv-2* locus is mediated within hematopoietic cell populations has come from studies utilizing *Fv-2* congenic mice. Such studies support the notion that the *Fv-2* locus is not a viral resistance gene per se, but rather is involved in controlling the behavior of hematopoietic cells in normal mice. First, using serological techniques, Risser (1979a) detected an antigen present on the surfaces of SFFV-infected cells, which was also present on normal hematopoietic cells of *Fv-2*^{ss} mice, but lacking in congenic *Fv-2*^{rr} mice. Second, using a radioactive cDNA probe specific for those sequences of the $SFFV_P$ genome not shared with Fr-MLV, Mak et al. (1979) demonstrated that the expression of these SFFV-specific sequences was controlled by the *Fv-2* locus in both normal and FV-P-infected mice. Marrow and spleen cells from *Fv-2*^{ss} mice have high levels of these sequences, whereas RNAs from hematopoietic cells of congenic *Fv-2*^{rr} mice contained very little, if any, SFFV-specific sequences. Third, Suzuki and Axelrad (1980) showed that the proportion of BFU-E (see Fig. 8.1) synthesizing DNA, as measured by their sensitivity to high-specific-activity [^{3}H]thymidine or [^{3}H]hydroxyurea, is controlled by *Fv-2*. Only a small proportion of BFU-E from congenic *Fv-2*^{rr} mice are engaged in DNA synthesis, whereas 30–50% of BFU-E from congenic *Fv-2*^{ss} mice are in the S phase. Finally, Yoosook et al. (1980) showed that spleen cells from infected *Fv-2*^{rr} mice produce SFFV, whereas the number of cells that could be transplanted as infectious centers was considerably reduced compared with that of congenic *Fv-2*^{ss} mice. From all of these observations, it has been suggested that the *Fv-2* gene locus is a regulatory gene involved in controlling normal hematopoiesis in uninfected mice.

The mechanism of regulation of hematopoietic cells by the *Fv-2* locus is not clear. A recent report by Axelrad and coworkers (1982) suggests that this control may function via a negative regulator in the form of a macromolecule excreted by a cell other than the BFU-E. On the other hand, in a study of the expression of resistance to FV-P using chimeras containing *Fv-2*^{rr} (B10.D2) and *Fv-2*^{ss} (DBA/2) bone-marrow cells, Silver and Teich (1981) have suggested that the intrinsic resistance to Friend-virus-stimulated erythropoiesis is not mediated by a soluble factor or by cell-cell interaction.

b. Fv-1. In the early genetic studies using the spleen focus assay for measuring host susceptibility to FV-P, it was noted that BALB/c mice homozygous at all autosomal loci shared an intermediate level of susceptibility to Friend virus similar to that observed in F_1 hybrids between C57BL/6 and DBA/2 mice. This observation suggested that a one gene: two alleles hypothesis at the *Fv-2* locus was inadequate to explain the host response to Friend virus (Odaka and Yamamoto 1965; Lilly 1967). Furthermore, Axelrad also noted in serial backcrosses of heterozygous mice to the resistant C57BL/6 strain that possibly another gene may be involved in the susceptibility to Friend virus infection (Axelrad and Van der Gaag 1969). This locus was subsequently identified to be a gene governing the relative resistance to Friend virus infection and was designated *Fv-1,* located on chromosome 4 of the mouse (Rowe et al. 1973; for review, see Lilly and Pincus 1973). The *Fv-1* locus has two alleles, $Fv\text{-}1^{n}$ and $Fv\text{-}1^{b}$, so designated because of the inherent differences in sensitivity of NIH-Swiss and BALB/c mice to various stocks of Friend virus. Viruses not restricted in $Fv\text{-}1^{nn}$ or $Fv\text{-}1^{bb}$ mice are termed N tropic or B tropic, respectively, whereas viruses not restricted in $Fv\text{-}1^{nn}$, $Fv\text{-}1^{bb}$, or $Fv\text{-}1^{nb}$ mice are NB tropic. Mice with an $Fv\text{-}1^{nb}$ genotype are resistant to infection by both N- and B-tropic viruses, indicating that resistance is dominant (Axelrad 1966; Pincus et al. 1971). The effect of the *Fv-1* locus on Friend virus has been studied by using the spleen focus assay. Although high levels of spleen foci can be titrated with single-hit kinetics in *Fv-1* permissive hosts, only a low titer with two-hit kinetics was observed in *Fv-1* restrictive hosts; this manifestation appears to be due to effect(s) on the replication of the helper viruses (Steeves 1975). The molecular basis for resistance conferred by the *Fv-1* locus is discussed in Chapters 4 and 5.

c. Fv-4. The *Fv-4* locus was first identified in the non-inbred mouse strain G. This locus restricts the growth of N-tropic, NB-tropic, and B-tropic MLVs and the development of splenomegaly by Friend virus complex (Kai et al. 1976). The locus is dominant for resistance and segregates independently of *Fv-1* and *Fv-2* (Odaka and Ikeda 1977). The mechanism of resistance is unknown. It is likely that it affects directly the replication of helper virus in fibroblasts as well as in hematopoietic tissue (Ikeda and Odaka 1979).

d. Fv-5. Host genes are also important in determining the type of modulations in erythropoiesis subsequent to infection by Friend virus. A newly described host gene called *Fv-5* controls whether the early erythroid response to FV-P infection is polycythemia or anemia. CBA and C3H mice (designated $Fv\text{-}5^{aa}$) develop a rapid and transient anemia instead of the polycythemia detected in DBA/2, BALB/c, or AKR mice (designated $Fv\text{-}5^{pp}$). The phenotype segregates as a single codominant locus. Despite the anemia observed in CBA and C3H mice infected with FV-P, the spleens of these mice still contain large numbers of Epo-independent erythroid colony-forming cells, the characteristic cellular feature of the early stages of FV-P disease (T. Shibuya and T. Mak, pers. comm.).

e. Fv-6. Host determinants are also important in determining the susceptibility of newborn mice to erythroleukemia induction after infection with the helper-virus Fr-MLV. Although newborn BALB/c, NIH-Swiss, and C3H/HcN mice are susceptible to disease induction, other mouse strains, including DBA/2 which is sensitive to $SFFV_A$ and $SFFV_P$, are resistant (Troxler and Scolnick 1978; MacDonald et al. 1980a; Ruscetti et al. 1981; T. Shibuya and T. Mak; F. Wendling and P. Tambourin; both pers. comm.). Studies with crosses between susceptible and resistant strains indicate that resistance to Fr-MLV-induced disease is dominant (Ruscetti et al. 1981). Backcrosses of F_1 mice to the susceptible BALB/c parent also suggest that susceptibility segregates as a single gene locus (T. Shibuya and T. Mak, pers. comm.).

Fr-MLV replicates to approximately equivalent titers in both resistant and susceptible strains, suggesting that resistance is not mediated by a block in replication of Fr-MLV. However, resistance correlates with the endogenous expression of an MCF gp70-related protein (Ruscetti et al. 1981). On the basis of this observation, i.e., that a Fr-MCF virus induces disease when injected into newborns as an amphotropic virus pseudotype, and of an earlier observation that MCF viruses can be isolated from the spleens of mice infected with Fr-MLV (Troxler and Scolnick 1978), it has been suggested that resistance of mice to Fr-MLV-induced erythroblastic disease is mediated by an interference phenomenon that blocks either the generation or the replication of MCF viruses after Fr-MLV infection (Ruscetti et al. 1981). An important aspect of this model is that these newly emerging MCF viruses play a central role in Fr-MLV disease.

f. Rfv-3. *Rfv-3* is a gene that affects the spontaneous recovery from erythroleukemia induced by the Friend leukemia virus complex. It appears to act in complement with the major histocompatibility complex (H-2) but is an independent, autosomal non-H-2-associated gene (Chesebro and Wehrly 1979). Mice that remain viremic after erythroleukemia induction are termed *Rfv-3*^{rr}, whereas mice that recover from their viremia are *Rfv-3*^{ss}. Resistance is dominant, so that *Rfv-3*^{rs} mice have a low incidence of viremia. The *Rfv-3* gene locus appears to affect viremia only, with no effect on the initial induction of leukemic splenomegaly. It is possible that this locus may act via the host immune response by influencing the level of anti-Friend virus antibody production (Chesebro et al. 1979).

7. Host Genes Affecting Normal Development and Susceptibility to Friend Virus

Several gene loci with known effects on development and differentiation in the mouse affect susceptibility to Friend-virus-induced erythroleukemia. These include three loci known to control directly hematopoietic progenitor cell function: steel (*Sl*), *W*, and flexed (*f*), all of which are associated with an anemia and affect different aspects of the hematopoietic differentiation process. These observations suggest that, in order for erythroleukemia induction to proceed, differentiation along the erythrocytic pathway must proceed normally or that abnormal erythropoiesis interferes with viral erythroleukemogenesis.

a. W. Mice carrying two mutant alleles at the *W* locus (W/W^v) exhibit a number of pleiotropic defects, including macrocytic anemia, sterility, and defective hair pigmentation (Russell and Bernstein 1966; Russell 1979). The hematopoietic defect in W/W^v mice appears to be intrinsic to the pluripotent stem cell, as the mice can be cured of their anemia by repopulation with normal +/+ bone marrow (Russell and Bernstein 1966). Furthermore, hematopoietic cells from W/W^v mice do not repopulate lethally irradiated +/+ mice, nor do W/W^v mice contain cells capable of forming macroscopic spleen colonies in irradiated mice (McCulloch et al. 1965a).

The *W* locus also controls susceptibility to spleen focus formation by FV-P. Steeves et al. (1968) noted that both homozygous +/+ and heterozygous $+/W^v$ mice were equally susceptible to spleen focus formation by $SFFV_P$. However, mice with the genotype $+/W$ had a reduced susceptibility, and anemic W/W^v animals were apparently completely refractory to $SFFV_P$. More recent studies, using virus preparations of higher titer, indicate that spleen focus formation in W/W^v mice is reduced approximately 100-fold compared with that in their +/+ littermates (MacDonald et al. 1980b).

The mechanism of resistance to FV-P mediated by the *W* locus is not known. However, in view of what is known about the nature of the cellular defect in the hematopoietic system of these mice, it is possible that mutation at the *W* locus reduces the number of functionally competent target cells available for Friend virus replication and/or transformation.

b. Sl. Mice carrying two mutant alleles at the steel locus (Sl/Sl^d) exhibit the same pleiotropic defects as do the W/W^v mice discussed above: They have a macrocytic anemia, are sterile, and have a defect in hair pigmentation (Russell and Bernstein 1966; Russell 1979). However, the *Sl* and *W* loci are clearly distinguished. The *W* locus is on chromosome 5, whereas *Sl* maps on chromosome 10. In addition, cellular transplantation experiments, analogous to those described above for the *W* locus, provide strong evidence that the cellular basis for the hematopoietic defects in Sl/Sl^d is extrinsic to the hematopoietic stem cell. Unlike W/W^v mice, Sl/Sl^d mice cannot be cured of their anemia by transplants of normal +/+ bone-marrow cells, nor do CFU-S form spleen colonies in irradiated Sl/Sl^d hosts. However, bone marrow from Sl/Sl^d mice contains cells capable of repopulating and forming spleen colonies in either irradiated +/+ or unirradiated W/W^v recipients (McCulloch et al. 1965b). These observations suggest that Sl/Sl^d stem cells can proliferate and differentiate when placed in a normal +/+ environment and, conversely, that stem cells from +/+ mice cannot function normally when placed in a Sl/Sl^d environment. Thus, the steel locus appears to regulate some aspect of the cellular environment in which stem cells divide and differentiate.

The steel defect, like *W*, also affects susceptibility to $SFFV_P$: Mice of genotype Sl/Sl^d have been reported to be completely resistant to spleen focus induction by SFFV (Bennett et al. 1968), although, as with W/W^v, more recent studies using a higher titer of $SFFV_P$ suggest that these mice are not absolutely resistant to $SFFV_P$ (McCool et al. 1979). The mechanism of resistance of Sl/Sl^d mice to Fr-$SFFV_P$ is not known, The *Sl* locus does not appear to control the replication of $SFFV_P$ in the spleens of infected animals (McCool et al. 1979), nor are the levels of SFFV-specific RNA sequences in the spleen decreased in SFFV-infected Sl/Sl^d mice, when compared with those in their infected +/+ littermates (Mak et al. 1980).

The *Sl* locus also does not regulate the growth of FV-P-transformed +/+ leukemic stem cells. These cells form spleen colonies with equal efficiency in both +/+ and Sl/Sl^d irradiated recipients (Mager et al. 1980). Thus, the development of these immortal cell clones, which occurs quite late after infection with FV-P, may be accompanied by autonomy from cell-cell intereactions such as those controlled by the steel locus.

c. f. The flexed-tail gene (*f*) of the mouse is situated on chromosome 13, and mutation at this locus is known to induce a transitory siderocytic anemia (Gruenberg 1942; Russell et al. 1968). The defect is manifested during periods of erythropoietic stress, such as during fetal life or in adult mice after bleeding. Mice of genotype *ff* have been reported to have a lower susceptibility to spleen focus induction by FV-P than do wild-type *FF* homozygotes (Axelrad and Van der Gaag 1969).

d. Major Histocompatibility Complex H-2. The influence of the *H-2* locus on susceptibility to viral leukemogenesis has been well documented (Lilly et al. 1964; Lilly 1968; Tennant and Snell 1968). An effect of the *H-2* locus on the susceptibility to Friend erythroleukemia has also been observed (Lilly 1968; Chesebro et al. 1974). These authors demonstrated that the *H-2* type influences the capacity of the mouse to recover from the initial stages of Friend disease. Using mice with a $Fv\text{-}2^{ss}$ or $Fv\text{-}2^{sr}$ background, it was found that, at low doses of Friend virus, mice with an $H\text{-}2^{b}$ haplotype were less susceptible to erythroleukemia induction than heterozygous $H\text{-}2^{d}/H\text{-}2^{b}$ mice. Furthermore, homozygous $H\text{-}2^{b}$ mice have a higher frequency of recovery or regression from the disease than do mice that are not homozygous $H\text{-}2^{b}$. Thus, the *H-2* locus appears to affect the incidence of Friend disease, as well as the incidence of recovery from the early phase of the disease.

More recent observations have also indicated that the H-2 complex plays a role in determining susceptibility to FV-P in mice homozygous for resistance at the *Fv-2* locus ($Fv\text{-}2^{rr}$). Using *Fv-2* mouse strains differing only at the *H-2* locus, Mak et al. (1980) observed that the *H-2* locus exerts an epistatic effect on the $Fv\text{-}2^{r}$ allele. For example, spleen focus induction, replication of $SFFV_P$, and expression of endogenous SFFV-specific RNA sequences in uninfected mice are almost totally inhibited in $Fv\text{-}2^{rr}$ mice with an $H\text{-}2^{b}$ haplotype. In contrast, $SFFV_P$ does induce low numbers of spleen foci and can replicate in the spleens of $Fv\text{-}2^{rr}$ congenic $H\text{-}2^{k}$, $H\text{-}2^{a}$, or $H\text{-}2^{d}$ mice. In addition, these mice express intermediate levels of SFFV-specific RNA sequences. These results indicate that the *H-2* locus has early, as well as late, effects on susceptibility to Friend leukemia virus.

8. Susceptibility to FV-A

Although most of the information accumulated on host control of erythroleukemia induction comes from studies on the polycythemia strain of Friend virus, recent experiments indicate that the susceptibility to infection by the anemia strain of Friend virus is also under the control of the same genes that affect FV-P, including the *W, Sl,* and *Fv-2* loci (MacDonald et al. 1980b).

B. Rauscher Leukemia Virus Complex

Rauscher leukemia virus complex (RV) (Rauscher 1962) was isolated from a transplantable ascites tumor derived from a virus-induced leukemia, originally described by Schoolman et al. (1957), first in adult Swiss mice and then in weanling BALB/c mice. The disease induced by the virus complex was recognized as having two pathological components. Within 14 days postinfection of either newborn or adult mice, RV induces splenomegaly and erythrocytopoiesis associated with anemia. Several weeks later, there is a second stage associated with the onset of lymphocytic leukemia.

Like Friend virus, RV appears to be composed of at least two virus components: a replication-competent helper virus (Ra-MLV) and a replication-defective spleen focus-forming virus (Ra-SFFV) (Pluznik and Sachs 1964). Although experiments to dissociate the roles of the two components have not been performed as they have been with Friend virus, it is likely that the Ra-SFFV component is responsible for the rapid erythropoietic changes (Hasthorpe and Bol 1979) associated with the early stages of Rauscher disease, whereas Ra-MLV is associated with lymphoid leukemia induction. Indeed, Reddy et al. (1980) recently reported the induction of lymphoid tumors of the B-cell lineage in NIH-Swiss mice infected as neonates with a biologically cloned isolate of Ra-MLV.

Ra-SFFV encodes an *env*-related glycoprotein of 54,000 daltons (Ruta and Kabat 1980; Van Griensven and Vogt 1980). Analysis of fibroblast nonproducer clones suggests that Ra-SFFV has intact *gag* and *pol* genes but does not have the complete *env* gene (Ruta and Kabat 1980).

Preparations of RV, derived after infection of SJL/J mice, also contain an MCF virus that replicates equally well in mink and mouse fibroblasts (Van Griensven and Vogt 1980). The origin of this component, Ra-MCF, is not clear. It may be an integral part of the RV complex, or like Fr-MCF (Troxler and Scolnick 1978), it may originate in vivo by recombination between either Ra-MLV or Ra-SFFV and endogenous virus sequences. The Ra-MCF component is of particular interest because it is pathogenic when injected into newborn NIH-Swiss mice (Van Griensven and Vogt 1980); hepatosplenomegaly occurs at 3–6 months postinfection, and the peripheral blood contains high numbers of morphologically immature erythroid cells (erythroblasts and normoblasts). Thus, Ra-MCF appears to have erythroblastic potential under these conditions and may share biological properties with Fr-MLV (see Section VIII.A.4). It will be of interest to determine whether the Ra-MCF present in RV preparations is necessary for the erythroleukemic activity of this complex in adult mice and whether Ra-SFFV and Ra-MCF induce erythroleukemia by similar mechanisms.

C. Myeloproliferative Sarcoma Virus Complex

1. Origin and Pathology

In 1968 Chirigos et al. reported the isolation of a variant of Moloney murine sarcoma virus (Mo-MSV), originally called plasma-passage MSV and now known as the myeloproliferative sarcoma virus (MPSV), from the plasma of BALB/c mice after multiple cellular passages in vivo of a MSV-induced sarcoma, followed by passage of cell-free filtrates. The history of the pathology of the disease induced by MPSV is strikingly similar to that of Friend virus. Like Friend virus, the disease induced by MPSV was classified as a highly undifferentiated tumor, in this case a sarcoma, characterized by a rapid increase in spleen weight in adult mice. Later, it became clear that MPSV can cause erythroleukemia and myeloid leukemia in adult mice (LeBousse-Kerdiles et al. 1980), as judged from its effects on the number and hormonal requirements of hematopoietic progenitor cells (Flagg et al. 1980). MPSV can also transform fibroblasts in vitro, a property it has presumably retained from its original parent Mo-MSV (Chirigos et al. 1968).

2. *Replication-defective MPSV-SFFV*

Uncloned MPSV obtained from extracts of the enlarged spleens of MPSV-infected DBA/2J mice contain high titers of a spleen focus-forming activity (MPSV-SFFV). Ostertag et al. (1980) obtained clonal isolates of this virus from MPSV-transformed nonproducer NRK rat cells. Superinfection of these nonproducer cells with either Mo-MLV or Fr-MLV resulted in the rescue of MPSV-SFFV, as determined by focus-forming ability in rat fibroblasts and by the ability to induce macroscopic spleen foci in DBA/2J mice. The natural helper virus present in the stocks of MPSV (MPSV-MLV) was also cloned and shown to have no focus-forming activity in vitro or in vivo. Thus, MPSV-SFFV, like Friend $SFFV_A$ and $SFFV_P$, appears to be replication-defective and requires a helper virus to provide replicative functions. Although the exact origin of MPSV-SFFV remains to be determined, molecular hybridization analysis indicates that the genome of this transforming virus includes sequences that are highly related to the *mos*-specific region of Mo-MSV (see Chapters 4, 7, and 9) and does not share sequences with Fr-$SFFV_P$ (Pragnell et al. 1981). The isolation of mutants of MPSV temperature-sensitive for transformation (W. Ostertag, pers. comm.) will facilitate the analysis of the transformation potentials of this virus.

3. *Cellular Aspects of MPSV Disease*

Infection of susceptible mice with MPSV leads to rapid alterations in hematopoietic progenitor cells that are similar to, but distinct from, those observed after infection with the various isolates of Friend virus. In addition to a marked increase in spleen weight and cellularity, the number of early erythroid progenitor cells (BFU-E) in the spleen increases, followed slightly later by a large increase in the CFU-E population. Both of these erythroid progenitor cells retain a requirement for Epo to proliferate and differentiate in cell culture, although it has been suggested that these BFU-E require less added Epo (Ostertag et al. 1980). Also, the proportion of nucleated cells containing spectrin, the erythroid-cell-membrane marker, increases in the bone-marrow and spleen after MPSV infection: MPSV can induce burst transformation of bone-marrow cells in vitro, similar to that observed with FV-P and FV-A (W.D. Hankins and I. Pragnell, pers. comm.).

Changes in the progenitor populations for granulocytes and macrophages (CFU-GM) (see Fig. 8.1) also occur. As discussed in Section III, normal CFU-GM require colony-stimulating factors (CSF) for their growth, whereas the CFU-GM observed 25 days after infection with MPSV appear to be CSF-independent (Klein et al. 1980).

D. Abelson Murine Leukemia Virus Complex

1. Origin and Pathology

The Abelson murine leukemia virus complex was isolated in 1970 from a steroid-treated BALB/c mouse infected with Mo-MLV (Abelson and Rabstein 1970a,b). It is of interest that treatment with the steroid, prednisolone, effectively leads to atrophy of the thymus (a chemical thymectomy) and hence to the loss of the presumptive target cell for Mo-MLV-induced leukemogenesis. When injected into neonatal or adult BALB/c mice, Abelson virus induces a lymphoid disease distinct from the typical thymic lymphoma induced by Mo-MLV, distinguished by its considerably shorter latent period (3–4 weeks), the pathology of the leukemia/lymphosarcoma, and the properties of the transformed cells derived in vivo or in vitro. The Abelson virus complex is composed of two components, the helper Mo-LMV and a replication-defective particle called Ab-MLV. More detailed discussions of the origin and defectiveness of the Ab-MLV genome are presented in Chapters 4 and 9.

Ab-MLV induces a nonthymic lymphoma similar to the original tumor from which it was isolated. Very soon after injection into neonatal mice, changes in lymph nodes and bone marrow can be observed (Abelson and Rabstein 1970b; Rabstein et al. 1971; Siegler et al. 1972; Risser et al. 1978a), although these may not all be specific for Ab-MLV. The tumor cells, presumably consisting of bone-marrow-derived lymphocytes, subsequently spread to the upper vertebral region and the skull. In adult mice, however, many tumors are found associated with the marrow of the lumbar vertebrae and spread to the vertebral muscle, often resulting in abnormal gait and paraplegia. In addition, marked lymphoadenopathy is commonly found and splenomegaly has been observed. Although thymic enlargement is occasionally observed, histological examination indicates that this is due to infiltrating tumor cells (Siegler et al. 1972). Furthermore, Abelson disease can be induced in athymic nude mice (Raschke et al. 1975), supporting the idea that Ab-MLV disease is thymus-independent. In addition, under certain circumstances (e.g., in mice inoculated with pristane, 2,6,10,14-tetramethylpentadecane), plasmacytic lymphomas and plasmacytomas (late B-lymphocyte tumors) can also be induced by Ab-MLV (Potter et al 1973; Aoki et al. 1975).

Histologically, the Abelson tumors consist of uniform populations of immature lymphocytes (Rabstein et al. 1971; Siegler et al. 1972; Risser et al. 1978a). They are generally large in size with a high nucleus-to-cytoplasm ratio, the cell nucleus is characterized by diffuse chromatin, and the cytoplasm contains abundant free ribosomes. Although these lymphoblasts are morphologically indistinguishable from other virus-induced lymphoma cells, the nature of their cell-surface markers indicates that, unlike tumors induced by Mo-MLV, they are derived from nonthymus (i.e., non-T)-related cells (see below).

2. Transformation In Vitro

The transformation of fibroblasts in vitro by Ab-MLV (Scher and Siegler 1975) has facilitated the studies of the genome of Ab-MLV and its mechanism of transformation. Similar to several other transforming viruses, Ab-MLV encodes a highly phosphorylated polyprotein that exhibits an associated tyrosine-specific protein kinase activity (Witte et al. 1978, 1980; Van de Ven et al. 1980), and transformed fibroblasts lose binding sites for epidermal growth factor (Blomberg et al. 1980). Interestingly, Ab-MLV appears to be unique among viruses that transform fibroblasts in vitro in that sarcomas have never been observed following infection of animals. However, it should be remembered that the fibroblast-transforming activity of Ab-MLV is apparently restricted to continuous lines like NIH-3T3 cells; transformation of primary embryo fibroblasts has not been achieved. Transformation of fibroblasts provides a means to quantitate Ab-MLV and allows the isolation of cell clones nonproductively infected with the replication-defective Ab-MLV genome. These nonproducer cells have been used to analyze the translational products encoded by Ab-MLV (see Chapters 4, 7, and 9) and the role of different helper viruses in leukemia induction (see Section VIII.D.4).

Direct transformation of hematopoietic cells in vitro by Ab-MLV has also been demonstrated. Infection of fetal liver, spleen, or bone-marrow cells, but not thymus or lymph node cells, in vitro with Ab-MLV results in the rapid proliferation of lymphoid cells from which continuous cell lines could be isolated (Sklar et al. 1974; Rosenberg et al. 1975; Rosenberg and Baltimore 1976). This assay provides a quantitative means of characterizing the target-cell population for transformation by Ab-MLV and of identifying possible host genes that regulate susceptibility to Ab-MLV at the cellular level. Moreover, lymphoid cell clones, either productively or nonproductively infected with Ab-MLV, have been established (Pratt et al. 1977; Witte et al. 1978; Rosenberg et al. 1979; Siden et al. 1979). All of the transformed lymphoid nonproducer cell clones contain the Ab-MLV genome, whereas only some of them are infected with the helper Mo-MLV. These observations suggest that transformation of hematopoietic cells, like fibroblast transformation, requires the Ab-MLV genome, but not the continuous replication or presence of Mo-MLV.

3. *Nature of Ab-MLV-transformed Cells*

Although it is generally agreed that the disease induced by Ab-MLV does not involve the thymus, the exact nature of the target-cell population involved in the in vitro-transformation experiments is not clear. Studies using the in vitro-transformation assay described above indicated that, at least in culture, the predominant cell types emerging from such a system are related to the B-cell lineage of the hematopoietic hierarchy (Teich and Dexter 1978; Boss et al. 1979; Siden et al. 1979). The hypothesis that Ab-MLV can affect or result in the transformation of cells in the B-cell lineage is supported by reports that cell lines with B-cell-specific markers can be obtained (Premkumar et al. 1975; Sklar et al. 1975; Pratt et al. 1977). Some of the Ab-MLV-transformed cell lines contain cytoplasmic immunoglobulin (Premkumar et al. 1975; Sklar et al. 1975; Pratt et al. 1977; Boss et al. 1979; Siden et al. 1979) and the surface B-cell-related Lyb-2 antigen (Sato and Boyse 1976; Silverstone et al. 1978), whereas they lack detectable levels of antigens associated with T lymphocytes, including Thy-1, TL, and Lyt-2,3 (Pratt et al. 1977; Silverstone et al. 1978). A high proportion (50–60%) of the transformed clones derived in vitro synthesize immunoglobulin in the form of the cytoplasmic μ-chain (Teich and

Dexter 1978; Boss et al. 1979; Siden et al. 1979), and a small proportion of these transformants also express a low level of IgM early after infection. Attempts to detect markers associated with more mature B cells, such as C′3 receptor, immune-associated antigen, and surface immunoglobulin, have been consistently negative (Sklar et al. 1975; Pratt et al. 1977; Silverstone et al. 1978). al. 1978).

There are several additional observations that suggest that pre-B or immature B lymphocytes are target cells for transformation by Ab-MLV. First, some of these tumor cell lines can be stimulated by the B-lymphocyte mitogen lipopolysaccharide to produce cytoplasmic or surface immunoglobulin (Boss et al. 1979; Rosenberg et al. 1979). Second, Ab-MLV can accelerate the induction of plasmacytomas in mice treated with pristane (Potter et al. 1973). Third, infection of long-term cultures of mixed populations of bone-marrow cells in the Dexter culture system (Dexter and Testa 1976) can result in transformed cultures of cells that synthesize cytoplasmic IgM (Teich and Dexter 1978). The immunoglobulin-gene structure characteristic of Ab-MLV-transformed lymphoid cells further supports the relationship of these cells to normal B-lymphocyte precursors. In one study in which 29 independently derived clonal isolates were examined (Alt et al. 1981), all had DNA rearrangements in the J_H region of the heavy-chain gene, with accompanying deletions of at least 5 kb 5′ to J_H. These rearrangements were identified in both alleles regardless of the immunoglobulin phenotype of the cells. In contrast, very few of the isolates (<10%) had rearrangements in any light-chain genes. Thus, most Ab-MLV-transformed lymphoid cells resemble an intermediate stage in B-lymphocyte development in which both heavy-chain genes, but not light-chain genes, are rearranged.

Although it appears that most of the cell lines derived in vitro and some derived in vivo possess characteristics of early pre-B lymphocytes, effects of Ab-MLV on hematopoietic cells from other lineages have also been reported. For example, Raschke et al. (1978) reported the establishment of tumor cell lines with macrophage characteristics after infection in vivo by Ab-MLV, whereas Greenberger et al. (1979) reported that infection of bone-marrow cells in vitro with Ab-MLV in a modified Dexter culture system in the presence of hydrocortisone results in the development of tumorigenic myeloid cell lines. Finally, infection of fetal liver cell cultures by Ab-MLV in vitro induces both lymphoid and erythroid colonies (Waneck and Rosenberg 1981). Thus, although the primary target population for transformation by Ab-MLV in vitro may be cells from the B-cell lineage, in vivo and in vitro infection with Ab-MLV may also result in the transformation of cells from a broad range of cells in the hematopoietic hierarchy.

The fact that Ab-MLV affects cells of different lineages led to speculation that Ab-MLV may directly transform the hematopoietic stem cell. The possibility is strengthened by the observation that Ab-MLV induces an antigen, termed Abelson antigen, that can be detected on both lymphoid cells transformed by Ab-MLV and uninfected cells from BALB/c bone marrow, spleen, and fetal liver (Risser et al. 1978b). In addition, approximately 50% of adult BALB/c CFU-S can be killed by antisera to Abelson antigen (Risser 1979). Furthermore, R. Risser and D. Grunwald (pers. comm.) report that one clonal Abelson-virus-transformed tumor cell line that possesses no detectable properties of B cells or T cells has the capacity to develop into a Thy-1-positive tumor cell line following passage in vivo. Shinefeld et al. (1980), however, have presented evidence suggesting that the CFU-S is not a target cell for transformation in vitro. Using a monoclonal rat anti-mouse brain antibody that is cytotoxic to Ab-MLV-transformed nonproducer lymphoid cells, but is not cytotoxic for CFU-S, they were able to eliminate target cells capable of being transformed by Ab-MLV in vitro. The antigen detected by this monoclonal antibody does not appear to be a virally encoded cell-surface constitutent, because absorption experiments show that Ab-MLV-transformed fibroblasts do not express this antigen on their cell surfaces, and the antigenic determinant recognized by this antibody is expressed in at least some normal pre-B cells (Paige et al. 1981). These observations are more consistent with the hypothesis that Ab-MLV directly affects a variety of committed progenitor cells from different lineages, rather than the uncommitted stem cell.

4. Role of Helper Virus in Ab-MLV Transformation

Studies on the transformation of fibroblasts by sarcoma viruses led to the conclusion that expression of the Ab-MLV oncogene (*abl*) protein is necessary, and probably sufficient in most instances, to maintain the transformed state. Defective sarcoma viruses require a helper virus only to provide virus functions necessary for replication, not transformation. However, studies by Rosenberg and Baltimore (1978) and Scher (1978) have demonstrated that, although fibroblast transformation by Ab-MLV is independent of the helper virus, the efficiency of transformation of hematopoietic cells both in vivo and in vitro by Ab-MLV is influenced by the helper virus. Only Ab-MLV stocks rescued from nonproducer cells with helper viruses that are themselves strongly oncogenic (Mo-MLV, Fr-MLV, or Ra-MLV) were efficient in inducing Abelson disease in vivo or colony formation in agarose after in vitro infection. In contrast, a number of weakly oncogenic or nononcogenic viruses, including Gross and Kirsten MLVs, were inefficient as helpers in the lymphoid transformation assays, whereas Ab-MLV pseudotypes made with these helper viruses transformed fibroblasts quite efficiently. The explanation of this helper-virus phenomenon in lymphoid transformation is unknown.

5. Host Control of Abelson Virus Lymphomagenesis

As with Friend virus, the induction of lymphomagenesis in mice by Ab-MLV is also under host control. Risser et al. (1978a) have examined 16 different mouse strains for susceptibility to Ab-MLV and have shown that only BALB/c and some of its derivative strains have high sensitivity. Using a series of recombinant inbred mice, they have determined that BALB/c carries dominant sensitivity alleles at two loci, designated *Av-1* and *Av-2.* These loci are unrelated to *Fv-1* and *Fv-2.* Using mouse strains on the C57BL/6 background and congenic at the *H-2* locus, it appears that the *H-2* locus may play a minor role in determining the sensitivity of mice to Ab-MLV. This effect is only seen in mice homozygous for resistance at both *Av-1* and *Av-2* (Risser et al. 1978b).

E. Harvey and Kirsten Murine Sarcoma Viruses

1. Origin and Pathology

The replication-defective Kirsten MSV (Ki-MSV) and Harvey MSV (Ha-MSV) were isolated following passage of MLV in rats: Ki-MSV from rats inoculated neonatally with cell-free filtrates from thymic lymphomas of old C3H mice (Kirsten and Mayer 1967) and Ha-MSV following inoculation of rats with Mo-MLV and injection of the rat-passaged virus into newborn BALB/c mice

(Harvey 1964) (see also Chapter 2). Both isolates contain related oncogene sequences (*ras;* see Chapters 4 and 9) acquired during the serial propagation in rats. Both viruses produce erythroleukemias, as well as sarcomas (Harvey 1964; Chesterman et al. 1966; Kirsten and Mayer 1967, 1969). Studies involving rescue of the MSV genomes from nonproducer cells with different helper viruses (Bassin et al. 1968; Scher et al. 1975) suggested that the capacity of MSV to induce both types of neoplasms was encoded within a single particle. In the case of Ha-MSV, the use of a molecular clone and constructed mutants thereof provided definitive evidence that the MSV genome encodes both properties (Wei et al. 1980). Although a similar experiment has not been reported for Ki-MSV, studies with the available temperature-sensitive mutants (see Chapter 7) or development of new mutants could be used to investigate this issue, particularly with regard to the in vitro-transformation assays described below.

Much of the pathology of Ha-MSV and Ki-MSV tumorigenesis has come from early studies, amply reviewed by Harvey and East (1971). Table 8.7 compares the prominent features of the disease symptoms with those observed following infection with Mo-MSV (Section VIII.F). The most notable difference is the lack of a major erythroid response to Mo-MSV.

The pathogenic spectrum is greatly influenced by (1) dose of MSV, (2) route of administration, and (3) age, strain, or species of animal inoculated. The dose of MSV is important in that too low a titer may lead to erythroid effects without concomitant sarcoma formation, local tumors that regress, or a latency period long enough so that the effects of the helper MLV become the predominant features. The route of injection determines mainly whether the sarcomas arise as widely disseminated tumors or whether they develop as localized well-circumscribed masses at the injection site; the latter condition arises particularly following intramuscular or subcutaneous routes. Animals more than a few weeks of age are relatively resistant to both sarcoma formation and erythroleukemia, presumably due to immunological competence. Strain differences are effected by host resistance genes, of which some are identifiable; for example, in mice, *Fv-1* regulates the replication of the helper MLV and *H-2* modifies immunological responses. Across species barriers, there are host restriction genes that control virus penetration (at the receptor level) or inhibit helper-virus

Table 8.7 Pathologic changes induced by MSV isolates

	Mice			Rats			Hamsters		
Lesions	Ha-MSV	Ki-MSV	Mo-MSV	Ha-MSV	Ki-MSV	Mo-MSV	Ha-MSV	Ki-MSV	Mo-MSV
Sarcomas	+++	+++	+++	+++	+++	+++	+++	+++	+++
Splenomegaly	+++	+++	+	+++	+++	±	–	n.d.	–
(erythroblastic)	+	+	–	+	+	–			
Severe anemia	+++	+++	±	+++	+++	n.d.	±	n.d.	±
Cystic and hemorrhagic lesions	++	++	±	+++	++	n.d.	+++	+	n.d.
Pleural effusions	+	n.d.	n.d.	+++	n.d.	+	++	n.d.	n.d.
Bone lesions	n.d.	–	n.d.	+	+++	++	+	n.d.	+

n.d. indicates no data. Data from Harvey and East (1971).

replication. This last feature is evident upon analysis of virus extracted from Ha-MSV-induced sarcomas in hamsters; MLV is not recoverable, but Ha-MSV may be found as a pseudotype bearing antigens and host-range properties of the endogenous hamster retrovirus (see Chapter 2).

The inoculation of newborn rats or mice with Ha-MSV leads to sarcoma formation within 2 weeks, and often death by 1 month. Simultaneously, the erythrogenic response leads to severe anemia and splenomegaly; death due to splenic rupture is not uncommon with Ha-MSV, whereas rupture does not occur with Ki-MSV. As with Friend virus, the spleen architecture becomes completely disorganized as the stroma is replaced by the proliferating erythroblast population, and abnormal erythrocytes may be discerned in the peripheral circulation.

Cystic swellings in the region of axillary and inguinal lymph nodes or lungs occur following infection with Ha-MSV (Harvey 1964; Chesterman et al. 1966). The cysts contain cells typical of inflammatory and neoplastic reactions. It is thought that rupture of these cysts may be the cause of the fatal pleural effusions detected primarily in rats and hamsters.

The sarcomas have been generally described as undifferentiated mesenchymal tumors. Histologically, they may also be classified sometimes as spindle-cell sarcomas (containing whorls of spindle-shaped cells), hemangiosarcomas and hemangioendotheliomas (because of the involvement of vascular tissue), or fibrosarcomas. Although invasion of muscle and bone also occurs, the tumors are not characterized as rhabdomyosarcomas or osteosarcomas. An intracranial tumor resembling an astrocytoma has been observed in one Ha-MSV-infected hamster (Harvey and East 1971).

2. *In Vitro-transformation Assays*

Transformation of fibroblasts in standard focus-induction assays and colony assays has helped to define the functions of the *ras* gene (see Chapter 9). Like Ab-MLV-transformed fibroblasts (Section VIII.D), Ki-MSV-transformed, as well as Mo-MSV- and FeSV-transformed, fibroblasts lose epidermal growth factor (EGF) binding sites (Todaro et al. 1976). Additionally, it has recently been demonstrated that both Ha-MSV and Ki-MSV induce proliferation of erythroid bursts in agar following infection in vitro of bone marrow cells (Hankins and Scolnick 1981). This property is also observed with Fr-SFFV (but not Fr-MLV) and MPSV (see Sections VIII.A and VIII.C), and thus may be considered a parameter for transient transformation of erythroid cells in vitro by most of the viruses capable of inducing erythroleukemia. This type of assay might be useful for dissecting the functions of the *ras* gene using temperature-sensitive or deletion mutants.

One interesting aspect of cells transformed by Ki-MSV and several other mammalian sarcoma viruses (including Mo-MSV and FeSVs) is the production of polypeptides capable of inducing morphological changes and anchorage-independent growth of nontransformed cells (see DeLarco and Todaro 1980 and references therein). These polypeptides have been called sarcoma growth factors (SGFs), and they appear to compete with EGF for the same membrane receptors. Thus, endogenous production of SGFs by MSV-transformed cells saturates receptors for EGF. However, SGFs and EGF can be distinguished by several biological and biochemical criteria. The role of SGFs in the initiation and maintenance of viral transformation has not been defined, but their potential significance has been underscored by the isolation of similar factors from several human tumor cells (Todaro et al. 1980).

One interesting feature regarding *ras*-gene expression is the finding of extremely high levels of $p21^{c\text{-}ras}$ in one hematopoietic cell line (Scolnick et al. 1981). This clonal cell line, 416B, was derived from a long-term bone marrow culture infected in vitro with the polycythemia strain of Friend virus (Dexter et al. 1979); it produces MLV, but not SFFV, and does not express the SFFV gp52 (N. Teich and J. Rowe, pers. comm.). More interesting, however, is the evolving nature of the cell with continued in vitro passage. Initially, the cells had bipotentiality for differentiation in vivo, forming spleen colonies of granulocytes and megakaryocytes (Dexter et al. 1979). Later, the cells also differentiated into erythroid cells in vivo and had the capability to repopulate mice that had been lethally irradiated, thus showing features of the multipotent stem cell, CFU-S (Fig. 8.1). Furthermore, none of the reconstituted animals developed tumors. Still later, the cells underwent erythroblastic differentiation in vivo but failed to repopulate mice (T.M. Dexter et al., pers. comm.). At this last stage, the 416B cells were examined and found to express five- to tenfold more $p21^{ras}$ than any other cell line tested, including fibroblasts transformed by Ha-MSV or Ki-MSV, or spleen or bone-marrow cells from uninfected mice (Scolnick et al. 1981). This study also showed that (1) p21 expression was due to an endogenous, nonamplified *c-ras* gene, (2) p21 was functionally active in the guanine nucleotide binding assay (Chapter 9), and (3) there was no apparent integration of the exogenously infected Fr-MLV in close proximity of *c-ras*. Scolnick et al. (1981) speculated that the very high expression of *c-ras* could be due to a mutation of the gene in 416B cells in such a way as to stimulate p21 production or, as a more interesting possibility, that hematopoietic differentiation requires elevated levels of p21 during some specific maturation process.

F. Moloney and Gazdar Murine Sarcoma Viruses

The Moloney strain of MSV was isolated from the plasma of a BALB/c mouse bearing a rhabdomyosarcoma induced with Mo-MLV (Moloney 1966), whereas the Gazdar MSV (Gz-MSV) was recovered from a spontaneously arising tumor in an (NZB × NZW)F_1 mouse (Gazdar et al. 1972). Both of these replication-defective viruses contain highly related oncogene (*mos*) sequences (see Chapter 9). However, the insertion of *mos* occurs at different locations in the genomes (see Chapter 4), suggesting the independent derivation of these two isolates. The pathologies of Mo-MSV and Gz-MSV are also similar (see Table 8.7).

Mo-MSV infection of neonates leads to detection of sarcomas within a few days and, following very rapid growth of the tumors, death can ensue within weeks. When low doses of MSV are used, or if older mice are inoculated, the appearance of the tumors is delayed. Tumors often regress and recur spontaneously, with tumors appearing at unrelated sites as well; this property is also influenced by strain variation (Fefer et al. 1967b; Law et al. 1968).

The constant association of the Mo-MSV-induced tumors with muscle tissue led to their designation as rhabdomyosarcomas (Moloney 1966; Perk and Moloney 1966), but other investigators have described the tumors variably as hemangiosarcomas, spindle-cell sarcomas, and undifferentiated sarcomas (Stanton et al. 1968; Chirigos et al. 1968; Berman and Allison 1969). There have been infrequent reports that inoculation of rats or hamsters with Mo-MSV induces osteogenic sarcomas (Berman 1967; Soehner and Dmochowski 1969; Fujinaga et al. 1970) and that intracerebral inoculation of newborn rats induces plasmacytomas as well as intracranial lesions (Ribacchi and Giraldo 1966). Around the site of injection, infiltration of granulocytes and lymphocytes characterizes the inflammatory response, and proximal lymph nodes become enlarged and may contain metastatic lesions (Lasneret 1967).

Splenomegaly occurs in mice inoculated as neonates, but unlike the situation with Ha-MSV and Ki-MSV, this is not due to erythroblastosis, but rather to hyperplasia. With Mo-MSV, the splenic architecture is maintained and there is no fatal spleen rupture (Perk and Moloney 1966; Stanton et al. 1968; Berman and Allison 1969). On the other hand, inoculation with Gz-MSV leads to replacement of the spleen stroma, marked by vascularization, inflammatory cells, and fibrosis of the spleen capsule (Gazdar et al. 1972). Whether this difference is due to the virus directly or to the use of different strains of mice has not been elucidated.

G. Hemangiosarcoma-inducing Virus

BALB-MSV (previously known as 138-MSV) is one of the few naturally occurring MSVs and was derived from a spontaneous chloroleukemia in an old BALB/c mouse. The initial cell-free filtrates produced undifferentiated and "MSV-like" sarcomas, lymphoreticular tumors, and lymphosarcomas. However, extracts obtained from an MSV-like sarcoma produced hemangiosarcomas (tumors of the blood vessels) within two passages and continued to produce this neoplasm predominantly thereafter, with a latency as short as 3 weeks (Peters et al. 1974).

The MSV isolate is replication-defective and appears to have been derived from a recombinational event between its associated B-tropic MLV helper and mouse cellular sequences (Andersen et al. 1981a). Different nonproducer transformed fibroblast lines synthesize some or all of the helper-virus-related *gag*-gene products, indicating that this viral gene has presumably remained intact during the generation of the MSV (Aaronson and Barbacid 1978). However, the most interesting point is that the BALB-MSV oncogene sequence and its product are highly related to those of Ha-MSV (i.e., *ras* and $p21^{ras}$) (Andersen et al. 1981b). Although this finding suggests that related sequences from different animal species (in this case, mice and rats) may function as oncogenes when expressed under retrovirus control, it is important to remember that the types of tumors produced by BALB-MSV are significantly different from those induced by *ras*-containing Ha-MSV and Ki-MSV.

Spontaneous hemangiomas and hemangiosarcomas occur at relatively low frequency in inbred mice (Altman and Katz 1979), although the various BALB/c substrains show a moderate incidence of this neoplasm. Such tumors can, however, be induced at high incidence in many inbred mouse strains following treatment with a variety of chemical carcinogens or inoculation with polyoma virus. Examination of these tumors for viruses related to BALB-MSV might provide insight as to whether there exists a common mechanism of hemangiosarcoma induction, a process about which little is yet known.

H. Osteosarcoma and Osteoma Viruses

Although spontaneous malignant bone tumors occur rarely in mice and other species, they can easily be induced following administration of osteotropic radioactive isotopes, such as strontium 90. In addition, selective inbreeding programs of descendants of mice bearing spontaneous tumors can generate strains with an incidence of bone tumors greater than 50%. In such strains, the latency period is approximately 15 months; the tumors frequently involve multiple sites and are identified as osteomas, osteosarcomas, chondro-osteosarcomas, and spindle-cell sarcomas (Pybus and Miller 1938a,b; for review, see Altman and Katz 1979).

1. FBJ Osteosarcoma Virus Complex

Prompted by the evidence for a virus etiology in many mouse tumors, Finkel and her colleagues searched for viruses in mouse osteogenic sarcomas (Finkel et al. 1966a). In their initial study, one virus isolate was obtained from a spontaneous osteosarcoma in a CF-1 mouse and was subsequently called FBJ virus.

The tumor-bearing animal from which the virus was isolated showed involvement of the thoracic vertebrae and a rib. Serial passage of tumor extracts in newborn mice led to a highly oncogenic virus stock that produced tumors after a latency period as short as 3 weeks. Notably, only bone tumors form and they may involve thoracic, pelvic and lumbar vertebrae, ribs, scapulae, and femurs. These tumors grow progressively and invade adjacent tissues, often resulting in bone fracture. Histologically, the tumors first appear as cortical thickenings and as small areas of increased density in the soft tissues adjacent to the bone (Fig. 8.7). Proliferation appears to begin at the periosteum, and growth proceeds peripherally with late involvement of the deep cortex. Microscopic examination reveals the presence of many cell types, including fibroblasts, giant cells, and osteocytes, associated with an abundant connective-tissue stroma (Ward and Young 1976).

FBJ-induced osteosarcomas are quite distinct radiographically and histologically from those produced by internal emitters, such as strontium 90. The latter originate in the endosteum or bone marrow cavity and show irregular density or abnormal structure within the bone (Finkel et al. 1966b). Since these two potent oncogenic agents seemed to affect different areas of bone, Finkel and her colleagues studied the effects of combined virus and isotope treatment and found no difference in the types of tumors or the latency period when inoculation with FBJ virus was followed by

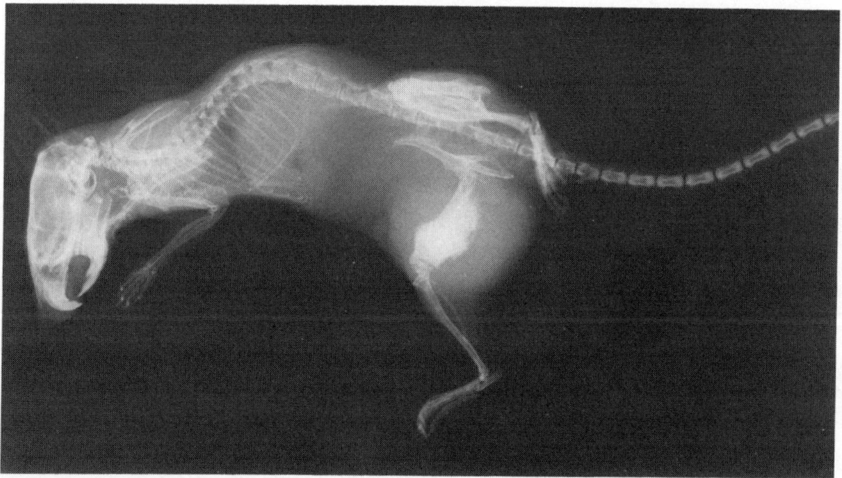

Figure 8.7 Osteosarcoma induced by the FBJ complex in a DBA mouse. Note the typical "sunburst" apperance of the tumor on the femur. (Photograph courtesy of N. Teich, Imperial Cancer Research Fund Laboratories, England.)

strontium-90 treatment (Finkel and Biskis 1968). More recently, viral particles have been observed in plutonium-239-induced osteosarcomas (Loutit and Lloyd 1977), and infectious osteosarcoma viruses have been obtained following radium-224 or thorium-227 treatment (Erfle et al. 1979, 1980); however, there is as yet no characterization of these viruses.

FBJ is a complex consisting of a helper virus and, as a minor population, a replication-defective, focus-forming sarcoma virus (Levy et al. 1978). Injection of the N-tropic helper virus into neonatal mice fails to invoke any tumors or detectable pathology (Levy et al. 1973, 1975a). On the other hand, the FBJ-MSV component induces osteosarcomas regardless of the helper virus provided (Levy et al. 1978; Curran and Teich 1982a).

The tumorigenicity of the FBJ virus complex has been tested in a number of mouse strains. Several strains appear to be highly susceptible, whereas C57BL and BALB/c are generally resistant (Finkel et al. 1966a; Kelloff et al. 1969; Yumoto et al. 1970). The incidence in resistant mice can be increased to virtually 100% when a B-tropic or NB-tropic helper virus is used to pseudotype the FBJ-MSV, thus indicating that the observed resistance may be totally or partly due to the influence of the *Fv-1* gene (Curran and Teich 1982a).

Transformed nonproducer cells have been used to elicit antisera specific for FBJ-MSV and have allowed the identification of two proteins, p39 and pp55, in FBJ-MSV tumor cells and in fibroblast cell lines transformed in vitro (Curran and Teich 1982a,b). Neither of these proteins is expressed in cells infected by the FBJ-MLV alone, nor are they precipitated by antisera to MLV structural protein antigens. However, only pp55 is found following translation of virion RNA in vitro. These data are most consistent with the hypothesis that p39 may be a virally induced cellular protein, whereas pp55 is most likely encoded by the MSV genome and thus is a candidate oncogene product.

2. FBR Osteosarcoma Virus Complex

FBR osteosarcoma virus was isolated from a strontium-90-induced steosarcoma in an X/Gf mouse (Finkel et al. 1973, 1975). X/Gf mice are particularly noted for their extremely low incidence of spontaneous tumors and their relatively high resistance to irradiation-induced carcinogenesis. FBR virus is highly oncogenic in newborn X/Gf mice; tumors appear as early as 3 weeks postinfection and the final incidence is 100%. On the other hand, FBR is poorly oncogenic for CF-1 mice (from which the FBJ virus complex was isolated) and vice versa (Lee et al. 1979); however, these data may reflect simply the *Fv-1* genotypes of the two mouse strains. The pathology of FBR virus resembles that induced by FBJ virus complex.

In vitro assays show that FBR stocks contain a B-tropic helper virus and a replication-defective focus-forming virus. This is consistent with the fact that X/Gf mice have the *Fv-1*^{bb} genotype. The kinetics of focus formation suggest that FBR-MSV occurs with a vast excess of FBR-MLV and that transformed foci arise by cell division rather than by cell recruitment (Lee et al. 1979).

3. RFB Osteoma Virus

A mixed extract from an FBJ-virus-induced osteosarcoma, a lymphosarcoma, and a spontaneous benign bone tumor (osteoma) in a CF-1 mouse (the same strain from which FBJ osteosarcoma virus was isolated) proved capable of inducing osteomas. Subsequent extracts from osteomas produced only the one type of neoplasm, and the associated virus was called RFB osteoma virus (Finkel et al. 1973). The isolate is highly oncogenic in CF-1, CBA, and NIH-Swiss mice but rarely induces tumors in X/Gf mice, perhaps related to *Fv-1* tropism.

The tumors induced by RFB virus in CF-1 mice resemble osteomas typical for this mouse strain, which has a relatively high incidence (10–20%) of benign bone tumors in mice living 18 months or more. They are characteristically well circumscribed, with no evidence of invasiveness, and consist of hard bone and osteocytes. As with FBJ virus, the tumors arise from the periosteum at about 2–3 months after inoculation of newborn mice, and multiple tumors are often found in a single animal. The osteomas grow rapidly for a few weeks, after which they progress very slowly. The tumors contribute to mortality only in those cases where they are located in a vital area, such as the spine, where they may cause paralysis, or in the jaw, where they interfere with eating.

If RFB virus is injected prior to or simultaneously with FBJ or FBR viruses, the time of appearance of osteosarcomas is delayed and the final incidence is decreased (Finkel et al. 1976); these findings suggest that the viruses are all immunologically related.

RFB can also interfere with FBJ-MSV focus formation in CF-1 embryo cells in vitro (Reilly and Finkel 1976). RFB virus does not induce transformation in vitro, and it is not known whether it is a single virus or a mixture.

I. Myeloid Leukemia Viruses

Several viruses capable of producing myeloid leukemias have been obtained following infection of mice with other retroviruses or passage of cell-free tumor filtrates. However, most of the studies have emphasized the pathogenic spectrum rather than the characterization of the virus(es) involved. Clearly, further study on this group of viruses is necessary. Experience gained from studies on other acute leukemia viruses indicates that the identification of the oncogenic agent will require biological and molecular cloning, as well as analysis of the complexity of infectious agents in virus stocks before and after passage in vivo.

1. Graffi Virus

Graffi (1957) obtained virus harvests that had a propensity to induce chloroleukemias (a form of myeloid leukemia characterized by a discernible greenish coloration of the involved lymph nodes) from a variety of transplantable mouse tumors: spontaneous reticulum cell sarcomas, the Ehrlich carcinoma (cf. Friend virus origin), and sarcoma 37 (cf. Mo-MSV origin). Preparations of each of these tumors induced a high incidence of leukemia (50–85%), of which 37–67% were chloroleukemias. The general pathological finding of Graffi-virus-induced leukemias, occurring after a latency of 4–6 months after inoculation of neonates or approximately 7 months after inoculation of adult mice, is massive enlargement of lymph nodes (up to 100-fold) and involvement of the spleen and extensive leukemic infiltration of liver, lungs, kidneys, and ovaries, with only rare involvement of the thymus. A 30-fold increase in the white-blood-cell count occurs (from the normal 10,000/mm^3 to 300,000/mm^3), and differential analysis of peripheral blood and bone-marrow smears reveals an increase in the number of immature myeloid cells, predominantly promyelocytes and myeloblasts.

One perplexing but quite interesting finding was that, depending on the mouse strain and the tissue of origin of the virus preparation, a variety of tumors developed that involved different hematopoietic lineages, suggesting the possibility that Graffi virus might indeed be a complex of several virus entities. Graffi and his colleagues (1966) noticed that, at least for the first passage, there was a marked tendency to breed true, i.e., reticulum cell tumor extracts gave rise to predominantly reticulum cell tumors and erythroblastic tumor extracts gave rise to erythroblastic tumors. They found that the organ from which the virus was isolated also seemed to influence the disease pattern, with spleen, bone marrow, and thymus giving rise to the highest frequency of chloroleukemias, whereas virus from other organs gave rise to a more random pattern. However, upon repeated cell-free passage in vivo, there was a decrease in this specificity, which Graffi termed hematological diversification.

From the limited number of studies on strain susceptibility, there do not appear to be any noticeably resistant strains (Graffi 1957; Graffi et al. 1966; Fiore-Donati and Chieco-Bianci 1964). A low incidence of myeloid and lymphoid leukemias and other hematological neoplasms was observed following inoculation of rats (Graffi and Gimmy 1957, 1959; Gimmy et al. 1960). It will be of interest in the future to delineate whether Graffi virus is endogenous or exogenous, of mouse or rat origin, and single or multiple virus entities.

2. *Stansly/Soule Myeloproliferative Virus*

This virus was isolated from BALB/c mice inoculated with Ehrlich ascites or cell-free extracts (cf. origin of Friend virus and Graffi) (Stansly and Soule 1962). Splenomegaly and lymph node enlargement, characterized by the prevalence of myeloid cells, occur about 3 months after inoculation of neonatal mice (Soule and Arnold 1970). Nooter and Bentvelzen (1976) reported that committed myelomonocytic progenitor cells (CFU-GM) from infected mice still require colony-stimulating factors for growth as agar colonies, although these colonies could grow in the absence of serum; the latter finding suggests that these cells may gain some properties of the transformed phenotype.

3. *Myeloid Leukemia Virus*

McGarry et al. (1974) sought to separate the components of FV-P (Mirand strain) by passaging the stock in vivo: once through

C57BL mice, once through weanling Swiss Ha/ICR, and ten times through neonatal Swiss mice. After this, it was passaged numerous times in newborn C57BL mice in which it induced hepatosplenomegaly at 2–3 months postinfection. Most of the infected mice died within 4 months from lymphatic leukemia involving spleen, liver, and often lymph nodes and thymus. However, a few mice survived beyond 6 months and these developed chloroleukemia (green coloration of the lymph nodes). At the tenth passage, chloroleukemic cells were serially transplanted and cell-free extracts from several passages induced myelogenous leukemias in newborn C57BL mice; the stock was referred to as myeloid leukemia virus (MyLV). No spleen foci were detectable in inoculated BALB/c mice, and hence it was concluded that the Fr-SFFV was lost.

Following inoculation with MyLV, the earliest signs of leukemia are palpable spleen and lymph nodes, whereas the peripheral white-blood-cell count is often normal, showing only a slight increase in the proportion of immature cells. As the disease progresses, early monocytes and erythroblasts become more numerous, but mature granulocytes predominate and leukemic cells infiltrate most organs. Approximately 50% of the animals die from chloroleukemia, whereas the remainder die from other myeloid leukemias. The incidence of mortality approaches 100% in C57BL mice inoculated as newborns. Myeloid leukemias are also induced in other strains of mice and in rats.

Preliminary data suggest that, although MyLV harvests from tumors contain replication-competent and replication-defective components, a single competent virus is sufficient to induce severe anemia, splenomegaly, and myeloid leukemia (J. Salles and N. Teich, pers. comm.). Thus, this virus appears to retain some features of Fr-MLV (and its associated disease; Section VIII.A.4) and additionally affects the white-blood-cell compartment.

IX. PATHOGENESIS OF MURINE LEUKEMIA VIRUSES

An extensive literature on the pathology of spontaneously arising mouse tumors, particularly the thymic lymphomas and leukemias, was developed during 1940–1960. The treatise by Gross (1970) described the histopathology of leukemias that arise spontaneously in high-incidence strains, as well as those tumors induced by

X-irradiation or from cell-free extracts of leukemic tissues. Not only was a virus etiology proved, and the importance of intact target tissue demonstrated, but also a number of contributing factors, such as age, diet, hormonal status, and host genes, were identified. In addition, transmission through the germ line (vertical, or more precisely genetic, transmission) was shown to be the primary, if not exclusive, mode of tumor induction. However, it is now patent that these early studies of cell-free transmission involved filtrates containing a mixture of distinct viruses derived from endogenous proviruses. Although this realization does not invalidate the previous results and attendant conclusions, the precise role of clonally isolated viruses from these filtrates has become an important field for examination. Most central to this issue was the discovery that viruses with an expanded (polytropic) host range could be isolated from preleukemic tissue of target organs. These MCF viruses, so named for their ability to produce cytopathic foci following infection of mink cells in vitro, have since been isolated from numerous strains of mice, from tumors involving different hematopoietic cell lineages, and from virus stocks that have long been passaged in vitro (see Chapter 2 and Section IX.B). Thus, the older experiments are summarized below only briefly in order to emphasize the conceptual conclusions, rather than to analyze the pleiomorphic responses that were often obtained with various virus filtrates.

A. A General Picture of Thymic Leukemias

For all intents and purposes (with the exception of natural transmission), the principles outlined below regarding virus isolation, experimental transmission with cell-free extracts, role of hormones, and role of the target organ are identical for the following four situations: (1) spontaneous thymomas in high-incidence strains (AKR and C58 mice), (2) X-radiation-induced thymomas in highly sensitive strains (C57BL and C3H mice), (3) thymomas induced by treatment with carcinogens such as 2-methylcholanthrene and 7,12-dimethylbenzanthracene, and (4) thymomas induced by exogenous MLV, such as Mo-MLV (Moloney 1960) and Gross passage-A virus (Gross 1957).

1. Transmission

The study of spontaneous leukemia and of the endogenous murine retroviruses was facilitated, and in a way initiated, by the development of inbred strains of mice with a high incidence of "spontaneous" leukemia. The C58 (Richter and MacDowell 1929) and AKR (Furth et al. 1933) strains each have an incidence approaching 90% by 6–10 months of age. Even with selective breeding, 10% of the mice who do not develop leukemia within this time span still produce offspring with the same 90% incidence (MacDowell and Richter 1935). As yet unidentified extrinsic and intrinsic factors presumably contribute to this phenomenon.

The spontaneous disease is often referred to as leukemia, but more precisely, it originates as a thymic lymphoma (thymoma or thymic leukemia) that may spread to other organs, most particularly to the spleen, and sometimes to the blood. Detailed histopathological analyses of preleukemic and leukemic thymuses are presented elsewhere (Metcalf 1966a; Gross 1970; Turusov 1979; Haran-Ghera 1980).

The initial success of Gross (1951a) in transmitting leukemia with AKR filtrates to C3H/Bi mice depended on his use of newborn animals as recipients. In addition, transmission to other C3H sublines (e.g., C3H/An) was often considerably diminished; the basis of these differences is still unexplained. The transmissibility of disease to C3H/Bi mice with AKR extracts was not always successful, and several serial passages of leukemic filtrates in vivo were required to develop a uniformly more potent stock, now known as Gross passage-A virus (Gross 1957). However, the use of neonatal animals for experimental tumor induction has remained a standard practice in recent years; the efficacy of this procedure may reflect the undeveloped immune responses of newborn animals or the existence of particular subsets of hematopoietic cells that may be in a more highly proliferative state at this stage in development, compared with a relatively quiescent state in adult animals.

Early studies on the natural transmission of thymic leukemias in AKR mice provided ample evidence that the disease was not transmitted through the milk, as with MMTV, or via intrauterine infection. First, foster nursing of AKR neonates on mothers from low-incidence strains generally did not decrease the incidence of tumor development (MacDowell and Richter 1935), although some studies showed a variable suppression (Barnes and Cole 1941) (all reviewed in Gross 1970). Conversely, mice of low-incidence strains foster-nursed on AKR females did not show a frequency of leukemia higher than that observed for their particular strain. Second, mice developed from fertilized AKR ova transplanted to pregnant females of low-incidence strains and subsequently nursed by their foster mothers did not have a diminished leukemia incidence, compared with that of conventionally bred AKR mice (Fekete and Otis 1954). Furthermore, reciprocal genetic crosses between AKR and low-incidence strains showed that the leukemia-prone trait was transmitted equally well by male or female AKR mice (MacDowell and Richter 1935; Gross 1970). These data led Gross (1951b) to coin the term vertical transmission. In the ensuing years, the possibility that the disease was due to infection of eggs or sperm has been definitively eliminated; additional evidence to support the model that endogenous leukemogenic proviruses are inherited as host genes has accumulated, and there is no question that the disease is genetically transmitted.

Low levels of MLV can be transmitted through the milk (of AKR or experimentally infected mice) to their offspring; however, the induction of leukemia by this route of administration is extremely low (Law and Moloney 1961), and infectious virus disappeared in succeeding generations. There is no evidence for germ-line integration following experimental infection by foster nursing or inoculation of neonatal animals leading to the conversion of a low-incidence strain into a high-incidence strain. However, as discussed in Chapter 10, MLV can be introduced into the germ line by inoculation of ova or preimplantation embryos; these manipulations can lead to the creation of mouse stains with altered genotypes and dramatically altered phenotypes.

2. *Virological Patterns*

Embryonic development is characterized by a plethora of MLV footprints. Intracisternal A-type particles and budding C-type particles have been observed by electron microscopy from the two-cell embryo stage through the entire gestation period; in most cases, these particles do not correlate with the phenotypic expression of leukemia in old age. However, Rowe and Pincus (1972) identified infectious ecotropic MLV in AKR-strain embryos as early as the fifteenth day of gestation, whereas embryos from strains with a low incidence of leukemia often do not have infectious MLV until several months after birth (Hartley et al. 1969; Peters et al. 1972). Thus, at a gross level, the presence of infectious ecotropic MLV in embryonic life seems to be a prognostic sign for the occurrence of leukemia. One of the enigmas of this situation is the very long latency between the detection of MLV and the development of overt leukemia (minimally 3 months, and often longer). To some extent, this discrepancy has been explained by the observation that the type of MLV produced during specific stages of life shows an identifiable, but changing, pattern (Hays and Vredevoe 1977). Early in life, the MLVs isolated are generally capable of inducing plaques in XC cells (but are nonleukemogenic); during the preleukemic phase, one isolates XC-negative, ecotropic viruses (some leukemogenic, some not) and XC-negative MCF viruses (some leukemogenic, some not; discussed in Section IX.B) (Kawashima et al. 1976; Hays and Vredevoe 1977; Nowinski and Doyle 1977; Nowinski and Hays 1978). Thus, there are very specific qualitative and quantitative changes in the spectrum of MLV expression and production.

3. *Intrinsic Factors Modulating Leukemogenesis*

Although most of the factors governing an animal's susceptibility or resistance to virally induced leukemogenesis can ultimately be traced back to the specific genetic constitution of that animal, only a few factors have been identified as defined gene loci. The inability to identify and control each variable places an enormous constraint on the task of resolving gene interactions and elucidating their individual consequences. However, a few salient features of the importance of genes modulating different aspects of the leukemogenic process have emerged (for review, see Lilly and Pincus 1973; Altman and Katz 1979; Pincus 1980).

a. Genetic Control. Most of the host genes influencing murine virus leukemogenesis described briefly below have been reviewed in more detail by Lilly and Pincus (1973) and Pincus (1980).

First, and most readily identifiable, are the endogenous proviruses that encode the ecotropic viruses themselves. The initial hybridization experiments (Chattopadhyay et al. 1974; Lowy et al. 1974) showed a clear correlation between the presence of sequences related to AKV and both spontaneous expression of infectious MLV and high incidence of spontaneous leukemia. However, early suggestions of a quantitative correlation between provirus number and disease incidence have not been borne out, and it seems that the number of proviruses is not as important as the qualitative differences between the strains. Whether the important differences are intrinsic to the different (but closely related) proviruses themselves, to the sites of residence of these proviruses, or to other genetic differences regulating virus expression and infection remains to be completely worked out (see Chapter 10).

Genes of the second category control expression of endogenous MLV antigens, e.g., *Tla* (control of TL antigen), *Gv-1* and *Gv-2* (expression of the ecotropic gp70-related G_{IX} antigen), and *Fv-6* (endogenous MCF expression in spleen and bone marrow). Some or all of these may also be endogenous proviruses, but this point has not yet been established.

Third, genes have been identified that specifically restrict virus replication. For example, the *Fv-1* locus controls the replication of ecotropic and MCF viruses (see Section VIII.A.6 and below) and thus may modulate responses in vivo to spontaneous virus expression. For example, BALB/c mice (*Fv-1*^{bb}) contain only one N-tropic ecotropic provirus, and little replicating virus can be detected early in life. Older animals, however, frequently yield high titers of B-tropic virus. Apparently, nonpermissivity due to *Fv-1* suppresses replication and consequent pathogenicity of the endogenous virus until the appearance of either a mutant or recombinant capable of replicating in B-type cells (see Chapter 10). Although the molecular basis for *Fv-1* is now partially understood (see Chapters 4 and 5), numerous other loci regulate virus replication by as yet unknown mechanisms (e.g., *Srv-1, Fv-2, Fv-4,* and *Rgv-2*).

Fourth, genes linked to the major histocompatibility (*H-2*) locus are thought to involve immunologically mediated responses to virion components or to virus-infected cells (e.g., *H-2* itself, *Rfv-1,* and *Rfv-2*). Some non-*H-2*-linked gene loci are also thought to involve immune response reactions (e.g., *hr, Fv-3,* and *Rfv-3*).

Fv-2 represents a fifth category, that of a gene believed to depress the cycling kinetics of a specific hematopoietic cell subset and thus reduce the numbers of the target-cell population. The *W, Sl, f,* and *nu* genes probably also relate to the target cells directly and/or to their microenvironment (see Section VIII.A.6).

Finally, the endogenous ecotropic provirus seems also to have an important regulatory influence, aside from its parental role. In crosses between AKR and the ecotropic-endogenous-virus-negative NFS mice, Cloyd et al. (1981) found that the sensitivity of mice to rapid tumor induction by MCF virus (in an acceleration assay, see Section IX.B.1) was correlated with the presence of Akv-1 or Akv-2. These authors suggested that this effect could be due to phenotypic mixing of the MCF genome with ecotropic *env* glycoprotein, thus permitting spread of the virus even in the presence of neutralizing antibody or other serum factors. A similar effect has also been observed following inoculation with deliberate mixtures of ecotropic and MCF viruses (Section IX.B.2).

b. Hormonal Influences. Hormonal effects on thymic leukemogenesis were suggested from the early observation that females of high-incidence strains had a higher incidence of leukemia and a shorter latency period, compared with that of their male siblings (Mercier 1937; Cole and Furth 1941). Experimental manipulation of hormonal balance confirmed this phenomenon; ovariectomy or treatment of females with testosterone reduced the incidence of leukemia (McEndy et al. 1944; Rudali et al. 1956), whereas orchidectomy increased the incidence in males (Murphy 1944; Law 1947). Chronic estrogen treatment also enhances the development of leukemia in low-incidence strains (Lacassagne 1937; Gardner et al. 1944). A corollary of these effects was the finding that spontaneous leukemia could be significantly reduced by limiting food intake to subsistence levels; the sexual organs of these mice were very undeveloped and thus hormonal imbalance was a likely contributory factor (Saxton et al. 1944). Furthermore, chronic administration of estrogens to low-incidence strains induces leukemia (Kunii et al. 1965). The influence of the glucocorticoid hormones is discussed in the next section.

4. *Target Cells*

First and foremost in the development of leukemia is the necessity for a specific target cell. Early experiments involving AKR mice thymectomized at 1–2 months of age demonstrated a significantly decreased incidence of leukemia (McEndy et al. 1944). Treatment of AKR mice with cortisone (which causes a chemical thymectomy) also diminished the incidence and increased the latency for the development of spontaneous leukemia (Woolley and Peters 1953). However, splenectomy had no effect on spontaneous disease (McEndy et al. 1944).

Similar findings were obtained in X-radiation-induced leukemias. Numerous strains are susceptible to X-radiation-induced thymomas, but the incidence varies considerably; C3H and C57BR mice are moderately susceptible, and C57BL and RF mice are highly susceptible. In all cases, thymectomy decreased the incidence of thymic leukemias (Kaplan 1950; Gross 1959). Interestingly, X-irradiation induces two types of leukemia in RF mice—thymic and myeloid (Upton et al. 1958). Thymectomy in RF mice before X-irradiation decreases the incidence of thymic leukemia, increases the incidence of lymphoid leukemias in extrathymic lymphoid tissues, and has no effect on the incidence of myeloid leukemia. Furthermore, splenectomy in RF mice resulted in a decrease of myeloid leukemia, whereas the incidence of thymic leukemia remained unchanged (Upton et al. 1958). Both the myeloid and thymic leukemias could be transmitted by cell-free extracts (Upton 1959). These data point out two major findings: strains differ in susceptibility to the type of leukemia induced by X-rays and X-radiation-induced tumors, depending on leukemia type, originate in different hematopoietic organs.

The requirement for a functional thymus is also indicated by the following results. First, ectopic thymus grafts restore the susceptibility of animals to spontaneous and X-radiation-induced leukemia (Law and Miller 1950; Kaplan et al. 1956). Second, shielding experiments show that protection of either bone marrow (Jacobson et al. 1949) or thymus (Toch et al. 1956) during the exposure of the animal to X-rays inhibits the development of X-radiation-induced leukemia. To a lesser extent, transplantation of normal unirradiated bone marrow also inhibits leukemia (Kaplan et al. 1953).

Thymectomy also decreases the susceptibility of animals to leukemogenesis by exogenous virus infection and, in some circumstances, changes the pattern of expression; for example, thymectomized C3H mice inoculated with Gross passage-A virus do not develop thymic leukemias, but they do develop a significant incidence of myeloid leukemia (Gross 1960). Restoration of susceptibility to exogenous virus infection also occurs with implantation of a normal thymus (Miller 1959; Gross 1960). Ectopic thymic tissue also restores susceptibility to carcinogen-induced leukemias (Law and Miller 1950).

Other corollaries of thymic manipulation involve the "masking" of leukemogenic properties of other viruses. For example, Graffi virus normally induces myeloid leukemia in many strains of mice, but infected AKR mice generally succumb to thymic leukemia, unless they were thymectomized, in which case they develop myeloid leukemias (Fiore-Donati et al. 1966). One of the most interesting corollaries, however, resulted from the injection of Mo-MLV into mice chronically treated with prednisolone (inducing a corticosteroid thymectomy); although a very rare occurrence, one mouse developed a nonthymic leukemia from which the novel Abelson virus was isolated (see Section VIII.D).

Absence of the target organ (spleen) in Friend-virus-infected mice can manifest the oncogenic potential of the helper virus (Fr-MLV) to induce lymphatic leukemia.

5. Chromosomal Changes in Thymic Leukemias

Karyologic analysis of tumors in man and other animals has often revealed the occurrence of discrete chromosomal abnormalities, including translocations, deletions, and duplications, that are characteristic of the particular tumor type. When a single chromosome is apparently involved in unique or multiple modifications, several questions are asked. Is the change prerequisite to, or caused by, the development of neoplasia? Is the change associated with cells showing phenotypic markers of a particular stage of maturation? Is the location of the chromosomal lesion(s) in close proximity to genes known to encode biochemical, immunological, or other properties that are expressed or altered (repressed or derepressed) in the tumor cells?

The consensus from karyotypic studies of murine thymomas induced intrinsically (from endogenous viruses) or extrinsically (mediated by exogenous virus infection, carcinogen administration, or X-irradiation) is the presence of chromosome-15 trisomies (Dofuku et al. 1975; Chang et al. 1977; Wiener et al. 1978a,b,c; Leonard and Decleve 1979). More sensitive techniques, using mice with genetically defined translocations, show that the distal portion of this chromosome is the involved segment, and in genetic crosses between sensitive and resistant strains (e.g., with regard to spontaneous leukemia or X-radiation-induced leukemia), it is the chromosome 15 of the sensitive strain that becomes duplicated (Spira et al. 1979, 1980; Wiener et al. 1980). Additionally, treatment of SJL mice with dimethylbenzanthracene induces thymic leukemias and, in thymectomized mice, nonthymic (non-T-cell) leukemias; only the thymic leukemias had the chromosome-15 trisomy. These data led Spira et al. (1980) to conclude that the cytogenetic abnormality was dependent on the target-cell type rather than on the carcinogen. The trisomy of the distal region of chromosome 15 also occurs following induction of thymomas in mice in which this region is genetically translocated onto other chromosomes (Robertsonian translocations) (Spira et al. 1979). Thus, the development of the cytogenetic change in thymomas induced by different initiating agents suggests that the trisomy may represent some requirement for a gene-dosage effect important to the growth of the tumor, although most likely not directly involved in the initial transforming event. Neither the genetic loci that influence thymoma development (see Section IX.A.3.a) nor the ecotropic MLV-inducing loci (e.g., *Akv-1, Akv-2;* see Chapter 10) map on chromosome 15. Furthermore, many of the loci governing antigens expressed during T-cell differentiation map on other chromosomes. Thus, there is as yet no obvious reason for this apparently specific chromosomal aberration.

6. *Immunotherapy*

Mice are not immunologically tolerant to antigenic determinants on their endogenous viruses, nor do they fail to mount an immune response to exogenous virus infections. In some cases, this response causes additional complications for the animal; for example, the chronic depositon of antigen-antibody complexes leads to glomerulonephritis in some strains of mice (Hanna et al. 1972; Oldstone et al. 1976). Antibodies to most of the viral proteins occur, although the major reactivities are directed against the viral envelope proteins, gp70 and p15(E), as expected (for review, see Ihle and Hanna 1977). More recently, antigens specific to the endogenous MCF viruses have also been identified, and humoral activities to them have been detected (Cloyd et al. 1979; Stockert et al. 1979; O'Donnell and Nowinski 1980; O'Donnell et al. 1980). However, there is as yet no defined role for autogenous humoral immunity in either suppression or enhancement of thymoma development.

Immunoprophylaxis has been accomplished in several murine

retrovirus diseases using either passive or active immunization procedures. Spontaneous AKR leukemia has been suppressed for extensive periods of time by treatment of neonatal mice with antiserum to ecotropic AKR MLV (Huebner et al. 1976) or even with antisera to the heterologous Friend virus gp70 (Schwarz et al. 1979). In these situations, the amount of infectious MLV circulating in the blood during the animal's lifetime is considerably reduced, MCF virus production is delayed, and autogenous antibody production is stimulated (Lee et al. 1977; Schwarz et al. 1979). Schwarz et al. (1979) also noted that treatment of pregnant mothers and further treatment of their offspring neonatally was even more efficacious in preventing spontaneous thymomas. On the basis of these data, Schwarz et al. (1979) proposed that during the first few days of life, there is transformation, by an ecotropic virus, of a thymus cell(s) at a distinct stage of differentiation such that it is primed as a preleukemic cell that would, only much later, develop its fully malignant character. However, more recent analyses (Yoshimura and Breda 1982; W. Herr and W. Gilbert, pers. comm.) indicate that most thymomas do not contain detectable newly integrated ecotropic proviruses and thus contradict a major prediction of this model. It seems likely, therefore, that continued replication and spread of ecotropic virus within the animal is a requirement for subsequent events.

Immunization by active or passive treatment prior to X-irradiation suppresses thymic leukemia development in C57BL/6 mice (Peters et al. 1977), and, similarly, active immunization has been shown to be effective against subsequent challenge with exogenous virus (Kelloff et al. 1976). Similar protocols involving both active and passive immunization prevent the acute Friend-virus-induced disease in adult mice (Hunsmann et al. 1975; Schafer et al. 1976; Collins et al. 1978).

B. MCF Viruses

Since the initial isolation of polytropic MCF viruses from the preleukemic thymuses of AKR mice (Hartley et al. 1977), considerable effort has been expended upon their characterization, and attempts have been made to decipher their roles in leukemogenesis. From the data obtained so far, it appears that MCF viruses act as the proximal carcinogens in the induction of a variety of hematopoietic neoplasms. Although the molecular events in the process remain largely unknown, the biological consequences of virus-virus and virus-host interactions are being identified.

MCF viruses have been isolated from naturally arising tumors and from experimentally induced tumors (involving exogenous virus infection, chemical or physical treatment, or graft-versus-host disease reactions) (see Chapter 2). Assays for oncogenic potential include two major tests: (1) the ability to accelerate the development of spontaneous leukemias in high-incidence strains (e.g., AKR or C58 mice), based on the initial study and protocol of Rudali et al. (1956), and (2) leukemogenicity in mice of low-incidence strains. Using these criteria, MCF isolates fall into four pathogenic categories: (1) those capable of inducing leukemia, (2) those capable of accelerating the appearance of leukemia in mouse strains predisposed to spontaneous disease, (3) those which are apparently apathogenic, and (4) one capable of preventing leukemia induction by other MCF isolates.

MCF viruses are not inherited as complete proviruses. They are generated de novo by recombination between ecotropic and endogenous viruses that are probably not identical with xenotropic viruses (Chattopadhyay et al. 1982); either endogenous or exogenous viruses may serve as the ecotropic parent (see Chapters 4 and 10). The most consistent finding is that recombination involves the gp70-coding portion of the *env* gene, as well as some portions further toward the 3′ (U_3) end of the genome, including the 3′-terminal portion of p15(E). These data are consistent with the host-range pattern in vitro. One important corollary of the recombinant *env*-gene product is the finding that normal mouse sera, which contain nonimmunoglobulin (apolipoprotein) factors capable of inactivating xenotropic MLV (Levy et al. 1975b; Fischinger et al. 1976; Kane et al. 1979; Montelaro et al. 1979), also inactivate MCF viruses (see below). Although the mechanism of this inactivation is unclear, the phenomenon may play a central role in considerations of the generation, spread, and infectivity of MCF viruses; their interactions with other viruses; and the long latency period sometimes observed between infection and overt leukemia (see Section IX.B.5).

As discussed below, MCF viruses exhibit a high degree of organotropism for replication, a finding that is closely correlated with the site of neoplastic transformation. Therefore, another corollary of the recombinant *env* gene involves the possibility for specific, and perhaps unique, recognition between the target cell and a particular MCF virus. M.S. McGrath et al. (1978) performed reciprocal binding assays using various thymic leukemias and the MCF viruses isolated from them. On the basis of these data they concluded that a defined cell-surface phenotype on a thymocyte predestines that cell to be the target of a specific thymomagenic MCF virus. Given the observed polymorphism of *env* phenotypes of MCF isolates, this theory predicts that spontaneous leukemias might be expected to be phenotypically diverse, whereas leukemias induced by a single virus isolate in several hosts should have identical surface properties. These predictions were verified by experimental analysis of cell-surface markers on spontaneous and MCF-induced leukemias (Zielinski et al. 1980). A similar study on Mo-MLV-induced thymomas showed phenotypic heterogeneity rather than identity (Pepersack et al. 1980); however, stocks of Mo-MLV are known to contain MCF viruses and to give rise to MCF viruses after infection, a finding that could explain this discrepancy. Diverse phenotypic expression of other spontaneous AKR thymomas (Krammer et al. 1976; Mathieson et al. 1978) supports the concept that the causative leukemogenic MCF viruses arise by random genetic recombination.

The recombination concept is also supported by the observation that each of the MCF viruses studied so far shows a different restriction endonuclease map and a distinctive oligonucleotide map, suggesting that many sites for recombination result in the production of viable progeny. Chattopadhyay et al. (1982), studying a number of strains of pathogenic and apathogenic MCF viruses by restriction enzyme mapping, found that the use of about 20 different enzymes distinguished only one enzyme site that was found exclusively in the pathogenic strains. More detailed analysis, described more fully in Chapter 10, has implied that a virus must have a specific pattern of *env* and 3′-terminal sequences to have the three characteristic features of leukemogenicity, thymus-specific replication (thymotropism), and polytropic host range. Viruses that violate this pattern have been isolated from a variety of sources (as described in the next section) and can be shown to lack one or more of the key characteristics. Analysis of these viruses by oligonucleotide mapping and nucleotide sequence determination (Lung et al. 1980; M. Lung et al., pers. comm.) has allowed a crude mapping of these characteristics (see Chapter 10); however, except for the association between polytropism and gp70, the functional basis for these differences remains unresolved.

1. Association with Thymic Leukemias

Cloyd et al. (1980) performed a detailed analysis of the oncogenicity of many MCF isolates from diverse sources and concluded that (1) the MCF isolates from spontaneously arising thymomas in AKR and C58 mice were the proximal cause of the disease and (2) the presence of high titers of ecotropic MLV in the thymus contributed, but was not essential, to the leukemogenic potential of MCFs. These conclusions were based on the following results. First, the oncogenic AKR-MCF (strain 247) induced leukemias in weanling AKR, C3H/Bi (low ecotropic MLV expression), and NIH-Swiss mice congenic for ecotropic MLV-inducing loci (*Akv-1* or *Akv-2*) but not in inbred NIH-Swiss (NFS), C57BR, C58, DBA/2, or BALB/c mice. A few other isolates from AKR thymomas also induced leukemias in the congenic *Akv* mice. All of these viruses are highly thymotropic. Second, isolates derived from leukemic lymphoid organs of *Akv* or *C58v* congenic mice were thymomagenic for such congenic mice, but not for other strains. These viruses generally did not function in the acceleration test and were classed as weakly oncogenic. Third, MCF isolates from nonthymic tumors (including leukemic spleens and lymph nodes) from strains of mice with a low incidence of leukemia were consistently negative in both leukemogenicity and AKR acceleration tests.

HRS/J mice carrying the mutant hairless (*hr;* chromosome 14) autosomal recessive allele in homozygous or heterozygous form are predisposed to the development of thymic leukemias, with incidences of about 75% and 20%, respectively, at 18 months of age (Meier et al. 1969). Two thymotropic MCF isolates from *hr/hr* mice, PTV-1 and PTV-2, accelerate leukemia in the homologous mouse and also are thymomagenic in the low-leukemia strain CBA/J (which, unlike other CBA substrains, has an ecotropic endogenous provirus), but not SWR/J or NIH-Swiss mice (Green et al. 1980). Schwartz and Khiroya (1981) analyzed the differential effects in CBA/J and inbred NIH (NFS) mice by comparing the titers of PTV-1 in thymic extracts. On the basis of genetic crosses between the two strains, they concluded that a single dominant gene for susceptibility occurred in CBA mice (*Ptv*^{s}), whereas the leukemia-resistant NFS mice possessed the recessive allele for resistance (*Ptv*^{r}).

BALB/Mo mice carry an integrated Mo-MLV provirus (*Mov-1*) and express a high incidence of thymic leukemias related to the amplification and expression of Mo-MLV sequences (see Chapter 10). An MCF virus (Mo-MCF-81) isolated from a BALB *mov-1* thymoma is weakly oncogenic in neonatal NIH-Swiss mice (Vogt 1979). In incidence and latency, Mo-MCF-81 is considerably less potent than its ecotropic Mo-MLV parent. In contrast, HIX virus, another Mo-MCF isolated from an in vitro-passaged stock of Mo-MLV, is as leukemogenic as its parent (Fischinger et al. 1975, 1978). Therefore, one must consider that, as with the generation of distinct MCF isolates in high-incidence strains, exogenous virus infection may also lead to the generation of numerous different MCF viruses. As with many of the other MCF isolates, cell cultures infected with Mo-MCF and Mo-MLV release most MCFs as pseudotypes with Mo-MLV envelopes (Fischinger et al. 1978; Vogt 1979), presumably analogous to the in vivo situation.

A virus etiology for thymic leukemias induced by X-irradiation in C57BL mice was first demonstrated by the experiments of Lieberman and Kaplan (1959), who successfully transmitted the disease to neonatal mice with cell-free tumor extracts. In the various C57BL substrains, virus expression in the thymomas is often absent (Ihle et al. 1976); however, explantation and culture of leukemic thymocytes or thymic reticulum cells often lead to a surfeit of distinct retroviruses (Lieberman et al. 1973; Haas and Hilgers 1975; Decleve et al. 1976, 1977; Haas 1978): (1) nonpathogenic ecotropic MLV, both N- and B-tropic isolates; (2) nonpathogenic xenotropic MLV; (3) a thymotropic thymomagenic virus that was reported to replicate in thymocytes but poorly, if at all, in fibroblasts in vitro; (4) a thymomagenic MCF virus; and (5) a B-cell lymphomagenic MCF virus (see Section IX.B.2). To complicate the situation even more, infection of nonproducer thymoma cell lines with a nonleukemogenic helper virus rescues a thymotropic thymomagenic virus (Lieberman et al. 1979), suggesting the existence of replication-defective precursors (possibly the unrecombined endogenous MCF sequences). Furthermore, infection of cultured thymus reticulum cell lines with the thymotropic isolate seems to lead to the recovery of an MCF-type particle (Haas et al. 1977; Haas 1978); presumably these represent analogous situations whereby pseudotype formation leads to an expanded host range and facilitates replication of the thymomagenic component in vivo. The formation of ecotropic pseudotypes of either the thymotropic or MCF isolates increases the incidence and decreases the latency for thymoma induction, possibly because such pseudotypes would be resistant to the inactivating effect of apolipoprotein.

Because T-cell lymphomas are the major type of neoplasm associated with MLV infection, several groups have proposed mechanisms of oncogenesis based on the special interactions that may occur between leukemogenic viruses and immune cells. Weissman and coworkers (Weissman and Baird 1977; Weissman and McGrath 1978, 1979) have shown that in comparison with other leukemogenic and nonleukemogenic viruses, lymphoma cells induced by a particular virus preferentially bind that virus. In addition, populations of preleukemic cells that are enriched for virus-binding cells transfer the leukemia to healthy recipients at a high frequency after a short latent period. On the basis of these data, they proposed a receptor-mediated model of leukemogenesis in which the oncogenic event is mediated by the binding of the leukemogenic virus to a subset of T lymphocytes that bear receptors specific for the viral glycoprotein. This mitogenlike interaction stimulates continued proliferation of the T cells and leads to leukemia. The nature of the receptors involved in virus binding has not been elucidated, but this model predicts that they would function as antigen receptors, rather than receptors for virus penetration. In fact, although infection of the virus-binding cells would increase the amount of viral glycoprotein available to provide a mitogenic stimulus, infection of the malignant cells by the virus is not an obligate requirement of this model.

Lee and Ihle (1981a,b) have shown that CBA/N mice, animals that carry an X-linked immunodeficiency gene, fail to display Mo-MLV-induced lymphomas even though the animals become viremic. Despite the presence of high levels of virus, these animals, in contrast to normal CBA mice, fail to develop a chronic cellular immune response to viral proteins. From these results, they have proposed that chronic immunostimulation plays an etiologic role in lymphomagenesis. According to this model, the chronic immunostimulation induces subpopulations of T lymphocytes to expand in the response to lymphokines produced during the immune response. This expanding population might provide additional target cells for virus infection. Alternatively, the presence of large numbers of binding cells might enhance the probability of somatic mutations that would lead to the development of leukemia. This theory, like that of Weissman and coworkers, does not require the infection of the tumor cells by leukemogenic virus.

2. Association with B-cell Lymphomas

Splenic extracts of C57BL/6 mice inoculated with the Latarjet and Duplan (1962) extracts (from X-radiation-induced thymic leukemias) can be shown to induce nonthymic lymphomas (reticulum cell sarcomas). An MCF isolate, designated MBC4, isolated from one leukemic spleen induced exclusively reticulum cell sarcomas in C57BL/6 mice with a latency period as short as 1 month (Haas and Patch 1980a; Haas and Reshef 1980); these tumors were further characterized as immunoglobulin-secreting B-cell lymphomas (unpublished data of P. Pattengale et al., cited in Haas and Patch 1980b). Preferential growth of MBC4 in spleen and lymph nodes, but not thymus, occurs in vivo (Haas and Meshorer 1979). Antigenic differences between MBC4 and other C57BL/6 retrovirus isolates could be distinguished (Haas and Patch 1980b). MBC4 could be effectively inactivated by normal mouse serum. Also, pseudotypes formed with an ecotropic MLV envelope induced tumors more rapidly in C57BL/6 mice than did MBC4 alone or mixed inocula containing nonpseudotyped MBC4 and an ecotropic MLV. These results led Haas and Patch (1980a) to speculate that pseudotyped virions escaped inactivation by serum factors in vivo and that the long latency period (about 5 months) observed between X-irradiation and overt leukemia in C57BL/6 mice could be accounted for in terms of the frequency of generating pseudotype particles and establishing a stable "carrier" state.

There are at least three instances in which MCF viruses have been isolated from B-cell tumors. MCF virus recovered from a pristane (mineral oil)-induced plasmacytoma was neither leukemogenic nor accelerating (Cloyd et al. 1980). Similarly, an MCF virus recently recovered from an Abelson-virus-induced pre-B leukemia was nonleukemogenic for BALB/c mice (Chang et al. 1982). The oncogenicity of the MCF virus isolated from a reticulum cell sarcoma induced by a chronic graft-versus-host response (Armstrong et al. 1980) has not been reported.

3. Association with Erythroproliferative Diseases

MCF virus has been recovered from the spleens of animals inoculated with the Rauscher virus complex (Van Griensven and Vogt 1980). Ra-MCF induces a slow erythroleukemia (3–6 months) in NIH-Swiss mice and does not have an SFFV-associated gp52 (see Section VIII.B). When injected into adult BALB/c mice as a pseudotype with the Ra-MLV envelope, distinct spleen focus formation is observed 10 days later; Ra-MCF is the only MCF virus with this property.

Spleens of susceptible mouse strains inoculated neonatally with Friend helper virus (Fr-MLV) produce MCF viruses (Troxler and Scolnick 1978; Ishimoto et al. 1981) (see Section VIII.A.4). Unlike Fr-MLV, Fr-MCF alone does not induce any erythroproliferative disease in neonatal or adult mice. However, inoculation with an amphotropic pseudotype of Fr-MCF produces the erythroproliferative disease. In addition, Fr-MLV pseudotypes of Fr-MCF accelerate the development of Fr-MLV disease (Ruscetti et al. 1981). Mice resistant to Fr-MLV disease are also resistant to disease induction by the Fr-MCF(Fr-MLV) pseudotypes. Serological analysis demonstrated that an MCF-specific *env*-related glycoprotein was expressed on the surfaces of spleen and bone marrow cells of resistant mice, and thus virus interference at the level of cell surface receptors was considered to be the basis for the genetically determined resistance (Ruscetti et al. 1981) (see also Sections VIII.A.4 and VIII.A.6.e).

4. A Leukemia-suppressing MCF Isolate

Among the many MCF isolates, so far only one isolate, SMX-1, is known to suppress both spontaneous and MCF-virus-induced leukemia (Stockert et al. 1980). SMX-1 was derived from Mo-MLV passaged in vivo and subsequently passaged and cloned in mouse and cat cells in vitro. Intrathymic inoculation of young adult AKR mice with SMX-1 prior to infection with a leukemogenic MCF virus (strain AKR-69L1) caused a dramatic decrease in the leukemia frequency and increased the latency period by 3–4 months. SMX-1 alone (intrathymically or intraperitoneally) has an even more marked suppression of spontaneous AKR leukemias: More than 6 months after all of the uninoculated controls had died, only 38% of SMX-1 virus-infected mice had developed leukemia. Another nonleukemogenic MCF virus (strain AKR-SC30) was not capable of producing these effects. This finding, together with analysis of the antigenic phenotypes of different MCF strains, suggested that interference was unlikely to be mediated by cross-immunization.

Stockert et al. (1980) also found that, although SMX-1 persisted in the thymus for long periods of time, it did not cause any gross morphological changes in the thymic architecture, nor did it modify the frequency of several T-cell subclasses. Thus, these authors concluded that elimination of the target cells (i.e., a virus-induced thymectomy or a virus-induced differentiation to more mature cells) was not involved in the protective mechanisms. On the other hand, the expected amplification of G_{IX} antigen and other MLV-related antigens on the surfaces of thymocytes, which occurs in preleukemic mice (Kawashima et al. 1976; O'Donnell et al. 1980), was not detected in mice infected with the SMX-1 virus, although the titers of endogenous ecotropic MLV in the thymus remained unchanged. Stockert et al. (1980) concluded that the most plausible explanation of the inhibitory effects of SMX-1 virus was a specific cross-interference, preventing superinfection of the target cells by the exogenous leukemogenic MCF virus and/or suppressing the generation or spread of an endogenous MCF.

5. *Overview*

The salient features of MCF lymphomagenesis described above may be presented in a few key points.

1. Isolates from nonneoplastic tissue are not leukemogenic and do not enhance in the acceleration test, unless they are derived from the preleukemic target tissues of high-incidence strains.
2. Isolates from neoplastic tissues other than leukemias or lymphomas are not leukemogenic, nor do they accelerate leukemia.
3. MCFs are regularly present in spontaneous thymomas and in X-radiation-induced thymomas in some strains.
4. MCF genomes apparently encode target specificity, i.e., those derived from thymomas induce thymomas, those from B-cell lymphomas induce B-cell lymphomas, and those from erythroleukemias induce erythroleukemias.

5. MCFs may be more or less leukemogenic than their ecotropic parent.
6. MCFs can be generated by exogenous MLV infection.
7. Host genes regulate the ability to generate MCF virus following exogenous infection.
8. Host-resistance genes regulate MCF attachment and penetration.
9. MCF viruses exhibit target-cell tropism for infection.
10. High ecotropic MLV expression in the host enhances the leukemogenicity of certain weakly oncogenic MCF viruses, although the latency period is prolonged, compared with that observed with potently leukemogenic MCF viruses.
11. The formation of pseudotype particles with ecotropic envelopes and MCF genomes generally increases the incidence and decreases the latency of leukemogenic MCF strains. This may be a function of protecting the virus from inactivation by serum factors that specifically bind to xenotropic MLV envelope antigenic determinants on MCF virions. Presumably, inhibition by these factors is circumvented in the target tissue by cell-to-cell spread of virus.
12. At least one nonleukemogenic MCF isolate can significantly inhibit spontaneous leukemia and interfere with exogenous leukemogenic MCF tumor induction.

The foregoing discussion has presented evidence that MCF viruses may be the proximal cause of T-cell leukemias in mice. Nevertheless, a number of unresolved questions remain. The success of immunotherapy during early postnatal life with antisera to ecotropic MLV components (see Section IX.A.6) suggests that critical events occur during a period in which no MCF-virus-specific gene expression is detected. This stage could involve the "preleukemic" transformation of a particular T-cell subset or a substantial period of ecotropic virus replication necessary to generate rare recombinants. Is it possible that chemical carcinogens and X-irradiation also function in this role? What happens during the latency period of several months? One can speculate that there is a requirement for the proliferation and expansion of the preleukemic clone or that several recombinational events must occur before a potently leukemogenic MCF virus is generated. Finally, the absence of identifiable *onc* genes in MCF genomes leaves us with the problem of how the MCF virus, with its virus-virus and virus-cell interactions, actually mediates leukemogenesis.

C. Leukemia and Neurological Disease in Wild Mice

For many years, Gardner and his associates have been studying the natural history of tumors and neurological disease among wild mice from several locâles in California (for review, see Gardner 1978; Gardner et al. 1980c). Early studies using cell-free filtrates from diseased tissue produced lymphomas and paralysis in neonatally infected inbred mice (Officer et al. 1973), but the later virological studies indicated that the inocula consisted of mixtures of ecotropic, xenotropic, and amphotropic MLVs that were distinct from MLVs of inbred strains. As discussed in Chapter 2, amphotropic viruses show the broad host range of the polytropic MCF viruses but do not cross-interfere with them and have so far been isolated only from feral mice (Hartley and Rowe 1976; Rasheed et al. 1976). For brevity the amphotropic and ecotropic isolates from wild mice are designated WMA-MLV and WME-MLV, respectively. The xenotropic wild-mouse isolates are apathogenic, like their counterparts from inbred strains of mice.

1. Natural History of Disease in Wild Mice

Mice derived from the Lake Casitas (LC) region are predisposed to both lymphoma and paralysis, whereas mice from other areas remain essentially free of these diseases; the major difference between the wild-mouse populations is the occurrence of viremia in the former group. LC mice also have a higher incidence of epithelial tumors; however, these are not thought to be associated with any retrovirus (Gardner et al. 1976b). LC mice can be divided into two classes: viremic and nonviremic. Among the viremic LC group, there is maternal transmission, mainly in the milk, of predominantly, if not exclusively, WMA-MLV. Early in life, persistent WMA-MLV viremia is established in about 65% of the mice, and the early infection leads to immunological tolerance (Gardner et al. 1976a, 1979b). The final incidences of lymphoma and paralysis are less than 20%, even in mice more than 2 years old. Cell-free extracts from lymphomas invariably contain WMA-MLV, and sometimes WME-MLV, whereas those from paralyzed animals contain WME-MLV only.

Selective inbreeding showed that offspring of nonviremic parents generally remained nonviremic; at 2 years of age, only 20% produce WMA-MLV, and the incidence of lymphoma is significantly reduced, whereas the latency period is increased (Gardner et al. 1979a). Most of the evidence supports the theory that WMA-MLV is endogenous (see Chapter 2); thus, this situation is analogous to the epigenetic milk transmission of MMTV in C3H mice, and the derivation of the nonviremic LC subline resembles that of the C3Hf substrain derived by foster nursing (see Section VII.C).

In crosses between AKR mice and LC mice, a gene was described that affects induction of endogenous ecotropic AKR-MLV without restricting expression of WMA-MLV (Gardner et al. 1980b). The gene, designated *Akvr-1,* is dominant for resistance (to AKR-MLV induction) and is polymorphic in the LC population, whereas AKR mice carry the recessive allele. Mice homozygous or heterozygous for the resistance allele show a marked suppression of spontaneous thymoma development and are also resistant to thymoma induction by exogenous MLV. *Akvr-1* appears to be identical with the *Fv-4* gene described for Japanese mice (see Section VIII.A.6.c). These data support the hypothesis that ecotropic MLV expression early in life is necessary for thymoma development (see Section IX.B.5).

2. Neurological Disease

Oldstone et al. (1977, 1980) have compared the efficacy of cloned isolates of WME-MLV and WMA-MLV in induction of the lower-limb paralysis. Neonatal infection of susceptible ($Fv\text{-}1^{nn}$) inbred mice with WME-MLV, but not WMA-MLV, leads to neurological disorders within 3 months. The major histopathological features of the slowly progressing disease include: (1) the absence of any inflammatory reactions in the involved neural tissue (a marked contrast with the immunopathological reaction in sheep infected with visna virus; see Section XIV), (2) demyelination of the neurons in the anterior horn of the spinal cord, ultimately resulting in neuronal death, and (3) lesions in the cerebellar oligodendrocytes and other brain cells. WME-MLV antigens can be detected in neural tissues at high titers. Viral particles are seen to bud from the plasma membrane of neurons into intracytoplasmic vacuoles, but not into the extracellular space; this is particularly interesting in that neuronal cells are believed to be incapable of cell division, although they can repair cellular DNA damage. Infection with WMA-MLV does not lead to any of these changes, nor can viral antigens be found in neural tissue. Oldstone et al. (1980) have suggested that neural cells may lack receptors for WMA-MLV adsorption/penetration. Passive immunization of neonatal LC mice with antisera to WME-MLV inhibits the development of the neurological syndrome (Gardner et al. 1980a).

3. Lymphoma

The lymphomas that develop in LC mice are probably null cells of B-cell origin (unpublished data of M. Bryant et al., cited in Gardner et al. 1980c); they arise primarily in the spleen and spread to lymph nodes and other organs, whereas the thymus is rarely involved.

Inoculation of neonatal NIH mice with a WME-MLV isolate (strain 4996) produces a 25% incidence of lymphomas at about 10 months postinfection; no paralysis was observed (Rasheed et al. 1977). Inoculation with WMA-MLV has a longer latency period (Gardner 1978). Comparison of these data with the results obtained with uncloned mixtures in earlier studies suggests that mixed virus inocula (perhaps containing pseudotype particles) may be more efficient in lymphoma induction.

X. PATHOGENESIS OF DISEASES INDUCED BY FELINE LEUKEMIA AND SARCOMA VIRUSES

A. Diseases Induced by FeLV and FeSV

Diseases due to the feline leukemia and sarcoma viruses are the most frequent nonaccidental cause of death among pet cats. FeLV can infect many different cell types, but it replicates best in rapidly dividing cells of the bone-marrow and lymphoid tissues, where it causes both neoplastic and nonneoplastic diseases (Table 8.8) (Hardy 1980b). For example, lymphosarcoma is an FeLV-induced neoplastic disease of lymphocytes, erythremic myelosis is a neoplastic disease of erythroid precursor cells, and myelogenous leukemia is a neoplastic disease of the granulocytes. However,

Table 8.8 Feline leukemia virus diseases

Cell type	Proliferative diseases (neoplastic)	Degenerative diseases (blastopenic)
	(a) *Diseases known to be caused by FeLV*	
Lymphoid cells	lymphosarcoma	thymic atrophy (kittens) primary lymphoid depletion diseases secondary immunosuppressive diseases
Bone-marrow cells	myeloproliferative diseases	myelodegenerative diseases
primitive mesenchymal cell	reticuloendotheliosis	
erythroblast	erythremic myelosis	erythroblastosis (regenerative anemia)
erythroblast → / myeloblast →	erythroleukemia	erythroblastopenia (nonregenerative anemia) pancytopenia
myeloblast	granulocytic leukemias (neutrophilic)	myeloblastopenia syndrome neutropenias
megakaryocyte	megakaryocytic leukemia	thrombocytopenia
fibroblast	myelofibrosis	—
osteoblast	medullary osteosclerosis	—
	osteochondromatosis	—
Kidney	—	FeLV immunocomplex glomerulonephritis
	(b) *Diseases thought to be caused by FeLV*	
Placenta and uterus	—	abortions and resorptions
Neural cells	—	neurologic syndrome
	(c) *FeSV disease*	
Skin fibroblasts	multicentric fibrosarcomas	—

FeLV causes more degenerative (blastopenic) diseases than neoplastic diseases of cells that replicate the virus, and more cats die from the nonneoplastic FeLV diseases than from FeLV-induced cancers. Thymic atrophy in kittens and immunosuppression in adult cats are degenerative diseases of the lymphocytes and granulocytes, FeLV-induced anemias are degenerative diseases of erythroid cells, and the FeLV myeloblastopenia is a nonneoplastic disease of granulocytic leukocytes. FeLV is also thought to cause fetal abortions and resorptions by damaging the maternal-fetal attachment. In rare cases, FeLV recombines with cellular genes to produce FeSV, a highly virulent virus that causes multicentric fibrosarcomas in young cats (see Chapters 4 and 9).

1. Neoplastic Diseases

a. Lymphosarcoma. Feline lymphosarcoma is the most frequent, naturally occurring mammalian lymphosarcoma and accounts for approximately one-third of all feline tumors (Dorn et al. 1968). Although FeLV causes lymphosarcomas in cats, seroepidemiological studies have shown that about 30% of all feline lymphosarcomas lack FeLV antigens (Hardy et al. 1980b; Francis et al. 1981). In a large study of 1612 pet cats, it was discovered that there is an epidemiologic association between exposure to FeLV and the development of FeLV-negative lymphosarcomas (Hardy et al. 1980b). The epidemiology of FeLV-negative lymphosarcoma is, in fact, remarkably similar to that of FeLV-positive lymphosarcoma. In one study of 528 FeLV-exposed cats, 389 were antigen-negative, and 11 of these 389 apparently uninfected cats developed FeLV-negative lymphosarcoma in a 3.5-year period, whereas none of the 1074 unexposed, uninfected cats developed lymphosarcoma during the same period. This difference in occurrence is statistically highly significant and suggests that FeLV causes FeLV-negative as well as FeLV-positive lymphosarcomas. It thus appears that the oncogenic function of FeLV is not dependent on continual replication of the virus in transformed cells.

Four major forms of feline lymphosarcoma can be distinguished according to the distribution of the major lesions (Crighton 1969). They are, in order of frequency of occurrence: (1) the multicentric form, in which the tumors occur in various lymphoid and nonlymphoid organs; (2) the thymic form, in which the tumors are located in the thymus of young cats; (3) the alimentary form, which often occurs in old cats and in which the primary tumor is found in the gastrointestinal tract and/or mesenteric lymph nodes; and (4) the unclassified form, which occurs only rarely and in which the tumors are found in nonlymphoid tissues such as the skin, eyes, and central nervous system. The frequencies of detection of FeLV antigen in the different forms of lymphosarcomas differ markedly. For example, approximately 76% of the cats with intestinal and skin lymphosarcomas are FeLV-negative, whereas about 80% of the cats with thymic and multicentric lymphosarcomas are FeLV-positive (Hardy 1980b). Most feline lymphosarcomas are T-cell tumors, although the intestinal form is predominantly a B-cell tumor (Hardy et al. 1978). All lymphosarcomas, regardless of their FeLV status, have been found to express the poorly defined feline oncovirus cell-membrane antigen (FOCMA) (see below) on their cell membranes (Essex et al. 1977; Hardy et al. 1977).

b. Myeloproliferative Diseases. FeLV replicates in all nucleated cells of the bone marrow of cats and induces a group of neoplastic diseases of bone-marrow cells known as myeloproliferative diseases (MPDs) that may involve any one or a combination of bone-marrow cell types (Table 8.8) (Cotter et al. 1975; Hardy 1980b, 1981a). There are four types of MPDs in cats: (1) erythremic myelosis, a marked proliferation of erythroid cells; (2) erythroleukemia, a neoplastic disease of both erythroid and granulocytic myeloid precursor cells; (3) granulocytic leukemia, a neoplastic disease of granulocytic myeloid cells (most often neutrophils); and (4) myelofibrosis, a proliferation of fibroblasts and cancellous bone resulting in medullary osteosclerosis and myelofibrosis. MPDs are characterized by the occurrence of abnormal cells in the blood and bone marrow and by profound nonregenerative anemias. The FeLV MPDs are very similar to those hematopoietic diseases that are induced by the acute transforming retroviruses of chickens.

c. FeSV Multicentric Fibrosarcomas. At the present time, six isolates of FeSV have been obtained from pet cats with multicentric fibrosarcomas (Snyder and Theilen 1969; Gardner et al. 1970; McDonough et al. 1971; Irgens et al. 1973; Hardy 1980c; Hardy et al. 1982). FeSVs are formed by the recombination of the FeLV genome with a cellular *onc* sequence (see Chapters 4 and 9). Fibrosarcomas account for between 6% and 12% of all cat tumors and usually occur in old cats as solitary tumors (Hardy 1980c). In young FeLV-infected pet cats, however, FeSV-induced fibrosarcomas occur very rarely as multiple subcutaneous tumors, which are anaplastic, rapidly growing, and often metastatic. One strain of FeSV can induce melanomas as well as fibrosarcomas (McCullough et al. 1972). There is no evidence that FeSV is contagious among pet cats, and each FeSV may arise de novo in any FeLV-infected cat.

FeSVs are found as pseudotypes with a defective FeSV genome in a virion derived from FeLV (see Chapter 4). Since the FeLV envelope governs the host range of the FeSV and since FeLV-B, with a wide host range, has been found in all natural FeSV isolates, FeSVs also have a wide host range (see Chapter 2). FeSVs can infect and transform mink, guinea pig, rabbit, dog, cat, pig, goat, sheep, bovine, primate, and human cells (Hardy 1980c).

2. FeLV Anemias

FeLV-induced anemias are very common FeLV-caused diseases in pet cats (Hardy 1980b). FeLV induces three distinct types of anemias (Hardy 1981b): (1) FeLV erythroblastosis (regenerative anemia), (2) FeLV erythroblastopenia (nonregenerative anemia), and (3) FeLV pancytopenia. FeLV erythroblastosis occurs in only about 15–18% of FeLV-infected cats with anemias (Mackey et al. 1975; Cotter 1979; Maggio 1979; Hardy 1981b; Hoover et al. 1974) and is characterized by the presence of immature erythrocytes in the blood in response to the anemia. This form of FeLV-induced anemia often progresses into the erythroblastopenia form. FeLV erythroblastopenia is also known as pure red-cell aplasia and is the most commonly occurring FeLV-induced anemia in pet cats. It is a nonregenerative anemia that is characterized by mature erythrocytes and few or no immature erythroid cells, progressing to profound anemias and death. FeLV pancytopenia is characterized by a marked reduction in all hematopoietic cells (profound anemias and leukopenia), and, in some cats, it is accompanied by myelofibrosis.

The mechanism by which FeLV induces anemias is not known. Possible mechanisms include an immune attack on viral antigens in red-cell membranes and an inhibition of erythroid cell growth or development by replicating virus.

3. FeLV Immunopathologic Diseases

FeLV-induced immunopathologic diseases can occur as a result of (1) immune-cell depletion, (2) immune-cell dysfunctions, and (3) pathogenic-antibody production (Perryman et al. 1972; Essex et al. 1975a; Cockerell et al. 1976; Hardy 1982b). These immune alterations can occur by at least four possible mechanisms. First, FeLV-infected lymphocytes and macrophages may, in some way, be damaged by FeLV replication, and their numbers may thus be reduced or their functions altered (Hoover et al. 1980; Hardy 1982b). In this regard, the FeLV p15(E) has been shown to abrogate feline lymphocyte blastogenesis in vitro, and the presence of soluble p15(E) in infected cats may induce immunosuppression in these cats (Mathes et al. 1978). Second, anti-FeLV antibody or sensitized lymphocytes or macrophages may react with FeLV antigens in the cell membranes of FeLV-infected lymphocytes and neutrophils, causing an immunologic impairment (Yoshiki et al. 1973; O'Brien et al. 1978). Third, persistently infected pet cats have a large amount of soluble FeLV antigen that may elicit an antibody response. Resulting FeLV-antigen–antibody immunocomplexes can then lead to immunocomplex diseases (Weksler et al. 1975; Day et al. 1980; Snyder et al. 1982). Finally, FOCMA antibody produced in infected cats may lyse transformed lymphoid or myeloid cells and result in immunosuppression due to lymphopenias and granulocytopenias (Grant et al. 1978).

a. Secondary FeLV-associated Immunosuppressive Diseases. Immunosuppressive diseases that are not directly caused by FeLV are frequently occurring diseases observed in FeLV-infected cats (Hardy 1982b). More pet cats die of FeLV-associated chronic secondary immunosuppressive diseases than die from lymphosarcoma. In these cats, there is no FeLV-induced lymphoid depletion, and the formation of immunocomplexes or the occurrence of soluble p15(E) may cause immunosuppression in these cats. FeLV-infected pet cats have been found to have circulating, infectious FeLV complexed with IgG (Hardy 1980b), and soluble FeLV gp70, p27, p15, and p12 antigens have been found as immunocomplexes with IgG in some infected cats (Snyder et al. 1982). Approximately 45% of pet cats with such chronic diseases as feline infectious peritonitis, chronic stomatitis and gingivitis, chronic nonhealing skin lesions and abscesses, and chronic upper respiratory diseases are infected with FeLV (Hardy 1980b).

b. FeLV-induced Immune-cell Deficiency Diseases. FeLV directly induces a fatal myeloblastopenia syndrome characterized by a severe reduction of all granulocytic leukocytes, anemia, hemorrhagic lymphadenopathy, and hemorrhagic enteritis (Hardy 1980b, 1982). In addition, the virus can induce specific lymphoid depletion diseases such as thymic atrophy in kittens and in adult cats (Anderson et al. 1971; Hoover et al. 1973; Hardy 1980b). The kittens develop a runting syndrome, intercurrent infection, and thymic and lymph node atrophy and die between 8 and 12 weeks of age. In adult cats, FeLV can induce depletion of T-lymphocyte-dependent areas in lymphoid tissues, leading to immunosuppression and death from secondary infectious agents (Hardy 1982b).

c. FeLV Immunocomplex Glomerulonephritis. Glomerulonephritis is thought to be a rare disease in pet cats. Cotter et al. (1975) reported that four out of five persistently FeLV-infected pet cats developed fatal glomerulonephritis without other concurrent FeLV diseases. In a larger study of cats from a single household, Jakowski et al. (1980) found that 29 of the 79 (36.7%) cats that died had glomerulonephritis. Of these 29 cats, 27 were tested for FeLV and 20 (74%) were found to be infected. The mean amount of FeLV proteins was higher in the sera of infected cats that had developed glomerulonephritis than in FeLV-infected healthy cats or infected cats that developed other diseases. Hardy et al. (1982) found FeLV internal antigens, IgG, and complement deposited in the kidneys of 3 of 12 (25%) infected cats with lymphosarcoma, and Anderson and Jarrett (1971) also found glomerulonephritis associated with leukemia in cats.

B. Immunology of FeLV-infected Cells

The cytoplasm of FeLV-infected cells contains large quantities of the FeLV internal p15, p12, p26, and p10 structural protein antigens (Hardy et al. 1973a). These antigens are useful markers of infection (Hardy et al. 1969), and their detection is the basis of the indirect immunofluorescent antibody (IFA) and enzyme-labeled immunoadsorbent assay (ELISA) tests for FeLV (Hardy et al. 1973a; Kahn et al. 1980). FeLV-infected cats can produce antibody to internal viral antigens and to viral reverse transcriptase (Jacquemin et al. 1978), but these antibodies serve no beneficial role. In fact, antibodies to FeLV internal-antigens can be harmful if they complex with FeLV antigens to form circulating immunocomplexes, which can have several deleterious effects, such as immunosuppression and kidney damage (Section X.A.3).

There are three different subgroups of FeLV envelope antigens that result in three immunologically distinct serotypes of FeLV: FeLV-A, FeLV-B, and FeLV-C (see Chapter 2) (Jarrett et al.

1973a; Sarma et al. 1973). Antibody to the envelope antigens can neutralize FeLV, and some pet cats are protected from FeLV infection by high titers of this antibody (Sarma et al. 1974; Hardy et al. 1976c; Russell and Jarrett 1978). The ability to produce FeLV-neutralizing antibody can thus be of great biological value to exposed cats, but it can also result in the formation of immunocomplexes and have detrimental effects in persistently infected cats (Snyder et al. 1982).

FeLV-infected tumor cells and FeSV-transformed cells, unlike FeLV-infected normal cells, express an antigen on their cell surfaces, i.e., the feline oncornavirus-associated cell-membrane antigen of FOCMA, which does not appear to be an FeLV subgroup-A or subgroup-B structural antigen (Essex et al. 1977; Hardy et al. 1977). Antibody to FOCMA prevents the development of lymphosarcoma and FeSV-induced multicentric fibrosarcomas in pet cats (Essex et al. 1971, 1975b). FOCMA is discussed in greater detail below.

C. Transmission

Many pet cats are exposed to FeLV at some time in their lives, but relatively few become persistently infected with the virus (Hardy 1980a). The most common vehicle of infection is the saliva, which can contain over 10^6 infectious viral particles per milliliter (Gardner et al. 1971; Francis et al. 1977). Since FeLV is also present in the blood of persistently infected cats, it is possible that blood-sucking insects, such as cat fleas, may act as vectors, and it has been shown that the virus can be spread iatrogenically via blood transfusions (Hardy 1980a). In the natural environment, it is probable that mutual grooming enables the virus to gain entry via the ocular, nasal, or respiratory membranes. The first organs in which FeLV replicates after infection are the tonsils and lymph nodes of the head and neck (Rojko et al. 1979). If the cat produces an adequate titer of neutralizing antibody at this stage of the infection, it will become immune to further infection by FeLV of the same serotype and will resolve the current virus infection. If no neutralizing antibody is produced, the virus will spread to the hematopoietic stem cells of bone marrow, where it replicates chronically. It is at this stage that large amounts of FeLV enter the bloodstream, both as free circulating virus and in the white blood cells. From the blood, the virus can spread to many different tissues, including the kidneys and salivary glands, and from these organs it is shed into the environment.

D. Pathogenesis by FeLV

1. Feline Leukemia Virus

FeLV is a replication-competent chronic leukemia virus, and, like other chronic leukemia viruses, it lacks a viral transforming gene (see Chapter 9). No acute FeLVs, such as the defective leukemia viruses of chickens, have been discovered. The mechanism by which FeLV induces leukemia is at present unknown. It has been suggested that the immunosuppression induced by viruses such as FeLV may permit spontaneously transformed cells to grow into a tumor (Dent 1972). Most FeLV-infected cats, however, die of immunosuppressive diseases before they develop lymphosarcomas (Hardy 1980b).

A major difficulty in the study of the FeLV-host interactions in cats is the presence of endogenous FeLV-related DNA sequences (Benveniste et al. 1975) (Chapter 10). These sequences occur at 8–10 copies per haploid genome, but FeLV cannot be induced as virus from uninfected cells (Benveniste et al. 1975; Koshy et al. 1979). The presence of these sequences in cat cells hinders molecular studies of exogenously acquired FeLV proviruses. Recently, Casey et al. (1981) prepared U_3- and U_5-specific probes of the FeLV LTRs. They found about 150 copies of the U_5 sequence in the DNA of uninfected cat cells, indicating that the U_5 region of the FeLV LTR is closely related to the endogenous proviruses and that LTRs may greatly outnumber full proviruses in the germ lines of domestic cats. In contrast, the U_3 region common to exogenous FeLV subgroups, A, B, and C anneals poorly to uninfected cat DNA, suggesting that (as in the avian system) endogenous and exogenous viruses differ markedly in the U_3 region.

Using the FeLV U_3 probe to detect exogenous FeLV sequences acquired by infection, Casey et al. (1981) found that, in some cases, exogenously acquired FeLV proviruses were present at the same sites in most or all of the cells of virus-positive cat lymphosarcomas, indicating a monoclonal origin of these tumors. However, the pattern of integration appeared different in each tumor. In other lymphosarcomas, the exogenous FeLV proviral sequences were present at different sites in cells from a single tumor, indicating that the tumors might be polyclonal. As discussed later in this section, approximately 30% of feline lymphosarcomas produce no FeLV antigens and no infectious FeLV (Hardy et al. 1980b; Francis et al. 1981). In recent studies, an epidemiological association between FeLV-negative lymphosarcomas and exposure to FeLV has been found (Hardy et al. 1980b; Francis et al. 1981). However, using the U_3 probe, no exogenous U_3 sequences were found in six FeLV-negative lymphosarcomas. Thus, although there is an epidemiologic association with exposure to FeLV in these virus-negative lymphosarcomas, there is no evidence of exogenous FeLV sequences in the tumor cells. If virus infection is required for oncogenic transformation, the viral DNA (or at least its U_3 region) must subsequently be lost. Alternatively, in these cases the virus may have contributed to the appearance of disease indirectly, e.g., by impairing the immune response to tumor cells.

E. Epidemiology

1. *Detection of FeLV Infection*

The IFA and ELISA tests for *gag* determinants are the most widely used methods for detecting FeLV in pet cats (Hardy et al. 1973a; Kahn et al. 1980). Studies using the IFA test have shown that FeLV is a contagious virus and that its spread can be prevented by removing infected cats from contact with other cats (Hardy et al. 1976a; Weijer and Daams 1978). These tests are now widely used to help prevent contagion and to aid in the diagnosis of the FeLV-induced diseases.

2. *FeLV Occurrence in Healthy Pet Cats*

The occurrence of FeLV in the natural cat population is dependent on the environment (Hardy 1980a). Less than 1% of healthy stray cats are persistently infected. However, in some environments where healthy cats are exposed to multiple FeLV-infected or -diseased cats for prolonged periods, an average of 30% of the exposed healthy cats are persistently infected. In households with multiple cats and no history of FeLV diseases, less than 1% of the cats are infected with the virus. These findings show that, unless there is prolonged direct contact between infected and uninfected cats, the occurrence of persistent FeLV infection is low.

F. Immune Response to FeLV

Cats can produce neutralizing antibody to the FeLV envelope antigens and antibodies to FOCMA that appear to be protective against lymphosarcoma (Table 8.9). Only approximately 30% of cats heavily exposed to FeLV become persistently infected (Hardy 1980a). Of the remainder, 30% remain susceptible to infection and 40% become immune to FeLV. Seroepidemiologic studies have shown that the production of both FeLV-neutralizing and FOCMA antibodies is dependent on environmental exposure to FeLV and that many cats producing FeLV-neutralizing antibody also produce FOCMA antibody. The immune response in these cats probably develops while the FeLV infection is localized and small numbers of FOCMA-bearing cells are present only in the lymph nodes of the head and neck. By determining the FeLV status, FeLV-neutralizing antibody titer, and FOCMA antibody titer, healthy pet cats have been classified into one of six immune categories (Table 8.9) (Hardy et al. 1976c; Hardy 1980a). Cats belonging to each of the six categories have been found in the natural environment. It is important to realize that the classification of a cat into one of the six categories is dynamic and may change with time because it depends on the environmental exposure to FeLV and on the immune response of the cat. For example, many susceptible (class 1) cats become immune to infection (class 4) after exposure. Furthermore, studies by McClelland et al. (1980) have shown that 83% of infected, but otherwise healthy, cats die within 3.5 years.

G. FOCMA

The feline oncornavirus-associated cell-membrane antigen, FOCMA, was first described by Essex and his coworkers (1971) as an antigen detected by an immunofluorescent antibody (IFA) reaction of certain cat sera with membranes of viable FL74 feline lymphosarcoma cells producing all three subgroups of FeLV (Theilen et al.

Table 8.9 Immune classes of healthy pet cats

Class	Exposure history	% Occurrence in cat population	FeLV status	Protective FeLV neutralizing antibody (≥1:10)	Protective FOCMA antibody (≥1:32)	Susceptibility or resistance to FeLV infection	Susceptibility or resistance to lymphosarcoma development
1	unexposed or exposed[a]	60.8	–	–	–	susceptible	susceptible
2	exposed	4.6	–	–	+	susceptible	resistant
3	exposed	5.4	–	+	–	resistant	susceptible
4	exposed	14.2	–	+	+	resistant	resistant
5	exposed	11.3	+	–	–	infected	very susceptible
6	exposed	3.7	+	–	+	infected	resistant

[a]Exposure in these cats was not enough to infect or to induce FeLV-neutralizing antibody or FOCMA antibody.

1969). The sera exhibiting FOCMA reactivity were obtained from cats that had been experimentally inoculated with FeSV(FeLV) and that had developed and rejected sarcomas. In addition to the apparent correlation between FOCMA antibody and regression of FeSV(FeLV)-induced sarcomas, Essex et al. (1975c) found a correlation between high titers of FOCMA antibody and resistance to development of lymphosarcoma in FeLV-inoculated cats (Essex et al. 1975d) and pet cats (Essex et al. 1975e). FOCMA antibody therefore appears to play a role in immunosurveillance of naturally occurring, feline-retrovirus-induced tumors (Essex et al. 1975a).

FOCMA can be detected on the surfaces of FeLV- and FeSV-(FeLV)-transformed cells by the original direct IFA test or by an antibody absorption test (Essex et al. 1971; Hardy et al. 1977, 1978). However, it should be noted that the antigens detected by direct versus absorption tests need not be serologically identical. In either test, serum from naturally exposed, persistently FeLV-infected cats, lacking detectable antibody to FeLV structural proteins, is used to assay for FOCMA. The antigens have been found on both FeLV-positive and apparently FeLV-negative cat lymphosarcoma cells, on FeSV(FeLV)-producing cat fibrosarcoma cells, and on FeLV-transformed lymphoid, myeloid, and erythroid cells of pet cats regardless of whether they contain replicating FeLV (Hardy et al. 1977; Essex et al. 1977; Hardy et al. 1978). FOCMA has not been detected on FeLV-infected normal fibroblasts. FOCMA antibody also appears distinct from neutralizing antibodies to FeLV subgroups A and B or from the internal FeLV virion proteins encoded by the viral *gag* gene (Charman et al. 1976; Hardy et al. 1976a; Essex et al. 1977; Stephenson et al. 1977; Snyder et al. 1980). FOCMA does not cross-react with antigens induced by the endogenous feline RD114 virus or with retroviral antigens from several other isolates, including MLV and ALV (Essex et al. 1976). Snyder and coworkers (1978) have isolated a 70,000-dalton protein from FeLV-producing FL74 cells that is distinct from the viral gp70 of FeLV subgroup A or B and that appears to contain FOCMA. It thus appears that FOCMA is tumor-specific and distinct from the viral structural proteins of the most prevalent FeLV subgroups.

Certain cat sera reactive to FL74 cells in the direct IFA test also exhibited viable cell immunofluorescence with mink cells nonproductively transformed by GA-FeSV, but not by several other mammalian sarcoma viruses (Sliski et al. 1977). Sera from viremic animals showed analogous end point titers whether tested on FeSV-transformed mink nonproducer cells or cat lymphosarcoma cells productively infected with FeLV (Sliski and Essex 1979). The lack of reactivity of these sera with FeLV-infected fibroblasts suggested the presence of an FeSV-associated, cross-reactive antigen, now designated FOCMA-S to distinguish it from the antigen (FOCMA-L) expressed on cat lymphosarcoma cells (Sherr et al. 1978a,b). Sera reactive to FOCMA-S, expressed on FeSV-transformed mink or rat cells, showed diminished IFA titers after absorption with FeSV pseudotype particles containing the FeSV-coded polyprotein $p85^{gag-fes}$) (Sherr et al. 1978a) or with the partially purified polyprotein itself (Sherr et al. 1978b). However, rats bearing tumors induced by FeSV produce sera that react strongly with *v-fes*-coded antigens but have not shown immunofluorescence with intact FeSV-transformed cells and do not specifically precipitate metabolically labeled products from cat FL74 cells (Ruscetti et al. 1980a; Sherr et al. 1980). Thus, FOCMA-L and FOCMA-S do not appear to be identical antigenic determinants. It is similarly unclear whether antibodies to FOCMA-S participate in immunosurveillance against tumors induced by the feline retroviruses.

H. Prevention of FeLV Infection

The spread of FeLV and the occurrence of FeLV diseases in the cat population can be prevented in two ways: (1) by removal of FeLV-infected carrier cats and (2) by vaccination (Jarrett et al. 1974; Hardy et al. 1976a; Hardy 1980a; Olsen et al. 1976, 1980).

1. FeLV Test and Removal Program

At present, the only readily available means for preventing the spread of FeLV is the removal method, using an FeLV test to identify the infected cats (Hardy et al. 1976a). All infected cats are removed from affected households and are isolated completely from other cats or subjected to euthanasia. The household is then cleaned with detergents and quarantined so that no new cats are allowed to enter or leave. After 3 months to allow any incubating virus in the remaining cats to become detectable in the FeLV test, the cats are retested. If they are all negative, the household is declared free of the virus; if some cats have become infected, they are removed, and the remaining cats are tested a third time 3 months later. This "test-and-removal" program has proved to be remarkably effective in protecting uninfected cats from FeLV infections and has reduced infection rates by as much as 40-fold (Hardy et al. 1976a; Weijer and Daans 1978).

2. FeLV Vaccines

The FeLV vaccine that would be the easiest to produce on a large scale, an attenuated live-virus vaccine, is not available. Furthermore, it may prove difficult to develop a live vaccine, since even a virus that did not induce relatively rapid disease might induce lymphosarcoma at some time after infection (Pedersen et al. 1979; Hardy et al. 1980b; Hardy 1981a). Vaccines produced from heat-, UV-, and formaldehyde-killed FeLVs have been studied by several groups, but they have generally not been found to be effective (Olsen et al. 1976; Yohn et al. 1976). In fact, in one study, kittens were found to be more susceptible to FeLV infection after inoculation with a combination of killed FeLV and FL74 lymphosarcoma cells (Yohn et al. 1976). An FeLV "subunit" vaccine composed of only the outer viral envelope components would be worth testing; unfortunately, such a vaccine would be the most difficult to produce (Salerno et al. 1978). A soluble tumor-cell vaccine containing FeLV gp70 and FOCMA appears promising (Olsen et al. 1980). Although an effective FeLV vaccine is still not available, recent advances in recombinant DNA technology may provide a means whereby the FeLV envelope components can be synthesized economically in relatively large amounts.

I. Treatment of Lymphosarcoma

Lymphosarcoma is the only FeLV disease—and probably the only retrovirus-induced disease—that has been frequently treated. Combined chemotherapy with vincristine, L-asparaginase, cyclophosphamide, and methotrexate has had only limited success (Hardy 1981a). Several different forms of immunotherapy have been attempted in cats with lymphosarcoma. Complete regression has been achieved by infusion of large quantities of whole blood, plasma, or serum from a normal cat, but not with the same material heat-inactivated at 56° C for 30 minutes (Hardy et al. 1976b). It was thus concluded that, as with serum therapy of AKR mice with leukemia (Kassel et al. 1973), complement played a major role in the antileukemic effect. In this regard, it should be noted that Kobilinsky et al. (1979) found that FeLV-infected cats with lymphosarcoma have reduced complement activity. In another study, cats with lymphosarcoma were treated with small quantities of cat serum that contained high titers of FOCMA antibody (Hardy et al. 1980a). Of 14 cats treated, 8 cats had complete regression of their disease and 3 cats had partial regression. Thus, it may be possible to lyse lymphosarcoma cells in vivo, as in vitro (Grant et al. 1978), by infusion of antibody to FOCMA.

Finally, a promising new form of immunotherapy has been reported in FeLV-infected cats with lymphosarcoma. This form of therapy involves removal of circulating immunocomplexes from the cat's plasma by passage of the cat's serum over a column containing *Staphylococcus aureus* Cowan I, followed by return of the clarified plasma to the cat (Jones et al. 1980a,b). Protein A on the surface of the bacterium removes free IgG, and IgG complexed as immunocomplexes, by attachment to the Fc fragment of the IgG molecule. Analyses of the immunocomplexes eluted from the *S. aureus* have shown that they contain FeLV gp70, p27, p15, and p12, with their corresponding antibodies (Snyder et al. 1982). Several pet cats treated with this ex vivo immunosorption therapy have had regression of their lymphosarcomas and complete reversal of their FeLV infections. After the cats became FeLV-negative, there was detectable FeLV gp70 antibody in their sera, along with a decrease in the amount of circulating immunocomplexes to normal levels. This form of therapy appears to hold promise for chronic virus infections and immunocomplex-mediated diseases.

XI. PATHOGENESIS OF BOVINE LEUKEMIA VIRUS

Bovine leukemia virus (BLV) is responsible for the disease known as enzootic bovine leukosis or lymphosarcoma in cattle. Historically, the disease seems to have been originally confined to eastern Europe (Bendixen 1963), but the exportation of cattle in this century from the endemic region to previously leukosis-free areas spread the disease worldwide and created a vast economic problem (for review, see Burny et al. 1980).

The recognition of clusters of high-incidence herds suggested that the disease was infectious, but evidence for a virus etiology awaited isolation of BLV from leukemic lymphocytes (Miller et al. 1969b) and detection of antibodies, in the serum of infected animals, that specifically reacted with viral antigens (Ferrer et al. 1972; Miller and Olson 1972). Virtually 100% of the cattle in multiple-case herds are BLV-positive (Ferrer et al. 1976; Piper et al. 1979).

The course of BLV infection and pathogenesis may be viewed as a multistage process: Infection can occur without clinical symptoms, then progress to "persistent lymphocytosis" (in which the number of circulating lymphocytes increases), and finally result in tumor production. Progression from one stage to the next shows extreme variation in both incidence and time course. Inoculation of newborn or young calves leads to detectable virus in the spleen and blood within 2 weeks, with humoral antibody production commencing anytime from 2 months after inoculation onward. These antibodies are reactive with *gag-*, *pol-*, and *env*-gene products (the last including neutralizing activity), and cell-mediated immunity can also be demonstrated. These immune responses could account, in part, for the finding that only a low but significant percentage of BLV-infected cattle develop lymphosarcoma or acute leukemia. The persistent lymphocytosis stage may begin within a few months after infection or only first occur as long as 10 years later, and the condition may remain stable for many years. Tumors are never seen in animals less than 2 years of age, with a mean value of about 6 years. The final incidence in any country is a reflection of the number of low-leukemia and high-leukemia herds; in some regions the frequency is 5–20/100,000 and in others, as high as 165/100,000 (for review, see Burny et al. 1980). Spread within herds occurs quite readily but does not extend to neighboring herds. Epidemiological evidence suggests that genetic and environmental factors influence the pace of progression through these stages, although none of these factors have yet been identified.

As discussed in Chapter 2, BLV is an exogenous virus, thus ruling out the possibility of genetic transmission. Natural transmission occurs via two routes: congenital infection involving transmission by the placenta (Piper et al. 1979) or by infected milk (Miller and Van Der Maaten 1979; Ferrer et al. 1981) and horizontal transmission. The latter is probably the more important mode of BLV infection. Healthy cattle brought into contact with BLV-infected animals soon show the presence of BLV-positive lymphocytes and develop antiviral antibodies. Horizontal transmission may occur through several means: exposure to BLV-infected excretions such as urine (Gupta and Ferrer 1980), mediation by blood-sucking insects (Bech-Nielsen et al. 1978), and contamination via artificial means (e.g., common equipment or instruments used by the handlers). However, congenital infection occurs as well, with about 15% of the calves in multiple-case herds showing evidence of being BLV carriers at birth (Piper et al. 1979). Physical isolation of calves born of BLV-infected cows after a few weeks of nursing shows that transplacental or milk-borne virus transmission is not very efficient for establishing infection (Ferrer and Piper 1981).

B-lymphocytes appear to be the major, and perhaps only, site of BLV replication within the animal (Kenyon and Piper 1977; Paul et al. 1977; Van Der Maaten and Miller 1978). In the acute phase of the disease, mature and immature B-cells increase in the peripheral blood. Many of these cells exhibit abnormal nuclear structures known as nuclear pockets (Miller et al. 1969a; Weber et al. 1969) and also have altered cytochemical and karyotypic characteristics (Marshak et al. 1962; Bendixen 1963; Urbaneck and Wittmann 1969). Tumors composed of mature B-lymphocytes bearing surface immunoglobulin develop most frequently in the pelvic lymph nodes, which are strikingly enlarged, with hemorrhagic and necrotic lesions. Other lymph nodes throughout the body may also be involved; leukemic infiltrates invade mammary glands, subcutaneous tissues, muscle, respiratory tract, and spinal cord, thus influencing the external symptoms of disease such as weight loss, listlessness, and nervous disorders.

Studies on the karyotypes of tumors (Hare et al. 1967) indicate that the tumors are monoclonal in origin. However, there is no consistent abnormality observed from one individual to another. More recently, restriction endonuclease mapping techniques have confirmed the monoclonality (Kettmann et al. 1980). In some animals with multiple tumors, the metastatic lesions are clearly derived from the primary clone, whereas in others it appears that several independently derived clones have become neoplastic. However, the endonuclease mapping technique, when applied to cells obtained during the persistent lymphocytotic stage, indicates that, although the majority of B cells carry the BLV genome, there is no evidence for a predominant clone (Kettmann et al. 1980). This finding is reminiscent of the bursal lymphomas induced in chickens by ALV (see Section IV).

The tumors in terminal cases apparently do not produce BLV particles or synthesize BLV structural proteins in vivo (Baliga and Ferrer 1977; Driscoll and Olson 1977). However, transfer of the lymphocytes to tissue culture, either in cocultures with susceptible cells or with mitogen stimulation, allows infectious BLV production (see Chapter 2). The mechanism of suppression of BLV gene expression in vivo is unknown. It is possible that cytotoxic cells sensitized for BLV antigens eliminate BLV-producing cells; as a result, latent infection would circumvent immunosurveillance processes.

BLV infection can be experimentally transmitted to heterologous hosts. Although inoculation of goats has generally proved apathogenic (Hoss and Olson 1974), one recent report documents the development of a lymphosarcoma in a goat 8 years after inoculation (Olson et al. 1981). The presence of integrated proviral BLV in the tumor substantiates the hypothesis of a BLV etiology. A second heterologous host is the chimpanzee; two animals infected with BLV-containing lymphocytes developed erythroleukemias (McClure et al. 1974). It has not been established whether the leukemic cells contain BLV proviruses.

Sheep are the most important heterologous hosts for BLV infection. Most sheep infected with BLV contain virus-positive lymphocytes and develop a humoral antibody response rapidly, and about 80% succumb with lymphosarcomas within months to several years following infection. However, there is no evidence for horizontal spread following experimental inoculation (Mammerickx et al. 1976; Van Der Maaten and Miller 1976). Thus, sheep provide a less expensive and more easily managed model for experimental studies. Interestingly, there are occasional outbreaks of leukemia in sheep associated with the retrovirus known as ovine leukemia virus (OLV) (Paulsen et al. 1974). OLV and BLV are virtually indistinguishable by serological parameters (see Chapter 2). These findings raise an interesting question: If BLV and OLV are actually one agent, why then do natural outbreaks suggest the occurrence of horizontal spread within sheep flocks? Several possibilities exist: congenital transmission is an important route of spread among sheep (Onuma et al. 1977), infected cattle act as reservoirs for transmitting the virus to sheep, or the clusters of ovine leukemia are due to accidental contamination (e.g., via vaccines from bovine sources).

Many countries prohibit the sale of organs from animals with detectable tumors, and thus disease control is of great commercial importance. To date, eradication programs have relied on detection of high-incidence herds and implementation of slaughter policies. In such instances, a dramatic decline in the incidence of enzootic bovine leukosis is observed within the first few years (Flensburg 1976). However, serological studies have shown that BLV persists in herds even when a long period has elapsed without an outbreak of tumors and that antibodies can be detected in herds with no history of lymphosarcoma (Olson et al. 1973; Baumgartener et al. 1975). For these reasons, vaccination using inactivated BLV has been explored. Although the studies have been based on few animals, this technique appears to be effective against subsequent challenge with virulent virus (Miller and Van Der Maaten 1978; Portetelle et al. 1978). The use of sensitive assays to detect carriers of latent BLV infections (see Chapter 2) should help in designing the most efficacious control protocol.

XII. PATHOGENESIS OF PRIMATE SARCOMA AND LEUKEMIA VIRUSES

Among the numerous isolates of retroviruses from various simian genera (see Chapter 2), only those belonging within the simian sarcoma virus/gibbon ape leukemia virus (SSV/GALV) family have as yet proved to be oncogenic. The Mason-Pfizer monkey virus (MPMV) isolated from a mammary carcinoma of a rhesus monkey and the baboon endogenous viruses (BaEV) readily isolated from tumor and normal tissues have been extensively assayed for oncogenicity, and the results clearly indicate that they are not oncogenic (for review, see Deinhardt 1980). Tests for tumor production by the remaining simian retroviruses have not been reported.

A. Simian Sarcoma Virus/Simian Sarcoma-associated Virus (SSV/SSAV)

The only known retrovirus isolates from a wooly monkey (*Lagothrix* sp.) are the SSV-SSAV complex from a fibrosarcoma that had developed in a young pet monkey in California (Thielen et al. 1971; Wolfe et al. 1971). As discussed in Chapter 2, SSV is a replication-defective fibroblast-transforming virus that was isolated in association with the replication-competent SSAV helper from which it was derived (Wolfe et al. 1972).

The pathological findings in the original animal included anemia, a solid neck tumor, and multiple tumor nodules scattered throughout the peritoneum. The tumors were classified as fibrosarcomas on the basis of the presence of fibroblasts, histiocytes, and occasional syncytia. In the bone marrow, there were focal necrosis, fibrosis, and myeloid metaplasia. Although some of the lymph nodes also showed signs of involvement, the spleen and liver remained normal.

The oncogenicity of the SSV/SSAV complex has been demonstrated in several nonhuman primate species. No effects are seen in galagos but, in squirrel monkeys, regressor nodules form at the site of injection and sometimes in the peritoneum. Histological examination of the nodules reveals an immunoreactive response rather than a neoplastic lesion (Rabin 1971; Theilen et al. 1973). However, the virus complex is oncogenic for neonatal animals in at least four species of marmosets (Wolfe et al. 1971; Deinhardt et al. 1972, 1973). In some cases, the tumors are fibromas that frequently regress within 3 to 6 months. In other cases, slow-growing, well-differentiated fibrosarcomas occur; metastases have been detected in only one animal whose clinical course was observed for more than 1 year. Even very-high-titer stocks of SSV (10^6 focus-forming units) are inefficient in inducing progressive tumors, and the latency period to tumor detection is generally 3 to 6 months (Deinhardt 1980). Chronic production of neutralizing antibodies has been detected (Wolfe and Deinhardt 1972) and could account for this phenomenon. To test this hypothesis, neonatal thymectomies were performed, but they appeared to have no significant effect (unpublished data of D. Johnson and A. Straus, cited in Wolfe and Deinhardt 1972). However, cell-mediated immunity is likely to be involved, since marmosets treated with antithymocyte serum

(ATS) after virus inoculation developed tumors more rapidly than untreated controls, and these tumors regressed when the ATS therapy was stopped. One animal treated with ATS prior to and following infection developed a massive tumor and metastases in lung and kidneys, suggesting that the immunosuppression increased the severity of the disease (unpublished data of D. Johnson and of L. Wolfe and F. Deinhardt, cited in Wolfe and Deinhardt 1972).

Intracerebral inoculation of newborn marmosets is more highly oncogenic than an equal dose of virus delivered by the intramuscular route. In one study, six out of ten animals inoculated intracerebrally developed generally lethal astrocytomas (Wolfe and Deinhardt 1978). The tumors contained pleiomorphic glial cells and were highly vascularized and edematous. Neutralizing antibodies were detected throughout the course of the disease. No tumorigenicity studies using SSAV alone or SSV pseudotyped by other helper viruses have been reported.

SSV is capable of inducing transformation of fibroblasts in vitro (Wolfe et al. 1972). However, a gene product of the putative oncogene (*sis*) has not been definitively identified (see Chapter 9). Markham et al. (1979) have shown that infection of fresh human peripheral blood leukocytes with SSV (or SSAV or GALV) enhances the frequency of obtaining EBV-positive B-lymphoblastoid cell lines. It is not known whether this finding results from a direct effect of these viruses upon B-cell differentiation or from an indirect effect, such as interaction with the latent herpesvirus genome or selective destruction of cytotoxic T cells in the blood-cell population.

B. Gibbon Ape Leukemia Viruses

The incidence of spontaneous malignancies in primates is apparently low (Lingeman et al. 1969) and therefore it was somewhat surprising that numerous hematopoietic tumors, including malignant lymphomas, lymphosarcomas, and granulocytic leukemias, were reported among gibbons (mainly *Hylobates lar*) maintained in captivity at different locations (Newberne and Robinson 1960; DiGiacomo 1967; De Paoli and Garner 1968; Johnson et al. 1971; Jones et al. 1972; De Paoli et al. 1973). The search for an infectious etiology resulted in numerous isolations of GALV from affected tissues. As discussed in Chapters 2 and 6, neither GALV nor SSAV is endogenous to its species of origin, and all of the isolates are highly related. Nonetheless, they can be distinguished on the basis of *env*- and *gag*-gene products and by nucleic acid hybridization. Using such criteria, the GALV isolates have been classified into four subgroups, which also reflect their location of origin.

The GALV-SF (San Francisco) isolates were obtained from two 3.5-year-old animals with lymphosarcomas that developed among six animals used in radiographic studies (Kawakami et al. 1972). The tumors were classified as prolymphocytic leukemias with infiltrations of spleen, liver, and bone marrow (De Paoli et al. 1973; Snyder et al. 1973).

The GALV-SEATO (Thailand) isolates were from tissues of five gibbons with granulocytic leukemia (Kawakami and Buckley 1974); there were also four cases of lymphomas in this colony in the preceding 2 years. All of the tumors developed in animals that had been inoculated with the malarial parasite *Plasmodium falciparum,* isolated from human blood (De Paoli et al. 1973; Kawakami and Buckley 1974; Kawakami et al. 1975). Additional GALV isolates were made from healthy animals (Kawakami et al. 1977), suggesting that infectious transmission occurs readily and that viremia does not necessarily lead to leukemia.

The GALV-Br (Louisiana) isolates were produced from brain tissues of three healthy gibbons that had been housed together in a single cage: two from animals inoculated with brain extracts of human Kuru patients (GBr-2 and GBr-3) and one from an uninoculated control animal (GBr-1) (Todaro et al. 1975).

The most recent isolate, GALV-H, was obtained from tissues of an animal kept on a free-ranging colony on Hall's Island off the coast of Bermuda (Gallo et al. 1978). This animal had disseminated lymphoma, with multifocal infiltration of most organs, from which virus was easily obtained.

The fact that these isolations were made from gibbons in direct contact with humans, and particularly from many inoculated with human materials, and the findings that GALV sequences were not endogenous to gibbon apes led to speculation that humans could be the source or reservoir for GALV. However, there is no seroepidemiological evidence to support this suggestion. It seems more likely that the incidence of tumors among captive animals may be enhanced because of the immunosuppressive effects elicited by the experimental treatments (e.g., irradiation and parasitic infection). For example, it has been demonstrated that mice concurrently infected with plasmodia and MLV show a dramatically increased incidence of virus-induced lymphomas, compared with those inoculated with MLV alone (Widderburn 1970). Nevertheless, it should be remembered that virological studies have not been conducted on gibbons in the wild, and therefore the pattern of natural transmission of the virus is unclear.

Despite the broad host range for infectivity of GALV (Chapter 2), attempts to induce disease in a wide range of unrelated neonatal primates (including marmosets) and nonprimates were not successful (unpublished data cited in Kawakami et al. 1980). However, a single GALV-SEATO isolate from a bone-marrow homogenate of a leukemic gibbon was injected into a few gibbons in a small breeding colony (Sun et al. 1978; Kawakami et al. 1980). Two 1-year-old gibbons developed chronic granulocytic leukemias within 14 months after inoculation, showing symptoms comparable with those reported for the original isolate. The serially passaged extracts were injected intraperitoneally into four young gibbons, ranging in age from 8 to 14 months. Two of these animals were reinoculated (within the medullary region of the femur) several months later. Initially, all infected animals developed transient viremia, followed by production of neutralizing antibody. Two animals remained normal for more than 3 years, whereas the other two showed a recurrence of chronic viremia with a concomitant decline in antibody titers. One of these animals developed myeloproliferative and osteoproliferative diseases 5 months after inoculation. The second animal developed chronic granulocytic leukemia and bone stromal proliferative lesions 11 months after inoculation.

The major hematological pathology included severe anemia (50% reduction) and a gradual increase, over several months, of the total leukocyte counts. At terminal stages, there was a predominant increase in mature granulocytes (25-fold) and monocytes (15-fold). The bone marrow also became cellular, with undifferentiated cells or immature granulocytes, and hepatosplenomegaly suggested evidence for infiltration of other hematopoietic organs. Metastatic lesions were found in the spleen and lung of one animal.

In addition to the myeloproliferative effects, the viremic gibbons developed bone lesions in the long bones of the arm. These lesions progressed with the development of the disease, with circumferential proliferation of the periosteum and areas of lysis within the cortex of the bone.

These results can be interpreted in relationship to other retrovirus-host systems. Unlike the situation with MLV in mice, animals beyond the neonatal stage are susceptible to viral leukemogenesis, and unlike the situation with FeLV in cats, neutralizing antibodies are protective against fulminating viremia and subsequent development of tumors. Furthermore, transmission of GALV between mother and offspring and among contacts can occur; this has been shown for a few breeding pairs (Kawakami et al. 1978a) and by studies of virus isolation and prevalence of humoral antibodies within gibbon colonies (Kawakami et al. 1978b; Krakower et al. 1978). Thus, the situation with GALV in gibbons most closely resembles that seen with BLV in cattle.

XIII. PATHOGENESIS OF EQUINE INFECTIOUS ANEMIA VIRUS

Equine infectious anemia virus (EIAV) causes a naturally occurring disease in all Equidae throughout the world, characterized by viral persistence, immunologically mediated lesions, and a variable clinical course.

In nature, transmission occurs from infected mares to their foals, although viremia can be detected in the absence of clinical symptoms (Kemen and Coggins 1972). Experimental disease is readily induced by the injection of infected blood or cell-free material by any parenteral route. The incubation period varies from 5 days to several months, and the same inoculum given to a group of horses will often result in acute deaths in some, and chronic disease, usually of an episodic nature, with minimal clinical manifestations, in others (Kemeny et al. 1971). The most prominent clinical feature is fever, often accompanied by weight loss, anemia, weakness, terminal depression, and edema (for review, see Henson and McGuire 1974).

The gross histological lesions include splenomegaly, lymphadenopathy, glomerulitis, and alterations in the architecture of the liver due to focal degeneration, including accumulation of lymphocytes and histiocytes (Ishii 1963; Henson et al. 1970; Ishitani 1970; Konno and Yamamoto 1970). Animals dying of the acute disease have lymphoid necrosis, with a lack of mature cells in the lymphoid germinal centers.

After inoculation, there is rapid virus proliferation to high titers in practically all tissues (Kono et al. 1971). Virus replication in circulating and resident macrophages appears to account for the episodic recurrence of viremia (McGuire et al. 1971). Concomitant antibody production occurs (anti-*env* and anti-*gag*) (Tanaka and Sakaki 1962), and most of the circulating virus is found as infectious complexes with antibody (Kono and Kobayashi 1966; Coggins et al. 1972; McGuire et al. 1972). Glomerulitis occurs in horses with active disease because of the deposition of circulating virus-antibody complexes (Banks et al. 1972). Thus, humoral responses are not able to eliminate infectious virus despite the vigorous and long-lasting production of antibody.

The erythrocytes in infected horses are coated with complement and antibodies (Kono 1969; McGuire et al. 1969). It is likely that the antiviral antibodies are responsible for the complement binding. These interactions at the cell surface result in decreased erythrocyte life span, active hemolysis, increased osmotic fragility, and erythrophagocytosis; all of these factors contribute to the severe anemia.

The necrotic lesions are most readily attributable to immunologic reactions resulting from persistence of the virus, deposition of immune reactants on cell surfaces or within tissues, and proliferation and infiltration of sensitized lymphocytes. An animal experiencing frequent exacerbations of disease will have severe lesions, whereas a horse that has been asymptomatic for months may have no lesions. Treatment of experimentally infected horses with immunosuppressants prevents the occurrence of lesions (Henson and McGuire 1971), suggesting that cell-mediated immunity is a major detrimental effect in this disease. Kono et al. (1970) have protected horses from challenge with homologous virus by vaccination with a presumably attenuated virus grown in tissue culture.

The mechanisms of virus persistence are fundamental problems in infectious disease research. The formation of complexes, with subsequent phagocytosis by macrophages, serves as a mechanism for perpetuating the infection rather than inactivating the virus. However, this supposition is not compatible with the protection of vaccinated horses against challenge by virulent virus. Other possible explanations include cell-to-cell spread of virus and antigenic drift at a sufficient rate to escape host mechanisms. The latter would also explain the occurrence of periodic attacks of clinical disease and fever. These possibilities are similar to those propounded for visna virus infections (described more fully in the next section).

XIV. PATHOGENESIS OF LENTIVIRUSES

Some retroviruses, particularly those in the subfamily Lentivirinae, are the cause of naturally occurring nonmalignant diseases of animals with the long incubation period and protracted symptomatic phase characteristic of "slow" infections (Sigurdsson 1954). Such viruses as EIAV (Section XIII) and some of the wild-mouse MLV isolates (Section IX) also fall into this category. The lentiviruses, of which visna is the prototype, comprise a subfamily defined basically on biological behavior (for reviews, see Haase 1975; Nathanson and Robinson 1979; Brahic and Haase 1981); the group includes visna/maedi (Sigurdsson et al. 1957; Gudnadottir and Palsson 1967), zwoegerziekte (DeBoer 1975), progressive pneumonia virus (Kennedy et al. 1968), and an arthritis-inducing virus (unpublished data from O. Narayan and J. Gorham, cited in Narayan et al. [1980]) from sheep, and caprine encephalitis-arthritis virus (CAEV) (Cork et al. 1974a) from goats. Visna, maedi, zwoegerziekte, and progressive pneumonia virus isolates are most likely variants of a single virus. Although various maedi isolates appear more closely related to one another than to visna isolates, and vice versa, there is as yet no correlation of the different disease syndromes (see below) with particular molecular variations. CAEV does exhibit some differences from the visna/maedi group (see Chapter 2), and as yet, little is known about the sheep arthritis isolate. These viruses are categorized together by criteria of morphology, structural composition, antigenic relatedness, and nucleotide sequence homology (see Chapter 2). In tissue-culture cells derived from their natural host, they replicate productively and lytically, typically causing formation of polykaryocytes. The viruses are nontransforming (the controversy regarding this issue is presented in Chapter 2). In their natural hosts in vivo, they are associated not with neoplasms, but with slowly progressive inflammatory destructive lesions. The interesting virus-host interactions involved in slow infections raise a number of novel issues of pathogenesis that are the subject of this section.

Four questions are central to understanding the pathogenesis of slow virus infections of any etiology: (1) How does a virus escape from the immunological surveillance mechanisms of its host over a period of years? (2) How is a virus disseminated in the animal in the face of these defense mechanisms? (3) How does the virus cause the pathological lesions? (4) Why does the infectious process evolve so slowly? Reasonably fundamental and satisfying answers can be put forward for the first two questions, but the last two remain subjects for continued investigation.

A. Lentivirus-induced Diseases

The following descriptions of slow infections caused by lentiviruses are intended to serve as illustrations of these themes and to provide information for a discussion of the mechanisms of disease. Visna-maedi first came to attention in Iceland, where introduction of the virus into a virgin population led to particularly widespread disease, but similar conditions are endemic throughout the world (Palsson 1976). The disease occurs primarily in sheep, but both experimental and natural transmission to goats also occurs. Natural infection of goats has been reported chiefly in India, with less frequent cases in Holland and Germany. In these cases, sheep seem to be the source of infection (Weinhold 1974; Weinhold and Triemer 1978). Attempts to transmit the disease to small animals have not been successful (Palsson 1976; Thormar 1976).

1. Visna

Visna (wasting) is primarily a neurological disease of the central nervous system (CNS). Visna virus affects animals of both sexes and at any age, although the disease is infrequent in sheep less than 2 years old; about 10% of infected animals may not show clinical symptoms at 8 years postinfection. The first symptoms include an aberration in gait, trembling of the lips, unnatural tilting of the head, and, infrequently, blindness. Progressive paralytic changes follow, especially of the hind limbs. The survival of the animal can be extended and the appearance of emaciation can be avoided for long periods of time if the animals are helped to obtain food and water. The only effective eradication program has proved to be slaughter of all animals from flocks showing infection.

The principal histopathological change is destruction of tissue in inflammatory foci in periventricular areas, choroid plexus, and meninges (Sigurdsson et al. 1962; Petursson et al. 1976). The inflammatory infiltrates consist of lymphocytes (at various stages of maturation, including mature plasma cells) and macrophages. These cells accumulate as a cuff around blood vessels and in discrete foci in the CNS; the cells may also infiltrate the septa between alveoli in the lung (see next section). In the CNS, tissue is destroyed in the inflammatory lesions, and when damage becomes extensive, paralysis ensues. Another early and persistent event is the infiltration of inflammatory cells into the cerebrospinal fluid. In animals with advanced lesions, demyelination may occur, but this is not a ubiquitous finding. Although visna virus induces syncytia formation in vitro, no syncytia have been observed in vivo (Georgsson et al. 1977), suggesting that this phenomenon is not important in the generation or progression of the lesions.

In nature, infection is transmitted horizontally from ewe to lamb via the milk (in which virus is excreted) or, in older animals, by respiratory aerosol or infected saliva (DeBoer et al. 1978). There is no evidence for transplacental infection (deBoer et al. 1978).

2. *Maedi*

Maedi (shortness of breath) is the name given to the pulmonary manifestations in virus-infected sheep. The clinical symptoms are respiratory difficulties and sometimes a dry cough. The clinical phase is quite prolonged and animals often die from acute bacterial pneumonia. The most marked change is a two- to threefold increase in the weight of the lung. Histopathological studies reveal thickening of interalveolar septa due to infiltration of inflammatory cells; eventually the alveolar spaces may be obliterated. Foci of inflammatory lesions occur throughout the lung parenchyma, with peribronchial and perivascular hyperplasia, and fibrosis (Palsson 1976). As the lesions in the lung enlarge, impairment of gaseous exchange ensues, thus leading to the shortness of breath.

Isolation of virus is most frequent from choroid plexus and lungs, although many other tissues are also productive. The disease occurs in sheep of both sexes, but rarely before 3 years of age. As with visna, transmission occurs through direct contact or by ingesting colostrum from infected ewes.

3. CAEV

Although goats in contact with visna/maedi-infected sheep can succumb to similar diseases, the appearance of an arthritic syndrome by CAEV warrants its classification as a separate entity.

Epidemiologically, the encephalomyelitis-arithritis syndrome in goats has been recognized in Germany (Stavrou et al. 1969), Australia (O'Sullivan et al. 1978), and the United States (Cork et al. 1974b; Sherman 1978; Williams 1979). Interestingly, visna/maedi is not found in Australia, providing further evidence for considering CAEV a distinct virus.

The clinical course shares several features with visna/maedi: interstitial pneumonia with shortness of breath, leukoencephaliltis, paralysis, and the diagnostic inflammatory lesions in the CNS and lung (Cork et al. 1974a,b). The principal hallmark of the syndrome that distinguishes it from visna/maedi is arthritis in the joints (Cork et al. 1974a; Crawford et al. 1980). Focal necrosis and hyperplasia of synovial membrane lining cells occur; the former can eventually progress to cause extreme fibrosis and destruction of surrounding cartilage. Edema is noted in surrounding tissues. In addition, the brain lesions show demyelination more frequently than is observed with visna.

Following experimental inoculation of goats, inflammatory lesions appear in the brain, joints, and lungs as early as 1 week postinfection and may persist for several years. Adult and newborn goats are equally susceptible. Virus can be recovered from many tissues, including choroid plexus, brain, synovial membrane, spleen, lymph nodes, thymus, and peripheral blood leukocytes (Cork and Narayan 1980). In nature, transmission occurs horizontally, either from ewe to kid or via other methods of direct contact.

B. Pathogenesis

The salient events in the course of infection can be reconstructed from experimental models. Following intracranial inoculation of virus, there is an acute phase of replication, but production of virus is restricted by several orders of magnitude vis-a-vis production in vitro. In the ensuing months and years of infection, virus production is even more restricted but continues despite a vigorous inflammatory and immune response mounted by the host. A cellular immune response is demonstrable in the first weeks of infection (Griffin et al. 1978a); readily detectable neutralizing antibodies appear later and are sustained at high levels throughout the course of the disease (Gudnadottir and Palsson 1965; Petursson et al. 1976), and there are immunoglobulin and nonimmunoglobulin components in serum and cerebrospinal fluid that neutralize virus as well (Griffin et al. 1978b; Thormar et al. 1979). These defense mechanisms undoubtedly suppress overall virus production without clearing the infection. In most animals, the continued production of virus with attendant pathology eventually leads to patent disease and death. The incubation period from the time of exposure to the overt appearance of symptoms is variable, ranging from months to several years; the clinically recognizable phase may also be extremely protracted, generally extending over several years.

Viruses ordinarily are eliminated by the concerted action of the host's macrophage/granulocyte phagocytic system, humoral and cellular immunity, and interferon. The persistence of the lentiviruses for periods of years implies that there are mechanisms that frustrate these defensive measures.

1. Virus Expression and Persistence

Considerable insight into the mechanism of persistence of lentiviruses has been gained by analysis of virus replication in individual cells by in situ hybridization refined to the point of detection of single copies of the viral genome (Brahic and Haase 1978). In the tissues of animals infected with visna virus, only a small proportion of the cells containing proviral DNA synthesize antigens or viral particles, detectable by immunofluorescence and electron microscopy, respectively (Haase et al. 1977). This restriction in vivo is imposed, at least in part, at a transcriptional level (Brahic et al. 1981). Some cells in the CNS of infected sheep contain virus-specific RNA corresponding quantitatively to levels in tissue culture of cells producing 0.1–1 plaque-forming units per cell or 0.1–1% of the full yield in permissive infections in vitro. These low levels of RNA synthesis may be responsible for the small amounts of virus always present in tissues that perpetuate and extend the infectious process.

The restriction of viral gene expression and the small proportion of cells synthesizing viral antigen provide a satisfying explanation for virus persistence at the molecular level, since the immunological surveillance system of the host will neither detect nor destroy most of the infected, but antigenically "silent," cells. Such cells are also not likely to be eliminated by other mechanisms such as interferon, since the lentiviruses are exceptionally resistant to its antiviral activity (Carroll et al. 1978). Thus, the animal is left with a burden of infected cells that can perpetuate the infection.

The factors that are of fundamental importance in regulating virus production in vivo are poorly understood and are the subject of continuing investigation. It is clear that the constraints on viral gene expression in vivo reflect diminished levels of RNA synthesis. There is now reason to believe that synthesis of virus and viral RNA under permissive conditions of growth is governed by the extent of DNA synthesis. In vitro, visna virus DNA is amplified in two phases to reach levels of 200–300 copies/cell, and little if any of the DNA is integrated, as demonstrated by restriction enzyme analysis. The first phase (about 50–100 copies/cell) is required for full virus production, since inhibition of viral DNA synthesis during this phase reduces both viral RNA and infectious progeny in a gene dosage-dependent manner (B. Traynor et al., pers. comm.). The extent to which gene dosage affects virus production and consequent tissue damage in vivo has yet to be determined.

2. *Virus Dissemination*

The spread of virus to distant sites in the presence of antibody can also be explained by latent dissemination in motile cell populations (peripheral blood leukocytes) with comparable limitations on gene expression in the cells that carry the virus. This hypothesis is substantiated by the observation that all of the cells in the hematopoietic system can be chronically infected with visna virus, although virus can be recovered from peripheral blood leukocytes at only a very low frequency (10^{-6}), presumably due to cell association of viral particles (Petursson et al. 1976). Conceivably, peripheral blood leukocytes, their precursors in the marrow, and other elements of the reticuloendothelial system might harbor the viral genome, with intermittent or continuous dissemination to distant sites. As long as antigen expression remained restricted in the blood leukocytes, circulating neutralizing antibody would have little effect in clearing the infection.

Antigenic variation is a second plausible explanation for the spread of virus. In visna-virus-infected sheep, variants arise that are not neutralized by antibody to the inoculated strain and therefore could replicate and spread temporarily unchecked (Narayan et al. 1977, 1978). There is good evidence for this mechanism in EIAV infections (Section XIII), leading to episodes of viremia and recurrent disease. Antigenic variants of visna virus probably arise by mutation and show alterations in the *env* gene that codes for the surface glycoprotein antigen(s) to which neutralizing antibody is directed (Scott et al. 1979; Clements et al. 1980). However, the role of the variants in dissemination is unclear for two reasons. First, parental and variant strains are not found extracellularly, but rather are always isolated from peripheral blood leukocytes. Second, despite equal replicative ability and the postulated selective advantage to the variant of temporary escape from immunolysis, the variants do not replace the parental strain or other variants in successive episodes. Instead, parental and variant strains are isolated contemporaneously (Narayan et al. 1978).

3. Slowness

Another striking feature of lentivirus infections is the protracted course of the disease. Slowness clearly refers to the pace of progression of disease in animals, not to the replication of these viruses, whose life cycles are completed in vitro in 3 or 4 days. Presumably, slowness reflects the interacting effects of the restricted viral gene expression and diminished production of infectious virus. Continuous reinfections enhance the pace of disease progression, as do conditions of stress (e.g., breeding, parasitic infections, and harsh climate).

4. Immunological Processes

In lentivirus infections, the basic pathological changes likely result from deleterious effects of the interaction between virus and the host defensive apparatus. Destruction of tissue in inflammatory foci provides evidence that the host's immune response is contributory to disease manifestations. Immunosuppressive treatment in these infections has the sparing effect predicted for immunologically mediated disease (Nathanson et al. 1976; Georgsson et al. 1977), whereas immunopotentiating treatment increases the severity of the lesions (Petursson et al. 1979).

C. Reprise

Visna/maedi virus and CAEV are paradigms of slow infections caused by retroviruses in animals. The restrained pace of disease is probably a reflection of both the diminished rate of virus production in vivo and the time required for tissue lesions to accumulate to symptomatic levels. Many cells that harbor the viral genome do not synthesize antigens or viral particles in detectable amounts, providing one explanation for the ability of the virus to escape elimination by the host's immune system. Tissue destruction is immunologically mediated, but the target antigen has not been identified.

REFERENCES

Aaronson, S.A. and M. Barbacid. 1978. Origin and biochemical properties of a new BALB/c mouse sarcoma virus. *J. Virol.* **27:** 366–373.

Abelson, H.T. and L.S. Rabstein. 1970a. Influence of prednisolone on Moloney leukemogenic virus in BALB/mice. *Cancer Res.* **30:** 2208–2212.

———. 1970b. Lymphosarcoma: Virus-induced thymic-independent disease in mice. *Cancer Res.* **30:** 2213–2222.

Abramson, S., R.G. Miller, and R.A. Phillips. 1977. The identification in adult bone marrow of pluripotent and restricted stem cells of the myeloid and lymphoid systems. *J. Exp. Med.* **145:** 1567–1579.

Adams, S., C. Alwine, G. de Crombrugge, and I. Pastan. 1979. Use of recombinant plasmids to characterize collagen RNAs in normal and transformed chick embryo fibroblasts. *J. Biol. Chem.* **254:** 4935–4938.

Alt, F.W., N.E. Rosenberg, S. Lewis, E. Thomas, and D. Baltimore. 1981. Organization and reorganization of immunoglobulin genes in Abelson murine leukemia virus-transformed cells: Rearrangement of heavy but not light chain genes. *Cell* **27:** 387–390.

Altman, P.L. and D.D. Katz, eds. 1979. *Inbred and genetically defined strains of laboratory animals.* Fed. Amer. Soc. Exp. Biol., Bethesda.

Ambros, V.R., L.B. Chen, and J.M. Buchanan. 1975. Surface ruffles as markers for studies of cell transformation by Rous sarcoma virus. *Proc. Natl. Acad. Sci.* **72:** 3144–3148.

Andersen, P.R., S.R. Tronick, and S.A. Aaronson. 1981a. Structural organization and biological activity (sic) of molecular clones of the integrated genome of a BALB/c mouse sarcoma virus. *J. Virol.* **40:** 431–439.

Andersen, P.R., S.G. Devare, S.R. Tronick, R.W. Ellis, S.A. Aaronson, and E.M. Scolnick. 1981b. Generation of BALB-MuSV and Ha-MSV by type C virus transduction of homologous transforming genes from different species. *Cell* **26:** 129–134.

Anderson, L.J. and W.F.H. Jarrett. 1971. Membranous glomerulonephritis associated with leukemia in cats. *Res. Vet. Sci.* **12:** 179–180.

Anderson, L.J., W.F.H. Jarrett, O. Jarrett, and H.M. Laird. 1971. Feline leukemia virus infection of kittens: Mortality associated with atrophy of the thymus and lymphoid depletion. *J. Natl. Cancer Inst.* **47:** 807–817.

Andervont, H.B. 1940. The influence of foster nursing upon the incidence of spontaneous mammary cancer in resistant and susceptible mice. *J. Natl. Cancer Inst.* **1:** 147–153.

———. 1945. Fate of the C3H milk influence in mice of strains C and C57 black. *J. Natl. Cancer Inst.* **5:** 383–390.

Andrews, J.M. and M.B. Gardner. 1974. Lower motor neuron degeneration associated with type-C RNA virus infection in mice: Neuropathological features. *J. Neuropathol. Exp. Neurol.* **33:** 285–307.

Aoki, T., M. Potter, M.M. Sturm, M. Liu, and M.J. Walling. 1975. Cell populations and known surface antigens of tumors induced by Abelson virus in pristane-primed BALB/c mice: An analysis by immunoelectron microscopy. *J. Natl. Cancer Inst.* **55:** 1097–1106.

Armitage, P. and R. Doll. 1961. Stochastic models for carcinogenesis. In *Proceedings of the 4th Berkeley Symposium on Mathematical Statistics and Probability: Biology and problems of health* (ed. J. Neyman), vol. 4, pp. 19–38. University of California Press, Berkeley.

Armstrong, M.Y.K., R.B. Weininger, D. Binder, C.A. Himsel, and F.F. Richards. 1980. Role of endogenous murine leukemia virus in immunologically triggered lymphoreticular tumors. II. Isolation of B-tropic mink cell focus-inducing (MCF) murine leukemia virus. *Virology* **104:** 164–173.

Arthur, L.O. and D.L. Fine. 1978. Naturally occurring humoral immunity to murine mammary tumor virus (MuMTV) and MuMTV gp52 in mice with low mammary tumor incidence. *Int. J. Cancer* **22:** 734–740.

Ash, J.F., P.K. Vogt, and S.J. Singer. 1976. Reversion from transformed to normal phenotype by inhibition of protein synthesis in rat kidney cells infected with a temperature-sensitive mutant of Rous sarcoma virus. *Proc. Natl. Acad. Sci.* **73:** 3603–3607.

Axel, R., S.C. Gulati, and S. Spiegelman. 1972. Particles containing RNA-instructed DNA polymerase and virus-related RNA in human breast cancers. *Proc. Natl. Acad. Sci.* **69:** 3133–3137.

Axelrad, A. 1966. Genetic control of susceptibility to Friend leukemia virus in mice: Studies with the spleen focus assay method. *Natl. Cancer Inst. Monogr.* **22:** 619–629.

Axelrad, A.A. and R.A. Steeves. 1964. Assay for Friend leukemia virus: Rapid quantitative method based on enumeration of macroscopic spleen foci in mice. *Virology* **24:** 513–518.

Axelrad, A. and H.C. Van der Gaag. 1969. Genetic and cellular basis of susceptibility or resistance to Friend leukemia virus infection in mice. *Can. Cancer Conf.* **8:** 313–343.

Axelrad, A.A., M. Ware, and H.C. Van der Gaag. 1972. Host cell susceptibility and resistance to murine leukemia viruses and their genetic control. In *RNA viruses and host genome in oncogenesis* (ed. P. Emmelot and P. Bentvelzen), pp. 239–254. North-Holland, Amsterdam.

Alexrad, A., H. Croizat, D. Eskinazi, S. Stewart, D. Vaithilingam, and H. Van der Gaag. 1982. Gene controlled negative regulation of DNA synthesis in erythropoietic progenitor cells. *J. Cell. Physiol.* (in press).

Balduzzi, P.C., M.F.D. Notter, H.R. Morgan, and M. Shibuya. 1981. Some biological properties of two new avian sarcoma viruses. *J. Virol.* **40:** 268–275.

Baliga, V. and J.F. Ferrer. 1977. Expression of the bovine leukemia virus and its internal antigen in blood lymphocytes. *Proc. Soc. Exp. Biol. Med.* **156:** 388–391.

Baltimore, D. 1975. Tumor viruses: 1974. *Cold Spring Harbor Symp. Quant. Biol.* **39:** 1187–1200.

Baluda, M.A. 1963. Properties of cells infected with avian myeloblastosis virus. *Cold Spring Harbor Symp. Quant. Biol.* **27:** 415–425.

Baluda, M.A. and I.E. Goetz. 1961. Morphological conversion of cell cultures by avian myeloblastosis virus. *Virology* **15:** 185–199.

Banks, K.L., J.B. Henson, and T.C. McGuire. 1972. Immunologically mediated glomerulitis of horses. I. Pathogenesis in persistent infection by equine infectious anemia virus. *Lab. Invest.* **26:** 701–707.

Barbacid, M., D.H. Troxler, E.M. Scolnick, and S.A. Aaronson. 1978. Analysis of translational products of Friend strain of spleen focus-forming virus. *J. Virol.* **27:** 826–830.

Barnes, W.A. and R.K. Cole. 1941. The effect of nursing on the incidence of spontaneous leukemia and tumors in mice. *Cancer Res.* **1:**99–101.

Bassin, R.H., P.J. Simons, F.C. Chesterman, and J.J. Harvey. 1968. Murine sarcoma virus (Harvey): Characteristics of focus formation in mouse embryo cell cultures, and virus production by hamster tumor cells. *Int. J. Cancer* **3:**265–272.

Battula, N. and H.M. Temin. 1977. Infectious DNA of spleen necrosis viruses is integrated at a single site in the DNA of chronically infected chicken fibroblasts. *Proc. Natl. Acad. Sci.* **74:**281–285.

———. 1978. Sites of integration of infectious DNA of avian reticuloendotheliosis viruses in different avian cellular DNAs. *Cell* **13:**387–398.

Baumgartener, L.E., C. Olson, J.M. Miller, and M.J. Van Der Maaten. 1975. Survey for antibodies to leukemia (C-type) virus in cattle. *J. Am. Vet. Med. Assoc.* **166:**249–251.

Beard, J.W. 1980. Biology of avian oncornaviruses. In *Viral oncology* (ed. G. Klein), pp. 55–87. Raven Press, New York.

Beaudreau, G.S., R.A. Bonar, D. Beard, and J.W. Beard. 1956. Virus of avian erythroblastosis. II. Influence of host age and route of inoculation on dose-response. *J. Natl. Cancer Inst.* **17:**91–100.

Beaudreau, G.S., C. Becker, R.A. Bonar, A.M. Wallbank, D. Beard, and J.W. Beard. 1960. Virus of avian myeloblastosis. XIV. Neoplastic response of normal chicken bone marrow treated with the virus in tissue culture. *J. Natl. Cancer Inst.* **24:**395–415.

Bech-Nielsen, S., C.E. Piper, and J.F. Ferrer. 1978. Natural mode of transmission of the bovine leukemia virus: Role of blood-sucking insects. *Am. J. Vet. Res.* **39:** 1089–1092.

Begg, A.M. 1927. A filtrable endothelioma of the fowl. *Lancet* **2:**912–915.

Bendixen, H.J. 1963. *Leukosis Enzootica Bovis. Diagnostik, Epidemiologi, Bekaempeise.* Mortensen, Copenhagen.

Bennett, M., R.A. Steeves, G. Cudkowicz, E.A. Mirand, and L.B. Russell. 1968. Mutant *Sl* alleles of mice affect susceptibility to Friend spleen focus-forming virus. *Science* **162:**564–565.

Bentvelzen, P. 1968. "Genetic control of the vertical transmission of the Muhlbock mammary tumor virus in the GR mouse strain." Ph.D. thesis. Hollandia, Amsterdam.

———. 1972. The biology of the mouse mammary tumor virus. *Int. Rev. Exp. Pathol.* **11:**259–297.

Bentvelzen, P. and J. Brinkhof. 1977. Organ distribution of exogenous murine mammary tumor virus as determined by bioassay. *Eur. J. Cancer* **13:**241–245.

Bentvelzen, P. and J.H. Daams. 1969. Hereditary infections with mammary tumor viruses in mice. *J. Natl. Cancer Inst.* **43:**1025–1035.

———. 1970. Mammary-tumor virus activity in brain and liver of GR strain mice. *Eur. J. Cancer* **6:**273–276.

Benveniste, R.E., C.J. Sherr, and G.J. Todaro. 1975. Evolution of type C viral genes: Origin of feline leukemia virus. *Science* **190:**886–888.

Ben-Zeév, A., A. Duerr, F. Solomon, and S. Penman. 1979. The outer boundary of the cytoskeleton: A lamina derived from plasma membrane proteins. *Cell* **17:**859–865.

Berman, L.D. 1967. Comparative morphologic study of the virus-induced solid tumors of Syrian hamsters. *J. Natl. Cancer Inst.* **39:**847–901.

Berman, L.D. and A.C. Allison. 1969. Studies on murine sarcoma virus; A morphological comparison of tumorigenesis by the Harvey and Moloney strains in mice, and the establishment of tumor cell lines. *Int. J. Cancer* **4:**820–836.

Bernhard, W. 1958. Electron microscopy of tumor cells and tumor viruses. A review. *Cancer Res.* **18:**491–509.

Bernhard, W., M. Guerlin, and C. Oberling. 1956. Mise en evidence de corpuscules d'aspect virusal dans differentes souches de cancers mammaires de la souris. Etude au microscope electronique. *Acta Unio Int. Contra Cancrum* **12:**545–557.

Bernstein, A., T.W. Mak, and J.R. Stephenson. 1977. The Friend virus genome: Evidence for the stable association of MuLV sequences and sequences involved in erythroleukemic transformation. *Cell* **12:** 287–294.

Beug, H., H. Muller, S. Grieser, G. Doederlein, and T. Graf. 1981. Hematopoietic cells transformed *in vitro* by REV_T avian reticuloendotheliosis virus express characteristics of very immature lymphoid cells. *Virology* **115:** 295–309.

Beug, H., A. von Kirchbach, G. Doderlein, J.-F. Conscience, and T. Graf. 1979. Chicken hematopoietic cells transformed by seven strains of defective avian leukemia viruses display three distinct phenotypes of differentiation. *Cell* **18:** 375–390.

Biggs, P.M., B.S. Milne, T. Graf, and H. Bauer. 1973. Oncogenicity of non-transforming mutants of avian sarcoma viruses. *J. Gen. Virol.* **18:** 399–403.

Bittner, J.J. 1936. Some possible effects of nursing on the mammary gland tumor incidence in mice. *Science* **84:** 162.

Blair, P.B. 1965. Immunology of the mouse mammary tumour virus (MTV): A qualitative *in vitro* assay for MTV. *Nature* **208:** 165–167.

Blomberg, J., F.H. Reynolds, Jr., W.J.M. Van de Ven, and J.R. Stephenson. 1980. Abelson murine leukaemia virus transformation involves loss of epidermal growth factor-binding sites. *Nature* **286:** 504–507.

Boettiger, D. and E.M. Durban. 1980. Progenitor-cell populations can be infected by RNA tumor viruses, but transformation is dependent on the expression of specific differentiated functions. *Cold Spring Harbor Symp. Quant. Biol.* **44:** 1249–1254.

Boettiger, D., K. Roby, J. Brumbaugh, J. Biehl, and H. Holtzer. 1977. Transformation of chicken embryo retinal melanoblasts by a temperature-sensitive mutant of Rous sarcoma virus. *Cell* **11:** 881–890.

Bollum, F.J. 1979. Terminal deoxynucleotidyl transferase as a hematopoietic cell marker. *Blood* **54:** 1203–1215.

Bonar, R.A. and D.F. Paulson. 1974. Response of chick-embryo kidney cells in vitro to two avian tumor viruses. *J. Natl. Cancer Inst.* **53:** 711–718.

Boot, L.M. 1970. Prolactin and mammary gland carcinogenesis. The problem of human prolactin. *Int. J. Cancer* **5:** 167–175.

Boot, L.M. and O. Muhlbock. 1956. The mammary tumor incidence in the C3H mouse-strain with and without the agent (C3H; C3Hf; C3He). *Acta Unio Int. Contra Cancrum* **12:** 569–581.

Bose, H.R., Jr. and A.S. Levine. 1967. Replication of the reticuloendotheliosis virus (strain T) in chicken embryo cell culture. *J. Virol.* **1:** 1117–1121.

Boss, M., M. Greaves, and N. Teich. 1979. Abelson virus-transformed haematopoietic cell lines with pre-B-cell characteristics. *Nature* **278:** 551–553.

Boyde, A., A.J. Banes, R.M. Dillaman, and G.L. Mechanic. 1978. A morphological study of an avian bone disorder caused by myeloblastosis-associated virus. *Metab. Bone Dis. Rel. Dis.* **1:** 235–242.

Bradley, T.R. and D. Metcalf. 1966. The growth of mouse bone marrow cells *in vitro. Aust. J. Exp. Biol. Med. Sci.* **44:** 287–300.

Brahic, M. and A.T. Haase. 1978. Detection of viral sequences of low reiteration frequency by *in situ* hybridization. *Proc. Natl. Acad. Sci.* **75:** 6125–6129.

———. 1981. Lentivirinae: Maedi/visna group infection. Comparative aspects and diagnosis. In *Comparative diagnosis of viral diseases* (ed. E. Kurstak), vol. 3, pp. 627–647. Academic Press, New York.

Brahic, M., L. Stowring, P. Ventura, and A.T. Haase. 1981. Gene expression in visna virus infection in sheep. *Nature* **292:** 240–242.

Brandes, D., B. Schofield, R. Slusser, and E. Anton. 1966. Studies of L1210 leukemia. I. Ultrastructure of solid and ascites cells. *J. Natl. Cancer Inst.* **37:** 467–485.

Breitman, M.L., M.M.C. Lai, and P.K. Vogt. 1980. The genomic RNA of avian reticuloendotheliosis virus REV. *Virology* **100:** 450–461.

Buffett, R.F. and J. Furth. 1959. A transplantable reticulum-cell sarcoma variant of Friend's viral leukemia. *Cancer Res.* **19:** 1063–1069.

Burgess, A.W., J. Camakaris, and D. Metcalf. 1977. Purification and properties of colony-stimulating factor from mouse lung-conditioned medium. *J. Biol. Chem.* **252:** 1998–2003.

Burmester, B.R. and N.F. Waters. 1956. Variation in the presence of the virus of visceral lymphomatosis in the eggs of the same hens. *Poultry Sci.* **35:** 939–944.

Burmester, B.R., R.F. Gentry, and N.F. Waters. 1955. The presence of the virus of visceral lymphomatosis in embryonated eggs of normal appearing hens. *Poultry Sci.* **34:** 609–617.

Burmester, B.R., M.A. Gross, W.G. Walter, and A.K. Fontes. 1959a. Pathogenicity of a viral strain (RPL12) causing avian visceral lymphomatosis and related neoplasms. II. Host-virus interrelations affecting response. *J. Natl. Cancer Inst.* **22:** 103–127.

Burmester, B.R., W.G. Walter, M.A. Gross, and A.K. Fontes. 1959b. The oncogenic spectrum of two "pure" strains of avian leukosis. *J. Natl. Cancer Inst.* **23:** 277–291.

Burnet, F.M. 1970. The concept of immunological surveillance. *Prog. Exp. Tumor Res.* **13:** 1–27.

Burny, A., C. Bruck, H. Chantrenne, Y. Cleuter, D. Dekegel, J. Ghysdael, R. Kettmann, M. Leclercq, J. Leunen, M. Mammerickx, and D. Portetelle. 1980. Bovine leukemia virus: Molecular biology and epidermiology. In *Viral oncology* (ed. G. Klein), pp. 231–289. Raven Press, New York.

Calafat, J. 1968. Virus particles of the B and C types associated with mouse mammary tumors. *J. Microscopie* **7:** 841–848.

Calafat, J., F. Buijs, P.C. Hageman, J. Links, J. Hilgers, and A. Hekman. 1974. Distribution of virus particles and mammary tumor virus antigens in mouse mammary tumors, transformed BALB/c mouse kidney cells, and GR ascites leukemia cells. *J. Natl. Cancer Inst.* **53:** 977–992.

Calnek, B.W. 1964. Morphological alteration of RIF-infected chick embryo fibroblasts. *Natl. Cancer Inst. Monogr.* **17:** 425–448.

Campbell, W.F., L.K. Baxter-Gabbard, and A.S. Levine. 1971. Avian reticuloendotheliosis virus (strain T). Virological characterization. *Avian Dis.* **15:** 837–849.

Carpenter, C.R., H.R. Bose, and A.S. Rubin. 1977. Contact-mediated suppression of mitogen induced responsiveness by spleen cells in reticuloendotheliosis virus-induced tumorigenesis. *Cell Immunol.* **33:** 392–401.

Carpenter, C.R., A.S. Rubin, and H.R. Bose, Jr. 1978a. Suppression of the mitogen-stimulated blastogenic response during reticuloendotheliosis virus-induced tumorigenesis: Investigations into the mechanism of action of the suppressor. *J. Immunol.* **120:** 1313–1320.

Carpenter, C.R., K.E. Kempf, H.R. Bose, and A.S. Rubin. 1978b. Characterization of the interaction of reticuloendotheliosis virus with the avian lymphoid system. *Cell. Immunol.* **39:** 307–315.

Carr, J.G. 1956. Renal adenocarcinoma induced by fowl leukaemia virus. *Br. J. Cancer* **10:** 379–383.

Carr, J.G. and J.G. Campbell. 1958. Three new virus-induced sarcomata. *Br. J. Cancer* **12:** 631–635.

Carroll, D., P. Ventura, A. Haase, C.R. Rinaldo, Jr., J.C. Overall, Jr., and L.A. Glasgow. 1978. Resistance of visna virus to interferon. *J. Infect. Dis.* **138:** 614–617.

Carroll, R.C., J.F. Ash, P.K. Vogt, and S.J. Singer. 1978. Reversion of transformed glycolysis to normal by inhibition of protein synthesis in rat kidney cells infected with temperature-sensitive mutant of Rous sarcoma virus. *Proc. Natl. Acad. Sci.* **75:** 5015–5019.

Casey, J.W., A. Roach, J.I. Mullins, K.B. Burck, M.O. Nicolson, M.B. Gardner, and N. Davidson. 1981. The U3 portion of the feline leukemia virus identifies horizontally acquired proviruses in leukemic cats. *Proc. Natl. Acad. Sci.* **78:** 7778–7782.

Chang, K.S.S., T. Log, and A.K. Bandyopadhyay. 1982. Characterization of xenotropic and dual-tropic type C retroviruses isolated from Abelson tumour. *J. Gen. Virol.* **58:** 115–125.

Chang, T.D., J.L. Biedler, E. Stockert, and L.J. Old. 1977. Trisomy of chromosome 15 in X-ray-induced mouse leukemia. *Proc. Am. Assoc. Cancer Res.* **18:** 225.

Charney, J., B.D. Pullinger, and D.H. Moore. 1969. Development of an infectivity assay for mouse mammary-tumor virus. *J. Natl. Cancer Inst.* **43:** 1289–1296.

Charyulu, V., M.M. Sigel, D.L. Durden, and D.M. Lopez. 1979. Mouse mammary tumor virus (MMTV) antigen(s) are present on B lymphocytes of BALB/c mice. *Int. J. Cancer* **24:** 813–818.

Chattopadhyay, S.K., D.R. Lowy, N.M. Teich, A.S. Levine, and W.P. Rowe. 1974. Evidence that the AKR murine-leukemia-virus genome is complete in DNA of the high-virus AKR mouse and incomplete in the DNA of the "virus-negative" NIH mouse. *Proc. Natl. Acad. Sci.* **71:** 167–171.

Chattopadhyay, S.K., M.W. Cloyd, D.L. Linemeyer, M.R. Lander, E. Rands, and D.R. Lowy. 1982. Cellular origin and role of mink cell focus-forming viruses in murine thymic lymphomas. *Nature* **295:** 25–31.

Chen, J.H., M.G. Moscovici, and C. Moscovici. 1980. Isolation of complementary DNA unique to the genome of avian myeloblastosis virus (AMV). *Virology* **103:** 112–122.

Chesebro, B. and K. Wehrly. 1979. Identification of a non-*H-2* gene (*Rfv-3*) influencing recovery from viremia and leukemia induced by Friend virus complex. *Proc. Natl. Acad. Sci.* **76:** 425–429.

Chesebro, B., K. Wehrly, and J. Stimpfling. 1974. Host genetic control of recovery from Friend leukemia virus-induced splenomegaly. Mapping of a gene with the major histocompatibility complex. *J. Exp. Med.* **140:** 1457–1467.

Chesebro, B., K. Wehrly, D. Doig, and J. Nishio. 1979. Antibody-induced modulation of Friend virus cell surface antigen decreases virus production by persistent erythroleukemia cells: Influence of the *Rfv-3* gene. *Proc. Natl. Acad. Sci.* **76:** 5784–5788.

Chesterman, F.C., J.J. Harvey, R.R. Dourmashkin, and M.H. Salaman. 1966. The pathology of tumors and other lesions induced in rodents by virus derived from a rat with Moloney leukemia. *Cancer Res.* **26:** 1759–1768.

Ching, L.-M. and R.G. Miller. 1980. Characterization of *in vitro* T lymphocyte colonies from normal mouse spleen cells: Colonies containing cytotoxic lymphocyte precursors. *J. Immunol.* **124:** 696–701.

Chirigos, M.A., D. Scott, W. Turner, and K. Perk. 1968. Biological, pathological and physical characterization of a possible variant of a murine sarcoma virus (Moloney). *Int. J. Cancer* **3:** 223–237.

Clarke, B.J., A.A. Axelrad, and D. Housman. 1976. Friend spleen focus-forming virus production in vitro by a nonerythroid cell line. *J. Natl. Cancer Inst.* **57:** 853–859.

Clarke, B.J., A.A. Axelrad, M.M. Shreeve, and D.L. McLeod. 1975. Erythroid colony induction without erythropoietin by Friend leukemia virus *in vitro. Proc. Natl. Acad. Sci.* **72:** 3556–3560.

Clements, J.E., F.S. Pedersen, O. Narayan, and W.A. Haseltine. 1980. Genomic changes associated with antigenic variation of visna virus during persistent infection. *Proc. Natl. Acad. Sci.* **77:** 4454–4458.

Cloyd, M.W., J.W. Hartley, and W.P. Rowe. 1979. Cell-surface antigens associated with recombinant mink cell focus-forming murine leukemia viruses. *J. Exp. Med.* **149:** 702–712.

———. 1980. Lymphomagenicity of recombinant mink cell focus-forming murine leukemia viruses. *J. Exp. Med.* **151:** 542–552.

Cloyd, M.W., J.W. Hartley, and W.P. Rowe. 1981. Genetic study of lymphoma induction by AKR mink cell focus-inducing virus in AKR × NFS crosses. *J. Exp. Med.* **154:** 450–458.

Cockerell, G.L., E.A. Hoover, S. Krakowka, R.G. Olsen, and D.S. Yohn. 1976. Lymphocyte mitogen reactivity and enumeration of circulating B- and T-cells during feline leukemia virus infection in the cat. *J. Natl. Cancer Inst.* **57:** 1095–1099.

Coggins, L., N.L. Norcross, and S.R. Nusbaum. 1972. Diagnosis of equine infectious anemia by immunodiffusion test. *Am. J. Vet. Res.* **33:** 11–18.

Cohen, J.C. 1980. Methylation of milk-borne and genetically transmitted mouse mammary tumor virus proviral DNA. *Cell* **19:** 653–662.

Cohen, J.C. and H.E. Varmus. 1979. Endogenous mammary tumor virus DNA varies among wild mice and segregates during inbreeding. *Nature* **278:** 418–423.

———. 1980. Proviruses of mouse mammary tumor viruses in normal and neoplastic tissues from GR and C3Hf mouse strains. *J. Virol.* **35:** 298–305.

Cohen, J.C., P.R. Shank, V.L. Morris, R.D. Cardiff, and H.E. Varmus. 1979. Integration of the DNA of mouse mammary tumor virus in virus-infected normal and neoplastic tissue of the mouse. *Cell* **16:** 333–345.

Cole, R.K. and J. Furth. 1941. Experimental studies on the genetics of spontaneous leukemia in mice. *Cancer Res.* **1:** 957–965.

Collins, J.J., F. Sanfilippo, L. Tsong-Chou, R. Ishizaki, and R.S. Metzgar. 1978. Immunotherapy of murine leukemia. I. Protection against Friend leukemia virus-induced disease by passive serum therapy. *Int. J. Cancer* **21:** 51–61.

Cook, M.K. 1969. Cultivation of a filterable agent associated with Marek's disease. *J. Natl. Cancer Inst.* **43:** 203–212.

Cooper, G.M. and P.E. Neiman. 1980. Transforming genes of neoplasms induced by avian lymphoid leukosis viruses. *Nature* **287:** 656–659.

———. 1981. Two distinct candidate transforming genes of lymphoid leukosis virus-induced neoplasms. *Nature* **292:** 857–858.

Cooper, M.D., H.G. Purchase, D.E. Bockman, and W.E. Gathings. 1974. Studies on the nature of the abnormality of B cell differentiation in avian lymphoid leukosis: Production of heterogeneous IgM by tumor cells. *J. Immunol.* **113:** 1210–1222.

Cooper, M.D., L.N. Payne, P.B. Dent, B.R. Burmester, and R.A. Good. 1968. Pathogenesis of avian lymphoid leukosis. I. Histogenesis. *J. Natl. Cancer Inst.* **41:** 373–389.

Copeland, N.G. and G.M. Cooper. 1980. Transfection by DNAs of avian erythroblastosis virus and avian myelocytomatosis virus strain MC29. *J. Virol.* **33:** 1199–1202.

Cork, L.C. and O. Narayan. 1980. The pathogenesis of viral leukoencephalomyelititis-arthritis of goats. I. Persistent viral infection with progressive pathological changes. *Lab. Invest.* **42:** 596–602.

Cork, L.C., W.J. Hadlow, T.B. Crawford, J.R. Gorham, and R.C. Piper. 1974a. Infectious leukoencephalomyelitis of young goats. *J. Infect. Dis.* **129:** 134–141.

Cork, L.C., W.J. Hadlow, J.R. Gorham, R.C. Piper, and T.B. Crawford. 1974b. Pathology of viral leukoencephalomyelitis of goats. *Acta Neuropathol.* **29:** 281–292.

Cotter, S.M. 1979. Anemia associated with feline leukemia virus infection. *J. Am. Vet. Med. Assoc.* **175:** 1191–1194.

Cotter, S.M., W.D. Hardy, Jr., and M. Essex. 1975. Association of feline leukemia virus with lymphosarcoma and other disorders in the cat. *J. Am. Vet. Med. Assoc.* **166:** 449–454.

Crawford, T.B., D.A. Adams, W.P. Cheevers, and L.C. Cork. 1980. Chronic arthritis in goats caused by a retrovirus. *Science* **207:** 997–999.

Crighton, G.W. 1969. Lymphosarcoma in the cat. *Vet. Res.* **84:** 329–331.

Crittenden, L.B., E.J. Smith, and A.M. Fadly. 1981. Influence of endogenous avian leukosis virus gene expression on response to RAV-1 and REV infection. (in press).

Crittenden, L.B., W.S. Hayward, H. Hanafusa, and A.M. Fadly. 1980. Induction of neoplasms by subgroup E recombinants of exogenous and endogenous avian retroviruses (Rous-associated virus type 60). *J. Virol.* **33:** 915–919.

Curran, T. and N.M. Teich. 1982a. Identification of a 39,000-dalton protein in cells transformed by the FBJ murine osteosarcoma virus. *Virology* **116:** 221–235.

———. 1982b. A candidate product of the FBJ murine osteosarcoma virus oncogene: Characterization of a 55,000 dalton phosphoprotein. *J. Virol.* **42:** 114–122.

Daams, J.H. 1970. Immunofluorescence studies on the biology of the mouse mammary tumour virus. In *Immunity and tolerance in oncogenesis* (ed. L. Severi), pp. 463–474. Division of Cancer Research, Perugia.

Daams, J.H., J. Calafat, E.Y. Lasfargues, B. Kramarsky, and P. Bentvelzen. 1970. Mammary tumor virus associated antigens on the membrane of infected mouse spleen cells. *Virology* **41:** 184–186.

Dalton, A.J., M. Potter, and R.M. Merwin. 1961. Some ultrastructural characteristics of a series of primary and transplanted plasma-cell tumors of the mouse. *J. Natl. Cancer Inst.* **26:** 1221–1267.

Datta, S.K., P.J. McConahey, N. Manny, A.N. Theofilopoulos, F.J. Dixon, and R.S. Schwartz. 1978. Genetic studies of autoimmunity and retrovirus expression in crosses of New Zealand black mice. II. The viral envelope glycoprotein, gp70. *J. Exp. Med.* **147:** 872–881.

Dawson, P.J., S.L. Dresler, and A.H. Fieldsteel. 1979. Erythroid leukemia induced by Friend lymphatic leukemia virus in T-cell-depleted mice. *Cancer Res.* **39:** 1611–1615.

Dawson, P.J., A.H. Fieldsteel, and W.L. Bostick. 1963. Pathologic studies of Friend virus leukemia and the development of a transplantable tumor in BALB/c mice. *Cancer Res.* **23:** 349–354.

Dawson, P.J., W.M. Rose, and A.H. Fieldsteel. 1966. Lymphatic leukaemia in rats and mice inoculated with Friend virus. *Br. J. Cancer* **20:** 114–121.

Day, N.K., C. O'Reilly-Felice, W.D. Hardy, Jr., R.A. Good, and S.S. Witkin. 1980. Circulating immune complexes associated with naturally occurring lymphosarcoma in pet cats. *J. Immunol.* **125:** 2363–2366.

DeBoer, G.F. 1975. Zwoegerziekte virus, the causative agent for progressive interstitial pneumonia (maedi) and meningo-leucoencephalitis (visna) in sheep. *Res. Vet. Sci.* **18:** 15–25.

DeBoer, G.F., C. Terfstra, and D.J. Houwers. 1978. Studies of zwoegerziekte (maedi) in the Netherlands, a review. *Bull. Off. Int. Epizoot.* **89:** 487–506.

Decleve, A., M. Lieberman, and H.S. Kaplan. 1977. *In vivo* interaction between RNA viruses isolated from the C57BL/Ka strain of mice. *Virology* **81:** 270–283.

Decleve, A., M. Lieberman, J.N. Ihle, and H.S. Kaplan. 1976. Biological and serological characterization of radiation leukemia virus. *Proc. Natl. Acad. Sci.* **73:** 4675–4679.

Deinhardt, F. 1980. Biology of primate retroviruses. In *Viral oncology* (ed. G. Klein), pp. 357–398. Raven Press, New York.

Deinhardt, F., L. Wolfe, R. Massey, J. Hoekstra, and R. McDonald. 1973. Simian sarcoma virus: Oncogenicity, focus assay, presence of associated virus, and comparison with avian and feline sarcoma virus-induced neoplasia in marmoset monkeys. In *Unifying concepts of leukemia* (ed. R.M. Dutcher and L. Chieco-Bianchi), pp. 258–262. Karger, Basel.

Deinhardt, F., L. Wolfe, R. Northrop, B. Marczynska, J. Ogden, R. McDonald, L. Falki, G. Shramek, R. Smith, and J. Deinhardt. 1972. Induction of neoplasms by viruses in marmoset monkeys. *J. Med. Primatol.* **1:** 29–50.

DeLarco, J.E. and G.J. Todaro. 1980. Sarcoma growth factor: Specific binding to and elution from membrane receptors for epidermal growth factor. *Cold Spring Harbor Symp. Quant. Biol.* **44:** 643–651.

Dent, P.B. 1972. Immunodepression by oncogenic viruses. In *Progress in medical virology* (ed. J.L. Melnick), pp. 1–35. Karger, Basel.

Dent, P.B., M.D. Cooper, L.N. Payne, J.J. Solomon, B.R. Burmester, and R.A. Good. 1968. Pathogenesis of avian lymphoid leukosis. II. Immunologic reactivity during lymphomagenesis. *J. Natl. Cancer Inst.* **41:** 391–401.

DeOme, K.B., L.J. Faulkin, Jr., H.A. Bern, and P.B. Blair. 1959. Development of mammary tumors from hyperplastic alveolar nodules transplanted into gland-free mammary fat pads of female C3H mice. *Cancer Res.* **19:** 515–520.

DeOme, K.B., S. Nandi, H.A. Bern, P.B. Blair, and D. Pitelka. 1962. The preneoplastic hyperplastic alveolar nodules as the morphologic precursor of mammary cancer in mice. In *The morphological precursors of cancer* (ed. L. Severi), pp. 349–369. Division of Cancer Research, Perugia.

De Paoli, A. and F.M. Garner. 1968. Acute lymphocytic leukemia in a white-cheeked gibbon (*Hylobates concolor*). *Cancer Res.* **28:** 2559–2561.

De Paoli, A., D.O. Johnsen, and W.W. Noll. 1973. Granulocytic leukemia in whitehanded gibbons. *J. Am. Vet. Med. Assoc.* **163:** 624–628.

Dexter, T.M. and N.G. Testa. 1976. Differentiation and proliferation of hemopoietic cells in culture. *Methods Cell Biol.* **14:** 387–405.

Dexter, T.M., T.D. Allen, and L.G. Lajtha. 1977. Conditions controlling the proliferation of haemopoietic stem cells in vitro. *J. Cell. Physiol.* **91:** 335–344.

Dexter, T.M., T.D. Allen, D. Scott, and N.M. Teich. 1979. Isolation and characterisation of a bipotential haematopoietic cell line. *Nature* **277:** 471–474.

Dexter, T.M., T.D. Allen, N.G. Testa, and E. Scolnick. 1981. Friend disease in vitro. *J. Exp. Med.* **154:** 594–608.

Dickson, C. and G. Peters. 1981. Protein-coding potential of mouse mammary tumor virus genome RNA as examined by in vitro translation. *J. Virol.* **37:** 36–47.

Dickson, C., R. Smith, and G. Peters. 1981. *In vitro* synthesis of polypeptides encoded by the long terminal repeat region of mouse mammary tumor virus DNA. *Nature* **291:** 511–513.

Dietz, M., S.P. Fouchey, C. Longley, M.A. Rich, and P. Furmanski. 1977. Spontaneous regression of Friend virus-induced erythroleukemia. I. The role of the helper murine leukemia virus component. *J. Exp. Med.* **145:** 594–606.

DiGiacomo, R.F. 1967. Burkitt's lymphoma in a white-handed gibbon (*Hylobates lar*). *Cancer Res.* **27:** 1178–1179.

DiStefano, H.S. and R.M. Dougherty. 1966. Mechanisms for congenital transmission of avian leukosis virus. *J. Natl. Cancer Inst.* **37:** 869–883.

Dmochowski. L. 1953. The milk agent in the origin of mammary tumors in mice. *Adv. Cancer Res.* **1:** 103–172.

Dmochowski, L., P.L. Langford, W.C. Williams, A.G. Liebelt, and R.A. Liebelt. 1968. Electron microscopy and bioassay studies of milk from mice of high and low mammary-cancer and high and low leukemia strains. *J. Natl. Cancer Inst.* **40:** 1339–1358.

Dofuku, R., J.L. Biedler, B.A. Spengler, and L.J. Old. 1975. Trisomy of chromosome 15 in spontaneous leukemia of AKR mice. *Proc. Natl. Acad. Sci.* **72:** 1515–1517.

Donehower, L.A., A.L. Huang, and G.L. Hager. 1981. Regulatory and coding potential of the mouse mammary tumor virus long terminal redundancy. *J. Virol.* **37:** 226–238.

Dorn, C.R., D.O.N. Taylor, R. Schneider, H.H. Hibbard, and M.R. Klauber. 1968. Survey of animal neoplasms in Alameda and Contra Costa Counties, California. II. Cancer morbidity in dogs and cats from Alameda County. *J. Natl. Cancer Inst.* **40:** 307–318.

Dougherty, R.M. and R. Rasmussen. 1964. Properties of a strain of Rous sarcoma virus that infects mammals. *Natl. Cancer Inst. Monogr.* **17:** 337–350.

Dresler, S., M. Ruta, M.J. Murray, and D. Kabat. 1979. Glycoprotein encoded by the Friend spleen focus-forming virus. *J. Virol.* **30:** 564–575.

Driscoll, D.M. and C. Olson. 1977. Bovine leukemia virus-associated antigens in lymphocyte cultures. *Am. J. Vet. Res.* **38:** 1897–1898.

Dudley, J.P., J.M. Rosen and J.S. Butel. 1978. Differential expression of poly(A)-adjacent sequences of mammary tumor virus RNA in murine mammary cells. *Proc. Natl. Acad. Sci.* **75:** 5797–5801.

Dunn, T.B. 1959. Morphology of mammary tumors in mice. In *The physiopathology of cancer,* 2nd edition (ed. F. Homburger), pp. 30–84. Hoeber-Harper, New York.

Durban, E.M. and D. Boettiger. 1981a. Replicating, differentiated macrophages can serve as in vitro targets for transformation by avian myeloblastosis virus. *J. Virol.* **37:** 488–492.

———. 1981b. Differential effects of transforming avian RNA tumor viruses on avian macrophages. *Proc. Natl. Acad. Sci.* **78:** 3600–3604.

Dux, A. 1972. Genetic aspects in the genesis of mammary cancer. In *RNA viruses and host genome in oncogenesis* (ed. P. Emmelot and P. Bentvelzen), pp. 301–308. Elsevier/North-Holland, Amsterdam.

Dux, A. and O. Muhlbock. 1968. Propagation of the mammary tumor agent (Bittner virus) in the absence of mammary glands in mice. *J. Natl. Cancer Inst.* **40:** 1309–1312.

Eckert, E.A., D. Beard, and J.W. Beard. 1955a. Dose-response relations in experimental transmission of avian erythromyeloblastic leukosis. V. Influence of host age and route of virus inoculation. *J. Natl. Cancer Inst.* **15:** 1195–1207.

Eckert, E.A., D.G. Sharp, D. Beard, I. Green, and J.W. Beard. 1955b. Neutralization and precipitation of the virus of avian erythromyeloblastosis with serum of hyperimmunized chicks. *Proc. Soc. Exp. Biol. Med.* **88:** 181–187.

Eckner, R.J. 1975. Continuous replication of Friend virus complex (spleen focus-forming virus—lymphatic leukemia-inducing virus) in mouse embryo fibroblasts. Retention of leukemogenicity and loss of immunosuppressive properties. *J. Exp. Med.* **142:** 936–948.

Eliason, J.F., N.G. Testa, and T.M. Dexter. 1979. Erythropoietin-stimulated erythropoiesis in long-term bone marrow culture. *Nature* **281:** 382–384.

Ellermann, V. and O. Bang. 1908. Experimentelle Leukamie bei Huhnern. *Zentralbl. Bakt.* **46:** 595–609.

———. 1909. Experimentelle Leukamie bei Huhnern. *Zeitschr. Hyg. Infekt.* **63:** 231–272.

Engelbreth-Holm, J. and A. Rothe Meyer. 1935. On the connection between erythroblastosis (haemocytoblastosis), myelosis and sarcoma in chicken. *Acta Pathol. Microbiol. Scand.* **12:** 352–365.

Ephrussi, B. and H.M. Temin. 1960. Infection of chick iris epithelium with the Rous sarcoma virus *in vitro*. *Virology* **11:** 547–552.

Erfle, V., R. Hehlmann, H. Schetters, A. Meier, and A. Luz. 1980. Time course of C-type retrovirus expression in mice submitted to osteosarcomagenic doses of ^{224}radium. *Int. J. Cancer.* **26:** 107–113.

Erfle, V., S. Schulte-Overberg, K.-H. Marquart, I.-D. Adler, and A. Luz. 1979. Establishment and characterization of C-type RNA virus-producing cell lines from radiation-induced murine osteosarcoma. *J. Cancer Res. Clin. Oncol.* **94:** 149–162.

Essex, M. 1975. Horizontally and vertically transmitted oncornaviruses of cats. *Adv. Cancer Res.* **21:** 175–248.

Essex, M., W.D. Hardy, Jr., S.M. Cotter, and R.M. Jakowski. 1975a. Immune response of healthy and leukemic cats to the feline oncornavirus-associated cell membrane antigen. In *Comparative leukemia research 1973* (ed. Y. Ito and R.M. Dutcher), pp. 483–488. Karger, Basel.

Essex, M., G. Klein, S.P. Snyder, and J.B. Harrold. 1971. Correlation between humoral antibody and regression of tumours induced by feline sarcoma virus. *Nature* **233:** 195–196.

Essex, M., S.M. Cotter, J.R. Stephenson, S.A. Aaronson, and W.D. Hardy, Jr. 1977. Leukemia, lymphoma and fibrosarcoma of cats as models for similar diseases of man. *Cold Spring Harbor Conf. Cell Proliferation* **4:** 1197–1214.

Essex, M., A. Sliski, S.M. Cotter, R.M. Jakowski, and W.D. Hardy, Jr. 1975b. Immunosurveillance of naturally occurring feline leukemia. *Science* **190:** 790–792.

Evans, L.H., P.H. Duesberg, and E.M. Scolnick. 1980. Replication of spleen focus-forming Friend virus in fibroblasts from C57BL mice that are genetically resistant to spleen focus formation. *Virology* **101:** 534–539.

Fagg, B., K. Vehmeyer, W. Ostertag, C. Jasmin, and B. Klein. 1980. Modified erythropoiesis in mice infected with anemia or polycythemia-producing strains of Friend virus or with myeloproliferative virus. In *In vivo and in vitro erythropoiesis: The Friend system* (ed. G.B. Rossi), pp. 163–172. Elsevier/North-Holand, Amsterdam.

Fanning, T.G., J.P. Puma, and R.D. Cardiff. 1980a. Identification and partial characterization of an endogenous form of mouse mammary tumor virus that is transcribed into the virion-associated RNA genome. *Nucleic Acids Res.* **8:** 5715–5723.

———. 1980b. Selective amplification of mouse mammary tumor virus in mammary tumors of GR mice. *J. Virol.* **36:** 109–114.

Fefer, A., J.L. McCoy, and J.P. Glynn. 1967. Induction and regression of primary Moloney sarcoma virus-induced tumors in mice. *Cancer Res.* **27:** 1626–1631.

Fekete, E. and H.K. Otis. 1954. Observations on leukemia in AKR mice born from transferred ova and nursed by low leukemic mothers. *Cancer Res.* **14:** 445–447.

Ferrer, J.F. and C.E. Piper. 1981. Role of colostrum and milk in the natural transmission of the bovine leukemia virus. *Cancer Res.* **41:** 4906–4909.

Ferrer, J.F., L. Avila, and N.D. Stock. 1972. Serological detection of type C viruses found in bovine cultures. *Cancer Res.* **32:** 1864–1870.

Ferrer, J.F., C.E. Piper, D.A. Abt, R.R. Marshak, and D.M. Bhatt. 1976. Natural mode of transmission of the bovine C type leukemia virus (BLV). In *Comparative leukemia research 1975* (ed. J. Clemmesen and D.S. Yohn), pp. 235–237. Karger, Basel.

Ferrer, J.F., S.J. Kenyon, and P. Gupta. 1981. Milk of dairy cows frequently contains a leukemogenic virus. *Science* **213:** 1014–1016.

Fieldsteel, A.H., P.J. Dawson, and W.L. Bostick. 1961. Quantitative aspects of Friend leukemia virus in various murine hosts. *Proc. Soc. Exp. Biol. Med.* **127:** 900–904.

Finkel, M.P. and B.O. Biskis. 1968. Experimental induction of osteosarcomas. *Prog. Exp. Tumor Res.* **10:** 72–111.

Finkel, M.P., B.O. Biskis, and P.B. Jinkins. 1966a. Virus induction of osteosarcomas in mice. *Science* **151:** 698–701.

Finkel, M.P., C.A. Reilly, Jr., and B.O. Biskis. 1975. Viral etiology of bone cancer. *Front. Radiat. Ther. Oncol.* **10:** 28–39.

———. 1976. Pathogenesis of radiation and virus-induced bone tumors. *Recent Results Cancer Res.* **54:** 92–103.

Finkel, M.P., P.B. Jinkins, J. Tolle, and B.O. Biskis. 1966b. Serial radiography of virus-induced osteosarcomas in mice. *Radiology* **87:** 333–339.

Finkel, M.P., C.A. Reilly, Jr., B.O. Biskis, and I.L. Greco. 1973. Bone tumor viruses. In *Bone—certain aspects of neoplasia* (ed. C.H.G. Price and F.G.M. Ross), pp. 353–366. Butterworths, London.

Fiore-Donati, L. and L. Chieco-Bianchi. 1964. Influence of host factors on development and type of leukemia induced in mice by Graffi virus. *J. Natl. Cancer Inst.* **32:** 1083–1107.

Fiore-Donati, L., L. Chieco-Bianchi, G. Tridente, and N. Pennelli. 1966. Studies on thymus-dependent mechanisms of mouse leukemogenesis by Graffi virus. *Natl. Cancer Inst. Monogr.* **22:** 587–603.

Fischinger, P.J., N.M. Dunlop, and C.S. Blevins. 1978. Identification of virus found in mouse lymphomas induced by HIX murine oncornavirus. *J. Virol.* **26:** 532–535.

Fischinger, P.J., S. Nomura, and D.P. Bolognesi. 1975. A novel murine oncornavirus with dual eco- and xenotropic properties. *Proc. Natl. Acad. Sci.* **72:** 5150–5155.

Fischinger, P.J., J.N. Ihle, D.P. Bolognesi, and W. Schafer. 1976. Inactivation of murine xenotropic oncornavirus by normal mouse sera is not immunoglobulin-mediated. *Virology* **71:** 346–351.

Fiszman, M.Y. and P. Fuchs. 1975. Temperature-sensitive expression of differentiation in transformed myoblasts. *Nature* **254:** 429–431.

Flensburg, J.C. 1976. Attempt to eradicate leukosis from a dairy herd by slaughter of cattle with lymphocytosis. Report over a ten year period. *Vet. Microbiol.* **1:** 301–305.

Foulds, L. 1956. The histological analysis of mammary tumors of mice. II. The histology of responsiveness and progression. The origins of tumors. *J. Natl. Cancer Inst.* **17:** 713–753.

Fourcade, A., T. Huynh, and F. Lacour. 1974. Transfection of chicken embryo cells with DNA extracted from avian virus-producing neoplastic cells. *J. Virol.* **14:** 407–411.

Francis, D.P., M. Essex, and W.D. Hardy, Jr. 1977. Excretion of feline leukaemia virus by naturally infected pet cats. *Nature* **269:** 252–254.

Francis, D.P., M. Essex, S.M. Cotter, N. Gutensohn, R. Jakowski, and W.D. Hardy, Jr. 1981. Epidemiologic association between virus-negative feline leukemia and the horizontally transmitted feline leukemia virus. *Cancer Lett.* **12:**37–42.

Franklin, R.B., R.L. Maldonado, and H.R. Bose. 1974. Isolation and characterization of reticuloendotheliosis virus transformed bone marrow cells. *Intervirology* **3:**342–352.

Friend, C. 1957. Cell-free transmission in adult Swiss mice of a disease having the character of a leukemia. *J. Exp. Med.* **105:**307–318.

Friend, C. and J.R. Haddad. 1960. Tumor formation with transplants of spleen or liver from mice with virus-induced leukemia. *J. Natl. Cancer Inst.* **25:**1279–1289.

Friend, C., W. Scher, J.G. Holland, and T. Sato. 1971. Hemoglobin synthesis in murine virus-induced leukemic cells in vitro: Stimulation of erythroid differentiation by dimethyl sulfoxide. *Proc. Natl. Acad. Sci.* **68:**378–382.

Fujinaga, S., W.E. Poel, and L. Dmochowski. 1970. Light and electron microscope studies of osteosarcomas induced in rats and hamsters by Harvey and Moloney sarcoma viruses. *Cancer Res.* **30:**1698–1708.

Fujinami, A. and K. Inamoto. 1914. Ueber Geswulste bei japanishen Haushuhnern insbesondere uber einen transplantablen Tumor. *Z. Krebsforsch.* **14:**94–119.

Fung, Y.-K.T., A.M. Fadly, L.B. Crittenden, and H.-J. Kung. 1981. One of the mechanism of retrovirus-induced avian lymphoid leukosis: Deletion and integration of the provirus. *Proc. Natl. Acad. Sci.* **78:**3418–3422.

Furth, J., H.R. Seibold, and R.R. Rathbone. 1933. Experimental studies on lymphomatosis of mice. *Am. J. Cancer* **19:**521–604.

Gallo, R.C., R.E. Gallagher, F. Wong-Staal, T. Aoki, P.D. Markham, H. Schetters, F. Ruscetti, M. Valeiro, M.J. Walling, R.T. O'Keeffe, W.C. Saxinger, R.G. Smith, D.H. Gillespie, and M.S. Reitz, Jr. 1978. Isolation and tissue distribution of type-C virus and viral components from a gibbon ape (*Hylobates lar*) with lymphocytic leukemia. *Virology* **84:**359–373.

Gardner, M.B. 1978. Type C viruses of wild mice: Characterization and natural history of amphotropic, ecotropic, and xenotropic MuLV. *Curr. Top. Microbiol. Immunol.* **79:**215–259.

Gardner, M.B., J.D. Estes, J. Casagrande, and S. Rasheed. 1980a. Prevention of paralysis and suppression of lymphoma in wild mice by passive immunization to congenitally transmitted murine leukemia virus. *J. Natl. Cancer Inst.* **64:**359–364.

Gardner, M.B., A. Chiri, M.F. Dougherty, J. Casagrande, and J.D. Estes. 1979a. Congenital transmission of murine leukemia virus from wild mice prone to the development of lymphoma and paralysis. *J. Natl. Cancer Inst.* **62:**63–70.

Gardner, M.B., S. Rasheed, B.K. Pal, J.D. Estes, and S.J. O'Brien. 1980b. *Akvr-1,* a dominant murine leukemia virus restriction gene, is polymorphic in leukemia-prone wild mice. *Proc. Natl. Acad. Sci.* **77:**531–535.

Gardner, M.B., R.W. Rongey, E.Y. Johnson, R. DeJournett, and R.J. Huebner. 1971. C-type virus particles in salivary tissue of domestic cats. *J. Natl. Cancer. Inst.* **47:**561–565.

Gardner, M.B., V. Klement, R.R. Rongey, P. McConahey, J.D. Estes, and R.J. Huebner. 1976a. Type C virus expression in lymphoma-paralysis-prone wild mice. *J. Natl. Cancer Inst.* **57:**585–590.

Gardner, M.B., B.K., Pal, S. Rasheed, M.L. Bryant, R.W. Rongey, and J.M. Andrews. 1979b. Murine retrovirus motor neuron disease. In *Slow transmissible diseases of the nervous system* (ed. S.B. Prusiner and W.J. Hadlow), vol. 2, pp. 187–207. Academic Press, New York.

Gardner, M.B., S. Rasheed, J.D. Estes, J. Casagrande, J.N. Ihle, and J.R. Stephenson. 1980c. The history of viruses and cancer in wild mice. *Cold Spring Harbor Conf. Cell Proliferation* **7:**971–987.

Gardner, M.B., P. Arnstein, R.W. Rongey, J.D. Estes, P.S. Sarma, C.F. Rickard, and R.J. Huebner. 1970. Experimental transmission of feline fibrosarcoma to cats and dogs. *Nature* **226:** 807–809.

Gardner, M.B., B.E. Henderson, J.D. Estes, R.W. Rongey, J. Casagrande, M. Pike, and R.J. Huebner. 1976b. The epidemiology and virology of C-type virus-associated hematological cancers and related diseases in wild mice. *Cancer Res.* **36:** 574–581.

Gardner, W.U., T.F. Dougherty, and W.L. Williams. 1944. Lymphoid tumors in mice receiving steroid hormones. *Cancer Res* **4:** 73–87.

Gazdar, A.F., H.C. Chopra, and P.S. Sarma. 1972. Properties of a murine sarcoma virus isolated from a tumor arising in an NZW/NZB F_1 hybrid mouse. I. Isolation and pathology of tumors induced in rodents. *Int. J. Cancer* **9:** 219–233.

Gazzolo, L., M.G. Moscovici, and C. Moscovici. 1974. Replication of avian sarcoma viruses in chicken macrophages. *Virology* **58:** 514–525.

Gazzolo, L., M.G. Moscovici, C. Moscovici, and P.K. Vogt. 1975. Susceptibility and resistance of chicken macrophages to avian RNA tumor viruses. *Virology* **67:** 553–565.

Gazzolo, L., C. Moscovici, M.G. Mosovici, and J. Samarut. 1979. Response of hemopoietic cells to avian acute leukemia viruses: Effects on the differentiation of the target cells. *Cell* **16:** 627–638.

Gazzolo, L., J. Samarut, M. Bouabdelli, and J.P. Blanchet. 1980. Early precursors in the erythroid lineage are the specific target cells of avian erythroblastosis virus in vitro. *Cell* **22:** 683–691.

Georgsson, G., P.A. Palsson, H. Panitch, N. Nathanson, and G. Petursson. 1977. The ultrastructure of early visna lesions. *Acta Neuropathol.* **37:** 127–135.

Ghysdael, J., J.C. Neil, A.M. Wallbank, and P.K. Vogt. 1981. Esh avian sarcoma virus codes for a *gag*-linked transformation-specific protein with an associated protein kinase activity. *Virology* **111:** 386–400.

Gillette, R.W., S. Robertson, R. Brown, and K.E. Blackman. 1974. Expression of mammary tumor virus antigen on the membranes of lymphoid cells. *J. Natl. Cancer Inst.* **53:** 499–505.

Gimmy, J., F. Fey, and A. Graffi. 1960. Hamatologische und histologische Untersuchungen an Rattenleukosen, die durch zellfreie Filtrate von Mauseleukamien erzeugt wurden. *Arch. Geschwulstforsch.* **16:** 118–128.

Golde, D.W., N. Bersch, C. Friend, D. Tsuei, and W. Marovitz. 1979. Transformation of DBA/2 mouse fetal liver cells infected in vitro by the anemic strain of Friend leukemia virus. *Proc. Natl. Acad. Sci.* **76:** 962–966.

Graf, T. 1972. A plaque assay for avian RNA tumor viruses. *Virology* **50:** 567–578.

———. 1973. Two types of target cells for transformation with avian myelocytomatosis virus. *Virology* **54:** 398–413.

———. 1975. *In vitro* transformation of chicken bone marrow cells with avian erythroblastosis virus. *Z. Naturforsch.* **30c:** 847–849.

Graf, T. and H. Beug. 1978. Avian leukemia viruses. Interaction with their target cells in vivo and in vitro. *Biochim. Biophys. Acta* **516:** 269–299.

Graf, T., H. Beug, and M.J. Hayman. 1980. Target cell specificity of defective avian leukemia viruses: Hematopoietic target cells for a given virus type can be infected but not transformed by strains of a different type. *Proc. Natl. Acad. Sci.* **77:** 389–393.

Graf, T., B. Royer-Pokora, and H. Beug. 1976a. *In vitro* transformation of specific target cells by avian leukemia viruses. In *Animal virology* (ed. D. Baltimore et al.), pp. 321–338. Academic Press, New York.

Graf, T., A. von Kirchbach, and H. Beug. 1981. Characterization of the hematopoietic target cells of AEV, MC29 and AMV avian leukemia viruses. *Exp. Cell Res.* **131:** 331-343.

Graf, T., D. Fink, H. Beug, and B. Royer-Pokora. 1977a. Oncornavirus-induced sarcoma formation obscured by rapid development of lethal leukemia. *Cancer Res.* **37:** 59–63.

Graf, T., N. Oker-Blom, T.G. Todorov, and H. Beug. 1979. Transforming capacities and defectiveness of avian leukemia viruses OK10 and E26. *Virology* **99:**431–436.

Graf, T., B. Royer-Pokora, G.E. Schubert, and H. Beug. 1976b. Evidence for the multiple oncogenic potential of cloned leukemia virus: *In vitro* and *in vivo* studies with avian erythroblastosis virus. *Virology* **71:**423–433.

Graf, T., B. Royer-Pokora, W. Meyer-Glauner, M. Claviez, E. Gotz, and H. Beug. 1977b. *In vitro* transformation with avian myelocytomatosis virus strain CMII: Characterization of the virus and its target cells. *Virology* **83:**96–109.

Graffi, A. 1957. Chloroleukemia of mice. *Ann. N.Y. Acad. Sci.* **68:** 540–558.

Graffi, A. and J. Gimmy. 1957. Erzeugung von Leukosen bei der Ratte durch ein leukamogenes Agens der Maus. *Naturwissenschaften* **44:** 518.

———. 1959. Rattenleukosen durch zellfreie Filtrate aus homologem leukamischem Gewebe. *Z. Naturforsch.* **146:** 747–748.

Graffi, A., F. Fey, and T. Schramm. 1966. Experiments on the hematologic diversification of viral mouse leukemias. *Natl. Cancer Inst. Monogr.* **22:** 21–31.

Granboulan, N. and M.R. Riviere. 1962. Etude au microscope electronique des particules virales presentes dan les lymphomatoses spontanees de la souris. *J. Microscopie* **1:**23–38.

Grant, C.K., M. Essex, N.C. Pedersen, W.D. Hardy, Jr., S.M. Cotter, and G. Theilen. 1978. Lysis of feline lymphoma cells by complement-dependent antibodies in feline leukemia virus contact cats. Correlation of lysis and antibodies to feline oncornavirus-associated cell membrane antigen. *J. Natl. Cancer Inst.* **60:** 161–166.

Green, N., H. Hiai, J.H. Elder, R.S. Schwartz, R.H. Khiroya, C.Y. Thomas, P.N. Tsichlis, and J.M. Coffin. 1980. Expression of leukemogenic recombinant viruses associated with a recessive gene in HRS/J mice. *J. Exp. Med.* **152:**249–264.

Greenberger, J.S., P.B. Davisson, P.J. Gans, and W.C. Moloney. 1979. In vitro induction of continuous acute promyelocytic leukemia cell lines by Friend or Abelson murine leukemia virus. *Blood* **53:**987–1001.

Griffin, D.E., O. Narayan, and R.J. Adams. 1978a. Early immune responses in visna, a slow viral disease of sheep. *J. Infect. Dis.* **138:**340–350.

Griffin, D.E., O. Narayan, J.F. Bukowski, R.J. Adams, and S.R. Cohen. 1978b. The cerebrospinal fluid in visna, a slow viral disease of sheep. *Ann. Neurol.* **4:**212–218.

Groner, B. and N.E. Hynes. 1980. Number and location of mouse mammary tumor virus proviral DNA in mouse DNA of normal tissue and of mammary tumors. *J. Virol.* **33:** 1013-1025.

Groner, B., E. Buetti, H. Diggelmann, and N.E. Hynes. 1980. Characterization of endogenous and exogenous mouse mammary tumor virus proviral DNA with site-specific molecular clones. *J. Virol.* **36:**734–745.

Gross, L. 1951a. "Spontaneous" leukemia developing in C3H mice following inoculation, in infancy, with AK-leukemic extracts, or AK-embryos. *Proc. Soc. Exp. Biol. Med.* **76:**27–32.

———. 1951b. Pathogenic properties, and "vertical" transmission of the mouse leukemia agent. *Proc. Soc. Exp. Biol. Med.* **78:**342–348.

———. 1957. Development and serial cell-free passage of a highly potent strain of mouse leukemia virus. *Proc. Soc. Exp. Biol. Med.* **94:**767–771.

———. 1959. Serial cell-free passage of a radiation-activated mouse leukemia agent. *Proc. Soc. Exp. Biol. Med.* **100:** 102–105.

———. 1960. Development of myeloid (chloro-) leukemia in thymectomized C3H mice following inoculation of lymphatic leukemia virus. *Proc. Soc. Exp. Biol. Med.* **103:**509–514.

———. 1970. *Oncogenic viruses,* 2nd edition. Pergamon Press. Oxford.

Groudine, M. and H. Weintraub. 1980. Activation of cellular genes by avian RNA tumor viruses. *Proc. Natl. Acad. Sci.* **77:**5351–5354.

Gruneberg, H. 1942. The anemia of flex-tailed mice. II. Siderocytes. *J. Genet.* **44:**246–271.

Gudnadottir, M. and P.A. Palsson. 1965. Host-virus interaction in visna infected sheep. *J. Immunol.* **95:** 1116–1120.

———. 1967. Transmission of maedi by inoculatin of a virus grown in tissue culture from maedi-affected lungs. *J. Infect. Dis.* **117:** 1–6.

Gupta, P. and J.F. Ferrer. 1980. Detection of bovine leukemia virus antigen in urine from naturally infected cattle. *Int. J. Cancer* **25:** 663–666.

Haas, M. 1978. Leukemogenic activity of thymotropic, ecotropic, and xenotropic radiation leukemia virus isolates. *J. Virol.* **25:** 705–709.

———. 1981. B-cell and T-cell malignant lymphomas in C57BL/6 mice induced by different recombinant retroviruses isolated from X-irradiated mice. *Cold Spring Harbor Conf. Cell Proliferation* **8:** 1073–1082.

Haas, M. and J. Hilgers. 1975. *In vitro* infection of lymphoid cells by thymotropic radiation leukemia virus grown in *vitro*. *Proc. Natl. Acad. Sci.* **72:** 3546–3550.

Haas, M. and A. Meshorer. 1979. Reticulum cell neoplasms induced in C57BL/6 mice by cultured virus grown in stromal hematopoietic cell lines. *J. Natl. Cancer Inst.* **63:** 427–439.

Haas, M. and V. Patch. 1980a. Genomic masking and rescue of dual-tropic murine leukemia viruses: Role of psueodtype virions in viral lymphomagenesis. *J. Virol.* **35:** 583–591.

———. 1980b. Cell-surface antigens associated with dualtropic and thymotropic murine leukemia viruses inducing thymic and nonthymic lymphomas. *J. Exp. Med.* **151:** 1321–1333.

Haas, M. and T. Reshef. 1980. Non-thymic malignant lymphomas induced in C57BL/6 mice by cloned dualtropic viruses isolated from hematopoietic stromal cell lines. *Eur. J. Cancer* **16:** 909–917.

Haas, M., T. Sher, and S. Smolinsky. 1977. Leukemogenesis *in vitro* induced by thymus epithelial reticulum cells transmitting murine leukemia viruses. *Cancer Res.* **37:** 1800–1807.

Haase, A.T. 1975. The slow infection caused by visna virus. *Curr. Top. Microbiol. Immunol.* **72:** 101–156.

Haase, A.T. and H.E. Varmus. 1973. Demonstration of a DNA provirus in the lytic growth of visna virus. *Nat. New Biol.* **245:** 237–239.

Haase, A.T., L. Stowring, O. Narayan, D. Griffin, and D. Price. 1977. Slow persistent infection caused by visna virus: Role of host restriction. *Science* **195:** 175–177.

Haase, A.T., M. Brahic, D. Carroll, J. Scott, L. Stowring, B. Traynor, and P. Ventura. 1978. Visna: An animal model for studies of virus persistence. In *Persistent viruses* (ed. J.G. Stevens et al.), pp. 643–654. Academic Press, New York.

Hageman, P.C., J. Links, and P. Bentvelzen. 1968. Biological properties of B particles from C3H and C3Hf mouse milk. *J. Natl. Cancer Inst.* **40:** 1319–1324.

Hageman, P., J. Calafat, and J.H. Daams. 1972. The mouse mammary tumor viruses. In *RNA viruses and host genome in oncogenesis* (ed. P. Emmelot and P. Bentvelzen), pp. 283–300. North-Holland, Amsterdam.

Hanafusa, H. 1977. Cell transformation by RNA tumor viruses. In *Comprehensive virology* (ed. H. Fraenkel-Conrat and R.P. Wagner), vol. 3, p. 401–483. Plenun Press, New York.

Hanafusa, T., L.-H. Wang, S.M. Anderson, R.E. Karess, W.S. Hayward, and H. Hanafusa. 1980. Characterization of the transforming gene of Fujinami sarcoma virus. *Proc. Natl. Acad. Sci.* **77:** 3009–3013.

Hankins, W.D. and E.M. Scolnick. 1981. Harvey and Kirsten sarcoma viruses promote the growth and differentiation of erythroid precursor cells in vitro. *Cell* **26:** 91–97.

Hankins, W.D. and D. Troxler. 1980. Erythroid bursts following *in vitro* infection of bone marrow cells with the anemia-inducing strains of Friend and Rauscher leukemia viruses. In *In vivo and in vitro erythropoiesis: the Friend system* (ed. G.B. Rossi), pp. 151–161. Elsevier/North-Holland, Amsterdam.

Hankins, W.D., T.A. Kost, M.J. Koury, and S.B. Krantz. 1978. Erythroid bursts produced by Friend leukaemia virus *in vitro*. *Nature* **276:**506–508.

Hanna, M.G., Jr., R.W. Tennant, J.M. Yuhas, N.K. Clapp, B.L. Batzing, and M.J. Snodgrass. 1972. Autologous immunity to endogenous RNA tumor virus antigens in mice with a low natural incidence of lymphoma. *Cancer Res.* **32:**2226–2234.

Haran-Ghera, N. 1980. Pathogenesis of murine leukemia. In *Viral oncology* (ed. G. Klein), pp. 161–185. Raven Press, New York.

Hardy, W.J., Jr. 1980a. The virology, immunology and epidemiology of the feline leukemia virus. In *Feline leukemia virus* (ed. W.D. Hardy, Jr. et al.), pp. 33–78. Elsevier/North-Holland, New York.

———. 1980b. Feline leukemia virus disease. In *Feline leukemia virus* (ed. W.D. Hardy, Jr. et al.), pp. 3–31. Elsevier/North-Holland, New York.

———. 1980c. The biology and virology of the feline sarcoma viruses. In *Feline leukemia virus* (ed. W.D. Hardy, Jr. et al.), pp. 79–118. Elsevier/North-Holland, New York.

———. 1981a. Hematopoietic tumors of cats. *J. Am. Anim. Hosp. Assoc.* **17:**921–940.

———. 1981b. Feline leukemia virus non-neoplastic diseases. *J. Am. Anim. Hosp. Assoc.* **17:**941–949.

Hardy, W.D., Jr. 1982. Immunopathology induced by the feline leukemia virus. In *Seminars in immunopathology* (ed. G. Klein). Springer Verlag, New York. (In press.)

Hardy, W.D., Jr., Y. Hirshaut, and P. Hess. 1973. Detection of the feline leukemia virus and other mammalian oncornaviruses by immunofluorescence. In *Unifying concepts of leukemia* (ed. R.M. Dutcher and L. Chieco-Bianchi), pp. 778–799, Karger, Basel.

Hardy, W.D., Jr., E.G. MacEwen, A.S. Hayes, and E.E. Zuckerman. 1980a. FOCMA antibody as specific immunotherapy for lymphosarcoma of pet cats. In *Feline leukemia virus* (ed. W.D. Hardy, Jr. et al.), pp. 227–233. Elsevier/North-Holland, New York.

Hardy, W.D., Jr., E.E. Zuckerman, M. Essex, E.G. MacEwen, and A.A. Hayes. 1978. Feline oncornavirus-associated cell-membrane antigen: An FeLV- and FeSV-induced tumor-specific antigen. *Cold Spring Harbor Conf. Cell Proliferation* **5:**601–623.

Hardy, W.D., Jr., E.E. Zuckerman, E.G. MacEwen, A.A. Hayes, and M. Essex. 1977. A feline leukemia virus-and sarcoma virus-induced tumor- specific antigen. *Nature* **270:**249–251.

Hardy, W.D., Jr., E. Zuckerman, R. Markovich, P. Besmer, and H.W. Snyder, Jr. 1982. Isolation of feline sarcoma viruses from pet cats with multicentric fibrosarcomas. In *Advances in comparative leukemia research 1981* (ed. D. Yohn and J. Blakeslee). Elsevier/North-Holland, New York. (In press.)

Hardy, W.D., Jr., G. Geering, L.J. Old, E. DeHarven, R.S. Brodey, and S. McDonough. 1969. Feline leukemia virus: Occurrence of viral antigen in the tissues of cats with lymphosarcoma and other diseases. *Science* **166:**1019–1021.

Hardy, W.D., Jr., A.J. McClelland, E.E. Zuckerman, P.W. Hess, E.G. MacEwen, and A.A. Hayes. 1976a. Prevention of the contagious spread of feline leukemia virus and the development of leukemia in pet cats. *Nature* **263:**326–328.

Hardy, W.D., Jr., A.J. McClelland, E.E. Zuckerman, H.W. Snyder, Jr., E.G. MacEwen, D. Francis, and M. Essex. 1980b. Development of virus nonproducer lymphosarcomas in pet cats exposed to FeLV. *Nature* **288:**90–92.

Hardy, W.D., Jr., P.W. Hess, E.G. MacEwen, A.A. Hayes, R.K. Kassell, N.K. Day, and L.J. Old. 1976b. Treatment of feline lymphosarcoma with feline blood constituents. In *Comparative leukemia research 1975* (ed. J. Clemmesen and D.S. Yohn), pp. 518–521. Karger, Basel.

Hardy, W.D., Jr., P.W. Hess, E.G. MacEwen, A.J. McClelland, E.E. Zuckerman, M. Essex, S.M. Cotter, and O. Jarrett. 1976c. Biology of feline leukemia virus in the natural environment. *Cancer Res.* **36:**582–588.

Hare, W.C.D., T.-J. Yang, and R.A. McFeely. 1967. A survey of chromosome findings in 47 cases of bovine lymphosarcoma (leukemia). *J. Natl. Cancer Inst.* **38:** 383–392.

Hartley, J.W. and W.P. Rowe. 1976. Naturally occurring murine leukemia viruses in wild mice: Characterization of a new "amphotropic" class. *J. Virol.* **19:** 19–25.

Hartley, J.W., W.P. Rowe, W.I. Capps, and R.J. Huebner. 1969. Isolation of naturally occurring viruses of the murine leukemia virus group in tissue culture. *J. Virol.* **3:** 126–132.

Hartley, J.W., N.K. Wolford, L.J. Old, and W.P. Rowe. 1977. A new class of murine leukemia virus associated with development of spontaneous lymphomas. *Proc. Natl. Acad. Sci.* **74:** 789–792.

Harvey, J.J. 1964. An unidentified virus which causes the rapid production of tumors in mice. *Nature* **204:** 1104–1105.

———. 1971. The murine sarcoma virus (MSV). *Int. Rev. Exp. Pathol.* **10:** 265–360.

Hasthorpe, S. and S. Bol. 1979. Erythropoietin responses and physical characterization of erythroid progenitor cells in Rauscher virus infected BALB/c mice. *J. Cell. Physiol.* **100:** 77–86.

Hays, E.F. and D.L. Vredevoe. 1977. A discrepancy in XC and oncogenicity assays for murine leukemia virus in AKR mice. *Cancer Res.* **37:** 726–730.

Hayward, W.S., B.G. Neel, and S.M. Astrin. 1981. Activation of a cellular *onc* gene by promoter insertion in ALV-induced lymphoid leukosis. *Nature* **290:** 475–480.

Henson, J.B. and T.C. McGuire. 1971. Immunopathology of equine infectious anemia. *Am. J. Clin. Pathol.* **56:** 306–314.

———. 1974. Equine infectious anemia. *Prog. Med. Virol.* **18:** 143–159.

Henson, J.B., T.C. McGuire, K. Kobayashi, K.L. Banks, W.C. Davis, and J.R. Gorham. 1970. Recent research on the virology, serology and pathology of equine infectious anemia. In *Proceedings of the 2nd International Conference on Equine Infectious Diseases,* pp. 178–199.

Heston, W.E. 1965. Genetic factors in the etiology of cancer. *Cancer Res.* **25:** 1320–1326.

Hilgers, J. and P. Bentvelzen. 1978. Interaction between viral and genetic factors in murine mammary cancer. *Adv. Cancer Res.* **26:** 143–195.

Hilgers, J.H.M., G.J. Theuns, and R. van Nie. 1973. Mammary tumor virus (MTV) antigens in normal and mammary tumor-bearing mice. *Int. J. Cancer* **12:** 568–576.

Hilgers, J., J. Haverman, R. Nusse, W.J. van Blitterswijk, F.J. Cleton, P.C. Hageman, R. van Nie, and J. Calafat. 1975. Immunologic, virologic, and genetic aspects of mammary tumor-induced cell-surface antigens: Presence of these antigens and the Thy 1.2 antigen on murine mammary gland and tumor cells. *J. Natl. Cancer Inst.* **54:** 1323–1333.

Hoelzer, J.D., R.B. Franklin, and H.R. Bose, Jr. 1979. Transformation by reticuloendotheliosis viruses: Development of a focus assay and isolation of a nontransforming virus. *Virology* **93:** 20–30.

Hoelzer, J.D., R.B. Lewis, C.R. Wasmuth, and H.R. Bose, Jr. 1980. Hematopoietic cell transformation by reticuloendotheliosis virus: Characterization of the genetic defect. *Virology* **100:** 462–474.

Holzer, H., J. Biehl, G. Yeoh, R. Meganath, and A. Kaji. 1975. Effects of oncogenic virus on muscle differentiation. *Proc. Natl. Acad. Sci.* **72:** 4051–4055.

Hooks, J.J. and C.J. Gibbs, Jr. 1975. The foamy viruses. *Bacteriol. Rev.* **39:** 169–185.

Hoover, E.A., L.E. Perryman, and G.J. Kociba. 1973. Early lesions in cats inoculated with feline leukemia virus. *Cancer Res.* **33:** 145–152.

Hoover, E.A., G.J. Kociba, W.D. Hardy, Jr., and D.S. Yohn. 1974. Erythroid hypoplasia in cats inoculated with feline leukemia virus. *J. Natl. Cancer Inst.* **53:** 1271–1276.

Hoover, E.A., J.L. Rojko, P.L. Wilson, and R.G. Olson. 1980. Macrophages and the susceptibility of cats to feline leukemia virus infection. In *Feline leukemia virus* (ed. W.D. Hardy, Jr. et al.), pp. 195–202. Elsevier/North-Holland, New York.

Horoszewicz, J.S., S.S. Leong, and W.A. Carter. 1975. Friend leukemia: Rapid development of erythropoietin-independent hematopoietic precursors. *J. Natl. Cancer Inst.* **54:** 265–267.

Hoss, H.E. and C. Olson. 1974. Infectivity of bovine C-type (leukemia) virus for sheep and goats. *Am. J. Vet. Res.* **35:** 633–637.

Huebner, R.J., R.V. Gilden, R. Toni, R.W. Hill, R.W. Trimmer, D.C. Fish, and B. Sass. 1976. Prevention of spontaneous leukemia in AKR mice by type-specific immunosuppression of endogenous ecotropic virogenes. *Proc. Natl. Acad. Sci.* **73:** 4633–4635.

Humphries, R.K., P.B. Jacky, F.J. Dill, A.C. Eaves, and C.J. Eaves. 1979. CFU-S in individual erythroid colonies derived *in vitro* from adult mice bone marrow. *Nature* **279:** 718–720.

Hunsmann, G., V. Moennig, and W. Schafer. 1975. Properties of mouse leukemia viruses. IX. Active and passive immunization of mice against Friend leukemia with isolated viral GP71 glycoprotein and its corresponding antiserum. *Virology* **66:** 327–329.

Hynes, R.O. 1974. Role of surface alterations in cell transformation: The importance of proteases and surface proteins. *Cell* **1:** 147–156.

Hynes, R.O. and A.T. Destree. 1978. Relationships between fibronectin (LETS protein) and actin. *Cell* **15:** 875–886.

Ihle, J.N. and M.G. Hanna, Jr. 1977. Natural immunity to endogenous oncornaviruses in mice. *Contemp. Top. Immunobiol.* **5:** 169–194.

Ihle, N.J., L.O. Arthur, and D.L. Fine. 1976a. Autogenous immunity to mouse mammary tumor virus in mouse strains of high and low mammary tumor incidence. *Cancer Res.* **36:** 2804–2844.

Ihle, J.M., D.R. Joseph, and N.H. Pazmino. 1976b. Radiation leukemia in C57BL mice. II. Lack of ecotropic virus expression in the majority of lymphomas. *J. Exp. Med.* **144:** 1406–1423.

Ikeda, H. and T. Odaka. 1979. Expression of $Fv\text{-}4^r$ allele in hematopoietic cells from G mice resistant to Friend leukemia virus. *Int. J. Cancer* **23:** 514–518.

Irgens, K., M. Wyers, A. Moraillon, A. Parodi, and V. Fortuny. 1973. Isolement d'un virus sarcomatogene feline a partir d'un fibrosarcome spontane du chat: Etude du pouvoir sarcomatogene *in vivo*. *C.R. Acad. Sci.* **276:** 1783–1786.

Iscove, N.N. 1978. Erythropoietin-independent stimulation of early erythropoiesis in adult marrow cultures by conditioned media from lectin-stimulated mouse spleen cell. In *Hematopoietic cell differentiation* (ed. D.W. Golde et al.), pp. 37–52. Academic Press, New York.

Ishii, S. 1963. Equine infectious anemia or swamp fever. *Adv. Vet. Sci.* **8:** 263–298.

Ishimoto, A., A. Adachi, K. Sakai, T. Yorifuji, and S. Tsuruta. 1981. Rapid emergence of mink cell focus-forming (MCF) virus in various mice infected with NB-tropic Friend virus. *Virology* **113:** 644–655.

Ishitani, R. 1970. Equine infectious anemia. *Natl. Inst. Anim. Health Q.* **10:** 1–28.

Ishizaki, R. and T. Shimizu. 1970. Heterogeneity of strain R avian (erythroblastosis) virus. *Cancer Res.* **30:** 2827–2831.

Ishizaki, R., A.J., Langlois, and D.O. Bolognesi. 1975. Isolation of two subgroup-specific leukemogenic viruses from standard avian myeloblastosis virus. *J. Virol.* **15:** 906–912.

Itohara, S., K. Hirata, M. Inoue, M. Hatsuoka, and A. Sato. 1978. Isolation of a sarcoma virus from a spontaneous chicken tumor. *Gann* **69:** 825–830.

Izui, S., P.J. McConahey, and F.J. Dixon. 1978. Increased spontaneous polyclonal activation of B lymphocytes in mice with spontaneous antoimmune disease. *J. Immunol.* **121:** 2213–2219.

Jacobs, S.W. and R.G. Miller. 1979. Characterization of *in vitro* T-lymphocyte colonies from spleens of nude mice. *J. Immunol.* **122:** 582–584.

Jacobson, L.O., E.K. Marks, M.J. Robson, E. Gaston, and R.E. Zirkle. 1949. The effect of spleen protection on mortality following X-irradiation. *J. Lab. Clin. Med.* **34:** 1538–1543.

Jacquemin, P.C., C. Saxinger, R.C. Gallo, W.D. Hardy, Jr., and M. Essex. 1978. Antibody response in cats to feline leukemia virus reverse transcriptase under natural conditions of exposure to the virus. *Virology* **91:**472–476.

Jakowski, R.M., M. Essex, W.D. Hardy, Jr., J.R. Stephenson, and S.M. Cotter. 1980. Membranous glomerulonephritis in a household of cats persistently viremic with feline leukemia virus. In *Feline leukemia virus* (ed. W.D. Hardy, Jr. et al.), pp. 141–149. Elsevier/North-Holland, New York.

Jarrett, O. 1981. Natural occurrence of subgroups of feline leukemia virus. *Cold Spring Harbor Conf. Cell Proliferation* **8:**603.

Jarrett, O., M. Laird, and D. Hay. 1973. Determinants of the host range of feline leukemia viruses. *J. Gen. Virol.* **20:**169–175.

Jarrett, W., L. Mackey, O. Jarrett, H. Laird, and C. Hood. 1974. Antibody response and virus survival in cats vaccinated against feline leukemia. *Nature* **248:**230–232.

D.O., W.L. Wooding, P. Tanticharoenyos, and C.H. Bourgeois, Jr. 1971. Malignant lymphoma in the gibbon. *J. Am. Vet. Med. Assoc.* **159:**563–566.

Johnson, G.R. and D. Metcalf. 1977. Pure and mixed erythroid colony formation stimulated by spleen conditioned medium with no detectable erythropoietin. *Proc. Natl. Acad. Sci.* **74:**3879–3882.

Jones, F.R., L.H. Yoshida, W.C. Ladiges, and M.A. Kenny. 1980a. Treatment of feline leukemia and reversal of FeLV by *ex vivo* removal of IgG. *Cancer* **46:**675–684.

Jones, F.R., L.H. Yoshida, W.C. Ladiges, N.S. Zeidner, M.A. Kenny, and A.J. McClelland. 1980b. Treatment of feline lymphosarcoma by extracorporeal immunosorption. In *Feline leukemia virus* (ed. W.D. Hardy, Jr. et al.), pp. 235–243. Elsevier/North-Holland, New York.

Jones, M.D., D.T. Lau, and J. Warthen. 1972. Lymphoblastic lymphosarcoma in two white-handed gibbons *(Hylobates lar). J. Natl. Cancer Inst.* **49:**599–601.

Kahn, D.E., A.S. Mia, and M.M. Tierney. 1980. Field evaluation of Leukassay F., and FeLV detection test kit. *Feline Pract.* **10:**41–45.

Kai, K., H. Ikeda, Y. Yuasa, S. Suzuki, and T. Odaka. 1976. Mouse strain resistant to N-, B-, and NB-tropic murine leukemia viruses. *J. Virol.* **20:**436–440.

Kaighn, M.E., J.D. Ebert, and P.M. Scott. 1966. The susceptibility of differentiating muscle clones to Rous sarcoma virus. *Proc. Natl. Acad. Sci.* **56:**133–140.

Kane, J.P., D.A. Hardman, J.C. Dimpfl, and J.A. Levy. 1979. Apolipoprotein is responsible for neutralization of xenotropic type C virus by mouse serum. *Proc. Natl. Acad. Sci.* **76:**5957–5961.

Kaplan, H.S. 1950. Influence of thymectomy, splenectomy, and gonadectomy on incidence of radiation-induced lymphoid tumors in strain C57 black mice. *J. Natl. Cancer Inst.* **11:**83–90.

Kaplan, H.S., M.B. Brown, and J. Paull. 1953. Influeunce of postirradiation thymectomy and of thymic implants on lymphoid tumor incidence in C57BL mice. *Cancer Res.* **13:**677–680.

Kaplan, H.S., W.H. Carnes, M.B. Brown, and. B.B. Hirsch. 1956. Indirect induction of lymphomas in irradiated mice. I. Tumor incidence and morphology in mice bearing nonirradiated thymic grafts. *Cancer Res.* **16:**422–425.

Kassel, R.L., L.J. Old, E.A. Carswell, N.C. Fiore, and W.D. Hardy, Jr. 1973. Serum-mediated leukemia cell destruction in AKR mice. *J. Exp. Med.* **138:**925–938.

Kawai, S. and H. Hanafusa. 1972. Plaque assay from some strains of avian leukosis virus. *Virology* **48:**126–135.

Kawakami, T.G. and P.M. Buckley. 1974. Antigenic studies on gibbon type-C viruses. *Transplant. Proc.* **6:**193–196.

Kawakami, T.G. and T.S. McDowell. 1980. Factors regulating the onset of chronic myelogenous leukemia in gibbons. *Cold Spring Harbor Conf. Cell Proliferation* **8:**719–727.

Kawakami, T.G., G.V. Kollias, Jr., and C. Holmberg. 1980. Oncogenicity of gibbon type-C myelogenous leukemia virus. *Int. J. Cancer* **25:**641–646.

Kawakami, T.G., L. Sun, and T.S. McDowell. 1977. Infectious primate type-C virus shed by healthy gibbons. *Nature* **268:**448–450.

———. 1978a. Distribution and transmission of primate type-C virus. In *Advances in comparative leukemia research 1977* (ed. P. Bentvelzen et al.), pp. 33–36. Elsevier/North-Holland, Amsterdam.

———. 1978b. Natural transmission of gibbon leukemia virus. *J. Natl. Cancer Inst.* **61:**1113–1115.

Kawakami, T.G., P.M. Buckley, A. DePaoli, W. Noll, and L.K. Bustad. 1975. Studies on the prevalence of type C virus associated with gibbon hematopoietic neoplasms. In *Comparative leukemia research 1973* (ed. Y. Ito and R.M. Dutcher), pp. 385–389. University of Tokyo Press, Tokyo.

Kawakami, T.G., S.D. Huff, P.M. Buckley, D.L. Dungworth, S.P. Snyder, and R.V. Gilden. 1972. C-type virus associated with gibbon lymphosarcoma. *Nat. New Biol.* **235:**170–171.

Kawashima, K., H. Ikeda, J.W. Hartley, E. Stockert, W.P. Rowe, and L.J. Old. 1976. Changes in expression of murine leukemia virus antigens and production of xenotropic virus in the late preleukemic period in AKR mice. *Proc. Natl. Acad. Sci.* **73:**4680–4684.

Keller, L.H., R. Rufner, and M. Sevoian. 1979. Isolation and development of a reticuloendotheliosis virus-transformed lymphoblastoid cell line from chicken spleen cells. *Infect. Immunol.* **25:**694–701.

Kelloff, G.J., W.T. Lane, H.C. Turner, and R.J. Huebner. 1969. *In vivo* studies of the FBJ murine osteosarcoma virus. *Nature* **223:**1379–1380.

Kelloff, G.J., R.L. Peters, R.M. Donahoe, I. Ghazzouli, B. Sass, R.M. Nims, and R.J. Huebner. 1976. An approach to C-type virus immunoprevention of spontaneously occurring tumors in laboratory mice. *Cancer Res.* **36:**622–630.

Kemen, M.J. and L. Coggins. 1972. Equine infectious anemia: Transmission from infected mares to foals. *J. Am. Vet. Med. Assoc.* **161:**496–499.

Kemeny, L.J., L.O. Mott, and J.E. Pearson. 1971. Titration of equine infectious anemia virus. Effect of dosage on incubation time and clinical signs. *Cornell Vet.* **61:**687–695.

Kennedy, R.C., C.M. Eklund, C. Lopez, and W.J. Hadlow. 1968. Isolation of a virus from lungs of Montana sheep affected with progressive pneumonia. *Virology* **35:**483–484.

Kenyon, S.J. and C.E. Piper. 1977. Cellular basis of persistent lymphocytosis in cattle infected with bovine leukemia virus. *Infect. Immun.* **16:**891–897.

Keshet, E. and H.M. Temin. 1979. Cell killing by spleen necrosis virus is correlated with a transient accumulation of spleen necrosis virus DNA. *J. Virol.* **31:**376–388.

Kettmann, R., Y. Cleuter, M. Mammerickx, M. Meunier-Rotival, G. Bernardi, A. Burny, and H. Chantrenne. 1980. Genomic integration of bovine leukemia provirus: Comparison of persistent lymphocytosis with lymph node tumor form of enzootic bovine leukosis. *Proc. Natl. Acad. Sci.* **77:**2577–2581.

Kirsten, W.H. and L.A. Mayer. 1967. Morphologic responses to a murine erythroblastosis virus. *J. Natl. Cancer Inst.* **39:**311–335.

———. 1969. Malignant lymphomas of extrathymic origin induced in rats by murine erythroblastosis virus. *J. Natl. Cancer Inst.* **43:**735–746.

Klein, B., C. LeBousse, B. Fagg, F. Smadja-Joffe, K. Vehmeyer, K.J. Mori, C. Jasmin, and W. Ostertag. 1981. Effects of myeloproliferative sarcoma virus on the pluripotential stem cell and granulocytic precursor cell population in DBA/2 mice. *J. Natl. Cancer Inst.* **66:**935–940.

Kletzien, R.F. and J.F. Perdue. 1975. Regulation of sugar transport in chick embryo fibroblasts infected with a temperature-sensitive mutant of RSV. *Cell* **6:**513–520.

Kobayashi, K. and Y. Kono. 1967. Propagation and titration of equine infectious anemia virus in horse leukocyte culture. *Inst. Anim. Hlth. Quart.* **7:**8–20.

Kobilinsky, L., W.D. Hardy, Jr., and N.K. Day. 1979. Hypocomplemententemia associated with naturally occurring lymphosarcoma in pet cats. *J. Immunol.* **122:**2139–2142.

Konno, S. and H. Yamamoto. 1970. Pathology of equine infectious anemia. Proposed classification of pathologic types of disease. *Cornell Vet.* **60:**393–449.

Kono, Y. 1969. Viremia and immunological response in horses infected with equine infectious anemia virus. *Natl. Inst. Anim. Health Q.* **9:**1–9.

Kono, Y. and K. Kobayashi. 1966. Complement fixation test of equine infectious anemia. II. Relationship between CF antibody response and the disease. *Natl. Inst. Anim. Health Q.* **6:**204–207.

Kono, Y., K. Kobayashi, and Y. Fukunaga. 1970. Immunization of horses against equine infectious anemia (EIA) with an attenuated EIA virus. *Natl. Inst. Anim. Health Q.* **10:**113–122.

———. 1971. Distribution of equine infectious anemia virus in horses infected with the virus. *Natl. Inst. Anim. Health Q.* **11:**11–20.

Korteweg. R. 1934. Proefondervindelijke onderzoekingen aangaandre erfelijkheid van kander. *Ned. Tijdschr. Geneesk.* **78:**240–245.

———. 1936. On the manner in which the disposition to carcinoma of the mammary gland is inherited in mice. *Genetics* **18:**350–371.

Koshy, R., F. Wong-Staal, R.C. Gallo, W.D. Hardy, Jr., and M. Essex. 1979. Distribution of feline leukemia virus DNA sequences in tissues of normal and leukemic domestic cats. *Virology* **99:**135–144.

Kost, T.A., M.J. Koury, W.D. Hankins, and S.B. Krantz. 1979. Target cells for Friend virus-induced erythroid bursts in vitro. *Cell* **18:**145–152.

Krakower, J.M., S.R. Tronick, R.E. Gallagher, R.C. Gallo, and S.A. Aaronson. 1978. Antigenic characterization of a new gibbon ape leukemia virus isolate: Seroepidemiologic assessment of an outbreak of gibbon leukemia. *Int. J. Cancer* **22:**715–720.

Krammer, P.H., R. Citronbaum, S.E. Read, L. Forni, and R. Lang. 1976. Murine thymic lymphomas as model tumors for T-cell studies. T-cell markers, immunoglobulin and Fc-receptors on AKR thymomas. *Cell. Immunol.* **21:**97–111.

Kunii, A., H. Takemoto, and J. Furth. 1965. Leukemogenic filterable agent from estrogen-induced thymic lymphoma in RF mice. *Proc. Soc. Exp. Biol. Med.* **119:**1211–1215.

Lacassagne, A. 1937. Sarcomes lymphoides apparus chez des souris longuement traitees par des hormones oesterogenes. *C.R. Soc. Biol.* **126:**193–195.

Lane, M.-A., A. Sainten, and G.M. Cooper. 1981. Activation of related transforming genes in mouse and human mammary carcinomas. *Proc. Natl. Acad. Sci.* **78:**5185–5189.

Langlois, A.J., S. Sankaran, P.-H.L. Hsiung, and J.W. Beard. 1967. Massive direct conversion of chick embryo cells by strain MC29 avian leukosis virus. *J. Virol.* **1:**1082–1084.

Langlois, A.J., R.B. Fritz, U. Heine, D. Beard, D.P. Bolognesi, and J.W. Beard. 1969. Response of bone marrow to MC29 avian leukosis virus *in vitro*. *Cancer Res.* **29:**2056–2074.

Langlois, A.J., R. Ishizaki, G.S. Beaudreau, J.F. Kummer, J.W. Beard, and D.P. Bolognesi. 1976. Virus-infected avian cell lines established *in vitro*. *Cancer Res.* **36:**3894–3904.

Lasfargues, E.Y., B. Kramarsky, J.C. Lasfargues, and D.H. Moore. 1974. Detection of mouse mammary tumor virus in cat kidney cells infected with purified B particles from RIII milk. *J. Natl. Cancer Inst.* **53:**1831–1833.

Lasfargues, E.Y., J.C. Lasfargues, A.S. Dion, A.E. Greene, and D.H. Moore. 1976. Experimental infection of a cat kidney cell line with the mouse mammary tumor virus. *Cancer Res.* **36:**67–72.

Lasneret, J. 1967. Etudes des tumeurs provoquees chez le rat par le virus de sarcome de Moloney. *Bull. Cancer* **53:**193–200.

Latarjet, R. and J.-F. Duplan. 1962. Experiment and discussion on leukaemogenesis by cell-free extracts of radiation-induced leukaemia in mice. *Int. J. Radiat. Biol.* **5:**339–344.

Law, L.W. 1947. Effect of gonadectomy and adrenalectomy on the appearance and incidence of spontaneous lymphoid leukemia in C58 mice. *J. Natl. Cancer Inst.* **8:**157–159.

Law, L.W. and J.H. Miller. 1950. The influence of thymectomy on the incidence of carcinogen-induced leukemia in strain DBA mice. *J. Natl. Cancer Inst.* **11:**425–437.

Law, L.W. and J.B. Moloney. 1961. Studies of congenital transmission of a leukemia virus in mice. *Proc. Soc. Exp. Biol. Med.* **108:**715–723.

Law, L.W., R.C. Ting, and M.F. Stanton. 1968. Some biologic, immunogenic, and morphologic effects in mice after infection with a murine sarcoma virus. I. Biological and immunogenic studies. *J. Natl. Cancer Inst.* **40:**1101–1112.

LeBousse-Kerdiles, M.C., F. Smadja-Joffe, B. Klein, B. Caillou, and C. Jasmin. 1980. Study of a virus-induced myeloproliferative syndrome associated with tumor formation in mice. *Eur. J. Cancer* **16:**43–51.

Lee, C.K., E.W. Chan, C.A. Reilly, Jr., V.A. Pahnke, G. Rockus, and M.P. Finkel. 1979. *In vitro* properties of FBR murine osteosarcoma virus. *Proc. Soc. Exp. Biol. Med.* **162:**214–220.

Lee, J.C. and J.N. Ihle. 1981a. Chronic immune stimulation is required for Moloney leukaemia virus-induced lymphomas. *Nature* **289:**407–409.

———. 1981b. Increased responses to lymphokines are correlated with preleukemia in mice inoculated with Moloney leukemia virus. *Proc. Natl. Acad. Sci.* **78:**7712–7716.

Lee, J.C., J.N. Ihle, and R. Huebner. 1977. The humoral immune response of NIH Swiss and SWR/J mice to vaccination with formalinized AKR or Gross murine leukemia virus. *Proc. Natl. Acad. Sci.* **74:**343–347.

Lee, W.-H., K. Bister, A. Pawson, R. Robins, C. Moscovici, and P.H. Duesberg. 1980. Fujinami sarcoma virus: An avian RNA tumor virus with a unique transforming gene. *Proc. Natl. Acad. Sci.* **77:**2018–2022.

Leonard, A. and A. Decleve. 1979. A chromosome marker for studies in the C57 black strain of mice. *Leuk. Res.* **3:**93–98.

Levy, J.A., J.W. Hartley, W.P. Rowe, and R.J. Huebner. 1973. Studies of FBJ osteosarcoma virus in tissue culture. I. Biologic characteristics of the "C"-type viruses. *J. Natl. Cancer Inst.* **51:**525–539.

———. 1975a. Studies of FBJ osteosarcoma virus in tissue culture. II. Autoinhibition of focus formation. *J. Natl. Cancer Inst.* **54:**615–619.

Levy, J.A., J.N. Ihle, O. Oleszko, and R.D. Barnes. 1975b. Virus-specific neutralization by a soluble nonimmunoglobulin factor found naturally in normal mouse sera. *Proc. Natl. Acad. Sci.* **72:**5071–5075.

Levy, J.A., P.L. Kazan, C.A. Reilly, Jr., and M.P. Finkel. 1978. FBJ osteosarcoma virus in tissue culture. III. Isolation and characterization of non-virus-producing FBJ-transformed cells. *J. Virol.* **26:**11–15.

Levy, S.B., L.A. Blankstein, E.C. Vinton, and T.J. Chambers. 1979. Biologic and biochemical characteristics of Friend leukemic cells representing different stages of a malignant process. In *Oncogenic viruses and host cell genes* (ed. Y. Ikawa and T. Odaka), pp. 409–428. Academic Press, New York.

Lewis, R.B., J. McClure, B. Rup, D.W. Niesel, F.R. Garry, J.D. Hoelzer, K. Nazerian, and H.R. Bose, Jr. 1981. Avian reticuloendotheliosis virus: Identification of the hematopoietic target cell for transformation. *Cell* **25:**421–431.

Liao, S.-K. and A.A. Axelrad. 1975. Erythropoietin-independent erythroid colony formation *in vitro* by hemopoietic cells of mice infected with Friend virus. *Int. J. Cancer* **15:**467–482.

Lieberman, M. and H.S. Kaplan. 1959. Leukemogenic activity of filtrates from radiation-induced lymphoid tumors of mice. *Science* **130:**387–388.

Lieberman, M., O. Niwa, A. Decleve, and H.S. Kaplan. 1973. Continuous propagation of radiation leukemia virus on a C57BL mouse-embryo line, with attenuation of leukemogenic activity. *Proc. Natl. Acad. Sci.* **70:**1250–1253.

Lieberman, M., A. Decleve, J.N. Ihle, and H.S. Kaplan. 1979. Rescue of a thymotropic, leukemogenic C-type virus from cultured, nonproducer lymphoma cells of strain C57BL/Ka mice. *Virology* **97:**12–21.

Lilly, F. 1967. Susceptibility to two strains of Friend leukemia virus in mice. *Science* **155:**461–462.

Lilly, F. 1968. The effect of histocompatibility-2 type on response to the Friend leukemia virus in mice. *J. Exp. Med.* **127:**465–473.

———. 1970. *Fv-2:* Identification and location of a second gene governing the spleen focus response to Friend leukemia virus in mice. *J. Natl. Cancer Inst.* **45:**163–169.

Lilly, F. and T. Pincus. 1973. Genetic control of murine viral leukemogenesis. *Adv. Cancer Res.* **17:**231–277.

Lilly, F., E.A. Boyse, and L.J. Old. 1964. Genetic basis of susceptibility to viral leukaemogenesis. *Lancet* **2:**1207–1209.

Lingeman, C.H., R.E. Reed, and F.M. Garner. 1969. Spontaneous hematopoietic neoplasms of nonhuman primates. Review, case report, and comparative studies. *Natl. Cancer Inst. Monogr.* **32:**157–170.

Linna, T.J., C. Hu, and K.D. Thompson. 1974. Development of systemic and local tumors induced by avian reticuloendotheliosis virus after thymectomy or bursectomy. *J. Natl. Cancer Inst.* **53:**847–854.

Loutit, J.F. and E.L. Lloyd. 1977. Tumours and viruses in mice injected with plutonium. *Nature* **266:**355–357.

Lowy, D.R, S.K. Chattopadhyay, N.M. Teich, W.P. Rowe, and A.S. Levine. 1974. AKR murine leukemia virus genome: Frequency of sequences in DNA of high-, low-, and non-virus-yielding mouse strains. *Proc. Natl. Acad. Sci.* **71:**3555–3559.

Ludford, G.G., H.G. Purchase, and H.W. Cox. 1972. Duck infectious anemia virus associated with *Plasmodium lophurae. Exp. Parasitol.* **31:**29–38.

Lung, M.L., C. Hering, J.W. Hartley, W.P. Rowe, and N. Hopkins. 1980. Analysis of the genomes of mark cell focus-inducing sarcoma type C viruses: A progress report. *Cold Spring Harbor Symp. Quant. Biol.* **44:** 1269–1274.

MacDonald, M.E., G.R. Johnson, and A. Bernstein. 1981. Different pseudotypes of Friend spleen focus-forming virus induce polycythemia and erythropoietin-independent colony formation in serum-free medium. *Virology* **110:** 231–236.

MacDonald, M.E., T.W. Mak, and A. Bernstein. 1980a. Erythroleukemia induction by replication-competent type C viruses cloned from the anemia- and polycythemia-inducing isolates of Friend leukemia virus. *J. Exp. Med.* **151:**1493–1503.

MacDonald, M.E., F.H. Reynolds, Jr., W.J.M. Van de Ven, J.R. Stephenson, T.W. Mak, and A. Bernstein. 1980b. Anemia- and polycythemia-inducing isolates of Friend spleen focus-forming virus. Biological and molecular evidence for two distinct viral genomes. *J. Exp. Med.* **151:**1477–1492.

MacDowell, E.C. and M.N. Richter. 1935. Mouse leukemia. IX. The role of heredity in spontaneous cases. *Arch. Pathol.* **20:**709–724.

Mackey, L.J., W. Jarrett, O. Jarrett, and H. Laird. 1975. Anemia associated with feline leukemia virus infection in cats. *J. Natl. Cancer Inst.* **54:**209–217.

Mager, D., T.W. Mak, and A. Bernstein. 1980. Friend leukemia virus-transformed cells, unlike normal stem cells, form spleen colonies in Sl/Sl^d mice. *Nature* **288:**592–594.

———. 1981a. Quantitative colony method for tumorigenic cells transformed by two distinct strains of Friend leukemia virus. *Proc. Natl. Acad. Sci.* **78:**1703–1707.

Mager, D., M.E. MacDonald, I.B. Robson, T.W. Mak, and A. Bernstein. 1981b. Clonal analysis of the late stages of erythroleukemia induced by two distinct strains of Friend leukemia virus. *Mol. Cell. Biol.* **1:**721–730.

Maggio, L. 1979. Anemia in the cat. *Comp. Cont. Ed.* **1:**114–122.

Mak, T.W., A.A. Axelrad, and A. Bernstein. 1979. *Fv-2* locus controls expression of Friend spleen focus-forming virus-specific sequences in normal and infected mice. *Proc. Natl. Acad. Sci.* **76:**5809–5812.

Mak, T.W., C.L. Gamble, M.E. MacDonald, and A. Bernstein. 1980. Host control of sequences specific to Friend erythroleukemia virus in normal and leukemic mice. *Cold Spring Harbor Symp. Quant. Biol.* **44:**893–899.

Mammerickx, M., D. Dekegel, A. Burny, and D. Portetelle. 1976. Study on the oral transmission of bovine leukosis to the sheep. *Vet. Microbiol.* **1:**347–350.

Manaker, R.A. and V. Groupé. 1956. Discrete foci of altered chicken embryo cells associated with Rous sarcoma virus in tissue culture. *Virology* **2:**838–840.

Marcelletti, J. and P. Furmanski. 1978. Spontaneous regression of Friend virus-induced erythroleukemia. III. The role of macrophages in regression. *J. Immunol.* **120:**1–8.

———. 1979. Infection of macrophages with Friend virus: Relationship to the spontaneous regression of viral erythroleukemia. *Cell* **16:**649–659.

Markham, P.D., F. Ruscetti, S.Z. Salahuddin, R.E. Gallagher, and R.C. Gallo. 1979. Enhanced induction of growth of B lymphoblasts from fresh human blood by primate type-C retroviruses (gibbon ape leukemia virus and simian sarcoma virus). *Int. J. Cancer.* **23:**148–156.

Marks, S.C. and D.L. Walker. 1976. Mammalian osteopetrosis: A model for studying cellular and humor factors in bone resorption. In *The biochemistry and physiology of bone* (ed. G.H. Bourne), vol. 4, pp. 227–301. Academic Press, New York.

Marshak, R.R., L.L. Coriell, W.C. Lawrence, J.E. Croshaw, Jr., H. Schryver, K.P. Altera, and W.W. Nichols. 1962. Studies on bovine lymphosarcoma. I. Clinical aspects, pathological alterations, and herd studies. *Cancer Res.* **22:**202–217.

Mathes, L.E., R.G. Olsen, L.C. Hebebrand, E.A. Hoover, and J.P. Schaller. 1978. Abrogation of lymphocyte blastogenesis by a feline leukemia virus protein. *Nature* **274:**687–689.

Mathieson, B.J., P.S. Campbell, M. Potter, and R. Asofsky. 1978. Expression of Ly 1, Ly 2, Thy 1, and TL differentiation antigens on mouse T-cell tumors. *J. Exp. Med.* **147:**1267–1279.

McCarter, J.A., J.K. Ball, and J.V. Frei. 1977. Lower limb paralysis induced in mice by a temperature-sensitive mutant of Moloney leukemia virus. *J. Natl. Cancer Inst.* **59:**179–183.

McClelland, A.J., W.D. Hardy, Jr., and E.E. Zuckerman. 1980. Prognosis of healthy feline leukemia virus infected cats. In *Feline leukemia virus* (ed. W.D. Hardy, Jr. et al.), pp. 121–126, Elsevier/North-Holland, New York.

McClure, H.M., M.E. Keeling, R.P. Custer, R.R. Marshak, D.A. Abt, and J.F. Ferrer. 1974. Erythroleukemia in two infant chimpanzees fed milk from cows naturally infected with the bovine C-type virus. *Cancer Res.* **34:**2745–2757.

McCool, D., T.W. Mak, and A. Bernstein. 1979. Cellular regulation in Friend virus induced erythroleukemia. Studies with anemic mice of genotype Sl/Sl^d. *J. Exp. Med.* **149:**837–846.

McCulloch, E.A., J.E. Till, and L. Siminovitch. 1965a. Genetic factors affecting the control of hemopoiesis. *Can. Cancer Conf.* **6:**336–356.

McCulloch, E.A., L. Siminovitch, J.E. Till, E.S. Russell, and S.E. Bernstein. 1965b. The cellular basis of the genetically determined hemopoietic defect in anemic mice of genotype Sl/Sl^d. *Blood* **26:**399–410.

McCullough, B., J. Schaller, J.A. Shadduck, and D.S. Yohn. 1972. Induction of malignant melanomas associated with fibrosarcoma in gnotobiotic cats inoculated with Gardner feline fibrosarcoma virus. *J. Natl. Cancer Inst.* **48:**1893–1896.

McDonough, S.K., S. Larsen, R.S. Brodey, N.D. Stock, and W.D. Hardy, Jr. 1971. A transmissible feline fibrosarcoma of viral origin. *Cancer Res.* **31:**953–956.

McEndy, D.P., M.C. Boon, and J. Furth. 1944. On the role of thymus, spleen, and gonads in the development of leukemia in a high-leukemia stock of mice. *Cancer Res.* **4:**377–383.

McGarry, M.P., R.A. Steeves, R.J. Eckner, E.A. Mirand, and P.J. Trudel. 1974. Isolation of a myelogenous leukemia-inducing virus from mice infected with the Friend virus complex. *Int. J. Cancer* **13:**867–878.

McGrath, C.M., E.J. Marineau, and B.A. Voyles. 1978. Changes in MuMTV DNA and RNA levels in Balb/c mammary epithelial cells during mailgnant transformation by exogenous MuMTV and by hormones. *Virology* **87:**339–353.

McGrath, M.S. and I.L. Weissman. 1978. A receptor-mediated model of viral leukemogenesis: Hypothesis and experiments. *Cold Spring Harbor Conf. Cell Proliferation* **5:**547–589.

———. 1979. AKR leukemogenesis: Identification and biological significance of thymic lymphoma receptors for AKR retroviruses. *Cell* **17:**65–75.

McGrath, M.S., A. Decleve, M. Lieberman, H.S. Kaplan, and I.L. Weissman. 1978. Specificity of cell surface virus receptors on radiation leukemia virus and radiation-induced thymic lymphomas. *J. Virol.* **28:**819–827.

McGuire, T.C., J.B. Henson, and S.E. Quist. 1969. Viral induced hemolysis in equine infectious anemia. *Am. J. Vet. Res.* **30:**2091–2097.

McGuire, T.C., T.B. Crawford, and J.B. Henson. 1971. Immunofluorescent localization of equine infectious anemia virus in tissues. *Am. J. Pathol.* **62:**283–292.

McGuire, T.C., T.B. Crawford, and J.B. Henson. 1972. Equine infectious anemia. Detection of infectious virus-antibody complexes in the serum. *Immunol. Commun.* **1:**545–551.

Meier, H., D.D. Myers, and R.J. Huebner. 1969. Genetic control by the *hr*-locus of susceptibility and resistance to leukemia. *Proc. Natl. Acad. Sci.* **63:**759–766.

Mellors, R.C. 1968. Autoimmune disease and neoplasia of NZB mice—Implication of murine leukemia-like virus. *Perspect. Virol.* **6:**239–258.

Mercier, L. 1937. Heredite du lymphosarcome de la souris dan les croisements d'heterozygotes pour le couple de facteurs cancer-noncancer. *C.R. Soc. Biol.* **124:**403–405.

———. 1966. *The thymus. Its role in immune responses, leukaemia development and carcinogenesis. Recent Results Cancer Res.* **5:**1–144.

———. 1977. *Hemopoietic colonies: In vitro cloning of normal and leukemic cells.* Springer-Verlag, New York.

Metcalf, D. and G.R. Johnson. 1978. Mixed hemopoietic colonies in vitro. In *Hematopoietic cell differentiation* (ed. D.W. Golde et al.), pp. 141–151. Academic Press, New York.

Metcalf, D., N.L. Warner, G.J.V. Nossal, J.F.A.P. Miller, K. Shortman, and E. Rabellino. 1975a. Growth of B lymphocyte colonies *in vitro* from mouse lymphoid organs. *Nature* **255:**630–632.

Metcalf, D., G.J.V. Nossal, N.L. Warner, J.F.A.P. Miller, T.E. Mandel, J.E. Layton, and G.A. Gutman. 1975b. Growth of B-lymphocyte colonies in vitro. *J. Exp. Med.* **142:**1534–1549.

Meyers, P., G.D. Ritts, and D.R. Johnson. 1976. Phytohemagglutinin-induced leukocyte blastogenesis in normal and avial leukosis virus-infected chickens. *Cell. Immunol.* **27:**140–146.

Michalides, R., G. Vlahakis, and J. Schlom. 1976. A biochemical approach to the study of the transmission of mouse mammary tumor viruses in mouse strains RIII and C3H. *Int. J. Cancer* **18:**105–115.

Michalides, R., L. Van Deemter, R. Nusse, and P.C. Hageman. 1979. Induction of mouse mammary tumor virus RNA in mammary tumors of BALB/c mice treated with urethane, X-irradiation, and hormones. *J. Virol.* **31:**63–72.

Michalides, R., L. van Deemter, R. Nusse, and R. van Nie. 1978a. Identification of the *Mtv*-2 gene responsible for the early appearance of mammary tumors in the GR mouse by nucleic acid hybridization. *Proc. Natl. Acad. Sci.* **75:**2368–2372.

Michalides, R., E. Wagenaar, B. Groner, and N.E. Hynes. 1981a. Mammary tumor virus proviral DNA in normal murine tissue and non-virally induced mammary tumors. *J. Virol.* **39:**367–376.

Michalides, R., L. van Deemter, R. Nusse, G. Ropcke, and L. Boot. 1978b. Involvement of mouse mammary tumor virus in spontaneous and hormone-induced mammary tumors in low-mammary-tumor mouse strains. *J. Virol.* **17:**551–559.

Michalides, R., R. van Nie, R. Nusse, N.E. Hynes, and B. Groner. 1981b. Mammary tumor induction loci in GR and DBAf mice contain one provirus of the mouse mammary tumor virus. *Cell* **23:**165–173.

Miller, J.M. and C. Olson. 1972. Precipitating antibody to an internal antigen of the C-type virus associated with bovine lymphosarcoma. *J. Natl. Cancer Inst.* **49:**1459–1462.

Miller, J.M. and M.J. Van Der Maaten. 1978. Evaluation of an inactivated bovine leukemia virus preparation as an immunogen in cattle. *Ann. Rech. Vet.* **9:**871–877.

———. 1979. Infectivity tests of secretions and excretions from cattle infected with bovine leukemia virus. *J. Natl. Cancer Inst.* **62:**425–428.

Miller, J.M., L.D. Miller, K.G. Gillette, and C. Olson. 1969a. Incidence of lymphocytic nuclear projections in bovine lymphosarcoma. *J. Natl. Cancer Inst.* **43:**719–727.

Miller, J.M., L.D. Miller, C. Olson, and K.G. Gillette. 1969b. Virus-like particles in phytohemagglutinin-stimulated lymphocyte cultures with reference to bovine lymphosarcoma. *J. Natl. Cancer Inst.* **43:**1459–1462.

Miller, J.F.A.P. 1959. Role of the thymus in murine leukaemia. *Nature* **183:**1069.

Mirand, E.A. 1967. Virus-induced erythropoiesis in hypertransfused-polycythemic mice. *Science* **156:**832–833.

Mirand, E.A., T.C. Prentice, J.G. Hoffmann, and J.T. Grace, Jr. 1961. Effect of Friend virus in Swiss and DBA/1 mice on Fe^{59} uptake. *Proc. Soc. Exp. Biol. Med.* **106:**423–426.

Mirand,, E.A., R.A. Steeves, R.D. Lange, and J.T. Grace, Jr. 1968a. Virus-induced polycythemia in mice: Erythropoiesis without erythropoietin. *Proc. Soc. Exp. Biol. Med.* **128:**844–849.

Mirand, E.A., R.A. Steeves, L. Avila, and J.T. Grace, Jr. 1968b. Spleen focus formation by polycythemic strains of Friend leukemia virus. *Proc. Soc. Exp. Biol. Med.* **127:**900–904.

Miskin, R., T.G. Easton, A. Maelicke, and E. Reich. 1978. Metabolism of acetylcholine receptor in chick embryo muscle cells: Effects of RSV and PMA. *Cell* **15:**1287–1300.

Moloney, J.B. 1960. Biological studies on a lymphoid-leukemia virus extracted from sarcoma 37. I. Origin and introductory investigations. *J. Natl. Cancer Inst.* **24:**933–951.

Moloney, J.B. 1966. A virus-induced rhabdomyosarcoma of mice. *Natl. Cancer Inst. Monogr.* **22:**139–142.

Montelaro, R.C., P.J. Fischinger, S.B. Larrick, N.M. Dunlop, J.N. Ihle, H. Frank, W. Schafer, and D.P. Bolognesi. 1979. Further characterization of the oncornavirus inactivating factor in normal mouse serum. *Virology* **98:**20–34.

Moore, D.H., J. Charney, and J.A. Holben. 1974. Titrations of various mouse mammary tumor viruses in different mouse strains. *J. Natl. Cancer Inst.* **52:**1757–1761.

Moore, D.H., J. Charney, and B.D. Pullinger. 1970. Mouse mammary tumor virus infectivity as a function of age at inoculation, breeding, and total lapsed time. *J. Natl. Cancer Inst.* **45:**561–565.

Moore, D.H., C.A. Long, A.B. Vaidya, J.B. Sheffield, A.S. Dion, and E.Y. Lasfargues. 1979. Mammary tumor viruses. *Adv. Cancer Res.* **29:**347–418.

Morris, V.L., W. Medeiros, G.M. Ringold, J.M. Bishop, and H.E. Varmus. 1977. Comparison of mouse mammary tumor virus-specific DNA in inbred, wild and asian mice, and in tumors and normal organs from inbred mice. *J. Mol. Biol.* **114:**73–91.

Moscovici, C. and P.K. Vogt. 1968. Effect of genetic cellular resistance on cell transformation and virus replication in chicken hematopoietic cell cultures infected with avian myeloblastosis virus (BAI-A). *Virology* **35:**487–497.

Moscovici, C. and M. Zanetti. 1970. Studies on single foci of hematopoietic cells transformed by avian myeloblastosis virus. *Virology* **42:**61–67.

Moscovici, C., L. Gazzolo, and M.G. Moscovici. 1975. Focus assay and defectiveness of avian myeloblastosis virus. *Virology* **68:**173–181.

Moscovici, C., R.W. Alexander, M.G. Moscovici, and P.K. Vogt. 1978. Transforming and oncogenic effects of MH-2 virus. In *Avian RNA tumor viruses* (ed. S. Barlati and C. deGiuli-Morghen), pp. 45–56. Piccin Medical Books, Padua.

Moscovici, C., D. Chi, L. Gazzolo, and M.G. Moscovici. 1976. A study of plaque formation with avian tumor viruses. *Virology* **73:**181–189.

Motta, J., L. Crittenden, H.G. Purchase, H. Stone, W. Okazaki, and R. Witter. 1975. Low oncogenic potential of avian endogenous RNA tumor virus infection or expression. *J. Natl. Cancer Inst.* **55:**685–689.

Muhlbock, O. 1965. Note on a new inbred mouse-strain GR/A. *Eur. J. Cancer* **1:**123–124.

Muhlbock, O. and P. Bentvelzen. 1968. The transmission of the mammary tumor viruses. *Perspect. Virol.* **6:**75–87.

Muhlbock, O. and L.M. Boot. 1959. Induction of mammary cancer in mice without the mammary tumor agent by isografts of hypophyses. *Cancer Res.* **19:**402–412.

Muhlbock, O. and A. Dux. 1974. Histocompatibility genes (the *H-2* complex) and susceptibility to mammary tumor virus in mice. *J. Natl. Cancer Inst.* **53:**993–996.

Munroe, J.S., F. Shipkey, R.A. Erlandson, and W.F. Windle. 1964. Tumors induced in juvenile and adult primates by chicken sarcoma virus. *Natl. Cancer Inst. Monogr.* **17:**365–390.

Murphy, J.B. 1944. The effect of castration, theelin, and testosterone on the incidence of leukemia in a Rockefeller Institute strain of mice. *Cancer Res.* **4:**622–624.

Mussman, H.C. and M.J. Twiehaus. 1971. Pathogenesis of reticuloendothelial virus disease in chickens—An acute runting syndrome. *Avian Dis.* **15:**483–502.

Nandi, S. 1963. New method for detection of mouse mammary tumor virus. I. Influence of foster nursing on incidence of hyperplastic mammary nodules in BALB/cCrgl mice. *J. Natl. Cancer Inst.* **31:**57–73.

———. 1974. Mechanism of resistance to mammary tumor development in C57BL and I strains of mice. II. Inherent differences between the two strains. *J. Natl. Cancer Inst.* **52:**1797–1804.

Nandi, S. and C. Helmich. 1974. Differential effect of ionizing radiation on mammary tumor virus activity associated with blood cells and mammary tumor cells. *J. Natl. Cancer Inst.* **52:**1271–1275.

Nandi, S. and C.M. McGrath. 1973. Mammary neoplasia in mice. *Adv. Cancer Res.* **17:**353–414.

Nandi, S., S. Haslam, and C. Helmich. 1972. Mechanism of resistance to mammary tumor development in C57BL and I strains of mice. I. Noduligenesis, tumorigenesis, and characteristics of nodules and tumors. *J. Natl. Cancer Inst.* **48:**1005–1012.

Nandi, S., C. Helmich, and S. Haslam. 1974. Hemic cell-associated mammary tumor virus activity in BALB/cfC3H mice. *J. Natl. Cancer Inst.* **52:**1277–1283.

Narayan, O., D.E. Griffin, and J. Chase. 1977. Antigenic shift of visna virus in persistently infected sheep. *Science* **197:**376–378.

Narayan, O., D.E. Griffin, and J.E. Clements. 1978. Virus mutation during "slow infection": Temporal development and characterization of mutants of visna virus recovered from sheep. *J. Gen. Virol.* **41:**343–352.

Narayan, O., J.E. Clements, J.D. Strandberg, L.C. Cork, and D.E. Griffin. 1980. Biological characterization of the virus causing leukoencephalitis and arthritis in goats. *J. Gen. Virol.* **50:**69–79.

Nathanson, N. and W. Robinson, eds. 1979. *Persistent viral infections,* vol. 3. DHEW Publication No. NIH 79-1833, pp.1-213. Department of Health, Education and Welfare, Washington, D.C.

Nathanson, N., H. Panitch, P.A. Palsson, G. Petursson, and G. Georgsson. 1976. Pathogenesis of visna. II. Effect of immunosuppression upon early central nervous system lesions. *Lab. Invest.* **35:**444-451.

Nazerian, K. 1980. Marek's disease: A herpesvirus-induced malignant lymphoma of the chicken. In *Viral oncology* (ed. G Klein), pp. 665-682. Raven Press, New York.

Neel, B.G., W.S. Hayward, H.L. Robinson, J. Fang, and S.M. Astrin. 1981. Avian leukosis virus-induced tumors have common proviral integration sites and synthesize discrete new RNAs: Oncogenesis by promoter insertion. *Cell* **23:**323-334.

Neiman, P., K. Beemon, and J.A. Luce. 1981. Independent recombination between avian leukosis virus terminal sequences and host DNA in virus-induced proliferative disease. *Proc. Natl. Acad. Sci.* **78:**1891-1900.

Neiman, P., L.N. Payne, and R.A. Weiss. 1980a. Viral DNA in bursal lymphomas induced by avian leukosis viruses. *J. Virol.* **34:**178-186.

Neiman, PE., L. Jordan, R.A. Weiss, and L.N. Payne. 1980b. Malignant lymphoma of the bursa of Fabricius: Analysis of early transformation. *Cold Spring Harbor Conf. Cell Proliferation* **8:**519-528.

Newberne, J.W. and V.B. Robinson. 1960. Spontaneous tumors in primates—A report of two cases with notes on the apparent low incidence of neoplasms in subhuman primates. *Am. J. Vet. Res.* **21:**150-155.

Niho, Y., T. Shibuya, and T.W. Mak. 1982. Modulation of erthropoiesis by the helper-independent Friend leukemia virus F-MuLV. *J. Cell. Physiol.* (in press).

Noon, M.C., R.G. Wolford, and W.P. Parks. 1975. Expression of mouse mammary tumor viral polypeptides in milks and tissues. *J. Immunol.* **115:**653-658.

Noori-Daloii, M.R., R.A. Swift, H.-J. Kung, L.B. Crittenden, and R.L. Witter. 1981. Specific integration of REV proviruses in avian bursal lymphomas. *Nature* **294:**574-576.

Nooter, K. and P. Bentvelzen. 1976. *In vitro* growth characteristics of virally transformed murine myeloid cells. *Cancer Res.* **36:**1246-1250.

Nowinski, R.C. and T. Doyle. 1977. Cellular changes in the thymuses of preleukemic AKR mice: Correlation with changes in the expression of murine leukemia viruses. *Cell* **12:**341-353.

Nowinski, R.C. and E.F. Hays. 1978. Oncogenicity of AKR endogenous leukemia viruses. *J. Virol.* **27:**13-18.

Nowinski, R.C., N.H. Sarkar, L.J. Old, D.H. Moore, D.I. Scheer, and J. Hilgers. 1971. Characteristics of the structural components of the mouse mammary tumor virus. II. Viral proteins and antigens. *Virology* **46:**21-38.

Nusse, R., R. Michalides, L.M. Boot, and G. Ropcke. 1980. Qualification of mouse mammary tumor virus structural proteins in hormone-induced mammary tumors of low mammary tumor mouse strains. *Int. J. Cancer* **25:**377-383.

Nusse, R., L. van der Ploeg, L. van Duijn, R. Michalides, and J. Hilgers. 1979. Impaired maturation of mouse mammary tumor virus precursor polypeptides in lymphoid leukemia cells, producing intracytoplasmic A particles and no extracellular B-type virions. *J. Virol.* **32:**251-258.

Oberling, C. and M. Guerin. 1934. La leucemie erythroblastique ou erythroblastose transmissible des poule. *Bull. Cancer* **23:**38-82.

O'Brien, S.J., J.M. Simonson, and S. Davis. 1978. Deposition of retrovirus associated antigens (p30 and gp70) on cell membranes of feline and murine leukemia virus infected cells. *J. Gen. Virol.* **38:**483-496.

Odaka, T. 1970. Inheritance of susceptibility to Friend mouse leukemia virus. VII. Establishment of a resistant strain. *Int. J. Cancer* **6:**18-23.

Odaka, T. and H. Ikeda. 1977. Genetic resistance to Friend leukemia virus in mice: Masking of *Fv-2* phenotype by an epistatic gene, *Fv-4*^{r}. *Jpn. J. Exp. Med.* **47:**515–521.

Odaka, T. and T. Yamamoto. 1962. Inheritance of susceptibility to Friend mouse leukemia virus. *Jpn. J. Exp. Med.* **32:**405–413.

———. 1965. Inheritance of susceptibility to Friend mouse leukemia virus. II. Spleen foci method applied to test the susceptibility of crossbred progeny between a sensitive and a resistant strain. *Jpn. J. Exp. Med.* **35:**311–314.

O'Donnell, P.V. and R.C. Nowinski. 1980. Serological analysis of antigenic determinants on the *env* gene products of dualtropic (MCF) murine leukemia viruses. *Virology* **107:**81–88.

O'Donnell, P.V., E. Stockert, Y. Obata, A.B. DeLeo, and L.J. Old. 1980. Murine-leukemia-virus-related cell-surface antigens as serological markers of AKR ecotropic, xenotropic, and dualtropic viruses. *Cold Spring Harb. Symp. Quant. Biol.* **44:**1255–1264.

Officer, J.E., N. Tecson, J.D. Estes, E. Fontanilla, R.W. Rongey, and M.B. Gardner. 1973. Isolation of a neurotropic type C virus. *Science* **181:**945–947.

Ogura, H., H. Gelderblom, and H. Bauer. 1974. Isolation of avian nephroblastoma virus from avian myeloblastosis virus by the infectious DNA technique. *Intervirology* **4:**69–76.

Oker-Blom, N., A. Kallio, and L. Hortling. 1975. Morphological changes in chick embryo cell cultures induced by avian leukosis viruses. *Intervirology* **5:**342–353.

Oker-Blom, N., L. Hortling, A. Kallio, E.-L. Nurmiaho, and H. Westermarck. 1978. OK 10 virus, an avian retrovirus resembling the acute leukaemia viruses. *J. Gen. Virol.* **40:**623–633.

Oldstone, M.B.A., B.C. Del Villano, and F.J. Dixon. 1976. Autologous immune responses to the major oncornavirus polypeptides in unmanipulated AKR/J mice. *J. Virol.* **18:**176–181.

Oldstone, M.B.A., P.W. Lampert, S. Lee, and F.J. Dixon. 1977. Pathogenesis of the slow disease of the central nervous system associated with WM 1504 E virus. I. Relationship of strain susceptibility and replication to disease. *Am. J. Pathol.* **88:**193–212.

Oldstone, M.B.A., F. Jensen, F.J. Dixon, and P.W. Lampert. 1980. Pathogenesis of the slow disease of the central nervous system associated with wild mouse virus. II. Role of virus and host gene products. *Virology* **107:**180–193.

Oliff, A., S. Ruscetti, E.C. Douglass, and E. Scolnick. 1981. Isolation of transplantable erythroleukemia cells from mice infected with helper-independent Friend murine leukemia virus. *Blood* **58:**244–254.

Oliff, A.I., G.L. Hager, E.H. Chang, E.M. Scolnick, H.W. Chan, and D.R. Lowy. 1980. Transfection of molecularly cloned Friend murine luekemia virus DNA yields a highly leukemogenic helper-independent type C virus. *J. Virol.* **33:**475–486.

Olsen, R.G., E.A. Hoover, L.E. Mathes, L.D. Heding, and J.P. Schaller. 1976. Immunization against feline oncornavirus disease using a killed tumor cell vaccine. *Cancer Res.* **36:**3642–3646.

Olsen, R.G., M. Lewis, L.E. Mathes, and W. Hause. 1980. Feline leukemia vaccine: Efficacy testing in a large multicat household. *Feline Pract.* **10:**13–16.

Olson, C., H.E. Hoss, J.M. Miller, and L.E. Baumgartener. 1973. Evidence of bovine C-type (leukemia) virus in dairy cattle. *J. Am. Vet. Med. Assoc.* **163:**355–357.

Olson, C., R. Kettmann, A. Burny, and R. Kaja. 1981. Goat lymphosarcoma from bovine leukemia virus. *J. Natl. Cancer Inst.* **67:**671–675.

Olson, L.D. 1967. Histologic and hematologic changes in moribund stages of chicks infected by T-virus. *Am. J. Vet. Res.* **28:**1501–1507.

Onuma, M., L.E. Baumgartener, C. Olson, and L.D. Pearson. 1977. Fetal infection with bovine leukemia virus in sheep. *Cancer Res.* **37:**4075–4081.

Ostertag, W., K. Vehmeyer, B. Fagg, I.B. Pragnell, W. Paetz, M.C. Le Bousse, F. Smadja-Joffe, B. Klein, C. Jasmin, and E. Eisen. 1980. Myeloproliferative virus, a cloned murine sarcoma virus with spleen focus-forming properties in adult mice. *J. Virol.* **33:**573–582.

O'Sullivan, B.M., F.W. Eaves, S.A. Baxendell, and K.J. Rowan. 1978. Leukoencephalomyelitis of goat kids. *Aust. Vet. J.* **54:**479–483.

Pacifici, M., D. Boettiger, K. Roby, and H. Holtzer. 1977. Transformation of chondroblasts by Rous sarcoma virus and synthesis of the sulfated proteoglycan matrix. *Cell* **11:**891–899.

Paige, C.J., P.W. Kincade, L.A. Shinefield, and V.L. Suto. 1981. Precursors of murine B lymphocytes: Physical and functional characterization and distinction of myeloid stem cells. *J. Exp. Med.* **153:** 154–165.

Palsson, P.A. 1976. Maedi and visna in sheep. In *Slow virus diseases of animals and man* (ed. R.H. Kimberlin), pp. 17–43. North-Holland, Amsterdam.

Parks, W., R.W. Gillette, K. Blackman, J.E. Verna, and L.R. Sibal. 1972. Mammary tumor virus expression in mice: Immunologic studies. In *Fundamental research on mammary tumours* (ed. J. Mouriquand), pp. 77–90. INSERM, Paris.

Paterson, R.W. and R.E. Smith. 1978. Characterization of anemia induced by an avian osteopetrosis virus. *Infect. Immunol.* **22:**891–900.

Paul, P.S., K.A. Pomeroy, D.W. Johnson, C.C. Muscoplat, B.S. Handwerger, F.S. Soper, and D.K. Sorensen. 1977. Evidence for the replication of bovine leukemia virus in the B-lymphocytes. *Am. J. Vet. Res.* **38:**873–876.

Pauley, R.J., D. Medina, and S.H. Socher. 1979. Murine mammary tumor virus expression during mammary tumorigenesis in BALB/c mice. *J. Virol.* **29:**483–493.

Paulsen, J., R. Rudolph, and J.M. Miller. 1974. Antibodies to common ovine and bovine C-type virus specific antigen in serum from sheep with spontaneous leukosis and from inoculated animals. *Med. Microbiol. Immunol.* **159:**105–114.

Payne, G.S., J.M. Bishop, and H.E. Varmus. 1982. Multiple arrangements of viral DNA and an activated host oncogene in bursal lymphomas. *Nature* **295:**209–214.

Payne, G.S., S.A. Courtneidge, L.B. Crittenden, A.M. Fadly, J.M. Bishop, and H.E. Varmus. 1981. Analysis of avian leukosis virus DNA and RNA in bursal tumors: Viral gene expression is not required for maintenance of the tumor state. *Cell* **23:**311–322.

Payne, L.N. and P.M. Biggs. 1970. Genetic resistance of fowl to MH2 reticulendothelioma virus. *J. Gen. Virol.* **7:**177–185.

Payne, L.N., A. Holmes, K. Howes, M. Pattison, and D.E. Walters. 1979. Studies on the associations between natural infection of hens, cocks and their progeny with lymphoid leukosis virus. *Avian Pathol.* **8:**411–424.

Pedersen, N.C., G.H. Theilen, and L.L. Werner. 1979. Safety and efficacy studies of live- and killed-feline leukemia virus vaccines. *Am. J. Vet. Res.* **40:**1120–1126.

Pepersack, L., J.C. Lee, R. McEwan, and J.N. Ihle. 1980. Phenotypic heterogeneity of Moloney leukemia virus-induced T cell lymphomas. *J. Immunol.* **124:**279–285.

Perek, M. 1960. An epizootic of histiocytic sarcoma in chickens induced by a cell-free agent. *Avian Dis.* **4:**85–94.

Perk, K. and J.B. Moloney. 1966. Pathogenesis of a virus-induced rhabdomyosarcoma in mice. *J. Natl. Cancer Inst.* **37:**581–599.

Perryman, L.E., E.A. Hoover, and D.S. Yohn. 1972. Immunologic reactivity of the cat: Immunosuppression in experimental feline leukemia. *J. Natl. Cancer Inst.* **49:**1357–1365.

Pessac, B. and G. Calothy. 1974. Transformation of chick embryo neuroretinal cells by Rous sarcoma virus *in vitro:* Induction of cell proliferation. *Science* **185:**709–710.

Peters, R.L., L.S. Rabstein, R. VanVleck, G.J. Kelloff, and R.J. Huebner. 1974. Naturally occurring sarcoma virus of the BALB/cCr mouse. *J. Natl. Cancer Inst.* **53:**1725–1729.

Peters, R.L., J.W. Hartley, G.J. Spahn, L.S. Rabstein, C.E. Whitmire, H.C. Turner, and R.J. Huebner. 1972. Prevalence of the group-specific (gs) antigen and infectious virus expressions of the murine C-type RNA viruses during the life span of BALB/cCr mice. *Int. J. Cancer* **10:**283–289.

Peters, R.L., B. Sass, J.R. Stephenson, I.K. Al-Ghazzouli, S. Hino, R.M. Donahoe, M.

Kende, S.A. Aaronson, and G.J. Kelloff. 1977. Immunoprevention of X-ray-induced leukemias in the C57BL mouse. *Proc. Natl. Acad. Sci.* **74:**1697–1701.

Peterson, R.D.A., H.G. Purchase, B.R. Burmester, M.D. Cooper, and R.A. Good. 1966. Relationships among visceral lymphomatosis, bursa of Fabricius, and bursa-dependent lymphoid tissue of the chicken. *J. Natl. Cancer Inst.* **36:**585–598.

Peto, R. 1977. Epidemiology, multistage models, and short-term mutagenicity tests. *Cold Spring Harbor Conf. Cell Proliferation* **4:**1403–1428.

Petursson, G., J.R. Martin, G. Georgsson, N. Nathanson, and P.A. Palsson. 1979. Visna. The biology of the agent and the disease. In *Aspects of slow and persistent virus infections* (ed. D.A.J. Tyrrell), pp. 165–197. Martinus Nijhoff, The Hague.

Petursson, G., N. Nathanson, G. Georgsson, H. Panitch, and P.A. Palsson. 1976. Pathogenesis of visna. I. Sequential virologic, serologic, and pathologic studies. *Lab. Invest.* **35:**402–412.

Pincus, T. 1980. The endogenous murine type C viruses. In *Molecular biology of RNA tumor viruses* (ed. J.R. Stephenson), pp. 77–130. Academic Press, New York.

Pincus, T., W.P. Rowe, and F. Lilly. 1971. A major genetic locus affecting resistance to infection with murine leukemia viruses. II. Apparent identity to a major locus described for resistance to Friend murine leukemia virus. *J. Exp. Med.* **133:**1234–1241.

Piper, C.E., J.F. Ferrer, D.A. Abt, and R.R. Marshak. 1979. Postnatal and prenatal transmission of the bovine leukemia virus under natural conditions. *J. Natl. Cancer Inst.* **62:**165–168.

Pitelka, D.R., H.A. Bern, S. Nandi, and K.B. DeOme. 1964. On the significance of virus-like particles in mammary tissues of C3Hf mice. *J. Natl. Cancer Inst.* **33:**867–885.

Pluznik, D.H. and L. Sachs. 1964. Quantitation of a murine leukemia virus with a spleen colony assay. *J. Natl. Cancer Inst.* **33:**535–546.

———. 1965. The cloning of normal "mast" cells in tissue culture. *J. Cell. Comp. Physiol.* **66:**319–324.

Ponten, J. 1964. The *in vivo* growth mechanism of avian Rous sarcoma. *Natl. Cancer Inst. Monogr.* **17:**131–145.

Portetelle, D., C. Bruck, A. Burny, D. Dekegel, and M. Mammerickx. 1978. Detection of complement-dependent lytic antibodies in sera from bovine leukemia virus-infected animals by the chromium-51 release assay. *Arch. Int. Physiol. Biochim.* **86:**955–956.

Potter, M., M.D. Sklar, and W.P. Rowe. 1973. Rapid viral induction of plasmacytomas in pristane-primed BALB/c mice. *Science* **182:**592–594.

Pourreau-Schneider, N., R.J. Stephens, and W.U. Gardner. 1968. Viral inclusions and other cytoplasmic components in a Leydig cell murine tumor: An electron microscopic study. *Int. J. Cancer* **3:**155–162.

Pragnell, I.B., A. Fusco, C. Arbuthnott, F. Smadja-Joffe, B. Klein, C. Jasmin, and W. Ostertag. 1981. Analysis of the myeloproliferative sarcoma virus genome: Limited changes in the prototype lead to altered target cell specificity. *J. Virol.* **38:**952–957.

Pragnell, I.B., G. Colletta, D. Frisby, B. Seliger, W. Ostertag, G. Warnecke, G. Koch, and J. Bilello. 1980. Genomic and subgenomic expression of the SFFV genome in infected and erythroleukemia cells. In *In vivo and in vitro erythropoiesis: the Friend system* (ed. G.B. Rossi), pp. 333–346. Elsevier/North-Holland, Amsterdam.

Pratt, D.M., J. Strominger, R. Parkman, D. Kaplan, J. Schwaber, N. Rosenberg, and C.D. Scher. 1977. Abelson virus-transformed lymphocytes: Null cells that modulate H-2. *Cell* **12:**683–690.

Premkumar, E., M. Potter, P.A. Singer, and M.D. Sklar. 1975. Synthesis, surface deposition, and secretion of immunoglobulins by Abelson virus-transformed lymphosarcoma cell lines. *Cell* **6:**149–159.

Purchase, H.G. and B.R. Burmester. 1978. Neoplastic diseases. Leukosis/sarcoma group. In *Diseases of poultry* (ed. M.S. Hofstad et al.), pp. 418–468. Iowa State University Press, Ames.

Purchase, H.G., R.C. Chubb, and P.M. Biggs. 1968. Effect of lymphoid leukosis and Marek's disease on the immunological responsiveness of the chicken. *J. Natl. Cancer Inst.* **40:**583–592.

Purchase, H.G., C. Ludford, K. Nazerian, and H.W. Cox. 1973. A new group of oncogenic viruses: Reticuloendotheliosis, chick syncytial, duck infectious anemia, and spleen necrosis viruses. *J. Natl. Cancer Inst.* **51:**489–499.

Purchase, H.G., W. Okazaki, P.K. Vogt, H. Hanafusa, B.R. Burmester, and L.B. Crittenden. 1977. Oncogenicity of avian leukosis viruses of different subgroups and of mutants of sarcoma viruses. *Infect. Immunol.* **15:**423–428.

Pybus, F.C. and E.W. Miller. 1938a. Spontaneous bone tumors of mice. *Am. J. Cancer* **38:**98–111.

———. 1938b. Multiple neoplasms in a sarcoma strain of mice. *Am. J. Cancer* **38:**252–254.

Quade, K. 1979. Transformation of mammalian cells by avian myelocytomatosis virus and avian erythroblastosis virus. *Virology* **98:**461–465.

Quesenberry, P. and L. Levitt. 1979. Hematopoietic stem cells. *N. Engl. J. Med.* **301:**755–760.

Quintrell, N., S.H. Hughes, H.E. Varmus, and J.M. Bishop. 1980. Structure of viral DNA and RNA in mammalian cells infected with avian sarcoma virus. *J. Mol. Biol.* **143:**363–393.

Rabin, H. 1971. Assay and pathogenesis of oncogenic viruses in nonhuman primates. *Lab. Anim. Sci.* **21:**1032–1041.

Rabstein, L.S., A.F. Gazdar, H.C. Chopra, and H.T. Abelson. 1971. Early morphological changes associated with infection by a murine nonthymic lymphatic tumor virus. *J. Natl. Cancer Inst.* **46:**481–491.

Racevskis, J. and G. Koch. 1977. Viral protein synthesis in Friend erythroleukemia cell lines. *J. Virol.* **21:**328–337.

Raschke, W.C., S. Baird, P. Ralph, and I. Nakoinz. 1978. Functional macrophage cell lines transformed by Abelson leukemia virus. *Cell* **15:**261–267.

Raschke, W.C., P. Ralph, J. Watson, M. Sklar, and H. Coon. 1975. Oncogenic transformation of murine lymphoid cells by in vitro infection with Abelson leukemia virus. *J. Natl. Cancer Inst.* **54:**1249–1253.

Rasheed, S., M.B. Gardner, and E. Chan. 1976. Amphotropic host range of naturally occurring wild mouse leukemia virus. *J. Virol.* **19:**13–18.

Rasheed, S., E. Toth, and M.B. Gardner. 1977. Characterization of purely ecotropic and amphotropic naturally occurring wild mouse leukemia viruses. *Intervirology* **8:**323–335.

Rauscher, F.J. 1962. A virus-induced disease of mice characterized by erythrocytopoiesis and lymphoid leukemia. *J. Natl. Cancer Inst.* **29:**515–543.

Reddy, E.P., C.Y. Dunn, and S.A. Aaronson. 1980. Different lymphoid cell targets for transformation by replication-competent Moloney and Rauscher mouse leukemia viruses. *Cell* **19:**663–669.

Reilly, C.A., Jr. and M.P. Finkel. 1976. *In vivo* interference of virus-induced osteosarcomas by a benign bone tumor virus. In *Comparative leukemia research 1975* (ed. J. Clemmensen and D.S. Yohn), pp. 441–444. Karger, Basel.

Revoltella, R., L. Bertolini, and C. Friend. 1979. *In vitro* transformation of mouse bone marrow cells by the polycythemic strain of Friend leukemia virus. *Proc. Natl. Acad. Sci.* **76:**1464–1468.

Ribacchi, R. and G. Giraldo. 1966. Plasmacytomas occurring in the bones of rats injected intracerebrally with murine sarcoma virus (MSV), Moloney's strain. *Lav. Ist. Anat. Istol. Patol. Univ. Studi Perugia* **26:**149–156.

Rich, M.A., R. Siegler, S. Karl, and R. Clymer. 1969. Spontaneous regression of virus induced murine leukemia. I. Host-virus system. *J. Natl. Cancer Inst.* **42:**559–570.

Richter, M.N. and E.C. MacDowell. 1929. The experimental transmission of leukemia in mice. *Proc. Soc. Exp. Biol. Med.* **26:**362–364.

———. 1935. Experiments with mammalian leukemia. *Physiol. Rev.* **15:**509–524.

Risser, R. 1979a. Friend erythroleukemia antigen. A viral antigen specified by spleen focus-forming virus and differentiation antigen controlled by the *Fv-2* locus. *J. Exp. Med.* **149:**1152–1167.

———. 1979b. Abelson antigen is expressed on hematopoietic spleen colony-forming cells from mice carrying the *Av-2*^{s} virus sensitivity gene. *Proc. Natl. Acad. Sci.* **76:**5350–5354.

Risser, R., M. Potter, and W.P. Rowe. 1978a. Abelson virus-induced lymphomagenesis in mice. *J. Exp. Med.* **148:**714–726.

Risser, R., E. Stockert, and L.J. Old. 1978b. Abelson antigen: A viral antigen that is also a differentiation antigen of BALB/c mice. *Proc. Natl. Acad. Sci.* **75:**3918–3922.

Robinson, F.R. and M.J. Twiehaus. 1974. Isolation of the avian reticuloendotheliosis virus (strain T). *Avian Dis.* **18:**278–288.

Robinson, H.L., B.M. Blais, P.N. Tsichlis, and J.M. Coffin. 1982. At least two regions of the viral genome determine the oncogenic potential of avian leukosis viruses. *Proc. Natl. Acad. Sci.* **79:** 1225–1229.

Robinson, H.L., M.N. Pearson, D.W. DeSimone, P.N. Tsichlis, and J.M. Coffin. 1980. Subgroup-E avian-leukosis-virus-associated disease in chickens. *Cold Spring Harbor Symp. Quant. Biol.* **44:**1133–1142.

Rojko, J.L., E.A. Hoover, L.E. Mathes, R.G. Olsen, and J.P. Schaller. 1979. Pathogenesis of experimental feline leukemia virus infection. *J. Natl. Cancer Inst.* **63:**759–768.

Rongey, R.W., A.H. Abtin, J.D. Estes, and M.B. Gardner. 1975. Mammary tumor virus particles in the submaxillary gland, seminal vesicle, and nonmammary tumors of wild mice. *J. Natl. Cancer Inst.* **54:**1149–1156.

Rosenberg, N. and D. Baltimore. 1976. A quantitative assay for transformation of bone marrow cells by Abelson murine leukemia virus. *J. Exp. Med.* **143:**1453–1463.

———. 1978. The effect of helper virus on Abelson virus-induced transformation of lymphoid cells. *J. Exp. Med.* **147:**1126–1141.

Rosenberg, N., D. Baltimore, and C.D. Scher. 1975. *In vitro* transformation of lymphoid cells by Abelson murine leukemia virus. *Proc. Natl. Acad. Sci.* **72:**1932–1936.

Rosenberg, N., E. Siden, and D. Baltimore. 1979. Synthesis of mu chains by Abelson virus-transformed cells and induction of light chain synthesis with lipopolysaccharide. In *B lymphocytes in the immune response* (ed. M. Cooper et al.), pp. 379–386. Elsevier/North-Holland, New York.

Rossi, G.B. and C. Peschle. 1980. Enhanced proliferation and migration of BFU-E, and erythropoietin-independence of CFU-E expression in FLV-infected mice: Comparative studies on anemic and plylcythemic strains. In *In vivo and in vitro erythropoiesis: The Friend system* (ed. G.B. Rossi), pp. 139–149. Elsevier/North-Holland, Amsterdam.

Rous, P. 1911. A sarcoma of the fowl transmissible by an agent separable from the tumor cells. *J. Exp. Med.* **13:**397–411.

Roussel, M., S. Saule, C. Lagrou, C. Rommens, H. Beug, T. Graf, and D. Stehelin. 1979. Three new types of viral oncogene of cellular origin specific for haematopoietic cell transformation. *Nature* **281:**452–455.

Rowe, W.P. 1973. Genetic factors in the natural history of murine leukemia virus infection. *Cancer Res.* **33:**3061–3068.

Rowe, W.P. and T. Pincus. 1972. Quantitative studies of naturally occurring murine leukemia virus infection of AKR mice. *J. Exp. Med.* **135:**429–436.

Rowe, W.P., J.B. Humphrey, and F. Lilly. 1973. A major genetic locus affecting resistance to infection with murine leukemia viruses. III. Assignment of the *Fv-1* locus to linkage group VIII of the mouse. *J. Exp. Med.* **137:**850–853.

Royer-Pokora, B., H. Beug, M. Claviez, H.-J. Winkhardt, R.R. Friis, and T. Graf. 1978. Transformation parameters in chicken fibroblasts transformed by AEV and MC29 avian leukemia viruses. *Cell* **13:**751–760.

Rubin, H., A. Cornelius, and L. Fanshier. 1961. The pattern of congenital transmission of an avian leukosis virus. *Proc. Natl. Acad. Sci.* **47:**1058–1069.
Rubin, H., L. Fanshier, A. Cornelius, and W.F. Hughes. 1962. Tolerance and immunity in chickens after congenital and contact infection with an avian leukosis virus. *Virology* **17:**143–156.
Rudali, G., J.F. Duplan, and R. Latarjet. 1956. Latence des leucoses chez des souris AN injectees avec un extrait leucemique acellulaire AK. *C.R. Acad. Sci.* **242:**837–839.
Rup, B.J., J.D. Hoelzer, and H.R. Bose. 1982. Helper viruses associated with avian acute leukemia viruses inhibit the cellular immune response. *Virology* **116:**61–71.
Rup, B.J., J.L. Spence, J.D. Hoelzer, R.B. Lewis, C.R. Carpenter, A.S. Rubin, and H.R. Bose, Jr. 1979. Immunosuppression induced by avian reticuloendotheliosis virus: Mechanism of induction of the suppressor cell. *J. Immunol.* **123:**1362–1370.
Ruscetti, S.K., L.P. Turek, and C.J. Sherr. 1980a. Three independent isolates of feline sarcoma virus code for three distinct *gag-x* polyproteins. *J. Virol.* **35:** 259–264.
Ruscetti, S., L. Davis, J. Feild, and A. Oliff. 1981. Friend murine leukemia virus-induced leukemia is associated with the formation of mink cell focus-inducing viruses and is blocked in mice expressing endogenous mink cell focus-inducing xenotropic viral envelope genes. *J. Exp. Med.* **154:**907–920.
Ruscetti, S., D. Troxler, D. Linemeyer, and E. Scolnick. 1980b. Three laboratory strains of spleen focus-forming virus: Comparison of their genomes and translational products. *J. Virol.* **33:**140–151.
Ruscetti, S.K., D. Linemeyer, J. Feild, D. Troxler, and E.M. Scolnick. 1979. Characterization of a protein found in cells infected with the spleen focus-forming virus that shares immunological cross-reactivity with the gp70 found in mink cell focus-inducing virus particles. *J. Virol.* **30:**787–798.
Russell, E.S. 1979. Hereditary anemias of the mouse: A review for geneticists. *Adv. Genet.* **20:**357–459.
Russell, E.S. and S.E. Bernstein. 1966. Blood and blood formation. In *Biology of the laboratory mouse* (ed. E.L. Green), pp. 351–372. McGraw-Hill, New York.
Russell, E.S., M.W. Thompson, and E.C. McFarland. 1968. Analysis of effects of *W* and *f* genic substitutions on fetal mouse hematology. *Genetics* **58:**259–270.
Russell, P.H. and O. Jarrett. 1978. The occurrence of feline leukemia virus neutralizing antibodies in cats. *Int. J. Cancer* **22:**351–357.
Ruta, M. and D. Kabat. 1980. Plasma membrane glycoproteins encoded by cloned Rauscher and Friend spleen focus-forming viruses. *J. Virol.* **35:**844–853.
Salerno, R.A., E.D. Lehman, V.M. Larson, and R.A. Hilleman. 1978. Feline leukemia virus envelope glycoprotein vaccine: Preparation and evaluation of immunizing potency in guinea pig and cat. *J. Natl. Cancer Inst.* **61:**1487–1494.
Sarma, P.S. and T. Log. 1973. Subgroup classification of feline leukemia and sarcoma viruses by viral interference and neutralization tests. *Virology* **54:**160–169.
Sarma, P.S., A. Sharar, V. Walters, and M. Gardner. 1974. A survey of cats and humans for prevalence of feline leukemia-sarcoma virus neutralizing serum antibodies. *Proc. Soc. Exp. Biol. Med.* **145:**560–564.
Sassa, S., F. Takaku, and K. Nakao. 1968. Regulation of erythropoiesis in the Friend leukemia mouse. *Blood* **31:**758–765.
Sato, H. and E.A. Boyse. 1976. A new alloantigen expressed selectively on B cells: The Lyb-2 system. *Immunogenetics* **3:**565–572.
Savin, K.W. and H. Beug. 1981. Cell-surface glycoprotein synthesis during differentiation of chicken erythroblasts transformed by temperature-sensitive avian erythroblastosis virus. *Cell Differ.* **10:**163–171.
Saxton, J.A., Jr., M.C. Boon, and J. Furth. 1944. Observations on the inhibition of development of spontaneous leukemia in mice by underfeeding. *Cancer Res.* **4:**401–409.

Schafer, W., H. Schwarz, H.-J. Thiel, E. Wecker, and D.P. Bolognesi. 1976. Properties of mouse leukemia viruses. XIII. Serum therapy of virus-induced murine leukemias. *Virology* **75**:401–418.

Scher, C.D. 1978. Effect of pseudotype on Abelson virus and Kirsten sarcoma virus-induced leukemia. *J. Exp. Med.* **147**:1044–1053.

Scher, C.D. and R. Siegler. 1975. Direct transformation of 3T3 cells by Abelson murine leukaemia virus. *Nature* **253**:729–731.

Scher, C.D., E.M. Scolnick, and R. Siegler. 1975. Induction of erythroid leukaemia by Harvey and Kirsten sarcoma viruses. *Nature* **256**:225–226.

Schlom, J., R. Michalides, D. Kufe, R. Hehlmann, S. Spiegelman, P. Bentvelzen, and P. Hageman. 1973. A comparative study of the biologic and molecular basis of murine mammary carcinoma: A model for human breast cancer. *J. Natl. Cancer Inst.* **51**:541–551.

Schmidt, E.V. and R.E. Smith. 1981. Avian osteopetrosis virus induces proliferation of cultured bone cells. *Virology* **111**:275–282.

Schmidt, E.V., J.D. Keene, M. Linial, and R.E. Smith. 1982. Association of unique 3′ terminal RNA sequences with avian leukosis viruses causing a high incidence of osteopetrosis. *Virology* **116**:163–180.

Schochetman, G., L.O. Arthur, C.W. Long, and R.J. Massey. 1979. Mice with spontaneous mammary tumors develop type-specific neutralizing and cytotoxic antibodies against the mouse mammory tumor virus envelope protein gp52. *J. Virol.* **32**:131–139.

Schoolman, H.M., W. Spurrier, S.O. Schwartz, and P.B. Szanto. 1957. Studies in leukemia. VI. The induction of leukemia virus in Swiss mice by means of cell-free filtrates of leukemic mouse brain. *Blood* **12**:694–700.

Schwartz, R.S. and R.H. Khiroya. 1981. A single dominant gene determines susceptibility to a leukaemogenic recombinant retrovirus. *Nature* **292**:245–246.

Schwarz, H., P.J. Fischinger, J.N. Ihle, H.-J. Thiel, F. Weiland, D.P. Bolognesi, and W. Schafer. 1979. Properties of mouse leukemia viruses. XVI. Suppression of spontaneous fatal leukemias in AKR mice by treatment with broadly reacting antibody against the viral glycoprotein gp 71. *Virology* **93**:159–174.

Scofield, V.L. and H.R. Bose, Jr. 1978. Depression of mitogen response in spleen cells from reticuloendotheliosis virus-infected chickens and their suppressive effect on normal lymphocyte response. *J. Immunol.* **120**:1321–1325.

Scofield, V.L., J.L. Spence, W.E. Briles, and H.R. Bose, Jr. 1978. Differential mortality and lesion responses to reticuloendotheliosis virus infection in Marek's disease-resistant and susceptible chicken lines. *Immunogenetics* **7**:169–172.

Scolnick, E.M., M.O. Weeks, T.Y. Shih, S.K. Ruscetti, and T.M. Dexter. 1981. Markedly elevated levels of an endogenous *sarc* protein in a hemopoietic precursor cell line. *Mol. Cell. Biol.* **1**:66–74.

Scott, J.V., L. Stowring, A.T. Hasse, O. Narayan, and R. Vigne. 1979. Antigenic variation in visna virus. *Cell* **18**:321–327.

Sevoian, M., R.N. Larose, and D.M. Chamberlain. 1964. Avian lymphomatosis. VI. A virus of unusual potency and pathogenicity. *Avian Dis.* **8**:336–347.

Sheiness, D. and J.M. Bishop. 1979. DNA and RNA from uninfected vertebrate cells contain nucleotide sequences related to the putative transforming gene of avian myelocytomatosis virus. *J. Virol.* **31**:514–521.

Sheiness, D.K., S.H. Hughes, H.E. Varmus, E. Stubblefield, and J.M. Bishop. 1980. The vertebrate homolog of the putative transforming gene of avian myelocytomatosis virus: Characteristics of the DNA locus and its RNA transcript. *Virology* **105**:415–424.

Sherman, D.N. 1978. Viral leucoencephalomyelitis in two Minnesota goats. *Vet. Med. Small Anim. Clin.* **73**:1439–1440.

Sherr, C.J., G.J. Todaro, A. Sliski, and M. Essex. 1978a. Characterization of a feline sarcoma virus-coded antigen (FOCMA-S) by radioimmunoassay. *Proc. Natl. Acad. Sci.* **75**:4489–4493.

Sherr, C.J., A. Sen, G.J. Todaro, A. Sliski, and M. Essex. 1978b. Pseudotypes of feline sarcoma virus contain an 85,000 dalton protein with feline oncornavirus-associated cell membrane antigen (FOCMA) activity.. *Proc. Natl. Acad. Sci.* **75:**1505–1509.

Sherr, C.J., L. Donner, L.A. Fedele, L. Turek, J. Even, and S.K. Ruscetti. 1980. Molecular structure and products of feline sarcoma and leukemia viruses: relationship to FOCMA expression. In *Feline leukemia virus* (ed. W.D. Hardy, Jr. et al.), pp. 293–307. Elsevier/North-Holland, Amsterdam.

Shibuya, T. and T.W. Mak. 1982a. Induction of erythroid tumorigenic colonies by Friend helper virus F-MuLV alone and isolation of a new class of Friend erythroleukemic cells. *J. Cell. Physiol.* (in press).

Shibuya, T. and T.W. Mak. 1982b. A host gene controlling early anaemia or polycythaemia induced by Friend erythroleukaemia virus. *Nature* **296:**577–579.

Shinefeld, L.A., V.L. Sato, and N.E. Rosenberg. 1980. Monoclonal rat anti-mouse brain antibody detects Abelson murine leukemia virus target cells in mouse bone marrow. *Cell* **20:**11–17.

Shiu, R.P.C., J. Pouyssegur, and I. Pastan. 1977. Glucose depletion accounts for the induction of two transformation-sensitive membrane proteins in Rous sarcoma virus-transformed chick embryo fibroblasts. *Proc. Natl. Acad. Sci.* **74:**3840–3844.

Siden, E.J., D. Baltimore, D. Clark, and N. Rosenberg. 1979. Immunoglobulin synthesis by lymphoid cells transformed in vitro by Abelson murine leukemia virus. *Cell* **16:**389–396.

Siegler, R., S. Zajdel, and I. Lane. 1972. Pathogenesis of Abelson-virus-induced murine leukemia. *J. Natl. Cancer Inst.* **48:**189–218.

Sigurdsson, B. 1954. Rida, a chronic encephalitis of sheep. *Br. Vet. J.* **110:**341–353.

Sigurdsson, B., P.A. Palsson, and H. Grimmson. 1957. Visna, a demyelinating transmissible disease of sheep. *J. Neuropathol. Exp. Neurol.* **16:**389–403.

Sigurdsson, B., P.A. Palsson, and L. van Bogaert. 1962. Pathology of visna. Transmissible demyelinating disease in sheep in Iceland. *Acta Neuropathol.* **1:**343–362.

Silver, J. and N. Teich. 1981. Expression of resistance to Friend virus-stimulated erythropoiesis in bone marrow chimeras containing *Fv-2*^{rr} and *Fv-2*^{ss} bone marrow *J. Exp. Med.* **154:**126–137.

Silverstone, A.E., N. Rosenberg, D. Baltimore, V.L. Sato, M.P. Scheid, and E.A. Boyse. 1978. Correlating terminal deoxynucleotidyl transferase and cell-surface markers in the pathway of lymphocyte ontogeny. *Cold Spring Harbor Conf. Cell Proliferation* **5:**433–453.

Singer, I. 1979. The fibronexus: A transmembrane association of fibronectin-containing fibers and bundles of 5 nm microfilaments in hamster and human fibroblasts. *Cell* **16:**675–685.

Singer, S.J., and G.L. Nicolson. 1972. The fluid mosaic model of the structure of cell membranes. *Science* **175:**720–731.

Sklar, M.D., B.J. White, and W.P. Rowe. 1974. Initiation of oncogenic transformation of mouse lymphocytes *in vitro* by Abelson leukemia virus. *Proc. Natl. Acad. Sci.* **71:**4077–4081.

Sklar, M.D., E.M. Shevach, I. Green, and M. Potter. 1975. Transplantation and preliminary characterisation of lymphocyte surface markers of Abelson virus-induced lymphomas. *Nature* **253:**550–552.

Sliski, A.H. and M. Essex. 1979. Sarcoma virus-induced transformation specific antigen: Presence of antibodies in cats that were naturally exposed to leukemia virus. *Virology* **95:**581–586.

Smith, G.H. 1966. Role of the milk agent in disappearance of mammary cancer in C3H/StWi mice. *J. Natl. Cancer Inst.* **36:**685–701.

Smith, R.E. and J. Ivanyi. 1980. Pathogenesis of virus-induced osteopetrosis in the chicken. *J. Immunol.* **125:**523–530.

Smith, R.E. and C. Moscovici. 1969. The oncogenic effects of nontransforming viruses from avian myeloblastosis virus. *Cancer Res.* **29:**1356–1366.
Smith, R.E. and J. van Eldik. 1978., Characterization of the immunosuppression accompanying virus-induced avian osteopetrosis. *Infect. Immunol.* **22:**452–461.
Smith, R.E, L.J. Davids, and P.E. Neiman. 1976. Comparison of an avian osteopetrosis virus with an avian lymphomatosis virus by RNA-DNA hybridization. *J. Virol.* **17:**160–167.
Snyder, H.W., Jr., F.R. Jones, N.K. Day, and W.D. Hardy, Jr. 1982. Isolation and characterization of circulating feline leukemia virus-immune complexes from plasma of persistently infected pet cats. *J. Immunol.* (in press).
Snyder, S.P. and G.H. Theilen. 1969. Transmissible feline fibrosarcoma. *Nature* **221:**1074–1075.
Snyder, S.P., D.L. Dungworth, T.G. Kawakami, E. Callaway, and D.T.-L. Lau. 1973. Lymphosarcomas in two gibbons *(Hylobates lar)* with associated C-type virus. *J. Natl. Cancer Inst.* **51:**89–94.
Soehner, R.L. and L. Dmochowski. 1969. Induction of bone tumours in rats and hamsters with murine sarcoma virus and their cell-free transmission. *Nature* **224:**191–192.
Soule, H.D. and W.J. Arnold. 1970. Murine myeloproliferative virus in cell culture. *J. Natl. Cancer Inst.* **45:**253–262.
Spencer, J.L., L.B. Crittenden, B.R. Burmester, W. Okazaki, and R.L. Witter. 1977. Lymphoid leukosis: Interrelations among virus infections in hens, eggs, embryos and chicks. *Avian Dis.* **21:**331–345.
Spira, J., F. Wiener, S. Ohno, and G. Klein. 1979. Is trisomy cause or consequence of murine T cell leukemia development? Studies on Robertsonion translocation mice. *Proc. Natl. Acad. Sci.* **76:**6619–6621.
Spira, J., M. Babonits, F. Wiener, S. Ohno, Z. Wirschubski, N. Haran-Ghera, and G. Klein. 1980. Nonrandom chromosomal changes in Thy-1-positive and Thy-1-negative lymphomas induced by 7,12-dimethylbenzanthracene in SJL mice. *Cancer Res.* **40:**2609–2616.
Sredni, B., Y. Kalechman, H. Michlin, and L.A. Rozenszajn. 1976. Development of colonies *in vitro* of mitogen-stimulated mouse T lymphocytes. *Nature* **259:**130–132.
Staff of the Roscoe B. Jackson Memorial Laboratory. 1933. The existence of non-chromosomal influence in the incidence of mammary tumors in mice. *Science* **78:**465–466.
Stanley, E.R., D.-M. Chen, and H.-S. Lin. 1978. Induction of macrophage production and proliferation by a purified colony stimulating factor. *Nature* **274:**168–170.
Stansly, P.G. and H.D. Soule. 1962. Transplantation and cell-free transmission of a reticulum-cell sarcoma in BALB/c mice. *J. Natl. Cancer Inst.* **29:**1083–1105.
Stanton, M.F., L.W. Law, and R.C. Ting. 1968. Some biologic, immunogenic, and morphologic effects in mice after infection with a murine sarcoma virus. II. Morphologic studies. *J. Natl. Cancer Inst.* **40:**1113–1129.
Stavrou, D., N. Deutschlander, and E. Dahme. 1969. Granulomatous encephalomyelitis in goats. *J. Comp. Pathol.* **79:**393–396.
Steeves, R.A. 1975. Spleen focus-forming virus in Friend and Rauscher leukemia virus preparations. *J. Natl. Cancer Inst.* **54:**289–297.
Steeves, R.A., M. Bennett, E.A. Mirand, and G. Cudkowicz. 1968. Genetic control by the *W* locus of susceptibility to (Friend) spleen focus-forming virus. *Nature* **218:**372–374.
Steeves, R.A., J.E. Bubbers, F. Plata, and F. Lilly. 1978. Origin of spleen colonies generated by Friend virus-infected cells in mice. *Cancer Res.* **38:**2729–2733.
Steeves, R.A., E.A. Mirand, A. Bulba, and P.J. Trudel. 1970. Spleen foci and polycythemia in C57BL mice infected with host-adapted Friend leukemia virus. *Int. J. Cancer* **5:**346–356.
Steeves, R.A., R.J. Eckner, M. Bennett, E.A. Mirand, and P.J. Trudel. 1971. Isolation and characterization of a lymphatic leukemia virus in the Friend virus complex. *J. Natl. Cancer Inst.* **46:**1209–1217.

Steffen, D. and R.A. Weinberg. 1978. The integrated genome of murine leukemia virus. *Cell* **15:**1003–1010.

Steinheider, G., H.J. Seidel, and L. Kreja. 1979. Comparison of the biological effects of anemia inducing and polycythemia inducing Friend virus complex. *Experientia* **35:**1173–1175.

Stephenson, J.R., A.A. Axelrad, and D.L. McLeod. 1972. Erythroid nature of the response to Friend leukemia virus infection in mice. *J. Natl. Cancer Inst.* **48:**531–539.

Stephenson, J.R., A.A. Axelrad, D.L. McLeod, and M.M. Shreeve. 1971. Induction of colonies of hemoglobin synthesizing cells by erythropoietin in vitro. *Proc. Natl. Acad. Sci.* **68:**1542–1546.

Stockert, E., A.B. DeLeo, P.V. O'Donnell, Y. Obata, and L.J. Law. 1979. $G_{(AKSL2)}$: A new cell surface antigen of the mouse related to the dualtropic mink cell focus-inducing class of murine leukemia virus detected by naturally occurring antibody. *J. Exp. Med.* **149:**200–215.

Stockert, E., P.V. O'Donnell, Y. Obata, and L.J. Old. 1980. Inhibition of AKR leukemogenesis by SMX-1, a dualtropic murine leukemia virus. *Proc. Natl. Acad. Sci.* **77:**3720–3724.

Stuck, B., E.A. Boyse, L.J. Old, and E.A. Carswell. 1964. *ML:* A new antigen found in leukaemias and mammary tumours of the mouse. *Nature* **203:**1033–1034.

Sun., L., T.G. Kawakami, and S.I. Matoba. 1978. Genomic stability of gibbon oncornavirus. *J. Virol.* **28:**767–771.

Suzuki, S. and A.A. Axelrad. 1980. *Fv-2* locus controls the proportion of erythropoietic progenitor cells (BFU-E) synthesizing DNA in normal mice. *Cell* **19:**225–236.

Svec, J., E. Hlavayova, J. Matoska, and V. Thurzo. 1979. Conditions for hormone-stimulated expression of endogenous C57Bl strain-associated mammary tumor virus genome. *Neoplasma* **26:**539–550.

Svoboda, J. 1964. Malignant interaction of Rous virus with mammalian cells *in vivo* and *in vitro*. *Natl. Cancer Inst. Monogr.* **17:**277–298.

Talal, N. and A.D. Steinberg. 1974. The pathogenesis of autoimmunity in New Zealand black mice. *Curr. Top. Microbiol. Immunol.* **64:**79–103.

Tambourin, P.E. 1978. Haemopoietic stem cells and murine viral leukaemogenesis. In *Stem cells and tissue homeostasis* (ed. B.I. Lord et al.), pp. 259–316. Cambridge University Press, Cambridge, England.

Tambourin, P.E., F. Wendling, C. Jasmin, and F. Smadja-Joffe. 1979. The physiopathology of Friend leukemia. *Leuk. Res.* **3:**117–129.

Tanaka, H. and D.H. Moore. 1967. Electron microscopic localization of viral antigens in mouse mammary tumors by ferritin-labelled antobody. I. The homologous system. *Virology* **33:**197–214.

Tanaka, H., A. Tamura, and D. Tsujimura. 1972. Properties of the intracytoplasmic A particles purified from mouse tumors. *Virology* **49:**61–78.

Tanaka, K. and K. Sakaki. 1962. Neutralization test on serum from horses infected with the virus of equine infectious anemia. *Natl. Inst. Anim. Health Q.* **2:**128–139.

Taylor, H.W. and L.D. Olson. 1973. Chronological study of the T-virus in chicks. I. Development of lesions. *Avian Dis.* **17:**782–794.

Teich, N.M. and T.M. Dexter. 1978. Effects of murine leukemia virus infection on differentiation of hematopoietic cells in vitro. *Cold Spring Harbor Conf. Cell Proliferation* **5:**657–670.

Teich, N.M. and J. Rowe. 1982. Preliminary studies on BSB: A virus complex that causes erythroleukemia in C57BL mice. In *Expression of differentiated functions in cancer cells* (ed. R.P. Revoltella and G. Pontieri). Raven Press, New York. (In press.)

Temin, H.M. and V.K. Kassner. 1974. Replication of reticuloendotheliosis viruses in cell culture: Acute infection. *J. Virol.* **13:**291–297.

———. 1975. Replication of reticuloendotheliosis viruses in cell culture: Chronic infection. *J. Gen. Virol.* **27:**267–274.

Temin, J.M. and H. Rubin. 1958. Characteristics of an assay for Rous sarcoma virus and Rous sarcoma cells in tissue culture. *Virology* **6:**669–688.

Tennant, J.R. and G.D. Snell. 1968. The *H-2* locus and viral leukemogenesis as studied in congenic strains of mice. *J. Natl. Cancer Inst.* **41:**597–604.

Theilen, G.H., R.F. Zeigel, and M.J. Twiehaus. 1966. Biological studies with RE virus (strain T) that induces reticuloendotheliosis in turkeys, chickens, and Japanese quail. *J. Natl. Cancer Inst.* **37:**731–743.

Theilen, G.H., D. Gould, M. Fowler, and D.L. Dungworth. 1971. C-type virus in tumor tissue of a woolly monkey (*Lagothrix* spp.) with fibrosarcoma. *J. Natl. Cancer Inst.* **47:**881–889.

Theilen, G.H., L.G. Wolfe, H. Rabin, F. Deinhardt, D.L. Dungworth, M.E. Fowler, D. Gould, and R. Cooper. 1973. Biological studies in four species of nonhuman primates with simian sarcoma virus (*Lagothrix*). In *Unifying concepts of leukemia* (ed. R.M. Dutcher and L. Chieco-Bianchi), pp. 251–257. Karger, Basel.

Thomson, S. and A.A. Axelrad. 1968. A quantitative spleen colony assay method for tumor cells induced by Friend leukemia virus infection in mice. *Cancer Res.* **28:**2105–2114.

Thormar, H. 1976. Visna-maedi infection in cell culture and in laboratory animals. In *Slow virus diseases of animals and man* (ed. R.H. Kimberlin), pp. 97–114. North-Holland, Amsterdam.

Thormar, H., H.M. Wisniewski, and F.H. Lin. 1979. Sera and cerebrospinal fluids from normal uninfected sheep contain a visna virus inhibiting factor. *Nature* **279:**245–246.

Till, J.E. and E.A. McCulloch. 1961. A direct measurement of the radiation sensitivity of normal mouse bone marrow cells. *Radiat. Res.* **14:**213–222.

———. 1980. Hemopoietic stem cell differentiation. *Biochim. Biophys. Acta* **605:**431–459.

Timmermans, A., P. Bentvelzen, P.C. Hageman, and J. Calafat. 1969. Activation of a mammary tumour virus in O20 strain mice by X-irradiation and urethane. *J. Gen. Virol.* **4:**619–621.

Toch, P., B.B. Hirch, M.B. Brown, C.S. Nagareda, and H.S. Kaplan. 1956. Lymphoid tumor incidence in mice treated with estrogen and X-radiation. *Cancer Res.* **16:**890–893.

Todaro, G.J., J.E. De Larco, and S. Cohen. 1976. Transformation by murine and feline sarcoma viruses specifically blocks binding of epidermal growth factor to cells. *Nature* **264:**26–31.

Todaro, G.J., C. Fryling, and J.E. DeLarco. 1980. Transforming growth factors produced by certain human tumor cells: Polypeptides that interact with epidermal growth factor receptors. *Proc. Natl. Acad. Sci.* **77:**5258–5262.

Todaro, G.J., M.M. Lieber, R.E. Benveniste, C.J. Sherr, C.J. Gibbs, Jr., and D.C. Gajdusek. 1975. Infectious primate type C viruses: Three isolates belonging to a new subgroup from the brains of normal gibbons. *Virology* **67:**335–343.

Tooze, J., ed. 1980. *The molecular biology of tumor viruses, part 2. DNA tumor viruses,* 2nd edition. Cold Spring Harbor Laboratory, Cold Spring Harbor, New York.

Trager, W. 1959. A new virus of ducks interfering with development of malaria parasite *(Plasmodium lophurae.) Proc. Soc. Exp. Biol. Med.* **101:**578–582.

Troxler, D.H. and E.M. Scolnick. 1978. Rapid leukemia induced by cloned Friend strain of replicating murine type-C virus. Association with induction of xenotropic-related RNA sequences contained in spleen focus-forming virus. *Virology* **85:**17–27.

Troxler, D.H., J.K. Boyars, W.P. Parks, and E.M. Scolnick. 1977a. Friend strain of spleen focus-forming virus: A recombinant between mouse type C ecotropic viral sequences and sequences related to xenotropic virus. *J. Virol.* **22:**361–372.

Troxler, D.H., W.P. Parks, W.C. Vass, and E.M. Scolnick. 1977b. Isolation of a fibroblast nonproducer cell line containing the Friend strain of the spleen focus-forming virus. *Virology* **76:**602–615.

Troxler, D.H., S.K. Ruscetti, D.L. Linemeyer, and E.M. Scolnick. 1980. Helper-independent and replication defective erythroblastosis-inducing viruses contained within anemia-inducing Friend virus complex (FV-A). *Virology* **102:**28–45.

Tsichlis, P.N. and J.M. Coffin. 1980. Recombinants between endogenous and exogenous avian tumor viruses: Role of the C region and other portions of the genome in the control of replication and transformation. *J. Virol.* **33:**238–249.

Turusov, V.S., ed. 1979. *Pathology of tumours in laboratory animals.* Volume II: Tumours of the mouse. International Agency for Research on Cancer, Lyon.

Unkeless, J.C., K. Danø, G.M. Kellerman, and E. Reich. 1974. Fibrinolysis associated with oncogenic transformation: Partial purification and characterization of the cell factor—A plasminogen activator. *J. Biol. Chem.* **249:**4295–4305.

Upton, A.C. 1959. Studies on mechanism of leukemogenesis by ionizing radiation. In *Carcinogenesis: Mechanisms of action,* pp. 249–268. Little Brown, Boston.

Upton, A.C., F.F. Wolff, J. Furth, and A.W. Kimball. 1958. A comparison of the induction of myeloid and lymphoid leukemias in X-radiated RF mice. *Cancer Res.* **18:**842–848.

Urbaneck, D. and W. Wittmann. 1969. Untersuchungen zur Pathologie und Pathogenese der enzootische Rinderleukose. IV. Blutmorphologische Befunde bei Fallen von Leukose und Praleukose. *Arch. Exp. Veterinaermed.* **23:**1141–1161.

Vaheri, A. and E. Ruoslahti. 1975. Fibroblast surface antigen molecules and their loss from virus-transformed cells: A major alteration in cell surface. *Cold Spring Harbor Conf. Cell Proliferation* **2:**967–975.

Vaidya, A.B., E.Y. Lasfargues, G. Heubel, J.C. Lasfargues, and D.H. Moore. 1976. Murine mammary tumor virus: Characterization of infection of non-murine cells. *J. Virol.* **28:**911–917.

Vaidya, A.B., C.A. Long, J.B. Sheffield, A. Tamura, and H. Tanaka. 1980. Murine mammary tumor virus deficient in the major glycoprotein: Biochemical and biological studies on virions produced by a lymphoma cell line. *Virology* **104:**279–293.

Van Der Maaten, M.J. and J.M. Miller. 1976. Induction of lymphoid tumors in sheep with cell-free preparations of bovine leukemia virus. In *Comparative leukemia research 1975* (ed. J. Clemmesen and D.S. Yohn), pp. 377–379. Karger, Basel.

———. 1978. Sites of *in vivo* replication of bovine leukemia virus in experimentally infected cattle. *Ann. Rech. Vet.* **9:**831–835.

Van de Ven, W.J.M., F.H. Reynolds, Jr., and J.R. Stephenson. 1980. The nonstructural components of polyproteins encoded by replication defective mammalian transforming retroviruses are phosphorylated and have associated protein kinase activity. *Virology* **101:**185–197.

Van Griensven, L.J.L.D. and M. Vogt. 1980. Rauscher "mink cell focus-forming" (MCF) virus causes erythroleukemia in mice: Its isolation and properties. *Virology* **101:**376–388.

van Nie, R. and J. de Moes. 1977. Development of a congeneic line of the GR mouse strain without early mammary tumors. *Int. J. Cancer* **20:**588–594.

van Nie, R. and A.A. Verstraeten. 1975. Studies of genetic transmission of mammary tumor virus by C3Hf mice. *Int. J. Cancer* **16:**922–931.

Varmus, H.E., N. Quintrell, E. Medeiros, J.M. Bishop, R. Nowinski, and N.H. Sarkar. 1973. Transcription of mouse mammary tumor virus genes in tissues from high and low tumor incidence mouse strains. *J. Mol. Biol.* **79:**663–679.

Verstraeten, A.A. and R. van Nie. 1978. Genetic transmission of mammary tumour virus in the DBAf mouse strain. *Int. J. Cancer* **21:**473–475.

Verstraeten, A.A., R. van Nie, H.G. Kwa, and P.C. Hageman. 1975. Quantitative estimation of mouse mammary tumor virus (MTV) antigens by radioimmunoassay. *Int. J. Cancer* **15:**270–281.

Vlahakis, G., W.E. Heston, and G.H. Smith. 1970. Strain C3H-A^{vy}fB mice: Ninety percent incidence of mammary tumors transmitted by either parent. *Science* **170:**185–187.

Vogt, M. 1979. Properties of "mink cell focus-inducing" (MCF) virus isolated from spontaneous lymphoma lines of BALB/c mice carrying Moloney leukemia virus as an endogenous virus. *Virology* **93:**226–236.

Wainberg, M.A., M. Yu, E. Schwartz-Luft, and E. Israel. 1977. Cellular and humoral antitumor immune responsiveness in chickens bearing tumors induced by avian sarcoma virus. *Int. J. Cancer* **19:**680–687.

Wallbank, A.M., F.G. Sperling, K. Hubben, and E.L. Stubbs. 1966. Isolation of a tumour virus from a chicken submitted to a poultry diagnostic laboratory—Esh sarcoma virus. *Nature* **209:**1265.

Waneck, G.L. and N. Rosenberg. 1981. Abelson leukemia virus induces lymphoid and erythroid colonies in infected fetal cell cultures. *Cell* **26:**79–89.

Wang, E. and A.R. Goldberg. 1979. Effects of the *src* gene product on microfilament and microtubule organization in avian and mammalian cells infected with the same temperature-sensitive mutant of Rous sarcoma virus. *Virology* **92:**201–210.

Wang, L.-H., R. Feldman, M. Shibuya, H. Hanafusa, M.F.D. Notter, and P.C. Balduzzi. 1981. Genetic structure, transforming sequences, and gene product of avian sarcoma virus UR1. *J. Virol.* **40:**258–267.

Ward, J.M. and D.M. Young. 1976. Histogenesis and morphology of periosteal sarcomas induced by FBJ virus in NIH Swiss mice. *Cancer Res.* **36:**3985–3992.

Weber, A., J. Andrews, B. Dickinson, V. Larson, R. Hammer, V. Dirks, D. Sorensen, and S. Frommes. 1969. Occurrence of nuclear pockets in lymphocytes of normal, persistent lymphocytic and leukemic adult cattle. *J. Natl. Cancer Inst.* **43:**1307–1315.

Wedderburn, N. 1970. Effect of concurrent malarial infection on development of virus-induced lymphoma in BALB/c mice. *Lancet* **2:**1114–1116.

Wei, C.-M., D.R. Lowy, and E.M. Scolnick. 1980. Mapping of transforming region of the Harvey murine sarcoma virus genome by using insertion-deletion mutants constructed *in vitro*. *Proc. Natl. Acad. Sci.* **77:**4674–4678.

Weijer, K. and J.H. Daams. 1978. The control of lymphosarcoma/leukemia and feline leukemia virus. *J. Small Anim. Pract.* **19:**631–637.

Weinhold, E. 1974. Visna-Virus-ahnliche Partikel in der Kultur von Plexus Choroideus-Zellen einer Ziege mit Visna-Symptomen. *Zent. Veterinaermed. (B)* **21:**32–36.

Weinhold, E. and B. Triemer. 1978. Visna bei der Ziege. *Z. Veterinaermed. B* **25:**525–538.

Weiss, R.A. and D.P. Frisby. 1981. Are avian endogenous viruses pathogenic? In *Leukemia and related diseases* (ed. D.S. Yohn). Elsevier/North-Holland, Amsterdam. (In press.)

Weissman, T.L. and S. Baird. 1977. Oncornavirus leukemogenesis as a model for selective neoplastic transformation. In *Neoplastic transformation: Mechanisms and consequences* (ed. H. Koprowski), pp. 135–152. Dahlem Konferenzen, Berlin.

Weksler, M.E., F.W. Ryning, and W.D. Hardy, Jr. 1975. Immune complex disease in cancer. *Clin. Bull.* **5:**109–113.

Weller, S.K., A.E. Joy, and H.M. Temin. 1980. Correlation between cell killing and massive second-round superinfection by members of some subgroups of avian leukosis virus. *J. Virol.* **33:**494–506.

Wendling, F. and P.E. Tambourin. 1978. Oncogenicity of Friend-virus-infected cells: Determination of origin of spleen colonies by the H-2 antigens as genetic markers. *Int. J. Cancer* **22:**479–486.

Wendling, F., F. Moreau-Gachelin, and P. Tambourin. 1981. Emergence of tumorigenic cells during the course of Friend virus leukemias. *Proc. Natl. Acad. Sci.* **78:**3614–3618.

Wendling, F., P. Tambourin, O. Gallien-Lartigue, and M. Charon. 1974. Comparative differentiation and numeration of CFUs from mice infected either by the anemia- or polycythemia-inducing strains of Friend viruses. *Int. J. Cancer* **13:**454–462.

Whittemore, A.S. 1978. Quantitative theories of oncogenesis. *Adv. Cancer Res.* **27:**55–88.

Wiener, F., S. Ohno, J. Spira, N. Haran-Ghera, and G. Klein. 1978a. Cytogenetic mapping of the trisomic segment of chromosome 15 in murine T-cell leukaemia. *Nature* **275:**658–660.

Wiener, F., S. Ohno, J. Spira, N. Haran-Ghera, and G. Klein. 1978b. Chromosome changes (trisomies) (#15 and 17) associated with tumor progression in leukemias induced by radiation leukemia virus. *J. Natl. Cancer Inst.* **60:**227–237.

Wiener, F., J. Spira, S. Ohno, N. Haran-Ghera, and G. Klein. 1978c. Chromosome changes (trisomy 15) in murine T-cell leukemia induced by 7,12-dimethylbenz(a)antracene (DMBA). *Int. J. Cancer* **22:**447–453.

Wiener, F., J. Spira, M. Babonits, N. Haran-Ghera, and G. Klein. 1980. Non-random duplication of chromosome 15 in murine T-cell leukemias: Further studies on translocation heterozygotes. *Int. J. Cancer* **26:**661–668.

Williams, C.S. 1979. Viral leucoencephalomyelitis in a goat in Michigan. *Vet. Med. Small Anim. Clin.* **74:**9–00.

Witte, O.N., A. Dasgupta, and D. Baltimore. 1980. Abelson murine leukaemia virus protein is phosphorylated in vitro to form phosphotyrosine. *Nature* **283:**826–831.

Witte, O.N., N. Rosenberg, M. Paskind, A. Shields, and D. Baltimore. 1978. Identification of an Abelson murine leukemia virus-encoded protein present in transformed fibroblast and lymphoid cells. *Proc. Natl. Acad. Sci.* **75:**2488–2492.

Witter, R.L. and L.B. Crittenden. 1979. Lymphomas resembling lymphoid leukosis in chickens inoculated with reticuloendotheliosis virus. *Int. J. Cancer* **23:**673–678.

Witter, R.L., H.G. Purchase, and G.H. Burgoyne. 1970. Peripheral nerve lesions similar to those of Marek's disease in chickens inoculated with reticuloendotheliosis virus. *J. Natl. Cancer Inst.* **45:**567–577.

Wolf, B.A. and A.R. Goldberg. 1976. Rous-sarcoma-virus-transformed fibroblasts having low levels of plasminogen activator. *Proc. Natl. Acad. Sci.* **73:**3613–3617.

Wolfe, L.G. and F. Deinhardt. 1972. Oncornaviruses associated with spontaneous and experimentally induced neoplasia in nonhuman primates. In *Medical primatology* (ed. E.I. Goldsmith and J. Moor-Jankowski), part III, pp. 176–196. Karger, Basel.

———. 1978. Overview of viral oncology studies in *Saguinus* and *Callithrix* species. *Primates Med.* **10:**96–118.

Wolfe, L.G., R.K. Smith, and F. Deinhardt. 1972. Simian sarcoma virus, type 1 (*Lagothrix*): Focus assay and demonstration of nontransforming associated virus. *J. Natl. Cancer Inst.* **48:**1905–1908.

Wolfe, L.G., F. Deinhardt, G.H. Theilen, H. Rabin, T. Kawakami, and L.K. Bustad. 1971. Induction of tumors in marmoset monkeys by simian sarcoma virus, type 1 (*Lagothrix*): A preliminary report. *J. Natl. Cancer Inst.* **47:**1115–1120.

Woolley, G.W. and B.A. Peters. 1953. Prolongation of life in high-leukemia AKR mice by cortisone. *Proc. Soc. Exp. Biol. Med.* **82:**286–287.

Wyke, J.A. and M. Linial. 1973. Temperature-sensitive avian sarcoma viruses: A physiological comparison of twenty mutants. *Virology* **53:**152–161.

Yamamoto, Y., C.L. Gamble, S.P. Clark, A. Joyner, T. Shibuya, M.E. MacDonald, D. Mager, A. Bernstein, and T.W. Mak. 1981. Clonal analysis of early and late stages of erythroleukemia induced by molecular clones of integrated spleen focus-forming virus. *Proc. Natl. Acad. Sci.* **78:**6893–6897.

Yohn, D.S., R.G. Olsen, J.P. Schaller, E.A. Hoover, L.E. Mathes, L. Heding, and G.W. Davis. 1976. Experimental oncornavirus vaccines in the cat. *Cancer Res.* **36:**646–651.

Yoosook, C., R. Steeves, and F. Lilly. 1980. *Fv-2*^{r}-mediated resistance of mouse bone-marrow cells to Friend spleen focus-forming virus infection. *Int. J. Cancer* **26:**101–106.

Yoshida, M. and H. Yoshikura. 1980. Analysis of spleen focus-forming virus-specific RNA sequences coding for spleen focus-forming virus-specific glycoprotein with a molecular weight of 55,000 (gp55). *J. Virol.* **33:**587–596.

Yoshiki, T., R.C. Mellors, and W.D. Hardy, Jr. 1973. Common cell-surface antigen associated with murine and feline C-type RNA leukemia viruses. *Proc. Natl. Acad. Sci.* **70:**1878–1882.

Yoshiki, T., R.C. Mellors, M. Strand, and J.T. August. 1974. The viral envelope glycoprotein of murine leukemia virus and the pathogenesis of immune complex glomerulonephritis of New Zealand Mice. *J. Exp. Med.* **140:**1011–1027.

Yoshiki, T., T. Hasyasaka, R. Fukatsu, T. Shirai, T. Itoh, H. Ikeda, and M. Katagiri. 1979. The structural proteins of murine leukemia virus and the pathogenesis of necrotizing arthritis and glomerulonephritis in SL/Ni mice. *J. Immunol.* **122:**1812–1820.

Yoshimura, F.K. and M. Breda. 1981. Lack of AKR ecotropic provirus amplification in AKR leukemic thymuses. *J. Virol.* **39:**808–815.

Yumoto, T., W.E. Poel, T. Kodama, and L. Dmochowski. 1970. Studies on FBJ virus-induced bone tumors in mice. *Texas Rep. Biol. Med.* **28:**145–165.

Zeigel, R.F., B.R. Burmester, and F.J. Rauscher. 1964. Comparative morphologic and biologic studies of natural and experimental transmission of avian tumor viruses. *Natl. Cancer Inst. Monogr.* **17:**711–731.

Zeilmaker, G.H. 1969. Transmission of mammary tumor virus by female GR mice: Results of egg transplantation. *Int. J. Cancer* **4:**261–266.

Zeller, N.K., L. Gazzolo, and C. Moscovici. 1980. A study of the epithelioid transformation of MC29-infected chicken embryo cells. *Virology* **104:**239–242.

Zielinski, C.C., S.D. Waksal, L.D. Tempelis, R.H. Khiroya, and R.S. Schwartz. 1980. Surface phenotypes in T-cell leukaemia are determined by oncogenic retroviruses. *Nature* **288:**489–491.

9

Functions and Origins of Retroviral Transforming Genes

- b. Two domains of *v-erb*
- c. Polyprotein product of *v-erb*-A
- d. Search for a product of *v-erb*-B

4. *myb*

D. *abl:* Oncogene of Abelson Murine Leukemia Virus
1. Oncogenesis and transformation by *v-abl*
2. Identifying the product of *v-abl*
3. *gag-abl* polyprotein is the sole product of the genome of Abelson virus
4. Composition and biological activities of *gag-abl* polyproteins
5. *gag-abl* polyprotein is an integral membrane protein
6. *gag-abl* polyprotein may be a tyrosine protein kinase
7. Is tyrosine phosphorylation responsible for neoplastic transformation by *v-abl*?

E. *mos:* Oncogene of Moloney and Gazdar murine sarcoma viruses
1. Structural definition of the gene
2. Nucleotide sequence of *mos*
3. Is the predicted product of *mos* related to other *onc* products?
4. Putative products of *mos* synthesized in vitro
5. What is the mRNA for *mos*?

F. *ras:* Oncogene of Harvey, Kirsten, and Rasheed Sarcoma Viruses
1. Classification of viruses containing *ras*
2. Identification of small phosphoproteins as the products of *ras* with antisera to nonstructural proteins
3. Structure of the *ras* proteins
4. $p21^{v-ras}$ is located in the plasma membrane
5. Biosynthesis of *ras* proteins
6. Functions of *ras* proteins: Binding of guanine nucleotides and a possible threonine kinase activity
7. Other candidate products of *ras*?

G. *fes* and *fms*: Oncogenes of Feline Sarcoma Viruses
1. Products of *fes* are *gag* fusion proteins
2. Products of *fes* are associated with tyrosine kinases
3. *fes* is related to *fps* and perhaps to other *onc* genes
4. Products of *fms*

H. *rel:* Oncogene of Reticuloendotheliosis Virus Strain T

I. *sis:* Oncogene of Simian Sarcoma Virus

III. The Origins of Viral Oncogenes

A. Emergence of the Thesis: First Clues and Hypotheses
B. Discovery of *c-onc* Genes
C. Characterizing *c-onc* Genes
D. *c-onc* Genes are Cellular Genes
E. Expression of *c-onc* Genes
F. Identifying the Proteins Encoded by *c-onc* Genes
G. How Similar are Viral Oncogenes and *c-onc* Genes?
H. The Family of *c-onc* Genes
I. Mechanisms of Genetic Mimicry: Genesis of Retroviral Oncogenes
J. Are *c-onc* Genes Useful to Normal Cells?
K. Paradox of Neoplastic Transformation by Retroviral Oncogenes
L. Does the Homology between *v-onc* Genes and *c-onc* Genes Dictate the Host Range of Viral Transformation?
M. Do *c-onc* Genes Provide a Common Pathway for Oncogenesis?

I. INTRODUCTION

Retroviruses first attracted the attention of experimentalists because of their ability to produce tumors in animals (Rous 1911; Gross 1970), and they were recognized by the late 1950s as useful reagents for analysis of the oncogenic process because of the efficiency with which transformation could be induced and scored in cell culture (Temin and Rubin 1958). Nevertheless, there was no genetic definition of virus components responsible for such biological effects until 1970 (Martin 1970; Vogt 1971; Bader 1972) and no biochemical or immunological definition of the products of retroviral oncogenes until 1977 (Brugge and Erikson 1977). However, during the past 4 years, there has been an extraordinary proliferation of new information about retroviral transforming genes. Several technical advances have propelled this fruitful activity: improved methods for biochemical analysis of viral genomes and mRNAs (Chapters 4 and 5); successful culturing of a variety of cell types, particularly hematopoietic cells (Chapter 8); cloning of retroviral DNA (Chapters 4 and 5); and the production of effective antisera combined with refined procedures for biochemical analysis of proteins (this chapter and Chapter 6). As tales unfolded about the nature and origins of transforming genes of widely used viruses, such as Rous sarcoma virus (RSV), many investigators turned to viruses that had been less commonly studied or even ignored since their original isolation.

A. Viruses with and without *onc*

As one consequence of this catholic approach, it is now possible to perceive a major division between two types of tumor-inducing retroviruses. On the one hand, there is a class of viruses believed to carry nucleotide sequences derived from normal cellular genes and capable of directing synthesis of all or part of a protein required for oncogenic transformation. Although formal genetic definition of such sequences is lacking in most cases, the sequences are generically termed *onc* for several reasons: they are associated with viruses capable of transforming cultured cells and inducing tumors rapidly in infected animals (Chapter 8); they are dispensable for virus replication and are unrelated to sequences found in the genomes of replication-competent viruses that lack transforming genes; and, in a few instances, conditional and nonconditional mutations affecting oncogenic properties have been mapped to these sequences. In most cases, the acquisition of cellular sequences which then serve as viral transforming genes involves the sacrifice of viral genes required for replication. Hence, most of the viruses in this class are replication-defective and can only be grown in the company of helper viruses; RSV is a notable exception to this rule.

The other class of oncogenic viruses includes those agents that do not carry sequences transduced from host-cell genomes and do not appear to contain coding sequences for proteins other than those normally implicated in virus replication. Oncogenic viruses lacking *onc* sequences are capable of inducing a variety of neoplasms, but the tumors generally appear after a long latency and the viruses have not been shown to transform cultured cells. The mechanisms by which such viruses effect oncogenic change are generally unknown, but some possibilities are considered in Section III.M and in Chapter 8.

B. Nomenclature for *onc* Sequences

Viruses possessing *onc* sequences have been isolated from at least six animal species. Comparisons of *onc* regions of these viruses by nucleic acid hybridization, oligonucleotide fingerprinting, and peptide mapping have shown that over a dozen apparently unrelated cellular genes have served as progenitors of viral *onc* genes. To distinguish conveniently among these several *onc* elements, a three-letter designation has been assigned to each definable element (Coffin et al. 1981) (Table 9.1 and Appendix A). This nomenclature has received general acceptance only recently, and reports published prior to 1980–1981 tend to refer to *onc* sequences either as sequences specific for the transforming component in a mixture of transforming and helper viruses or as "*src* sequences," based on the precedent of RSV for which the transforming gene (*src*) had been defined by classic genetic criteria. The names for transforming sequences are derived from the names of the viruses in which the sequences were first encountered, and they are intended to be trivial, not implying target-cell specificity or function of the transforming protein. Since related, but nonidentical, *onc* sequences are often found in independent virus isolates, the names are often prefixed with the name or abbreviation of a virus strain. The distinction between the viral and cellular versions of related sequences is maintained by using *v-* and *c-* as prefixes; names without a prefix are understood to designate the viral sequence. *c-onc* sequences are usually highly conserved through evolution and hence can be found in species other than the original host for the transforming virus; the animal source of a cellular sequence is therefore often indicated in parentheses, e.g., *c-src* (chicken) or *c-src* (mouse).

In the first part of this chapter we describe what is known about the protein products of *v-onc* genes. The organization of genomes containing *onc* is presented in Chapter 4, the mutations affecting *onc* are reviewed in Chapter 7, and the biological consequences of infection with viruses containing *onc* are described in Chapter 8. The remainder of this chapter is devoted to a consideration of the origins of viral transforming genes: the structure, distribution, and function of *c-onc* genes; the nature of their protein products; and the possible mechanisms by which *c-onc* genes may have been transduced by retroviruses.

C. General Properties of *v-onc* Sequences

Different strategies are used to express *onc* sequences, depending primarily on the structure of the viral genome: (1) Most of the *v-onc* sequences identified to date are translated to form part of a fusion protein in which the aminoterminal domain is encoded by viral replicative genes (*gag* or *gag* and *pol*). This implies that the viral transforming protein and the product of the homologous *c-onc* may exhibit major differences in structure and function, since *c-onc* genes are not linked to endogenous viral genes. (2) Some *v-onc* genes appear to be expressed as proteins encoded entirely by the transforming sequence, either by translation of subgenomic mRNA (e.g., *src*, *erb*-B, *myb*, and probably *mos*) or by translation of genome-size mRNA (e.g., *ras*).

Unequivocal identification of the products of *onc* genes in infected cells has been greatly facilitated by the production of appropriate antisera. *gag-onc* fusion proteins can be readily identified by immunoprecipitation with antisera to the viral structural gene components of the polyproteins, but only in a few instances (e.g., *fes*, *erb*-A, and *abl*) have antibodies to *onc* determinants in these proteins been obtained. Without activity against *onc* determinants, it is obviously

Table 9.1 Viral *onc* genes and their protein products

Name	*v-onc*	Virus strain	Probable animal of origin	Protein product
src	RSV-*src*	Rous sarcoma virus	chicken	$pp60^{src}$
	B77-*src*	B77 avian (or Rous) sarcoma virus	chicken	$pp60^{src}$
	rASV-*src*	recovered avian sarcoma virus	chicken, Japanese quail	$pp60^{src}$
	PR-RSV-*src*	Prague strain Rous sarcoma virus	chicken	$pp60^{src}$
fps	FuSV-*fps*	Fujinami sarcoma virus	chicken	$P140^{gag\text{–}fps}$
	PRCII-*fps*	PRCII sarcoma virus	chicken	$P105^{gag\text{–}fps}$
	PRCIV-*fps*	PRCIV sarcoma virus	chicken	$P170^{gag\text{–}fps}$
	UR1-*fps*	Rochester sarcoma virus 1	chicken	$P150^{gag\text{–}fps}$
	16L-*fps*	16L recovered avian sarcoma virus	chicken	$P142^{gag\text{–}fps}$
yes	Y73-*yes*	Y73 avian sarcoma virus	chicken	$P90^{gag\text{–}yes}$
	ESV-*yes*	Esh sarcoma virus	chicken	$P80^{gag\text{–}yes}$
ros	*ros*	UR-2 virus	chicken	$P68^{gag\text{–}ros}$
myc	MC29-*myc*	avian myelocytomatosis virus MC29	chicken	$P110^{gag\text{–}myc}$
	CMII-*myc*	avian myelocytomatosis virus CMII	chicken	$P90^{gag\text{–}myc}$

	MH2-*myc*	avian myelocytomatosis and carcinoma virus MH2	chicken	$P100^{gag-myc}$
	OK10-*myc*	avian myelocytomatosis virus OK10	chicken	$P200^{gag-pol-myc,?}$
erb-A	AEV-*erb*-A	avian erythroblastosis virus	chicken	$P75^{gag-erb-A}$
erb-B	AEV-*erb*-B	avian erythroblastosis virus	chicken	$p44^{erb-B}$
myb	AMV-*myb*	avian myeloblastosis virus strain BAI-A	chicken	?
	E26-*myb*	avian leukemia virus strain E26	chicken	$P130^{gag-myb}$
rel	*rel*	avian reticuloendotheliosis virus T	turkey	?
abl	*abl*	Abelson murine leukemia virus	mouse	$P120^{gag-abl}$
mos	Moloney-*mos*	Moloney murine sarcoma virus	mouse	?
	Gazdar-*mos*	Gazdar murine sarcoma virus	mouse	?
bas	*bas*	BALB murine sarcoma virus	mouse	$p21^{bas}$
ras	Kirsten-*ras*	Kirsten murine sarcoma virus	rat	$p21^{ras}$
	Harvey-*ras*	Harvey murine sarcoma virus	rat	$p21^{ras}$
	Rasheed-*ras*	Rasheed rat sarcoma virus	rat	$P29^{gag-ras}$
fes	ST-*fes*	Snyder-Theilen feline sarcoma virus	cat	$P85^{gag-fes}$
	GA-*fes*	Gardner-Arnstein feline sarcoma virus	cat	$P95^{gag-fes}$
fms	SM-*fms*	McDonough feline sarcoma virus	cat	$P180^{gag-fms}$
sis	*sis*	Simian sarcoma virus	woolly monkey	?

not possible to identify products of the corresponding *c-onc*. It has also been difficult to raise antisera to *onc* proteins encoded entirely by transforming genes. After protracted efforts, antisera to the products of *src* (Brugge and Erikson 1977) and *ras* (T. Y. Shih et al. 1979a) have been obtained; but insights into the products and the mode of expression of *erb*-B and *myb* are derived mostly from nucleotide sequencing, in vitro translation, and physical characterization of mRNAs, since antisera to the proteins encoded by those genes are not available.

Although the mechanisms by which *v-onc* proteins transform cells and the functions of *c-onc* proteins are not known, several of these proteins display (or are closely associated with) a protein kinase activity capable of phosphorylating tyrosine residues. These putative protein kinases (the products of *src, fps, yes, ros, abl,* and *fes*) are all phosphoproteins, containing phosphotyrosine and usually other phosphoamino acids. In addition, it is possible that the products of retroviral transforming genes have similar locations within cells. Three examples studied to date, the products of *src, ras,* and *abl*, appear to be associated with plasma membranes. The significance of these functional homologies among *onc* products is considered in detail in subsequent sections.

II. VIRAL TRANSFORMING GENES AND THEIR PRODUCTS

A. *src*: The Oncogene of RSV

1. First Revelations: Identification of $pp60^{src}$

RSV was the first retrovirus to be isolated and characterized, and the product of its oncogene (*src*) likewise became the first retroviral transforming protein to be identified. The successful pursuit of the *src* product owed much to a powerful alliance between genetics and biochemistry. RSV represented the sole *onc*-containing retrovirus that could be propagated in large quantities without the requirement for a helper virus; a versatile suite of conditional and nonconditional mutations affecting *v-src* were available; the gene had been mapped with some precision on the viral genome; and the mRNA by which *src* is expressed had been identified.

The product of *src* was sought with two parallel strategies that ultimately proved to be mutually reinforcing: (1) the development of tumor antisera that might react with the *src* product as well as with structural proteins of the virus (Brugge and Erikson 1977) and (2) the translation of the gene in vitro, using fragments derived from the 3′ third of the viral genome (Purchio et al. 1978). The serological strategy proved decisive. Antisera obtained from rabbits bearing sarcomas induced by RSV could be used to immunoprecipitate a 60,000-dalton protein (pp60$^{v\text{-}src}$) that was found only in cells infected with RSV and that could be precipitated only by tumor antisera, not by antisera to structural proteins of RSV (Brugge and Erikson 1977; Levinson et al. 1978; Sefton et al. 1978). The same protein could be recognized in the products of translation from *src* in vitro (Beemon and Hunter 1978; Purchio et al. 1978; Weiss et al. 1981), thus placing the genetic origin of pp60$^{v\text{-}src}$ virtually beyond doubt.

The efforts to translate *src* in vitro unearthed the then surprising finding that neither the 5′ cap nor the leader sequence of authentic mRNA was required for initiation of translation from retroviral genes (Beemon and Hunter 1977; Purchio et al. 1977; 1978) (see also Chapter 5). Instead, it was sufficient to fragment the genome so as to place the appropriate initiation codon near the 5′ terminus of the RNA to be translated. This approach is treacherous, however, because it also permits initiation at methionine codons that do not represent the beginning of a coding element. As a consequence, the first reports of *src* products failed to identify the complete protein (Beemon and Hunter 1977; Kamine and Buchanan 1977), and the errors were corrected only with the development of the tumor antisera that reacted with pp60$^{v\text{-}src}$ (Purchio et al. 1977; Beemon and Hunter 1978).

Several kinds of polymorphisms have been recognized in pp60$^{v\text{-}src}$. First, some batches of tumor antisera are not cross-reactive among the forms of pp60$^{v\text{-}src}$ encoded by different strains of RSV (Sefton et al. 1978; Brugge et al. 1979; Oppermann et al. 1979). For example, most of the antisera produced to date have been raised with the Schmidt-Ruppin (SR) strain of RSV; only some of these antisera react with the pp60$^{v\text{-}src}$ of B77-RSV or Prague (PR)-RSV-C. Second, the *src* products of different strains of RSV are distinguishable by both size and the patterns of peptides produced when the proteins are hydrolyzed with trypsin (Beemon et al. 1979; Brugge et al. 1979). These polymorphisms had not been anticipated by previous analyses with molecular hybridization (Stehelin et al. 1976a), but they do conform to differences found by the mapping of oligonucleotides within *v-src* (Wang et al. 1975, 1976).

Is pp60$^{v\text{-}src}$ the sole product of *v-src*? The question was not easily answered at first. It seemed quite possible that the tumor antisera failed to recognize other proteins encoded by the gene; in addition, translation of genome fragments in vitro produced a relatively complex pattern of polypeptides that might obscure products of *src* other than pp60$^{v\text{-}src}$ (Kamine et al. 1978; Purchio et al. 1978; Sefton et al. 1978). Nevertheless, the size of the protein was in approximate accord with the estimated coding capacity of the gene, and translation from the purified mRNA of *src* produced only pp60$^{v\text{-}src}$ (Bishop et al. 1980; Weiss et al. 1981). The issue was laid to rest when the nucleotide sequence of *src* became available (Czernilofsky et al. 1980; D. Schwartz, pers. comm.). The sequence revealed a single open reading frame within the *src* locus with the capacity to generate a 60,000-dalton protein.

DNA fragments bearing *src*, but no other viral gene, were shown to transform fibroblasts in culture (Copeland et al. 1980; P. Luciw, pers. comm.); the transformed cells contained pp60$^{v\text{-}src}$ and were tumorigenic when injected into syngeneic animals (P. Luciw and H. Oppermann, pers. comm.). These findings address an immensely important issue: One gene, by means of a single protein, may induce the entire tumorigenic phenotype. No other conclusion can speak quite as effectively to the value of retroviral oncogenes for the experimental analysis of tumorigenesis. (A second open reading frame within the 60,000-dalton domain of *src* could encode a protein of about 20,000 daltons. The potential coding sequence for this protein does not begin with a methionine codon and would therefore require splicing to establish a unit suitable for translation. Since the necessary splice has not been explicitly sought, it remains possible that two proteins actually arise from *src*. The likelihood that this occurs is impossible to assess at present.)

2. *The Product of* v-src *Is a Phosphoprotein*

Phosphorylation is now recognized as a widely used device for regulating the activities of proteins (Rubin and Rosen 1975; Weller 1979). It was only natural, therefore, that the early analyses of pp60$^{v\text{-}src}$ included tests for phosphorylation (Brugge et al. 1978; Levinson et al. 1978). The tests were positive and contained the makings of a novel and important observation. Initial descriptions reported that pp60$^{v\text{-}src}$ contained phosphoserine and phosphothreonine (Collett et al. 1979a,b), the two common forms of phosphoamino acids in proteins (Krebs and Beavo 1979). But serendipity intervened to revise this description when Hunter and his colleagues discovered that reactions with immunoprecipitates in vitro phosphorylated the middle T antigen of polyoma virus on tyrosine—a heretofore unrecognized phosphoamino acid that has figured largely in all subsequent examinations of viral oncogenesis (Eckhart et al. 1979). Similar analyses were then quickly applied to pp60$^{v\text{-}src}$, and they revealed that what had been previously identified as phosphothreonine was, in reality, phosphotyrosine (Hunter and Sefton 1980).

By what means is pp60$^{v\text{-}src}$ phosphorylated? The question has not been answered in full. On the one hand, there is little doubt that the phosphorylation of serine in pp60$^{v\text{-}src}$ is carried out by a cyclic AMP (cAMP)-dependent protein kinase of the host cell (Collett et al. 1979a). In contrast, there is disagreement regarding the mechanism that phosphorylates tyrosine in pp60$^{v\text{-}src}$. Some investigators have reported that the protein phosphorylates itself (Erikson et al. 1979) in an autocatalytic manifestation of the tyrosine protein kinase activity attributed to pp60$^{v\text{-}src}$ (see below). Other efforts have failed to perceive autocatalytic phosphorylation of pp60$^{v\text{-}src}$ (Levinson et al. 1980). The issue is far from arcane. It is widely and justifiably assumed that phosphorylation of pp60$^{v\text{-}src}$ regulates the function of the protein. The origin of this regulatory influence is a matter of considerable import; the activity of pp60$^{v\text{-}src}$ may not be entirely autonomous.

Phosphorylation of pp60$^{v\text{-}src}$ is affected by conditional and nonconditional mutations in *v-src* (Levinson et al. 1978; Oppermann et al. 1981a). Virtually all temperature-sensitive mutations in *v-src* reduce the phosphorylation of pp60$^{v\text{-}src}$ by perceptible or even large degrees at the restrictive temperature (Levinson et al. 1978; Rübsamen et al. 1979; Bishop et al. 1980). These effects were important in early efforts to document the genetic origin of pp60$^{v\text{-}src}$. The synthesis and stability of the mutant protein went unperturbed when infected cells were maintained at the restrictive temperature (Levinson et al. 1978), a disquieting finding for those who wished to conclude that *src* encoded pp60$^{v\text{-}src}$. The striking effects of the mutations on phosphorylation of the protein saved the day and provided a valuable genetic link between *src* and pp60$^{v\text{-}src}$.

Ironically, we remain uncertain as to why the mutations affect phosphorylation of pp60$^{v\text{-}src}$. The problem is particularly vexing in the case of tyrosine phosphorylation, which is generally more strongly affected by the mutations than is serine phosphorylation (Collett et al. 1979a; Bishop et al. 1980). Phosphorylation of tyrosine in the mutant proteins might fail because the substrate site has been shielded by an alteration in the configuration of the protein or because the phosphorylation truly is autocatalytic and the kinase activity itself has been affected by the mutation. The enigma is circular. Conditional mutations in pp60$^{v\text{-}src}$ generally have a perceptible effect on the kinase activity of the protein (see below). Should we attribute this to a direct effect on the active site of the molecule or to the failure of tyrosine phosphorylation? The tangle will probably be unraveled only by the use of purified enzymes and fully characterized mutants.

3. Where Does pp60$^{v\text{-}src}$ Act in the Cell?

Efforts to locate pp60$^{v\text{-}src}$ within the infected cell have produced an embarrassment of riches. By one account or another, the protein has been found on the exterior of the nuclear envelope, gathered around centrioles, in the juxtanuclear endoplasmic reticulum, in the cytoskeletal framework of the cytoplasm, in focal adhesion plaques, adjacent to tight junctions between cells, and bound to the plasma membrane. The absence of the nucleus from this list would have come as a surprise until quite recently. T antigens of papovaviruses were first found in the nuclei of transformed cells, and it soon became conventional to attribute the oncogenicity of these viruses to direct effects of the T antigens on cellular DNA replication (Weinberg 1977; Martin 1981). This view has now been revised. The role of the nuclear T antigens in transformation is now suspect, and other viral proteins located in the plasma membrane and the cytoplasm have emerged as potential mediators of transformation (Crawford 1980). The findings with pp60$^{v\text{-}src}$ have added impetus to these evolving views.

The preponderance of evidence indicates that the bulk of pp60$^{v\text{-}src}$ in infected cells is bound to the plasma membrane. Evidence for this conclusion has come from three diverse techniques: immunofluorescence microscopy (Willingham et al. 1979; Rohrschneider 1980), immunoelectron microscopy (Willingham et al. 1979), and biochemical fractionation of subcellular organelles (Courtneidge et al. 1980; Krueger et al. 1980a). The image that has emerged places pp60$^{v\text{-}src}$ in tight affiliation with the cytoplasmic aspect of the plasma membrane, particularly at tight junctions between adjacent cells (Willingham et al. 1979; Levinson et al. 1981). A portion of the protein may be embedded within the lipid bilayer of the membrane, but the evidence for this remains indecisive (Levinson et al. 1981) despite the very hydrophobic nature of pp60$^{v\text{-}src}$ (Levinson et al. 1980). Efforts to detect pp60$^{v\text{-}src}$ on the external surface of cells have failed (Sefton et al. 1978; S. Courtneidge and A. D. Levinson, pers. comm.) unless the cells were first treated with formaldehyde (R. Friis, pers. comm.), a maneuver whose effects on the permeability of the plasma membrane are difficult to assess. For the present, therefore, it is impossible to deduce whether any portion of pp60$^{v\text{-}src}$ might span the entire lipid bilayer of the plasma membrane. Substantial quantities of pp60$^{v\text{-}src}$ are included in, or attached to, the lipid envelopes of RSV (Bunte et al. 1981) and vesicular stomatitis virus (VSV) (G. Clinton, pers. comm.) produced by *src*-transformed cells, providing further manifestation of the affinity of pp60$^{v\text{-}src}$ for the plasma membrane. The finding of pp60$^{v\text{-}src}$ in association with the plasma membrane and the inference that the protein exerts its principal effects there are not entire heresies. It has been known for several years that enucleated cells can still display phenotypic effects of pp60$^{v\text{-}src}$ (Beug et al. 1978). Moreover, some cell biologists have long argued that the control of cell growth and division is effected at the plasma membrane (Edelman 1976).

The synthesis of pp60$^{v\text{-}src}$ takes place on soluble polyribosomes, rather than on membrane-bound polyribosomes (Lee et al. 1979; Purchio et al. 1980; Levinson et al. 1981). The protein then reaches the plasma membrane within 5 to 10 minutes (Levinson et al. 1981), but the route and means by which this occurs are unknown. Precedents exist, however, in the coat protein of phage M13 and a number of other proteins whose attachment to, or insertion into, a membrane occurs after completion of their synthesis (Wickner 1980). An early report suggested that newly synthesized pp60$^{v\text{-}src}$ could be cleaved to a smaller form by a protease in the endoplasmic reticulum, as if a “signal sequence” might direct pp60$^{v\text{-}src}$ to the plasma membrane (Kamine and Buchanan 1978). These findings have not been confirmed. In other hands, newly completed pp60$^{v\text{-}src}$ (whether synthesized in vitro or in vivo) and the protein labeled to steady state in vivo have been indistinguishable by size (Sefton et al. 1978; Levinson et al. 1981; Weiss et al. 1981).

Several of the prominent morphological changes that accompany transformation have been attributed to the dismantling of focal adhesion plaques—specialized regions of the plasma membrane that apparently anchor normal cells to solid surfaces (David-Pfeuty and Singer 1980). Combined analyses by interference electron microscopy and fluorescence microscopy have demonstrated accumulations of pp60^{v-src} in adhesion plaques of RSV-infected cells (Rohrschneider 1980), as if the protein might be acting directly to disrupt the structure and function of the plaques. The finding is in one sense paradoxical, since fully transformed cells are said to be virtually devoid of adhesion plaques (David-Pfeuty and Singer 1980). It appears that occasional lines of RSV-transformed cells retain sufficient vestiges of the normal phenotype to permit the visualization of adhesion plaques; the presence of pp60^{v-src} in these vestigial structures can only be supposed to reflect what is otherwise a transient location of the viral protein. A correlative finding has been made, however, in the search for protein substrates of pp60^{v-src}: Tyrosine phosphorylation in the 130,000-dalton protein vinculin is enhanced by almost tenfold in cells transformed by RSV (Sefton et al. 1981b). Vinculin is a component of focal adhesion plaques that is rearranged into a more diffuse distribution in transformed cells, presumably as a concomitant of the dismantling of the plaques (David-Pfeuty and Singer 1980), perhaps as a result of tyrosine phosphorylation (Sefton et al. 1981b).

Reports of membranous locations for pp60^{v-src} were followed almost immediately by the seemingly contradictory claim that the protein is associated with the cytoskeleton of infected cells (Burr et al. 1980). Treatment of cells with nonionic detergent under specialized conditions disrupts the plasma membrane, dissolves about 75% of the cellular proteins, but leaves the cytoskeletal framework of the cell intact (Ben-Ze'ev et al. 1979; Fulton et al. 1980). In preparations of this kind, the phosphorylated forms of pp60^{v-src} as well as the *src*-specific protein kinase activity are found in the cytoskeletal residue, rather than among the soluble proteins (Burr et al. 1980). The paradoxical nature of these findings may be illusory. A substantial domain of pp60^{v-src} is exposed at the cytoplasmic aspect of the plasma membrane (see below) and might well be anchored to the cytoskeleton. The transforming protein encoded by *gag-abl* appears to be similarly disposed. One domain traverses the lipid bilayer of the plasma membrane (Witte et al. 1979a) and another domain is anchored to the cytoskeletal framework (D. Baltimore, pers. comm.).

An early report based on fluorescence microscopy suggested that large concentrations of pp60^{v-src} could be found in a perinuclear focus of uncertain nature (Rohrschneider 1979). Other investigators have been more explicit in such descriptions, claiming that certain mammalian cells (but not avian cells) transformed by RSV do not have significant quantities of $pp60^{v-src}$ attached to the plasma membrane (Krueger et al. 1980b). Instead, the protein is found mainly in the juxtanuclear endoplasmic reticulum and on the exterior of the nuclear envelope. Peptide analysis indicated that the $pp60^{v-src}$ in these cells is altered from the wild-type form in the aminoterminal domain of the protein (A. R. Goldberg, pers. comm.), which is thought to be responsible for anchoring the protein to the plasma membrane (see below). These are puzzling observations that cannot be easily dismissed, because the cells containing the variant $pp60^{v-src}$ are allegedly transformed by the action of *src*.

Some transformed cells and tumors secrete growth factors that bind to receptors on the surfaces of normal cells and elicit phenotypic aspects of neoplastic transformation (Todaro et al. 1980). The discovery of this "autocrine" production of growth factors excited interest in the possibility that viral transforming proteins might also act on cell surfaces subsequent to secretion. To date, no retroviral transforming protein has been found to follow this scheme. In particular, several searches for $pp60^{v-src}$ among the proteins secreted by RSV-transformed cells have been unavailing (Sefton et al. 1978; R. Hynes and H. Oppermann, pers. comm.).

In summary, $pp60^{v-src}$ appears to act mainly at the periphery of the cell: in specialized regions of the plasma membrane (such as adhesion plaques), perhaps at other sites within or on the cytoplasmic surface of the membrane, and even beyond the confines of the membrane (at nearby sites in the cytoplasm, cytoskeleton, etc.). However, these are largely circumstantial inferences. The techniques used so far to locate $pp60^{v-src}$ have limited resolving power and sensitivity; trace amounts of $pp60^{v-src}$ in presently unappreciated locations might cause major effects. It is nevertheless true that one of the two alleged substrates for $pp60^{v-src}$ whose identities are known (vinculin [Sefton et al. 1981b]) is associated with the plasma membrane in uninfected cells.

4. Possible Mechanism for Viral Oncogenesis: Tyrosine Phosphorylation by $pp60^{v-src}$

Confronted with an identified transforming protein, how might we deduce its function? The problem is daunting, because we know so little of how the growth and division of cells are controlled. However, one theme pervades the puzzle: the changes in the neoplastic cell are myriad. If these changes are caused by a single protein, the action of the protein must be formidably pleiotropic. Only a few mechanisms of pleiotropic change within cells are known, and prominent among these is protein phosphorylation (Rubin and Rosen 1975). It nevertheless required an inspired guess to prompt the testing of pp60^{v-src} for protein kinase activity, particularly since the first (and successful) tests were performed before purification of the protein had even been initiated (Collett and Erikson 1978; Levinson et al. 1978). In one instance, a fortuitous observation emboldened the guess: When pp60^{v-src} was phosphorylated in crude extracts of infected cells, the rate and extent of the reaction proved to be independent of the concentration of the protein in the extracts, as if pp60^{v-src} might be phosphorylating itself (Levinson et al. 1978). Ironically, the ability of pp60^{v-src} to phosphorylate itself has remained the subject of controversy long after the kinase activity of the protein seems well established (see below).

The assay used to test pp60^{v-src} for kinase activity was unorthodox in design and results (Fig. 9.1), but it nevertheless uncovered the first indications that pp60^{v-src} is indeed a protein kinase; it has since served to test the same issue for a number of other retroviral transforming proteins (see below). Immunoprecipitates containing pp60^{v-src} were used in phosphotransfer reactions with [^{32}P]ATP in the hope that added substrate proteins (such as histone and casein) might be phosphorylated. Instead, the heavy chain of the immunoglobulin in the precipitates was phosphorylated (Collett and Erikson 1978; Levinson et al. 1978) on tyrosine (Hunter and Sefton 1980), located in the variable region of the Ig molecule (Maness et al. 1979).

These findings alone would not warrant the conclusion that pp60^{v-src} has kinase activity. Other evidence was therefore sought and obtained: (1) Phosphorylation of the Ig molecule was observed only when pp60^{v-src} was present in the immunoprecipitate; the use of nor did extracts of normal cells react with tumor antisera specific for pp60^{v-src} (Collett and Erikson 1978; Levinson et al. 1978). (However, it was later found that certain tumor antisera can precipitate from extracts of normal cells small quantities of a protein whose structure and function are very similar to those of pp60^{v-src} [see below].) (2) Synthesis of pp60^{v-src} by translation in vitro also produced a precipitable kinase activity resembling that obtained from infected cells

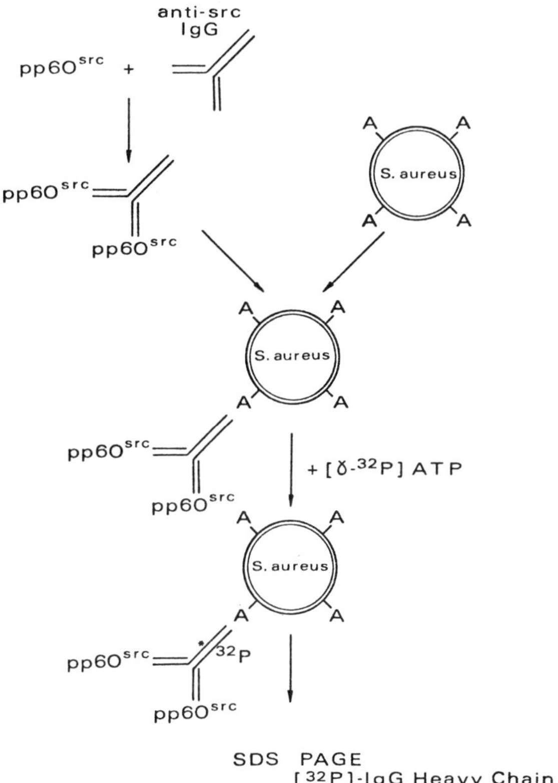

Figure 9.1 Illustration of the immune complex assay for protein kinase activity associated with pp60^{src}. Extracts of cells containing pp60^{src} are prepared and mixed with antiserum from tumor-bearing rabbits and the immune complexes are collected with protein A-bearing *S. aureus*. After extensive washing, the *S. aureus*-immune complex is suspended in 5 mM $MgCl_2$, 10 mM Tris (pH 7.2), and 1 μM [γ-^{32}P]ATP. After incubation to allow phosphorylation to proceed, the IgG and all adsorbed proteins are eluted with SDS-containing buffer and analyzed by polyacrylamide gel electrophoresis.

(Erikson et al. 1978; Sefton et al. 1979). (3) The kinase activity in cells infected with a temperature-sensitive mutant of *src* was substantially more thermolabile than the activity in cells infected with wild-type virus (Collett and Erikson 1978; Levinson et al. 1978; Rübsamen et al. 1979; Sefton et al. 1980a). Taken together, these findings made it seem likely that pp60^{v-src} itself possessed the enzymic activity of a protein kinase, although the possibility that a separate protein kinase was tightly bound to pp60$^{v\text{-}src}$ could not be rigorously excluded.

The kinase activity in immunoprecipitates containing pp60$^{v\text{-}src}$ transferred phosphorus from either ATP or GTP, and it displayed no response to cAMP (Collett and Erikson 1978; Levinson et al. 1978). These are hallmark properties of cyclic-nucleotide-independent protein kinases (Rubin and Rosen 1975). The enzymic activity also used an unexpected variety of other nucleoside triphosphates as phosphate donors, including CTP and several deoxyribonucleoside triphosphates (Richert et al. 1979). These novel observations prompted the suggestion that protein phosphorylation was an anomalous manifestation of the true function of pp60$^{v\text{-}src}$, i.e., the protein might in fact be a kinase of a different sort, perhaps a polynucleotide kinase. The capability of nucleoside triphosphates other than ATP and GTP to serve as phosphate donors has since been substantiated with purified pp60$^{v\text{-}src}$ (Levinson et al. 1980), but extensive testing has failed to detect phosphorylation of any substrates other than proteins (A. D. Levinson, pers. comm.).

The kinase reaction in immunoprecipitates was completed instantaneously, and its rate appeared independent of the concentration of the protein reactants (Levinson et al. 1978; Richert et al. 1979). It was therefore concluded that the kinase was phosphorylating the antibody to which it was bound and that the active site of the enzyme must be held in close proximity to the substrate site in the Ig molecule. Although it might have been reasonable to expect that at least some antibodies to pp60$^{v\text{-}src}$ would inactivate the protein, rather than serve as substrates for its activity, no inactivating antisera have been described to date, either from rabbits or from several other species that also produce anti-pp60$^{v\text{-}src}$ as a result of tumorigenesis by RSV (H. Oppermann and J. Brugge, pers. comm.).

The discovery that tyrosine was the target amino acid for phosphorylation in the immunoprecipitates containing pp60$^{v\text{-}src}$ came some time after the initial descriptions of the enzymic activity (Hunter and Sefton 1980), but it nevertheless provided a persuasive addition to the mounting evidence that protein phosphorylation is the agency by which *src* induces neoplastic transformation. Phosphotyrosine is an extremely rare amino acid in normal cells (~0.01% of the total phosphoamino acids in proteins) (see Hunter and Sefton 1980). The amount increases about tenfold in cells transformed by *src*, but not in cells transformed by chemicals or viral oncogenes to which no protein kinase activity has been attributed (Sefton et al. 1980c). Here was tangible evidence that a rare form of protein phosphorylation was augmented by infection with RSV. Moreover, the amounts of phosphotyrosine reflected the relative activity of pp60$^{v\text{-}src}$ in cells infected with temperature-sensitive mutants of *src*. At the permissive temperature, the quantities were elevated to the levels found in cells infected with wild-type virus, and, at the restrictive temperature, the quantities were those found in normal cells; shifts from one temperature to the other were followed in short order by changes in the amounts of phosphotyrosine (Sefton et al. 1980c). It now seemed clear that the activity of pp60$^{v\text{-}src}$ was required to induce and sustain the elevation of phosphotyrosine in cells transformed by RSV. But a more persuasive demonstration that the responsible kinase activity might be a property of pp60$^{v\text{-}src}$ itself awaited purification of the protein.

5. *Purification of pp60*$^{v\text{-}src}$

Substantial technical obstacles confronted attempts to purify pp60$^{v\text{-}src}$, including its hydrophobic nature, its tight association with the plasma membrane, and its vulnerability to the action of cellular proteases. Several tactics were employed to overcome these obstacles (Erikson et al. 1979; Levinson et al. 1980). The protein was extracted from infected cells and kept in solution by the use of nonionic detergents. Protease inhibitors were employed in profuse varieties and amounts; immunoaffinity chromatography was used to separate pp60$^{v\text{-}src}$ rapidly from other cellular constituents. The results have not been entirely satisfactory.

When purified in large quantities by standard chromatographic procedures, at least a portion of pp60$^{v\text{-}src}$ is reduced in size by a protease activity that acts on the aminoterminal domain of the molecule (Erikson et al. 1979; Levinson et al. 1980). A 52K protein has been obtained as ostensibly homogeneous preparations and retains kinase activity that phosphorylates tyrosine in protein substrates (Levinson et al. 1980). These findings sustain the view that the kinase activity is an intrinsic property of pp60$^{v\text{-}src}$, but one would obviously prefer to have a native, rather than a partially degraded, protein for purposes of further structural and enzymological analyses. In contrast, immunoaffinity chromatography has more readily provided intact pp60$^{v\text{-}src}$ with evident tyrosine protein kinase activity (Erikson et al. 1979; Levinson et al. 1980). However, the amounts of material obtained by this means have been small, precluding rigorous evaluation of purity and limiting the variety of further experiments that can be undertaken.

Purification of pp60$^{v\text{-}src}$ provided further evidence that pp60$^{v\text{-}src}$ and its attendant protein kinase activity are encoded by *src*. When prepared from cells infected with a temperature-sensitive mutant of *src*, the kinase activity of the purified pp60$^{v\text{-}src}$ is appreciably more thermolabile than the wild-type protein prepared in parallel (Erikson et al. 1979; Levinson et al. 1980).

The enzymic properties of the purified enzyme are much the same as those of the activity demonstrated in immunoprecipitates containing pp60$^{v\text{-}src}$. In particular, phosphate donors for the enzyme include ATP, GTP, and other nucleoside triphosphates (such as CTP and several deoxyribonucloside triphosphates), and cyclic nucleotides have no effect on the kinase activity (Erikson et al. 1979; Levinson et al. 1980).The purified protein displays high levels of ATPase activity (A. Levinson, pers. comm.), much as described for the large T antigen of SV40 virus (Tjian and Robbins 1979); the significance of these findings is not known. In contrast to T antigen, however, pp60$^{v\text{-}src}$ does not bind appreciably to either single- or double-stranded DNA (A. Levinson, pers. comm.).

Little has been learned by examining the substrate specificity of the purified enzyme. A number of proteins have been phosphorylated in vitro by purified pp60$^{v\text{-}src}$, including several that are demonstrably not tyrosine phosphoproteins in vivo (e.g., tubulin, casein, and actin) (Erikson et al. 1979; Levinson et al. 1980). Moreover, the range of protein substrates used successfully has varied from one laboratory to another. These findings are not surprising, since the apparent substrate specificity of protein kinases can be greatly distorted by the use of isolated acceptor proteins in vitro (Weller 1979).

Kinetic parameters have not been extensively studied with the purified enzyme; moreover, the protein acceptor (tubulin) employed in the few measurements made to date is probably not a substrate of pp60$^{v\text{-}src}$ in vivo (Levinson et al. 1980; Sefton et al. 1981b). In any event, the results were disquieting. The rate of phosphate transfer was at least 100-fold lower than the values usually obtained with authentic protein kinases operating on bona fide substrates (Levinson et al. 1980). These findings can be rationalized, but they nevertheless cast modest doubt on the physiological significance of the kinase activity observed in vitro with pp60$^{v\text{-}src}$ and call for corroborative evidence that phosphotransfer is an authentic activity of the protein. Reassurance of a sort has been obtained very recently by producing pp60$^{v\text{-}src}$ from molecular clones of *src* DNA inserted into *E. coli* (so far as we know, the bacteria themselves do not possess tyrosine protein kinase activity). The pp60$^{v\text{-}src}$ obtained in this manner is not phosphorylated on either serine or tyrosine, yet displays at least small amounts of tyrosine protein kinase activity that is likely to be intrinsic to the viral protein (R.D. Erikson and A.D. Levinson, pers. comm.).

6. *Molecular Topography of pp60*$^{v\text{-}src}$

Physical studies indicated that pp60$^{v\text{-}src}$ is an elongated rather than a globular molecule (Levinson et al. 1980). We have now achieved a relatively detailed image of how functionally important landmarks are distributed along the length of the molecule. Two major technical strategies have given form to this image. First, partial hydrolysis with proteases can be used to divide the protein into recognizable domains. In particular, the initial cleavage of pp60$^{v\text{-}src}$ by the V8 protease of *Staphylococcus aureus* in the presence of SDS produces a 36,000-dalton fragment that includes the amino terminus of pp60$^{v\text{-}src}$ and a 24,000-dalton fragment representing the carboxyterminal domain of the protein (Collett et al. 1979a). The ability to generate these geographically specific fragments has been a principal underpinning of efforts to locate structural and functional domains on pp60$^{v\text{-}src}$ and to define the structural changes in genetic variants of the protein. Second, we now have the nucleotide sequence of *src* from both SR-RSV (Czernilofsky et al. 1980) and PR-RSV (D. Schwartz, pers. comm.) and, hence, a deduced amino acid sequence for pp60$^{v\text{-}src}$. These data provide reference points for all structural studies of the protein, since they define with great precision the chemical compositions of the various domains of the molecule, potential sites of phosphorylation, and points of attack by site-specific proteases.

The technical strategies just described provided the points of departure that produced the following geographical description of pp60$^{v\text{-}src}$ (Fig. 9.2):

1. There are probably two major sites of serine phosphorylation in pp60$^{v\text{-}src}$. The exact amino acid residues phosphorylated have not been identified with any assurance. One may be at position 17 in

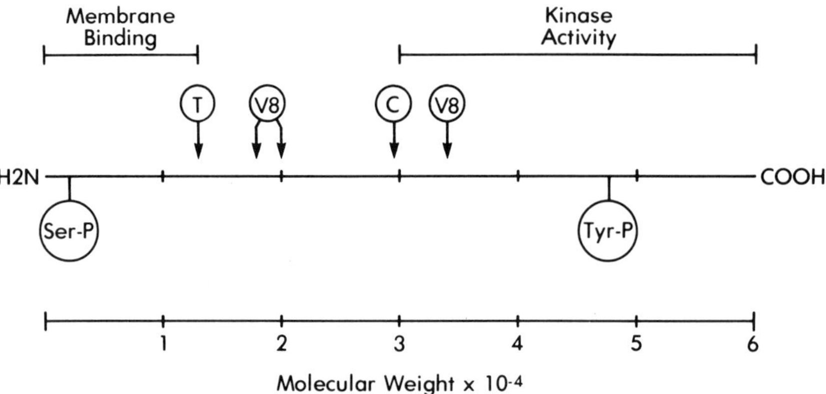

Figure 9.2 The molecular topography of pp60^{v-srv}. The topographical features illustrated here were located as described in the text. The domains for membrane binding and protein kinase activity are shown in their maximum possible extents; in reality, either or both domains may be smaller. The figure shows one phosphoserine residue (at position 17); there may be a second site for serine phosphorylation located between 16,000 and 18,000 daltons from the amino terminus of the molecule. The phosphotyrosine is located at residue 416 in pp60^{v-src} of the Prague strain of RSV. Preferred sites for cleavage are illustrated for trypsin (T), chymotrypsin (C), and the V8 protease of *Staphylococcus aureus* (V8).

the sequence of amino acids that composes the amino terminus of the protein; the other is less well defined but apparently lies between 16,000 daltons and 18,000 daltons from the amino terminus of the protein (R. Erikson and H. Oppermann, pers. comm.). In contrast, the single identified phosphotyrosine residue has been located precisely at position 419 of the published sequence for the SR-RSV or at position 416 in the sequence for PR-RSV-C. (This apparent discrepancy is probably not significant; it may be due to an error in the sequence of the SR-RSV *src* gene. In any event, the amino acid sequence that surrounds the phosphorylated tyrosine is identical in the two strains of virus ([Smart et al. 1981; T. Patchinsky, pers. comm.]). The amino acid sequence located to the amino terminal side of the phosphotyrosine (arg-leu-ile-glu-asp-asn-glu-*tyr*; see Smart et al. 1981) displays several features that have since been found at sites of tyrosine phosphorylation in other proteins (including retrovirus transforming proteins, the middle T antigen of polyoma virus, and proteins phosphorylated by pp60^{v-src}): arg at the seventh residue removed from the phosphotyrosine; a predominance of acidic amino acids; and the recurrence of glu, especially—but not inevitably—in the configuration glu-X-X-glu-*tyr* (Smart et al. 1981; Neil et al. 1981d; T. Hunter et al., pers. comm.; also, see below Section B.7). It appears that these features may typify sites of tyrosine phosphorylation by at least one major class of protein kinase (in most instances, the enzyme responsible for the tyrosine phosphorylation has yet to be identified), just as the configurations arg-arg-X-*ser* and lys-arg-X-X-*ser* are frequent sites of serine phosphorylation by cAMP-dependent protein kinases (Krebs and Beavo 1979).

2. A domain of about 8000 daltons at the amino terminus of $pp60^{v-src}$ anchors the protein to the plasma membrane (Krueger et al. 1980b; Levinson et. al. 1981). Neither the precise portion of this domain required for anchorage nor the nature of the anchorage is presently known. A variant of SR-RSV has been described in which the aminoterminal domain is present but chemically altered (as judged from peptide maps). The $pp60^{v-src}$ of this variant apparently does not attach in significant quantities to the plasma membrane, yet cells infected with the variant possess a transformed phenotype (A. R. Goldberg, pers. comm.). The significance of these findings is for the moment moot, since other mutants of *src* that lack the membrane-attachment domain fail to transform cells (Oppermann et al. 1981b). It is clear, however, that considerable latitude in structure at the amino terminus of $pp60^{v-src}$ is compatible with full function. Variants of the protein as short as 55,000 daltons and as long as 68,000 daltons have been described (Karess and Hanafusa 1981; Oppermann et al. 1981b). The variations in all of these versions of $pp60^{v-src}$ occur in the aminoterminal domain of the protein, and all of the variants transform cells.
3. The active site for phosphotransfer resides in the carboxyterminal half of $pp60^{v-src}$. Mutants lacking as much as 15,000 daltons from the aminoterminal portion of the protein retain protein kinase activity (Oppermann et al. 1981b). Moreover, partial cleavage with trypsin generates a fragment of 30,000 daltons that represents the carboxyterminal half of the protein, contains the phosphotyrosine residue, and is more active as a protein kinase than is the native form of $pp60^{v-src}$ (Levinson et al. 1981). The substrate specificity of this isolated domain of $pp60^{v-src}$ has

not been assessed; indeed, it could not be properly assessed at the moment for want of suitable parameters. It is quite possible that certain aspects of the aminoterminal domain of pp60$^{v\text{-}src}$ (e.g., the serine phosphorylation) regulate both kinetic features and substrate specificity of the kinase activity, perhaps by allosteric effects.

7. *Reprise: Is pp60$^{v\text{-}src}$ a Protein Kinase?*

The enzymic activity of an isolated protein is never easily proven. Copurification of activity and protein (as apparently achieved for pp60$^{v\text{-}src}$) can be a deception attributable to tight binding between the protein in view and the true, but unidentified, source of the enzymic activity. The kinetic performance of pp60$^{v\text{-}src}$ has also raised eyebrows: The rate of phosphotransfer by purified preparations of the protein is at least tenfold below what is generally observed with better-studied kinases. These caveats have been answered as follows:

1. The protein kinase activity attributed to pp60$^{v\text{-}src}$ accompanies the monomeric form of the viral protein precisely during careful measurement of molecular weight and configuration (Levinson et al. 1980); if an unidentified kinase is bound to pp60$^{v\text{-}src}$, it must be quite small.
2. The kinase activity found with temperature-sensitive mutants of *src* is thermolabile in infected cells (Collett and Erikson 1978; Sefton et al. 1980a), in crude extracts of infected cells (Levinson et al. 1978), in the products of translation from viral RNA in vitro (Sefton et al. 1979), and in purified preparations of pp60$^{v\text{-}src}$ (Erikson et al. 1979; Levinson et al. 1980).
3. Protein kinase activity survives the treatment of pp60$^{v\text{-}src}$ with trypsin and accompanies the isolated carboxyterminal half of the molecule (Levinson et al. 1981; A. Levinson, pers. comm.).
4. The amount of phosphotyrosine increases in cells transformed by *src* but not in a substantial number of cells transformed by other means (Sefton et al. 1981c). Moreover, in cells infected with temperature-sensitive mutants of *src*, the concentration of phosphotyrosine fluctuates in accord with the measurable activity of the mutant pp60$^{v\text{-}src}$ (Sefton et al. 1981c).
5. Protein kinase activety is affiliated with pp60$^{v\text{-}src}$ even if the protein is produced in *E. coli* (see above, Section A.5).

All of these observations cojoin to sustain the conclusion that pp60^{v-src} is a tyrosine protein kinase and that this enzymic activity is central to (indeed, may be exclusively responsible for) neoplastic transformation induced by the activity of *src*. Two possible schemes come to mind. Either phosphorylation of a single protein precipitates a cascade of events that together give rise to the neoplastic phenotype, or the kinase activity of pp60^{v-src} is itself pleiotropic, i.e., it acts on numerous proteins, directly affecting each of their activities, and perhaps precipitating secondary events or even cascades in turn. What little we know at the moment makes it seem likely that the pleiotropic alternative is correct. For example, there exist mutations in *src* that affect only a portion of the phenotypic response to the gene: some aspects of neoplastic transformation become manifest when *src* is expressed, others do not (Anderson et al. 1981). These findings are most easily explained by assuming that pp60^{v-src} acts independently on multiple "targets" within the cell. With these issues in view, the experimentalist will turn quickly to the search for cellular proteins whose phosphorylation by pp60^{v-src} might mediate the phenotypic changes displayed by a transformed cell. The search has become a feverish activity that is in its formative period, that has yet to identify changes responsible for the malignant growth of transformed cells, and that promises insight into the control of growth in normal as well as in neoplastic cells.

8. Search for Targets: Proteins That Bind to pp60^{v-src}

Affinity for substrates provides a potentially powerful means by which to purify enzymes and identify their substrates. Thus, any cellular protein that binds to pp60^{v-src} would perforce attract attention. Two such proteins, with molecular weights of 89,000 and 50,000 daltons, have been identified by virtue of the fact that they immunoprecipitate with pp60^{v-src} (Hunter and Sefton 1980; Oppermann et al. 1981c; J. Brugge, pers. comm.). Both proteins appear to be in physical complex with pp60^{v-src}, at least in extracts of infected cells (it cannot yet be said whether the complex exists within the intact cell) (Oppermann et al. 1981c; J. Brugge, pers. comm.). The functional significance of the complex is uncertain. There is provisional evidence to suggest that the complex may be the first, but transient, destination of pp60^{v-src} following its synthesis (J. Brugge, pers. comm.); that while in the complex, pp60^{v-src} is phosphorylated only on serine and has no kinase activity (J. Brugge, pers. comm.); and that the 50K protein may be one of the much sought substrates for the viral enzyme, thus accounting for its interaction with pp60$^{v\text{-}src}$ (Hunter and Sefton 1980; G.S. Martin, pers. comm.).

The 89K protein is a major constituent of the cytoplasmic fraction in every vertebrate cell examined; has a highly conserved structure, with peptide maps that are virtually indistinguishable across broad evolutionary distances; is phosphorylated only on serine; and is among a handful of proteins whose synthesis is substantially augmented when cells are exposed to a variety of noxious influences, such as unphysiologically high temperatures (so-called heat shock) and chelating agents (Hunter and Sefton 1980; Oppermann et al. 1981a). The function of the 89K protein is not known, and we cannot explain either its participation in the heat-shock response or its apparent binding to pp60$^{v\text{-}src}$. The same protein may also bind to the protein encoded by Fujinami sarcoma virus (FuSV)-*fps* (J. Brugge, pers. comm.) and PRC-II-*fps* (B. Adkins, pers. comm.). Neoplastic transformation by a variety of agents (including RSV) has no effect on the amounts of the 89K protein in the cell (Oppermann et al. 1981a).

The 50K protein is a relatively minor constituent of vertebrate cells and, unless immunoprecipitated with pp60$^{v\text{-}src}$, can be found only by diligent searching among the very large number of proteins that are resolved by two-dimensional electrophoresis of cellular extracts (G.S. Martin, pers. comm.). In contrast to the 89K protein, the structure of the 50K protein is not conserved among different species; in fact, the forms of this protein isolated from avian and mammalian cells yield entirely different peptide maps and would not be considered kindred but for their sizes and shared property of binding to pp60$^{v\text{-}src}$ (Oppermann et al. 1981c). In avian cells transformed by RSV, the 50K protein is phosphorylated on serine and tyrosine (Hunter and Sefton 1980; Oppermann et al. 1981c). The tyrosine phosphorylation naturally prompted the suggestion that the protein might be a substrate for the *v-src* protein kinase. The suggestion has not been simple to test because of the following: (1) Phosphorylation of the 50K protein recovered from transformed chicken cells in complex with pp60$^{v\text{-}src}$ is unaffected when the kinase activity of temperature-sensitive mutants of *src* is modulated (Oppermann et al. 1981c; J. Brugge, pers. comm.); from this, one might conclude that the 50K protein is not a substrate of $pp60^{v\text{-}src}$. (2) When examined directly, rather than by immunoprecipitation, phosphorylation of tyrosine in the 50K protein is clearly a concomitant of transformation by *src*—the protein is phosphorylated only on serine in uninfected chicken cells. Paradoxically, however, the tyrosine phosphorylation is not affected by temperature-sensitive mutations in *src*. Even infection at the restrictive temperature in a manner that precludes the initiation of cellular transformation leads to phosphorylation of tyrosine in the 50K protein (G.S. Martin, pers. comm.). (3) The 50K protein found in complex with $pp60^{v\text{-}src}$ in RSV-transformed mammalian cells displays no detectable tyrosine phosphorylation under any circumstances (Oppermann et al. 1981c).

These contrasting findings are not easy to reconcile, but at least one conclusion seems reasonable: Tyrosine phosphorylation in the 50K protein of avian cells appears to be a consequence of infection by RSV and may represent an activity of $pp60^{v\text{-}src}$ that is not affected by any of the conditional mutations tested to date. Moreover, provisional evidence indicates that phosphorylation of tyrosine in the avian 50K protein is also induced by the activity of the *fps* and *yes* oncogenes (J. Brugge, pers. comm.). There seems little doubt that further study of the 50K protein (its subcellular location, function, and interaction with sundry viral transforming proteins) will prove fruitful.

9. Search for Targets: Proteins Phosphorylated on Tyrosine in Infected Cells

The discovery that $pp60^{v\text{-}src}$ can phosphorylate proteins on tyrosine aided subsequent efforts to decipher the events that occur within cells transformed by RSV. Two main strategies have been developed: (1) examine infected cells for proteins in which the phosphorylation of tyrosine is augmented as a consequence of cellular transformation by *src* and (2) use purified $pp60^{v\text{-}src}$ to test individual proteins for their susceptibility to tyrosine phosphorylation. Neither of these strategies is sufficient when used alone. On the one hand, it is unlikely that all tyrosine phosphorylations in RSV-transformed cells are directly mediated by $pp60^{v\text{-}src}$. On the other hand, it is generally acknowledged that the phosphorylation of protein in vitro can utilize inauthentic substrate sites. But if the two approaches are combined, i.e., if identical tyrosine phosphorylations can be identified by parallel studies in vivo and in vitro, then the experimentalist has done the best that is presently possible to identify potential targets of pp60$^{v\text{-}src}$.

Two-dimensional gel fractionation procedures permit the resolution of perhaps 10% of all of the proteins in a mammalian cell (O'Farrell et al. 1977). If these procedures are applied to proteins derived from RSV-transformed cells that have been labeled with radioactive phosphate, it is possible to search for individual proteins whose phosphorylation has been augmented as a consequence of transformation by *src*. The use of this approach soon identified a 34,000–36,000-dalton protein (pp36) that qualified as a potential "target" for pp60$^{v\text{-}src}$ (Radke and Martin 1979; Erikson and Erikson 1980; Radke et al. 1980). This protein is present, but not phosphorylated, in uninfected avian and mammalian cells (Radke and Martin 1979; Erikson and Erikson 1980; Radke et al. 1980). Transformation of cells by RSV leads to phosphorylation of tyrosine and serine on perhaps 15% of the molecules of pp36, without changing the total amount of the protein (Radke et al. 1980). Several findings indicate that pp36 is phosphorylated directly by pp60$^{v\text{-}src}$: (1) Phosphorylation of pp36 does not occur in all transformed cells but, instead, has been observed only in cells transformed by either RSV or other retroviruses whose oncogenes apparently encode tyrosine protein kinases (Pawson et al. 1980; Radke et al. 1980; Cooper and Hunter 1981a,b; Erikson et al. 1981). (2) Phosphorylation of pp36 in cells infected with a temperature-sensitive mutant of *src* responds to shifts in temperature as if pp60$^{v\text{-}src}$ were the responsible enzyme (Radke and Martin 1979; Radke et al. 1980). Serine phosphorylation in pp36 also responds to temperature in these experiments, an unexpected and presently unexplained finding. (3) Phosphorylation of tyrosine in vivo occurs at a single site in avian pp36 (Erikson and Erikson 1980; Radke et al. 1980). The same site on purified pp36 is phosphorylated in vitro by purified pp60$^{v\text{-}src}$ (Erikson and Erikson 1980).

We can therefore conclude that pp36 is likely to be a substrate for pp60$^{v\text{-}src}$ within the infected cell. Moreover, the same cellular protein may be phosphorylated by tyrosine protein kinases encoded by other retroviral oncogenes, such as *fps* and *abl* (Pawson et al. 1980; Cooper and Hunter 1981b; Erikson et al. 1981; T. Hunter, pers.

comm.). Little else is known of pp36. Although it is a major constituent of both avian and mammalian cells (~0.25–0.5% of the total cellular protein), there is as yet no clear picture of where pp36 might be located within the cell (other than general agreement that it is probably not a nuclear protein) and no indication as to its function.

The analyses that uncovered pp36 failed to reveal any other proteins that might qualify as targets for $pp60^{v\text{-}src}$ (Radke and Martin 1979); the fractionation scheme had apparently been taxed to the limits of its potential. The capability of this approach has recently been improved, however, by exploiting the relative stability of phosphotyrosine in alkali to eliminate preferentially phosphate residues from serine and threonine following fractionation of proteins. This procedure reduces the background in the analysis and has brought to light several more cellular proteins whose tyrosine phosphorylation may be attributable to the action of $pp60^{v\text{-}src}$ (Cooper and Hunter 1981a,b). The identity, subcellular location, and function of these proteins are all unknown, and there is as yet no rigorous evidence that the proteins are direct targets for $pp60^{v\text{-}src}$. The results nevertheless give further impetus to the idea that $pp60^{v\text{-}src}$ acts on more than one cellular protein, i.e., that $pp60^{v\text{-}src}$ is a pleiotropic effector in its own right.

Efforts to conduct comprehensive searches for tyrosine phosphorylations in infected cells have been supplemented by analyses directed to specific consequences of neoplastic transformation. For example, numerous changes occur in the cytoskeleton of the cell as a result of the action of *src* and other transforming agents (Hanafusa 1977). Individual components of the cytoskeleton have therefore been examined by immunoprecipitation in an effort to detect tyrosine phosphorylation that might be mediated by $pp60^{v\text{-}src}$ (Sefton et al. 1981b). The analyses have of necessity been limited to a few cytoskeletal proteins for which antisera were available (actin, tubulin, myosin, α-actinin, filamin, vimentin, and vinculin), and of these, only vinculin has been implicated as a potential target for $pp60^{v\text{-}src}$.

Vinculin is a 130,000-dalton protein whose presence in focal adhesion plaques may be essential to certain morphological features of normal cells (David-Pfeuty and Singer 1980). Neoplastic transformation dismantles the adhesion plaques and redistributes vinculin within the cell. In cells transformed by RSV, these changes may be due to the protein kinase activity of $pp60^{v\text{-}src}$ (Sefton et al. 1981b).

Tyrosine phosphorylation in vinculin increases by almost tenfold; the change reflects both additional phosphorylation of a tyrosine residue that is also phosphorylated in uninfected cells and phosphorylation of a new residue in the transformed cells. The use of temperature-sensitive mutants of *src* has linked the augmented phosphorylation of vinculin to the action of $pp60^{v-src}$. However, there is as yet no direct demonstration that vinculin is a substrate for $pp60^{v-src}$ and no direct evidence that phosphorylation of vinculin is responsible for the redistribution of the protein in transformed cells. Moreover, the increase in tyrosine phosphorylation affects only 1% of the total population of vinculin in the cell. This finding is at first glance disquieting but can be rationalized by arguing that only a small and perhaps specific subset of vinculin molecules need be modified in order to disrupt the adhesion plaque (Sefton et al. 1981b).

Altered phosphorylation of vinculin is not an inevitable concomitant of the neoplastic phenotype. For example, tyrosine phosphorylation in vinculin is unchanged in cells transformed by a chemical carcinogen, a DNA tumor virus, and the PRCII retrovirus (Sefton et al. 1981b). The last of these exceptions is particularly notable, since the oncogene of PRCII (*fps*) is thought to encode a tyrosine protein kinase (see Section II.B.3). The apparent failure of this enzyme to phosphorylate vinculin has been invoked as an explanation for the fusiform morphology of cells transformed by PRCII virus (Sefton et al. 1981b) (Section II.B.4). The findings with vinculin exemplify the pleiotropic nature of the action of $pp60^{v-src}$ and other transforming proteins: Phosphorylation of vinculin provides an explanation for several of the prominent morphological changes that accompany transformation by *src*, but it is probably not required for the loss of growth control that typifies the transformed cell.

Considerable recent attention has been given to the possibility that the products of *src* and other oncogenes might be involved in a protein kinase cascade that ultimately affected the activity of membrane-associated Na^+/K^+ ATPase (Spector et al. 1980a,b; 1981a,b; Racker and Spector 1981). However, these claims have now been questioned (Racker 1981; P.K. Vogt et al., in prep.), and readers are advised to view the published experiments with caution unless they are successfully reproduced.

B. *fps, yes,* and *ros:* Oncogenes of Defective Avian Sarcoma Viruses

1. Discovery and Classification of Defective Avian Sarcoma Viruses

Until 1980, the only avian retroviruses with transformation potential confined to fibroblasts were believed to be the various strains of RSV, all of which carried closely related versions of *src*. However, a highly productive reversal of this position occurred with the discovery that FuSV, a sarcomagenic virus of chickens (Fujinami and Inamoto 1914), previously believed to bear *src* (Stehelin et al. 1976a; Wang et al. 1980), in fact contained a novel set of sequences unrelated to *src* or to any replicative genes of avian leukosis viruses (Hanafusa et al. 1980; Lee et al. 1980). (The initial misconception about the transforming gene of FuSV appears to have resulted from confusion of some FuSV stocks with RSV.) In the following 2 years, there has been an unexpected proliferation of new strains of avian sarcoma viruses lacking *src*, each defective for all three replication genes and capable of transforming only fibroblasts in culture and inducing only fibrosarcomas in animals.

The most extensively studied isolates of defective avian sarcoma viruses have been placed into three groups, based on the nature of genomic sequences believed to be responsible for the oncogenic properties of the viruses. One group is composed of FuSV, three closely related isolates from the Poultry Research Center (PRCII, PRCIIp, and PRCIV [Carr and Campbell 1958]), and two less completely studied viruses (UR-1 [Balduzzi et al. 1981; Wang et al. 1981] and 16L [B. Neel et al., pers. comm.]) and is united by a transforming sequence called *fps*. As discussed below (Section II.G.3), *fps* is closely related to the transforming sequence (*fes*) of certain feline sarcoma viruses (Shibuya et al. 1980), and the products of *fps* and *fes* are related structurally, immunologically, and functionally (Barbacid et al. 1981; Beemon 1981b). A second group, containing thus far only Yamaguchi 73 virus (Y73; Itohara et al. 1978) and Esh sarcoma virus (ESV; Wallbank et al. 1966), is identified by a transforming sequence called *yes*. (Viruses with *fps* have been called class-II viruses and those with *yes* have been called class-III viruses by Vogt and associates [Neil et al. 1981b].) A third group is so far represented only by UR-2 (Balduzzi et al. 1981) with a unique trans-

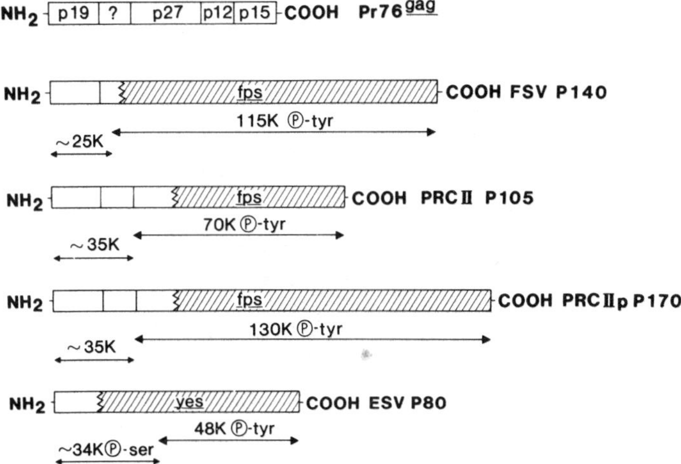

Figure 9.3 The polyproteins of defective avian sarcoma viruses. The structures of three products of *gag-fps* and one of *gag-yes* gene fusions were determined by peptide mapping of the cleavage fragments generated with $p15^{gag}$ (Ghysdael et al. 1981b). For comparison, the organization of $Pr76^{gag}$ of RSV is presented on the top line; the box with a question mark is thought to correspond to $p10^{gag}$ (see Chapter 6).

forming sequence designated *ros* (L. H. Wang et al., M. Shibuya et al; both in prep.).

It is convenient to discuss *fps, yes,* and *ros* together because of their functional similarities, despite the lack of apparent nucleotide sequence homology. All of the well-studied isolates bearing any of these three genes appear to synthesize only a single polyprotein, varying in size from 68,000 daltons to 170,000 daltons. The amino terminus of these polyproteins is encoded by residual *gag* sequences (the p19 region in all cases, with a portion of the p27 region in some), and the remainder is encoded by *onc* sequences (Fig. 9.3). Thus far, detection of these proteins has depended primarily on the use of antisera with activity against appropriate *gag* determinants, although the antisera have been obtained both from animals immunized against viral structural proteins (anti-*gag* serum) and from rabbits bearing RSV-induced tumors (TBR serum). All of the polyproteins contain phosphoserine and phosphotyrosine (albeit in differing ratios), all have exhibited a phosphotransferase activity associated with immune complexes, and all are capable of transferring phosphate from ATP to tyrosine residues on the viral polyprotein or on heavy chains of immunoglobulins. The potential significance of the protein kinase activity has been supported by finding elevated levels of phosphotyrosine in fibroblasts transformed by *fps* and *yes* (Beemon 1981) and by the identification of *ts fps* and *ros* mutants displaying thermolability of both the kinase activity and the transformed phenotype (Pawson et al. 1980; Beemon 1981; Hanafusa et al. 1981, and pers. comm.; Hirano and Vogt 1981, and pers. comm.) (see Chapter 7). Several of the polyproteins encoded by these viruses are susceptible to cleavage by p15^{gag} (Ghysdael et al. 1981b; T. Pawson et al., pers. comm.) (Fig. 9.3), and cleavage appears to remove most or all of the *gag* region from the polyprotein. This may offer a useful approach to dissection of the structure and function of these polyproteins although such cleavages do not occur in the infected cell.

2. The Protein Product of FuSV (P140$^{gag-fps}$) Is a Phosphoprotein Associated with Tyrosine Kinase Activity

The first of the uniquely sarcomagenic *gag-onc* polyproteins to be identified was the 140,000-dalton product of FuSV, P140$^{gag-fps}$ (Bister et al. 1980b; Feldman et al. 1980; Hanafusa et al. 1980, 1981; Lee et al. 1980; Beemon 1981). As anticipated from genomic structure (Chapter 4), P140$^{gag-fps}$ has structural and immunological determinants of p19^{gag}. Some initial confusion about the sites of phosphorylation of P140$^{gag-fps}$ and the amount of associated protein kinase activity was clarified by the surprising finding that at least one of the unselected and apparently unmutagenized stocks of FuSV used for some studies was dominated by a mutant temperature-sensitive for transformation (Pawson et al. 1980; Beemon 1981). Wild-type virus (or temperature-sensitive virus grown at the permissive temperature) produces P140$^{gag-fps}$ phosphorylated predominantly at tyrosine residues in the *fps* portion of the protein; phosphorylation also occurs at serine residues in the *gag* portion and at threonine residues in the *fps* portion (T. Pawson and G. S. Martin; both pers. comm.). Similarities among the sites of tyrosine phosphorylation in the products of *src, fps,* and *yes* are discussed in Section II.B.7.

The protein kinase activity associated with immune complexes of FuSV P140$^{gag-fps}$ exhibits some unusual properties, many of which are shared with other viruses carrying *fps, yes,* or *ros* (Feldman et al. 1980, and pers. comm.; Pawson et al. 1980; Beemon 1981). When the activity is elicited with TBR sera, most or all of the phosphate is transferred to tyrosine residues on heavy chains, with little or no transfer to P140$^{gag\text{-}fps}$. In contrast, when the activity is elicited with antibodies to *gag* proteins, all of the tyrosine phosphorylation appears to occur on P140$^{gag\text{-}fps}$ itself, at the site (or sites) phosphorylated in P140$^{gag\text{-}fps}$ in vivo. Presumably, sera from the rabbits bearing RSV-induced tumors contain immunoglobulins that can function more efficiently as targets for the *fps* (and *yes*) kinases, but a satisfactory explanation for this phenomenon is not yet available. The kinase activity associated with P140$^{gag\text{-}fps}$, unlike that associated with pp60$^{v\text{-}src}$, utilizes ATP, but not GTP, as phosphate donor. It shares with the *gag-fps* polyprotein of PRCII a strong preference for Mn^{++} over Mg^{++} as a divalent cation during the reaction. This proclivity for Mn^{++} is not shared by the products of *src* or *yes* (Levinson et al. 1978; Ghysdael et al. 1981a).

The belief that the kinase activity is present in P140$^{gag\text{-}fps}$ itself, rather than in an associated protein, rests primarily on studies of spontaneous and induced temperature-sensitive mutants of FuSV-*fps* (Pawson et al. 1980; Hanafusa et al. 1981; cf. Chapter 7). Immune complexes prepared with P140$^{gag\text{-}fps}$ from cells grown at the nonpermissive temperature demonstrate little or no kinase activity, and the loss of activity coincides with morphological changes toward normal functions, i.e., decreased glucose uptake, decreased production of plasminogen activator, reduced phosphorylation of P140$^{gag\text{-}fps}$, and a return to normal levels of total cellular phosphotyrosine. Thus far, there have been no reports of the purification of P140$^{gag\text{-}fps}$ or of the synthesis of enzymically active P140$^{gag\text{-}fps}$ in vitro.

3. Protein Products of PRC Viruses

Of the three PRC viruses, PRCII has been the most closely studied; but it now appears likely that PRCII was derived from PRCIIp (or from PRCIV, which is virtually indistinguishable from PRCIIp) by a genetic deletion (Breitman et al. 1981b). The putative parental viruses, PRCIIp and PRCIV, produce a *gag-fps* polyprotein of 170,000 daltons (P170$^{gag\text{-}fps}$), whereas the product of PRCII is 105,000 daltons (P105$^{gag\text{-}fps}$) (Breitman et al. 1981a,b; Neil et al. 1981a). The PRC polyproteins contain antigenic determinants and methionine-labeled peptides of p27^{gag}, as well as p19^{gag}, validating the assumption that the major *fps* viruses, FuSV and PRCII, represent independent recombination events between viral genomes and *c-fps*. Tryptic peptide maps do not distinguish between P170$^{gag\text{-}fps}$ of PRCIIp and PRCIV, but a comparison of the maps of P170$^{gag\text{-}fps}$

and $P105^{gag\text{-}fps}$ reveals two peptides specific to the PRCIIp product and one specific to the PRCII product, in addition to at least four shared peptides (Ghysdael et al. 1981b).

Immunoprecipitates of the PRCII $P105^{gag\text{-}fps}$ exhibit a tyrosine-specific protein kinase activity similar to that observed for the FuSV $P140^{gag\text{-}fps}$ (Beemon 1981; Neil et al. 1981c). As for $P140^{gag\text{-}fps}$, the conclusion that the kinase activity is virus-coded rests primarily on the analysis of temperature-sensitive mutants of *fps* mutants of PRCII (Hirano and Vogt 1981, and pers. comm.) (Chapter 7). However, $P105^{gag\text{-}fps}$ has recently been synthesized in a reticulocyte lysate programmed with PRCII virion RNA (B. Atkins, pers. comm.). A tyrosine-specific protein kinase activity was elicited upon immunoprecipitation of the in vitro product with TBR serum; demonstration of the kinase activity was blocked by preincubation of the serum with RSV structural proteins.

4. Oncogenic Properties of fps *Proteins*

The several strains of PRC viruses and of FuSV display some unusual biological properties that may prove to be useful points of departure for studying the mechanisms of transformation by these agents. In general, agents bearing *fps* produce myxomatous tumors in animals and fusiform rather than round cell transformation of fibroblasts in culture, sometimes with excessive production of mucinous material (Breitman et al. 1981a). These properties could reflect the cellular targets chosen for phosphorylation by products of *fps*. However, comparison of the proteins containing phosphotyrosine in cells transformed by *src, fps,* and *yes*, using two-dimensional gel systems, reveals a surprisingly similar set of seven putative target proteins (Cooper and Hunter 1981b). A major specific target of $pp60^{v\text{-}src}$, the 36K protein of Radke and Martin (1979), is also highly phosphorylated in FuSV-transformed cells (Pawson et al. 1980). On the other hand, cells transformed by PRCII, unlike cells transformed by RSV (*src*) and Y73 (*yes*), do not manifest enhanced tyrosine phosphorylation of vinculin (Sefton et al. 1981b) (see Section II.A.9); the relationship of this difference to phenotypic differences (e.g., fusiform morphology) is only speculative.

5. Additional Isolates Containing fps

Protein products of two other *fps*-containing viruses have recently been subjected to preliminary characterization. The UR-1 virus, isolated from a spontaneous fibrosarcoma and capable of inducing myxosarcomas in animals and small foci of round cells in culture (Balduzzi et al. 1981), encodes a 150,000-dalton *gag-fps* polyprotein, with an associated tyrosine kinase activity, similar in several respects to that associated with other *gag-fps* proteins (L.H. Wang et al. 1981). Another virus, 16L, was isolated from a fibrosarcoma induced by infection with the temperature-independent deletion *src* mutant 107A of SR-RSV (Kawai et al. 1977; B. Neel et al., pers. comm.). Cells transformed by 16L contain a polyprotein of 142,000 daltons with an associated protein kinase activity; the polyprotein is presumed to be encoded by residual *gag* sequences and by sequences in the 6.2-kb genome shown to be homologous to *fps*.

6. *Protein Products of Y73 and ESV, P90$^{gag-yes}$ and P80$^{gag-yes}$ Are Closely Related Phosphoproteins*

Two avian viruses bearing the putative transforming sequences called *yes* have recently been studied in detail. The Y73 virus, isolated in 1973 from a transplantable tumor in a white leghorn chicken in Yamaguchi, Japan (Itohara et al. 1978), encodes a 90,000-dalton phosphoprotein (P90$^{gag-yes}$); ESV, isolated by Wallbank et al. (1966) from a spontaneous sarcoma in a Pennsylvania farm chicken, induces nonmetastatic fibrosarcomas in chickens and encodes a phosphoprotein of 80,000 daltons (P80$^{gag-yes}$). Mapping of tryptic peptides and characterization of associated protein kinase activities have revealed strong similarities between P80$^{gag-yes}$ and P90$^{gag-yes}$, as well as several differences between them and the products of *src* and *fps* (Kawai et al. 1980; Ghysdael et al. 1981a,c). Both of the *gag-yes* polyproteins contain peptides and immunological determinants of p19^{gag}, but not of p27^{gag}. However, p15^{gag} cleaves the ESV product, but not the Y73 product, suggesting that the site within *gag* at which recombination has occurred with *yes* sequences differs in the two isolates (Ghysdael et al. 1981b). The patterns of phosphorylation in vivo also differ, P80$^{gag-yes}$ being equally well phosphorylated at tyrosine and serine residues and P90$^{gag-yes}$ being more heavily phosphorylated at serine than at tyrosine residues (Kawai et al. 1980; Beemon 1981; Ghysdael et al. 1981a). In both cases, however, there is a serine phosphorylation site that appears to lie outside the *gag* region, presumably in the *yes* portion of the polyprotein, but closer than the phosphotyrosine residue to the amino terminus (Ghysdael et al. 1981a,b). P90$^{gag-yes}$ and P80$^{gag-yes}$ share all four of their methionine-containing *yes* peptides and at least seven of their cysteine-containing *yes* peptides, but there are also a few cysteine-containing peptides unique to poly protein. The methionine peptide maps of P80$^{gag\text{-}yes}$ and P90$^{gag\text{-}yes}$ bear no relationship to those of pp60^{src} or to the *fps* portions of P105$^{gag\text{-}fps}$ or P140$^{gag\text{-}fps}$, although there are intergenic homologies at the tyrosine phosphorylation sites (see Section II.B.7).

7. Protein Kinase Activity Associated with Products of yes

Immunoprecipitates containing either of the *gag-yes* polyproteins display a protein kinase activity specific for tyrosine residues (Kawai et al. 1980; Ghysdael et al. 1981a,c). As also observed with products of *fps*, the kinase activity is directed principally toward immunoglobulin heavy chains when TBR sera are used, but only the *gag-yes* protein itself is phosphorylated using sera raised against viral structural proteins (Kawai et al. 1980; Ghysdael et al. 1981c). Curiously, preabsorption of TBR sera with disrupted RAV-2 did not appreciably affect labeling of the heavy chains in a subsequent immune-complex assay with P90$^{gag\text{-}yes}$, although the modest labeling of P90$^{gag\text{-}yes}$ itself was eliminated by the preabsorption step. Immune complexes containing either P90$^{gag\text{-}yes}$ or P80$^{gag\text{-}yes}$ can phosphorylate added targets, such as α-casein, but they phosphorylate tyrosine residues exclusively, regardless of substrate. The kinase activities affiliated with *gag-yes* and *src* proteins exhibit a sharp difference from that of *gag-fps* proteins with respect to divalent cation response (see Section II.B.2).

The single phosphotyrosine peptide from either P90$^{gag\text{-}yes}$ or P80$^{gag\text{-}yes}$ labeled in vitro is the same as that found in the phosphoprotein isolated from infected cells (Ghysdael et al. 1981a), and the implicated peptides from the two proteins behave identically in two-dimensional gel analyses. Moreover, the phosphotyrosine peptides from P90$^{gag\text{-}yes}$ and P80$^{gag\text{-}yes}$ comigrate with the phosphotyrosine peptide from pp60^{src} in multiple fractionation procedures, indicating a high degree of homology between the phosphorylation sites in these proteins (Neil et al. 1981c,d; Patchinsky and Sefton 1981). Digestion with *S. aureus* V8 protease, which cleaves on the carboxyl side of glutamic acid residues, and partial amino acid sequencing reveal that the tyrosine phosphorylation site in the *gag-yes* proteins contains the sequence -glu-X-X-glu-*tyr*-, very similar to (and possibly identical with) the probable phosphotyrosine site in pp60^{src} (-glu-asp-asn-glu-*tyr*-ala-arg-) (Smart et al. 1981; Neil et al. 1981d, and pers. comm.; T. Patchinsky, pers. comm.). Although the phosphotyrosine-containing peptide from the *gag-fps* proteins is readily differentiated from those of *src* and *gag-yes* proteins by conventional mapping procedures (Neil et al. 1981d), the tyrosine phosphorylation site again appears to be enriched for the acidic amino acid, glutamic acid, in the tentative configuration -glu-X-X-(glu)-*tyr*- (J. C. Neil et al., pers. comm.). These results suggest that the target sites for phosphorylation by tyrosine kinases may be generally related by the presence of neighboring acidic residues. However, it should be emphasized that the enzymes that phosphorylate the sites on these putative transforming proteins may not be the transforming proteins themselves, since rigorous evidence for autophosphorylation is not yet available (see Section II.A.2).

The apparent similarities in tyrosine phosphoacceptor sites in these proteins may, however, be reflected in the very similar arrays of major phosphotyrosine-containing proteins observed after transformation by *yes, fps, src,* and *abl* (Cooper and Hunter 1981a). Few of the proteins phosphorylated on tyrosine residues after transformation by *yes* have been specifically identified, but at least one, vinculin, is similarily affected after transformation by *src* and *yes*, although not (as noted earlier) after transformation by *fps* (Sefton et al. 1981b). The relevance of these findings to the mechanism of transformation is uncertain. Localization of *yes*- and *fps*-transforming proteins within the cell, isolation and characterization of viral (and host) mutants, and better definition of the target proteins for tyrosine phosphorylation will be required for mechanistic interpretations.

8. Other Fibroblast-transforming Genes?

There is reason to believe that additional genetic elements have been isolated in replication-defective, fibroblast-transforming agents of birds. Balduzzi et al. (1981) have identified an agent called UR-2 that encodes a 68,000-dalton *gag-onc* protein with associated tyrosine kinase activity, but the transforming sequence (*ros*) of UR-2 lacks apparent homology with other avian *onc* sequences (L.H. Wang et al.; M. Shibuya et al.; both in prep.) The product of the *ros* gene, $P68^{gag-ros}$, is phosphorylated in vivo both at serine and tyrosine residues. Immunoprecipitates of $P68^{gag-ros}$ are associated with a cyclic nucleotide-independent kinase activity which preferentially phosphorylates $P68^{gag-ros}$ itself but also phosphorylates rabbit IgG in the immune complexes and α-casein, an added, soluble protein substrate. The phosphorylation is specific for tyrosine residues in the substrate proteins. UR-2 P68$^{gag-ros}$, like P140$^{gag-fps}$ and P90$^{gag-yes}$, has a marked preference for Mn^{++} over Mg^{++} ions. However, P68$^{gag-ros}$ differs from P90$^{gag-yes}$ in that it cannot use GTP as a phosphate donor and differs from P140$^{gag-fps}$ in the pH dependence of the reaction. Thus, the product of *ros* may be another tyrosine-specific protein kinase with unique enzymatic properties (T. Feldman et al., pers. comm.).

Stavnezer et al. (1981) have characterized three replication-defective viruses (SK770, SK780, and SK790) derived after passage of *td* B77-RSV in tissue culture; these agents transform only fibroblasts, synthesize polyproteins of 110,000–125,000 daltons with *gag* or *gag-pol* determinants, and lack homology with the transforming genes of other avian viruses. With the SK viruses, however, protein kinase activity has yet to be observed in the conventional immune-complex assay, and the level of phosphotyrosine is unaltered in transformed cells (E. Stavnezer, pers comm.).

C. *myc, erb, and myb:* Oncogenes of Defective Avian Leukemia Viruses

1. Patterns and Themes

Viral leukemia was first recognized at the turn of this century, when Ellerman and Bang (1908) attributed an erythroleukemia in chickens to a transmissible agent. Their discovery was soon eclipsed by the work of Rous on chicken sarcoma virus, and decades passed before the possibility of leukemogenesis by viruses came under close scrutiny. We now realize that retroviruses cause leukemias in mammals and fowl, we have learned that there are viral genes whose unassisted action may be leukemogenic, and we are even willing to entertain the possibility that some forms of human leukemia are caused by viruses. Leukemia viruses may be our best hope to achieve an understanding of the mechanisms by which hematopoietic cells become malignant.

The most diverse set of leukemogenic retroviruses presently available were isolated from tumors of chickens. These viruses all require a helper virus to assist their replication and are therefore known as defective leukemia viruses (DLVs). However, the term is something of a misnomer; many of the viruses can cause neoplastic disease other than leukemia, and in some instances, the hematological disease may be a solid tumor rather than leukemia. It is nevertheless as leukemogenic agents that these viruses first came into view. It is their ability to transform hematopoietic cells in culture that most effectively unites the viruses into a taxonomic group, and it is their effects on hematopoietic cells that may have the most far-ranging implications.

Each DLV generally transforms cells in culture that are representative of the tissues affected by tumorigenesis in the same host species. The correlations are not entirely perfect; e.g., E26 virus transforms myeloid cells in culture and may also induce phenotypic changes in fibroblasts, yet the virus usually causes erythroblastosis in chickens and has not been reported to induce sarcomas (Graf and Beug 1978; Graf et al. 1979; Moscovici et al. 1981; and Sotirov 1981). (Similarly, to anticipate subsequent discussion [see Section II.D.1], the transformation of NIH-3T3 fibroblasts by the Abelson murine leukemia virus [Ab-MLV] appears to be an experimental peculiarity that is not manifest in the tumorigenicity of the virus.) Many of the DLVs display pluripotent oncogenicity and accordingly transform more than one type of cell in culture, whereas the tumorigenicity and transforming potential of other DLVs are limited to a single type of cell. The pathogenicities of DLVs are sufficiently characteristic of individual viruses to have permitted the formation of taxonomic subdivisions; these classifications are consonant with biochemical analyses of *v-onc* genes (see below).

The *v-onc* sequences of DLVs were first recognized as nucleotide sequences that replace portions of viral replicative genes (see Chapter 4). The role of these sequences in oncogenesis has not been easy to prove. In particular, the application of genetic strategies has been thwarted by several large difficulties, including the requirement for complementation merely to replicate the viruses, the failure of suitable mutants to arise in response to a variety of mutagenic manipulations, and the relatively demanding nature of the bioassays for the leukemogenic potential of these viruses. A few exceptions exist (see Chapter 7). Valuable conditional and nonconditional mutations have been identified in *v-erb* (Graf et al. 1978; Beug et al. 1980), deletions that affect *v-myc* have been described (Ramsay et al. 1980), and a single temperature-sensitive mutation in *v-myb* has recently been isolated (C. Moscovici et al., pers. comm.). Otherwise, it is by two circumstantial arguments that the *v-onc* genes of DLVs have been identified. First, each of the presumed *v-onc* genes is associated with a characteristic pattern of pathogenicity. For example, the nucleotide sequence of *v-myc* is different from the sequences of *v-src, v-erb,* or *v-myb* present in viruses with different pathogenic potential (Roussel et al. 1979; Bister and Duesberg 1980) (Chapter 8). Moreover, if independent isolates of DLVs bear the same *v-onc* (e.g., MC29, MH2, CMII, and OK10), they display the same set of pathogenicities (Rousell et al. 1979; Bister and Duesberg 1980; Sheiness et al. 1980a). Second, each of the alleged *v-onc* genes is distinguished from the remainder of the viral genome by homology with conserved nucleotide sequences in vertebrate DNA presumed to be *c-onc* genes (Roussel et al. 1979; Sheiness and Bishop 1979) (see Section III). These rather frail arguments have served remarkably well, but they should soon be eclipsed by the manipulation of cloned viral DNAs to generate site-specific mutations in *v-onc* genes.

The *v-onc* genes of DLVs are constructed and expressed in at least three distinct ways: (1) as fusions between the *onc* domain and a portion of *gag*, so that a single protein is produced from a genomic-length mRNA (e.g., MC29); (2) as an independently expressed gene, with protein produced from a subgenomic mRNA in the manner of *v-src* (e.g., avian myeloblastosis virus [AMV]); and (3) as two separately expressed domains, one fused with a portion of *gag* and the other expressed independently. In the last instance, the *gag-onc* protein is produced from a genomic-length mRNA and the second *onc* protein is produced from a subgenomic mRNA (e.g., avian erythroblastosis virus [AEV]). In a further variation on these themes, the same class of *v-onc* can be expressed as a polyprotein with *gag* in some virus isolates and as a separate *onc* protein in others. Examples include *v-myc* in MC29 (polyprotein produced from a genomic mRNA) or OK10 (unidentified *onc* protein produced from a subgenomic mRNA) and *v-myb* in either AMV (separate *onc* protein, subgenomic mRNA) or E26 (polyprotein, genomic-length mRNA).

Identification and characterization of *v-onc* products for DLVs have been halting exercises to date. Efforts to raise tumor antisera similar to those that proved so valuable in the study of *src* have generally failed and, where successful, have yielded antisera that proved to be less useful than those raised against $pp60^{v\text{-}src}$. Polyproteins that include a portion of *gag* can be recovered by immunoprecipitation with antibodies to viral structural proteins. This approach has been the mainstay of most efforts to study the transforming proteins of DLVs, but it naturally fails when *v-onc* is expressed partly or entirely as a separate genetic domain unlinked to a viral replicative gene. Translation of viral RNA in vitro has been used to substantiate the origins of polyproteins and to obtain first glimpses of transforming proteins for which no antisera are available. Few of these exercises have employed authentic mRNA, and they are therefore at risk of the pitfalls outlined above in the description of *src* (Section II.A.1). Two new technical strategies may soon provide antigens to raise the all important antisera. The molecular cloning of *v-onc* genes should facilitate production of large quantities of the protein products in bacterial or other hosts. Alternatively, knowledge of the nucleotide sequence of *v-onc* genes permits the synthesis of peptides that represent small domains within the *v-onc* products, and these peptides can be rendered antigenic by coupling to suitable carrier proteins (Walter et al. 1980; Lerner et al. 1981).

How do the transforming proteins of DLVs act? We know very little of their possible functions, partly because none of the proteins have been purified to date and partly because some of the proteins have yet to be recovered in their native state from transformed cells. The polyprotein products studied to date are generally phosphorylated in both the *gag* and *onc* domains, but phosphotyrosine has not been found, the proteins have as yet no demonstrable kinase activity, and there is no measurable change in the amount of phosphotyrosine in cells transformed by DLVs.

It is presently popular to view leukemogenesis as the consequence of a block to differentiation in one or another hematopoietic lineage (Greaves and Janossy 1978). For example, recent work has engendered the hypothesis that *v-erb* arrests erythropoiesis in a specific compartment of the erythroid developmental pathway and that the arrest suffices to explain leukemogenesis (Graf et al. 1978). According to this view, the immature cells that constitute the compartment continue to divide, as is their nature, and become a continuously expanding population, a tumor composed of ostensibly normal cells. This proposal has never seemed entirely sound. We have no rigorous definition of the compartment in which the *erb*-transformed erythroid cells are allegedly arrested, and the tumor cells elicited by *v-erb* display an autonomy and longevity of growth in culture that cannot be achieved with untransformed erythroid cells (Graf et al. 1978; Beug et al. 1979). The scheme has now come under more direct criticism. Either early stem cells or terminally differentiated cells in the myelomonocytic lineage (macrophages) can be transformed by *v-myb* (Boettiger and Durban 1980; Durban and Boettiger 1981a,b). In either case, the transformed cells display phenotypic properties that are characteristic of multiple compartments within the lineage: in some properties, the cells are more mature than the stem cell and in most properties, they are less mature than the terminally differentiated cell (Durban and Boettiger 1981a,b). According to these findings, the phenotype of the transformed cell is chaotic and does not indicate a simple block in differentiation.

2. myc

a. Identification of v-myc. Viruses carrying *v-myc* are exemplified by MC29, first isolated from a rare tumor composed of relatively mature myeloid cells (myelocytomatosis). Three other related, but independent, isolates have since been added to the roster: MH2, CMII, and OK10 (Graf and Beug 1978). Interest in these viruses quickened with the appreciation that they characteristically induce carcinomas, a common malignancy for which tumor virology had not previously provided an experimental model more malleable than the mouse mammary tumor virus (Chapter 8). We now know that the oncogene of MC29 (*v-myc*) is a versatile and highly virulent tumorigenic agent, capable of inducing carcinomas and sarcomas with great speed and reliability (Moscovici et al. 1978); ironically, the hematological tumor occurs only rarely unless the virus is administered in the egg (C. Moscovici, pers. comm.). The effects of *v-myc* on cells in culture are similarly broad and predictable from the pathogenicities observed in birds: fibroblasts, cells of myeloid lineage, and epithelial cells can all be transformed (Graf and Beug 1978).

Efforts to identify *v-myc* exploited the distinctive pathogenicity of MC29 virus and its kin. Parallel studies employing oligonucleotide mapping (Bister et al. 1979; Bister and Duesberg 1979a) and molecular hybridization (Roussel et al. 1979; Sheiness et al. 1980) demonstrated that these viruses shared not only portions of retroviral replicative genes, but also a nucleotide sequence of about 1.5 kb not found in any other retrovirus examined. Moreover, closely related nucleotide sequences were found in both the DNA and RNA of fowl and mammals (Roussel et al. 1979; Sheiness and Bishop 1979), in contradistinction to the viral replicative genes and in close analogy with *src* (Stehelin et al. 1976b; Spector et al. 1978a) (see Section III). Thus, *v-myc* was brought into view—the first DLV oncogene to be identified by any criterion and the eventual prototype for all oncogenes constructed by fusing *onc* to a portion of a replicative gene.

b. Polyproteins of MC29, MH2, and CMII. The exploration of viral proteins in cells transformed by MC29 uncovered a protein ($P110^{gag\text{-}myc}$) unlike any previously identified retroviral gene product (Bister et al. 1977). The protein contained antigenic determinants of *gag* and hence could be immunoprecipitated by antibodies to the structural proteins of the virus. But neither *pol* nor *env* determinants were represented, despite the size of the protein. By reference to the emerging physical map of the MC29 genome, it was deduced that $P110^{gag\text{-}myc}$ represented a fusion between *gag* and *v-myc*. Exhaustive analyses of tryptic peptides in $P110^{gag\text{-}myc}$ confirmed this formulation and defined the *gag* constituents with considerable precision (p19, p10, and a portion of p27) (Rettenmeier et al. 1979; Kitchener and Hayman 1980).

The precedent of $P110^{gag\text{-}myc}$ led easily to identification of similar proteins for MH2 ($P100^{gag\text{-}myc}$) (Hu et al. 1978) and CMII ($P90^{gag\text{-}myc}$) (Hayman et al. 1979a). Peptide analysis revealed that the proteins differed mainly in the fraction of *gag* constituting the amino-terminal domains (see Fig. 9.4). Moreover, the *myc* portions of $P110^{gag\text{-}myc}$, $P100^{gag\text{-}myc}$, and $P90^{gag\text{-}myc}$ were closely related and could be reckoned to constitute about 60,000 daltons of each of the proteins. The commonality of this domain among the three proteins added further weight to the conclusion that *v-myc* is essential to the oncogenic potential of the viruses (Kitchener and Hayman 1980).

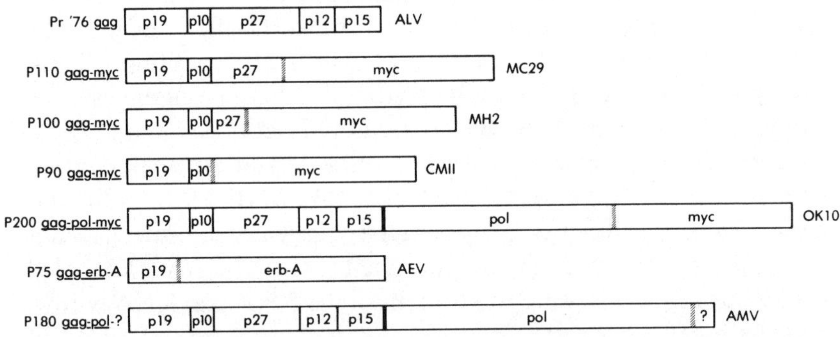

Figure 9.4 The polyproteins of defective avian leukemia viruses. The illustration should be taken as an approximation only. Many of the proteins have not been analyzed in detail. Diagonal shading indicates uncertainty in the position of fusion between *gag* and *onc*.

c. gag-myc *Polyproteins Are the Sole Gene Products of MC29, MH2, and CMII.* The broad-ranging pathogenicity of *v-myc* raised the possibility that the oncogene might encode more than one protein. All available evidence speaks against this possiblity for MC29, MH2, and CMH viruses: (1) In each instance, the polyprotein is large enough to account for the entirety of *gag* and *v-myc* found in the viral genome. (2) All of the *v-myc*-specific mRNA in cells transformed by these viruses is the same length as the viral genome (Sheiness et al. 1981; D. Stehelin, pers. comm.), from which the polyproteins can be translated in vitro (Mellon et al. 1978). (3) Antisera that react with the *v-myc* portion of MC29 $P110^{gag-myc}$ have not uncovered a second gene product in cells transformed by MC29 (H. Oppermann, pers. comm.). It therefore appears that oncogenesis by MC29 and its kindred viruses can be attributed entirely to the *gag-myc* polyproteins. Moreover, there is no evidence that these proteins are metabolized into smaller products in the infected cell (Bister et al. 1977). All of the oncogenic potentials of *v-myc* may therefore be effected by a single, pleiotropic protein.

The singular nature of the MC29 *v-myc* product was not always so clear. In vitro translation of RNA obtained from virions of MC29 produced not only $P110^{gag-myc}$, but also an abundance of two smaller proteins with molecular weights of approximately 56,000 and 37,000 daltons (Mellon et al. 1978). Until the strategy of MC29 *v-myc* expression became clear from analyses of the viral mRNA, it seemed possible that one or both of these smaller proteins were also products of *v-myc*. Instead, they are almost certainly telling examples of the prospects for artifact when fragments of retroviral RNA are translated in vitro (see Section II.A.1).

d. gag-myc *Polyproteins Are Phosphoproteins without Demonstrable Kinase Activity.* The polyprotein products representing *v-myc* are phosphorylated on serine at the usual sites of phosphorylation within *gag* proteins and on both serine and threonine within the *myc* region (H. Oppermann et al., pers. comm.). The domains of phosphorylation have been dissected by using the specific proteolytic activity of $p15^{gag}$ to cleave the polyproteins at positions where Pr76 is normally divided into the mature *gag* products (Vogt et al. 1979; A. D. Levinson and M. Hayman, pers. comm.). This procedure generates several of the expected *gag* products, and a 60,000-dalton fragment representing *v-myc* (and the small residue of p27 that remains in $P110^{gag-myc}$). The 60,000-dalton fragment is heavily phosphorylated (A. D.Levinson, pers. comm.), but the precise sites of modifications have yet to be explored.

None of the *gag-myc* proteins have been purified in their native forms. Descriptions of their possible enzymic activities therefore rest on the unsatisfactory procedure of testing immunoprecipitates that contain the protein. Kinase activities are detectable in these immunoprecipitates but are easily washed away and are unlikely to be intrinsic properties of the viral polyproteins (Bister et al. 1980a). As noted above, attempts to implicate phosphorylation of tyrosine in transformation by *v-myc* have failed. The polyprotein products contain no phosphotyrosine, and transformation by *v-myc* has no effect on the amounts of phosphotyrosine in the affected cells (Sefton et al. 1980c).

Although the mechanism by which $P110^{gag-myc}$ transforms cells is unknown, a clue may be provided by recent effects to define its intracellular location. Standard cellular fractionation procedures and immunofluorescence tests have both revealed $P110^{gag-myc}$ to be predominantly in the nucleus of MC29-transformed quail cells (H. Abrams et al., in prep.).

e. Genetic Evidence That $P110^{\mathrm{gag-myc}}$ *of MC29 Is Involved in Transformation.* A protracted search has turned up several spontaneous deletion mutants of MC29 whose properties sustain the conclusion that *v-myc* and its polyprotein product are required for neoplastic transformation (Ramsay et al. 1980). Peptide mapping and oligonucleotide mapping demonstrated that the deletions affect a region of *myc* within the polyprotein. The mutants have suffered severe reductions in their capacity to transform macrophages, whereas their ability to transform fibroblasts is undiminished, compared with that of wild-type virus. These findings further implicate *v-myc* in oncogenesis and raise the possibility that the functions that transform cells of different types may be distributed among different domains of $P110^{gag-myc}$.

f. v-myc *of OK10 May Be Expressed as a Separate Genetic Domain.* As investigators pursued the apparent similarities among the various viruses bearing *v-myc*, the curious case of OK10 virus emerged. In striking contrast to MC29, the genome of OK10 contains the entirety of *gag*, most or all of *pol*, and *v-myc* inserted in place of portions of *pol* and *env* (Bister et al. 1980b). Cells transformed by OK10 (and containing no helper-virus genome) produce noninfectious viral particles, contain Pr76^{gag} (processing the protein to mature *gag* products), and produce P200 (a protein with antigenic determinants and tryptic peptides of *gag* and *pol*) (Ramsay and Hayman 1980). It was therefore originally deduced that P200 might be the transforming protein, generated by the uninterrupted translation from an intact *gag*, a nearly intact *pol*, and *v-myc*. Examination of the mRNAs for OK10 has revised the possibilities appreciably, because the virus generates a spliced subgenomic mRNA that represents the portion of the genome bearing *v-myc* (Chiswell et al. 1981). Although the product of the subgenomic mRNA has yet to be identified, it appears likely that the *v-myc* of OK10 is expressed independently of the replicative genes and that the role of P200 in transformation has become moot. These will be useful findings, if correct, because independent expression of *v-myc* would remove *gag* as a necessary constituent of the *myc* transforming protein and would help define the functional limits of both the viral oncogene and its cellular homolog, *c-myc*.

3. erb

a. Defining the Oncogene of AEV. The genetic locus of neoplastic transformation by AEV is the best defined of all the DLV oncogenes. We have this exceptional definition by virtue of parallel genetical and biochemical attacks. First, the molecular strategies developed to achieve a provisional physical definition of *v-myc* were applied to the search for *v-erb* with an analogous outcome. A 3.0-kb region of the AEV genome was identified that proved to be unrelated to replicative genes (Bister and Duesberg 1979a; Lai et al. 1979), absent from retroviral genomes with transforming potentials different from those of AEV (Bister and Duesberg 1979; Roussel et al. 1979), and related to the conserved and expressed vertebrate nucleotide sequences denoted *c-erb* (Roussel et al. 1979; Saule et al. 1981; B. Vennstrom, pers. comm.). Second, a diligent search turned up conditional and nonconditional mutations that affected the transforming capacity of AEV. The conditional mutants elicit temperature-sensitive transformation of both erythroid cells and fibroblasts, although the effect of the mutations appears to be only partially penetrant in fibroblasts (Graf et al. 1978; Beug and Graf 1980). These findings provide rigorous evidence that AEV possesses a genetic locus directly responsible for neoplastic transformation and make it likely that the locus encodes one or more proteins. The nonconditional mutant (there is only one report to date) fails to transform erythroid cells, transforms fibroblasts in the manner of wild-type virus, and apparently bears a deletion in *v-erb*, too small to affect the measured length of the viral genome but perceptible by peptide mapping of a protein encoded in *v-erb* (Royer-Pokora et al. 1979; Beug et al. 1980).

b. Two Domains of v-erb. Neither the conditional nor the nonconditional mutants just described affect the transformation of erythroid cells and fibroblasts in an entirely coordinate manner. These findings raised the possibility that *v-erb* might be divided into two domains of expression and/or function. Pursuit of the *v-erb* products, mapping of the viral genome, and examination of viral mRNAs combined to realize this possibility: (1) The first *v-erb* product identified was P75$^{gag\text{-}erb\text{-}A}$, a polyprotein containing elements of both *gag* and *erb* (see below). Attempts to map this protein to the viral genome immediately indicated that as much as half of the *v-erb* locus might not be represented in the protein (Lai et al. 1979). (2) Cells transformed by AEV contain two mRNAs carrying at least portions of *v-erb*. One mRNA is the length of the viral genome and contains the entirety of *v-erb*; the other is a spliced subgenomic mRNA representing the 3′ two-thirds of *v-erb* (Anderson et al. 1980; Sheiness et al. 1981). (3) In vitro translation established that the genomic-length RNA of AEV gives rise to P75$^{gag\text{-}erb\text{-}A}$ (Anderson et al. 1980; Lai et al. 1980; Pawson and Martin 1980; Yoshida and Toyoshima 1980). The presumption that the subgenomic mRNA produces a second *erb* protein has been subjected to provisionally successful but nonrigorous tests (see below).

Together, these findings engendered the formal definition of two domains within *erb*, v-*erb*-A and v-*erb*-B (Coffin et al. 1981). Further quests for products of *v-erb* have proceeded on the assumption that at least two proteins are involved in tumorigenesis by AEV.

c. Polyprotein Product of v-erb-*A*. Antibodies to viral structural proteins react with a single product of the AEV genome, P75$^{gag\text{-}erb\text{-}A}$ (Hayman et al. 1979b). The same protein can be precipitated by antisera obtained from chickens during their spontaneous recovery from transient erythroleukemia induced by AEV (Beug et al. 1981). These antisera react with both *gag* determinants and determinants within the *v-erb*-A domain of the protein, but their use has added disappointingly little to our knowledge of the AEV gene products. P75$^{gag\text{-}erb\text{-}A}$ is encoded by a portion of *gag* and the 5′ domain of *v-erb* now known as *v-erb*-A (Hayman et al. 1979b; Rettenmeier et al. 1979; M. Privalsky, pers. comm.). Peptide mapping has defined the *gag* constituents of the protein (p19 and perhaps a portion of p10) and has identified a domain of the protein that is apparently unique to *v-erb*-A (Eisenman et al. 1979; Hayman et al. 1979b; Rettenmeier et al. 1979). The protein is phosphorylated, but phosphoamino acids and their distribution within the protein have not been satisfactorily explored.

d. Search for a Product of v-erb-*B.* Alert to the likelihood that *v-erb* is composed of two separately expressed domains and hampered by the lack of suitable tumor antisera, investigators turned to in vitro translation hoping to identify a second product of *v-erb*. Repeated efforts using RNA from virions of AEV produced two proteins: $P75^{gag\text{-}erb\text{-}A}$, translated from genomic-length RNA, and a smaller protein (~44,000 m.w.), translated from RNA representing the 3′ half of the viral genome (Anderson et al. 1980; Lai et al. 1980; Pawson and Martin 1980; Yoshida and Toyoshima 1980). It was at first assumed that fragments of the genome were serving as messenger for the smaller protein (known provisionally as $p44^{erb\text{-}B}$), but we now know that virions of AEV contain perceptible and sometimes substantial amounts of the spliced subgenomic mRNA (B. Vennstrom and M. Privalsky, pers. comm.), and we presume that this RNA generates $p44^{erb\text{-}B}$ during translations in vitro.

The evidence that $p44^{erb\text{-}B}$ is an authentic product of the AEV genome is far from complete. On the one hand, hybrid-arrested translation has mapped the coding regions for the protein with considerable precision to the domain of *erb*-B, substantiating the genetic origins of the protein (M. Privalsky, pers. comm.). On the other hand, spliced mRNA free of genomic fragments has yet to be used to produce $p44^{erb\text{-}B}$; the chicken tumor antisera to *v-erb* do not react with the protein (Beug et al. 1981); and we have no evidence that $p44^{erb\text{-}B}$ is either present in infected cells or involved in oncogenesis by AEV.

e. What Is the Mechanism of Transformation by v-erb*?* Our division of *v-erb* into two domains seems well founded. Moreover, the separation between the domains is complete: mapping of $P75^{gag\text{-}erb\text{-}A}$ and $p44^{erb\text{-}B}$ onto the genome by hybrid-arrested translation established that the coding regions of the two domains do not overlap (M. Privalsky, pers. comm.). Is one of these domains responsible for transformation of erythroid cells and the other, for transformation of fibroblasts? Or do the two domains work in concert to transform both types of cells? The fragmentary evidence available to us provides conflicting answers to the question: (1) Temperature-sensitive mutations in *v-erb* affect the transformation of both erythroid cells and fibroblasts, although the latter effect is only partially penetrant (Graf et al. 1978; Beug and Graf 1980). The mutations have not been mapped within *erb*, but it seems unlikely that both domains have incurred conditional lesions in each of the several mutants now in hand. Hence, we are led to the inference that at least one of the two domains is required for both types of transformation by *v-erb*. (2) The deletion mutant that shortens $P75^{gag\text{-}erb\text{-}A}$ cannot transform erythroid cells but transforms fibroblasts just as easily as does wild-type virus (Royer-Pokora et al. 1979). The superficial conclusion would be that $P75^{gag\text{-}erb\text{-}A}$ is not required for transformation of fibroblasts by AEV. But perhaps an unaffected and still active domain in the mutant protein participates in transformation of fibroblasts.

We know nothing of the mechanisms by which *v-erb* transforms cells. Phosphorylation of tyrosine has not been persuasively implicated in either erythroid or fibroblastic transformation (although increases of 1.5-fold have been reported for total phosphotryosine and for phosphotyrosine in pp36 [see Radke and Martin 1979; Sefton et al. 1980c]). Moreover, no kinase activity has been detected (although there is at present no means by which to test $p44^{erb\text{-}B}$ for any enzymic activity). Neither of the *erb* products has been tracked to a specific subcellular location.

4. myb

Two independent isolates of retroviruses contain *v-myb*: AMV and E26 virus (Graf and Beug 1978; Graf et al. 1979; Roussel et al. 1979). The two isolates are distinguished by unexpected differences in pathogenicity and transforming abilities. AMV causes myeloid leukemia, described variously as myeloblastosis or monocytic leukemia (Moscovici 1975; Graf and Beug 1978; Durban and Boettiger 1981a), whereas E26 causes erythroblastosis or, less frequently, a mixed leukemia of erythroid and myeloid cells (Graf and Beug 1978; Moscovici et al. 1981; Sotirov 1981). Both AMV and E26 transform macrophages in culture; E26, but not AMV, exerts effects on quail fibroblasts that mimic, in part, the transformed phenotype; and neither virus has been reported to transform erythroid cells

(Graf et al. 1979; C. Moscovici, pers. comm.). These contrasting findings herald and perhaps reflect the fact that the genomes of AMV and E26 are topographically different.

AMV came under biochemical scrutiny only lately, and it was assumed that the virus would prove to have an *onc* element fused to a replicative gene, as is the usual style for DLVs. The assumption proved incorrect. AMV possesses an intact and functioning *gag* gene, most (if not all) of *pol*, and *v-myb* (in place of *env*) (Duesberg et al. 1980; Chen et al. 1981; Gonda et al. 1981). As a consequence of this genomic structure, cells infected with AMV (but not with a helper virus) produce noninfectious particles, $Pr76^{gag}$ that may be processed into mature *gag* proteins, and a protein that is virtually indistinguishable from $Pr180^{gag\text{-}pol}$ but fails to generate enzymically active reverse transcriptase (Duesberg et al. 1980; Silva and Baluda 1980; H. Oppermann, pers. comm.). The expression of *v-myb* is relegated entirely to a spliced subgenomic mRNA whose protein product awaits identification (Chen et al. 1981; Gonda et al. 1981). The use of tumor antisera has proved unproductive to date, and efforts to translate *v-myb* in vitro have produced only tenuous candidates for the transforming protein.

E26 possesses *v-myb* that appears to be closely related to the analogous locus in the AMV genome (Roussel et al. 1979). But in contradistinction to AMV, the *v-myb* of E26 is fused with a portion of *gag*, and the hybrid gene is probably expressed from a genomic-length mRNA. The polyprotein product of the E26 *gag-myb* unit ($P130^{gag\text{-}myb}$) has not been studied in any detail, and we cannot explain the differences between the transforming potentials of AMV and E26.

D. *abl*: Oncogene of Abelson Murine Leukemia Virus

1. Oncogenesis and Transformation by v-abl

The discovery of Ab-MLV and the pursuit of its oncogenic mechanisms led to a fruitful marriage between tumor virology and immunology (Baltimore et al. 1979; Rosenberg and Baltimore 1980). The oncogene (*v-abl*) of the virus can be used to establish continuous lines of lymphoid tumor cells whose phenotype may represent an early stage in the development of immunoglobulin-producing B lymphocytes. Analysis of these cell lines has uncovered new aspects of immunocyte maturation and amended our knowledge of how antibody diversity is generated.

Infection of mice with Ab-MLV induces lymphosarcomas whose cellular origins have been difficult to discern (Baltimore et al. 1979). A clearer picture emerged, however, from studies with cell cultures. Adult bone marrow and fetal liver of mice contain cells that can be transformed by *v-abl* to continuous growth and tumorigenicity (Rosenberg et al. 1975; Rosenberg and Baltimore 1976; Baltimore et al. 1979) (Chapter 8). The identity of the cells that undergo transformation is unknown, but the phenotype of the cells subsequent to transformation has been examined in great detail, and it is generally assumed that the transformed cells are not too far removed from their normal progenitors. This is an important assumption, because the transformed cells appear to represent a heretofore unrecognized stage in the development of B cells (Baltimore et al. 1979). It is assumed that the phenotype of the cells was frozen in place by the action of *v-abl*; alternatively, however, transformation might induce anomalous immunological properties that bear no relationship to the pathway of normal B-cell development.

The tumorigenicity of *v-abl* is restricted to hematopoietic cells (Rosenberg and Baltimore 1980). In cell culture, however, *v-abl* can transform certain established lines of murine fibroblasts (NIH-3T3 mouse cells are most commonly used) (Scher and Siegler 1975). Although transformation of fibroblasts by *v-abl* is limited to artificial settings, it has nevertheless been a valuable adjunct to the experimental analysis of Ab-MLV. Clones of the virus can be readily isolated, and the transforming genome can be segregated from the genome of the helper virus.

2. *Identifying the Product of* v-abl

The genome of Ab-MLV contains *v-abl* fused to a portion of the *gag* gene of MLV (Reynolds et al. 1978; Witte et al. 1978; Shields et al. 1979; Goff et al. 1981). Polyprotein produced from this hybrid genetic element has been identified by three means. First, antibodies to structural proteins of MLV can precipitate *gag-abl* polyprotein by reacting with its *gag* constituents (Reynolds et al. 1978; Witte et al. 1978). Second, antisera that react with the *v-abl* portion of a polyprotein have been obtained by immunizing C57L/Jb mice with Ab-MLV-transformed cells (Witte et al. 1979a). Successful immunization appeared to depend on the ability of the mice to reject the resulting tumors within a period of a few weeks. Production of the antisera was not an easy task because most strains of mice succumb to the tumors without raising detectable antibodies to the *v-abl* polypeptide; the utility of the C57L/J strain was recognized only after a lengthy search. Third, translation of the Ab-MLV genome in vitro produced the polyprotein, providing further evidence of its genetic origin (Shields et al. 1979).

3. gag-abl *Polyprotein Is the Sole Product of the Ab-MLV Genome*

Cells transformed by *v-abl* contain a genomic-length mRNA that is presumed to be the source of *gag-abl* polyprotein, and no other mRNA bearing any portion of *v-abl* has been identified (Baltimore et al. 1980). From these findings, it was concluded that the polyprotein is probably the sole product of the Ab-MLV genome. Other points of evidence support this conclusion: No gene other than the *gag-abl* unit has been identified in the Ab-MLV genome, and *gag-abl* polyproteins are the only proteins that can be detected by the use of the two types of antisera described above.

4. Composition and Biological Activities of gag-abl *Polyproteins*

The *gag-abl* product of the most widely used strain of Ab-MLV displayed a molecular weight of approximately 120,000 daltons ($P120^{gag\text{-}abl}$), but detailed study of several independent clones of Ab-MLV has uncovered an informative set of variants whose polyproteins range in size from 90,000 daltons to 160,000 daltons (Rosenberg and Witte 1980; Goff et al. 1981). All of these proteins contain the same portion of *gag* (p15, p12, and part of p30); only the *v-abl* constituent varies in size and composition. The variant proteins arise from genomes of three different lengths (Fig. 9.5): (1) $P160^{gag\text{-}abl}$ derives from the largest Ab-MLV genome identified to date (6.3 kb) and appears to terminate well before the 3′ boundary of *v-abl.* (2) Three variants of different sizes ($P90^{gag\text{-}abl}$, $P100^{gag\text{-}abl}$, and $P120^{gag\text{-}abl}$) are encoded by genomes whose lengths have each been reduced to about 5.5 kb by a deletion in *v-abl.* The differences among the proteins have been attributed to premature termination of translation induced by point mutations. (3) A fifth protein ($P92^{gag\text{-}abl}$) is produced from an even smaller genome (about 4.6 kb) which has suffered a second deletion, also within *v-abl.*

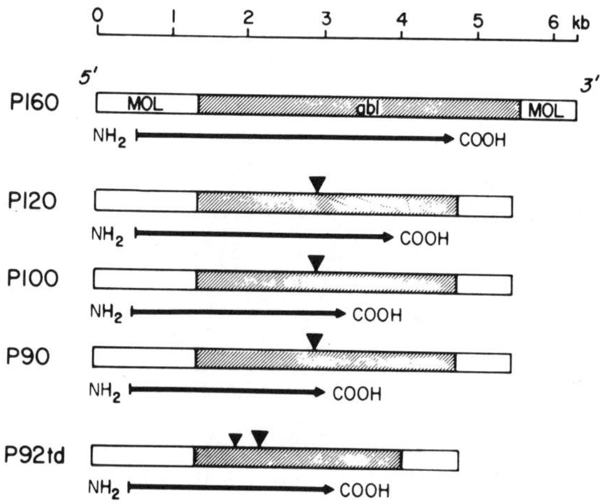

Figure 9.5 Structure of Abelson murine leukemia virus (Ab-MLV) genomes. (▧) M-MLV-specific regions (MOL); (■) the *abl* sequences for five different Ab-MLV strains; the dark line under each represented genome shows the region encoding the Ab-MLV polypeptide; (▽) the position, which is not known accurately, of the sequence missing in all strains except the the Ab-MLV; (▼) the position of the additional deletion found in the Ab-MLV(P92td) strain.

The utility of these variants derives from differences in their oncogenicity and transforming potential (Rosenberg and Baltimore 1980; Rosenberg and Witte 1980; Goff et al. 1981). The virus that produces $P92^{gag-abl}$ is completely defective in transformation. It fails to induce tumors in mice and cannot transform either fibroblasts or hematopoietic cells in culture. The deletion that reduced the genome of this virus from 5.5 kb to 4.6 kb probably removes a vital region of *v-abl.* The strains that produce $P90^{gag-abl}$ and $P100^{gag-abl}$ are poorly oncogenic, transform hematopoietic cells in culture at a very low efficiency, but are fully capable of transforming fibroblasts. Production of either $P120^{gag-abl}$ or $P160^{gag-abl}$ leads to oncogenesis and to transformation of both fibroblasts and hematopoietic cells. Hence, there is appreciable latitude in the portion of *v-abl* that must be expressed in order to achieve the properties of wild-type Ab-MLV.

5. gag-abl *Polyprotein Is an Integral Membrane Protein*

In other sections we describe the evidence that $pp60^{v-src}$ and $p21^{v-ras}$ are associated with the plasma membrane of the transformed cell (see Sections II.A.2 and II.F.4). A similar location for the *gag-abl* protein was deduced from the discovery that a portion of the *abl* polypeptide is exposed on the external surface of the cell (Witte et al. 1979a). Since the *gag* component of the polyprotein could not be detected in the same location, it was further inferred that the protein was probably inserted into the lipid bilayer of the membrane. The *gag* component has now been found to be anchored tightly to the cytoskeletal matrix of the cytoplasm (D. Baltimore, pers. comm.). These findings have led to the conclusion that the *gag-abl* protein spans the lipid bilayer of the plasma membrane; some portion of the carboxyterminal *abl* domain is exposed on the external surface of the membrane, whereas the aminoterminal *gag* domain protrudes into the cytoplasm. An extensive portion of *v-abl* may lie outside the confines of the membrane, since antigenic determinants of *v-abl* are detectable on the surfaces of cells containing either $P160^{gag-abl}$ or $P90^{gag-abl}$ (D. Baltimore, pers. comm.). As noted above, these proteins differ solely in the sizes of their *v-abl* domains. Despite its transmembrane disposition, the *gag-abl* polyprotein appears not to be glycosylated (Witte et al. 1979a).

6. gag-abl *Polyprotein May Be a Tyrosine Protein Kinase*

The *gag-abl* polyprotein recovered from infected cells was initially reported to contain phosphoserine, but no phosphotyrosine (Witte et al. 1980a). (A subsequent independent analysis has found phosphotyrosine in the *gag-abl* protein [Sefton et al. 1981a]). It was therefore surprising to learn that $P120^{gag-abl}$ can be phosphorylated exclusively on tyrosine in reactions carried out with either immunoprecipitates or soluble, partially purified *gag-abl* protein (Witte et al. 1980a). The phosphotransfer was tentatively attributed to the *v-abl* product, particularly because it can occur in *trans*. Protein that is itself inactive in phosphotransfer (such as heated $P120^{gag-abl}$ or the variant $P92^{gag-abl}$) is phosphorylated on tyrosine when mixed with active $P160^{gag-abl}$ (Witte et al. 1980a,b). The paucity of other demonstrable substrates for the *abl* enzyme is puzzling, and the attribution of kinase activity to the *gag-abl* protein remains provisional.

7. Is Tyrosine Phosphorylation Responsible for Neoplastic Transformation by v-abl*?*

The similarities between the apparent enzymic activities of $pp60^{v-src}$ and the *gag-abl* protein were strong enough to evoke the hypothesis that both proteins may transform cells by the same mechanism: phosphorylation of tyrosine in key cellular substrates. The argument that sustains this hypothesis for *v-abl* follows the precedents established with *v-src*: (1) A transformation-defective variant of Ab-MLV has been described (see above). The protein P92$^{gag-abl}$ encoded by this virus has no demonstrable kinase activity (Witte et al. 1980b). (2) Similarly, P90$^{gag-abl}$ and P100$^{gag-abl}$ possess attenuated transforming potentials (see above) and relatively feeble kinase activity (Rosenberg and Witte 1980; Rosenberg et al. 1980). (3) Both hematopoietic cells and fibroblasts transformed by *v-abl* contain more phosphotyrosine than do their normal counterparts (Sefton et al. 1981a). (4) Transformation of cells by *v-abl* augments the tyrosine phosphorylation of two of the suspected substrates for pp60^{v-src}, pp36 and vinculin (Cooper and Hunter 1981b; Sefton et al. 1981b; G.S. Martin, pers. comm.).

These are not conclusive points of evidence, by any means. In particular, the argument is crippled by the lack of conditional mutations in *v-abl* that might permit closer scrutiny of the relationship between the activity of the oncogene and tyrosine phosphorylation in infected cells, and parallel studies of potential substrates in vitro and in vivo have not progressed very far. Nevertheless, the actions of *v-src* and *v-abl* appear quite similar, and it therefore seems likely that tyrosine phosphorylation will prove to be central to the oncogenic mechanisms of Ab-MLV.

E. *mos*: Oncogene of Moloney and Gazdar Murine Sarcoma Viruses

1. Structural Definition of the Gene

The transformation-specific genetic sequence (*mos*) of Moloney murine sarcoma virus (Mo-MSV) and Gazdar murine sarcoma virus (Gz-MSV) has been defined genetically with mutants, as described in Chapter 7, and its physical location has been mapped approximately 1.0–2.2 kb from the 3′ terminus of the 5.8-kb genome of Mo-MSV clone 124 (isolated by Ball et al. [1973]) on the basis of comparisons between the Mo-MSV genome and that of its Mo-MLV helper virus (Hu et al. 1977) (see Chapter 4). Subgenomic Mo-MSV DNA fragments which include the *v-mos* region lead to transformation (Andersson et al. 1979; Canaani et al. 1979; Blair et al. 1980). Thus, the transforming virus-specific sequences have been directly shown to induce transformation. The Mo-MSV clone-124 genome has been shown, by comparison between nucleic acid and protein sequences, to contain the entire *gag* gene of Mo-MLV (Van Beveren et al. 1981a), despite several earlier reports that a deleted *gag* precursor protein was encoded by Mo-MSV. Unlike the majority of retroviral transforming genes, *mos* is not usually fused to one of the viral structural genes. Therefore, immunoprecipitation from Mo-MSV-transformed cells with antibodies to viral structural proteins has not resulted in immunoprecipitation of the *mos*-gene product (Wood et al. 1980). However, there is at least one possible exception to the general rule that the *mos* gene of Mo-MSV is not expressed as a *gag-mos* fusion protein. Cells infected with *ts*110, a mutant of Mo-MSV clone 349 temperature-sensitive for the maintenance of transformation (Blair et al. 1979) (Chapter 7), produce p58^{gag} and a fusion protein P85, which contains both *gag* and putative *mos* sequences (Horn et al. 1981). P85$^{gag-mos}$ is synthesized predominantly at the permissive temperature for transformation, whereas P58^{gag} is synthesized at both temperatures. This mutant packages two MSV RNA species of 5.0 kb and 5.9 kb, in contrast to the 6.8-kb virion RNA of the wild-type parent. Thus, it appears that either deletion or removal through RNA processing of the sequences between the *gag* and *mos* genes has allowed expression of a fusion protein in cells infected by this mutant. However, it is not clear whether expression of P85 is sufficient or necessary for transformation. Expression of any unfused *mos* products, possibly encoded by one of the RNA species present in virions, would not have been observed.

2. Nucleotide Sequence of mos

Recently, two different groups have reported nucleotide sequences for the entire *v-mos* gene (Appendix C). Both sequences have open reading frames large enough to code for a protein of approximately 40,000 daltons, consisting of either 374 amino acids (Van Beveren et al. 1981b) or 408 amino acids (Reddy et al. 1980). Both predicted *mos*-gene products are initiated at an AUG in the region of MSV derived from the MLV *env* gene, 14–16 nucleotides upstream from the junction between MLV and *mos* sequences. The sequence data of Van Beveren et al. (1981a,b) predict that the *mos* product terminates within the *mos* sequence, whereas those of Reddy et al. (1980) predict that the carboxyterminal region of the protein is in a different reading frame and that the protein terminates after extending 58 nucleotides into MLV-derived sequences. Sequence data from both groups reveal two potential poly(A) addition signals downstream from the *mos* gene in the MSV genome.

3. Is the Predicted Product of mos *Related to Other* onc *Products?*

A surprising finding was made as a result of comparison of the amino acid sequence of the predicted 40K *mos*-gene product with that of RSV pp60^{src}. Significant homology was observed between the *mos* product and the carboxyterminal region of pp60^{src}, particularly in the region of pp60^{src} residues 387–468 (out of a total of 530) and *mos* amino acids 227–309 (out of 374) (Van Beveren et al. 1981b). This result suggests that *mos* and *src* are derived from a common ancestor, even though no homology is observed at the nucleic acid level. It is interesting to note that the region of homology lies in that half of pp60^{src} shown to be sufficient for protein kinase activity (Levinson et al. 1981) and that the homology brackets, but does not include, pp60^{src} amino acid 419, which is a tyrosine specifically phosphorylated in transformed cells (T. Hunter; H. Oppermann, both pers. comm.).

However, there is evidence to suggest that the *mos*-gene product does not function as a tyrosine-specific protein kinase in transformed cells in a manner similar to that of pp60^{src}. Analysis of phosphotyrosine levels in cellular proteins of Mo-MSV-transformed mouse cells shows no elevation above levels in the untransformed parent cells, whereas RSV-transformed cells, in contrast, show six- to tenfold elevations in similar assays (Sefton et al. 1980c). Similarly, transformation by Mo-MSV is not associated with phosphorylation of the 36K protein phosphorylated after transformation by several other retroviruses (Cooper and Hunter 1981b). A serine-specific protein kinase with a molecular weight of 15,000 is packaged in virions of Mo-MSV, but not in Mo-MLV helper virions. Furthermore, *ts*110, a Mo-MSV mutant temperature-sensitive for transformation, packages a protein kinase that is four times more thermolabile than that found in wild-type virions (Sen et al. 1979). However, there is no direct evidence that these kinase acitivities represent a virus-coded transforming protein.

4. Putative Products of mos *Synthesized In Vitro*

In vitro translation studies of Mo-MSV clone-124 virion RNA led to the observation of a class of MSV-specific products with overlapping sequences and approximate molecular weights of 37,000,

33,000, 24,000, and 18,000 (Papkoff et al. 1980). These products formed a nested set, with common carboxyl termini and different amino termini. However, all appeared to be translated from RNA containing *mos* sequences, deduced on the basis of sizing poly(A)-containing RNA fragments. The 37K class of proteins did not react immunologically or share methionine tryptic peptides with any of the Mo-MLV structural gene products. It appears that these products are the result of initiation in vitro at each of the methionine residues identified in the open reading frame of *v-mos*. In vitro translation products of Mo-MSV RNA with similar molecular weights were also reported by Philipson et al. (1978) and Lyons et al. (1980), and very similar in vitro translation products were observed using virion RNA from the independently isolated Gz-MSV (Gazdar et al. 1972; J. Papkoff, pers. comm.), despite its slightly different genomic organization from Mo-MSV clone 124 (Donoghue et al. 1979a). Hybridization of Mo-MSV virion RNA with *mos*-specific DNA fragments specifically inhibited in vitro synthesis of the 37K class of products (Cremer et al. 1981; J. Papkoff, pers. comm.). Similar products were synthesized in vitro from RNA isolated from cells transformed with Mo-MSV clone 124 by hybridization with *mos*-specific DNA, whereas the HT-1 and S^+L^- strains of Mo-MSV encoded slightly smaller *mos*-specific polypeptides (Cremer et al. 1981).

Rabbit antiserum has been raised recently against a synthetic peptide containing 11 amino acids from the C-terminus of the putative *mos* product according to the sequence of Van Beveren et al. (1981b) and using the method of Walter et al. (1980). This serum immunoprecipitates the 37K and related in vitro translation products of MSV 124 virion RNA (Papkoff et al. 1981). MSV 124-infected NIH-3T3 cells contain a specifically immunoprecipitable protein doublet with a molecular weight of approximately 37,000. Precipitation of this doublet was blocked by an excess of the C-terminal peptide. A slightly smaller protein was immunoprecipitated from cells infected with the HT-1 strain of MSV with this same antiserum (J. Papkoff and M. Lai, pers. comm.). Further characterization of these proteins will be necessary to ascertain whether they are the long-sought *mos* products.

5. *What Is the mRNA for* mos?

Several different subgenomic RNAs containing *mos* sequences have been detected in cells transformed by Mo-MSV, although in producer cells these RNAs are much less abundant than the genomic-length RNA species. Donoghue et al. (1979b) observed a 3.1-kb subgenomic RNA, which included a 0.4-kb sequence derived from the 5′ end of the MSV genome, in a clone of Mo-MSV 124-transformed cells. However, it has not been ruled out that such an RNA represents the genome of a deleted provirus, rather than a subgenomic mRNA of intact Mo-MSV 124. Two smaller RNAs with approximate lengths of 2.0 kb and 2.3 kb have also been observed by hybridization with *mos*-specific DNA probes (Dina and Nadel-Ginand 1980; J. Papkoff, pers. comm.). However, the data are contradictory concerning whether or not any of these RNAs are spliced to 5′ leader sequences. It is not clear which of these three RNAs are translated to *mos* products. Current data suggest that *mos* mRNA may be transcribed from a promoter independent of that for the genomic RNA, rather than arising as a spliced product of a genomic-sized precursor RNA.

F. *ras*: Oncogene of Harvey, Kirsten, and Rasheed Sarcoma Viruses

1. Classification of Viruses Containing ras

A number of transforming viruses of rodents, including the Harvey and Kirsten strains of murine sarcoma virus (Ha-MSV and Ki-MSV) and several apparently identical isolates of Rasheed rat sarcoma virus, are related by a viral oncogene termed *ras*. All of these viruses are replication-defective, transform cultured fibroblasts, and produce sarcomas in rodents; in addition, Ki-MSV and Ha-MSV can induce erythroleukemia in vivo and erythroid bursts in cultured marrow cells (Chapter 8) (D. Hankin and E. Scolnick, pers. comm.).

Discussion of *ras* is complicated because, unlike most other viral oncogenes, *ras* sequences in the various virus isolates are derived from a small family of cellular genes, rather than from a unique gene. Harvey-*ras* is derived from one of two closely related *c-ras* genes and is readily distinguished by molecular hybridization under conventional conditions from Kirsten-*ras*; the latter, in turn, appears to be derived from a third *c-ras* gene that is partially homologous to the predecessor of Harvey-*ras* (DeFeo et al. 1981; D.R. Lowy et al., pers. comm.) (see Section III.C). Rasheed-*ras* seems to be more closely related to Harvey-*ras* than to Kirsten-*ras* (H. Young et al., pers. comm.).

To complicate matters further, Ha-MSV and Ki-MSV were generated during propagation of MLVs in rats, and their genomes are composed of three parental components. The terminal sequences were provided by the MLV genomes; about 1 kb of *ras* sequences is located in the 5′ half of the RNA, and sequences from a replication-defective, endogenous virus-like (VL) genome of rats (rat VL30) flank both sides of *ras* (Ellis et al. 1980) (see Chapter 4). Thus, at least two independent recombinational events must have been required in the unique process that generated Ha-MSV and Ki-MSV. In contrast, a single event that joins sequences from an endogenous rat leukemia virus RNA to *c-ras* suffices to produce rat sarcoma virus, and this event can be recapitulated under certain conditions in cell culture (Rasheed et al. 1978; Young et al. 1981) (see Section III.C).

2. Identification of Small Phosphoproteins as the Products of ras *with Antisera to Nonstructural Proteins*

Persuasive evidence for the assignment of the transforming genes of Ki-MSV, Ha-MSV, and rat sarcoma virus to a single category has emerged from study of the protein products of their genomes. Like $pp60^{src}$, but unlike the products of many other *v-onc* genes, the products of Harvey-*ras* and Kirsten-*ras* are not fusion proteins containing immunological determinants of viral structural proteins, nor do the products appear to be found in appreciable amounts in viral particles. Therefore, convincing identification of *ras*-gene products required the development of antisera to these nonstructural proteins. Suitable sera were first obtained by T. Y. Shih et al. (1979a) following syngeneic transplantation of Ha-MSV-transformed rat (NRK) cells. Sera from rats bearing progressively expanding tumor masses precipitated a phosphoprotein of 21,000 daltons ($p21^{ras}$) from mouse and dog cells transformed by the same virus strain and from mink cells transformed by Ki-MSV. In subsequent studies, it was shown that these antisera also precipitated a protein of 29,000 daltons from cells transformed by rat sarcoma virus (Young et al. 1979) and proteins of approximately 21,000 daltons from a wide variety of uninfected vertebrate cells (Langbeheim et al. 1980) (see Section III.C).

A murine sarcoma virus isolated from BALB/c mice (BALB-MSV) carries a putative transforming sequence closely related to Harvey-*ras* (Andersen et al. 1981). Although termed *bas,* this sequence is similar if not identical to the Harvey-*ras* sequence present in the mouse genome.

Several kinds of evidence support the contention that p21^{ras} immunoprecipitated from extracts of Ha-MSV or Ki-MSV-transformed cells is the product of a viral transforming gene: (1) the cells employed in the initial studies were nonproducer cells from a number of animal species; hence, they did not contain the genomes of endogenous or coinfecting rodent leukemia viruses. (2) The antisera also precipitated a 21,000-dalton polypeptide whose synthesis was programmed in vitro by genomic RNA of Ha-MSV and Ki-MSV (Parks and Scolnick 1977; T. Y. Shih et al. 1979a). (3) Transfection studies with subgenomic fragments of cloned Ha-MSV DNA and with deletion and insertion mutants of cloned Ha-MSV DNA demonstrated that an intact region corresponding to about 1–2 kb near the 5′ end of viral RNA confers upon cells both the transformed phenotype and the ability to synthesize immunoprecipitable p21^{ras} (Chang et al. 1980; Wei et al. 1980; Goldfarb and Weinberg 1981a). (4) Little or no p21^{ras} is immunoprecipitable from extracts of cells infected with a temperature-sensitive transformation mutant of Ki-MSV (*ts*371) when the cells are propagated at the nonpermissive temperature (T. Y. Shih et al. 1979b).

3. Structure of the ras *Proteins*

Both immunological and biochemical criteria support the idea that the products of Harvey and Kirsten transforming genes are closely related and devoid of *gag* determinants (T. Y. Shih et al. 1979a; Langbeheim et al. 1980; Young et al. 1981). In contrast, the product of the transforming gene of rat sarcoma virus is immunoprecipitable by antisera to the p15^{gag} determinants in rat leukemia virus, as well as by antisera to products of Harvey-*ras* or Kirsten-*ras* (Young et al. 1979, 1981). The Rasheed-*ras* product, at 29,000 daltons, is significantly larger than the products of Harvey-*ras* and Kirsten-*ras* and appears to be synthesized from fused *gag* and *ras* genes. Since antisera to other *gag* proteins (p12, p10, and p30) are unable to precipitate P29$^{gag\text{-}ras}$, it is likely that only the aminoterminal peptides of *gag* are encoded in the fused gene. The *gag* peptides do not, however, appear to be required for the transforming function of the protein, since a spontaneous transformation-competent mutant rat sarcoma virus lacks most or all of the *gag* determinants (H. Young et al., pers. comm.).

Immunoprecipitated *ras* proteins from cells transformed by Ha-MSV and Ki-MSV migrate as a doublet in SDS-polyacrylamide gels, with an average apparent molecular weight of 21,000. The components of the two bands are closely related, as judged by mapping with proteases, but the protein with reduced mobility is heavily phosphorylated, primarily at threonine residues (T. Y. Shih et al. 1979a).

4. p21^{ras} *Is Located in the Plasma Membrane*

Fluorescent and ferritin-tagged antisera have been used to localize p21^{ras} to the inner surfaces of plasma membranes in dog, mink, rat, and mouse cells transformed by Ha-MSV (Willingham et al. 1980). The vast majority of the protein appears to be membrane-associated, but it is not exposed on the cell surface (as judged by the absence of surface fluorescence, using fixed cells); *ras* protein is not concentrated in close junctions or desmosomes, as observed by the same workers for pp60^{src} (Willingham et al. 1979). Thus, *ras* products, like those of *src* and *abl*, may act predominantly at the periphery of the cell.

5. Biosynthesis of ras *Proteins*

From the position of the *ras* gene near the 5′ terminus of viral RNA in all three isolates, it might be predicted that translation of P29$^{gag-ras}$ and p21^{ras} would occur from genomic RNA in infected cells as well as in vitro. To date, only a single species of genomic-size RNA has been identified in cells transformed by these viruses (Chien and Lai 1980; Goldfarb and Weinberg 1981b), confirming the suggestion that *ras* is not expressed via subgenomic mRNAs.

In recent pulse-chase labeling studies by T. Y. Shih et al. (pers. comm.), Harvey p21^{ras} was found in the cytosol within 15 minutes after addition of [^{35}S]methionine to transformed cells. After a 4-hour chase, the protein comigrated with the faster species of the p21 doublet in electrophoresis, and, after an 18-hour chase, it comigrated with the slower species, was heavily phosphorylated, and was found principally in the plasma membrane. These results suggest that *ras*, like *src*, is expressed on free polyribosomes and that subsequent steps (membrane association and phosphorylation) can be examined individually.

6. Functions of ras *Proteins: Binding of Guanine Nucleotides and a Possible Threonine Kinase Activity*

Two biochemical properties have been associated with the products of *ras*, efficient binding to guanine nucleotides (Scolnick et al. 1979) and an apparent autophosphorylation at threonine residues (Shih et al. 1980), but neither function has been clearly implicated in the mechanism by which p21^{ras} (or P29$^{gag\text{-}ras}$) transforms cells. The capacity of Harvey p21^{ras} to bind labeled guanine nucleotides (particularly GDP, GTP, and dGTP) has been used to monitor partial purification of the protein (Shih et al. 1980). A preparation enriched about 265-fold for p21^{ras} after chromatography on hydroxyapatite and phenyl-Sepharose demonstrates strong binding for only GTP, dGTP, and GDP (half-maximal binding at about 8×10^{-9} M); the only other nucleotide to exhibit significant binding (dATP) was bound at least three logs less efficiently. Comigration of the binding activity and immunoprecipitable p21^{ras} throughout the chromatographic procedures supports the claim that p21^{ras} itself is responsible for the binding. Furthermore, the binding activity is impaired when cells infected with the transformation mutant of Ki-MSV, *ts*371 are grown at the nonpermissive temperature (Scolnick et al. 1979), suggesting that the binding activity is encoded in *ras* and perhaps influential in determining the transformed phenotype. (A more complete description of the behavior of this interesting mutant is presented in Chapter 7.) However, the close association of p21^{ras} with a cellular protein capable of binding guanine nucleotides has not been rigorously excluded as an explanation for these phenomena.

The protein kinase activity associated with p21^{ras} appears to differ in virtually all properties from that associated with other *onc* products, such as pp60^{src}, or from that of common cellular kinases. The enzymic activity was first observed in the partially purified preparation of Harvey p21^{ras} described above (Shih et al. 1980). The enzyme uses GTP or dGTP, but not ATP or dATP, as donors to transfer phosphate to threonine residues on p21^{ras}. The phosphorylated product of this reaction is immunoprecipitable with anti-*ras* antisera and comigrates with the phosphorylated upper band of the characteristic p21^{ras} doublet in polyacrylamide gels. The major site of phosphorylation in vitro appears from peptide mapping to be the site of threonine phosphorylation in infected cells. The activity is unaffected by cAMP and does not phosphorylate casein, phosvitin, histones, or other common substrates for kinases. Moreover, the reaction with p21 is insensitive to EDTA, EGTA, *N*-ethyl maleimide, and calcium. Although guanine binding occurs rapidly at 4°C, the kinase reaction is relatively slow, even at 30°C or 37°C. These unusual features strongly suggest that the activity is probably an inherent property of p21^{ras}, although the relationship of the activity to cell transformation is unknown.

7. *Other Candidate Products of* ras?

Although p21^{ras} is generally accepted as the product of the Ki-MSV transforming gene, G. R. Andersson and colleagues (1979) have argued that the product is instead associated with lactate dehydrogenase (LDH) activity; it is uncertain whether this hypothesis can be reconciled with the prevailing view for which such strong support exists by proposing that the p21^{ras} serves as a subunit in an LDH complex (Anderson and Kovacik 1981). Scheinberg and Strand (1980) have described a 20,000-dalton protein in normal cells that is phosphorylated and associated with the plasma membrane; however, this protein is shed into the culture medium after transformation with Ki-MSV and precipitated by antisera to structural proteins of a rat leukemia virus. For these reasons and others, it seems unlikely to be closely related to the products of *ras*.

G. *fes* and *fms*: Oncogenes of Feline Sarcoma Viruses

1. *Products of* fes *Are* gag *Fusion Proteins*

Three different feline sarcoma viruses (FeSVs) have been isolated from spontaneous sarcomas in cats (Snyder and Theilen 1969; Gardner et al. 1970; McDonough et al. 1971). The Snyder-Theilen (ST) isolate of FeSV encodes a *gag*-related protein, P85$^{gag\text{-}fes}$, which includes the feline leukemia virus (FeLV) *gag* proteins p15, p12, and a portion of p30, fused to *fes*-specific sequences (Barbacid et al. 1980b; Van de Ven et al. 1980). Since this is the only known gene product of this defective virus, it is likely to be the ST-FeSV transforming protein. The Gardner-Arnstein (GA) isolate of FeSV also encodes a *gag*-related protein whose molecular weight is approximately 95,000 (P95$^{gag\text{-}fes}$) (Barbacid et al. 1980b). This protein is closely related to ST-FeSV P85$^{gag\text{-}fes}$, as demonstrated by immunological and tryptic peptide mapping techniques, as well as by nucleic acid hybridization with *fes* DNA (Frankel et al. 1979; Barbacid et al. 1980b; Van de Ven et al. 1980). Both of these proteins are phosphorylated at multiple sites in vivo and contain phosphorylated serine, threonine, and tyrosine residues (Barbacid et al. 1980a; Reynolds et al. 1980). Glycosylated forms of these proteins have also been observed (Sherr et al. 1980).

2. *Products of* fes *Are Associated with Tyrosine Kinases*

Both $P85^{gag\text{-}fes}$ and $P95^{gag\text{-}fes}$, isolated by immunoprecipitation, are associated with protein kinase activity resulting in transfer of phosphate from ATP to tyrosine residues on the virus-coded proteins. With some antisera, phosphate is also transferred to the IgG heavy chain (Barbacid et al. 1980a; Reynolds et al. 1980). When serum from rabbits bearing SR-RSV-D-induced tumors was incubated with immune complexes of ST-FeSV-coded P85 precipitated with anti-FeLV p30, a large increase in the amount of phosphate transferred to the IgG was observed with a concomitant decrease in the phosphorylation of $P85^{gag\text{-}fes}$ (K. Beemon, pers. comm.). Cells transformed by ST-FeSV and GA-FeSV show a five-to tenfold elevation in levels of tyrosine phosphorylation in protein (Barbacid et al. 1980a; Reynolds et al. 1980). Transformation-defective, nonconditional mutants of ST-FeSV have been isolated that have lost their associated protein kinase activity, although they encode proteins the same size as wild-type $P85^{gag\text{-}fes}$ (Barbacid et al. 1981a; Reynolds et al. 1981a). By these criteria, ST-FeSV and GA-FeSV proteins appear to be functionally similar to the RSV transforming protein $pp60^{src}$. However, purification of the FeSV proteins will be required to determine whether the tyrosine-specific protein kinase activity is an intrinsic property of these viral proteins.

3. fes *Is Related to* fps *and Perhaps to Other* onc *Genes*

The *fes* sequences of both ST-FeSV and GA-FeSV have been shown to be homologous to the *fps* transformation-specific regions of the defective avian sarcoma viruses, FuSV and PRCII, by nucleic acid hybridization with a *fps*-specific probe (Shibuya et al. 1980) and by immunological and peptide-mapping studies of the four viral polyproteins (Barbacid et al. 1981b; Beemon 1981). Furthermore, the ST-FeSV genome has been sequenced, and some amino acid sequence homology has been observed between proteins encoded by *fes, mos,* and *src* (A. Hampe, pers. comm.)

4. *Products of* fms

A third FeSV isolate, SM-FeSV, obtained by McDonough et al. (1971), does not contain the *fes* sequences of ST-FeSV and GA-FeSV but instead has an apparently unrelated transformation-specific region termed *fms*. SM-FeSV encodes a 180,000-dalton *gag*-related protein and a 120,000-dalton protein without *gag* sequences ($P180^{gag-fms}$ and $p120^{fms}$). $P120^{fms}$ and $P180^{gag-fms}$ are clearly related in sequence to each other, and pulse-chase studies suggest that the smaller protein is at least in part derived from the other (Barbacid et al. 1980b). It is not known which of the virus-coded proteins is necessary for transformation.

Antisera that recognize antigenic sites in *fms* as well as in the *gag* domains of $P180^{gag-fms}$ have been raised in goats inoculated with cells nonproductively infected with SM-FeSV. When SM-FeSV-coded $P120^{fms}$ and $P180^{gag-fms}$ were immunoprecipitated with such antisera, protein kinase activity was detected, leading to specific phosphorylation of both $P120^{gms}$ and $P180^{gag-fms}$, predominantly on tyrosine residues (Barbacid and Lauver, 1981). However, the proteins encoded by SM-FeSV are very different from those encoded by ST-FeSV and GA-FeSV in that $P120^{fms}$ and $P180^{gag-fms}$ are not phosphorylated at tyrosine residues in vivo. Furthermore, protein kinase assays with $P180^{gag-fms}$ immunoprecipitated with antisera to *gag* determinants resulted in only barely detectable activity. SM-FeSV-transformed cells also failed to show elevated levels of phosphotyrosine in cellular protein (Barbacid and Lauver 1981; Reynolds et al. 1981b). Therefore, it appears likely that transformation by *fms* differs mechanistically from transformation by *fes*.

H. *rel*: Oncogene of Reticuloendotheliosis Virus Strain T

Molecular hybridization, oligonucleotide fingerprinting, and restriction-mapping techniques have been used to define a region unique to the genome of an avian replication-defective virus, known as reticuloendotheliosis virus strain T (REV-T), believed to be responsible for fibroblast and hematopoietic cell transformation and for rapid induction of lymphoreticular neoplasms arising from the B-cell lineage (Breitman et al. 1980; Gonda et al. 1980; Cohen et al. 1981; Lewis et al. 1981; I. S. Chen et al., pers. comm.) (see Chapters 4 and 8). Approximately 1.5–2.0 kb positioned near the 3′ end of the 5.5-kb REV-T genome are composed of sequences unrelated to replication genes of helper REV or to the transforming genes of other avian transforming viruses (Breitman et al. 1980; Cohen et al. 1981). These sequences, termed *rel*, are homologous to single-copy sequences in the genomes of turkeys and other birds. Although such observations conform to those made with other, well-documented viral oncogenes, as yet there is little genetic or biochemical evidence for the function of *rel*. A subgenomic mRNA containing *rel* sequences has recently been observed in REV-T-infected cells, implying that the product of *rel* may be unlinked to the products of viral structural genes. In the absence of *rel*-specific antisera, the only available clue to the nature of the *rel*-gene product is the provisional finding of a 58,000-dalton, in vitro translation product of the fragmented genome of REV-T (M. Lai, pers. comm.). For reasons stated earlier (Section II.A.1), it is necessary to exercise caution before ascribing this protein to *rel*.

I. *sis*: Oncogene of Simian Sarcoma Virus

Simian sarcoma virus (SSV), the only transforming retrovirus isolated from primates to date, has been difficult to characterize because of the great excess of helper virus (SSAV) over SSV in conventional stocks. Application of recombinant DNA methods to the study of SSV has recently provided a physical definition of a segment of the viral genome derived from a conserved cellular sequence and apparently unique to SSV. This region of the SSV genome has been called *sis*, but there is no biochemical or genetic definition of its products or functions.

Identification of *sis* has proceeded by the molecular cloning of either unintegrated closed circular DNA (Gelmann et al. 1981) or proviral DNA (Robbins et al. 1981). Using restriction maps in concert with R-loop studies, both groups have judged the ~5.5-kb genome of SSV to be defective for most or all of the replication genes of SSAV, with a substitution of about 1 kb (*v-sis*) positioned close to the 3′ end of viral RNA. Attempts to anneal *v-sis* DNA to a variety of other *onc* sequences have been unsuccessful, sustaining the premise that *sis* is a novel oncogene, unrelated to those described previously (F. Wong-Staal et al., pers. comm.). The position of *sis* within the SSV genome can be construed as a likely indicator that the gene will be expressed independently, not as a component of fused genes; experience with other oncogenes suggests that the product of *v-sis* may therefore be particularly difficult to identify.

III. THE ORIGINS OF VIRAL ONCOGENES

The oncogenes of retroviruses are genetic luxuries. In no known instance is the function of an oncogene required for virus replication, and numerous strains of retroviruses have survived the hazards of evolutionary selection without benefit of an oncogene. How then, and from where, did these genes arise? The quest for answers to these ostensibly abstruse questions has led retrovirologists to what could be the heart of malignant transformation. It now appears that retroviral oncogenes originated from normal genes of vertebrate cells (designated here by the generic term *c-onc*), that oncogenes and their vertebrate progenitors remain closely related if not identical, and that the functions of *c-onc* genes presage the effects of viral oncogenes on infected cells. The discovery of *c-onc* genes has unveiled a family of cellular genes whose alteration or anomalous expression may underlie many forms of oncogenesis (Table 9.2).

A. Emergence of the Thesis: First Clues and Hypotheses

The virus isolated from a chicken sarcoma by Rous did not spring quickly or easily into view. Rather, an infectious tumorigenic agent was obtained from extracts of tumor tissue only after the original sarcoma had been passaged repeatedly from one bird to another (Rous 1911). It seems possible, in retrospect, that the original tumor was not the consequence of virus infection; the sarcoma virus that eventually emerged may not have been present in the tissue with which Rous began his work. The isolation of MSVs (Harvey 1964; Moloney 1966) and Ab-MLV (Abelson and Rabstein 1970a,b) decades later raised these issues in a more explicit manner: The new viruses appeared during the passage of leukemia viruses in rodents, as if new capabilities for pathogenesis could be acquired from the host animal.

The discovery of endogenous retroviruses in chickens (Robinson 1978) and mice (Aaronson and Stephenson 1976) (see Chapter 10), and the development of inbred lines of mice whose predisposition to leukemia appeared to involve genetically transmitted retroviruses (Rowe 1973), added appreciably to these inferences and engendered the "oncogene hypothesis" of Huebner and Todaro (1969; Todaro and Huebner 1972). According to this hypothesis, carcinogens of

Table 9.2 The *c-onc* genes of retroviruses

v-onc[a]	Probable species of origin[b]	*c-onc*	References	*c-onc* expressed[c]	Protein product of *c-onc*[d]
v-src	chicken/quail[e]	*c-src*	Stehelin et al. (1976b)	yes	$pp60^{c\text{-}src}$
v-rel	turkey	*c-rel*	Wong and Lai 1981	yes	?
v-myc	chicken	*c-myc*	Roussel et al. (1979); Sheiness and Bishop (1979)	yes	?
v-erb-A	chicken	*c-erb*-A[f]	Roussel et al. (1979); Vennstrom and Bishop 1982	yes	?
v-erb-B	chicken	*c-erb*-B[f]	Roussel et al. (1979); Vennstrom and Bishop 1982	yes	?
v-myb	chicken	*c-myb*	Roussel et al. (1979); Souza et al. (1980)	yes	?
v-fps	chicken	*c-fps*[g]	Shibuya et al. (1980); H. Hanafusa (pers. comm.)	?	?
v-yes	chicken	*c-yes*	Yoshida et al. (1980)	?	?
v-mos	mouse	*c-mos*	Frankel and Fischinger (1977)	n.d.[h]	?[i]
v-abl	mouse	*c-abl*	Goff et al. (1980)	yes	$p150^{c\text{-}abl}$

v-bas	mouse	*c-bas*[k]	Andersen et al. (1981)	yes	$p21^{c\text{-}bas}$
v-ras	rat	*c-ras*[j]	Ellis et al. (1980)	yes	$p21^{c\text{-}ras}$
v-fes	cat	*c-fes*	Frankel et al. (1979)	yes	$p92^{c\text{-}fes}$
v-fms	cat	*c-fms*	C. Sherr (pers. comm.)	?	?
v-sis	woolly monkey	*c-sis*	Favera et al.(1981)	?	?

[a]The names of viral genes are treated here as generic terms, although in most instances several separate virus isolates are known (see Table 9.1).

[b]The probable species of origin is inferred from the host in which the particular oncovirus first emerged.

[c]Expression is defined as either detection of transcription from the *c-onc* or detection of a protein encoded by the locus.

[d]Question marks indicate that suitable analyses have not been completed.

[e]Some strains of RSV have been generated experimentally in quail (Wang et al. 1979), but all field isolates of *v-src* have come from chickens.

[f]The separate domains of *erb* (A and B) are represented by similarly separate domains in the chicken genome.

[g]The *c-fps* of chicken is apparently related to *c-fes* of cats (Shibuya et al. 1980).

[h]Fairly extensive efforts have failed to detect transcription of *c-mos* (Frankel and Fischinger 1976).

[i]Failure to detect transcription from *c-mos* raises the possibility that *c-mos* is inactive unless transferred into a retroviral genome.

[j]Rat DNA contains at least two small distinct gene families related to *v-ras*. One family is apparently the source of Harvey and Rasheed *v-ras;* the other family is the source of Kirsten *v-ras* (DeFeo et al. 1981).

[k]The *c-bas* of mice is closely related to *c-ras* of rats (Andersen et al. 1981).

many types act by inducing the expression of otherwise cryptic retroviral genes already resident in the genomes of the target cells. The oncogene hypothesis is no longer regarded as strictly correct, but it fueled two lines of inquiry. On the one hand, numerous efforts have been made to implicate the induction of retroviruses in the oncogenic mechanisms of chemical and physical carcinogens (Freeman et al. 1973). These experiments have produced enigmatic results, at best. More importantly, however, the oncogene hypothesis was a major heuristic stimulus that prompted experimentalists to ask whether normal cellular DNA might contain retroviral oncogenes. We now know that vertebrate cells do harbor genetic loci homologous to retroviral oncogenes, but these loci are cellular, not viral, genes, and the oncogene hypothesis has been eclipsed by even more sweeping views of the nature of these cellular genes.

B. Discovery of *c-onc* Genes

The search for oncogenes in cellular DNA began with the use of molecular hybridization, following the strategy illustrated by Figure 9.6. The strategy exploited naturally occurring deletions that remove most or all of *v-src* (but no other viral gene) from the genome of RSV and render the virus transformation defective (Duesberg and Vogt 1970; Martin and Duesberg 1972; Lai et al. 1973). Viral RNA bearing this class of deletions could be employed to isolate radioactive DNA (cDNA$_{src}$) that hybridized only with nucleotide sequences encoding (or related to) *src* (Stehelin et al. 1976a). The result was a

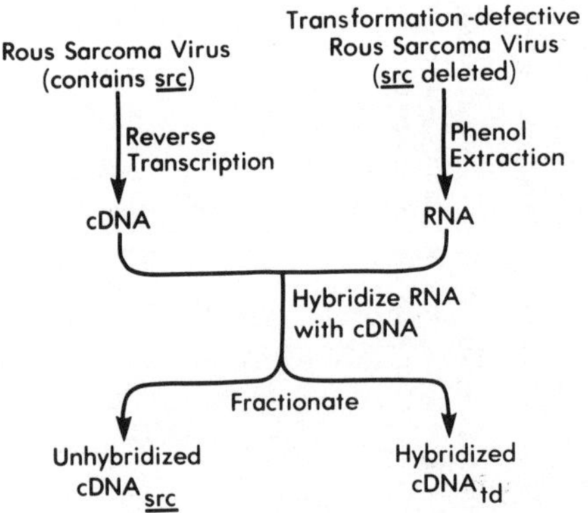

Figure 9.6 Strategy for the preparation of cDNA$_{src}$. The figure outlines the preparation of cDNA$_{src}$. (For details, see Stehelin et al. 1976a).

reagent that provided specificity and sensitivity sufficient to detect a single genetic locus among the immense complexity of vertebrate DNA. Similar cDNAs were prepared for replication-defective MSVs (Scolnick et al. 1973, 1975; Frankel et al. 1976), but the genetic definition of these reagents was less rigorous because suitable deletion mutants were not available for isolation of the cDNAs. As a consequence, the experimental strategies had to rely on the assumption that nucleotide sequences not present in the genome of the helper virus must perforce represent portions of the oncogene, an assumption that proved useful, but not inevitably correct (see below).

The initial findings with $cDNA_{src}$ for RSV prefigured subsequent conclusions for virtually all retroviral oncogenes. Each family of vertebrates examined, including fish, birds, and mammals, displayed evidence of both DNA and RNA related to the *src* gene (Stehelin et al. 1976b; Spector et al. 1978a). The DNA related to *v-src* appeared to occur as only one or very few copies in each haploid portion of vertebrate genomes. Retrovirologists had obtained their first glimpse of the cellular gene we now know as *c-src*.

The mere fact that homologous DNA could be detected across such large phylogenetic distances indicated that the genetic locus or loci in question were highly conserved during the course of evolution. More recent findings have dramatized the extent of this conservation by demonstrating homology with *v-src* (and several other *v-oncs*) in the DNA of *Drosophila* (Shilo and Weinberg 1981b). Conservation of *c-src* was also explored by evaluating the thermal stability of molecular hybrids formed between $cDNA_{src}$ and DNAs from various sources. The results indicated that the nucleotide sequences of *c-src* might diverge by no more than 10–15% from fish to chicken genomes, on the one hand, and from chicken to human genomes on the other hand (Stehelin et al. 1976b; Spector et al. 1978a). The full implications of these findings were not easily sustained at the outset, largely because no assay was available for the protein product of *src*. Nevertheless, it appeared that vertebrate species possessed a highly conserved and expressed (i.e., transcribed) gene that is closely related to a viral oncogene. The strong evolutionary conservation of this gene, and the fact that it was found to be expressed in every tissue and every species examined, signified an essential function in cellular metabolism. These early deductions were later validated and extended by the identification and characterization of a protein encoded by *c-src* (and known as pp60$^{c\text{-}src}$; see below).

Difficulties did arise, however, from the use of a less-well-defined cDNA for the oncogene of Ha/Ki-MSV (*v-ras*). Initial results indicated that *v-ras* was related to (and presumably derived from) nucleotide sequences in the genome of an endogenous retroviruslike element of rats (Scolnick et al. 1973; Scolnick and Parks 1974), a troubling deduction, since it stood in striking contrast to the mounting evidence that other retroviral oncogenes are derived from conserved cellular genes. The advent of molecular cloning to the study of retroviral genomes quickly resolved the apparent anomaly. It now appears that the genome of Ha/Ki-MSV was constructed with three distinct components (Ellis et al. 1980) (Chapter 4). One component was derived from the murine helper virus that was used to initiate recovery of the sarcoma virus and was isolated together with the sarcoma virus; a second was derived from an endogenous virus of rats; and a third, the oncogene proper, was derived true to form from a cellular gene of the rat in which the sarcoma virus originally arose.

The principles first enunciated for *src* have since been shown to be widely applicable to retroviral oncogenes (Table 9.2): homologs of these genes (i.e., *c-onc* genes) can be found in vertebrate DNA, many (but apparently not all) of which are expressed in phenotypically normal cells. The sole exception at present is the oncogene of spleen focus-forming virus (SFFV), which appears to be a recombinant form of the retroviral *env* gene, rather than the derivative of a cellular gene (Oliff et al. 1980). All of the identified *c-onc* genes are found in more than one vertebrate species, but the extent of evolutionary conservation varies from one *c-onc* to another: Some are readily detectable only in closely related species, whereas others appear to have taken form in the earliest vertebrates and to have evolved thereafter in concert with speciation. However, these variations may be only matters of degree; it is now reasonable to suppose that every *c-onc* represents a genetic lineage that extends throughout the vertebrate phyla and, in at least some instances, farther down the phylogenetic hierarchy.

The kinship between retroviral oncogenes and cellular genes is certain. But how can we discern parent from progeny? Phylogenetic patterns provide a clue. In contrast to the evolutionary conservation of the cellular genes, the viral oncogenes are usually (although not inevitably; see below) restricted to single strains of retroviruses that were isolated from particular species. Moreover, the homology between the viral oncogene and cellular DNA is greatest for the species in which the oncogene allegedly originated. The most straightforward interpretation of these findings is that retroviral oncogenes are derived from cellular genes. The widespread acceptance of this scheme and the remarkable similarity between retroviral oncogenes and their cellular homologs (described below) have engendered a standard nomenclature described in the introduction to this chapter. The nomenclature is only a convenience, however, and should not be construed as indicating that homologous viral and cellular genes are necessarily identical in either structure or function. The precise relationship between cellular progenitor and viral progeny has yet to be fully explored for any retroviral oncogene.

C. Characterizing *c-onc* Genes

Enumeration of *c-onc* genes by molecular hybridization and by mapping with restriction endonucleases has revealed that many may be unique loci within a given species. However, apparent exceptions exist: (1) the DNA of chickens may contain a second, possibly incomplete locus (a pseudogene) related to *c-src* (Parker et al. 1981); (2) *c-ras* for Ha-MSV is represented by two distinctive loci in rats, one with introns and one without (DeFeo et al. 1981); (3) *v-ras* of the Ki-MSV apparently derives from another cellular gene that is related only distantly to the Harvey *c-ras* (Ellis et al. 1981); and (4) the Rasheed form of *v-ras* apparently derived from a representative of the Harvey *c-ras* family (E. Scolnick, pers. comm.). The last of these findings was unexpected because the relationship of the Rasheed oncogene to the other forms of *v-ras* originally seemed quite distant and was perceived only by serological analyses (Young et al. 1979).

c-onc genes behave as classical Mendelian loci. They occupy constant positions within the genomes of particular species (Hughes et al. 1979a), and they segregate in a predictable fashion when breedings are analyzed with the assistance of structural polymorphisms that have been identified by restriction mapping (D. Spector; B. Vennstrom; both pers. comm.). The loci are recognized by virtue of homology with a viral oncogene, but in most (if not all) instances, the homologous nucleotide sequences do not comprise the entire cellular gene. Three major considerations prompt this statement. First, heteroduplex analysis and restriction mapping have demonstrated that the homology between several viral oncogenes and their *c-onc* genes is interrupted by one or more intervening sequences (or introns) in the cellular locus (Goff et al. 1980; DeFeo et al. 1981; Franchini et al. 1981; Parker et al. 1981; Shalloway et al. 1981; Takeya et al. 1981). An example is provided in Figure 9.7, which illustrates a heteroduplex formed by hybridizing DNA representing *v-src* to a portion of *c-src* from chicken DNA; six loops of various sizes are visible, each representing an intron in the cellular locus. The *c-onc* for *v-mos* provides an interesting exception to this rule: The murine and human forms of *c-mos* display uninterrupted homology with *v-mos* in heteroduplex analysis (Jones et al. 1980; Oskarsson et al. 1980; G. Vande Woude, pers. comm.) and by nucleotide sequencing (Van Beveral et al. 1981a). The same is true of at least one of the several rat loci representing *c-ras* (DeFeo et al. 1981). Second, transcription from at least several *c-onc* genes generates RNAs that, even in their mature forms, are appreciably more complex than the homologous viral oncogene (Table 9.2). For example, the mature form of RNA produced from *c-src* is 3.9 kb (Parker et al. 1981), a complexity almost three-fold greater than that of *v-src*. Yet both *v-src* and *c-src* give rise to a protein of 60,000 daltons (Brugge and Erikson 1977; Collett et al. 1978; Oppermann et al. 1979). It appears that large portions of the mRNA for *c-src* may not be translated and that the boundaries of this (or any other) *c-onc* can only be located by applying the definitions that demarcate a transcriptional unit in eukaryotic DNA (i.e., the sites of initiation and polyadenylation). Third, many retroviral oncogenes have been formed by fusing a portion of a replicative gene (typically, *gag*) (see Chapter 4) to nucleotide sequences of a *c-onc*. It seems unlikely that this fusion always incorporates the entirety of the *c-onc* locus into the viral genome. In particular, sequences in the 5′ domain of the *c-onc* may be missing from the viral oncogene.

D. *c-onc* Genes Are Cellular Genes

The oncogene hypothesis portrayed cellular oncogenes as components of retroviral genomes—a conceptual predisposition that proved difficult to override. But we are now certain that *c-onc* genes are cellular genes, not viral genes in disguise. The conclusion rests on three major points of evidence: (1) the location of *c-onc* genes at constant genetic loci in every member of a species (in striking contrast to the diverse distribution and positioning of endogenous retroviral genes) (see, e.g., Hughes et al. 1979a, 1980);

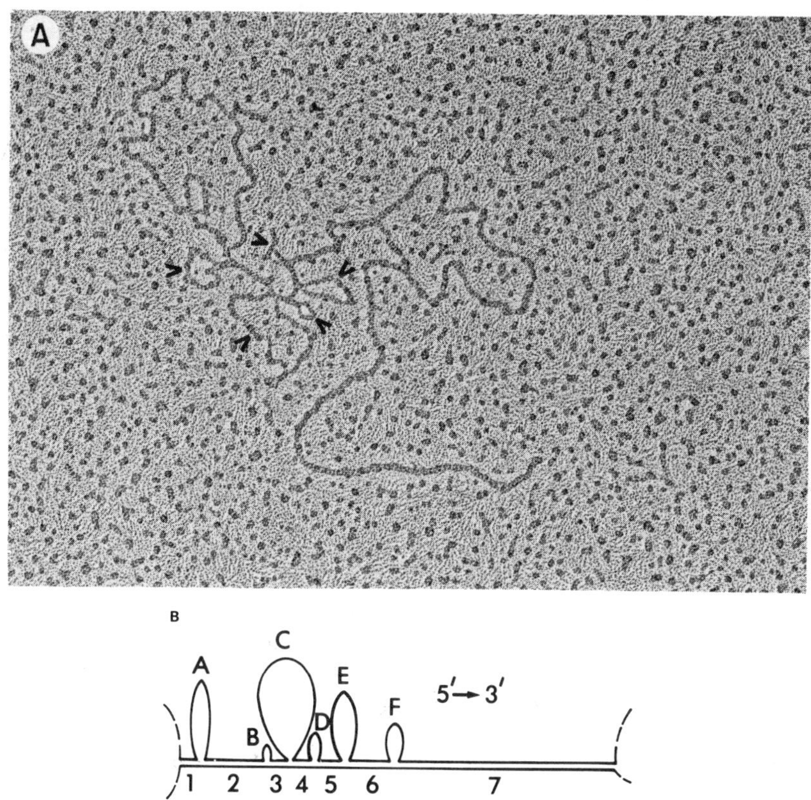

Figure 9.7 Introns in *c-src*. Electron microscopy was used to examine a heteroduplex formed between DNA containing *v-src* and DNA containing *c-src*. The DNAs were prepared by molecular cloning. (*A*) Each loop marked with an arrowhead represents an "intron"—DNA present in *c-src* but not in *v-src* (and presumably not in the mRNA representing *c-src*). (For details, see Parker et al. 1981.) (*B*) Diagramatic representation of the heteroduplex. Dashed lines at each end represent vector DNA. Introns are designated by letters, exons by numbers. The polarity given as 5′→3′ relates the DNA to the plus strand of viral RNA.

(2) the presence of intervening sequences within many of the *c-onc* genes (a hallmark of eukaryotic genes, and, again, in telling contrast to the organization of retroviral genes); and (3) the fact that no *c-onc* has been found within or even linked to a complete or defective provirus of an endogenous retrovirus (Hughes et al. 1979a, 1980; Sheiness et al. 1980b). It seems unlikely that *c-onc* genes were introduced into vertebrate genomes by infection of ancestral species with retroviruses; instead, we must explain how complex cellular genes have made their way partly or entirely into the genomes of preexistent retroviruses.

E. Expression of *c-onc* Genes

The possibility that *c-onc* genes might be expressed in phenotypically normal cells emerged from the discovery of RNA homologous to *v-src* in uninfected fibroblasts of several avian species (Wang et al. 1977; Spector et al. 1978b,c). Similar findings were made subsequently for other *c-onc* genes and other species (Roussel et al. 1979; Sheiness and Bishop 1979; Chen 1980; Bishop et al. 1981). However, some *c-onc* genes may not be expressed; e.g., a thorough-going search has failed to detect transcription from *c-mos* (Frankel and Fischinger 1976; D. Dina, pers. comm.). Efforts to detect transcription from *c-fes* were also unsuccessful (Frankel et al. 1979), but a more recent report described a protein ($pP92^{c\text{-}fes}$) that may be encoded by *c-fes* and that was found in a number of mammalian species (Barbacid et al. 1980a).

Transcription from *c-onc* genes has not been widely studied, but a reasonably coherent set of data is available for four *c-onc* genes representative of avian retroviruses: *c-src, c-myc, c-erb,* and *c-myb.* Several principles are apparent that may endure even after a greater variety of *c-onc* genes have been studied (Bishop et al. 1981): (1) Each of the *c-onc* genes is transcribed in a variety of tissues and in every species that has been satisfactorily examined (Table 9.3). (2) Transcription from each *c-onc* appears to be independently controlled from one tissue to another (Table 9.4) (Chen 1980; D. Sheiness and B. Vennstrom; D. Stehelin; both pers. comm.); thus, the *c-onc* genes are not coordinately expressed as a group, and the function of each gene may be required only in certain tissues. (3) There is no evidence that transcription from *c-onc* genes is ever coordinated with the expression of endogenous retrovirus genes

Table 9.3 RNAs transcribed from the *c-onc* genes of several avian retroviruses

	RNA size in kilobases						
	c-src	*c-myc*	*c-myb*	*c-erb*			
Chick embryos	3.9	2.5	4.0	12	9.0	4.5	3.0
Chick fibroblasts	3.9	2.5	—	12	9.0	4.5	3.0
Chick bone marrow	3.9	2.5	4.0	—	—	4.5	3.0
Chick yolk sac	3.9	2.5	4.0	—	—	4.5	3.0
Chick brain	3.9	2.5	—				
Chick muscle	3.9	2.5	—				
Chick liver	3.9	2.5	—				
Chick thymus	3.9	2.5	4.0				
Chick bursa	3.9	2.5	4.0				
Chick spleen	3.9	2.5	—				
Duck embryo	3.9	2.5					
Quail embryo	3.9	2.5	4.0				
Mouse fibroblasts	3.9	2.5					
Rat fibroblasts	3.9	2.5					

Data from T. Gonda, D. Sheiness, and B. Vennstrom (all unpubl.). — denotes not detected; blank spaces indicate that data are not available.

(Wang et al. 1977; Spector et al. 1978c). (4) The *c-onc* genes give rise to distinctive RNAs whose sizes have so far proved to be identical in various types of cells and even in different species (Table 9.3). The constancy of these RNAs among widely diverged species testifies to the selective pressures that have apparently preserved the structure and function of *c-onc* genes. As discussed above, most of the transcripts are appreciably larger than would be required to encode the nucleotide sequences that are shared by the homologous viral and cellular genes. (5) Three of the *c-onc* genes (*c-src, c-myb,* and *c-myc*) give rise to single mature transcripts (Table 9.3), in accord with the expectation that each locus represents but one gene. Transcription from *c-erb* provides a striking contrast, however, because at least four (and perhaps five) different mature RNAs have been identified, and the distribution of these RNAs varies among different tissues (Table 9.3) (Vennstrom and Bishop 1982). Two of the RNAs are derived from one domain of *c-erb* and the others are from a separate domain; this pattern mirrors the organization of *v-erb* (Sheiness et al. 1981), which is also composed of two independently expressed domains (*v-erb*-A and *v-erb*-B) (see Sheiness et al. 1981; and Chapter 4).

Table 9.4 Transcription of *c-onc* genes in different tissues of the chicken

Tissue or cells	Relative amount of RNA transcribed from *c-onc* genes[a]			
	c-erb	*c-myb*	*c-myc*	*c-src*
Liver	2	<0.2	0.5	0.6
Brain	2	<0.2	0.5	0.7
Embryonic fibroblasts	2	0.2	5	2
Bone marrow	2	30	4	0.4
Yolk sac	4	60	5	<0.3
Macrophages	0.7	<0.2	1	6
Thymus	1	90	5	2
Isolated thymic lymphocytes	0.3	30	15	0.4
Bursa	1	5	2	1
Isolated bursal lymphocytes	0.3	20	10	n.t.
Spleen	1	2	5	6
Isolated splenic lymphocytes	0.3	20	15	n.t.

Data from T. Gonda and D. Sheiness (both unpubl.).
[a]n.t. denotes not tested.

F. Identifying the Proteins Encoded by *c-onc* Genes

RNA transcribed from several *c-onc* genes has been found in polyribosomes and is therefore presumably translated into proteins (Spector et al. 1978b; B. Vennstrom, pers. comm.). The search for these proteins has not been easy. Most cells contain only small amounts of *c-onc* mRNAs and proteins, and the identification of *c-onc* proteins has so far depended on the development of antisera that react with the product(s) of the corresponding viral oncogenes, an undertaking that is itself unpredictable and technically demanding.

Four proteins encoded by *c-onc* genes have been identified to date: pp60$^{c\text{-}src}$, a 60,000-dalton phosphoprotein specified by *c-src* (Collett et al. 1978, 1979b; Oppermann et al. 1979; Rohrschneider et al. 1979); p21$^{c\text{-}ras}$, a 21,000-dalton phosphoprotein encoded by the Harvey *c-ras* (Langbeheim et al. 1980); p150$^{c\text{-}abl}$, a 150,000-dalton protein apparently derived from *c-abl* and formerly called NCP150 (Witte et al. 1979b), and p92$^{c\text{-}fes}$, a 92,000-dalton protein presumed to be encoded by *c-fes* and formerly called NCP92 (Barbacid et al. 1980a). Both pp60$^{c\text{-}src}$ and p21$^{c\text{-}ras}$ have been extensively studied, both are remarkably similar to their viral counterparts in structure and apparent function (Collett et al. 1978, 1979b; Karess et al. 1979; Oppermann et al. 1979; Rohrschneider et al. 1979; Langbeheim et al. 1980; Sefton et al. 1980b; Karess and Hanafusa 1981); and both are found in a large variety of cells and are distributed across wide phylogenetic distances (Oppermann et al. 1979; Rohrschneider et al. 1979; Langbeheim et al. 1980). Much less is known of $p150^{c\text{-}abl}$ (Witte et al. 1979b). Its size and composition are different from those of any of the proteins encoded by the several variants of *v-abl,* it has been found in appreciable (but very small) amounts only in thymocytes and other lymphoid cells, its phylogenetic distribution has not been reported, and nothing is known of its function. Surprisingly, RNA transcribed from *c-abl* has been found widely distributed among tissues and cells of many sorts, most of which contain no detectable $p150^{c\text{-}abl}$ (D. Baltimore, pers. comm.). This discrepancy cannot presently be explained.

The apparent product of *c-fes* ($p92^{c\text{-}fes}$) has been found in the cells of rats and related mammals, but not in rodents or primates (Barbacid et al. 1980a). Little else is known of the protein: the extent of its relationship to products of *v-fes* has not been critically assessed; no function has been identified, and there is no explanation for the failure to find RNA transcribed from *c-fes* in species known to produce $p92^{c\text{-}fes}$.

G. How Similar Are Viral Oncogenes and *c-onc* Genes?

Assessment of the similarities between *c-onc* genes and their viral derivatives has taken two general forms: comparison of the nucleotide sequences that embody the genes and comparison of the proteins encoded by the genes. Early studies with molecular hybridization raised the possibility of a substantial kinship between the *c-onc* and viral oncogene, but satisfactory tests of the issue awaited the isolation of the genes by molecular cloning, on the one hand, and identification and characterization of the proteins encoded by the genes, on the other. With either or both of these chores now accomplished in several instances, the evidence mounts for remarkable similarity, if not identity, between the viral and cellular forms of oncogenes:

1. Coding sequences shared by viral and cellular oncogenes have so far been indistinguishable by heteroduplex analysis (Jones et al. 1980; Oskarsson et al. 1980; DeFeo et al. 1981; Parker et al. 1981; Shalloway et al. 1981; Takeya et al. 1981), although ambiguities arise whenever the cellular locus is punctuated by introns.
2. DNA sequencing has permitted an extensive comparison of *v-mos* and *c-mos* (Van Beveren et al. 1981a,b). The first few codons of *v-mos* in Mo-MSV are vestiges of the *env* gene into which *c-mos* was inserted. Otherwise, only occasional nucleotide substitutions distinguish *v-mos* from *c-mos.*
3. The *c-erb* locus is extraordinarily complex, extending over at least 40 kb of chicken-cell DNA and containing a minimum of 12 introns (Vennstrom and Bishop 1982). Nevertheless, when the exons of the locus were mapped against *v-erb,* close homology was observed. The viral gene encodes two proteins in separate domains (Anderson et al. 1980; Sheiness et al. 1981) and the cellular locus displays the same structural organization (Vennstrom and Bishop 1982).
4. The viral and cellular forms of $pp60^{src}$ are remarkably similar (Collett et al. 1978, 1979b; Karess et al. 1979; Oppermann et al. 1979; Rohrschneider et al. 1979; Sefton et al. 1980b; Karess and Hanafusa 1981). They share size, display antigenic cross-reactivities, and yield closely related peptide maps. Both are principally affiliated with the plasma membrane of the cell (Courtneidge et al. 1980). Both are phosphorylated and have similarly disposed phosphoamino acids, with phosphoserine in the proximity of the amino terminus (Collett et al. 1979a,b) and phosphotyrosine within a carboxyterminal domain (Hunter and Sefton 1980; Karess and Hanafusa 1981). Both are protein kinases that phosphorylate tyrosine in substrate proteins (Collett et al. 1979b, 1980; Oppermann et al. 1979; Rohrschneider et al. 1979; Hunter and Sefton 1980; Levinson et al. 1980). The two proteins can be distinguished only by very subtle criteria: Some antisera react with the viral protein, but not the cellular protein, presumably reflecting the fact that the antisera were raised against the viral protein, rather than the cellular protein (Oppermann et al. 1979); the peptide maps of the two proteins differ in a few respects (Sefton et al. 1980b; Karess and Hanafusa 1981); and the phosphotyrosine may be contained within different tryptic peptides in

the two proteins (Karess and Hanafusa 1981; Smart et al. 1981). It also remains possible that the viral and cellular proteins respond differently to controlling influences in the cell and that the kinase activities of the two proteins have different substrate specificities. Definitive tests of these important potential distinctions are not presently available.

5. The possibility that *v-src* and *c-src* are functionally similar has received dramatic support from the claim that recombination between *c-src* (in chickens) and deletion mutants of *v-src* can apparently reconstitute a functional oncogene (Hanafusa et al. 1977; Wang et al. 1978, 1979; Karess et al. 1979; Vigne et al. 1980; Karess and Hanafusa 1981). In the most telling examples, the allegedly reconstituted oncogene retains a 3′-terminal portion of *v-src* (~25% of the gene) but is otherwise apparently constructed entirely of nucleotide sequences derived from *c-src* (Wang et al. 1979; Karess and Hanafusa 1981). The protein encoded by the reconstituted *v-src* is so similar to both $pp60^{v\text{-}src}$ and $pp60^{c\text{-}src}$ that its genetic origins are difficult to discern, although peptide maps suggest that $pp60^{v\text{-}src}$ of the recombinant virus is indeed a hybrid of both cellular and viral origins (Vigne et al. 1980; Karess and Hanafusa 1981). Even these findings cannot assure us that $pp60^{c\text{-}src}$ and $pp60^{v\text{-}src}$ are functionally equivalent, however; in every instance, the recombinant viral protein has derived at least 20% of its carboxyterminal domain from the parental virus in the recombination (Wang et al. 1979; Karess and Hanafusa 1981), and it is the carboxyterminal domain of $pp60^{v\text{-}src}$ that bears the protein kinase activity (Levinson et al. 1981; Oppermann et al. 1981b). Moreover, an extensive analysis of oligonucleotides from *src* in different strains of RSV failed to find any evidence that could trace the origins of the reconstituted viruses to *c-src* (Lee et al. 1981). It therefore remains conceivable that the reconstituted RSVs arose from recombination among defective viruses or from other forms of RSV contaminating the stocks of deletion mutants used to initiate the experiments.
6. The proteins encoded by Harvey *v-ras* and one of the two closely related *c-ras* genes have been compared in considerable detail and appear to be quite similar. They each have a molecular weight of approximately 21,000, they react with the same antisera, they yield related peptide maps, and they display the same

biochemical function, i.e., the capacity to bind guanine nucleotides with high affinity (Scolnick et al. 1979; Shih et al. 1980). However, they may differ in one regard; $pp21^{v\text{-}ras}$ is phosphorylated on threonine residues, whereas phosphorylation of $p21^{c\text{-}ras}$ has yet to be detected (T.Y. Shih et al. 1979a; Langbeheim et al. 1980; Shih et al. 1980).

7. Functional similarities between *v-onc* and *c-onc* have been demonstrated most persuasively by work with *c-mos* and *c-ras*. Both of these *c-onc* genes have been isolated by molecular cloning (*c-mos* from mouse DNA, *c-ras* from rat DNA) and coupled to a retrovirus long terminal repeat (LTR) in order to favor vigorous expression. Some of the cells that receive these hybrid genetic units by transfection become transformed to a neoplastic phenotype (Oskarsson et al. 1980; DeFeo et al. 1981), as if the *c-onc*s might carry out the same functions as their homologous *v-onc*s (see also Section K.3).

None of the preceding examples provide a definitive demonstration of identity between the viral oncogene and *c-onc*. But the weight of the evidence now suggests that retroviral oncogenes encode functions also found in normal vertebrate cells. If correct, this conclusion may have significance that reaches far beyond the confines of tumor virology (see below).

H. The Family of *c-onc* Genes

We presently know of at least a dozen retroviral oncogenes, each distinguished by its nucleotide sequence and each with a corresponding oncogene (see Table 9.1). Moreover, ostensibly similar oncogenes may be the products of related but separate cellular loci. For example, the apparently homologous oncogenes of Ha-MSV and Ki-MSV (*v-ras*), formerly believed to have originated from the same *c-onc,* are now known to be the progeny of two different (albeit related) cellular genes (DeFeo et al. 1981). The total number of *c-onc* genes is therefore likely to grow as efforts to identify novel isolates of retroviruses continue. On the other hand, the number of these genes may not be inordinately large: the *c-onc* genes for *src, myc, erb, myb, yes,* and *fps* are each represented at least twice among the handful of independently isolated avian retroviruses, *c-fes* is a feline counterpart of *c-fps* that appears in two strains of feline sarcoma virus (Shibuya et al. 1980) and *c-bas* is a murine counterpart of *c-ras* that appears in sarcoma viruses isolated from rats (Andersen et al. 1981). The reiterative emergence of *c-onc* genes in different virus isolates and from different species suggests that we may have the majority of these genes already in view.

Whatever their number, *c-onc* genes might comprise a family of genes whose interrelationships are akin to those found in the multigene families that encode immunoglobulins, histocompatibility antigens, etc. This suggestion stems from the fact that all *c-onc* genes, however diverse in structure, give rise to viral genes with the dramatic property of oncogenicity in common. In fact, there are reasons to believe that the apparent structural diversity of *c-onc* genes may obscure common origins and related functions: (1) The nucleotide sequences of *v-src* and *v-mos* are very different, yet the amino acid sequence encoded by these genes reveals significant homologies that indicate a common ancestor (Van Beveren et al. 1981a); (2) several different *v-onc* genes (and so far as we know, their *c-onc* genes as well) encode tyrosine protein kinases (Feldman et al. 1980; Reynolds et al. 1980; Witte et al. 1980a; Neil et al. 1981c), and these enzymes may affect similar sets of cellular proteins (Cooper and Hunter 1981a,b; T. Hunter, pers. comm.).

Given the apparent functional relationships among the identified *c-onc* genes, it is of interest to know whether these genes might be clustered or linked in the cellular genome. The available data are in conflict. Fractionation of chicken chromosomes by rate-zonal centrifugation has located *c-src* on one of the smaller macrochromosomes (Padgett et al. 1977; Hughes et al. 1979b), *c-myc* on one of the two or three largest chromosomes (Sheiness et al. 1980b), and *c-erb* on a chromosome of intermediate size (B. Vennstrom, pers. comm.). In contrast, hybridization in situ indicated that *c-src, c-myc, c-myb,* and *c-erb* are all located on one or another of the chicken microchromosomes (Tereba et al. 1979; A. Tereba, pers. comm.). The discrepancies may arise from the fact that the cells used for chromosome fractionation are neoplastic and contain at least one chromosomal translocation. On the other hand, it may not be necessary that all *c-onc* genes be genetically linked. For example, demonstrably related genes (such as α- and β-globin genes and genes whose functions are coordinately induced by estrogen) are located on different chromosomes in the chicken (Hughes et al. 1979b).

I. Mechanisms of Genetic Mimicry: Genesis of Retroviral Oncogenes

By what means have *c-onc* genes been acquired by viral genomes? Two competing answers to this question have emerged:

1. It is possible that each retrovirus arises fully grown from the rearrangement and permutation of cellular genes (Temin 1980). This account is a restatement of Temin's original "protovirus hypothesis" (Temin 1974) and suggests that oncogenes may be present from the inception of certain retroviral genomes.
2. It is more generally assumed that preexistent retroviruses assimilate *c-onc* genes by recombination (Bishop 1981). Several lines of evidence conform to (but do not prove) this explanation. First, large (but never complete) deletions in *v-src* can be repaired by recombination with *c-src* in chickens (see above). It is by no means certain, however, that the mechanism of this recombination provides a general explanation for the transduction of *c-onc* genes. Second, the oncogenes of several murine retroviruses (*v-ras, v-mos,* and *v-abl*) appeared during the passage of leukemia viruses in rodent hosts (Harvey 1964; Moloney 1966; Abelson and Rabstein 1970a,b). We presume, but cannot prove, that here the experimentalist may have reproduced the events that give rise to *v-onc* genes in the wild. Third, several investigators have reported deliberate and apparently successful efforts to transduce *c-onc* genes by infection of cells in tissue culture with retroviruses that do not initially contain oncogenes (Rapp and Todaro 1978, 1980; Rasheed et al. 1978; Stavnezer et al. 1981). These efforts have produced retroviruses with varied and novel oncogenic potentials, but the genetic bases of most of these potentials have yet to be elucidated.

Neither of the preceding views offers a persuasive account of the mechanism by which the transduction of *c-onc* genes actually occurs. The protovirus hypothesis now relies mainly on the possibility that retroviruses are produced by the antics of ancestral transposable elements (Temin 1980). The evidence for this possibility is limited and circumstantial. But we can do little better at suggesting how *c-onc* genes might be recombined into preexistent retroviral genomes. In particular, homologous regions that could facilitate the putative cross have not been identified, and we need to explain how the introns of *c-onc* genes are removed to generate the uninterrupted coding units of *v-onc* genes. Recent work by Goldfarb and Weinberg (1981b) may have provided a pertinent experimental model, however, by demonstrating that retroviruses may participate in illegitimate recombination, so long as RNAs representing the genetic elements to be recombined are first encapsidated and rendered infectious for susceptible host cells.

Other puzzles remain, as well. Is the seizure of *c-onc* genes a unique event, or might retroviruses be generalized transducing agents whose acquisition of more prosaic genes is merely less likely to be perceived? Are there selective pressures that favor the transduction of *c-onc* genes and their retention by retroviral genomes? When oncogenes are formed by fusing *c-onc* to a portion of a viral structural gene (as is frequently the case; see Chapter 4), what portion of the cellular locus actually joins the viral genome and what influence does the hybrid nature of the resulting oncogene essential for oncogenicity? (The hybrid genetic structure appears not to be necessary for tumorigenesis: at least two oncogenes—*v-myc* and *v-myb*—occur as both hybrid genes and as independently expressed loci not fused with *gag*.) And how are we to interpret the unusual nature of the oncogene for SFFV? Is it an exception to an otherwise pervasive rule or does it signify that the origins of retroviral oncogenes are more diverse and more complex than we presently realize?

J. Are *c-onc* Genes Useful to Normal Cells?

It has become an article of faith that *c-onc* genes serve essential purposes in uninfected cells. Why else would these genes have been conserved over long periods of evolutionary time and why else would many of their numbers be expressed in both embryonic and adult tissues? The inference is easy to draw but difficult to explore, and the difficulty lies less with biochemical function than with cellular physiology. Once $pp60^{v\text{-}src}$ was known to be a protein kinase, the demonstration of a similar enzymic activity associated with pp60^{c-src} followed in short order (Collett et al. 1979b; Oppermann et al. 1979; Rohrschneider et al. 1979). But how does this enzymic activity, or for that matter, the biochemical function of any other *c-onc,* serve the metabolism of the normal cell? The question is usually answered by reasoning that the actions of *v-onc* genes mirror the functions of *c-onc* genes. The cell transformed by a retroviral oncogene divides incessantly. Might the homologous proto-oncogene therefore be a normal effector of cell division? Many (perhaps all) retroviral oncogenes arrest, reverse, or otherwise disturb the normal course of cellular differentiation (Graf and Beug 1978; Boettiger and Durban 1980; Maltzman and Levine 1981). Might their counterparts in normal cells be regulators of growth and development and, if so, might the lineages in which they are normally active dictate the kinds of cells that are vulnerable to transformation by the homologous viral oncogenes? Experimental data that relate to these issues are sparse and enigmatic:

1. Since *v-src* transforms fibroblasts, it is conceivable that expression of the cellular homolog *c-src* might vary in concert with changes in cell growth. To date, efforts to sustain this expectation have failed. For example, the expression of *c-src* remained unchanged throughout the course of experiments in which the growth of fibroblasts was first arrested for as long as 2 weeks by serum deprivation and then stimulated by restoration of serum to the growth medium (Spector et al. 1978a).

2. Efforts to discern preferential expression of *c-onc* genes in specific tissues have so far failed to yield coherent results. Some loci (such as *c-src, c-myc,* and *c-erb*) are active at low or intermediate levels across a broad spectrum of tissues, whereas the activities of others (e.g., *c-myb*) are more restricted in their distribution (Table 9.4). In most instances, the distribution of activity does not conform to predictions based on the pathogenicities of the corresponding oncogenes. The most provocative finding at present comes from Scolnick et al. (1981): Primitive hematopoietic cells (pluripotent CFU-S cells), but not cells of other origins, contain large amounts of p21^{c-ras}, a protein whose viral homolog is apparently capable of inducing erythroleukemias as well as sarcomas.

K. Paradox of Neoplastic Transformation by Retroviral Oncogenes

If retroviral oncogenes embody functions found also in normal vertebrate cells, why do the oncogenes induce abnormal phenotypes in infected cells? Two possible answers come to mind. First, transformation by retroviruses may be a consequence of dosage. The virus may overload cells with otherwise normal gene products; sustained and abundant expression of the genes, rather than anomalous properties of their products, may lie at the root of tumorigenesis by *v-onc* genes. Alternatively, *v-onc* genes and *c-onc* genes may differ in subtle but important ways. For example, the protein kinase activity of $pp60^{v\text{-}src}$ might have unique substrate specificities that could account for neoplastic transformation by RSV.

Although the extent of resemblance between *c-onc* genes and *v-onc* genes has yet to be fully measured, several points of evidence suggest that retroviral oncogenes transform cells by means of dosage:

1. The dosage of *v-onc* products is indeed large, when compared with the amounts of *c-onc* products found in most cells; fibroblasts transformed by RSV contain about 100-fold more $pp60^{v\text{-}src}$ than $pp60^{c\text{-}src}$ (Collett et al. 1978; Oppermann et al. 1979), and similar differences have been found for other oncogene and *c-onc* products (Witte et al. 1979b; Langbeheim et al. 1980). The vigor of oncogene expression may be attributable in large measure to the efficacy of the retrovirus promoter for transcription (see Chapter 5).
2. The relatively large dosages of oncogene products are essential to maintain the neoplastic phenotype. On occasion, presently unidentified events in the infected cell can attenuate the synthesis of retroviral RNA and, hence, the expression of viral genes (see Chapter 5). The amounts of oncogene product fall by 10- to 100-fold, and the cell reverts to an ostensibly normal phenotype (Macpherson 1965; Boettiger 1974; Deng et al. 1977; Porzig et al. 1979; Bishop et al. 1980).
3. Molecular clones of two *c-onc* genes (*c-mos* and *c-ras*) have been linked to portions of the MLV genome that encourage viral gene expression (in particular, the LTR). The chimeric DNAs, bearing no portion of a viral oncogene, can transform fibroblasts to a

neoplastic phenotype (Oskarsson et al. 1980; Blair et al. 1981; DeFeo et al. 1981; G. Vande Woude; E. Scolnick; both pers. comm.). Cells transformed in this manner by *c-ras* contain relatively large quantities of the gene product, p21$^{c\text{-}ras}$ (DeFeo et al. 1981; E. Scolnick, pers. comm.), thus sustaining the view that amplification of *c-ras* expression suffices to induce the neoplastic phenotype.

L. Does the Homology between *v-onc* Genes and *c-onc* Genes Dictate the Host Range of Viral Transformation?

Neoplastic transformation by retroviral oncogenes is remarkably specific. Pathogenicity for specific tissues is a distinctive property of each strain of retrovirus. In cell culture, oncogenes display a similarly predictable and generally limited range of susceptible cells that correlates well with the actions of the oncogene in infected animals (Graf and Beug 1978). The origins of target-cell specificity, as this phenomenon is known, are uncertain. It is first of all possible that transformation is merely a reflection of susceptibility to infection by different strains of virus. Inference speaks against this possibility. Viral genes that determine the host range of infectivity (such as *gag* and *env*) are shared among families of retroviruses whose spectra of oncogenicities are very different. Moreover, experimental data indicate that cells can be infected by and produce retroviruses bearing oncogenes without necessarily being transformed (Graf et al. 1980; Durban and Boettiger 1981a). These findings have led to the more subtle suggestion that only certain cells are vulnerable to the effects of each oncogene.

What factors could determine cellular vulnerability to transformation by *v-onc* genes? We do not know, but it has been suggested that the kinship of *v-onc* genes and *c-onc* genes might be responsible. The deleterious effects of oncogene dosage might be restricted to cells in which the homologous *c-onc* is normally expressed and effective; alternatively, cells in which the *c-onc* is not usually active might be more vulnerable to the actions of the oncogene. The available (and admittedly provisional) data do not sustain these views. For example, the pattern of *c-onc* expression illustrated in Table 9.4 in no way reflects the spectrum of susceptibility to the homologous viral oncogenes.

M. Do *c-onc* Genes Provide a Common Pathway for Oncogenesis?

The action of viral oncogenes may provide useful analogs for the enzymic mechanisms that give rise to and sustain the malignant phenotype. But it appears that viruses bearing oncogenes are not usually responsible for tumorigenesis in human beings (Pimentel 1979). We should therefore look to the cell itself if we are ever to discern common origins of malignancy. In particular, we need to identify the events that spark the onset of oncogenesis, and we must determine whether a particular cellular gene (or set of genes) always mediates progression to and maintenance of the malignant phenotype.

We do not know how oncogenesis initiates. The matter has elicited great controversy, with some investigators arguing for mutations (Ames 1979; Epstein and Swartz 1981) and others for chromosomal rearrangements, transpositions of DNA, or even reversible epigenetic events (Rubin 1980; Cairns 1981). In contrast, the discovery of *c-onc* genes may have brought to view genes whose actions can mediate oncogenesis, once the cell has sustained an initiating lesion. We have diverse reasons to suspect the existence of such "cancer genes":

1. A number of malignancies have appeared as heritable traits in human pedigrees (Knudson 1981), and it has even been suggested that each of the roughly 100 types of malignancies will eventually be attributable to abnormalities affecting a specific genetic locus (Knudson 1979, 1981).
2. Several efforts have been made to enumerate the genetic loci that might mediate neoplastic transformation by chemical carcinogens. In most instances, the results implicate no more than a few dozen or a few hundred genes as potential mediators of chemical carcinogenesis (Parodi and Brambilla 1977).
3. DNAs extracted from some lines of chemically transformed cells and from certain tumors induce neoplastic transformation when transferred into cells in culture (C. Shih et al. 1979; Krontiris and Cooper 1981; Shilo and Weinberg 1981a). Caveats are necessary: The efficiency of transformation is generally quite low; transformation occurs reliably in only a few (and empirically recognized) line of recipient cells (e.g., mouse NIH-3T3); and only a limited number of transformed cell lines or tumors have so far yielded DNA capable of inducing neoplastic transformation. But the

data do suggest that DNAs from at least some forms of neoplastic cells contain stable and heritable changes that are responsible for the malignant phenotype. Moreover, provisional studies with restriction endonucleases indicate that the same domain of DNA may be affected in independent tumors of common type and/or common cause (Shilo and Weinberg 1981a).

4. If first sheared to molecular weights of approximately 0.3×10^6 to 3×10^6, even DNA from normal cells can transform NIH-3T3 cells at a very low frequency, and the transformed mouse cells, in turn, yield DNA that can induce transformation at much higher efficiencies (Cooper et al. 1980), as if the original shearing of normal DNA unleashed a potentially oncogenic gene whose action is now stably established in the transformed mouse cells. Activation of the gene has been attributed to disruption of linkage between the oncogenic gene and a *cis*-active regulator (Cooper et al. 1980).

Are *c-onc* genes the cancer genes of normal cells? Is it the induction of their activities that lies at the root of all forms of oncogenesis? Answers to these questions may come eventually from exhaustive surveys of *c-onc* expression in naturally occurring tumors. At present, we have a single but immensely provocative clue, derived from an unexpected source: the study of tumorigenesis by avian leukosis viruses (ALVs).

As explained in detail in Chapter 8, most of the ALV-induced bursal tumors examined to date contained viral DNA integrated in the vicinity of *c-myc,* and as a seeming consequence of the insertions, the expression of the *c-onc* appeared to have been greatly augmented. Detailed analysis of the bursal tumors has produced three conclusions that are important in the present context: Oncogenesis by retroviruses may not always require viral gene products; the frequency with which ALV proviruses are found in the vicinity of *c-myc* implies that the site of insertion figures in the oncogenic mechanism; and it is likely (but by no means proven) that the heightened expression of *c-myc* provokes and/or sustains the chain of events that eventuates in lymphoid leukosis or renal carcinoma. However, the following questions remain:

1. In a few ALV-induced tumors, viral DNA is not inserted near *c-myc* and expression of *c-myc* has not been induced (Hayward et al. 1981; W. Hayward, pers. comm.). Nevertheless, single (or

very few) sites have been used for integration of the ALV provirus in each of these tumors, and it is therefore possible that the insertion of viral DNA has induced the expression of nearby cellular DNA representing an as yet unidentified *c-onc.*

2. The viral oncogene (*v-myc*) derived from *c-myc* has never been reported to cause lymphomas (Moscovici et al. 1978). The implication of *c-myc* in the genesis of B-cell tumors therefore came as a surprise that remains unexplained. However, the induction of lymphomas by ALV follows a protracted course of events that may not spring immediately from the effects of a single gene; the roles of *c-myc* and *v-myc* in oncogenesis may differ greatly. There is evidence to sustain this view (Cooper and Neiman 1980). DNA from lymphoid tumors induced by ALV elicits the neoplastic phenotype when introduced into mouse fibroblasts by transfection. Contrary to expectations, however, the transformed mouse cells contain neither ALV DNA nor *c-myc* derived from the lymphoid tumors (G. Cooper, pers. comm.). Transformation of the fibroblasts must therefore be due to another oncogene, activated in the infected B cells (perhaps by the effects of *c-myc*), and more effective than *c-myc* itself in the transformation of fibroblasts. In this formulation, *c-myc* can be viewed as the initiator of tumorigenesis, the oncogene responsible for transformation of fibroblasts as a potential maintenance function.
3. Is the alleged tumorigenic effect of *c-myc* limited to cells in the B-lymphocyte lineage? Possibly not; for example, provisional data also implicate *c-myc* in the genesis of renal tumors induced by ALV (Cooper and Neiman 1981). It is perhaps significant that these tumors are analogous to the renal carcinomas commonly induced by the action of *v-myc* (Moscovici et al. 1978).
4. Is *c-myc* an inevitable participant in the genesis of B-cell (and perhaps renal) tumors, whatever their initiating cause? The induction of *c-myc* expression has been implicated in lymphomagenesis by another retrovirus that lacks an oncogene, the chicken syncytial virus (CSV) (H.-J. Kung, pers. comm.). Although the CSV genome is not homologous to that of ALV, the similarities of the two viruses are too great to provide a compelling test of the larger issue. The question may be answered properly, however, by forthcoming surveys of *c-myc* expression (as well as expression of other *c-onc* genes) in tumors of various origins.

Do the findings with ALV reveal how other viruses devoid of

oncogenes might cause tumors? The induction of *c-onc* expression by the integration of ALV DNA is a form of insertional mutagenesis, and other integrative viruses are in principal capable of the same. For example, provisional evidence indicates that the integration of RAV-1 DNA in the vicinity of one or both *c-erb* loci may be involved in the genesis of avian erythroblastosis induced by this virus (H.-J. Kung, pers. comm.); and a number of mouse mammary carcinomas induced by mouse mammary tumor virus (MMTV) carry viral DNA integrated in the same domain of cellular DNA (R. Nusse, pers. comm.). Other potential examples abound: the nephroblastoma induced by some strains of MAV-2 (Watts and Smith 1980); the thymic leukemia induced by murine leukemia virus (MLV); the leukemias induced by feline, bovine, and ape leukemia viruses; and further afield, leukemogenesis by SV40 virus, the hepatitis-B virus that has been implicated in the genesis of hepatic carcinoma, and even oncogenesis by herpesviruses. If any of these sundry viruses acts by means of insertional mutagenesis, the sites of integration in the DNA of the tumor cells may finger cancer genes not yet identified by other means. Virologists are in hot pursuit of these possibilities, hoping to expand the catalog of cancer genes and to gain insight into the apparent tissue specificity of their actions.

REFERENCES

Aaronson, S.A. and J.R. Stephenson. 1976. Endogenous type-C RNA viruses of mammalian cells. *Biochim. Biophys. Acta* **458:** 323–354.

Abelson, H.T. and L.S. Rabstein. 1970a. Influence of prednisolone on Moloney leukemogenic virus in BALB/c mice. *Cancer Res.* **30:** 2208–2212.

———. 1970b. Lymphosarcoma: Virus-induced thymic-independent disease in mice. *Cancer Res.* **30:** 2213–2222.

Ames, B.N. 1979. Identifying environmental chemicals causing mutations and cancer. *Science* **204:** 587–593.

Andersen, P.R., S.G. Devare, S.R. Tronick, R.W. Ellis, S.A. Aronson, and E.M. Scolnick. 1981. Generation of BALB-MuSV and Ha-MuSV by type C virus transduction of homologous transforming genes from different species. *Cell* **26:** 129–134.

Anderson, D.D., R.P. Beckman, E.H. Harms, K. Nakamura, and M.J. Weber. 1981. Biological properties of "partial" transformation mutants of Rous sarcoma virus and characterization of their pp60^{src} kinase. *J. Virol.* **37:** 445–458.

Anderson, G.R. and W.P. Kovacik, Jr. 1981. LDH$_K$, an unused oxygen-sensitive lactate dehydrogenase expressed in human cancer. *Proc. Natl. Acad. Sci.* **78:** 3209–3213.

Anderson, G.R., K.R. Marotti, and P.A. Whitaker-Dowling. 1979. A candidate rat-specific gene product of the Kirsten murine sarcoma virus. *Virology* **99:** 31–48.

Andersson, P., M.P. Goldfarb, and R.A. Weinberg. 1979. A defined subgenomic fragment of in vitro synthesized Moloney sarcoma virus DNA can induce cell transformation upon transfection. *Cell* **16:**63–75.

Anderson, S.M., W.S. Hayward, B.G. Neel, and H. Hanafusa. 1980. Avian erythroblastosis virus produces two mRNA's. *J. Virol.* **36:**676–683.

Bader, J.P. 1972. Temperature-dependent transformation of cells infected with a mutant of Bryan Rous sarcoma virus. *J. Virol.* **10:**267–276.

Balduzzi, P.C., M.F.D. Notter, H.R. Morgan and M. Shibuya. 1981. Some biological properties of two new avian sarcoma viruses. *J. Virol.* (in press).

Ball, J.K., J.A. McCarter, and S.M. Sunderland. 1973. Evidence for helper independent murine sarcoma virus. I. Segregation of replication-defective and transformation-defective viruses. *Virology* **56:**268–284.

Baltimore, D., N. Rosenberg, and O.N. Witte. 1979. Transformation of immature lymphoid cells by Abelson murine leukemia virus. *Immunol. Rev.* **48:**3–22.

Baltimore, D., A. Shields, G. Otto, S. Goff, P. Besmer, O. Witte, and N. Rosenberg. 1980. Structure and expression of the Abelson murine leukemia virus genome and its relationship to a normal cell gene. *Cold Spring Harbor Symp. Quant. Biol.* **44:** 849–854.

Barbacid, M. and A.V. Laver. 1981. The gene products of McDonough felme sarcoma virus have an in vitro associated protein kinase that phosphorylates tyrosine residues; lack of detection of this enzymatic activity in vivo. *J. Virol.* (in press).

Barbacid, M., K. Beemon, and S.G. Devare. 1980a. Origin and functional properties of the major gene product of the Snyder-Theilen strain of feline sarcoma virus. *Proc. Natl. Acad. Sci.* **77:**5158–5162.

Barbacid, M., A.V. Lauver, and S.G. Devare. 1980b. Biochemical and immunological characterization of polyproteins coded for by the McDonough, Gardner-Arnstein, and Snyder-Theilen strains of feline sarcoma virus. *J. Virol.* **33:**196–207.

Barbacid, M., L. Donner, S.K. Ruscetti, and C.J. Sherr. 1981a. Transformation-defective mutants of Snyder-Theilen feline sarcoma virus lack tyrosine-specific protein kinase activity. *J. Virol.* **39:**246–254.

Barbacid, M., M.L. Breitman, A.V. Lauver, L.K. Long, and P.K. Vogt. 1981b. The transformation-specific protein of avian (Fujinami and PRC-II) and feline (Snyder-Theilen and Gardner-Arnstein) sarcoma viruses are immunologically related. *Virology* **110:**411–419.

Beemon, K. 1981. Transforming proteins of some feline and avian sarcoma viruses are related structurally and functionally. *Cell* **24:**145–153.

Beemon, K. and T. Hunter. 1977. *In vitro* translation yields a possible Rous sarcoma virus *src* gene product. *Proc. Natl. Acad. Sci.* **74:**3302–3306.

———. 1978. Characterization of Rous sarcoma virus *src* gene products synthesized in vitro. *J. Virol.* **28:**551–566.

Beemon, K., T. Hunter, and B.M. Sefton. 1979. Polymorphism of avian sarcoma virus *src* proteins. *J. Virol.* **30:**190–200.

Ben-Ze'év, A., A. Duerr, F. Solomon, and S. Penman. 1979. The outer boundary of the cytoskeleton: A lamina derived from plasma membrane proteins. *Cell* **17:**859–865.

Beug, H. and T. Graf. 1980. Transformation parameters of chicken embryo fibroblasts infected with the *ts*34 mutant of avian erythroblastosis virus. *Virology* **100:**348–356.

Beug, H., T. Graf, and M.J. Hayman. 1981. Production and characterization of antisera specific for the *erb*-portion of p75, the presumptive transforming protein of avian erythroblastosis virus. *Virology* **111:**201–210.

Beug, H., M. Claviez, B.M. Jockusch, and T. Graf. 1978. Differential expression of Rous sarcoma virus-specific transformation parameters in enucleated cells. *Cell* **14:**843–856.

Beug, H., G. Kitchener, G. Doederlein, T. Graf, and M.J. Hayman. 1980. Mutant of avian erythroblastosis virus defective for erythroblast transformation: Deletion in the *erb* portion of p75 suggests function of the protein in leukemogenesis. *Proc. Natl. Acad. Sci.* **77:**6683–6686.

Beug, H., A. von Kirchbach, G. Doderlein, J.-F. Conscience, and T. Graf. 1979. Chicken hematopoietic cells transformed by seven strains of defective avian leukemia viruses display three distinct phenotypes of differentiation. *Cell* **18:**375–390.

Bishop, J.M. 1981. Enemies within: The genesis of retrovirus oncogenes. *Cell* **23:**5–6.

Bishop, J.M., T. Gonda, S.H. Hughes, D.K. Sheiness, E. Stubblefield, B. Vennstrom, and H.E. Varmus. 1981. The genesis of avian retrovirus oncogenes. *Miami Winter Symp.* **12:**261–273.

Bishop, J.M., S.A. Courtneidge, A.D. Levinson, H. Oppermann, N. Quintrell, D.K. Sheiness, S.R. Weiss, and H.E. Varmus. 1980. Origin and function of avian retrovirus transforming genes. *Cold Spring Harbor Symp. Quant. Biol.* **44:**919–930.

Bister, K. and P.H. Duesberg. 1979a. Structure and specific sequences of avian erythroblastosis virus RNA: Evidence for multiple classes of transforming genes among avian tumor viruses. *Proc. Natl. Acad. Sci.* **76:**5023–5027.

———. 1980. Genetic structure of avian acute leukemia viruses. *Cold Spring Harbor Symp. Quant. Biol.* **44:**801–822.

Bister, K., M.J. Hayman, and P.K. Vogt. 1977. Defectiveness of avian myelocytomatosis virus MC29: Isolation of long-term nonproducer cultures and analysis of virus-specific polypeptide synthesis. *Virology* **82:**431–448.

Bister, K., W.-H. Lee, and P.H. Duesberg. 1980a. Phosphorylation of the nonstructural proteins encoded by three avian acute leukemia viruses and by avian Fujinami sarcoma virus. *J. Virol.* **36:**617–621.

Bister, K., H.C. Loliger, and P.H. Duesberg. 1979. Oligoribonucleotide map and protein of CM II: Detection of conserved and nonconserved genetic elements in avian acute leukemia viruses CMII, MC29, and MH2. *J. Virol.* **32:**208–219.

Bister, K., G. Ramsay, M.J. Hayman, and P.H. Duesberg. 1980b. OK10, an avian acute leukemia virus of the MC29 subgroup with a unique genetic structure. *Proc. Natl. Acad. Sci.* **77:**7142–7146.

Blair, D.G., M.A. Hull, and E.A. Finch. 1979. The isolation and preliminary characterization of temperature-sensitive transformation mutants of Moloney sarcoma virus. *Virology* **95:**303–316.

Blair, D.G., W.L. McClements, M.K. Oskarsson, P.J. Fischinger, and G.F. Vande Woude. 1980. Biological activity of cloned Moloney sarcoma virus DNA: Terminally redundant sequences may enhance transformation efficiency. *Proc. Natl. Acad. Sci.* **77:**3504–3508.

Blair, D.G., M. Oskarsson, T.G. Wood, W.L. McClements, P.J. Fischinger, and G.G. Vande Woude. 1981. Activation of the transforming potential of a normal cell sequence: A molecular model for oncogenesis. *Science* **212:**941–943.

Boettiger, D. 1974. Reversion and induction of Rous sarcoma virus expression in virus-transformed baby hamster kidney cells. *Virology* **62:**522–529.

Boettiger, D. and E.M. Durban. 1980. Progenitor-cell populations can be infected by RNA tumor viruses, but transformation is dependent on the expression of specific differentiated functions. *Cold Spring Harbor Symp. Quant. Biol.* **44:**1249–1254.

Breitman, M.L., M.M.C. Lai, and P.K. Vogt. 1980. The genomic RNA of avian reticuloendotheliosis virus REV. *Virology* **100:**450–461.

Breitman, M.L., J.C. Neil, C. Moscovici, and P.K. Vogt. 1981a. The pathogenicity and defectiveness of PRCII: A new type of avian sarcoma virus. *Virology* **108:**1–12.

Breitman, M.L., A. Hirano, T. Wong, and P.K. Vogt. 1981b. Characteristics of avian sarcoma virus strain PRCIV and comparison with strain PCRII.p. *Virology* (in press).

Brugge, J.S. and R.L. Erikson. 1977. Identification of a transformation-specific antigen induced by an avian sarcoma virus. *Nature* **269:**346–348.

Brugge, J.S., E. Erikson, M.S. Collett, and R.L. Erikson. 1978. Peptide analysis of the transformation-specific antigen from avian sarcoma virus-transformed cells. *J. Virol.* **26:**773–782.

Brugge, J.S., M.S. Collett, A. Siddiqui, B. Marczynska, F. Deinhardt, and R.L. Erikson. 1979. Detection of the viral sarcoma gene product in cells infected with various strains of avian sarcoma virus and of a related protein in uninfected chicken cells. *J. Virol.* **29:**1196–1203.

Bunte, T., M.K. Owada, P. Donner, C.B. Boschek, and K. Moelling. 1981. Association of the transformation-specific protein pp60^{src} with the membrane of an avian sarcoma virus. *J. Virol.* **38:**1034–1047.

Burr, J.G., G. Dreyfuss, S. Penman, and J.M. Buchanan. 1980. Association of the *src* gene product of Rous sarcoma virus with cytoskeletal structures of chicken embryo fibroblasts. *Proc. Natl. Acad. Sci.* **77:**3484–3488.

Cairns, J. 1981. The origin of human cancers. *Nature* **289:**353–357.

Canaani, E., K.C. Robbins, and S.A. Aaronson. 1979. The transforming gene of Moloney murine sarcoma virus. *Nature* **282:**378–383.

Carr, J.G. and J.G. Campbell. 1958. Three new virus-induced fowl sarcomata. *Br. J. Cancer* **12:**631–635.

Chang, E.H., J.M. Maryak, C.-M. Wei, T.Y. Shih, R. Shober, H.L. Cheung, R.W. Ellis, G. Hager, E.M. Scolnick, and D.R. Lowy. 1980. Functional organization of the Harvey murine sarcoma virus genome. *J. Virol.* **35:**76–92.

Chen, J.H. 1980. Expression of endogenous avian myeloblastosis virus information in different chicken cells. *J. Virol.* **36:**162–170.

Chen, J.H., W.S. Hayward, and C. Moscovici. 1981. Size and genetic content of virus-specific RNA in myeloblasts transformed by avian myeloblastosis virus (AMV). *Virology* **110:**128–136.

Chien, Y.-H. and M.M.C. Lai. 1980. Virus RNA species in Kirsten murine sarcoma virus-transformed mink cells. *J. Gen. Virol.* **51:**195–199.

Chiswell, D.J., G. Ramsay, and M.J. Hayman. 1981. Two virus specific RNA species are present in cells transformed by defective leukemia virus OK10. *Virology* (in press).

Coffin, J.M., H.E. Varmus, J.M. Bishop, M. Essex, W.D. Hardy, G.S. Martin, N.E. Rosenberg, E.M. Scolnick, R.A. Weinberg, and P.K. Vogt. 1981. A proposal for naming host cell-derived inserts in retrovirus genomes. *J. Virol.* (in press).

Cohen, R.S., T.L. Wong, and M.M.C. Lai. 1981. Characterization of transformation- and replication-specific sequences of reticuloendotheliosis virus. *Virology* **113:**672–685.

Collett, M.S. and R.L. Erikson. 1978. Protein kinase activity associated with the avian sarcoma virus *src* gene product. *Proc. Natl. Acad. Sci.* **75:**2021–2024.

Collett, M.S., J.S. Brugge, and R.L. Erikson. 1978. Characterization of a normal avian cell protein related to the avian sarcoma virus transforming gene product. *Cell* **15:**1363–1369.

Collett, M.S., E. Erikson, and R.L. Erikson. 1979a. Structural analysis of the avian sarcoma virus transforming protein: Sites of phosphorylation. *J. Virol.* **29:**770–781.

Collett, M.S., A.F. Purchio, and R.L. Erikson. 1980. Avian sarcoma virus-transforming protein pp60^{src} shows protein kinase activity specific for tyrosine. *Nature* **285:** 167–169.

Collett, M.S., E. Erikson, A.F. Purchio, J.S. Brugge, and R.L. Erikson. 1979b. A normal cell protein similar in structure and function to the avian sarcoma virus transforming gene product. *Proc. Natl. Acad. Sci.* **76:**3159–3163.

Cooper, G.M. and P.E. Neiman. 1980. Transforming genes of neoplasms induced by avian lymphoid leukosis viruses. *Nature* **287:**659–660.

———. 1981. Two distinct candidate transforming genes of lymphoid leukosis virus-induced neoplasms. *Nature* **292:**857–858.

Cooper, G.M., S. Okenquist, and L. Silverman. 1980. Transforming activity of DNA of chemically transformed and normal cells. *Nature* **284:**418–421.

Cooper, J.A. and T. Hunter. 1981a. Changes in protein phosphorylation in Rous sarcoma virus-transformed chicken embryo cells. *Mol. Cell. Biol.* **1:**165–178.

———. 1981b. Four different classes of retroviruses induce phosphorylation of tyrosines present in similar cellular proteins. *Mol. Cell. Biol.* **1:**394–407.

Copeland, N.G., A.D. Zelenetz, and G.M. Cooper. 1980. Transformation by subgenomic fragments of Rous sarcoma virus DNA. *Cell* **19:**863–870.

Courtneidge, S.A., A.D. Levinson, and J.M. Bishop. 1980. The protein encoded by the transforming gene of avian sarcoma virus ($pp60^{src}$) and a homologous protein in normal cells ($pp60^{proto-src}$) are associated with the plasma membrane. *Proc. Natl. Acad. Sci.* **77:**3783–3787.

Crawford, L.V. 1980. Transforming genes of DNA tumor viruses. *Cold Spring Harbor Symp. Quant. Biol.* **44:**9–11.

Cremer, K., E.P. Reddy, and S.A. Aaronson. 1981. Translational products of Moloney murine sarcoma virus RNA: Identification of proteins encoded by the murine sarcoma virus *src* gene. *J. Virol.* **38:**704–711.

Czernilofsky, A.P., A.D. Levinson, H.E. Varmus, J.M. Bishop, E. Tischler, and H.M. Goodman. 1980. Nucleotide sequence of an avian sarcoma virus oncogene (*src*) and proposed amino acid sequence for gene product. *Nature* **287:**198–203.

David-Pfeuty, T. and S.J. Singer. 1980. Altered distributions of the cytoskeletal proteins vinculin and α-actinin in cultured fibroblasts transformed by Rous sarcoma virus. *Proc. Natl. Acad. Sci.* **77:**6687–6691.

DeFeo, D., M.A. Gonda, H.A. Young, E.H. Chang, D.R. Lowy, E.M. Scolnick, and R.W. Ellis. 1981. Analysis of two divergent rat genomic clones homologous to the transforming gene of Harvey murine sarcoma virus. *Proc. Natl. Acad. Sci.* **78:**3328–3332.

Deng, C.-T., D. Stehelin, J.M. Bishop, and H.E. Varmus. 1977. Characteristics of virus-specific RNA in avian sarcoma virus-transformed BHK-21 cells and revertants. *Virology* **76:**313–330.

Dina, D. and B. Nadal-Ginard. 1980. Moloney murine sarcoma virions contain subgenomic-length mRNA-like molecules that direct the synthesis of sarcoma-specific polyproteins in vitro. *Cold Spring Harbor Symp. Quant. Biol.* **44:**901–905.

Donoghue, D.J., P.A. Sharp, and R.A. Weinberg. 1979a. Comparative study of different isolates of murine sarcoma virus. *J. Virol.* **32:**1015–1027.

———. 1979b. An MSV-specific subgenomic mRNA in MSV-transformed G8-124 cells. *Cell* **17:**53–63.

Duesberg, P.H. and P.K. Vogt. 1970. Differences between the ribonucleic acids of transforming and nontransforming avian tumor viruses. *Proc. Natl. Acad. Sci.* **67:**1673–1680.

Duesberg, P.H., K. Bister, and C. Moscovici. 1980. Genetic structure of avian myeloblastosis virus, released from transformed myeloblasts as a defective virus particle. *Proc. Natl. Acad. Sci.* **77:**5120–5124.

Durban, E.M. and D. Boettiger. 1981a. Differential effects of transforming avian RNA tumor viruses on avian macrophages. *Proc. Natl. Acad. Sci.* **78:**3600–3604.

———. 1981b. Infection of hematopoietic stem cells by avian myeloblastosis virus results in neo-differentiation of the target cells. *Cell* (in press).

Eckhart, W., M.A. Hutchinson, and T. Hunter. 1979. An activity phosphorylating tyrosine in polyoma T antigen immunoprecipitates. *Cell* **18:**925–933.

Edelman, G.M. 1976. Surface modulation in cell recognition and cell growth. *Science* **192:**218–226.

Eisenman, R.N., M. Linial, M. Groudine, R. Shackh, S. Brown, and P.E. Nieman. 1980. Recombination in the avian oncovirus as a model for the generation of defective transforming viruses. *Cold Spring Harbor Symp. Quant. Biol.* **44:**1235–1247.

Ellerman, V. and O. Bang. 1908. Experimentelle Leukamie bei Huhnern. *Centralbl. Bakteriol.* **46:**595–609 (Abstr.).

Ellis, R.W., D. DeFeo, J.M. Maryak, H.A. Young, T.Y. Shih, E.H. Chang, D.R. Lowy, and

E.M. Scolnick. 1980. Dual evolutionary origin for the rat genetic sequences of Harvey murine sarcoma virus. *J. Virol.* **36:**408–420.

Ellis, R.W., D. DeFeo, T.Y. Shih, M.A. Gonda, H.A. Young, N. Tsvchida, D.R. Lowy, and E.M. Scolnick. 1981. The p21 *src* genes of Harvey and Kirsten sarcoma viruses originate from divergent members of a family of normal vetebrate genes. *Nature* **292:**506–511.

Epstein, S.S. and J.B. Swartz. 1981. Fallacies of lifestyle cancer theories. *Nature* **289:** 127–130.

Erikson, E. and R.L. Erikson. 1980. Identification of a cellular protein substrate phosphorylated by the avian sarcoma virus-transforming gene product. *Cell* **21:**829–836.

Erikson, E., M.S. Collett, and R.L. Erikson. 1978. *In vitro* synthesis of a functional avian sarcoma virus transforming-gene product. *Nature* **274:**919–921.

Erikson, E., R. Cook, G.J. Miller, and R.L. Erikson. 1981. The same normal cell protein is phosphorylated after transformation by avian sarcoma viruses with unrelated transforming genes. *Mol. Cell. Biol.* **1:**43–50.

Erikson, R.L., M.S. Collett, E. Erikson, and A.F. Purchio. 1979. Evidence that the avian sarcoma virus transforming gene product is a cyclic AMP-independent protein kinase. *Proc. Natl. Acad. Sci.* **76:**6260–6264.

Favera, R.D., E.P. Gelmann, R.C. Gallo, and F. Wong-Staal. 1981. A human *onc* gene homologous to the transforming gene (v-*sis*) of simian sarcoma virus. *Nature* **292:**31–35.

Feldman, R.A., T. Hanafusa, and H. Hanafusa. 1980. Characterization of protein kinase activity associated with the transforming gene product of Fujinami sarcoma virus. *Cell* **22:**757–765.

Franchini, G., J. Even, C.J. Sherr, and F. Wong-Staal. 1981. *onc* sequences (v-*fes*) of Snyder-Theilen feline sarcoma virus are derived from noncontiguous regions of a cat cellular gene (c-*fes*). *Nature* **290:**154–157.

Frankel, A.E. and P.J. Fischinger. 1976. Nucleotide sequences in mouse DNA and RNA specific for Moloney sarcoma virus. *Proc. Natl. Acad. Sci.* **73:**3705–3709.

———. 1977. Rate of divergence of cellular sequences homologous to segments of Moloney sarcoma virus. *J. Virol.* **21:**153–160.

Frankel, A.E., R.L. Neubauer, and P.J. Fischinger. 1976. Fractionation of DNA nucleotide transcripts from Moloney sarcoma virus and isolation of sarcoma virus-specific complementary DNA. *J. Virol.* **18:**481–490.

Frankel, A.E., J.H. Gilbert, K.J. Porzig, E.M. Scolnick, and S.A. Aaronson. 1979. Nature and distribution of feline sarcoma virus nucleotide sequences. *J. Virol.* **30:**821–827.

Freeman, A.E., R.V. Gilden, M.L. Vernon, R.G. Wolford, P.E. Hugunin, and R.J. Huebner. 1973. 5-bromo-2′-deoxyuridine potentiation of transformation of rat-embryo cells induced *in vitro* by 3-methylcholanthrene: Induction of rat leukemia virus gs antigen in transformed cells. *Proc. Natl. Acad. Sci.* **70:**2415–2419.

Fulton, A.B., K.M. Wan, and S. Penman. 1980. The spatial distribution of polyribosomes in 3T3 cells and the associated assembly of proteins into the skeletal framework. *Cell* **20:**849–857.

Fujinami, A. and K. Inamoto. 1914. Ueber Geschwulste bei japanischen Haushuhern, insbesondere uber einen transplantablen Tumor. z. *Krebsforsch.* **14:**94–119.

Gardner, M.B., R.W. Rongey, P. Arnstein, J.B. Estes, P. Sarma, R.J. Huebner, and C.G. Rickard. 1970. Experimental transmission of feline fibrosarcoma to cats and dogs. *Nature* **226:**807–809.

Gazdar, A.F., H.C. Chopra, and P.S. Sarma. 1972. Properties of a murine sarcoma virus isolated from a tumor arising in an NZW/NZB F_1 hybrid mouse. I. Isolation and pathology of tumors induced in rodents. *Int. J. Cancer* **9:**219–233.

Gelmann, E.P., F. Wong-Staal, R.A. Kramer, and R.G. Gallo. 1981. Molecular cloning and comparative analyses of the genomes of simian sarcoma virus and its associated helper virus. *Procl. Natl. Acad. Sci.* **78:**3373–3377.

Ghysdael, J., J.C. Neil, and P.K. Vogt. 1981a. A third class of avian sarcoma viruses, defined by related transformation-specific proteins of Yamaguchi 73 and Esh sarcoma virus. *Proc. Natl. Acad. Sci.* **78:**2611–2615.

———. 1981b. Cleavage of four avian sarcoma virus polyproteins with virion protease p15 removes *gag* sequences and yields large fragments that function as tyrosine phosphoacceptors *in vitro. Proc. Natl. Acad. Sci.* (in press).

Ghysdael, J., J.C. Neil, A.M. Wallbank, and P.K. Vogt. 1981c. Esh avian sarcoma virus codes for a *gag*-linked transformation-specific protein with an associated protein kinase activity. *Virology* **111:**386–400.

Goff, S.P., E. Gilboa, O.N. Witte, and D. Baltimore. 1980. Structure of the Abelson murine leukemia virus genome and the homologous cellular gene: Studies with cloned viral DNA. *Cell* **22:**777–785.

Goff, S.P., O.N. Witte, E. Gilboa, N. Rosenberg, and D. Baltimore. 1981. Genome structure of Abelson murine leukemia virus variants: Proviruses in fibroblasts and lymphoid cells. *J. Virol.* **38:**460–468.

Goldfarb, M.P. and R.A. Weinberg. 1981a. Structure of the provirus within NIH 3T3 cells transfected with Harvey sarcoma virus DNA. *J. Virol.* **38:**125–135.

———. 1981b. Generation of novel, biologically active Harvey sarcoma virus via apparent illegitimate recombination. *J. Virol.* **38:**136–150.

Gonda, M.A., N.R. Rice, and R.V. Gilden. 1980. Avian reticuloendotheliosis virus: Characterization of the high-molecular-weight viral RNA in transforming and helper virus populations. *J. Virol.* **34:**743–751.

Gonda, T.J., D.K. Sheiness, L. Fanshier, J.M. Bishop, C. Moscovici, and M.G. Moscovici. 1981. The genome and the intracellular RNAs of avian myeloblastosis virus. *Cell* **23:**279–290.

Graf, T. and H. Beug. 1978. Avian leukemia viruses. Interaction with their target cells in vivo and in vitro. *Biochim. Biophys. Acta* **516:**269–299.

Graf, T., N. Ade, and H. Beug. 1978. Temperature-sensitive mutant of avian erythroblastosis virus suggests a block of differentiation as mechanism of leukeamogenesis. *Nature* **257:**496–501.

Graf, T., H. Beug, and M.J. Hayman. 1980. Target cell specificity of defective avian leukemia viruses: Hematopoietic target cells for a given virus type can be infected but not transformed by strains of a different type. *Proc. Natl. Acad. Sci.* **77:**389–393.

Graf, T., N. Oker-Blom, T.G. Todorov, and H. Beug. 1979. Transforming capacities and defectiveness of avian leukemia viruses OK10 and E26. *Virology* **99:**431–436.

Greaves, M. and G. Janossy. 1978. Patterns of gene expression and the cellular origins of human leukaemias. *Biochim. Biophys. Acta* **516:**193–230.

Gross, L. 1970. *Oncogenic viruses.* Pergamon Press, New York.

Hanafusa, H. 1977. Cell transformation by RNA tumor viruses. In *Comprehensive virology* (ed. H. Fraenkel-Conrat and R.P. Wagner), vol. 10, pp. 401–483. Plenum Press, New York.

Hanafusa, H., C.C. Halpern, D.L. Buchhagen, and S. Kawai. 1977. Recovery of avian sarcoma virus from tumors induced by transformation-defective mutants. *J. Exp. Med.* **146:**1735–1747.

Hanafusa, T., L.-H. Wang, S.M. Anderson, R.E. Karess, W.S. Hayward, and H. Hanafusa. 1980. Characterization of the transforming gene of Fujinami sarcoma virus. *Proc. Natl. Acad. Sci.* **77:**3009–3013.

Hanafusa, T., B. Mathey-Prevot, R.A. Feldman, and H. Hanafusa. 1981. Mutants of Fujinami sarcoma virus which are temperature-sensitive for cellular transformation and protein kinase activity. *J. Virol.* **38:**347–355.

Harvey, J.J. 1964. An unidentified virus which causes the rapid production of tumours in mice. *Nature* **204:**1104–1105.

Hayman, M.J., G. Kitchener, and T. Graf. 1979a. Cells transformed by avian myelocytomatosis virus strain CMII contain a 90K *gag*-related protein. *Virology* **98:**191–199.

Hayman, M.J., B. Royer-Pokora, and T. Graf. 1979b. Defectiveness of avian erythroblastosis virus: Synthesis of a 75K *gag*-related protein. *Virology* **92:**31–45.

Hayward, W.S., B.G. Neel, and S.M. Astrin. 1981. Activation of a cellular *onc* gene by promoter insertion in ALV-induced lymphoid leukosis. *Nature* **290:**475–480.

Hirano, A. and P.K. Vogt. 1981. Avian sarcoma virus PRCII: Conditional mutants temperature sensitive in the maintenance of fibroblast transformation. *Virology* **109:**193–197.

Horn, J.P., T.G. Wood, E.C. Murphy, D.G. Blair, and R.B. Arlinghaus. 1981. A selective temperature-sensitive defect in viral RNA production in cells infected with a ts mutant of murine sarcoma virus. *Cell* **25:**37–46.

Hu, S., N. Davidson, and I.M. Verma. 1977. A heteroduplex study of the sequence relationships between the RNAs of M-MSV and M-MLV. *Cell* **10:**469–477.

Hu, S.S.F., C. Moscovici, and P.K. Vogt. 1978. The defectiveness of Mill Hill 2, a carcinoma-inducing avian oncovirus. *Virology* **89:**162–178.

Huebner, R.J. and G.J. Todaro. 1969. Oncogenes of RNA tumor viruses as determinants of cancer. *Proc. Natl. Acad. Sci.* **64:**1087–1094.

Hughes, S.H., P.K. Vogt, E. Stubblefield, H. Robinson, J.M. Bishop and H.E. Varmus. 1980. Organization of endogenous and exogenous viral and linked non viral sequences. *Cold Spring Harbor Symp. Quant. Biol.* **44:**1077–1089.

Hughes, S.H., F. Payvar, D. Spector, R.T. Schimke, H.L. Robinson, G.S. Payne, J.M. Bishop, and H.E. Varmus. 1979a. Heterogeneity of genetic loci in chickens: Analysis of endogenous viral and nonviral genes by cleavage of DNA with restriction endonucleases. *Cell* **18:**347–359.

Hughes, S.H., E. Stubblefield, F. Payvar, J.D. Engel, J.B. Dodgson, D. Spector, B. Cordell, R.T. Schimke, and H.E. Varmus. 1979b. Gene localization by chromosome fractionation: Globin genes are on at least two chromosomes and three estrogen-inducible genes are on three chromosomes. *Proc. Natl. Acad. Sci.* **76:**1348–1352.

Hunter, T. and B.M. Sefton. 1980. Transforming gene product of Rous sarcoma virus phosphorylates tyrosine. *Proc. Natl. Acad. Sci.* **77:**1311–1315.

Itohara, S., K. Hirata, M. Inoue, M. Hatsuoka, and A. Sato. 1978. Isolation of a sarcoma virus from a spontaneous chicken tumor. *Gann* **69:**825–830.

Jones, M., R.A. Bosselman, V.J.F. Houtin, A. Berub, H. Fan, and I.M. Verma. 1980. Identification and molecular cloning of Moloney mouse sarcoma virus-specific sequences from uninfected mouse cells. *Proc. Natl. Acad. Sci.* **77:**2651–2655.

Kamine, J. and J.M. Buchanan. 1977. Cell-free synthesis of two proteins unique to RNA of transforming virions of Rous sarcoma virus. *Proc. Natl. Acad. Sci.* **74:**2011–2015.

———. 1978. Processing of 60,000-dalton *sarc* gene protein synt hesized by cell-free translation. *Proc. Natl. Acad. Sci.* **75:**4399–4403.

Kamine, J., J.G. Burr, and J.M. Buchanan. 1978. Multiple forms of *sarc* gene proteins from Rous sarcoma virus RNA. *Proc. Natl. Acad. Sci.* **75:**366–370.

Karess, R.E. and H. Hanafusa. 1981. Viral and cellular *src* genes contribute to the structure of recovered avian sarcoma virus transforming protein. *Cell* **24:**155–164.

Karess, R.E., W.S. Hayward, and H. Hanafusa. 1979. Cellular information in the genome of recovered avian sarcoma virus directs the synthesis of transforming protein. *Proc. Natl. Acad. Sci.* **76:**3154–3158.

Kawai, S., P.H. Duesberg, and H. Hanafusa. 1977. Transformation-defective mutants of Rous sarcoma virus with *src* gene deletions of varying length. *J. Virol.* **24:**910–914.

Kawai, S., M. Yoshida, K. Segawa, H. Sugiyama, R. Ishizaki, and K. Toyoshima. 1980. Characterization of Y73, an avian sarcoma virus: A unique transforming gene and its product, a phosphopolyprotein with protein kinase activity. *Proc. Natl. Acad. Sci.* **77:**6199–6203.

Kitchener, G. and M.J. Hayman. 1980. Comparative tryptic peptide mapping studies suggest a role in cell transformation for the *gag*-related proteins of avian erythroblastosis virus and avian myelocytomatosis virus strains CMII and MC29. *Proc. Natl. Acad. Sci.* **77:** 1637–1642.

Knudson, A.G. Jr. 1979. Persons at high risks of cancer. *N. Engl. J. Med.* **301:** 606–607.

———. 1981. Human cancer genes. In *Genes, chromosomes, and neoplasia* (ed. F.E. Arrighi et al.), pp. 453–462. Raven Press, New York.

Krebs, E.G. and J.A. Beavo. 1979. Phosphorylation-dephosphorylation of enzymes. *Annu. Rev. Biochem.* **48:** 923–959.

Krontiris, T.G. and G.M. Cooper. 1981. Transforming activity of human tumor DNAs. *Proc. Natl. Acad. Sci.* **78:** 1181–1184.

Krueger, J.G., E. Wang, and A.R. Goldberg. 1980a. Evidence that the *src* gene product of Rous sarcoma virus is membrane associated. *Virology* **101:** 25–40.

Krueger, J.G., E. Wang, E.A. Garber, and A.R. Goldberg. 1980b. Differences in intracellular location of $pp60^{src}$ in rat and chicken cells transformed by Rous sarcoma virus. *Proc. Natl. Acad. Sci.* **77:** 4142–4146.

Lai, M.M.C., S.S.F. Hu, and P.K. Vogt. 1979. Avian erythroblastosis virus: Transformation-specific sequences from a contiguous segment of 3.25 kb located in the middle of the 6-kb genome. *Virology* **97:** 366–377.

Lai, M.M.C., J.C. Neil, and P.K. Vogt. 1980. Cell-free translation of avian erythroblastosis virus RNA yields two specific and distinct proteins with molecular weights of 75,000 and 40,000. *Virology* **100:** 475–483.

Lai, M.M.C., P.H. Duesberg, J. Horst, and P.K. Vogt. 1973. Avian tumor virus RNA: A comparison of three sarcoma viruses and their transformation-defective derivatives by oligonucleotide fingerprinting and DNA-RNA hybridization. *Proc. Natl. Acad. Sci.* **70:** 2266–2270.

Langbeheim, H., T.Y. Shih, and E.M. Scolnick. 1980. Identification of a normal vertebrate cell protein related to the p21 *src* of Harvey murine sarcoma virus. *Virology* **106:** 292–300.

Lee, J.S., H.E. Varmus, and J.M. Bishop. 1979. Virus-specific messenger RNAs in permissive cells infected by avian sarcoma virus. *J. Biol. Chem.* **254:** 8015–8022.

Lee, W.-H., M. Nunn, and P.H. Duesberg. 1981. *src* genes of ten Rous sarcoma virus strains, including two reportedly transduced from the cell, are completely allelic; putative markers of transduction are not detected. *J. Virol.* **39:** 758–766.

Lee, W.-H., K. Bister, A. Pawson, T. Robins, C. Moscovici, and P.H. Duesberg. 1980. Fujinami sarcoma virus: An avian RNA tumor virus with a unique transforming gene. *Proc. Natl. Acad. Sci.* **77:** 2018–2022.

Lerner, R.A., J.G. Sutcliffe, and T.M. Shinnick. 1981. Antibodies to chemically synthesized peptides predicted from DNA sequences as probes of gene expression. *Cell* **23:** 309–310.

Levinson, A.D., S.A. Courtneidge, and J.M. Bishop. 1981. Structural and functional domains of the Rous sarcoma virus transforming protein ($pp60^{src}$). *Proc. Natl. Acad. Sci.* **78:** 1624–1628.

Levinson, A.D., H. Oppermann, H.E. Varmus, and J.M. Bishop. 1980. The purified product of the transforming gene of avian sarcoma virus phosphorylates tyrosine. *J. Biol. Chem.* **255:** 11973–11980.

Levinson, A.D., H. Oppermann, L. Levintow, H.E. Varmus, and J.M. Bishop. 1978. Evidence that the transforming gene of avian sarcoma virus encodes a protein kinase associated with a phosphoprotein. *Cell* **15:** 561–572.

Lewis, R.B., J. McClure, B. Rup, D.W. Neisel, R.F. Garvey, J.D. Hoelzer, K. Nazarian, and H.R. Bose, Jr. 1981. Avian reticuloendotheliosis virus: Identification of the hematopoietic target cell for transformation. *Cell* **25:** 421–431.

Lyons, D.D., E.C. Murphy, Jr., S.-M. Wong, and R.B. Arlinghaus. 1980. The translation products of Moloney murine sarcoma virus-124 RNA. *Virology* **105:**60–70.

Macpherson, I.A. 1965. Reversion in hamster cells transformed by Rous sarcoma virus. *Science* **148:**1731–1733.

Maltzman, W. and A.J. Levine. 1981. Viruses as probes for development and differentiation. *Adv. Virus Res.* **26:**65–116.

Maness, P.F., H. Engeser, M.E. Greenberg, M. O'Farrell, W.E. Gall, and G.M. Edelman. 1979. Characterization of the protein kinase activity of avian sarcoma virus *src* gene product. *Proc. Natl. Acad. Sci.* **76:**5028–5032.

Martin, G.S. 1970. Rous sarcoma virus: A function required for the maintenance of the transformed state. *Nature* **227:**1021–1023.

Martin, G.S. and P.H. Duesberg. 1972. The *a* subunit in the RNA of transforming avian tumor viruses: I. Occurence in different virus strains. II. Spontaneous loss resulting in nontransforming variants. *Virology* **47:**494–497.

Martin, R.G. 1981. The transformation of cell growth and transmogrification of DNA synthesis by simian virus 40. *Adv. Cancer Res.* **34:**1–68.

McDonough, S.K., S. Larsen, R.S. Brodey, N.D. Stock, and W.D. Hardy Jr. 1971. A transmissible feline fibrosarcoma of viral origin. *Cancer Res.* **31:**953–956.

Mellon, P., A. Pawson, K. Bister, G.S. Martin, and P.H. Duesberg. 1978. Specific RNA sequences and gene products of MC29 avian acute leukemia virus. *Proc. Natl. Acad. Sci.* **75:**5874–5878.

Moloney, J.B. 1966. A virus-induced rhabdomyosarcoma of mice. *Natl. Cancer Inst. Monogr.* **22:**139–142.

Moscovici, C. 1975. Leukemic transformation with avian myeloblastosis virus: Present status. *Curr. Top. Microbiol. Immunol.* **71:**79–101.

Moscovici, C., R.W. Alexander, M.G. Moscovici, and P.K. Vogt. 1978. Transforming and oncogenic effects of MH-2 virus. In *Avian RNA tumor viruses* (ed. S. Barlati and C. De Giuli-Morghen), pp. 45–56. Piccin, Padua.

Moscovici, C., J. Samurat, L. Gazzolo, and M.G. Moscovici. 1981. Myeloid and erythroid responses to avian defective leukemia viruses in chickens and quail. *Virology* **113:**765–768.

Neil, J.C., M.L. Breitman, and P.K. Vogt. 1981a. Characterization of a 105,000 molecular weight *gag*-related phosphoprotein from cells transformed by the defective avian sarcoma virus PRCII. *Virology* **108:**98–110.

Neil, J.C., J.F. Delamarter, and P.K. Vogt. 1981b. Evidence for three classes of avian sarcoma viruses: Comparison of the transformation-specific proteins of PRCII, Y73, and Fujinami viruses. *Proc. Natl. Acad. Sci.* **78:**1906–1910.

Neil, J.C., J. Ghysdael, and P.K. Vogt. 1981c. Tyrosine-specific protein kinase activity associated with p105 of avian sarcoma virus PRCII. *Virology* **109:**223–228.

Neil, J.C., J. Ghysdael, P.K. Vogt, and J.E. Smart. 1981d. Homologous tyrosine phosphorylation sites in transformation-specific gene products of distinct avian sarcoma viruses. *Nature* **291:**675–677.

O'Farrell, P.Z., H.M. Goodman, and P.H. O'Farrell. 1977. High resolution two-dimensional electrophoresis of basic as well as acidic proteins. *Cell* **12:**1133–1142.

Oliff, A., D. Linemeyer, S. Ruscetti, R. Lowe, D.R. Lowy, and E. Scolnick. 1980. Subgenomic fragment of molecularly cloned Friend murine leukemia virus DNA contains the gene(s) responsible for Friend murine leukemia virus-induced disease. *J. Virol.* **35:**924–936.

Oppermann, H., W. Levinson, and J.M. Bishop. 1981a. A cellular protein that associates with the transforming protein of Rous sarcoma virus is also a heat-shock protein. *Proc. Natl. Acad. Sci.* **78:**1067–1071.

Oppermann, H., A.D. Levinson, and H.E. Varmus. 1981b. The structure and protein kinase activity of proteins encoded by nonconditional mutants and back mutants in the *src* gene of avian sarcoma virus. *Virology* **108:**47–70.

Oppermann, H., A.D. Levinson, H.E. Varmus, L. Levintow, and J.M. Bishop. 1979. Uninfected vertebrate cells contain a protein that is closely related to the product of the avian sarcoma virus transforming gene (*src*). *Proc. Natl. Acad. Sci.* **76:**1804–1808.

Oppermann, H., A.D. Levinson, L. Levintow, H.E. Varmus, J.M. Bishop, S. Kawai. 1981c. Two cellular proteins that immunoprecipitate with the transforming protein of Rous sarcoma virus. *Virology* **113:**736–751.

Oskarsson, M., W.L. McClements, D.G. Blair, J.V. Maizel, and G.F. Vande Woude. 1980. Properties of a normal mouse cell DNA sequence (sarc) homologous to the src sequence of Moloney sarcoma virus. *Science* **207:**1222–1224.

Padgett, T.G., E. Stubblefield, and H.E. Varmus. 1977. Chicken macrochromosomes contain an endogenous provirus and microchromosomes contain sequences related to the transforming gene of ASV. *Cell* **10:**649–657.

Papkoff, J., T. Hunter, and K. Beemon. 1980. *In vitro* translation of virion RNA from Moloney murine sarcoma virus. *Virology* **101:**91–103.

Papkoff, J., M.H.T. Lai, T. Hunter, and I.M. Verma. 1981. Analysis of transforming gene products of Moloney murine sarcoma virus. *Cell* (in press).

Parker, R.C., H.E. Varmus, and J.M. Bishop. 1981. The cellular homologue (c-*src*) of the transforming gene of Rous sarcoma virus: Isolation, mapping, and transcriptional analysis of c-*src* and flanking regions. *Proc. Natl. Acad. Sci.* (in press).

Parks, W.P. and E.M. Scolnick. 1977. In vitro translation of Harvey murine sarcoma virus RNA. *J. Virol.* **22:**711–719.

Parodi, S. and G. Brambilla. 1977. Relationship between mutation and transformation frequencies in mammalian cells treated *in vitro* with chemical carcinogens. *Mutat. Res.* **47:**53–74.

Patchinsky, T. and B.M. Sefton. 1981. Evidence that there exist four classes of RNA tumor viruses which encode proteins with associated protein kinase activities. *J. Virol.* **38:**104–144.

Pawson, T. and G.S. Martin. 1980. Cell-free translation of avian erythroblastosis virus RNA. *J. Virol.* **34:**280–284.

Pawson, T., J. Guyden, T.-H. Kung, K. Radke, T. Gilmore, and G.S. Martin. 1980. A strain of Fujinami sarcoma virus which is temperature-sensitive in protein phosphorylation and cellular transformation. *Cell* **22:**767–775.

Philipson, L., P. Andersson, U. Olshevsky, R. Weinberg, D. Baltimore, and R. Gesteland. 1978. Translation of MuLV and MSV RNAs in nuclease-treated reticulocyte extracts: Enhancement of the gag-pol polypeptide with yeast suppressor tRNA. *Cell* **13:**189–199.

Pimentel, F. 1979. Human oncovirology. *Biochim. Biophys. Acta* **560:**169–216.

Porzig, K.J., K.C. Robbins, and S.A. Aaronson. 1979. Cellular regulation of mammalian sarcoma virus expression: A gene regulation model for oncogenesis. *Cell* **16:**875–884.

Purchio, A.F., E. Erikson, and R.L. Erikson. 1977. Translation of 35S and of subgenomic regions of avian sarcoma virus RNA. *Proc. Natl. Acad. Sci.* **74:**4661–4665.

Purchio, A.F., S. Jovanovich, and R.E. Erickson. 1980. Sites of synthesis of viral proteins in avian sarcoma virus-infected chicken cells. *J. Virol.* **35:**629–636.

Purchio, A.F., E. Erikson, J.S. Brugge, and R.L. Erikson. 1978. Identification of a polypeptide encoded by the avian sarcoma virus *src* gene. *Proc. Natl. Acad. Sci.* **75:**1567–1571.

Racker, E. 1981. Letter: Working effect revisited. *Science* **213:**1313.

Racker, E. and M. Spector. 1981. Warburg effect revisited: Merger of biochemistry and molecular biology. *Science* **213:**303–307.

Radke, K. and G.S. Martin. 1979. Transformation by Rous sarcoma virus: Effects of *src* gene expression on the synthesis and phosphorylation of cellular polypeptides. *Proc. Natl. Acad. Sci.* **76:**5212–5216.

Radke, K., T. Gilmore, and G.S. Martin. 1980. Transformation by Rous sarcoma virus: A cellular substrate for transformation-specific protein phosphorylation contains phosphotyrosine. *Cell* **21:**821–828.

Ramsay, G. and M.J. Hayman. 1980. Analysis of cells transformed by defective leukemia virus OK 10: Production of non infectious particles and synthesis of $Pr76^{gag}$ and an additional 200,000-dalton protein. *Virology* **106:**71–81.

Ramsay, G., T. Graf, and M.J. Hayman. 1980. Mutants of avian myelocytomatosis virus MC29 with smaller *gag* gene-related proteins have an altered transforming ability. *Nature* **288:**170–172.

Rapp, U.R. and G.J. Todaro. 1978. Generation of new mouse sarcoma viruses in cell culture. *Science* **201:**821–824.

———. 1980. Generation of oncogenic mouse type-C viruses: *In vitro* selection of carcinoma-inducing variants. *Proc. Natl. Acad. Sci.* **77:**624–628.

Rasheed, S., M.G. Gardner, and R.I. Huebner. 1978. In vitro isolation of stable rat sarcoma viruses. *Proc. Natl. Acad. Sci.* **75:**2972–2976.

Reddy, E.P., M.J. Smith, E. Canaani, K.C. Robbins, S.R. Tronick, S. Zain, and S.A. Aaronson. 1980. Nucleotide sequence analysis of the transforming region and large terminal redundancies of Moloney murine sarcoma virus. *Proc. Natl. Acad. Sci.* **77:**5234–5238.

Rettenmeier, C.W., S.M. Anderson, M.W. Riemen, and H. Hanafusa. 1979. *gag*-related polypeptides encoded by replication-defective avian oncoviruses. *J. Virol.* **32:**749–761.

Reynolds, F.H., Jr., T.L. Sacks, D.N. Deobagkar, and J.R. Stephenson. 1978. Cells nonproductively transformed by Abelson murine leukemia virus express a high molecular weight polyprotein containing structural and nonstructural components. *Proc. Natl. Acad. Sci.* **75:**3974–3978.

Reynolds, F.H., Jr., W.J.M. Van de Ven, and J.R. Stephenson. 1980. Feline sarcoma virus P115-associated protein kinase phosphorylates tyrosine. Identification of a cellular substrate conserved during evolution. *J. Biol. Chem.* **255:**11040–11047.

Reynolds, F.H., Jr., W.J.M. Van de Ven, J. Blomberg, and J.R. Stephenson. 1981a. Involvement of a high-molecular-weight polyprotein translational product of Snyder-Theilen feline sarcoma virus in malignant transformation. *J. Virol.* **37:**643–653.

Reynolds, F.H., W.J.M. Vande Ven, J. Blomberg, and J.R. Stephenson. 1981b. Differences in mechanisms of transformation by independent feline sarcoma virus isolates. *J. Virol.* **38:**1084–1089.

Richert, N.D., P.J.A. Davies, G. Jay, and I.H. Pastan. 1979. Characterization of an immune complex kinase in immunoprecipitates of avian sarcoma virus-transformed fibroblasts. *J. Virol.* **31:**695–706.

Robbins, K.C., S.G. Devare, and S.A. Aaronson. 1981. Molecular cloning of integrated simian sarcoma virus: Genome organization of infectious DNA clones. *Proc. Natl. Acad. Sci.* **78:**2918–2922.

Robinson, H.L. 1978. Inheritance and expression of chicken genes that are related to avian leukosis sarcoma virus genes. *Curr. Top. Microbiol. Immunol.* **83:**1–36.

Rohrschneider, L.R. 1979. Immunofluorescence on avian sarcoma virus-transformed cells: Localization of the *src* gene product. *Cell* **16:**11–24.

———. 1980. Adhesion plaques of Rous sarcoma virus-transformed cells contain the *src* gene product. *Proc. Natl. Acad. Sci.* **77:**3514–3518.

Rohrschneider, L.R., R.N. Eisenman, and C.R. Leitch. 1979. Identification of a Rous sarcoma virus transformation-related protein in normal avian and mammalian cells. *Proc. Natl. Acad. Sci.* **76:**4479–4483.

Rosenberg, N. and D. Baltimore. 1976. A quantitative assay for transformation of bone marrow cells by Abelson murine leukemia virus. *J. Exp. Med.* **143:**1453–1463.

———. 1980. Abelson virus. In *Viral oncology* (ed. G. Klein), pp. 187–203. Raven Press, New York.

Rosenberg, N. and O.N. Witte. 1980. Abelson murine leukemia virus mutants with alterations in the virus-specific P120 molecule. *J. Virol.* **33:**340–348.

Rosenberg, N., D. Baltimore, and C.D. Scher. 1975. *In vitro* transformation of lymphoid cells by Abelson murine leukemia virus. *Proc. Natl. Acad. Sci.* **72:**1932–1936.

Rosenberg, N.E., D.R. Clark, and O.N. Witte. 1980. Abelson murine leukemia virus mutants deficient in kinase activity and lymphoid cell transformation. *J. Virol.* **36:**766–774.

Rous, P. 1911. A sarcoma of the fowl transmissible by an agent separable from the tumor cells. *J. Exp. Med.* **13:**397–411.

Roussel, M., S. Saule, C. Lagrou, C. Rommens, H. Beug, T. Graf, and D. Stehelin. 1979. Three new types of viral oncogene of cellular origin specific for haematopoietic cell transformation. *Nature* **281:**452–455.

Rowe, W.P. 1973. Genetic factors in the natural history of murine leukemia virus infection. *Cancer Res.* **33:**3061–3068.

Royer-Pokora, B., S. Grieser, H. Beug, and T. Graf. 1979. Mutant avian erythroblastosis virus with restricted target cell specificity. *Nature* **282:**750–752.

Rubin, C.S. and O.M. Rosen. 1975. Protein phosphorylation. *Annu. Rev. Biochem.* **44:**831–887.

Rubin, H. 1980. Is somatic mutation the major mechanism of malignant transformation? *J. Natl. Cancer Inst.* **64:**995–1000.

Rübsamen, H., R.R. Friis, and H. Bauer. 1979. *src* gene product from different strains of avian sarcoma virus: Kinetics and possible mechanism of heat inactivation of protein kinase activity from cells infected by transformation-defective, temperature-sensitive mutant and wild-type virus. *Proc. Natl. Acad. Sci.* **76:**967–971.

Saule, S., M. Roussel, C. Lagrou, and D. Stehelin. 1981. Characterization of the oncogene *(erb)* of avian erythroblastosis virus and its cellular progenitor. *J. Virol.* **38:**409-419.

Scheinberg, D.A. and M. Strand. 1980. Transformation-related proteins associated with Kirsten sarcoma virus. *Virology* **106:**335–348.

Scher, C.D. and R. Siegler. 1975. Direct transformation of 3T3 cells by Abelson murine leukaemia virus. *Nature* **253:**729–731.

Scolnick, E.M. and W.P. Parks. 1974. Harvey sarcoma virus: A second murine type C sarcoma virus with rat genetic information. *J. Virol.* **13:**1211–1219.

Scolnick, E.M., A.G. Papageorge, and T.Y. Shih. 1979. Guanine nucleotide-binding activity as an assay for *src* protein of rat-derived murine sarcoma viruses. *Proc. Natl. Acad. Sci.* **76:**5355–5359.

Scolnick, E.M., E. Rands, D. Williams, and W.P. Parks. 1973. Studies on the nucleic acid sequences of Kirsten sarcoma virus: A model for formation of a mammalian RNA-containing sarcoma virus. *J. Virol.* **12:**458–463.

Scolnick, E.M., M.O. Weeks, T.Y. Shih, S.K. Ruscetti, and T.M. Dexter. 1981. Markedly elevated levels of an endogenous *sarc* protein in a hematopoietic precursor cell line. *Mol. Cell. Biol.* **1:**66–74.

Scolnick, E.M., R.S. Howk, A. Anisowicz, P.T. Peebles, C.D Scher, and W.P. Parks. 1975. Separation of sarcoma virus-specific and leukemia virus-specific genetic sequences of Moloney sarcoma virus. *Proc. Natl. Acad. Sci.* **72:**4650–4654.

Sefton, B.M., K. Beemon, and T. Hunter. 1978. Comparison of the expression of the *src* gene of Rous sarcoma virus in vitro and in vivo. *J. Virol.* **28:**957–971.

Sefton, B.M., T. Hunter, and K. Beemon. 1979. Product of in vitro translation of the Rous sarcoma virus *src* gene has protein kinase activity. *J. Virol.* **30:**311–318.

———. 1980a. Temperature-sensitive transformation by Rous sarcoma virus and temperature-sensitive protein kinase activity. *J. Virol.* **33:**220–229.

———. 1980b. Relationship of polypeptide products of the transforming gene of Rous sarcoma virus and the homologous gene of vertebrates. *Proc. Natl. Acad. Sci.* **77:**2059–2063.

Sefton, B.M., T. Hunter, and W.C. Raschke. 1981a. Evidence that the Abelson virus protein functions *in vivo* as a protein kinase that phosphorylates tyrosine. *Proc. Natl. Acad. Sci.* **78:**1552–1556.

Sefton, B.M., T. Hunter, E.H. Ball, and S.J. Singer. 1981b. Vinculin: A cytoskeletal target of the transforming protein of Rous sarcoma virus. *Cell* **24:**165–174.

Sefton, B.M., T. Hunter, K. Beemon, and W. Eckhart. 1980c. Evidence that the phosphorylation of tyrosine is essential for cellular transformation by Rous sarcoma virus. *Cell* **20:**807–816.

Sen, A., G.J. Todaro, D.G. Blair, and W.G. Robey. 1979. Thermolabile protein kinase molecules in a temperature-sensitive murine sarcoma virus pseudotype. *Proc. Natl. Acad. Sci.* **76:**3617–3621.

Shalloway, D., A.D. Zelenetz, and G.M. Cooper. 1981. Molecular cloning and characterization of the chicken gene homologous to the transforming gene of Rous sarcoma virus. *Cell* **24:**531–541.

Sheiness, D. and J.M. Bishop. 1979. DNA and RNA from uninfected vertebrate cells contain nucleotide sequences related to the putative transforming gene of avian myelocytomatosis virus. *J. Virol.* **31:**514–521.

Sheiness, D., B. Vennstrom, and J.M. Bishop. 1981. Virus-specific RNAs in cells infected by avian myelocytomatosis virus and avian erythroblastosis virus: Modes of oncogene expression. *Cell* **23:**291–300.

Sheiness, D., K. Bister, C. Moscovici, L. Fanshier, T. Gonda; and J.M. Bishop. 1980a. Avian retroviruses that cause carcinoma and leukemia: Identification of nucleotide sequences associated with pathogenicity. *J. Virol.* **33:**962–968.

Sheiness, D.K., S.H. Hughes, H.E. Varmus, E. Stubblefield, and J.M. Bishop. 1980b. The vertebrate homolog of the putative transforming gene of avian myelocytomatosis virus: Characteristics of the DNA locus and its RNA transcript. *Virology* **105:**415–424.

Sherr, C.J., L. Donner, L.A. Fedele, L. Turek, J. Even, and S.K. Ruscetti. 1980. Molecular structures and products of feline sarcoma and leukemia viruses: Relationship to FOCMA expression. In *Feline leukemia viruses* (ed. W.D. Hardy, Jr. et al.) pp. 293–307. Elsevier/North-Holland, New York.

Shibuya, M., T. Hanafusa, H. Hanafusa, and J.R. Stephenson. 1980. Homology exists among the transforming sequences of avian and feline sarcoma viruses. *Proc. Natl. Acad. Sci.* **77:**6536–6540.

Shields, A., S. Goff, M. Paskind, G. Otto, and D. Baltimore. 1979. Structure of the Abelson murine leukemia virus genome. *Cell* **18:**955–962.

Shih, C., L.C. Padhy, M. Murray, and R.A. Weinberg. 1981. Transforming genes of carcinomas and neuroblastomas introduced into mouse fibroblasts. *Nature* **290:**261–263.

Shih, C., B.-Z. Shilo, M.P. Goldfarb, A. Dannenberg, and R.A. Weinberg. 1979. Passage of phenotypes of chemically transformed cells via transfection of DNA and chromatin. *Proc. Natl. Acad. Sci.* **76:**5714–5718.

Shih, T.Y., M.O. Weeks, H.A. Young, and E.M. Scolnick. 1979a. Identification of a sarcoma virus-coded phosphoprotein in nonproducer cells transformed by Kirsten or Harvey murine sarcoma virus. *Virology* **96:**64–79.

———. 1979b. p21 of Kirsten murine sarcoma virus is thermolobile in a viral mutant temperature sensitive for the maintenance of transformation. *J. Virol.* **31:**546–556.

Shih, T.Y., A.G. Papageorge, P.E. Stokes, M.O. Weeks, and E.M. Scolnick. 1980. Guanine nucleotide-binding and autophosphorylating activities associated with the $p21^{src}$ protein of Harvey murine sarcoma virus. *Nature* **287:**686–691.

Shilo, B.-Z., and R.A. Weinberg. 1981a. Unique transforming gene in carcinogen-transformed mouse cells. *Nature* **289:**607–609.

———. 1981b. Genes homologous to vertebrate oncogenes are conserved in *Drosophila melanogaster*. *Proc. Natl. Acad. Sci.* (in press).

Silva, R.F. and M.A. Baluda. 1980. Avian myeloblastosis virus proteins in leukemic chicken myeloblasts. *J. Virol.* **35:**766–774.

Smart, J.E., H. Oppermann, A.P. Czernilofsky, A.F. Purchio, R.L. Erikson, and J.M. Bishop. 1981. Characterization of sites for tyrosine phosphorylation in the transforming protein of Rous sarcoma virus ($pp60^{src}$) and its normal cellular homologue ($pp60^{c-src}$). *Proc. Natl. Acad. Sci.* (in press).

Snyder, S.P. and G.H. Theilen. 1969. Transmissible feline fibrosarcoma. *Nature* **221:**1074–1075.

Sotirov, N. 1981. Histone H5 in the immature blood cells of chickens with leukosis induced by avian leukosis virus strain E26. *J. Natl. Cancer Inst.* **66:**1143–1147.

Souza, L.M., J.N. Strommer, R.L. Hillyard, M.C. Komaromy, and M.A. Baluda. 1980. Cellular sequences are present in the presumptive avian myeloblastosis virus genome. *Proc. Natl. Acad. Sci.* **77:**5177–5181.

Spector, D.H., H.E. Varmus, and J.M. Bishop. 1978a. Nucleotide sequences related to the transforming gene of avian sarcoma virus are present in the DNA of uninfected vertebrates. *Proc. Natl. Acad. Sci.* **75:**4102–4106.

Spector, D.H., B. Baker, H.E. Varmus, and J.M. Bishop. 1978b. Characteristics of cellular RNA related to the transforming gene of avian sarcoma viruses. *Cell* **13:**381–386.

Spector, D.H., K. Smith, T. Padgett, P. McCombe, D. Roulland-Dussoix, C. Moscovici, H.E. Varmus, and J.M. Bishop. 1978c. Uninfected avian cells contain RNA related to the transforming gene of avian sarcoma viruses. *Cell* **13:**371–379.

Spector, M., S. O'Neal, and E. Racker. 1980a. Reconstitution of the Na^+K^+ pump of Ehrlich ascites tumor and enhancement of efficiency by Quercetin. *J. Biol. Chem.* **255:**5504–5507.

———. 1980b. Phosphorylation of the β subunit of Na^+K^+-ATPase in Ehrlich ascites tumor by a membrane-bound protein kinase. *J. Biol. Chem.* **255:**8370–8373.

———. 1981a. Regulation of phosphorylation of the β-subunit of the Ehrlich ascites tumor Na^+K^+-ATPase by a protein kinase cascade. *J. Biol. Chem.* **256:**4219–4227.

Spector, M., R.B., Pepinsky, V.M. Vogt, and E. Racker. 1981b. A mouse homologue to the avian sarcoma virus *src* protein is a member of a protein kinase cascade. *Cell* **25:**9–21.

Stavnezer, E., D.S. Gerhard, R.C. Binari, and I. Balazs. 1981. Generation of transforming viruses in cultures of chicken fibroblasts infected with an avian leukosis virus. *J. Virol.* **39:**920–934.

Stehelin, D., R.V. Guntaka, H.E. Varmus, and J.M. Bishop. 1976a. Purification of DNA complementary to nucleotide sequences required for neoplastic transformation of fibroblasts by avian sarcoma viruses. *J. Mol. Biol.* **101:**349–365.

Stehelin, D., H.E. Varmus, J.M. Bishop and P.K. Vogt. 1976b. DNA related to the transforming gene(s) of avian sarcoma viruses is present in normal avian DNA. *Nature* **260:**170–173.

Takeya, T., H. Hanafusa, R. Junghans, G. Ju, and A.M. Skalka. 1981. Comparison between the viral transforming gene (*src*) of recovered avian sarcoma virus and its cellular homologue. *Mol. Cell. Biol.* (in press).

Temin, H.M. 1974. On the origin of RNA tumor viruses. *Annu. Rev. Genet.* **8:**155–177.

———. 1980. Origin of retroviruses from cellular moveable genetic elements. *Cell* **21:**599–600.

Temin, H.M. and H. Rubin. 1958. Characteristics of an assay for Rous sarcoma virus and Rous sarcoma cells in tissue culture. *Virology* **6:**669–688.

Tereba, A., M.M.C., Lai, and K.G. Murti. 1979. Chromosome 1 contains the endogenous RAV-0 retrovirus sequences in chicken cells. *Proc. Natl. Acad. Sci.* **76:**6486–6490.

Tjian, R. and A. Robbins. 1979. Enzymatic activities associated with a purified simian virus 40 T antigen-related protein. *Proc. Natl. Acad. Sci.* **76:**610–614.

Todaro, G.J. and R.J. Huebner. 1972. The viral oncogene hypothesis: New evidence. *Proc. Natl. Acad. Sci.* **69:** 1009–1015.

Todaro, G.J., C. Fryling, and J.E. DeLarco. 1980. Transforming growth factors produced by certain human tumor cells: Polypeptides that interact with epidermal growth factor receptors. *Proc. Natl. Acad. Sci.* **77:** 5258–5262.

Van Beveren, C., F. Van Straaten, J.A. Galleshaw, and I.M. Verma. 1981a. Nucleotide sequence of the genome of a murine sarcoma virus. *Cell* (in press).

Van Beveren, C., J.A. Galleshaw, V. Jonas, A.J.M. Berns, R.F. Doolittle, D.J. Donoghue, and I.M. Verma. 1981b. Nucleotide sequence and formation of the transforming gene of a mouse sarcoma virus. *Nature* **289:** 258–262.

Van de Ven, W.J.M., A.S. Khan, F.H. Reynolds, Jr., K.T. Mason, and J.R. Stephenson. 1980. Translational products encoded by newly acquired sequences of independently derived feline sarcoma virus isolates are structurally related. *J. Virol.* **33:** 1034–1045.

Vennstrom, B. and J.M. Bishop. 1982. Isolation and characterization of chicken DNA homologous to the two putative oncogenes of avian erythroblastosis virus. *Cell* (in press).

Vigne, R., J.C. Neil, M.L. Breitman, and P.K. Vogt. 1980. Recovered *src* genes are polymorphic and contain host markers. *Virology* **105:** 71–85.

Vogt, P.K. 1971. Spontaneous segregation of nontransforming viruses from cloned sarcoma viruses. *Virology* **46:** 939–946.

———. 1977. Genetics of RNA tumor viruses. In *Comprehensive virology* (ed. H. Fraenkel-Conrat and R.R. Wagner), vol. 9, pp. 341–455. Plenum Press, New York.

Vogt, V.M., A. Wight, and R. Eisenman. 1979. *In vitro* cleavage of avian retrovirus *gag* proteins by viral protease p15. *Virology* **98:** 154–167.

Wallbank, A.M., F.G. Sperling, K. Hubben, and E.L. Stubbs. 1966. Isolation of a tumor virus from a chicken submitted to a Poultry Diagnostic Laboratory: Esh sarcoma virus. *Nature* **209:** 1265.

Walter, G., K.-H. Scheidtmann, A. Carbone, A. Landano, and R.A. Doolittle. 1980. Antibodies specific for the carboxy- and amino-terminal regions of simian virus 40 large tumor antigen. *Proc. Natl. Acad. Sci.* **77:** 5197–5200.

Wang, L.-H., P. Duesberg, K. Beemon, and P.K. Vogt. 1975. Mapping RNase T_1-resistant oligonucleotides of avian tumor viruses RNAs: Sarcoma-specific oligonucleotides are near the poly(A) end and oligonucleotides common to sarcoma and transformation-defective viruses are at the poly(A) end. *J. Virol.* **16:** 1051–1070.

Wang, L.-H., P.H. Duesberg, S. Kawai, and H. Hanafusa. 1976. Location of envelope-specific and sarcoma-specific oligonucleotides in RNA of Schmidt-Ruppin Rous sarcoma virus. *Proc. Natl. Acad. Sci.* **73:** 447–451.

Wang, L.-H., C.C. Halpern, M. Nadel, and H. Hanafusa. 1978. Recombination between viral and cellular sequences generates transforming sarcoma virus. *Proc. Natl. Acad. Sci.* **75:** 5812–5816.

Wang, L.-H., C. Moscovici, R.E Karess, and H. Hanafusa. 1979. Analysis of the *src* gene of sarcoma viruses generated by recombination between transformation-defective mutants and quail cellular sequences. *J. Virol.* **32:** 546–556.

Wang, L.-H., P. Snyder, T. Hanafusa, C. Moscovici, and H. Hanafusa. 1980. Comparative analysis of cellular and viral sequences related to sarcomagenic cell transformation. *Cold Spring Harbor Symp. Quant. Biol.* **44:** 755–764.

Wang, L.-H., R. Feldman, M. Shibuya, H. Hanafusa, M.F.P. Notter, and P.C. Balduzzi. 1981. Genetic structure, transforming sequence and gene product of avian sarcoma virus, UR1. *J. Virol.* (in press).

Wang, S.Y., W.S. Hayward, and H. Hanafusa. 1977. Genetic variation in the RNA transcripts of endogenous virus genes in uninfected chicken cells. *J. Virol.* **24:** 64–73.

Watts, S.L.and R.E. Smith. 1980. Pathology of chickens infected with avian nephroblastoma virus MAV-2(N). *Infection and Immunity* **27:**501–512.

Wei, C.-M., D.R. Lowy, and E.M. Scolnick. 1980. Mapping of transforming region of the Harvey murine sarcoma virus genome by using insertion-deletion mutants constructed *in vitro. Proc. Natl. Acad. Sci.* **77:**4674–4678.

Weinberg, R.A. 1977. How does T antigen transform cells? *Cell* **11:**243–246.

Weiss, S.R., H.E. Varmus, and J.M. Bishop. 1981. Cell-free translation of purified avian sarcoma virus *src* mRNA. *Virology* **110:**476–478.

Weller, M. 1979. *Protein phosphorylation.* Pion, London.

Wickner, W. 1980. Assembly of proteins into membranes. *Science* **210:**861–868.

Willingham, M.C., G. Jay, and I. Pastan. 1979. Localization of the ASV *src* gene product to the plasma membrane of transformed cells by electron microscopic immunocytochemistry. *Cell* **18:**125–134.

Willingham, M.C., I. Pastan, T.Y. Shih, and E.M. Scolnick. 1980. Localization of the *src* gene product of the Harvey strain of MSV to the plasma membrane of transformed cells by electron microscopic immunocytochemistry. *Cell* **19:**1005–1014.

Witte, O.N., A. Dasgupta, and D. Baltimore. 1980a. Abelson murine leukaemia virus protein is phosphorylated *in vitro* to form phosphotyrosine. *Nature* **283:**826–831.

Witte, O.N., N. Rosenberg, and D. Baltimore. 1979a. Preparation of syngeneic tumor regressor serum reactive with the unique determinants of the Abelson murine leukemia virus-encoded P120 protein at the cell surface. *J. Virol.* **31:**776–784.

———. 1979b. A normal cell protein cross-reactive to the major Abelson murine leukaemia virus gene product. *Nature* **281:**396–398.

Witte, O.N., S. Goff, N. Rosenberg, and D. Baltimore. 1980b. A transformation-defective mutant of Abelson murine leukemia virus lacks protein kinase activity. *Proc. Natl. Acad. Sci.* **77:**4993–4997.

Witte, O.N., N. Rosenberg, M. Paskind, A. Shields, and D. Baltimore. 1978. Identification of an Abelson murine leukemia virus-encoded protein present in transformed fibroblast and lymphoid cells. *Proc. Natl. Acad. Sci.* **75:**2488–2492.

Wong, T.C., and M.M.C. Lai. 1981. Avian reticuloendotheliosis virus contains a new class of oncogene of turkey origin. *Virology* **111:**289–293.

Wood, T.G., D.D. Lyons, V.L. Ng, E.C. Murphy, Jr., and R.B. Arlinghaus. 1980. Characterization of viral polyproteins in cells transformed and producing Moloney murine sarcoma virus-124. *Biochim. Biophys. Acta* **608:**215–231.

Yoshida, M. and K. Toyoshima. 1980. *In vitro* translation of avian erythroblastosis virus RNA: Identification of two major poplypeptides. *Virology* **100:**484–487.

Yoshida, M., S. Kawai, and K. Toyoshima. 1980. Uninfected avian cells contain structurally unrelated progenitors of viral sarcoma genes. *Nature* **287:**653–654.

Young, H.A., S. Rasheed, R. Sowder, C.V. Benton, and L.E. Henderson. 1981. Rat sarcoma virus: Further analysis of individual viral isolates and the gene product. *J. Virol.* **38:**286–293.

Young, H.A., T.Y. Shih, E.M. Scolnick, S. Rasheed, and M.B. Gardner. 1979. Different rat-derived transforming retroviruses code for an immunologically related intracellular phosphoprotein. *Proc. Natl. Acad. Sci.* **76:**3523–3527.

10

Endogenous Viruses

I. INTRODUCTION

One of the most striking features that distinguishes retroviruses from all other animal viruses is the presence, in the chromosomes of normal uninfected cells, of genomes closely related to, or identical with, those of infectious viruses. Endogenous viruses are extremely widespread in animal populations and have been described in species as diverse as reptiles, birds, and many mammals, quite possibly including man. Their study has occupied a major portion of RNA tumor virus research, with the result that it has recently been possible to reconcile very complex biological and genetic observations into a quite clear virological picture of the phenomenon. We begin with a brief historical background of the subject. More detail can be found in numerous excellent reviews (Gross 1970; Aaronson and Stephenson 1976; Levy 1978; Robinson 1978; Pincus 1980; Todaro 1980; Weinberg 1980).

A. Historical Survey

Endogenous viruses were postulated to be elements of importance in cancer long before their existence was conclusively demonstrated. Although this rationale stimulated research in the area, it should be emphasized that evidence for such a connection presently exists only in some laboratory mouse systems, which may represent special cases. Andrewes (1939) speculated on the possible activation of latent viral infections in cancerous tissues, and it was postulated by Darlington (1948) that such viruses could arise from cellular genetic elements, which he named proviruses. Gross (1958) and Lieberman and Kaplan (1959) observed that lymphoid tumors induced in mice by X rays contained murine leukemia virus (called radiation leukemia virus [RadLV]), which induced similar tumors when injected into unirradiated mice. The induction of RNA tumor viruses following treatment of animals (usually mice) with physical or chemical carcinogens has been reported many times (see Gross 1970). In parallel, genetic studies with GR mice (Muhlbock 1955) led to the observation that spontaneous mammary tumor induction could be transmitted genetically as well as by milk-borne virus.

On the basis of these kinds of observations, it was suggested (Lwoff 1960; Latarjet and Duplan 1962; Bentvelzen et al. 1968) that the viruses may exist in a proviral state that can be activated by carcinogens or X rays in the same way that temperate bacteriophages are activated in lysogenic bacteria.

The concepts of endogenous viruses as components of normal-cell genomes were developed in parallel in the avian and murine tumor virus systems. The first hint that viral information might be expressed in normal cells came from observations that leukosis-free chick embryos contained an antigen that reacted in the complement-fixation test for group-specific (gs) antigens of the avian RNA tumor viruses (Dougherty and Di Stefano 1966; Dougherty et al. 1967). In studies of gs antigens in leukosis-free, inbred lines of chickens, Payne and Chubb (1968) found that the Reaseheath C-line was consistently negative, whereas the Reaseheath I-line was consistently positive for the gs antigen, although no mature virus could be detected. In cross-breeding experiments, they found that the F_1 hybrids were all gs^+ and backcrosses to the C-line were 50% gs^+. Moreover, the gs^+ trait was not sex-linked. These results showed that the gs antigen was determined by a single, autosomal, Mendelian locus with a dominant allele for gs-antigen expression, and Payne and Chubb (1968) suggested that this autosomal locus might represent the site of an integrated avian leukosis virus (ALV) genome, possibly a defective genome because complete virus was not released. The ability of some normal uninfected chick cells to complement defective Rous sarcoma virus (RSV) with an endogenous evelope antigen called chick helper factor (chf) (Vogt 1967; Weiss 1967, 1969; H. Hanafusa et al. 1970) was also found to be inherited in the Reaseheath I-line as a dominant Mendelian train (Weiss and Payne 1971).

In an attempt to find evidence to support the provirus hypothesis, Temin (1964) looked for viral DNA in infected cells using the technique of nucleic acid hybridization. He claimed that viral DNA was present in infected cells, but when investigators in other laboratories (Harel et al. 1966; Bader 1967; Wilson and Bauer 1967) examined the problem, they showed that viruslike DNA was present not only in infected cells, but also in uninfected cells. These results did not seem to lend support to the provirus hypothesis, and their real significance was not immediately appreciated. With the introduction of more sophisticated hybridization techniques, it was realized that several DNA genomes or partial genomes of ALV exist in normal uninfected cells, integrated into the host-cell genome (Rosenthal et al. 1971; Baluda 1972; Varmus et al. 1972b; Neiman 1973a).

Final proof came with the isolation of infectious virus from uninfected cells. Vogt and Friis (1971) found spontaneous production of RAV-0 in embryo cells of line-7 chickens. Crittenden et al. (1973, 1974) subsequently showed that there is a high incidence of RAV-0 viremia in certain line-7 and line-100 chickens. These chickens carry a dominant gene predisposing the cells to spontaneous activation of the genomes of endogenous viruses. This gene was later identified as the RAV-0 provirus itself.

The heritable nature of the viral genome specifying gs antigen and chf led Weiss and Payne (1971) to attempt to activate virus production by X-irradiation, which activates bacteriophages in lysogenic bacteria. Their results, based on a helper-virus assay, were inconclusive, but with the discovery that RAV-0 replicates efficiently in pheasant cells, Weiss et al. (1971) used these cells to amplify the titer of virus that might be released from gs^+ nonproducer cells following X-ray treatment. They found that chemical mutagens and carcinogens, as well as ionizing radiation, could induce release of ALV belonging to subgroup E for some gs^+ and gs^- cells; this virus was named induced leukosis virus (ILV).

Evidence for the existence of endogenous murine leukemia virus (MLV) in normal cells and tissues of the mouse was gathered from experiments similar to those done with chicken cells. The presence of viruslike sequences in the DNA of uninfected murine cells was reported by Harel et al. (1967). Viral gs antigens were found in embryonic and adult tissues (Huebner et al. 1970; Taylor et al. 1971), and another MLV-associated antigen (G_{IX}) was detected in certain normal mouse strains (Stockert et al. 1971). The spontaneous appearance in vivo of MLV in strains with a high incidence of leukemia had been described, but the first convincing evidence that the MLV was released as a result of the activation of inherited viral genomes came from experiments that showed the spontaneous or induced appearance of MLV in previously nonproducing cultures of fibroblasts (Aaronson et al. 1969; Rowe et al. 1971). Lowy et al. (1971) found that the halogenated analogs of thymidine, 5-bromodeoxyuridine (BrdU) and 5-iododeoxyuridine (IdU), were the most efficient inducing agents in cells from AKR mice.

The first evidence for genetically transmitted mouse mammary tumor virus (MMTV) genomes emerged from studies of tumorigenesis in the unusual European mouse strain, GR. Unlike the American mice, which had been studied up to that time, females of the GR strain were shown by Bentvelzen, Muhlbock, and their colleagues to develop virus-associated mammary carcinomas at an early age even after foster nursing by virus-negative females (Muhlbock 1955; Bentvelzen 1969; Bentvelzen and Daams 1969; Bentvelzen et al. 1970). Similar experiments with some American strains revealed another genetic element responsible for mammary tumor formation in the absence of milk-borne virus. Sublines of C3H and DBA mice (called C3Hf and DBAf) were freed of milk-borne virus by foster nursing on low-incidence strains of mice, yet still showed a high incidence of virus-producing mammary carcinoma, albeit quite late in life. This phenotype is distinguished from that of GR mice by the time of appearance of the tumor and other pathological characteristics; however, in both cases single dominant alleles, termed *mtv-2* in GR and *mtv-1* in C3Hf, were found to be responsible for the phenotypes (DeOme et al. 1967; Nandi and McGrath 1973; van Nie and Verstraeten 1975; van Nie and de Moes 1977; and Verstraeten and van Nie 1978).

B. Overview of Endogenous Viruses

In this chapter, we discuss several features of endogenous viruses, including mode of expression and inheritance, genomic and proviral structures, pathogenicity, and distribution among various animal species. At this point a brief overview is presented to orient the reader to the more detailed discussion that follows. Unfortunately, the older literature on the subject contains numerous interpretations later proved to be incorrect and can therefore be very difficult to read. The following generalizations have been found to hold true for all endogenous viruses analyzed in sufficient detail.

1. Endogenous Viruses Behave as Stable Mendelian Genes in Genetic Experiments

In numerous crosses to test segregation of endogenous proviruses (with both mice and chickens), endogenous proviruses or their associated phenotypes have been found to behave as reasonably stable elements, with a consistent site of residence in a host chromosome. Such loss, acquisition, or rearrangement of proviruses as may occur is too infrequent to be seen in this type of experiment. Phenotypes directly associated with endogenous viruses (inducibility of virus or antigen expression, for example) are invariably dominant over their absence. Furthermore, endogenous viruses are not linked to one another or to the *c-onc* genes (see Chapters 4 and 9) any more than to any other genes. Thus, endogenous viruses are not intermediates in the generation of transforming viruses and are not due to integration of such viruses into the germ line.

2. Endogenous Viruses Are Evolutionarily Unstable

Within all but highly inbred strains of animals, the number and distribution of endogenous proviruses can vary greatly from individual to individual. For example, some 14 different endogenous proviruses of white leghorn chickens have been characterized, with individuals containing between 0 and 6 of these. Even sublines or individuals of some highly inbred lines of mice can vary somewhat in their content of endogenous proviruses, apparently a result of new germ-line integration during the breeding program. It is therefore not surprising that the situation becomes even more chaotic when related species are compared. The wild relative of domestic chickens (*Gallus*), for example, contains RAV-0-related proviruses, but other species of the same genus do not. Nevertheless, related viruses reappear in some species of the more distantly related pheasants. Thus, endogenous viruses have not been stably associated with their hosts over evolutionary history and have apparently spread by mechanisms other than evolutionary divergence.

3. Endogenous Viruses Resemble Normal Proviruses

In their gross structure, endogenous proviruses have exactly the structure of proviruses acquired by infection (Chapter 5), i.e., they have the order cell-LTR-*gag-pol-env*-LTR-cell. Furthermore, in the one case that has been examined in detail, the sequences at either virus-cell junction have undergone rearrangements identical with those found after integration of infecting viruses, i.e., a loss of two nucleotides from the ends of viral DNA and a duplication of 6 bases of host DNA at the integration site. Additionally, introns, found in most cellular genes, have not been found in endogenous proviruses. These features, along with their individual variability and evolutionary instability, distinguish endogenous proviruses from normal-cell genes.

4. Endogenous Viruses Vary Greatly in Expression

A great deal of phenotypic variation encoded by endogenous viruses is frequently encountered, ranging from apparently complete silence through expression of only one viral gene product to production of infectious virus. Although early proposals suggested that partial repression of complete genomes might be responsible for this variation, much or all of the qualitative differences observed can be attributed to mutations—often significant deletions—in the proviruses themselves. Differences in levels of expression, in contrast, appear to be due largely to chemical modifications (methylation has been recently implicated) in the proviruses themselves, a phenomenon that has also been occasionally observed after exogenous infection of cells. Expression of infectious endogenous viruses in the whole animal seems to be most commonly regulated at the level of inhibition of replication. Thus, animals that inherit complete proviruses do not exhibit significant production of infectious virus unless their cells are susceptible to infection by this virus.

5. Most Endogenous Viruses Are Nonpathogenic

With the exception of some laboratory strains of mice, no evidence associating endogenous viruses with increased mortality from neoplastic or other disease has been found. In the best-studied case, chickens viremic with RAV-0 have been maintained for many years and have shown no higher incidence of disease attributable to the virus than controls.

6. *At Least Some Endogenous Viruses Are Nonessential to the Host*

When it was first recognized that endogenous proviruses were widespread in many animal species, it was proposed that they might represent normal cellular elements, related to infectious virus, that carried out some important role in development. This view gained further support with the finding of development-specific expression of certain endogenous virus antigens in mice. More recently, however, chickens completely lacking in known endogenous viruses have been bred with no obvious ill effects. Similarly, strains of mice with no endogenous MMTV or ecotropic MLV exist and remain completely healthy relative to virus-positive animals. Furthermore, tissue-specific expression of endogenous viruses is not consistent from one strain of mouse to another. Therefore, it is unlikely that endogenous viruses mediate essential developmental processes. It is, of course, possible that endogenous viruses may confer more subtle selective advantages on their hosts, e.g., protection against pathogenesis by exogenous viruses.

II. INHERITANCE AND EXPRESSION OF ENDOGENOUS PROVIRUSES

Soon after it was realized that endogenous proviruses were present in chickens and mice, it became apparent that expression of these proviruses differed substantially from that found in exogenously infected cells. In some cases, expression of only some genes (particularly *gag* or *env*) could be observed; in others, complete proviruses could be demonstrated by various treatments that led to the activation of infectious virus; and in still others, spontaneous production of infectious virus was frequently observed. This complexity was further confused by the early nucleic acid hybridization experiments, which suggested that there was little or no difference in endogenous virus content between different individuals with different types of endogenous virus expression (see, e.g., Rosenthal et al. 1971; Baluda 1972; Varmus et al. 1972a,b; Gelb et al. 1973; Neiman 1973a). The mechanisms behind the phenotypic complexity have only gradually been unraveled over the last decade, and it is now apparent that there are two underlying phenomena. First, endogenous viruses are frequently mutants capable of expressing only a portion of the genome (of the 14 well-characterized endogenous proviruses of chickens, 10 are such mutants). Second, most inherited proviruses are subject to cellular controls that render them transcriptionally silent. These controls can be abrogated either by infection of susceptible cells with the virus produced (having the effect of moving the provirus to another location) or by treatment with certain inducing agents that significantly increase transcriptional rates. In this section, we consider the general features of inheritance and induction of endogenous viruses of chickens and mice; specific proviruses and their phenotypes are discussed in a later section.

A. Inheritance of Proviruses

1. Genetic Studies

Clearly, the most important feature "regulating" endogenous virus phenotypes is the inheritance of the appropriate provirus. Even before the discovery of RAV-0, it was observed that the inheritance of ALV-*gag*-related (group-specific or gs antigens) and *env*-related (chicken helper factor or chf) proteins was by simple Mendelian genetics, with each behaving as a dominant locus (Payne and Chubb 1968; Weiss and Payne 1971). Similarly, G_{IX} antigen (Stockert et al. 1971), representing a slightly modified MLV *env*-gene product (Rosner et al. 1980) (see Chapters 4 and 6), was associated with two semidominant loci (Boyse and Old 1971). Shortly after the discovery of spontaneous RAV-0 production by cells from line-7 chickens (Vogt and Friis 1971), a detailed genetic study revealed that the spontaneous virus production in line-7 and related line-100 chickens was also inherited as a single dominant Mendelian locus (Crittenden et al. 1974), initially called *V* and now known as *ev*-2 (Astrin et al. 1980a). In the mouse, two independent dominant loci in the AKR strain were found to confer spontaneous ecotropic virus release in young mice. These were initially called V_1 and V_2 (Rowe 1972; Rowe and Hartley 1972) and are now known as *Akv-1* and *Akv-2.* These loci have been mapped to chromosomes 7 and 16, respectively (Rowe 1972; Kozak and Rowe 1980b). The actual situation in AKR mice has turned out to be more complex (discussed later). A similar locus, known as *Cv*, which confers inducibility of N-tropic ecotropic virus, was identified in BALB/c mice (Stephenson and Aaronson 1972) and mapped to chromosome 5 (Kozak and Rowe 1979). A locus conferring inducibility of xenotropic virus, termed *Bxv-1*, was also identified in BALB/c mice (Stephenson and Aaronson 1972) and later found to be widespread in many diverse strains of mice (Kozak and Rowe 1980a); and two loci conferring spontaneous xenotropic virus expression, *Nzv-1* and *Nzv-2*, were found in NZB mice (Datta and Schwartz 1977). The locus responsible for the MMTV-associated tumors in GR mice segregates in a Mendelian dominant fasion (Bentvelzen 1969, 1972; van Nie and Hilgers 1976) and has recently been mapped on chromosome 18 (R. van Nie, unpubl.).

2. Physical Identification of Proviruses

In genetic experiments of the type described above, investigators could study only those loci conferring characteristic phenotypes, usually spontaneous expression or inducibility of complete virus. Recent advances in nucleic acid hybridization technology have demonstrated that most or all of the genetic elements discussed above are endogenous proviruses and have revealed the presence of many more loci than were previously recognized. The first experiments of this sort were those of Chattopadhyay et al. (1974, 1975a,b), who were able to prepare a hybridization probe from labeled cDNA complementary to the AKR virus (AKV) genome with partial specificity for the ecotropic AKV-like proviruses of AKR mice. With this probe, it was possible to demonstrate that specific sequences segregated with the genetically defined *Akv* loci.

The application of restriction mapping and DNA-transfer hybridization (according to the method of Southern [1975]) to the analysis of the genomes of endogenous viruses has drastically changed the way in which these genomes are viewed. The principle of the approach is that described in Chapter 5 for analysis of integration sites. If cellular DNA containing an integrated provirus is digested with a restriction enzyme, two classes of fragments will be detected after gel electrophoresis, transfer to membrane filters, and hybridization with a virus-specific probe: (1) internal fragments containing only viral DNA and (2) junction fragments containing both viral and nonviral DNA. The number of internal fragments can vary depending on the number of cleavage sites the provirus contains; there can, at most, be two junction fragments per provirus (assuming the absence of introns in the endogenous proviruses, which seems to be the case). The size and number of internal fragments vary from individual to individual, with variations in the provirus itself; the size of the junction fragments depends on the content of neighboring cell sequences, i.e., with its location within the cell genome. Thus, comparison of patterns obtained from different individuals allows one to determine the way in which the genomes of endogenous viruses vary in structure and location from one animal to the next. When such an analysis is done with probes specific for the "usual" types of genes, such as globin, ovalbumin, or even *src* or other *onc* genes, essentially no variation is found from one individual to the next in either internal structure, copy number, or (in accord with the principles of Mendelian genetics) location (Hughes et al. 1979). Thus, these genes must have been fixed in the population at some distant time, probably prior to speciation. In contrast, a quite different pattern was found when endogenous proviruses were sought in this way. Using digestion with two enzymes, *Eco*RI and *Bam*HI, whose cleavage sites had been mapped in the RAV-0 genome (see Chapters 4 and 5), Hughes et al. (1979) examined a large number of individuals, both from commercial and laboratory flocks. A great variability was found in the number of endogenous proviruses (from one to more than seven), in their location in the cellular DNA, and, to a lesser extent, in their structure. (Many of the endogenous proviruses so identified yielded internal fragments identical with those of RAV-0; however, a number of apparently deleted genomes were found.) Clearly, the genes of endogenous viruses are not fixed in chickens and most have undergone considerable variation by addition of new proviruses and (possibly) by deletion of others, subsequent to speciation and even to the development of present day strains. The situation is not completely chaotic, however, since, in a number of cases, apparently identical endogenous proviruses were found at identical sites in individuals of somewhat different backgrounds, and some of these seemed to be associated with certain endogenous virus phenotypes.

A somewhat more practical approach was taken by Astrin (Astrin 1978; Astrin et al. 1980b), who examined a group of chickens with a number of restriction enzymes and decided on one enzyme, *Sst*I, for further analysis, since it gave the simplest patterns. (As it happens, *Sst*I cleaves the RAV-0 provirus twice in *gag* [Shank et al. 1981], but the left-hand fragments contain too little proviral DNA to have been readily detectable with the ^{32}P RNA probe used; therefore, the characteristic fragment detected is usually the 3′ junction fragment.)

Each of the characteristic fragments observed was termed *ev* followed by a number. Since all the different fragments segregated independently of one another in appropriate crosses, they must represent distinct genetic loci. If all chickens were considered, the number of different *ev* loci would probably be extremely high. However, only about 12 were found in the strains of chickens commonly used for virological purposes.

There is no doubt that the different *ev* loci are the endogenous proviruses responsible for the various phenotypes previously observed in different chickens. First, there is correlation between the presence of a given locus in chickens and the associated phenotype. For example, *ev*-2 was present in 20 out of 20 RAV-0 positive (V^+) birds of line 7 and absent in 125 out of 125 V^- birds (Astrin et al. 1980a). This correlation also held true when birds of different lines were examined. *ev*-3 is associated with the gs^+chf^+ phenotype in SPAFAS, K16, and 6_3 chickens, and both line-15 chickens and Reaseheath line-C chickens contain the nondefective *ev*-10 locus and, after induction, give a virus with the same oligonucleotide map (J. M. Coffin et al., unpubl.). Second, each phenotype is completely linked to a particular *ev* locus in genetic crosses (Astrin 1978; Astrin and Robinson 1979; Astrin et al. 1979b, 1980b). Third, in all cases where it has been possible to test, the expression of a phenotype associated with one *ev* locus is not influenced by the presence of another locus (Hayward et al. 1980; Baker et al. 1981). For example, the presence of *ev*-1 and *ev*-3, both associated with high levels of 21S virus-specific mRNA, did not increase the expression of other RNAs associated with each locus or of 35S RNA of *ev*-1 in the same cell. Also, the expression of endogenous loci is not affected by infection with exogenous virus (Hayward and Hanafusa 1976). Finally, as discussed in more detail later, the structure of each *ev* provirus is consistent with the structure of virus-specific RNA found in cells that contain it.

This analysis also resolved the old paradox of phenotype variation in the face of apparently constant copy number. One provirus, designated as the *ev*-1 locus, was found to be present in more than 99% of the white leghorn chickens examined (Astrin 1978; Tereba and Astrin 1980). Although it has no major deletions, the *ev*-1 provirus is expressed at a very low level (Hayward et al. 1980; Baker et al. 1981), does not encode infectious virus (K. F. Conklin et al., in prep.), and therefore has no readily detectable phenotype. In addition, many lines of chickens contain several additional inactive proviruses. Early hybridization methodology was insufficiently precise to detect the small variation in copy number provided by the biologically relevant proviruses. The finding of a few birds of line 7_2 that were lacking *ev*-1 (Astrin 1978) made it possible to develop a line of chickens that contained no detectable endogenous proviruses at all (Astrin et al. 1979a).

Similar, although less extensive, analyses have been applied to the ecotropic endogenous (AKV-related) proviruses of mice. It was found that laboratory strains of mice have a variability similar to that of the ALV-related proviruses of chickens, except that, being highly inbred individuals of a given strain are usually identical to one another. Different strains of mice contain between zero and about seven AKV-related proviruses. This analysis, however, is substantially more complicated because all strains contain upward of 15 other closely related proviruses, presumably xenotropic or defective (Steffen and Weinberg 1978; Canaani and Aaronson 1979; Dolberg et al. 1980). To detect the ecotropic proviruses, it is therefore necessary to use carefully selected probes, with the most useful being one derived from the subgroup-coding portion of *env* (Chan et al. 1980; Chattopadhyay et al. 1980; see Chapter 4). The nonecotropic background precludes obtaining detailed restriction maps without first isolating infectious virus or preparing molecular clones of each provirus to be studied. Also, although it has been observed that the composition of nonecotropic proviruses varies considerably from strain to strain and even among wild mice trapped in nearby locations (Steffen and Weinberg 1978), none of these have yet been associated with the genetically defined xenotropic or partial expression phenotypes.

The endogenous proviruses of MMTV, when examined in the same way, were found to display a variability similar to that of endogenous ALV; i.e., mice of different strains varied in their content from three to roughly ten distinct proviruses, and some wild mice have been found that contain no detectable MMTV-related DNA (Cohen and Varmus 1979). The MMTV-related sequences were originally identified as "units" characterized by distinctive internal and junction fragments created by cleavage with specific restriction endonucleases (*Pst*I and *Eco*RI, respectively, were found to be most useful (Shank et al. 1978; Cohen and Varmus 1979). Subsequently, Unit V of Cohen and Varmus (1979) was found to cosegregate with genetically identified *mtv-1* alleles of some C3H and DBA sublines (Michaelides et al. 1981). Thus, the characteristic phenotype of late mammary tumor appearance in these mice was almost certainly due to this specific MMTV provirus.

In no other species besides chickens and mice have similar genetic analyses been performed. However, restriction mapping and DNA-transfer techniques have revealed that many species contain numerous copies of proviruses (or at least sequences related to infectious viruses of the same or other species). Such species include other rodents (rats, for example), cats, several primates, and quite possibly humans. Again, these are discussed in subsequent sections.

B. Activation of Endogenous Virus Expression

Although structurally distinguishable from usual cellular genes, endogenous proviruses do resemble cellular genes in one significant respect: occasionally much of the time they are transcriptionally silent, yet can be shown to have significant levels of expression in certain developmental stages. Most of the time, this transcriptional silence (and also probably the development-specific activation) is not a consequence of structural features of the provirus itself, but rather of regulatory controls imposed upon it by the cell. For this reason, study of spontaneous and induced activation of endogenous proviruses has been intensively pursued with the hopes of using them as probes for underlying basic regulatory mechanisms in the cell. To be frank, endogenous viruses have not yet proved very useful in this regard, although some principles determined for other genes have recently been confirmed and extended in this system.

1. Spontaneous Expression

a. Production of Infectious Virus. (i) AVIAN TUMOR VIRUSES. Chicken cells that inherit complete proviruses do not necessarily produce readily detectable infectious virus or even detectable levels of viral antigen (Weiss et al. 1971; Robinson et al. 1976). Levels of viral RNA are generally very low in such cells (~0.2 copies/cell for *ev*-2) (Wang et al. 1977; Hayward et al. 1980). In contrast, cells from related birds with identical endogenous provirus content will often produce respectable levels of infectious virus (Vogt and Friis 1971) and have levels of RNA of around 1000 copies per cell (Wang et al.

1977; Hayward et al. 1980). Detailed genetic analysis of this phenomenon (Payne et al. 1971; Pani and Payne 1973; Crittenden et al. 1973, 1974, 1977) revealed that the important factor governing whether a tissue culture (or a whole animal) spontaneously expresses high levels of infectious virus was the ability of a cell to be infected with virus of subgroup E (the subgroup of RAV-0 and all other endogenous ALVs; see Chapter 3). Two types of loci affecting this susceptibility were found. The first was identified as the dominant allele of *tv-b* conferring susceptibility to infection by subgroup-E virus, presumably by encoding the appropriate receptor (Chapter 3). The second was an unlinked locus, termed an epistatic inhibitor (or I^e), whose dominant allele confers a partial (100- to 1000-fold) resistance to infection by subgroup-E virus. Because preliminary evidence suggested a linkage to spontaneous expression of gs antigen, it was postulated that the I^e effect was the result of blocking of cell-surface receptors by an endogenously synthesized *env*-gene product (Payne et al. 1971). Consistent with this idea, it was found that preinfection of I^e C/O cells with subgroup-A or subgroup-C ALV could abrogate the I^e restriction of infection with subgroup-E virus (Ishizaki and Shimizu 1970; Weiss 1973), presumably by "clearing" the cell surface of *env* glycoproteins as a result of their incorporation into virions. Definitive evidence for the association of I^e with chf has recently been obtained by H. L. Robinson et al. (pers. comm.), who observed that three endogenous loci associated with spontaneous high expression of chf (*ev*-3, *ev*-6, and *ev*-9) segregate completely with the partial resistance to infection by subgroup-E virus.

The presence of three different types of genetic loci involved in spontaneous RAV-0 production clearly created a very complex genetic situation that was difficult to sort out. Once clarified, however, it was found that the system was easily explicable in terms of the straightforward virological principles of inheritance of proviruses, presence of cell-surface receptors, and superinfection resistance. But an underlying puzzle remained: Why should features that control the ability of a cell to be exogenously infected with a virus regulate the expression of an endogenous virus? The genetic observations could be reconciled into a fairly simple model for endogenous virus production (Payne et al. 1971; Crittenden et al. 1974; Cooper and Temin 1976). Complete endogenous proviruses, such as *ev*-2, contain all sequences necessary to produce infectious virus and are themselves expressed at a very low rate, but sufficient to synthesize an occasional infectious virion. The control of virus production is *cis* to the endogenous provirus and is not inherited by the virus progeny. Therefore, cells that are susceptible to subgroup-E virus will be reinfected by the progeny of the provirus they contain, and the provirus acquired by infection will be expressed at a high level, leading to the rapid spread of virus through the animal or cell culture. Several observations strongly support this model. First, by reannealing kinetics, *ev*-2 C/O cells have more copies of proviral DNA than do *ev*-2 C/E cells (Cooper and Temin 1976). Second, analysis of proviral DNAs from the two types of cells also reveals the presence of additional proviruses at random integration sites in C/O cells, as compared with C/E cells, as well as some differences in restriction enzyme digestion patterns (discussed in more detail later) (Humphries et al. 1979). Third, Cooper and Temin (1976) found that the DNA from RAV-0-producing *ev*-2 C/O cells was infectious for C/O cells, but that DNA from poorly producing C/E cells was not. Therefore, the provirus of the low-producer cells, although genetically identical with that obtained from high-producer cells, must be different in some way that affects its ability to be expressed when introduced into cells as pure DNA.

The model of a *cis*-acting repressor gained support from the finding that infectivity of *ev*-2 DNA could be somewhat enhanced by shearing, suggesting that the removal of neighboring DNA sequences could at least partially relieve the block in expression (Cooper and Silverman 1978). A more complicated situation exists with the endogenous virus expression by line-15B birds. These birds contain the *ev*-7 and *ev*-1 loci and are generally C/O and highly susceptible to infection with RAV-0 (Robinson et al. 1976). Unlike line-100 C/O chickens, which always produce high levels of RAV-0 by 10 days of embryonic life, cell cultures and birds of line 15B only sporadically become virus-producing, and generally rather late in life (Robinson et al. 1979). No infectious virus whatever can be detected in nonproducing embryos, but a low level of production of noninfectious virions can be detected (by reverse transcriptase assay) following BrdU treatment of cell cultures. Typically, this virus disappears within a short time after BrdU is removed, and, after several weeks, the culture begins to produce high levels of infectious virus and continues to do so thereafter. The appearance of infectious virus following BrdU induction is greatly accelerated in F_1 hybrid birds that are heterozygous for the *ev*-7 and a locus conferring *env* expression, such as *ev*-3 or *ev*-9 (Robinson et al. 1979).

The most probable explanation for the interesting behavior of the *ev*-7 locus is that it encodes a genome capable of making reverse-transcriptase-containing virions that are noninfectious (perhaps due to an *env* defect, although this point is not established). Induction of this provirus allows the production of virions and, as a rare event, recombination between the progeny of the *ev*-7 locus and other defective loci (such as *ev*-1) in the same cell. Analysis of the infectious 15B-E virus supports this model. The apparent molecular weights of p19 of different isolates of such viruses are variable from one isolate to the next (Robinson et al. 1979), a feature of many viruses isolated as recombinants involving endogenous virus (Shaikh et al. 1978) and probably acquired from *ev*-1 (K. F. Conklin et al., in prep.). Oligonucleotide maps of the viruses support this conclusion (J. M. Coffin et al., unpubl.). This situation may be analogous to the more recalcitrant case of the polytropic viruses of mice (see Section III.B.1.d).

(ii) C-TYPE ENDOGENOUS MLV. The factors regulating spontaneous MLV release in cell culture and in animals seem similar in principle to those established for ALV, although somewhat different in detail. Again, the most important feature regulating infectious virus production seems to be the susceptibility of the cells or the whole animal to spread of the virus. Loci controlling surface receptors for MLV, analogous to *tv* loci in chickens, have not been described in mice (or other mammals), but a similar effect is observed in mice with *Fv-1* restriction (see Chapter 8). For example, both AKR (*Fv-1*^{nn}) and BALB/c (*Fv-1*^{bb}) mice inherit N-tropic endogenous proviruses (Rowe 1972; Stephenson and Aaronson 1972; Ihle et al. 1979; Kozak and Rowe 1979), yet only AKR mice contain high titers of N-tropic infectious virus expressed at an early age, whereas in BALB/c mice, there is only a very low level of expression of N-tropic virus and a high level of infectious virus is not observed until late in life, and then the virus is B tropic. Similarly, N-tropic virus can be induced from cell cultures of both types of mice. AKR cells so treated become permanently virus-producing, presumably as a result of reinfection (Lowy et al. 1971), whereas the production of virus by BALB/c cells is transient (Aaronson et al. 1971; Stephenson and Aaronson 1972). This cessation of virus production presumably reflects either a turnoff of expression or an overgrowth of nonexpressing cells, combined with an inability of the induced N-tropic virus to replicate in the B-type cells. The late expression of B-tropic virus in BALB/c mice may well represent a phenomenon analogous to that of the 15B chicken discussed above, since the B-tropic determinant seems to arise as a result of a rare recombination between the N-tropic endogenous virus and some unidentified locus encoding xenotropic virus (Gautsch et al. 1978, 1980).

Interestingly, unlike chickens in which virtually all susceptible *ev-2* animals produce large amounts of RAV-0 from early embryonic life (Crittenden et al. 1974), AKR mice do not begin to express AKV until shortly before birth (Rowe 1972). Also, AKR embryo-cell cultures are generally virus-negative when prepared and only sporadically become spontaneously producing. Clones of these cells can be prepared that are stable nonproducers and only become virus-producing when treated with an inducer (Rowe et al. 1971). Thus, control of endogenous *Akv* loci in the mouse seems to be somewhat different from that of *ev-2* in the chicken.

In addition to effects on infectibility of cells by virus, a number of loci in the mouse have been identified that affect expression of virus and attendant development of leukemia in the whole animal. Some of these, like certain *H-2* alleles, may act by modifying the immune response (Lilly 1970). A detailed discussion of these phenomena is beyond the scope of this chapter; refer to Chapter 8 and to Pincus (1980) and Steeves and Lilly (1977) for a more thorough review.

As with ecotropic viruses, in the nonpermissive case, induction of xenotropic viruses from mouse cells is transient (Aaronson and Stephenson 1973), and these viruses are rarely expressed at high levels in most strains of mice. There are a few interesting exceptions to the low expression of these viruses, such as in NZB mice (Levy 1973), and in leukemic and preleukemic AKR thymus (Kawashima et al. 1976). Presumably, contrary to the usual case, such animals contain a significant number of cells in which the usual block in expression has been largely relieved, although the presence of a special population of cells sensitive to xenotropic virus infection has not been conclusively excluded.

b. Partial Virus Expression.

In addition to spontaneous expression of complete infectious virus, there are numerous phenotypes involving high-level spontaneous expression of some viral gene products, but not others. Proviruses responsible for such phenotypes include *ev*-3, *ev*-6, and *ev*-9 in the chicken, all three of which confer high levels of chf activity. In contrast to the situation with the other *ev* loci, both complete and defective, these are characterized by relatively high transcriptional activity (at least in fibroblasts), and the amount of virus-related RNA has been estimated at 50–150 copies per cell (Wang et al. 1977; Hayward et al. 1980). In the mouse, there is striking tissue-specific partial expression of certain endogenous proviruses. This type of expression is best exemplified by the gp70-associated G_{IX} antigen, which was initially described for thymocytes (Stockert et al. 1971). More recent immunofluorescent studies have shown a highly specific localization of G_{IX} antigen to epithelial cells of mouse epididymus (Lerner et al. 1976). Similarly, the *mtv-3* allele encodes the expression of MMTV-related *gag* but not *env* antigens in the mammary glands of GR mice (Nusse et al. 1980). Studies of this sort led to hypotheses of a direct specific role of these virus-related proteins in normal developmental processes, but, in view of the precedent with chickens and the variability in such expression from strain to strain, it seems quite difficult to infer a major role for these antigens in the life of the animal. It is not yet known whether tissue-specific expression reflects features of the provirus itself or chance integration into an area of the genome that is itself under some developmental control. Nevertheless, in both the mouse and the chicken, it is striking that the most highly expressed endogenous proviruses are those that express *env* and little else. Conceivably, these confer some subtle selective advantage on the host, perhaps in inhibiting infection by exogenous virus or reducing its pathogenic effects (L. Crittenden, pers. comm.).

2. Induction

Since the initial descriptions of induction of endogenous ALV by X-irradiation and chemical carcinogens (Weiss et al. 1971) and of MLV by halogenated pyrimidines (Lowy et al. 1971), the phenomenon has been intensively studied in mouse cells in tissue culture. (Except for the study of Robinson et al. [1976] and the recent work of Groudine et al. [1981] and K. F. Conklin et al. [in prep.], discussed later, the avian system has been largely ignored for this sort of analysis.) The studies have involved both analysis of a large variety of agents and testing of a variety of experimental protocols and cell types in not altogether successful attempts to infer the underlying mechanism of control of endogenous provirus (and, perhaps by extension, expression of any cellular gene). A selection of the agents and protocols tested and the results are presented in Table 10.1. We will not discuss specific experiments here; rather, we will present a

Table 10.1 Agents that induce endogenous virus expression

Agent	Virus induced	Comment	References
IdU, BrdU	ecotropic, xenotropic MLV	effect enhanced by near-UV light; incorporation into DNA appears to be required	Lowy et al. (1971); Teich et al. (1973); Aaronson et al. (1971)
IdU, BrdU	endogenous ALV ecotropic MLV		Robinson et al. (1976) Rowe et al. (1971)
UV-, X-irradiation	endogenous ALV		Weiss et al. (1971)
γ-Irradiation	endogenous MLV	inefficient compared with IdU, BrdU	Rowe et al. (1971); Tennant and Rascati (1980)
5-Methylcholanthrene	endogenous ALV	inefficient compared with IdU, BrdU	Weiss et al. (1971)

Inhibitors of protein synthesis (puromycin, pactamycin, cycloheximide)	xenotropic but not ecotropic BALB/c virus	transient effect; DNA synthesis not required	Aaronson and Dunn (1974)
L-Canavanine	endogenous MLV	arginine analog	Aksamit and Long (1977)
Hydroxyurea	endogenous MLV	inhibitor of DNA synthesis	Rascati and Tennant (1978)
Graft-vs.-host reaction and mixed lymphocyte reaction	xenotropic MLV	lymphocyte proliferation required	Scherr et al. (1974); Levy et al. (1977)
B-cell mitogens (e.g., lipopolysaccharide)	xenotropic MLV	T-cell mitogens ineffective	Moroni and Schumann (1975)
Herpesvirus infection	xenotropic MLV	transient	Reed and Rapp (1976)
5-Azacytidine	endogenous ALV, including *ev*-1 and *ev*-2	demethylates DNA	Groudine et al. (1981); K.F. Conklin et al. (in prep.)

very brief overview of the types of experiments and their conclusions. (For more detail, see Pincus [1980] and Aaronson and Stephenson [1976]). It is apparent from Table 10.1 that a wide range of treatments will lead to induction of endogenous viruses. Agents as diverse as inhibitors of DNA and protein synthesis, deoxynucleoside and amino acid analogs, and immunological reagents all lead to the appearance of endogenous viruses. Measurements of viral RNA levels suggest that the effect is on transcription (Besmer et al. 1975). It is, however, extremely difficult to infer a consistent underlying mechanism from these observations. The common effects of nucleoside analogs and inhibitors of protein synthesis are consistent with the existence of a short-lived repressor, whose binding to DNA could be imagined to be inhibited by incorporation of the analogs into DNA. However, there is no independent evidence for the existence of such a repressor, and if one does exist it must act only indirectly on the provirus, since the replication of exogenous AKV, for example, in the same cells is unaffected by the same treatments. Also, the results of Lowy (1978) are inconsistent with a simple repressor model, since he found that infectivity of DNA from nonproducer AKR mouse cells was greatly enhanced by pretreatment of the recipient cells with IdU, whereas IdU-substituted AKR DNA, obtained by pretreatment of the donor cells, did not have enhanced infectivity. These experiments imply an indirect effect through the cell, as opposed to its inability to repress substituted DNA.

3. Methylation of Endogenous Proviruses

A possible entry into the puzzle of low expression of inherited proviruses has been provided by recent studies of the extent to which the DNA of the inherited provirus is methylated. Eukaryotic DNA is methylated almost exclusively at ^{m5}C in the dinucleotide CpG (for review, see Razin and Riggs 1980), and a large fraction of this particular dinucleotide is methylated in all eukaryotic cells examined. The overall extent of methylation of specific genes can be readily probed by use of restriction endonucleases whose cleavage is inhibited by the presence of ^{m5}CpG in the cleavage site. Particularly useful is the enzyme pair *Hpa*II and *Msp*I, both of which recognize the sequence CCGG. Since only *Hpa*II is sensitive to inhibition by methylation at this site, a difference in band patterns observed after DNA-transfer hybridization following digestion of parallel samples with the two enzymes is evidence for methylation of the sequence being examined

(Waalwijk and Flavell 1978). By use of this technique, it was demonstrated that there is a good correlation between the extent of methylation of certain cellular genes and their transcriptional activity. Globin genes, for example, were found to be demethylated only in tissues or cells actively synthesizing globin mRNA (Mandel and Chambon 1979; Van der Ploeg and Flavell 1980). It has been proposed that methylation may be a mechanism used by the organism to silence more or less permanently genes not in use, except at particular developmental stages. It has also been suggested that methylation is inherited during DNA synthesis. Since the methylated dinucleotide is palindromic (i.e., its complement is also CG), the methylase responsible has been postulated to recognize the presence of ^{m5}dC on one strand of newly replicated DNA and to methylate the complement (Holliday and Pugh 1975; Riggs 1975).

The first suggestion of involvement of methylation in endogenous provirus expression was a comparison of the restriction maps of *ev*-2 in C/E cells that did not synthesize detectable virus with that of the amplified RAV-0 provirus in *ev*-2 C/O cells (Humphries et al. 1979). With a number of enzymes, identical patterns were found, but with *Hha*I (which is inhibited by methylation), quite different patterns were observed between the two cell types. In a more extensive study, Cohen (1980) used the *Hpa*II/*Msp*I system to show that endogenous MMTV proviruses in mice are extensively methylated, compared with exogenously acquired proviruses in infected cells or in tumors. Similarly, Moloney MLV (Mo-MLV) proviruses experimentally introduced into the germ line (as the *mov* loci [Section III.B.4]) are both extensively methylated and transcriptionally silent. Only in tissues that contain additional unmethylated proviruses acquired as a result of reinfection can virus RNA be detected (Stuhlmann et al. 1981). Additionally, inherited *mov* proviruses are not infectious if added to cells as DNA from nonproducing cells, but infectivity is restored by molecular cloning, which leads to loss of methylation (Harbers et al. 1981). Most recently, Groudine et al. (1981) found that the transcriptionally silent *ev*-1 provirus in chicken cells was largely methylated, in comparison with the much more active *ev*-3 provirus. Furthermore, a variant chicken embryo culture with a very high spontaneous expression of *ev*-1 was found to have at least partial demethylation of *ev*-1, in comparison with nonexpressing siblings (K. F. Conklin et al., in prep.). In both these latter cases, there was also a correlation with the presence of sites in the provirus hypersensitive to cleavage by DNase-I treatment of chromatin, another feature previously associated with high transcriptional activity (Weintraub and Groudine 1976). Interestingly, the hypersensitive sites were located in or very near both the 5′ long terminal repeat (LTR) and the 3′ LTR of *ev*-1.

More definitive evidence in support of the idea of methylation as inhibiting transcription of endogenous proviruses comes from use of the inhibitor 5-azacytidine. This analog of cytidine was found to induce extensive and permanent demethylation of dC residues in DNA, presumably by being converted to the deoxy form and incorporated into DNA in place of deoxycytidine. Since the N atom at the 5 position cannot be methylated, the model presented above for the heritability of methylation would predict that a sequence into which 5-azadeoxycytidine residues were incorporated would become permanently demethylated (Jones and Taylor 1980). Consistent with this prediction, brief treatment of growing chicken cells with 5-azacytidine was found to lead to rapid, extensive, and permanent (for at least 10–20 generations) demethylation of the *ev*-1 provirus (Groudine et al. 1981; K. F. Conklin et al., in prep.), accompanied by an equally permanent and very high induction of expression of *ev*-1. The level of expression of *ev*-1 in such cells approached that of RAV-0 production by fully infected C/O cells and far exceeded that obtainable with BrdU. Similar induction of *ev*-2 (R. Eisenman, pers. comm.) and some endogenous MLV (R. Weinberg; O. Niwa and T. Sugahara; both pers. comm.) has also been found. It is possible that halogenated pyrimidines and other analogs operate through the same mechanism, although this point remains to be tested. In any case, these experiments provide very good evidence that at least one important mechanism involved in the silence of inherited proviruses is methylation of the provirus itself or the region in which it is found.

III. ENDOGENOUS VIRUSES OF VARIOUS ANIMAL SPECIES

In this section, we describe specific endogenous viruses, their genomes and phenotypes, and other phenomena associated with them. The biology and taxonomy of many of these viruses were covered in Chapter 2 and elsewhere; therefore, most detailed description of the viruses is omitted here.

A. Endogenous Viruses of Chickens

All endogenous-virus-related information identified in chickens is closely related to the genomes of avian oncoviruses (for review, see Robinson 1978), and the various endogenous genomes are even more closely related to one another. Nevertheless, there are substantial variations in the endogenous virus phenotypes among chickens. These are characterized by the presence or absence of complete virus production, either spontaneously or after induction, and by proteins related to *gag*-gene or *env*-gene products. The identified endogenous proviruses and their associated phenotypes are listed in Table 10.2.

1. Phenotypes of Avian Endogenous Viruses

a. gs. The first description of endogenous viruses was the finding by Dougherty and Di Stefano (1966) that some uninfected chicken cells contain antigens that cross-react with antibody to gs antigens (i.e., viral *gag*-gene products) in the absence of infectious virus production. Such cells are referred to as gs^+. The gs^+ phenotype is encoded by only one known locus, *ev*-3, and is due to a mutant *gag-pol* precursor.

Table 10.2 The *ev* loci of white leghorn chickens

Locus	Pseudonym	Molecular weight of major *Sst*I (*Sac*I) fragment (kbp)	Phenotype	Products
ev-1	none	10.7	$gs_L chf_L$	*gag* proteins, $gPr92^{env}$
ev-2	V-E7	6.5	V^+	infectious virus (RAV-0)
ev-3	Gs	6.9	gs^+chf^+	$P120^{gag-pol}$, gp85, gp37
ev-4	none	9.6	—	—
ev-5	none	18.0	—	—
ev-6	H-E	18.0	gs^-chf^+	gp85, gp37
ev-7	V-15B	14.0	V^+	noninfectious virus (15B-ILV)
ev-8	none	16.5	—	—
ev-9	H-E	21.0	gs^-chf^+	gp85, gp37
ev-10	V-EC	19.5	V^+	infectious virus (C-ILV)
ev-11	V	12.0	V^+	infectious virus
ev-12	V	7.5	V^+	infectious virus
ev-15	none	4.2	—	none (LTR only?)
ev-16	none	5.4	—	none (LTR only?)

The pseudonym refers to the designations of Robinson (1976). Data from Astrin (1978), Tereba and Astrin (1980), and Hughes et al. (1981a). (The molecular weights given are mostly those of Hughes et al. 1981a.)

b. chf. Cells of some chickens can complement the *env*-gene defect of RSV(−) to allow the production of infectious virus in the absence of helper virus (Vogt 1967; Weiss 1967, 1969; H. Hanafusa et al. 1970). The complementing factor was named chicken helper factor (chf) and identified as an envelope glycoprotein of endogenous virus (Hanafusa et al. 1973; Halpern et al. 1975). chf pseudotypes of RSV(−) have a host range and antigenicity distinct from those of exogenous viruses of subgroups A–D and were designated subgroup E (Weiss 1969; Vogt and Friis 1971). Resistance to subgroup-E virus is very common (but not universal) among strains of chickens used in the laboratory, but cells of other avian species, such as Japanese quail, turkeys, and pheasants, are susceptible (Weiss 1969). chf appears to be a structurally normal envelope glycoprotein. In addition to complementing the RSV(−) *env* defect, it can be readily detected by its ability to form pseudotypes with vesicular stomatitis virus (VSV) (Love and Weiss et al. 1974), and, as described previously (Section II.B.1 and Chapter 3), its presence in chicken cells confers at least partial resistance to infection with subgroup-E virus.

Three phenotypes of chickens involving gs and chf have been identified. gs^+chf^+ chickens express both coordinately. In crosses with negative birds, both characters segregate together as a single dominant allele (Hanafusa et al. 1974), termed *Gs* by Robinson (1978), and identified as *ev*-3 (see below).

gs^-chf^+, also called gs_Lh_E (for low gs and helper extremely high), or simply h-e, is characterized by low to undetectable levels of gs antigen and high levels of chf activity (Weiss and Payne 1971;Hanafusa et al. 1974). Two 1independent loci (*ev*-6 and *ev*-9) each give rise to variations of the gs^-chf^+ phenotype (Astrin et al. 1980b).

gs^-chf^- chickens are, in fact, not usually completely negative but have small but detectable amounts of chf and gs activity (Hanafusa et al. 1974). This characteristic is due to the *ev*-1 locus, which is common in many lines of white leghorn chickens (Astrin 1978; Astrin et al. 1980b).

c. RAV-60. The *env*-related information in all three phenotypes can participate not only in phenotypic mixing to yield infectious (but replication-defective) virus, but also in recombination to yield replication-competent virus. T. Hanafusa et al. (1970a) found that passage of RAV-2 (subgroup B) in chf^+ chicken cells, followed by passage in Japanese quail cells that are resistant to subgroup-B virus, led to the isolation of a replication-competent virus of subgroup E, with envelope properties similar to those of RSV (chf). They designated this virus RAV-60 and proposed that it was a recombinant between RAV-2 and the information giving rise to chf. The recombinant nature of RAV-60 was demonstrated by cross-hybridization with RAV-2-, RAV-0-, and RAV-60-specific cDNA probes, in which RAV-60 was shown to be intermediate in hybridization properties between RAV-0 and RAV-2 (Hayward and Hanafusa 1975), and by oligonucleotide mapping, which demonstrated the substitution in RAV-60 of the RAV-2 *env* region with a set of oligonucleotides closely related to, but not identical with, the *env* gene of RAV-0 (Coffin et al. 1978a; Robinson et al. 1980b). This type of recombination is not limited to the case just discussed. RAV-60 viruses can be isolated from ALV of any subgroup and from chicken cells of all three chf phenotypes, although the efficiency of isolation of RAV-60 from chf^- cells is lower (Hanafusa et al. 1972). This phenomenon is not limited to nontransforming viruses. Weiss et al. (1973) showed that subgroup-E nondefective transforming viruses could be isolated in an analogous manner from chf^+ cells starting with PR-RSV or SR-RSV. When the same experiment is attempted with RSV(−), nondefective transforming virus is not isolated (as with attempted recombination between RSV[−] and RAV); rather a typical RAV-60 arises (Weiss 1969; Kawai and Hanafusa 1973) apparently by replacement of *src* with the env^E gene. It should be kept in mind that, unlike RAV-0, RAV-1, RAV-2, etc., which (in principle) denote single strains of virus, RAV-60 is a class of viruses. Separate strains must be designated with a trivial isolate number to distinguish them.

RAV-60s and the analogous subgroup-E transforming viruses provide a convenient means of examining the relationship among the proviruses that encode chf and other endogenous-virus-related elements. Coffin et al. (1978a) compared oligonucleotide maps of the genomes of a set of RAV-60s from gs^+chf^+ cells with those of exogenous parents and were able to infer that the subgroup coding region of *env* (as identified by recombinants between exogenous viruses) was derived from endogenous information. A number of recombinants, however, also acquired additional information toward the 3′ end of *env*, but the U_3 region was always derived from the exogenous parent (Robinson et al. 1980b). As with recombinants involving RAV-0 (see later and Chapter 4), the retention of the U_3 regions of exogenous viruses most likely confers a significant growth advantage to the recombinant (Tsichlis and Coffin 1979, 1980a,b). Recombination in the 5′ part of the genome was only rarely observed, and then only in the *gag* region (Rettenmier and Hanafusa 1977; K. Conklin, unpubl.). This selectivity could reflect the defectiveness of the endogenous parent in this region. Comparison of oligonucleotide maps of subgroup-E recombinants from chicken cells of the three different phenotypes shows that the endogenous *env* genes associated with each are very closely related to one another, and to that of RAV-0, yet differ slightly (Coffin et al. 1978a; Robinson et al. 1980b). Such differences, although small, serve as markers to show that the different *env* genes are derived from different endogenous proviruses.

d. RAV-0 and ILV. As discussed in Section II.B.1, cells of certain chickens have the property that they can spontaneously release infectious virus of subgroup E (Vogt and Friis 1971; Crittenden et al. 1974) or that they can be induced to release infectious virus with agents such as BrdU, chemical carcinogens, or ionizing radiation (Weiss et al. 1971; Robinson et al. 1976). The spontaneous production or inducibility of infectious virus has been associated with 4 of the 12 characterized *ev* loci (*ev*-2, *ev*-10, *ev*-11, and *ev*-12) (Astrin et al. 1980a,b; Tereba and Astrin 1980). Vogt and Friis (1971) named the virus spontaneously released from line-7 cells RAV-0, and the virus that was induced was termed ILV (Weiss et al. 1971). These viruses had a host range of subgroup E, identical with one another and with RAV-60. (A few isolates of ILV of different subgroup were found and later attributed to generation of subgroup-F virus endogenous to the pheasant cells used to amplify the induced virus [Hanafusa and Hanafusa 1973; Fujita et al. 1974].)

2. *The Genome of RAV-0*

RAV-0 closely resembles exogenous ALV in structure, but there are some interesting differences in biology. The subgroup-E host range has not been found in any exogenous virus strain isolated from animals. Unlike all exogenous ALV strains, RAV-0 has not been shown to cause any disease, either following injection into susceptible birds or when it is spontaneously produced in high levels in V^+ C/O birds (Motta et al. 1975; Robinson et al. 1980a). In addition, it has a growth rate distinctly less than those of exogenous viruses in cell culture (Hanafusa et al. 1975; Linial and Neiman 1976; Robinson et al. 1976; Coffin et al. 1981). Except for subgroup, these properties are not shared with RAV-60 isolates, which have growth rates similar to those of exogenous viruses and induce lymphoid leukosis (and some other diseases) in susceptible chickens (Crittenden et al. 1980; Robinson et al. 1980a,b). These differences in biological properties have induced particular interest in the RAV-0 genome as a test system for analysis of features that control replication rate and oncogenicity by ALV.

The genome of RAV-0 has been compared to that of exogenous ALV by hybridization competition (Neiman et al. 1977; Neiman 1978), oligonucleotide mapping (Coffin et al. 1978b), restriction mapping (Shank et al. 1981), and heteroduplex mapping (Chien et al. 1980). A schematic representation of the results is shown in Chapter 4 (Fig. 4.6). The 5′ half of the RAV-0 genome is nearly identical with that of typical strains of ALV, with only scattered single-base differences and a small insert in *gag* that is perhaps reflected as a slightly larger apparent molecular weight for p27 (Shaikh et al. 1978). The *env* genes of RAV-0 and exogenous viruses of subgroups B and C differ in the same way that *env* genes of different subgroups vary from one another (see Chapter 4), i.e., with a central region of greater divergence (the *S* region marking the central subgroup-specific region of gp85) flanked by more conserved sequences. The greatest sequence differences are found near the 3′ end. The sequence to the left of *src* in nondefective RSV genomes is either not present or substantially diverged in the RAV-0 genome; the U_3 region, highly conserved among exogenous viruses, is quite different. The nucleotide sequences of the U_3 region of RAV-0 and of the *ev*-1 provirus have recently been determined (Hishinuma et al. 1981; S. Hughes, pers. comm.) and have been found to be quite similar to one another and distinctly different from that of exogenous ALV (Fig. 10.1). Most notably, the endogenous (U_3^n) region is substantially shorter—167 nucleotides as compared with 248 nucleotides in the corresponding region (U_3^x) of exogenous ALV (see Chapter 4). In spite of these differences, there are regions of similarity. The two regions most strongly implicated in control of gene expression, the AAUAAA "polyadenylation signal" and the putative promoter signal (Hogness box), are preserved in both sequence and location relative to the end of the genome. Also strongly preserved is the region around the plus-strand primer-binding site (PB+) at the 5′ end of U_3. In between these conserved regions, there is substantial

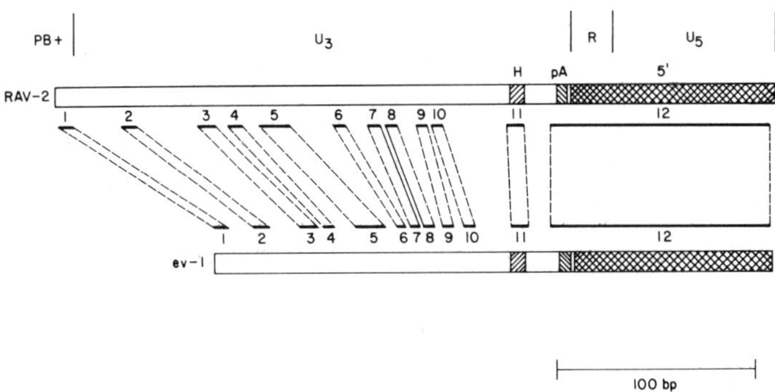

Figure 10.1 Relationship between the LTRs of endogenous and exogenous ALVs. The numbered lines show areas of identical sequences and their relative locations. Note that the 5′ (R-U_5) regions are closely related; the U_3 region much less so. (Adapted from Hishinuma et al. 1981.)

divergence, yet nine small regions of homology could be detected, giving a total of about 35% homology (relative to U_3^x) for the entire region. As predicted from nucleic acid hybridization results (Coffin et al. 1978b), R and U_5 (the remainder of the LTR) were virtually identical in sequence, with only scattered single-base differences.

Another approach to comparison of the genomes of endogenous and exogenous viruses was taken by Tsichlis and Coffin (1979, 1980a,b), who prepared recombinants between RAV-0 and several ALV and RSV strains, selecting from subgroup E and either transformation or rapid growth. The only region of the exogenous virus genome inherited by all recombinants was the U_3 region, implying that the U_3-region difference is responsible for the difference in growth rate. In particular, a recombinant whose genome was identical (by oligonucleotide mapping) with that of RAV-0, except for the U_3 region, had a growth rate typical of exogenous viruses (Tsichlis and Coffin 1980a; Coffin et al. 1981; H. L. Robinson et al., unpubl.). Interestingly, although this virus also had a high growth rate in vivo, it was weakly oncogenic compared either with RAV-60 or with its transformation-defective RSV parent, which had a distinct pathology. The recombinant was, however, significantly more pathogenic than RAV-0 (Coffin et al. 1981; H. L. Robinson et al., unpubl.). Thus, although the U_3-region difference seems to be the only major determinant affecting growth, some other region(s) of the genome must be involved in oncogenicity. The high oncogenicity of RAV-60 viruses shows that this region is not the part of *env* involved in host range, and a comparison of the structures of the various recombinants tentatively implicates a region 5′ of U_3 extending partway into the gp37 coding region.

Other endogenous ALVs closely resemble RAV-0 in biology and genomic structure, but there are small differences in nucleotide sequence detectable by oligonucleotide mapping (J. M. Coffin et al., unpubl.). For example, C-ILV (the product of *ev*-10) contains four (out of 30) oligonucleotides not found in RAV-0 and lacks four RAV-0 oligonucleotides. These differences probably reflect less than 1% sequence divergence between these genomes, with no known biological significance, but serve as markers for the different *ev* loci. For this reason, it is recommended that the suggestions of Robinson (1978) be followed and that RAV-0 be reserved as the name for the product of *ev*-2; C-ILV, for the product of *ev*-10; and 15B-E virus, for the infectious virus occasionally produced by line-15 cells (*ev*-7 × *ev*-1; see Section II.B.1.a).

3. The ev *loci*

As discussed above (Section II.A.2), the description of the *ev* loci and correlation with phenotypes of endogenous viruses was a major advance in clarifying the analysis of endogenous ALV. A substantial amount of work has subsequently provided detailed descriptions of the structures of these proviruses, as well as their transcripts and gene products, and of their relationships to one another and to exogenous ALV. These are summarized in Table 10.2 and Figure 10.2. The following major points have become clear. First, the *ev* proviruses closely resemble exogenous proviruses in structure, with LTRs, the same gene order, and (in the one case studied) similar alterations at the integration site. Second, the variety of phenotypes observed is completely explicable in terms of either mutational variation in the proviruses themselves (frequently involving deletions) or variations in overall levels of expression. Third, the *ev* loci are found on numerous chromosomes and are not linked to *onc* genes. Fourth, the *ev* proviruses are closely related to exogenous ALV, yet are much more closely related to one another and therefore form a distinct lineage of virus.

a. ev-*1.* *ev*-1 is almost ubiquitous in all strains of white leghorn chickens examined, although it is not as widely distributed in other

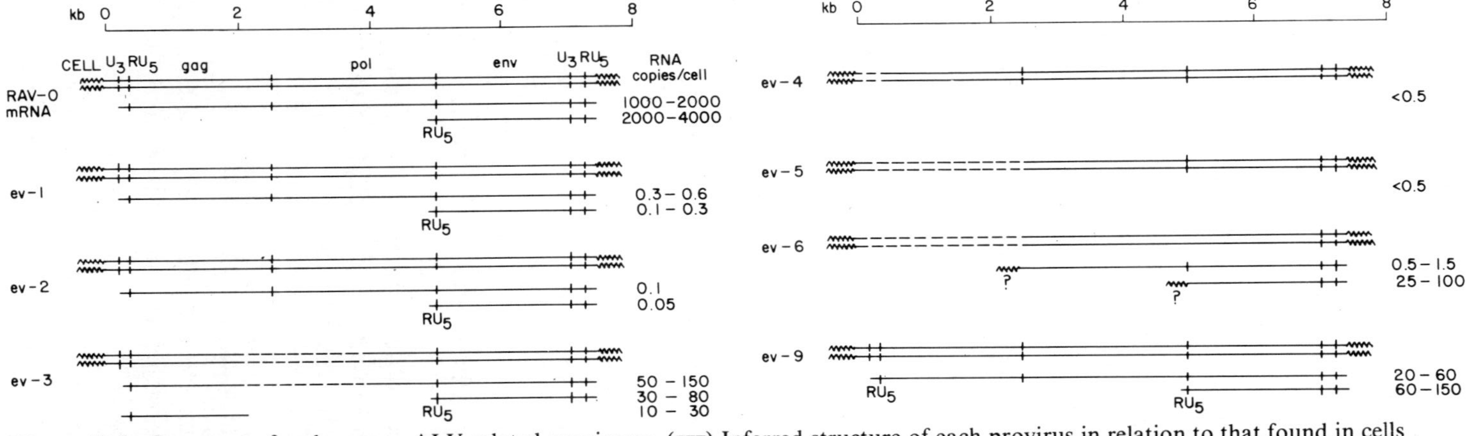

Figure 10.2 Structure of endogenous ALV-related proviruses. (===) Inferred structure of each provirus in relation to that found in cells infected with RAV-0 (first set of lines); (-----) deletions; (——) stable transcripts attributed to each provirus with the approximate copy number shown on the right. Data from Hayward et al. (1980), Skalka et al. (1980), Baker et al. (1981), and Hughes et al. (1981a).

breeds (Astrin 1978; Tereba and Astrin 1980; Hughes et al. 1981b) and is responsible for the gs_Lchf_L phenotype usually found in chicken cells. It encodes low levels (about 0.2–0.5 copies/cell, respectively) of apparently structurally normal viral RNA of 7.5 kb (genome) and 3 kb (*env* mRNA) (Wang et al. 1977; Hayward et al. 1980; Baker et al. 1981), but no infectious virions can be found. DNA of the *ev*-1 provirus has been studied in detail following molecular cloning and partial-nucleotide-sequence analysis (Skalka et al. 1980; Hishinuma et al. 1981) (see Appendix D), and again no gross defects have been found. It was found that the provirus is flanked by an LTR of identical sequence at each end, closely related to that of RAV-0 (Hishinuma et al. 1981) (Fig. 10.1), and has a restriction map very similar to that of exogenous ALV. The availability of *ev*-negative chickens (Astrin et al. 1979a) made it possible to obtain molecular clones of the unoccupied integration site, and it was found that a 6-base sequence present once in the cellular DNA was duplicated at each end of the provirus (Hishinuma et al. 1981). This feature is identical with that found in integration of exogenous viruses (Chapter 5) and strongly implies that the *ev*-1 provirus was inserted into the chicken germ line by processes similar to or identical with those involved in the usual replication cycle. The *ev*-1 provirus has been localized to chromosome 1 by in situ hybridization (Tereba and Astrin 1980).

Considering that *ev*-1-containing cells have, on average, somewhat more virus-specific RNA than *ev*-2-containing cells, which produce low levels of infectious RAV-0 (Hayward et al. 1980), the defect in *ev*-1 for virus production cannot be explained simply on quantitative grounds. A resolution of this issue was made possible by the recent observations of a variant chicken-cell culture with high spontaneous expression of *ev*-1 (K. F. Conklin et al., in prep.) and by the finding that 5-azacytidine could efficiently induce high-level *ev*-1 production in chicken cells (Groudine et al. 1981; K. F. Conklin et al., in prep.) (see Section II.B.3). Such cells were found to produce noninfectious virions that contained a genome closely related to, but not identical with, that of RAV-0. The lack of infectivity could be attributed to a complete absence of reverse transcriptase activity and polypeptides, as well as to improper processing of $gPr92^{env}$. The lack of reverse transcriptase was apparently due to a failure to synthesize $Pr180^{gag\text{-}pol}$ (see Chapter 6), since no *gag*-related translation product larger than Pr76 could be found, and the synthesis and processing of *gag* proteins was apparently normal. Interestingly, the p19 encoded by *ev*-1 had a substantially lower molecular weight than that of other exogenous or endogenous ALVs, perhaps accounting for the frequency with which low-molecular-weight p19s are observed in recombinants involving endogenous viruses (Shaikh et al. 1978; Robinson et al. 1979).

b. ev-*2.* *ev*-2 is the inducible locus responsible for the V^+ phenotype of lines 7 and 100 and is therefore the endogenous provirus of RAV-0 (Astrin 1978; Astrin et al. 1980a). Cells that contain *ev*-2 alone have only very small quantities of virus-related RNA, about 0.1 and 0.05 copies per cell of 7.5-kb and 3-kb RNAs, respectively (Hayward et al. 1980). Considering that it encodes infectious virus, the *ev*-2 locus is presumably a structurally normal provirus, in agreement with the structure deduced from restriction mapping (Hughes et al. 1981a; Shank et al. 1981).

c. ev-*3.* *ev*-3 is responsible for the gs^+chf^+ phenotype in several lines of chickens (Astrin and Robinson 1979). It encodes three polyadenylated RNA species of 6.5 kb, 2.7 kb, and 3.0 kb at levels of about 60, 100, and 20 copies per cell, respectively (Wang et al. 1977; Hayward et al. 1980; Baker et al. 1981). The gs antigenicity is due to a 120,000-dalton protein (P120), with sequences related to p19, p27, and p12, and reverse transcriptase (Eisenman et al. 1978). This protein has the properties expected for the translation product of a viral RNA, with a deletion including p15, the *gag-pol* boundary, and the left end of *pol.* This, in fact, is the structure of the 6.5-kb RNA (Baker et al. 1981). A corresponding deletion is also found in the DNA encompassing about 1.5 kb around the *gag-pol* junction (Hayward et al. 1980; Hughes et al. 1981a). The 3-kb species is indistinguishable from normal *env* mRNA (see Chapter 5) and must encode the chf activity. The 2.7-kb species represents only the 5′ portion of the genome and has not been seen in other endogenous or exogenous viruses. It is too small to encode the P120, and it has not been further characterized.

d. ev-*4,* ev-*5, and* ev-*8.* *ev*-4, *ev*-5, and *ev*-8 have no known associated phenotypes (Astrin et al. 1980b). They have been found in several lines of chickens. Their presence does not increase the amount of viral RNA above the level typical of *ev*-1 in the same cell (Hayward et al. 1980; Baker et al. 1981), and any associated RNAs, if present, must be at the level of less than 0.5 copies per cell. By hybridization with specific cDNA probes, *ev*-4 lacks the 5′ copy of the LTR and *ev*-5 seems not to contain *gag* or the 5′ copy of the LTR (Hayward et al. 1980; Hughes et al. 1981a). This deletion could account for the lack of expression of those proviruses, since the virus-specified promoter, present in the 5′ copy of the U_3 region in the integrated provirus (Chapter 5), would be missing. No such deletion was found in *ev*-8 (Hughes et al. 1981a), and its lack of expression is unexplained. Interestingly, all these highly defective loci seem to be located on the same chromosome (chromosome 1) as is the defective *ev*-1 provirus (A. Tereba, pers. comm.).

e. ev-*6.* *ev*-6 is one of two proviruses responsible for the gs^-chf^+ phenotype (Astrin et al. 1980b). Cells containing *ev*-6 have about 100 copies of a 3-kb *env* RNA and about 1 copy of a 28S RNA with *env* and some *pol* sequences (Hayward et al. 1980; Baker et al. 1981). No *gag*-containing RNAs were found. Unlike virus-specific mRNAs either in infected cells or associated with all other loci tested, the 3-kb RNA species associated with *ev*-6 does not contain sequences capable of hybridizing to DNA specific for the U_5 region (Hayward et al. 1980; Baker et al. 1981) and therefore apparently lacks at least part of the spliced-on leader sequence of the typical 3-kb *env* mRNA, yet is capable of functioning as an mRNA as evidenced by the high level of chf. Like *ev*-5, the *ev*-6 provirus does not appear to have sequences related to *gag* or to the 5′ LTR, thus explaining the absence of these sequences in the RNAs. Hayward et al. (1980) have proposed that *ev*-6 utilizes cellular sequences to the left of the provirus both as promoter for transcription and possibly to provide a leader sequence for splicing onto the *env* mRNA.

f. ev-*7.* *ev*-7 is found in chickens of line 15B and segregates in genetic crosses with the V-15 phenotype (Robinson et al. 1979). It is therefore the provirus encoding the inducible, noninfectious virions discussed in Section II.B.1.a. The provirus does not contain major deletions (Hughes et al. 1981a), and the structure of *ev*-7-associated RNAs has not been studied. The ability of *ev*-7 cells to produce polymerase-containing particles after induction implies the presence of a functional *pol* gene, as does the ability to recombine with the progeny of *ev*-1 (defective in *pol*) to form infectious virus (Robinson et al. 1979). The lack of infectivity of these particles and their failure to complement RSV(−) (Robinson et al. 1979) suggest an *env*-gene defect. Other possible defects (in terminal regions, for example) have not been excluded. Unlike the other *ev* loci, *ev*-7 was found to behave as a sex-linked locus in appropriate genetic crosses, and must therefore be located on the Z chromosome (Smith and Crittenden 1981), a result in agreement with the in situ hybridization studies of Tereba and Astrin (1980).

g. ev-*9.* *ev*-9 is a second locus encoding the gs^-chf^+ phenotype (Astrin et al. 1980b). The provirus itself appears structurally normal by restriction mapping, (Baker et al. 1981) and the 7.5-kb and 3-kb virus-specific RNAs are found in *ev*-9 cells at levels of about 40 and 100 copies per cell, respectively (Hayward et al. 1980). The 7.5-kb RNA appears structurally normal, yet must have some defect affecting processing, since it is found only in nuclei of *ev*-9 cells (Baker et al. 1981). This defect could easily explain the failure of this RNA to be translated into *gag* proteins.

h. ev-*10,* ev-*11, and* ev-*12.* *ev*-10 is found in Reaseheath C-line and in some line-15 chickens. It closely resembles *ev*-2 in that it is an inducible locus that encodes infectious virus, in this case C-ILV (Weiss et al. 1971; Astrin et al. 1980b). *ev*-11 is found in RPRL line-$15I_4$ chickens (Tereba and Astrin 1980) and also encodes infectious virus, as does *ev*-12 of line-15_1 chickens (Tereba and Astrin 1980).

i. ev-*15 and* ev-*16.* *ev*-15 and *ev*-16 are interesting elements found in a variety of chickens. They seem to consist only of an LTR, although the complete absence of other viral information remains to be verified (Hughes et al. 1981a). Such a structure could conceivably be generated by recombination between the two LTRs, with a resultant loss of all sequences in between.

4. Distribution and Origin of Endogenous Virus Loci

As discussed above, DNA-transfer hybridization allows the detection, enumeration, and structural and genetic analyses of the endogenous proviruses of chickens. With this kind of methodology, it has also been possible to draw some conclusions about their origin and possible function. Early experiments based on hybridization of cellular DNAs from various species to RAV-0-specific probes suggested that some avian species contained virus-related information whose extent of relationship to RAV-0 was roughly proportional to the evolutionary relationship of the various species to chickens (Kang and Temin 1974; Shoyab and Baluda 1975; Tereba et al. 1975). No related sequences were detected in distantly related birds, such as ducks, and a little homology (5–15%) was found in pheasants. The presence of related sequences in pheasants was not surprising in view of the presence of chf-like activity and the ability to form RAV-60-like viruses in ring-necked pheasant cells (Hanafusa and Hanafusa 1973; Fujita et al. 1974). Yet, the complex patterns of endogenous virus loci in chickens and the absence of any locus common to all chickens are suggestive of acquisition of these loci, most likely by germ-line infection, subsequent to speciation (Hughes et al. 1979).

To resolve this issue, Frisby et al. (1979) examined the DNAs of some individuals of other members of the *Gallus* genus, most closely related to the domestic chicken (*Gallus gallus*). In the four species tested, both by hybridization under stringent and nonstringent conditions and by DNA transfer RAV-0-related sequences were found only in the red jungle fowl, which is the wild relative of the domestic chicken. More distantly related sequences were found in ring-necked and Japanese green pheasants (both of genus *Phasianus*), partridges, and grouses, but not in pheasants of six other genera or in quails (Frisby et al. 1979, 1980; Hughes et al. 1981b). Since the different *Gallus* species are separated from one another by some 6 million years of evolution and from pheasants by some 30 million years, this pattern is clearly inconsistent with endogenous proviruses behaving as normal-cell genes. Rather, it is more likely that the endogenous proviruses arose by germ-line infection with a RAV-0-like virus of some ancestor of the red jungle fowl and with a related virus of some *Phasianus* ancestor (and ancestors of patridges and grouses as well), but that related species escaped such infection.

The diversity of the structures and integration sites of endogenous virus loci suggests that germ-line infection has taken place repeatedly in chickens and is probably still occurring (although it has not been observed directly). Such reinfection could occur by the usual mechanisms of the virus or, less likely, by some more direct movement of the provirus itself from site to site. Considering the diversity of integration sites, the sequences of endogenous proviruses themselves are remarkably highly conserved and differ from one another principally by deletions. All inducible infectious viruses of chickens and even of red jungle fowl are indistinguishable biologically (Weiss and Biggs 1972) and differ only by a few scattered point mutations, as revealed by oligonucleotide mapping (Coffin et al. 1981). Similarly, the *env* genes (and their products) of the genomes of defective endogenous virus (*ev*-1, *ev*-3, *ev*-6, *ev*-7, and *ev*-9) differ only slightly from one another and from RAV-0. As a group, the endogenous viruses of chickens are more closely related to one another than the exogenous viruses and are a distinct lineage from exogenous viruses, with specific conserved oligonucleotide markers scattered throughout their genomes, but concentrated in the *env* and U_3 regions (J. M. Coffin et al., unpubl.). On the basis of such analyses, it is possible to infer the relationship scheme shown in Figure 10.3. Assuming that the oligonucleotide differences represent randomly distributed base differences, the greatest divergence observed (between *ev*-1 and *ev*-10) represents less than 2% of sequence difference.

None of a large number of endogenous proviruses in different chickens contains an exogenous-virus-related U_3 region as marked by the absence of a common *Eco*RI site and by hybridization with U_3-region-specific probes (Hughes et al. 1981a,b). Thus, the endogenous viruses of chickens are descended from one another, rather than from reintroduction of exogenous virus. This result is some-

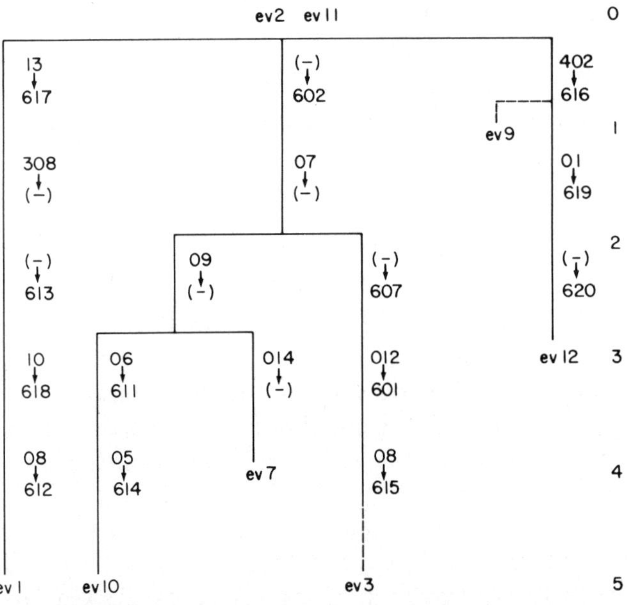

Figure 10.3 Possible relationships among endogenous ALV proviruses. The numbers at the right of each line signify detectable point mutations leading to altered oligonucleotides (see Chapter 4, Fig. 4.6, for a map of RAV-0). If randomly distributed, each change corresponds to about 1 base change per 600 nucleotides. (Data from J. Coffin et al., unpubl.)

what surprising in view of the much greater prevalence of infectious exogenous viruses, as compared with endogenous viruses in domestic chickens, and the frequency of the C/E phenotype among these chickens. Whether the propensity for the RAV-0-related viruses to become "endogenized" is somehow greater than that of exogenous viruses or whether the failure to find germ-line integration of exogenous viruses represents selection against such birds (due to a high rate of leukemia, for example, as occurs in mice that have acquired an endogenous provirus for Mo-MLV [Section III.B.4]), remains to be determined. It is also possible that there is greater access to the germ line of viruses already present there.

B. Endogenous Viruses of Mice

The endogenous viruses of laboratory mice comprise one of the most complicated systems in all of virology (for review, see Aaronson and Stephenson 1976; Levy 1978; Pincus 1980). There are no less than four distinct types of endogenous "viral" loci—including proviruses of C-type and B-type viruses, A-type particles, and VL30 RNAs— most of which are found in multiple copies in the germ line. As a consequence of their presence in multiple copies, restriction enzyme digests of mouse-cell DNA's give very complex patterns when analyzed by hybridization with viral DNA probes and (using enzymes that do not cleave the provirus probe) more bands are detected than can be easily counted (Steffen and Weinberg 1978; Canaani and Aaronson 1979). It has been estimated that as much as 0.05% of the total mouse genome consists of endogenous-virus-related information (Callahan and Todaro 1978). In spite of this complexity, it seems likely that the same general principles for the endogenous viruses of chickens will also apply to those of mice, i.e., that each mode of virus expression will be due to a distinct endogenous provirus, which is a fairly recent acquisition into the germ line of the mouse. In the two cases where it has been possible to study the endogenous proviruses directly by hybridization (the endogenous ecotropic C-type viruses and MMTV), it has been found that inheritance of the virus-producing phenotype is the same as inheritance of specific proviral DNA sequences. Also, there is significant variation in the patterns of virus-specific restriction enzyme fragments between different inbred strains of mice but relatively little between individuals of a given strain, suggesting divergence subsequent to speciation and prior to the origin of the strains.

Of the distinguishable endogenous "viruses" of mice, at least two are demonstrably viruses: C type and MMTV. Two other types have been related to viruses in various ways but have not been shown to be authentic viral genomes. These include the genes encoding 30S RNA and A-type particles. In the sections that follow, each of these entities is discussed with respect to its genetics and genomic structure. More information on their biology can be found in other chapters.

1. C-type Viruses

The endogenous ecotropic and xenotropic viruses are quite closely related to one another, since their genomes share many restriction enzyme cleavage sites (Chattopadhyay et al. 1981), they have numerous antigenic determinants in common (Barbacid et al. 1978), and they can recombine with one another to yield viable virus. Nucleic acid hybridization with specific probes (Chattopadhyay et al. 1981) and heteroduplex mapping (Chien et al. 1978) show greatest variation in the region of *env* that can be expected (from the precedent of avian tumor viruses; Chapter 4) to encode host range. In these respects, ecotropic and xenotropic endogenous viruses are probably more closely related to one another than ecotropic endogenous virus is to ecotropic exogenous virus (such as Mo-MLV) (D. Steffen pers. comm.). However, because their biological properties are quite different, as are their distributions in mice, we consider the ecotropic and xenotropic viruses separately.

a. Ecotropic Viruses. Viruses capable of infecting mouse cells are produced spontaneously or can be induced from many strains of mice, including AKR, BALB/c, C57BL/10, and HRS, but a number of strains, such as NIH-Swiss (and the inbred NFS mice derived from them), SWR, NZB, and 129, have been found to be negative in all tests (see Levy 1978; Pincus 1980). The genetics of the ecotropic endogenous virus in AKR mice has been studied by Rowe and collaborators (Rowe 1972; Rowe and Hartley 1972; Kozak and Rowe 1979, 1980b). In crosses between AKR and NIH Swiss mice, two independently segregating dominant loci for virus production were identified and named *Akv-1* and *Akv-2* and were mapped on chromosomes 7 and 16, respectively. That these loci correspond to the endogenous proviruses themselves is shown by two lines of evidence. Chattopadhyay et al. (1975a,b) examined in detail the reassociation kinetics of cellular DNA from a number of strains of mice using cDNA complementary to the AKV genome. Two classes of virus-related sequences were identified. One class, found in all mice examined, was only partially homologous to the probe and found in multiple copies. This class probably contained endogenous xenotropic or other unidentified viruses. The second class was found only in mice from which ecotropic virus could be isolated and had substantial homology with the probe. Such sequences were approximately twice as abundant in AKR mice as in (NIH × AKR)F_1 hybrids or in NIH-Swiss mice congenic for *Akv-1*.

The second line of evidence identifying the *Akv-1* and *Akv-2* loci as independent endogenous proviruses comes from the observation that the genomes of viruses induced from *Akv-1* and *Akv-2* cogenic mice have T1 fingerprints identical to each other and to virus induced from AKR mice (Rommelaere et al. 1977). Viruses isolated from other strains of mice, e.g., BALB/c, HRS, and C57BL/6, have very similar, yet distinct, fingerprints in that their genomes share 70–90% of the large oligonucleotides (Rommelaere et al. 1977; Faller and Hopkins 1978a; Green et al. 1980). Thus, inheritance of an ecotropic locus corresponds to inheritance of a specific viral genome, marked by a specific fingerprint.

In BALB/c mice, only a single dominant locus (termed *Cv*) for the production of endogenous virus was found (Stephenson and Aaronson 1972; Ihle et al. 1979; Kozak and Rowe 1979), yet two endogenous ecotropic viruses can be identified: an N-tropic virus, which replicates only very poorly in B-type BALB/c cells, and a B-tropic virus, which replicates well (Pincus et al. 1971a,b). Treatment of BALB/c cells with BrdU results in the induction of the N-tropic virus, which decreases soon after removal of the inducer (Stephenson and Aaronson 1972; Besmer et al. 1975). A B-tropic virus is not induced in such experiments but can be found in older mice. The genomes of N-tropic and B-tropic viruses are closely related to each other but differ by the presence of a number of oligonucleotides specific for each isolate, including the markers for tropism and G_{IX} antigen (see Chapter 4). Since one provirus seems to encode both viruses, it is likely that the B-tropic virus arises from the N-tropic virus by some rare event involving either recombination or mutation and is strongly selected, since replication of the N-tropic endogenous virus is restricted in BALB/c cells. Peptide mapping of p30s of the N-tropic and B-tropic viruses shows that the p30 of the B-tropic virus closely resembles those of some xenotropic viruses (Gautsch et al. 1978, 1980), implying recombination with an as yet unidentified xenotropic-related virus as the source of B tropism. Interestingly, an H-2 congenic strain, B10.BR, yields only B-tropic virus either in vivo or following induction of cell cultures. The responsible locus has been mapped to chromosome 11, distinct from parental strains. This result implies reintegration into the germ line of a B-tropic virus which most likely arose as the result of a somatic recombination event (Moll et al. 1979). A recent analysis of the endogenous ecotropic loci in a number of mouse strains has been performed (D. Steffen et al., in prep.; N. Jenkins et al., unpubl.). A compilation of these results is shown in Tables 10.3 and 10.4.

The genomes of the endogenous ecotropic viruses of mice are related to those of exogenous MLV, although the relationship is rather more distant than between endogenous and exogenous viruses of chickens. Considerable cross-hybridization between, for example, Mo-MLV and AKR virus probes can be detected, but

Table 10.3 Endogenous ecotropic proviruses found in various strains of mice

	Cell-virus DNA junction fragments (kb)			Internal viral DNA fragments (kb)		
Provirus	*Pvu*II	*Hin*dIII	*Xba*I	*Kpn*I	*Bam*HI	*Pst*I
emv-1	4.3	7.0	10.5	4.4	3.3	8.2
emv-2	5.2	7.0	11.5	4.4	3.3	8.2
emv-3	5.4	6.4	8.4	4.4	3.3	8.2
emv-4	4.8	8.4	8.4	4.4	3.3	8.2
emv-5	6.4	15.0	9.0	4.4	3.3	8.2
emv-6	13.0	19.0	5.3	3.8	2.1	5.1
emv-7	5.6	6.0	9.8	4.4	3.3	8.2
emv-8	5.8	8.4	8.0	4.4	3.3	8.2
emv-9	4.8	6.6	6.3	3.8	2.1	5.1
emv-10	4.1	11.0	11.5	4.4	3.3	8.2
Akv-1 (*emv*-11)	4.8	5.9	13.5	4.4	3.3	8.2
Akv-2 (*emv*-12)	5.0	7.0	11.5	4.4	3.3	8.2
Akv-3 (*emv*-13)	3.9	21.0	13.5	4.4	3.3	8.2
Akv-4 (*emv*-14)	8.3	6.0	13.5	4.4	3.3	8.2

The fragments indicated are only those that react with a short probe specific for ecotropic virus and are derived from the *env* region of AKV DNA (Chattopadhyay et al. 1980). Data courtesy of N. Jenkins, N. Copeland, B. Lee, and B. Taylor, Jackson Laboratories.

Table 10.4 Ecotropic proviruses in various inbred mice

Strain	*emv* loci	Strain	*emv* loci
A/HeJ	1	C58/J	multiple
A/J	1	DA/HuSn	7
A/WySnJ	1	DBA/1J	3
AKR/N	11, 12, 13	DBA/2J	3
AKR/J	11, 13, 14	DBA/2DeJ	3
AU/SsJ	none	FS/Ei	1
BALB/cByJ	1	HRS/J	1, 3
BALB/cGnEi	1	I/LnJ	multiple
BALB/cJ	1	LG/J	4
BALB/cWtEi	1	LP/J	5
BDP/J	3	LT/SV	multiple
BUB/BnJ	none	MA/MyJ	8, 9
CBA/CaJ	none	NFS	none
CBA/H-T6J	none	NZB/B1NJ	none
CBA/J	1	P/J	3
CBA/N	none	PL/J	multiple
CE/J	none	RF/J	multiple
C3H/HeBFeJ	1	RIIIS/J	none
C3H/HeJ	1	SEA/GnJ	1, 3
C3H/HeSnJ	1	SEC/1ReJ	1
C57BL/KsJ	2	SJL/J	9, 10
		SJL/Wt	9, 10
C57BL/6ByJ	2	SM/J	1
C57BL/6J	2	ST/bJ	6
C57BL/10J	2	SWR/J	none
C57BL/10SnJ	2	129/J	none
C57BR/cdJ	2	129/SvJ	none
C57L/J	none		

The content of *emv* loci (Table 10.3) for each of 53 strains of inbred mice is shown courtesy of N. Jenkins, N. Copeland, B. Lee, and B. Taylor, Jackson Laboratories.

there are no large T1 oligonucleotides shared between the two genomes (Rommelaere et al. 1977; Coffin et al. 1978c; Faller and Hopkins 1978b). Heteroduplex mapping shows four substitution loops that distinguish this pair of viruses, one in the 5′ half near the *gag-pol* boundary and three in the 3′ half, probably within *env* (Chien et al. 1980). The significance of these differences remains to be investigated.

b. Variation in Endogenous Ecotropic Proviruses. Genetically transmitted proviruses coding for the AKV strain of ecotropic MLV are sufficiently stable that they behave in a Mendelian fashion in genetic crosses and can be mapped to specific linkage groups in the mouse genome. It has recently been demonstrated, however, that this stability is not absolute. Among viremic mice, the provirus copy number increases over time.

An increase in AKV provirus copy number has been observed in three systems: NFS/N congenic mice carrying the *Akv-1* provirus from AKR mice, recombinant inbred strains derived from AKR × C57BL, and mice of the AKR strain. A genetic analysis revealed that some lines of *Akv-1* congenic mice had acquired new proviruses during their inbreeding (Rowe and Kozak 1980). Animals were observed to have acquired up to three additional proviruses. In these experiments, it was also shown that acquisition of new AKV proviruses occurred only if the provirus was acquired from the maternal parent, suggesting that novel germ-line integrations are the result of infection in utero, infection by milk-borne virus, or infection of the oocyte.

Amplification of provirus copy number has also been demonstrated using solution or DNA-transfer hybridization. Using such approaches, introduction of new genetically transmitted AKV proviruses was shown to have occurred during the generation of AKR × C57BL/10 and AKR × C57L recombinant inbred lines (Datta et al. 1978b; D. Steffen et al., in prep.) and during maintenance of the AKR strain (D. Steffen et al.; W. Herr; both in prep.).

Several different sublines of the AKR mouse strain currently exist (see Fig. 10.4). These all derive from the Ak strain inbred by Fürth et al. (1933) and selected for a high incidence of leukemia. Sublines were independently maintained by inbreeding and became separated from one another at various times, beginning in 1935. When the AKV provirus-containing restriction endonuclease fragments of the DNA from these sublines were compared, considerable variability was observed (Quint et al. 1981; D. Steffen et al., in prep.). Only one locus is occupied by a provirus in all of these sublines. In addition to this one common locus, AKV proviruses are present at 13 additional loci in one or more of the sublines (see Fig. 10.4).

The variability in number and sites of residence of AKV proviruses among the AKR sublines is almost certainly not the result of residual heterozygosity of the AKR strain at the times of subline divergence. Instead, the observed pattern is quite consistent with sequential acquisition of AKV proviruses during inbreeding of the sublines, rather than loss or movement of proviruses. Thus, the

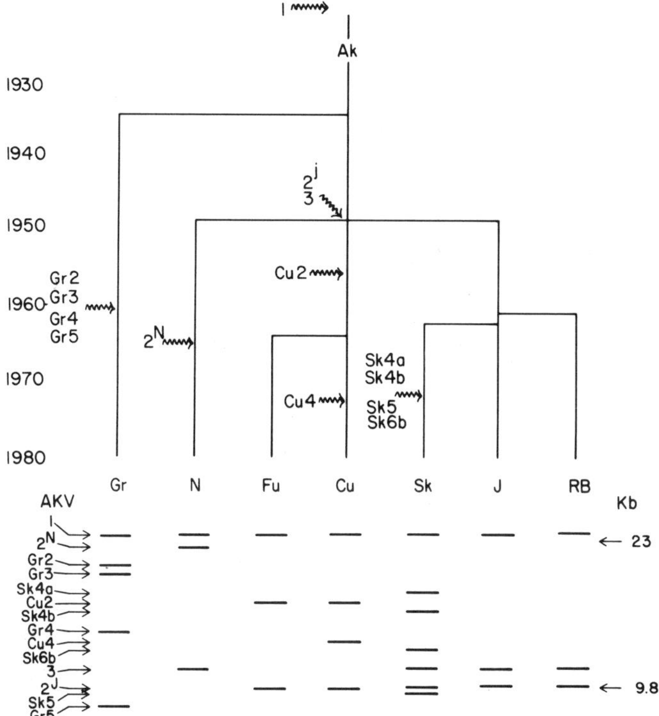

Figure 10.4 Genealogy of the AKR sublines and their endogenous AKV-like viruses. The genealogy of the AKR sublines is diagramed at the top. Beneath each lineage is the name of each subline, e.g., AKR/Gr and AKR/N. Points in the genealogies at which provirus integration may have occurred are indicated by wavy lines. At the bottom is a schematic of the mobility of the provirus in gel electrophoresis. At either side of the figure, the mobility of the *Eco*RI fragment containing each provirus is indicated by arrows. (Adapted from D. Steffen et al., in prep.)

ancestral Ak strain is presumed to have carried only the one AKV provirus common to all sublines. It was this one ancestral provirus that was responsible for the high incidence of leukemia of the Ak strain. Subsequently, the AKR sublines have each acquired two to five additional proviruses.

This instability of AKV proviruses is both interesting and a potential source of experimental difficulty. The *Akv-1* provirus identified by Rowe (1972) happens to be the ancestral provirus and thus is present in all AKR sublines. In contrast, the *Akv-2* provirus is unique to the AKR/N subline; it is absent from other sublines, in particular from the commonly used AKR/J subline (Steffen et al. 1979).

The process of provirus amplification presently continues. The AKR/J subline is now in the process of acquiring new proviruses. Previous to 1975, the AKR/J subline transmitted three AKV proviruses. An AKR/J mouse purchased in 1980 might have three, four, or five AKV proviruses, with the two new proviruses being either homozygous or heterozygous. In the future, either or both of the new proviruses might be fixed or lost during continuing inbreeding of the AKR/J stocks (W. Herr, in prep.).

Amplification of provirus copy number is dependent on viremia. Both the AKR and C3H strains of mice genetically transmit AKV proviruses. Both strains are permissive for replication of the AKV virus, and AKV expression occurs early in the life of both strains. In general, the C3H strains, although they contain complete MLV proviruses, do not become viremic. When DNAs from five sublines of C3H mice were examined for AKV proviruses, four of them were found to carry only one AKV provirus (D. L. Steffen et al., in prep.) (see Table 10.4). The one exception, the C3H/Fg subline, transmits several AKV proviruses and is also the only subline that exhibits lifelong viremia.

The amplification of AKV provirus copy number helps explain the origin of the AKV proviruses genetically transmitted in laboratory strains of mice. When DNAs from 22 wild mice were examined for AKV proviruses, such proviruses were observed only in Japanese mice (Steffen et al. 1980). Since Japanese mice were present in the stocks from which laboratory mice were derived (Potter 1978), it was hypothesized that AKV proviruses entered the laboratory strains via this route. The genetic contribution of Japanese mice to laboratory strains has, however, been quite small as measured by isozyme markers, whereas at least half of the laboratory strains of mice transmit AKV proviruses. Amplification of the number of AKV proviruses, coupled with segregation during outbreeding, would maintain AKV proviruses in the gene pool from which laboratory strains were drawn, even as other Japanese alleles were being lost by dilution.

When the rate at which AKV proviruses have become fixed in AKR sublines and in the AKR × C57L recombinant inbred lines was determined, it was found that one provirus was fixed per line every 15 to 30 years (D. Steffen et al., in prep.). This rate is quite slow on the time scale of an experiment, but it is astonishingly rapid on an evolutionary time scale. Such a result would predict that mice should have acquired an enormous number of proviruses. It seems likely that evolutionary selection must limit the process of provirus amplification.

It would seem that, in spite of natural selection, a considerable degree of provirus amplification has occurred during the evolution of *Mus musculus*. As described above, mice genetically transmit four unrelated kinds of proviruslike information: the C-type provirus (including ecotropic and xenotropic proviruses), MMTV proviruses, A-type particle information, and the VL30 RNA information. Of these, three are present as multiple copies in all strains and subspecies of *M. musculus*: the MLV proviruses at about 50 copies, the VL30 information at about 30 copies, and the A-type particle information at about 500 copies. These multiple proviruses might be the result of provirus amplification analogous to that which is presently occurring with AKV proviruses.

Considering the evolutionarily rapid rate with which new proviruses can be acquired in the germ line, and their ability to interrupt cellular sequences, it is possible that they could be a significant source of spontaneous mutations in animals with large numbers. An intriguing suggestion that endogenous viruses might be important mutagens comes from recent observations by Jenkins et al. (1981), who found that an endogenous AKV-like provirus, *emv*-3 (Tables 10.3 and 10.4), is very closely linked to an identified genetic marker of DBA mice. This allele, called *d*, is responsible for the "dilute-brown" hair color of DBA and some other strains of mice. Five different inbred and two mutant strains of mice that carry the *d* allele also have *emv*-3, and *emv*-3 segregated concordantly with the *d* allele in 53 out of 53 recombinant inbred strains derived from DBA. In addition, analysis of DNA of a spontaneous *d*-allele revertant of DBA/2J mice indicated that ecotropic-specific proviral DNA sequences were no longer present in the genome. This very close linkage suggests that integration of the *emv*-3 provirus at the *d* locus may have been the mutagenic event responsible for the coat-color change.

c. Xenotropic Viruses. Unlike the ecotropic viruses of mice, which are found in some but not all strains, endogenous xenotropic viruses are widespread in mice (for review, see Levy 1978). These viruses are characterized by a host range that includes many species of mammals and even some birds (such as ducks), but not mice. Because the xenotropic viruses grow relatively poorly and individual isolates are frequently mixtures of related species, relatively little biochemical or genetic characterization of the genomes of these viruses has been done. Prior to 1980, for example, no fingerprints or restriction maps of the genomes of xenotropic viruses had been published. Nevertheless, a substantial amount of work has been done to classify the xenotropic viruses of mice and study the genetics of their expression.

The expression of xenotropic viruses varies considerably from strain to strain. Three different phenotypes of infectious virus production can be identified. A few strains of mice, most notably NZB, produce relatively high levels of virus throughout life, which can be detected in all organs tested (Levy and Pincus 1970; Levy et al. 1975). Other strains, such as BALB/c and AKR mice, do not generally express virus, yet the production of infectious viruses can be induced in fibroblast cultures with a number of agents, such as BrdU or cycloheximide (Aaronson and Stephenson 1973). In some of these strains, a high degree of tissue specificity of spontaneous xenotropic virus production can be observed. In AKR and HRS/J mice, for example, significant amounts of xenotropic-virus-related antigen production can be found in the preleukemic thymus (Kawashima et al. 1976). The third phenotype of xenotropic virus production is found in some strains, such as NIH-Swiss and C57L, in which attempts to induce virus production in tissue culture have been usually negative, but the presence of endogenous proviruses can be shown by the occasional isolation of virus from animals (Levy 1973).

Comparison of type-specific antigenic determinants (Stephenson et al. 1974; Barbacid et al. 1978) and cross-hybridization experiments suggest a division into two classes; the "noninducible" class-III viruses of NIH and NZB mice are more closely related to one another than the inducible class-II viruses of BALB/c and other mice. These latter viruses show a close relationship in the *gag* proteins to endogenous ecotropic viruses (Barbacid et al. 1978). Interestingly, the inducible xenotropic viruses are found in mice that also carry ecotropic endogenous virus loci. Barbacid et al. (1978) have suggested that viruses of this type are recombinants between endogenous ecotropic virus and xenotropic virus information, with the *gag* gene donated by the ecotropic virus. Consistent with this observation is the presence of a number of T1 oligonucleotides in *gag* and *pol* shared between the ecotropic and xenotropic viruses of HRS/J mice (Green et al. 1980). Peptide mapping of the gp70s of the various viruses, however, suggests that the *env* gene of the NIH virus is more closely related to that of the inducible class than to the *env* gene of the NZB virus (Elder et al. 1977).

An extensive analysis of restriction maps of nine different endogenous xenotropic viruses (Chattopadhyay et al. 1981) (see Appendix B) suggests a somewhat more complex picture. A rough division, perhaps corresponding to class II and class III, could be seen, but the two classes were not as distinct and seemed to intergrade into one another. It is possible that these represent the progeny of many different proviruses or that extensive recombination between the progeny of a few proviruses gives the variety of genomes observed. Most endogenous nonecotropic proviruses seem to be closely related to one another, since cleavage of mouse DNA with enzymes that cut within the LTR greatly reduces the complexity to a few bands (Dolberg et al. 1980), which must be internal fragments common to the majority of endogenous proviruses.

The inheritance of the predominant xenotropic virus in BALB/c and NZB mice has been analyzed in crosses and backcrosses with appropriate expression-negative strains such as NIH-Swiss and SWR. The ability of BALB virus-2 (the inducible xenotropic virus) to be induced segregates as a single dominant locus (*Bxv-2*) in crosses with NIH-Swiss mice, independent of the inducibility of ecotropic virus (Stephenson and Aaronson 1972). Thus, (BALB/c × NIH)F_1 mice are all inducible for both viruses, and F_1 + NIH backcross mice can be divided into four groups of roughly equal size: one inducible for ecotropic virus alone, one for xenotropic virus alone, one for both viruses, and one for neither. This locus has been mapped to chromosome 1 (Kozak and Rowe 1978) and has subsequently been identified in a number of strains (Kozak and Rowe 1980a). Inheritance of both the virus spontaneously produced by culture NZB fibroblasts and the chemically inducible virus involves primarily one dominant locus (Levy 1973; Stephenson and Aaronson 1974). Using a more sensitive infectious center assay that reflected in vivo expression of virus in spleen cells, Datta and Schwartz (1977) identified two loci dominant for expression of xenotropic virus. These two loci have been termed *Nzv-1* and *Nzv-2*, and they segregate independently of each other. The viruses produced as a consequence of the presence of *Nzv-1* or *Nzv-2* are quite similar, but the amount of virus production is quite different, such that *Nzv-1* mice contain 10^3 to 10^4 infectious centers per 10^7 spleen cells and *Nzv-2* mice contain about 10 to 100. Analogy to the endogenous chicken and ecotropic mouse viruses would suggest that these loci correspond to the proviruses themselves, but there is as yet no direct evidence on this point.

d. Endogenous C-Type Viruses and Disease. As far as is known, the laboratory mouse is unique in that its endogenous viruses participate in certain disease processes. In all other cases analyzed (most notably the chicken), endogenous viruses seem to be completely benign. It is unlikely that this association in the genetically best-studied laboratory animal is fortuitous; rather, it is highly probable that selection of lines with high tumor incidence (such as AKR) was accompanied by selection of a complex and otherwise very rare set of phenomena involving endogenous provirus expression. From this standpoint, the virological events of such "spontaneous" disease may be of questionable relevance to natural tumors, either nonviral or virus-induced. Nevertheless, these diseases present a fascinating puzzle involving basic issues of virus expression and interaction, which still await complete solution.

(i) SPONTANEOUS LYMPHOMA AND POLYTROPIC VIRUSES. Several strains of mice, including AKR, C58, C3H/Fg, and HRS, exhibit a high incidence of spontaneous T-cell lymphoma at 6 months to 1 year of age. It was from one of these strains that Gross (1958) isolated the first MLV and demonstrated that it could induce the same disease following injection into low-leukemia C3H mice. As the endogenous viruses of AKR mice were described, many attempts were made to repeat Gross's observation with isolates of AKV from young mice or from cell cultures. These attempts were uniformly negative. A solution to this paradox was first described by Hartley et al. (1977), who proposed that the endogenous viruses themselves were not directly leukemogenic. Rather, the leukemogenic virus itself was the product of recombination between the progeny of two or more different endogenous proviruses. Such viruses have been obtained from leukemic or preleukemic animals of all strains with high leukemia incidence (Hartley et al. 1977; Cloyd et al. 1980; Green et al. 1980; Rowe et al. 1980). Many, but not all, such viruses are characterized by a unique host range, relative to the known endogenous viruses, in that they can infect both mouse and non-mouse cells with equal efficiency. Such a host range is referred to as dualtropic or (to avoid mixing Latin and Greek roots) polytropic. The original isolates from AKR mice were called MCF, for mink-cell focus-forming virus, due to their ability to form cytopathic "foci" on mink cells (Hartley et al. 1977). There is strong evidence that these viruses are recombinants between endogenous ecotropic virus and another endogenous virus. First, oligonucleotide maps of the viral genome (Rommelaere et al. 1978; Green et al. 1980; Lung et al. 1980), restriction maps of the provirus (Chattopadhyay et al. 1981), and peptide maps of their proteins (Elder et al. 1977) show that these viruses contain some markers characteristic of the ecotropic virus and lack others that have been replaced by markers related to those of xenotropic virus. Second, such viruses are found only in mice that have a provirus encoding endogenous ecotropic virus. In particular, they are not found in NFS mice but have been isolated from NFS congenic mice that contain the *Akv-1* locus. Interestingly, the MCF viruses isolated from these mice are not strongly leukemogenic (Rowe et al. 1980). Third, although different MCF isolates from a single strain of mice share common features, such as the replacement of a set of oligonucleotides in the *env* gene, they show considerable variation from one another in other portions of the genome, such that it is highly improbable that there is a distinct endogenous provirus for each particular isolate. Although one of the parents of the MCF viruses can be identified as the ecotropic virus, the other parent or parents have not been found. The *env* gene and gp70 of MCF-like viruses of AKR and HRS/J mice are related to the prevalent xenotropic viruses of the same mice, but there are enough different markers to make it apparent that none of these are the parent itself (Rommelaere et al. 1978; Green et al. 1980; Chattopadhyay et al. 1981). For example, two isolates of MCF-like leukemogenic virus from HRS/J mice share four *env* oligonucleotides not found in the ecotropic virus, but only two of these were found in any one of three isolates of xenotropic virus from the same mice (Green et al. 1980) and none are shared with the prevalent xenotropic virus of NZB mice (C. Thomas, pers. comm.). Thus, although this *env* alteration is almost certainly responsible for the different host range of the virus, it cannot be determined whether the nonecotropic parent *env* gene encoded a xenotropic or polytropic host range, and an analogy to the sort of crossovers observed to the *env* gene of ALV (Chapters 3 and 4) implies that the parent may already be polytropic in host range.

Since many of the MCF viruses cause the accelerated appearance of leukemia in AKR mice (Hartley et al. 1977; Nowinski and Hays 1978), the recombinant *env* gene has been proposed to play a relatively direct role in leukemogenesis (Chapter 8), perhaps either by some direct effect of the gp70 on the infected cell or by donating to the virus a host range that allows it to infect the target cell. In support of this conclusion is the observation that lymphomas induced by exogenous MLV, either due to injected Mo-MLV or virus expression in BALB/Mo mice, also contain newly integrated recombinant proviruses with a similar substitution in *env* (Van der Putten et al. 1981), whereas other tissues contain only the parental type virus. Thus, formation of *env* recombinant viruses seems also to be important in induction of thymoma by exogenous viruses. However, viruses from NFS *Akv-1* congenic mice with similar *env* genes seem to be only very weakly leukemogenic. Two consistent differences between the genomes of strongly leukemogenic and weakly leukemogenic viruses were found by oligonucleotide mapping. The first is near the 3′ end (including both the U_3 region and the 3′ end of the p15[E] coding region), where the more highly leukemogenic AKR-derived MCF viruses have an alteration relative to AKV not found in the NIH viruses. The second difference is in the length of the substitution in *env*, where the AKR viruses have a shorter region derived from the nonecotropic parent (Lung et al. 1980). Determination of the nucleotide sequence of the 3′-terminal region of AKV and MCF 247 (a prototype polytropic leukemogenic virus) allows the relative precise localization of the crossovers involved in the generation of the MCF viruses (N. Hopkins; J. Lenz and W. Haseltine; both pers. comm.). From this analysis (shown in Fig. 10.5), it can be concluded that three regions of the genome are important in lymphomagenesis: the polytropic gp70 region, the AKV amino-terminal region of p15(E), and the nonecotropic carboxyterminal region of p15(E) and U_3 region. A similar conclusion has been derived from analysis of restriction maps of a similar series of viruses, although the U_3 and carboxyterminal p15(E) differences are not seen (Chattopadhyay et al. 1981). The specific roles of these regions in leukemia remains a mystery.

Not all leukemogenic viruses from AKR mice are polytropic; some isolates with an ecotropic host range have been found (Nowinski and Hayes 1978). Oligonucleotide mapping of several

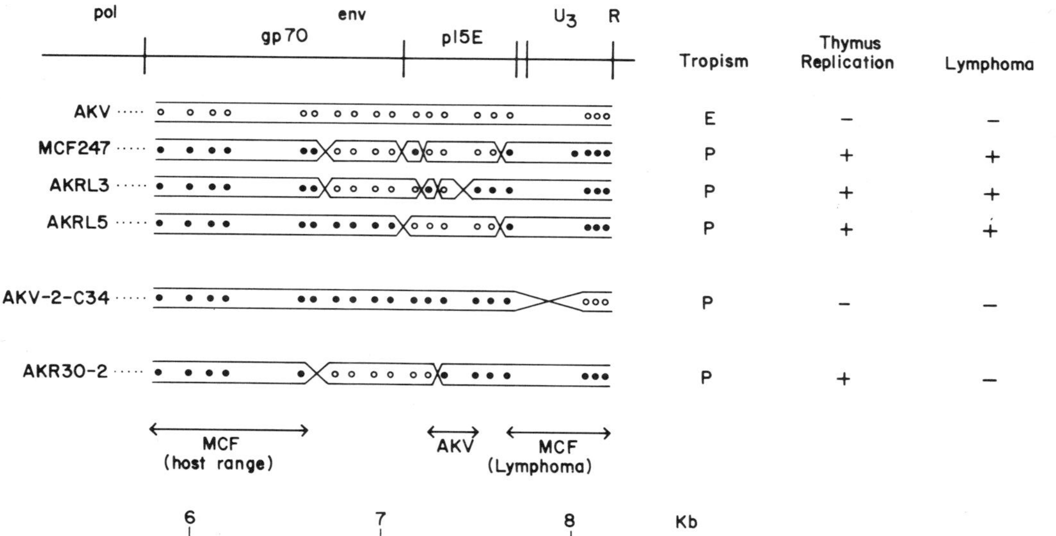

Figure 10.5 Genomes of viruses of AKR mice. The scale at the top shows the 3′ terminal region of AKV, with schematic representations of AKV and some recombinant viruses derived from it. The maps are based on representative samples of oligonucleotide maps of numerous isolates (Lung et al. 1980; N. Hopkins, pers. comm.), with the properties of host range (E, ecotropic; P, polytropic), ability to replicate well in the thymus (O'Donnell et al. 1980), and lymphomagenicity shown at the right. The oligonucleotides are mapped according to the nucleotide sequence of the *env* region of AKV (J. Lenz and W. Haseltine, pers. comm.) and the p15(E) and U_3 region of AKV and MCF 247 (N. Hopkins, pers. comm.). (○) AKV-specific markers; (●) the absence of an AKV-specific marker or the presence of an MCF-specific marker. The boxes interrupted by crosses indicate the minimal crossovers that could give rise to the recombinants shown; the arrows at the bottom show important regions for leukemogenicity and whether or not they are AKV-specific sequences. (Courtesy of N. Hopkins.)

such viruses, including the original Gross passage-A strain isolated from AKR mice (Gross 1958), shows that the major differences between this isolate and AKV lie near the 3′ end of the genome and are similar to, although not identical with, the 3′ differences in MCF viruses (Buchhagen et al. 1980). This difference is reminiscent of the difference between RAV-0 and RAV-60 (Section III.A.2), but whether the underlying principles are the same remains to be decided.

(ii) RADIATION LEUKEMIA VIRUS. It has been more than 20 years since Gross (1958) and Lieberman and Kaplan (1959) described the isolation of highly leukemogenic viruses following X-irradiation of C57BL or C3H mice, yet there is very little known about the genome of this virus. It seems probable that induction of endogenous viruses accompanied by formation of some sort of recombinant is involved (Decleve et al. 1977; Haas 1978), but the relevant virus seems to grow poorly in fibroblasts and pure biologically active isolates have not been obtained. In contrast to the spontaneous lymphoma of AKR mice, polytropic viruses do not appear to be involved in the X-ray-induced lymphomas of BALB/c mice (Ellis et al. 1980). There is a recent suggestion of a component structurally resembling a defective transforming virus in a highly passaged RadLV isolate (Manteuil-Brutlag et al. 1980) (see Chapter 4), but the significance of this species remains to be determined.

(iii) XENOTROPIC VIRUSES AND AUTOIMMUNE DISEASE. NZB mice and hybrids derived from them have a high spontaneous incidence of an autoimmune disease characterized by nephritis resulting from deposition of antigen-antibody complexes in the kidney. Since these mice spontaneously express high levels of xenotropic virus (Levy 1973) and viral antigens are a major component of the immune complex (Dixon et al. 1971), a causal role of xenotropic virus was postulated. However, in a series of genetic crosses, Datta et al. (1978a) found that the disease segregated independently of xenotropic virus expression. Thus, it seems that the underlying defect is immunological, not virological, and that the virus provides a convenient antigen for immune-complex formation but is hardly essential to the disease (see Chapter 3).

2. Endogenous Proviruses of MMTV

Both genetic and physical techniques have been used to study the distribution and function of DNA related to MMTV RNA in the germ lines of mice. In concept, the conclusions drawn from these studies are similar to those derived from studies of other types of endogenous proviruses: (1) Germinally transmitted MMTV DNA is generally arranged in the form of proviruses, with replicative genes flanked by terminally repeated sequences (LTRs); (2) these proviruses are distributed in various numbers and at various sites in the genomes of all laboratory mice, many wild mice, and probably in other species of *Mus*; (3) endogenous MMTV proviruses differ with respect to oncogenic potential and levels of gene expression; and (4) most, if not all, can be distinguished physically by restriction mapping techniques.

Current evidence favors the idea that the endogenous MMTV proviruses were acquired by multiple, independent infections of mouse germ lines long after speciation, with integration occurring on several chromosomes. Once integrated, the proviruses appear to behave like stable genetic elements; they segregate in a Mendelian fashion and can even serve as useful markers for the success of inbreeding programs. Two important features of the milk-borne (horizontally transmitted) strains of MMTV are also exhibited by at least some endogenous viruses: the ability to induce mammary carcinomas in the host (see Chapter 8) and regulation of gene expression by glucocorticoid hormones (see Chapter 5). Endogenous proviruses may also display tissue-dependent regulation of gene expression that may be instrumental in oncogenesis.

a. Genetic Studies. Early genetic experiments had shown that female GR mice developed mammary carcinomas even after foster nursing on females of virus-free strains (Muhlbock 1955; Bentvelzen 1969; Bentvelzen and Daams 1969; Bentvelzen et al. 1970). This phenotype—production of oncogenic virus in the milk and the production of early mammary tumors—was believed to reflect the carriage of a "germinal provirus" (Bentvelzen et al. 1970), a hypothesis that depended initially on elaborate transplantation experiments designed to exclude the posibility of transmission of virus epigenetically, in the egg or sperm or via the placenta (Bentvelzen 1969). The results of recent experiments strongly support the original claims that the GR phenotype is a manifestation of an MMTV provirus at a single locus. Segregation tests argue in favor of a single genetic determinant of the phenotype (Bentvelzen 1969, 1972; van Nie and Hilgers 1976); in one set of experiments in which this view was contested (Heston et al. 1976; Heston and Parks 1977), one of the scored markers (expression of MMTV antigens) could have been produced by other MMTV proviruses. One other set of crosses, which suggested two tumor-inducing loci (Nandi and Helmich 1974), has not been satisfactorily reconciled with the prevailing view. By performing successive backcrosses, van Nie and her colleagues (van Nie and de Moes 1977; van Nie et al. 1977) have established a congenic GR strain that does not exhibit the characteristic phenotype and lacks a single endogenous MMTV provirus among the several present in the parent strain (Michalides et al. 1976; Fanning et al. 1980a). This same provirus is present in animals with the GR phenotype that were derived from crosses between GR mice and mice with low tumor incidence (Michalides et al. 1981). A provirus in the GR germ line has restriction sites characteristic of the proviruses found in cells after experimental infection with the GR strain of MMTV (Cohen and Varmus 1980; Drohan et al. 1980; Fanning et al. 1980b). The responsible allele has been termed *Mtv-2* (van Nie and de Moes 1977) and has been assigned to chromosome 18 (R. van Nie, unpubl.). Features of this and other endogenous MMTV proviruses are summarized in Table 10.5.

At least two other endogenous proviruses have been postulated on the basis of classical genetic criteria. The *Mtv-1* allele was proposed to explain the observation that certain American mouse strains dependent on milk-borne infection for a high incidence of early mammary tumors (e.g., DBA and sublines of C3H) still developed virus-associated tumors late in life if deprived of virus-containing milk (DeOme et al. 1967; Nandi and McGrath 1973; van Nie and Verstraeten 1975; Bentvelzen et al. 1978; Verstraeten and van Nie 1978). Physical techniques have identified a single provirus that segregates with (and is probably equivalent to) the *Mtv-1* allele (Michalides et al. 1981), and *Mtv-1* has been assigned to chromosome 7, as determined by the results of linkage tests (A. A. Verstraeten and R. van Nie, unpubl.) (Table 10.5). The virus produced by animals bearing this allele has been variously termed MMTV-L (for low lethality; Bentvelzen 1974), NIV (for nodule-inducing virus; Nandi and McGrath 1973), and MMTV (C3Hf) or MMTV (DBAf); the virus has also been introduced into a BALB/c colony in which it is transmitted as a milk-borne agent (Blair 1968; Ringold et al. 1976). Tumors induced by this virus in either infected BALB/c mice or mice carrying the *Mtv-1* allele contain proviruses with a restriction map indistinguishable from that of the endogenous provirus, called unit V (see below), which segregates with the *Mtv-1* allele (Cohen and Varmus 1980; Michalides et al. 1981).

Mtv-3 is an allele identified in the GR strain in the absence of *Mtv-2*; the phenotype associated with *Mtv-3* is the expression of *gag* polypeptides in mammary glands, without detectable *env* determinants (Nusse et al. 1980). Although the *mtv-3* allele has been mapped genetically to chromosome 11 (Nusse et al. 1980), the physical composition of *Mtv-3* has not yet been determined. From experience with avian endogenous proviruses (see above), it seems probable that an *env*-defective provirus constitutes the *Mtv-3* allele, but it is possible that *Mtv-3* is a regulatory locus governing noncoordinate expression of proviruses at other loci.

b. Biochemical Studies. Although it has been recognized for several years that multiple copies of MMTV DNA are present in all inbred strains of mice, including some with little or no evidence of MMTV gene expression (Varmus et al. 1972a; Michalides et al. 1976; Morris et al. 1977), classification of this endogenous virus DNA was impossible prior to the introduction of techniques for DNA mapping. In the earlier studies, labeled virus-specific DNA or viral DNA was used as a probe to measure the rates of annealing of virus-specific cellular sequences in solution; the first estimates of 50–90 copies per diploid cell (Varmus et al. 1972a) were gradually reduced to about 5–15 copies per diploid cell as reagents and techniques improved (Michalides and Schlom 1975; Drohan et al. 1977; Morris et al. 1977). But even in these later studies, only the GR strain could be clearly distinguished from the others with respect to its content of endogenous MMTV DNA.

Application of restriction endonucleases and the DNA-transfer technique to this problem dramatically altered perceptions of the viral DNA content of mouse strains. Cohen and Varmus (1979) used *Eco*RI (which generally cleaves once within MMTV proviruses) and *Pst*I (which usually cleaves at multiple internal sites) (Shank et al. 1978) to examine MMTV DNA endogenous to a large number of mouse colonies derived from a cross (performed in 1920) between a Bagg albino mouse and a DBA mouse. They were able to identify at least six separate units of viral DNA, distributed variously among the strains; however, all members of each colony were indistinguishable, reflecting the success of the inbreeding program. The distri-

Table 10.5 Characteristics and distribution of some endogenous MMTV proviruses

Genetic designation	Other designation	Phenotype	Implicated mouse strains	Chromosomal location	Size of *Eco*RI fragments	References
Mtv-1	unit V	virus production; late tumors	DBA, C3H/HeN, C3H/An	7	6.5, 4.5	1–5
Mtv-2	—	virus production; early tumors (pregnancy dependent)	GR	18	11.0, 6.9	5–9
Mtv-3	—	*gag* antigen expression; no *env* antigen	GR	11	?	10
Mtv-4	—	virus expression; early tumor	SHN	—	—	14
Mtv-5	—	virus expression	SL/NiA	—	—	14
Mtv-6	unit I	?	DBA/2, BALB/c, CBA/J, CBA/St, C3H/St, C3H/Bi, C3H/An, C3H/He	?	16.7	2, 11
Mtv-7	unit Ia		C3H/Bi, DBA/2, CBA/J, CBA/St	1	16.7	4

Mtv-8	unit II	?	Same as for unit I + CBA/N, CBA/CaJ, C57BL, C57BL/6, C57BL/10	?	8.5, 6.7	2, 4, 11, 13
Mtv-9	unit III	?	BALB/c, CBA/N, CBA/CaJ, CBA/J, C3H/Bi, C3H/St, C57BL, C57BL/6, C57BL/10	?	10.0, 7.8	2, 4, 11, 13
Mtv-10	unit IV	?	DBA/2, CBA/St, C3H/St, C3H/Bi, CBA/J	1	11.7, 10.0	2, 4
Mtv-11	unit VII	?	DBA/2	?	5.8	4
Mtv-12	unit VI	?	DBA/2J	?	15.0	2, 4
Mtv-13	unit VIII	?	DBA/2J	?	9.0	4
Mtv-14	unit IX	?	DBA/2	6	1.7	4
Mtv-15	unit X	?	DBA/2 or C57BL, C57BL/6, C57BL/10	?	10.0	4, 13
?	—	steroid-responsive RNA synthesis	GR	?	7.8, 6.4	12
Mtv-16	—	?	C57BL	?	13.0, 5.3	15

References: [1]van Nie and Verstaeten (1975); [2]Cohen and Varmus (1979); [3]Cohen and Varmus (1980); [4]Traina et al. (unpubl.); [5]Michalides et al. (1981); [6]van Nie et al. (1977); [7]van Nie and DeMoes (1977); [8]Michalides et al. (1980); [9]Fanning et al. (1980b); [10]Nusse et al. (1980); [11]Cohen et al. (1979a); [12]Hynes et al. (1981); [13]Long et al. (1980); [14]J. Hilgers (unpubl.); [15] Vaidya (unpubl.).

bution of these units (termed units I through VI; see Table 10.5) suggested that they had segregated as stable genetic elements during the 60 years of inbreeding. A number of additional units have subsequently been identified in this lineage (Table 10.5) and some of the same and other units of viral DNA have been found in unrelated mouse strains (Table 10.6).

What is the relationship between these endogenous proviruses and the genomes of viruses horizontally transmitted via milk in some of the same mouse strains? In two instances discussed earlier, it is apparent that endogenous provirus(es) can be assigned to alleles (*Mtv-1* and *Mtv-2*) that govern virus production and oncogenesis; hence, it is likely that these proviruses encode viral genomes competent to replicate and induce tumors. Although type-specific antigens (Massey et al. 1980; Arthur et al. 1981a) and cell-surface receptors (Altrock et al. 1981) can be used to distinguish between the *env* proteins of MMTV (C3Hf), the product of *Mtv-1* (unit V), and the *env* proteins of MMTV (C3H), a milk-borne virus, the first 46 amino acids at the amino terminus of the major glycoprotein (gp52) of these two viruses are identical (Arthur et al. 1981b). In other cases in which the virus encoded by the endogenous provirus has not been isolated, physical mapping studies strongly suggest a close relationship between endogenous DNA and DNA acquired by experimental infection with milk-borne strains of MMTV. For example, Cohen et al. (1979a) constructed physical maps of two units (II and III) endogenous to BALB/c mice and showed that these units had the complexity and LTRs characteristic of proviruses (see Chapter 5). On the other hand, restriction maps have distinguished these two units and others from proviruses of milk-borne virus (Cohen et al. 1979a,b; Donehower et al. 1980; Groner et al. 1980). Hynes et al. (1981) cloned an apparently complete endogenous provirus (other than the *Mtv-2* allele) from GR mouse DNA; again the physical map showed structural relatedness but nonidentity with proviruses acquired during experimental infection. L. A. Donehower and G. L. Hager (unpubl.) have determined the sequence of most of the LTR of unit II (cloned from C3H/HeN DNA) and have found it to be very similar to that of the LTR of MMTV (C3H) DNA; the sequence includes an open reading frame of about 340 codons, as does the LTR of MMTV (C3H) (Dickson and Peters 1981; Donehower et al. 1981; J. Majors, unpubl.), although a protein product from this region has yet to be identified in cells.

Table 10.6 Endogenous MMTV proviruses in some common laboratory strains of *M. musculus*

Mouse strains	No. of endogenous proviruses	Identified proviruses[a]	Unassigned *Eco*RI fragments (kb)	References
GR	5	*Mtv-2*	6.6, 6.7, 7.8, 7.9, 9.0, 13, 18, 23	Michalides et al. (1981)
DBA/2J	8	*Mtv-1, -7,* -8, -9, -11, -12 -13, -14, -15	—	Cohen and Varmus (1979); Traina et al. (unpubl.)
C3H/He	3	*Mtv-16*, -8	—	Cohen and Varmus (1979)
C3H/Bi	4	*Mtv-7*, -8, -9, -10	—	Cohen and Varmus (1979)
BALB/c	3	*Mtv-6*, -8, -9	—	Cohen and Varmus (1979)
C57BL	3	*Mtv-8*, -9, -15, -16	—	A. Vaidya (unpubl.)
C57BL/6 and 10	3	*Mtv-8*, -9, -15	—	Long et al. (1980)
A	4		3.8, 4.5, 5.4, 6.2, 6.8, 9, 15	Morris et al. (1979)

[a]See Table 10.5

Although most endogenous MMTV proviruses can be distinguished from proviruses of known virus strains by physical mapping, there are exceptions other than the proviruses assigned to *Mtv-1* and *Mtv-2*. For example, unit IV, widely distributed among progeny of the Bagg albino × DBA mating (Cohen and Varmus 1979), yields *Pst*I fragments characteristic of the proviruses of MMTV (C3H) and MMTV (GR); however, the functional capacity of unit IV has not been established. Schlom and his colleagues have prepared a hybridization reagent capable of distinguishing between proviruses present endogenously in C3H/HeN DNA and those acquired by milk-borne infection with MMTV (C3H) (Drohan et al. 1977). This reagent (labeled viral RNA selected for inefficient annealing to the proviruses endogenous to C3H/HeN liver DNA) detects proviral DNA presumably closely related to the genome of MMTV (C3H) in liver DNA from GR mice and from strains shown to carry unit IV (Drohan and Schlom 1979a). Although there is as yet no indication that MMTV encodes a transforming gene, it is possible that some of the sequences detected by this probe are specifically implicated in oncogenesis by MMTV. However, this probe is apparently from widespread regions of the genome (Drohan and Schlom 1979a); it is thus difficult to examine the mechanism of oncogenesis from this perspective (see Chapter 8).

c. Expression. Information about the mode and level of expression of endogenous MMTV proviruses is rudimentary compared, for example, with the correlations between proviral structure and function that have been made for endogenous chicken proviruses (see above). It has been recognized for several years that inbred mouse strains, even those that do not transmit virus in milk, invariably express MMTV-related genes at the transcriptional level (Varmus et al. 1972a) but that concentrations of viral RNA vary among tissues and among mouse strains. It is simplest to assume that such differences among strains are related to the strengths of promoters associated with the endogenous provirus(es) in each strain, but a full evaluation of this problem has yet to be made. C57BL mice, for example, have about 100-fold more viral RNA in their lactating mammary glands than do BALB/c mice, and this trait is dominant in F_1 hybrids. However, about 85% of the BALB/c × (BALB/c × C57BL)F_1 backcross progeny also displayed the high level of viral RNA, indicating that the high level of expression is likely to derive from multiple proviruses (A. Vaidya and C. Long, pers. comm.). This is surprising, since two of the three endogenous proviruses in C57BL mice appear indistinguishable in tests with *Eco*RI and *Pst*I from proviruses in BALB/c mice (Table 10.6). Variation in expression of MMTV proviruses among tissues is not understood. The high degree of methylation of most endogenous MMTV DNA (Cohen 1980) may be implicated in control.

It is apparent that those proviruses at the alleles *Mtv-1* and *Mtv-2* must occasionally be transcribed into full-sized RNA, since these alleles are associated with virus production. However, the efficiency of transcription from these two endogenous proviruses is not known. This issue is of some importance in relation to the mechanism of oncogenesis under the influence of these alleles. Most of the evidence to date suggests that insertion of new proviruses made by virus produced from endogenous loci is necessary for tumor formation (Cohen and Varmus 1980; Fanning et al. 1980a; V. Morris, unpubl.), but at least one group of investigators has argued that expression of *Mtv-2* itself may be sufficient for the induction of mammary tumors in GR mice (Michalides et al. 1981).

There is, in general, little information about the question of whether endogenous MMTV proviruses, like those introduced by infection of cultured cells or found in mammary tumors with elevated numbers of proviruses, are regulated at the transcriptional level by glucocorticoid hormones (for review, see Ringold 1979; Varmus et al. 1979; also Chapter 5). Hynes et al. (1981) have recently cloned an entire endogenous provirus from GR-mouse cellular DNA in a prokaryotic host-vector system and found, upon reintroducing the cloned DNA into mammalian cells, that the provirus was expressed at a low constitutive level, which could be augmented severalfold by addition of dexamethasone to the culture medium. It is not known whether the cloned provirus is normally expressed in GR mice or whether it exhibits steroidal control in its usual context. Similar observations have been made with a complete cloned copy of unit V (G. Hager, unpubl.). Stallcup et al. (1979) have examined MMTV RNA synthesis in lymphoma cell lines from AKR, BALB/c, and C57BL/6 mice; these lines appear to contain only endogenous MMTV DNA, yet some exhibit glucocorticoid-sensitive production of MMTV RNA. Assignment of transcripts to specific proviral elements has not yet been possible.

There are now several examples of anomalous expression of *gag* and *env* functions from endogenous proviruses, although the explanations for these anomalies are not yet known: (1) As noted earlier, the *Mtv-3* allele in GR mice is manifest by production of *gag* products in the absence of *env* products (Nusse et al. 1980). (2) Teramoto et al. (1980b) have observed much higher concentrations of *gag* proteins than of *env* proteins in tissues and tumors of certain BALB/c and Swiss mice. (3) A. Vaidya and C. Long (unpubl.) have found that C57BL mice (and progeny of crosses between BALB/c and C57BL mice) have undetectable levels of MMTV proteins despite a moderately high concentration of MMTV RNA in polyribosomes. Furthermore, the putative mRNA is translatable in vitro, but the nature of this apparent translational (or posttranslational) control has not been elucidated.

d. Origins, Distribution, and Function. Nucleotide sequences related to the MMTV genome have been detected in all inbred mouse strains and in many closely related animals, including feral *M. musculus* and *M. musculus molossinus* (Varmus et al. 1972a; Michalides and Scholm 1975; Morris et al. 1977; Cohen and Varmus 1979). Solution-hybridization tests have also revealed MMTV-related DNA in Asian mice (*M. caroli* and *M. cervicolor*), although thermal-denaturation studies indicate a high degree of mismatching of these hybrids (Morris et al. 1977). An MMTV-related B-type virus has been recovered from *M. cervicolor* (Schlom et al. 1978), and its proteins have been used in immunological tests to detect MMTV-related proteins in normal tissues of *M. musculus, M. cervicolor, M. cookii,* and *M. caroli* (Horan-Hand et al. 1980; Teramoto et al. 1980a). A low level of homology has also been reported between a subset of MMTV sequences and the DNAs of laboratory rats (Drohan and Schlom 1979b). However, there is no convincing evidence for homology between the MMTV genome and the DNAs of other vertebrates, despite suggestions that MMTV-related agents might be implicated in human mammary neoplasia (see Chapter 11).

Several kinds of experiments favor the notion that the homologous sequences represent proviruses introduced into the germ lines of these animals by MMTV-related agents postspeciation. Examination of the DNA from individual wild mice (*M. musculus*) with restriction endonucleases has provided the most compelling argument, since each mouse appears to carry a distinctive set of endogenous proviruses at various integration sites, and some animals (most commonly from the Lake Casitas area of southern California) are completely devoid of MMTV DNA (Cohen and Varmus 1979). Inbred strains are likewise quite heterogeneous with respect to their endogenous proviruses (Table 10.2); however, individuals within a strain are identical, indicating that the proviruses are not highly unstable (Cohen and Varmus 1979). The presence of MMTV proviruses on several different chromosomes (Morris et al. 1979) (Table 10.5), as well as variation in physical maps of flanking cellular DNA, indicates that the multiple proviruses did not arise by simple amplification.

The absence of endogenous MMTV proviruses in some American wild mice suggested that such proviruses are not necessary for viability (Cohen and Varmus 1979). This has been further documented by the development of a strain of mice, bred in captivity from Lake Casitas mice, that lacks endogenous MMTV DNA (J. C. Cohen and M. Gardner, unpubl.), and by the identification of enclaves of mice from Morocco (*M. domestica brevirostris*) and Czechoslovakia (*M. musculus musculus*) devoid of MMTV proviruses (W. Drohan, unpubl.). In view of these results, the widespread distribution of endogenous MMTV proviruses is unexplained, particularly since it is apparent from work with *Mtv-1* and *Mtv-2* that endogenous proviruses can have a detrimental effect in the form of tumors in some instances. Whether such proviruses can also provide subtle advantages to their hosts is a matter of conjecture.

3. Other Endogenous Virus-like Elements of Mice

In addition to the endogenous viruses just described, two additional types of elements resembling the genome of endogenous virus can be detected in mice by various tests, although neither of these has been shown to be capable of encoding infectious virions. For this reason, the genetic and functional properties of these elements are obscure. This class of elements includes the genes encoding VL30 RNA and intracisternal A-type particles.

a. VL30 RNA. Preparations of C-type viruses grown on mouse or rat cells often contain substantial amounts of RNA with a sedimentation coefficient of about 30S (Howk et al. 1978; Sherwin et al. 1978; Besmer et al. 1979), corresponding to a size of about 6.5 kb. This RNA species, also referred to as VL30 (VL for viruslike) RNA (Besmer et al. 1979) or 30S DRV (for defective retrovirus) RNA (Scolnick et al. 1979), has several properties similar to those of endogenous retroviruses. (The mouse and rat VL30 RNAs are not detectably related to one another, but they seem highly similar in most properties and are considered together.)

1. In cells producing a helper virus, VL30 RNA is efficiently packaged into helper virions as a complex (presumably a dimer) of about 55S (Besmer et al. 1979) and can also be found in a 70S complex with helper-virus genomes (Scolnick et al. 1979).
2. When pseudotyped in a virion, it can be copied in an endogenous reverse transcriptase reaction in vitro (Scolnick et al. 1979).
3. When rat VL30 pseudotypes are used to infect unrelated cells (e.g., bat cells), the RNA can be shown to be copied into proviral DNA, integrated into the cellular genome, and transcribed into RNA as though it were a typical viral genome (Scolnick et al. 1979).
4. Sequences related to VL30 RNA are found in multiple copies (20–50 copies/cell) in the mouse or rat genome (Scolnick et al. 1976; Besmer et al. 1979; Keshet et al. 1980).
5. The expression of VL30 RNA varies considerably from one cell line to another (Young et al. 1978) and can be enhanced by treatment of cells with BrdU (Besmer et al. 1979). In BrdU-treated JLS-V9 cells (a continuous line of BALB/c bone marrow cells), the 30S species forms the major RNA in the induced virions. Although the virion proteins are encoded by the C-type proviruses, the virion RNA contains only a minor contribution from them (Besmer et al. 1979).
6. At least in the case of the rat, recombination can occur between rat or mouse leukemia virus and 30S RNA, as evidenced by the generation of Kirsten and Harvey sarcoma viruses discussed in Chapter 4 (see Young et al. 1980). Whether such recombination occurs at a high frequency is uncertain.
7. Molecular clones of several VL30-related sequences from mouse DNA have recently been obtained (Keshet et al. 1980). Analysis of these has shown that the sequences form a closely related family, differing by short insertions and substitutions. Furthermore, they resemble endogenous proviruses in being integrated at multiple different sites in the mouse genome and by being flanked by a LTR (Keshet and Shaul 1981).

In spite of the similarities to endogenous proviruses, the VL30 RNAs of mice and rats are not detectably related to the genomes of any known replication-competent viruses (or to each other) either by hybridization or by oligonucleotide analysis (Scolnick et al. 1979). Furthermore, they do not encode any known proteins. In uninduced JLS-V9 cells, for example, VL30 RNA can be found in polysomes, yet there is no detectable synthesis of virions or virus-related proteins (Besmer et al. 1979). In addition, a subgenomic polysomal RNA species (analogous to *env* mRNA) cannot be found.

On the basis of these findings, it is most probable that the VL30 "genome" is an RNA molecule that contains sequences analogous to retroviral sequences required for replication (i.e., terminal redundancy, primer-binding site, etc.) and packaging and that is capable of being so utilized by a variety of mammalian retrovirus systems but is otherwise unrelated. There are at least two possibilities for the origin of this element. First, it may represent the germ-line integration of a defective unrelated retrovirus from some other source. Second, it may have been derived from a nonvirus-related cellular sequence by acquisition of viruslike "replication" signals, possibly by recombination with a viral genome or perhaps even by chance combination of appropriate sequences of nonviral origin. Note that a cellular sequence that acquired such signals might well tend to become reiterated in the cellular genome as a consequence of repeated infections.

Whatever its origin or function, the VL30 RNA of rats and mice (and possibly other mammals as well) can be a significant nuisance for biochemical studies. Nucleic acid probes prepared from viruses grown in cells containing VL30 RNA may be substantially contaminated with VL30-related species, and experiments involving such reagents must be carefully controlled to ensure the absence of consequent artifacts.

b. Intracisternal A-type Particles. These particles are frequently found in cells of embryos, tumors, and in cell lines of mice (deHarven and Friend 1958; Dalton et al. 1961). Morphologically, the particles resemble retroviral nucleocapsids, in particular the immature form of B-type viruses. In contrast to the usual viruses, there is no evidence that A-type particles are ever released from the cell in virions. Some mouse tumor cell lines, however, contain sufficient amounts of these particles for their purification and biochemical characterization (Kuff et al. 1968, 1972). The "genomes" contained within these particles resemble retroviral genomes in size, presence of poly(A), association with reverse transcriptase, and ability to be translated in vitro to yield a polypeptide of 73,000 daltons, identical with the major structural protein of the particle (Wilson and Kuff 1972; Wong-Staal et al. 1975; Lueders et al. 1977; Paterson et al. 1978).

Three genomelike RNA species are found associated with A-type particles with sizes of roughly 9 kb, 7.6 kb, and 5.2 kb. These species are closely related in sequence and ability to be translated (Paterson et al. 1978), and the basis for the different sizes is unknown. The RNAs and proteins of the A-type particles are unrelated to those of any known endogenous viruses of *M. musculus*, but a partial (about 25%) sequence homology with M432, an infectious endogenous virus of *M. cervicolor* (Callahan et al. 1976), has been reported (Kuff et al. 1978). It is possible that this relationship may be a consequence of germ-line infection of *M. musculus* with a defective variant of the *M. caroli* virus or of the fact that an ancestor common to both the M432 virus and the A-type particle was present in a common ancestor to the two *Mus* species.

Proviruses of A-type particles are one of the most abundant (if not the most abundant) transcribed sequences in the mouse genome. Copy numbers between 650 and 1800 have been estimated by reassociation kinetics (Lueders and Kuff 1977; Ono et al. 1980). Expression of these proviruses is especially high in tumors, most notably plasmacytomas. In an attempt to isolate immunoglobulin genes from plasmacytoma cells, Ono et al. (1980) obtained molecular clones of DNA sequences that were selected on the basis of (1) their encoding abundant mRNAs and (2) their being well represented in mouse DNA without regard to their particular sequence. Of 11 such clones, 10 were A-type-particle proviruses. These were found to resemble other endogenous proviruses by being flanked by LTRs and embedded within unrelated flanking sequences (Cole et al. 1981). As with VL30 proviruses, heteroduplex analysis showed a significant variability in internal sequences.

4. Experimental Introduction of New Endogenous Viruses into the Germ Line

Exogenous retroviruses are endemic in populations of many animals, including chickens and mice, and are transmitted frequently, if not primarily, by vertical infection as egg- or milk-borne virus.

Nevertheless, germ-line integration of these viruses has never been observed. As discussed in section III.B.1.b, occasional reintegration of endogenous viruses has been observed but is quite rare, and it has not been possible to isolate the events for experimental study. This rarity may reflect the existence of relatively specific barriers to germ-line infection; germ-line cells are resistant to infection, and transplacental transmission does not seem to occur (Jaenisch 1980a,b). It may also reflect a frequent detrimental effect of such integrations.

A system for addressing these issues and examining the nature and effects of exogenous virus infection of the germ line has recently been developed by Jaenisch and colleagues (Jaenisch 1976, 1977, 1979, 1980a; Breindl et al. 1979, 1980; Jaenisch et al. 1980; for review, see Jaenisch 1980b). Preimplantation 4-8 cell embryos of BALB/c mice were treated with protease to remove the zona pellucida (which blocks virus penetration), incubated with Mo-MLV, and reimplanted in foster mothers. Surprisingly, a large percentage of these embryos developed normally, and some of these were viremic throughout life, developing a typical Mo-MLV lymphoma late in life. Unlike animals infected shortly after birth, these mice had detectable replicating virus and additional MLV DNA in all organs tested, not just in the usual targets. This comparison suggested that integration of the infecting provirus had occurred at a very early stage of development and implied that germ-line cells of these animals might also have integrated proviruses.

That such germ-line integration had in fact occurred was shown by several lines of evidence. First, 50% of the offspring of a male mouse so treated inherited a phenotype of acquiring spontaneous viremia and active virus replication specifically in target organs (thymus and spleen) shortly after birth. Second, the spontaneously appearing virus was shown to be biologically and biochemically indistinguishable from Mo-MLV. Third, more extensive genetic analysis showed a straightforward Mendelian inheritance of this trait and has permitted mapping of the dominant locus involved to chromosome 6. This locus was named *mov*-1. Finally, the *mov*-1 locus was found to cosegregate with sequences in the mouse DNA detectable with an Mo-MLV-specific probe and characterized by unique junction fragments. Thus, the introduced Mo-MLV provirus behaves very much like a usual endogenous provirus, except that it seems to induce directly a disease very similar to the disease induced by injected Mo-MLV.

Mice carrying the *mov*-1 provirus are referred to as BALB/Mo mice. Several additional strains of such mice carrying Mo-MLV as endogenous provirus at distinct integration sites have been developed (Jähner and Jaenisch 1980; Jaenisch et al. 1981). These mice show an interesting phenotypic variation in the time of appearance of infectious virus and of disease. Mice with *mov*-13 show a very early onset of virus replication and develop lymphoma and die at 2–4 months of age. Interestingly, these mice also tend to develop gray hair at an early age, a phenomenon probably due to extensively early virus replication, since it is also seen in mice inoculated with Mo-MLV as midgestation embryos. Another interesting feature of *mov*-13 is that among numerous progeny of two heterozygous parents, homozygous mice have not been found (R. Jaenisch, pers. comm.), suggesting either that the *mov*-13 interupts an essential gene or, less likely, that the double gene dosage and attendant higher virus production is lethal to the embryo. Mice with *mov*-1 become viremic a few weeks after birth and develop leukemia at a later age; only 20% of mice with *mov*-2 become viremic and these very late in life. An additional group of loci (such as *mov*-4) that induce neither viremia nor leukemia was also found. Those loci probably either contain defective proviruses (as shown for *mov*-4) or are in completely silent regions of the genome. As determined biochemical or biological tests, *mov*-1, *mov*-2, and *mov*-13, and other loci encode identical viruses. Although these tests do not exclude that the phenotype variation is due to undetected viral mutations, it seems quite likely that the variability is a consequence of different integration sites.

Recent experiments with these mice have revealed a further similarity of the *mov* provirus to endogenous viruses in that they are heavily methylated (Harbers et al. 1981; Stuhlman et al. 1981). Furthermore, even in animals with extensive replication of virus in target tissues, the endogenous provirus remains extensively methylated and transcriptionally inactive (as judged by resistance of the chromatin to DNase-I digestion; see Section II.B.3). Thus, it seems that the apparent activation of virus in the target organs is due to proviruses acquired by infection, that the initial activation of the virus may occur elsewhere in the mouse, and that the specificity seen is a consequence of tissue-specific replication, not activation. These results also show that methylation and transcriptional inactivity are not special features of the endogenous viruses but seem to be controls imposed by the host on any provirus brought into the germ line. Nevertheless, the different phenotypes of the distinct loci do suggest some specificity of activation, and these loci, as well as other endogenous proviruses, may provide useful probes for the mechanism of such activation.

E. Endogenous Viruses of Other Species

There are numerous other isolates of endogenous viruses from other species, ranging from vipers to primates, and many more reports of related sequences and antigens in species from which no infectious virus has yet been isolated. In general, the molecular biology and genetics of these viruses are underdeveloped when compared with those of the viruses of chickens and mice, and few new principles have been uncovered with them. Many of the endogenous viruses of other mammals were described in Chapter 2, and we will not present another such list here. We will, however, use a few examples to point up some of the interesting relationships that have emerged through their study (for review, see Todaro 1980).

1. Endogenous viruses of Cats

a. RD114/CCC Virus. The genome of the domestic cat (*Felis catus*) contains at least two different types of endogenous proviruses. One of these, the RD114 type, encodes complete infectious virus, and it was discovered in RD cells (a human rhabdomyosarcoma line) following tumor passage in the brain of a kitten (McAllister et al. 1972). RD 114 was originally thought to be a human virus. However, it was subsequently shown to be an endogenous cat virus by induction of the virtually identical CCC virus from a line of cat cells (Fischinger et al. 1973; Livingston and Todaro 1973) and by demonstration of extensive homology with uninfected cat DNA (Baluda and Roy-Burman 1973; Neiman 1973b). Analogous to xenotropic MLV and many other endogenous viruses of mammals, this virus is noninfectious for cat cells. It shows no detectable relationship to exogenous feline leukemia virus (FeLV) (Livingston and Todaro 1973) but is partially related to endogenous viruses isolated from baboons (Sherr et al. 1974). Furthermore, probing of DNA from nine species in the genus *Felis* with labeled DNA of RD114 showed related sequences only in the four species most closely related to the domestic cat (Todaro 1980). These results suggest that the RD114-type endogenous virus was first introduced to a common ancestor of the four positive species after its divergence from the five negative species (Benveniste and Todaro 1974).

b. FeLV-related Proviruses. The other endogenous virus of cats consists of sequences related to exogenous FeLV. Such sequences can be readily detected by solution or DNA-transfer hybridization with labeled FeLV cDNA (Gillespie et al. 1973; Quintrell et al. 1974; Benveniste et al. 1975; Koshy et al. 1980) and are found in multiple copies (at least ten) in the cat genome. Restriction enzyme analysis and DNA-transfer hybridization (Koshy et al. 1980; Mullins et al. 1981) reveal the same sort of heterogeneity of these endogenous proviruses as was seen with chickens and mice; i.e., although each individual animal has about the same number of such bands, no two individuals have the same pattern. Thus, the endogenous FeLV-related proviruses exhibit the same type of evolutionary instability as seen with other endogenous proviruses.

Although closely related to exogenous FeLV, it has not yet been possible to isolate or induce infectious endogenous FeLV or to associate any particular phenotype with it. This situation is hardly unique to cats; many species of mammals contain detectable virus-related sequences but have not yet yielded infectious virus (see Todaro 1980). This situation may reflect defects in the proviruses themselves, an extremely tight "repression" of endogenous proviruses, or a very narrow host range of the induced virus. Application of molecular cloning techniques, combined with transfection studies and marker-rescue experiments, should allow resolution of this issue.

A partial analysis of the relationship between endogenous FeLV and exogenous FeLV has been performed (Mullins et al. 1981; J. Mullins, pers. comm.). The two types of genomes were found to be most closely related in a central conserved region of 3.2 kb including parts of *pol* and *env*, with greater divergence toward the ends. In particular, the U_3 regions of the two viruses seem to be substantially unrelated, a situation highly reminiscent of the relationship between exogenous ALV and RAV-0 (Section II.A.2). As with other endogenous proviruses, there seem to be significant and variable rearrangements of the endogenous FeLV proviruses relative to exogenous FeLV.

As with RD114 sequences, endogenous FeLV-related sequences

are found in the four species most closely related to the domestic cat (Benveniste et al. 1975), suggesting that these two viruses were introduced into the population at about the same time. Again, sequences related to FeLV are found in much more distantly related species—in this case, the endogenous C-type viruses of rodents (Benveniste et al. 1975).

2. *Endogenous Viruses of Primates*

Because of their close relationship to man, primates have been intensively studied for endogenous viruses and virus-related information (for review, see Todaro 1980), and a number of such viruses have been obtained (see Chapter 2), mostly by patient cocultivation of primate cell cultures with cells of candidate permissive host species. In some cases, cocultivation periods exceeding 6 months were required before infectious virus was isolated (Sherwin and Todaro 1979). To date, infectious virus has been isolated from more than six species of primates, most readily from baboons. Most of these are typical C-type viruses, yet some D-type viruses have also been isolated from squirrel monkeys and langurs (Colcher et al. 1977; Heberling et al. 1977; Todaro et al. 1978b). The majority of the C-type endogenous virus isolates fall into two groups: those related to the baboon endogenous viruses (BaEV) (Todaro et al. 1973; Goldberg et al. 1974) and those related to the macaque virus (MAC-1) (Todaro et al. 1978a). Neither of these groups is closely related to the exogenous viruses of primates. However, as mentioned before, BaEV is related to the RD114 endogenous viruses of cats. Interestingly, the MAC-1 group of viruses is most closely related to the reticuloendotheliosis viruses (REVs)—exogenous viruses of birds—as measured by homologies in the RU_5 (strong-stop) portion of the genome (Lovinger et al. 1981), in the major *gag* protein p28 (Oroszlan et al. 1981), and by the presence of cross-hybridizing sequences in *gag* and *pol* (Rice et al. 1981).

The most extensive analysis of relationships of endogenous viruses in various primate species has been carried out with BaEV. There are several closely related or identical isolates of this virus, which was first described by Todaro et al. (1973). Sequences related to BaEV can be found in all species of baboon in multiple copies (on the order of 100 or more per cell) (Benveniste and Todaro 1976; Donehower et al. 1977; Gallo and Wong-Staal 1980). These endogenous proviruses are closely related in the different species, since the majority yield identical internal restriction fragments (Gallo and Wong-Staal 1980); however, some variability was detected, particularly in the *gag* region (Cohen et al. 1980). Surveys using BaEV cDNA as a probe have revealed the presence of related sequences in most Old World primates. An extensive series of experiments (Benveniste et al. 1974; Benveniste and Todaro 1976; Bonner and Todaro 1980) comparing the degree of cross-hybridization of BaEV cDNA to cellular DNA with the extent of evolutionary divergence (as measured by cross-hybridization of cellular DNA) yielded the results shown in Figure 10.6. There seems to be a good correlation of the

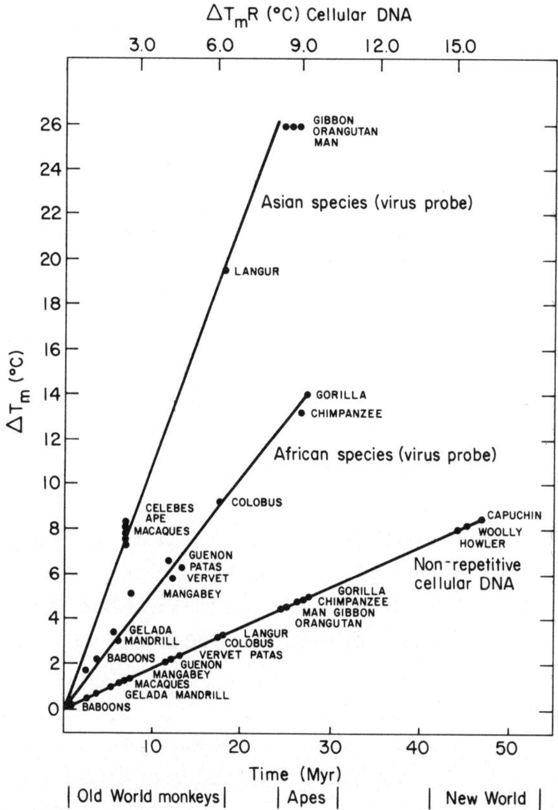

Figure 10.6 Relationships among the DNAs of primates and their endogenous-virus-related sequences. The ΔT_m represents the thermal stability of either BaEV probe or single-copy cellular DNA hybrids with genomic DNA from the species shown. The evolutionary divergence is estimated from the single-copy DNA results. (Adapted from Benveniste and Todaro 1976.)

extent of relatedness of viral DNA with the relatedness of each species to baboons, although, clearly, the genomes of endogenous viruses have diverged more rapidly than the unique-sequence cellular DNA. Interestingly, the data seemed to fall on two distinct curves, divided according to whether the species compared was Asian or African. Thus, there seems to be a relationship between the geographical location and the extent to which these sequences have diverged. From the position of human DNA on this curve, it was argued that man more likely originated in Asia, rather that in Africa (as generally believed). However, more careful studies have failed to reveal a significantly greater relationship of human DNA to BaEV than DNA from unrelated species such as pig and dog (Bonner and Todaro 1980). Furthermore, the variation in location of endogenous proviruses in different individuals of other species would suggest that the maintenance of endogenous viruses in the germ line over evolutionary time is not due to stability of integrated proviruses. Rather, it would seem to suggest a more fluid situation involving frequent loss of old proviruses and reintegration of new ones until some sort of steady state is reached. The selective pressures governing such a process are difficult to assess, but it is unlikely that they are similar to those affecting total cellular DNA, and it is not hard to imagine that they could be easily altered by more subtle differences than continental distribution.

IV. CONCLUSIONS

Since their first accurate description about 10 years ago, endogenous viruses have been the subject of intensive research and equally intensive speculation. These elements have been variously put forth as entities ancestral to horizontally transmitted infectious retroviruses (and even unrelated groups of viruses); as agents important in the etiology of naturally occurring tumors; as genes encoding important normal-cell functions; and as messengers mediating information transfer from cell to cell during the normal life span of an organism or in the course of evolutionary processes. As shown in the preceding sections, detailed studies of endogenous viruses have not provided strong evidence in support of any of these contentions in any general way. Rather, we have seen that endogenous viruses are highly variable in distribution among closely related species and even among individuals within species, in sites of integration, in structural and functional features, and in level and specificity of expression. In many of these respects, the endogenous provirus content of animals resembles the same variety of phenomena seen in exogenously acquired proviruses of cells infected in culture. In spite of this resemblance, however, it is clear that endogenous proviruses are not simply random remnants of exogenous virus infections that happened to involve the germ line of some ancestral animal. On the other hand, exogenous retroviruses endemic to a species of animal are not rescued endogenous viruses. Rather, the two types of viruses seem to be distinct from each other in significant ways. The endogenous viruses seem to be distinct from each other in significant ways. The endogenous viruses of primates, for example, bear little relationship to exogenous viruses of the same species. The endogenous viruses of chickens, although closely related to exogenous ALV, are distinct in several regions of the genome from their exogenous relatives. Thus, endogenous viruses clearly are a special group, although perhaps not as special as once perceived. Given this perspective, it is worth speculating on the phenomenon of the origin of endogenous viruses and on their persistence as a significant fraction of the genome of many animal species.

A. Origins of Endogenous Viruses

As with most evolutionary problems, the origins of endogenous viruses are not accessible to direct experimentation. However, two lines of evidence argue strongly that most or all endogenous viruses were introduced into the germ line by exogenous infection of relatively recent ancestors of modern animal species. The first argument involves their distribution. Endogenous ALV-related proviruses are found only in one species of gallinaceous fowl and are not found in related species, but they are found again in some pheasants. Similarly, endogenous RD-114-like sequences are found in some species of cats but not in others, and the most closely related sequences are found in baboons. Although either selective loss of preexisting proviruses from some species but not others or highly variable rates of divergence could have led to the same observations, these seem unlikely in the face of the simpler possibility of exogenous infection of an ancestor or ancestors at some given time in the distant past.

The second argument centers around the structures of endogenous proviruses. Although often defective in one way or another, these sequences are still highly related to replication-competent viruses and often retain at least some genes (e.g., *env*) that are completely intact and usable for virus replication. The only conceivable way these genes could have arisen is by selection for their ability to replicate as a virus. Thus, all endogenous viruses that have been studied are not elements evolving toward viruses but must have had a virus ancestor at some time in the past. (The VL30 sequences might represent a special sort of exception to this generalization, but that remains to be determined.)

It has been suggested (Temin 1980) that retroviruses, in general, arose from other sorts of cellular transposable elements. If such ancestral elements exist, they remain to be found; they are most likely not represented by the endogenous proviruses that have been analyzed, although it should be noted that it may be very difficult to distinguish endogenous transposable elements from defective endogenous viruses. In any case, the origin by exogenous infection implied by the apparent sudden appearance of endogenous proviruses suggests that if retroviruses are derived from endogenous elements these elements are no longer available to us for analysis.

The germ line seems to present substantial barriers to infection by exogenous retroviruses, at least in experimental time, yet endogenous viruses have managed to gain access to it repeatedly over evolutionarily very short periods. It is clear that endogenous viruses form lineages distinct from those of prevalent exogenous viruses in the same species, i.e., one endogenous provirus is descended from another endogenous provirus. Thus, either endogenous viruses as a group have special features that allow them to infect germ-line cells or animals that have acquired other types of proviruses have a selective disadvantage, e.g., due to a high rate of spontaneous leukemia. In either case, the genomes of endogenous viruses must have special adaptive features that permit their particular life-style. At the very least, they must not be sufficiently pathogenic to confer a selective disadvantage on their host. The distinctive U_3 region of endogenous ALV and the low replication rate associated with it most likely reflect this constraint. In the case of RAV-0, there may be additional features limiting pathogenicity as well. The presence of special regions of the genome relating to ability to infect germ-line cells remains to be demonstrated.

B. How Do Endogenous Proviruses Persist?

The widespread presence, in many animal species, of often unrelated endogenous proviruses indicates that the endogenous life-style of retroviruses is a highly successful one. Clearly, endogenous infections must have been independently established multiple times in different animals, and, once established, such infections have been maintained and even amplified within the germ line so that they are available to us for study today. The variability in structure and location of endogenous proviruses even among related individuals implies that, unlike cellular genes, there is relatively little continuity of inheritance of an endogenous provirus at a specific locus. Rather, the situation resembles a steady state in which proviruses are constantly being gained and lost, but the total number remains roughly constant. The acquisition of new proviruses in sublines of AKR mice suggests that the gain occurs by apparently normal infection processes, the loss most likely by random deletion. Whether such infections occur from virus arising elsewhere within the animal or even exogenously from another individual is not known. This distinction is important, because if reinfection were limited to the germ line, then individuals with only defective endogenous proviruses (such as chickens with *ev*-1) would be unable to acquire more, and it would seem that the high mutation frequency of these viruses would lead to their eventual loss altogether, unless there is a selective advantage to their presence. The accessibility of the germ line to exogenous infection would allow even the genomes of most defective endogenous viruses to move as pseudotypes with infecting exogenous viruses. It should be emphasized that there is no evidence for movement of endogenous proviruses, or indeed of any provirus, in the absence of a complete infection cycle.

The success of endogenous proviruses requires that they do no significant harm to their hosts; it is not known whether they also do good. It is not necessary to invoke a selective advantage to account for their existence; endogenous viruses could persist as benign parasites, with their ability to spread to new locations in the host genome, and even from individual to individual, outweighing their tendency to be lost by random deletion. In this context, they could be considered as a sort of "selfish" genetic element, which need not justify its existence by benefiting its host, as proposed for transposable elements (Doolittle and Sapienza 1980; Orgel and Crick 1980). Clearly, such elements cannot multiply unchecked. There must come a point at which significantly high numbers impose a severe burden on their host either by adding significantly to the amount of DNA to be replicated or by mutational effects of interrupting essential genes. The case of laboratory mice, which may carry as many as 1000 endogenous proviruses, suggests that at least some animals can stand a substantial load without harmful effects. Nevertheless, there must be a limit. Limitation of the number of proviruses could be due to special features of the proviruses themselves, which retard the reintegration rate to roughly balance the rate of loss, or to adaptation of the host to limit endogenous virus replication. The widespread phenomenon of "xenotropism" (i.e., the resistance of many animal cells to infection by their own endogenous viruses, while related species are susceptible to the same viruses) may well reflect an adaptive response of the host to limit the spread of endogenous viruses. The inability of endogenous virus to replicate in somatic cells may also have the effect of reducing or eliminating pathogenicity by these viruses.

In this chapter we have seen that endogenous viruses represent a unique, complex, and fascinating aspect of virology. Intensive work in the past decade has led to a clear understanding of many of the phenomena involved and to a realization that, in most cases, they are explicable in terms of what has been learned from studies with exogenous infections in vitro. Nevertheless, interesting issues remain, including the special features that allow endogenous viruses to adapt to their special environments, the regulation of their expression, and the possible benefits they may confer on their hosts.

REFERENCES

Aaronson, S.A. and C.Y. Dunn. 1974. Endogenous C-type viruses of BALB/c cells: Frequencies of spontaneous and chemical induction. *J. Virol.* **13:** 181–185.

Aaronson, S.A. and J.R. Stephenson. 1973. Independent segregation of loci for activation of biologically distinguishable RNA C-type viruses in mouse cells. *Proc. Natl. Acad. Sci.* **70:** 2055–2058.

———. 1976. Endogenous type-C RNA viruses of mammalian cells. *Biochim. Biophys. Acta* **458:** 323–354.

Aaronson, S.A., J.W. Hartley, and G.J. Todaro. 1969. Mouse leukemia virus: "Spontaneous" release by mouse embryo cells after long-term in vitro cultivation. *Proc. Natl. Acad. Sci.* **64:** 87–94.

Aaronson, S.A., G.J. Todaro, and E.M. Scolnick. 1971. Induction of murine C-type viruses from clonal lines of virus-free BALB/3T3 cells. *Science* **174:** 157–159.

Aksamit, R.R. and C.W. Long. 1977. Induction of endogenous murine type C virus by an arginine analog: L-canavanine. *Virology* **78:** 567–570.

Altrock, B.W., L.O. Arthur, R.J. Massey, and G. Schochetman. 1981. Common surface receptors on both mouse and rat cells distinguish different classes of mouse mammary tumor viruses. *Virology* **109:** 257–266.

Andrewes, C.H. 1939. Latent virus infections and their possible relevance to the cancer problem. *Proc. R. Soc. Med.* **33:** 75–86.

Armstrong, M.Y.K., N.H. Ruddle, M.B. Lipman, and F.F. Richards. 1973. Tumor induction by immunologically activated murine leukemia virus. *J. Exp. Med.* **137:** 1163–1179.

Arthur, L.O., B.W. Altrock, and G. Schochetman. 1981a. Type-specific determinants on proteins of an endogenous C3H mouse mammary tumor virus (MMTV) distinguish this virus from highly oncogenic MMTVs. *Virology* **110:** 270–280.

Arthur, L.O., T.D. Copeland, S. Oroszlan, and G. Schochetman. 1981b. Processing and amino acid sequence analysis of the mouse mammary tumor virus *env* gene product. *J. Virol.* (in press).

Astrin, S.M. 1978. Endogenous viral genes of white leghorn chickens: Common site of residence and sites associated with specific phenotypes of viral gene expression. *Proc. Natl. Acad. Sci.* **75:** 5941–5945.

Astrin, S.M. and H.L. Robinson. 1979. *Gs,* an allele of chickens for endogenous avian leukosis viral antigens, segregates with *ev* 3, a genetic locus that contains structural genes for virus. *J. Virol.* **31:** 420–425.

Astrin, S.M., E.G. Buss, and W.S. Hayward. 1979a. Endogenous viral genes are nonessential in the chicken. *Nature* **282:** 339–341.

Astrin, S.M., L.B. Crittenden, and E.G. Buss. 1979b. *ev*-3, a structural gene locus for endogenous virus, segregates with the gs^+chf^+ phenotype in matings of line 6_3 chickens. *Virology* **99:** 1–9.

———. 1980a. *ev*-2, a genetic locus containing structural genes for endogenous virus, codes for Rous-associated virus type 0 produced by line 7_2 chickens. *J. Virol.* **33:** 250–255.

Astrin, S.M., H.L. Robinson, L.B. Crittenden, E.G. Buss, J. Wyban, and W.S. Hayward. 1980b. Ten genetic loci in the chicken that contain structural genes for endogenous avian leukosis viruses. *Cold Spring Harbor Symp. Quant. Biol.* **44:** 1105–1109.

Bader, J.P. 1967. Metabolic requirements for infection by Rous sarcoma virus. In *Subviral carcinogenesis* (ed. Y. Ito), p. 144–155. Nagoya, Japan.

Baker, B., H.L. Robinson, H.E. Varmus, and J.M. Bishop. 1981. Analysis of endogenous avian retrovirus DNA and RNA: Viral and cellular determinants of retrovirus gene expression. *Virology* **144:** 8–22.

Baluda, M.A. 1972. Widespread presence, in chickens, of DNA complementary to the RNA genome of avian leukosis viruses. *Proc. Natl. Acad. Sci.* **692:** 576–580.

Baluda, M.A. and P. Roy-Burman. 1973. Partial characterization of RD114 virus by DNA-RNA hybridization studies. *Nat. New Biol.* **244:** 59–62.

Barbacid, M., K.C. Robbins, S. Hino, and S.A. Aaronson. 1978. Genetic recombination between mouse type C RNA viruses: A mechanism for endogenous viral gene amplification in mammalian cells. *Proc. Natl. Acad. Sci.* **75:** 923–927.

Bentvelzen, P. 1969. *Genetic control of the vertical transmission of the Muhlbock mammary tumor virus in the GR mouse strain.* Hollandia, Amsterdam.

———. 1972. Hereditary infections with mammary tumor viruses in mice. In *RNA viruses and host genome in oncogenesis* (ed. P. Emmelot and P. Bentvelzen), pp. 309–337. North-Holland, Amsterdam.

———. 1974. Host-virus interactions in murine mammary carcinogenesis. *Biochim. Biophys. Acta* **355:** 236–259.

Bentvelzen, P. and J.H. Daams. 1969. Hereditary infections with mammary tumor viruses in mice. *J. Natl. Cancer Inst.* **43:** 1025–1035.

Bentvelzen, P., J. Brinkhof, and J.J. Haaijman. 1978. Genetic control of endogenous murine mammary tumour viruses reinvestigated. *Eur. J. Cancer.* **14:** 1137–1147.

Bentvelzen, P., J.H. Daams, P. Hageman, and J. Calafat. 1970. Genetic transmission of viruses that incite mammary tumor in mice. *Proc. Natl. Acad. Sci.* **67:** 377–384.

Bentvelzen, P., A. Timmermans, J.H. Daams, and A. van der Gugten. 1968. Genetic transmission of mammary tumor inciting viruses in mice: Possible implications for murine leukemia. *Bibl. Haematol.* **31:** 101–103.

Benveniste, R.E. and G.J. Todaro. 1974. Evolution of C-type viral genes: Inheritance of exogenously acquired viral genes. *Nature* **252:** 456–459.

———. 1976. Evolution of type C viral genes: Evidence for an Asian origin of man. *Nature* **261:** 101–108.

Benveniste, R.E., C.J. Sherr, and G.J. Todaro. 1975. Evolution of type C viral genes: Origin of feline leukemia virus. *Science* **190:** 886–888.

Benveniste, R.E., R. Heinemann, G.L. Wilson, R. Callahan, and G.J. Todaro. 1974. Detection of baboon type C viral sequences in various primate tissues by molecular hybridization. *J. Virol.* **14:** 56–67.

Besmer, P., U. Olshevsky, D. Baltimore, D. Dolberg, and H. Fan. 1979. Virus-like 30S RNA in mouse cells. *J. Virol.* **29:** 1168–1176.

Besmer, P., D. Smotkin, W. Haseltine, H. Fan, A.T. Wilson, M. Paskind, R. Weinberg, and D. Baltimore. 1975. Mechanism of induction of RNA tumor viruses by halogenated pyrimidines. *Cold Spring Harbor Symp. Quant. Biol.* **39:** 1103–1107.

Blair, P.B. 1968. The mammary tumor virus (MTV) *Curr. Top. Microbiol. Immunol.* **45:** 1–69.

Bonner, T.I. and G.J. Todaro. 1980. The evolution of baboon endogenous type C virus: Related sequences in the DNA of distant species. *Virology* **103:** 217–227.

Boyse, E.A. and L.J. Old. 1971. A comment on the genetic data relating to expression of TL antigens. *Transplantation* **11:** 561–562.

Breindl, M., L. Bacheler, H. Fan, and R. Jaenisch. 1980. Chromatin conformation of integrated Moloney leukemia virus DNA sequences in tissue of BALB/Mo mice and in virus-infected cell lines. *J. Virol.* **34:** 373–382.

Breindl, M., J. Doehmer, K. Willecke, J. Dausman, and R. Jaenisch. 1979. Germ line integration of Moloney leukemia virus: Identification of the chromosomal integration site. *Proc. Natl. Acad. Sci.* **76:** 1938–1942.

Buchhagen, D.L., F.S. Pedersen, R.L. Crowther, and W.A. Haseltine. 1980. Most sequence differences between the genomes of the Akv virus and a leukemogenic Gross A virus passaged *in vitro* are located near the 3′ terminus. *Proc. Natl. Acad. Sci.* **77:** 4359–4363.

Callahan, R. and G.J. Todaro. 1978. Four major endogenous retrovirus classes each genetically transmitted in various species of *Mus*. In *Origins of inbred mice* (ed. H.C. Morse, III), p. 689–713. Academic Press, New York.

Callahan, R., R.E. Benviniste, M.M. Lieber, and G.J. Todaro. 1976. A new class of genetically transmitted retrovirus from *Mus cervicolor*. *Proc. Natl. Acad. Sci.* **73:** 3579–3583.

Canaani, E. and S.A. Aaronson. 1979. Restriction enzyme analysis of mouse cellular type C viral DNA: Emergence of new viral sequences in spontaneous AKR/J lymphomas. *Proc. Natl. Acad. Sci.* **76:** 1677–1681.

Chan, H.W., T. Bryan, J.L. Moore, S.P. Staal, W.P. Rowe, and M.A. Martin. 1980. Identification of ecotropic proviral sequences in inbred mouse strains with a cloned subgenomic DNA fragment. *Proc. Natl. Acad. Sci.* **77:** 5779–5783.

Chattopadhyay, S.K., M.R. Lander, E. Rands, and D.R. Lowy. 1980. Structure of endogenous murine leukemia virus DNA in mouse genomes. *Proc. Natl. Acad. Sci.* **77:** 5774–5778.

Chattopadhyay, S.K., W.P. Rowe, N.M. Teich, and D.R. Lowy. 1975a. Definitive evidence that the murine C-type virus inducing locus *Akv-1* is viral genetic material. *Proc. Natl. Acad. Sci.* **72:** 906–910.

Chattopadhyay, S.K., M.R. Lander, S. Gupta, E. Rands, and D.R. Lowy. 1981. Origin of mink cytopathic focus-forming (MCF) viruses: Comparison with ecotropic and xenotropic murine leukemia virus genomes. *Virology* **113:** 465–483.

Chattopadhyay, S.K., D.R. Lowy, N.M. Teich, A.S. Levine, and W.P. Rowe. 1974. Evidence that the AKR murine-leukemia-virus genome is complete in DNA of the high-virus AKR mouse and incomplete in the DNA of the "virus-negative" NIH mouse. *Proc. Natl. Acad. Sci.* **71:** 167–171.

———. 1975b. Qualitative and quantitative studies of AKR-type murine leukemia virus sequences in mouse DNA. *Cold Spring Harbor Symp. Quant. Biol.* **39:** 1085–1101.

Chien, Y.-H., R.P. Junghans and N. Davidson. 1980. Electron microscopic analysis of the structure of RNA tumor virus nucleic acids. In *Molecular biology of RNA tumor viruses* (ed. J.H. Stephenson), pp. 395–446. Academic Press, New York.

Chien, Y.-H., I.M. Verma, T.Y. Shih, E.M. Scolnick, and N. Davidson. 1978. Heteroduplex analysis of the sequence relations between the RNAs of mink cell focus-inducing and murine leukemia viruses. *J. Virol.* **28:** 352–360.

Cloyd, M.W., J.W. Hartley, and W.P. Rowe. 1980. Lymphomagenicity of recombinant mink cell focus-inducing virus. *J. Exp. Med.* **151:** 542–552.

Coffin, J.M., M.A. Champion, and F. Chabot. 1978a. Genome structure of avian RNA tumor viruses: Relationships between exogenous and endogenous viruses. In *Avian RNA tumor viruses* (ed. S. Barlati and C. deGiuli-Morghen), pp. 68–87. Piccin Medical Books, Padua.

———. 1978b. Nucleotide sequence relationships between the genomes of an endogenous and an exogenous avian tumor virus. *J. Virol.* **28:** 972–991.

Coffin, J.M., P.N. Tsichlis, and H.L. Robinson. 1981. Genetics of leukemogenicity of avian leukosis viruses. In *Modern trends in human leukemia IV* (eds. R. Neth et al.) pp. 432–438. Springer-Verlag, Berlin.

Coffin, J.M., T.C. Hageman, A.M. Maxam, and W.A. Haseltine. 1978c. Structure of the genome of Moloney murine leukemia virus: A terminally redundant sequence. *Cell* **13:** 761–773.

Cohen, J.C. 1980. Methylation of milk-borne and genetically transmitted mouse mammary tumor virus proviral DNA. *Cell* **19:** 653–662.

Cohen, J.C. and H.E. Varmus. 1979. Endogenous mammary tumour virus DNA varies among wild mice and segregates during inbreeding. *Nature* **278:** 418–423.

———. 1980. Proviruses of mouse mammary tumor virus in normal and neoplastic tissues from GR and C3Hf mouse strains. *J. Virol.* **35:** 298–305.

Cohen, J.C., J.E. Majors, and H.E. Varmus. 1979a. Organization of mouse mammary tumor virus-specific DNA endogenous to BALB/c mice. *J. Virol.* **32:** 483–496.

Cohen, J.C., P.R. Shank, V.L. Morris, R. Cardiff, and H.E. Varmus. 1979b. Integration of the DNA of mouse mammary tumor virus in virus-infected normal and neoplastic tissues of the mouse. *Cell* **16:** 333–345.

Cohen, M., N. Davidson, R.V. Gilden, R.M. McAllister, M.O. Nicolson, and R.M. Stephens. 1980. The baboon endogenous virus genome. II. Provirus sequence variations in baboon cell DNA. *Nucleic Acids Res.* **8:** 4423–4440.

Colcher, D., R.L. Heberling, S.S. Kalter, and J. Schlom. 1977. Squirrel monkey retroviruses: An endogenous virus of a New World primate. *J. Virol.* **23:** 294–301.

Cole, M.D., M. Ono, and R.C.C. Huang. 1981. Terminally redundant sequences in cellular intracisternal A-particle genes. *J. Virol.* **38:** 680–687.

Cooper, G.M. and L. Silverman. 1978. Linkage of the endogenous avian leukosis virus genome of virus-producing chicken cells to inhibitory cellular DNA sequences. *Cell* **15:** 573–577.

Cooper, G.M. and H.M. Temin. 1976. Lack of infectivity of the endogenous avian leukosis virus-related genes in the DNA of uninfected chicken cells. *J. Virol.* **17:** 422–430.

Crittenden, L.B., J.V. Motta, and E.J. Smith. 1977. Genetic control of RAV-0 production in chickens. *Virology* **76:** 90–97.

Crittenden, L.B., E.J. Wendel, and J.V. Motta. 1973. Interaction of genes controlling resistance to RSV (RAV-0). *Virology* **52:** 373–384.

Crittenden, L.B., W.S. Hayward, H. Hanafusa, and A.M. Fadly. 1980. Induction of neoplasms by subgroup E recombinants of exogenous and endogenous avian retroviruses (Rous-associated virus type 60). *J. Virol.* **33:** 915–919.

Crittenden, L.B., E.J. Smith, R.A. Weiss, and P.S. Sarma. 1974. Host gene control of endogenous avian leukosis virus production. *Virology* **57:** 128–138.

Dalton, A.J., M. Potter, and R.M. Merwin. 1961. Some ultrastructural characteristics of a series of primary and transplanted plasma-cell tumors of the mouse. *J. Natl. Cancer Inst.* **26:** 1221–1267.

Darlington, C.D. 1948. The plasmagene theory of the origin of cancer. *Br. J. Cancer.* **2:** 118–126.

Datta, S.K. and R.S. Schwartz. 1977. Mendelian segregation of loci controlling xenotropic virus production in NZB crosses. *Virology* **83:** 449–452.

Datta, S.K., N. Manny, C. Andrzejewski, J. Andre-Schwartz, and R.S. Schwartz. 1978a. Genetic studies of autoimmunity and retrovirus expression in crosses of New Zealand black mice. I. Xenotropic virus. *J. Exp. Med.* **147:** 854–871.

Datta, S.K., P.N. Tsichlis, R.S. Schwartz, S.K. Chattopadhyay, and C.J.M. Melief. 1978b. Genetic differences unrelated to H-2 in H-2 congenic mice. *Immunogenetics* **7:** 359–365.

Decleve, A., M. Lieberman, and H.S. Kaplan. 1977. *In vivo* interaction between RNA viruses isolated from the C57BL/Ka strain of mice. *Virology* **81:** 270–283.

deHarven, E. and C. Friend. 1958. Electron microscope study of a cell-free induced leukemia of the mouse: A preliminary report. *J. Biophys. Biochem. Cytol.* **4:** 151–156.

DeOme, K.B., L. Young, and S. Nandi. 1967. Comparison of the behavior of nodule-inducing virus (NIV) in C3Hf(F) and BALB/c (C) mice. *Proc. Am. Assoc. Cancer Res.* **8:** 13 (Abstr.).

Dickson, C. and G. Peters. 1981. Protein-coding potential of mouse mammary tumor virus genome RNA as examined by in vitro translation. *J. Virol.* **37:** 36–47.

Dixon, F.J., M.B.A. Oldstone, and G. Tonietti. 1971. Pathogenesis of immune complex-glomerulonephritis of New Zealand mice. *J. Exp. Med.* **134** (Suppl.): 65s–71s.

Dolberg, O., L.T. Bacheler, and H. Fan. 1980. A study of the endogenous Moloney related sequences of mice. *ICN-UCLA Symp. Mol. Cell. Biol.* **18:** 187–195.

Donehower, L.A., A.L. Huang, and G.L. Hager. 1981. Regulatory and coding potential of the mouse mammary tumor virus long terminal redundancy. *J. Virol.* **37:** 226–238.

Donehower, L., F. Wong-Staal, and D. Gillespie. 1977. Divergence of baboon endogenous type C virogenes in primates: Genomic viral RNA in molecular hybridization experiments. *J. Virol.* **21:** 932–941.

Donehower, L.A., J. Andre, D.S. Berard, R.G. Wolford, and G.L. Hager. 1980. Construction and characterization of molecular clones containing integrated mouse mammary tumor virus sequences. *Cold Spring Harbor Symp. Quant. Biol.* **44:** 1153–1159.

Doolittle, W.F. and C. Sapienza. 1980. Selfish genes, the phenotype paradigm and genome evolution. *Nature* **284:** 601–603.

Dougherty, R.M. and H.S. Di Stefano. 1966. Lack of relationship between infection with avian leukosis virus and the presence of COFAL antigen in chick embryos. *Virology* **29:** 586–595.

Dougherty, R.M., H.S. Di Stefano, and F.K. Roth. 1967. Virus particles and viral antigens in chicken tissues free of infectious avian leukosis virus. *Proc. Natl. Acad. Sci.* **58:** 808–817.

Drohan, W. and J. Schlom. 1979a. Diversity of mammary tumor viral genes within the genes of *Mus*, the species *Mus musculus*, and the strain C3H. *J. Virol.* **31:** 53–62.

———. 1979b. Differential distribution of mouse mammary tumor virus-related sequences in the DNAs of rats. *J. Natl. Cancer Inst.* **62:** 1279–1286.

Drohan, W., J. Young, and J. Schlom. 1980. Correlation between the development of murine mammary cancer and the segregation of endogenous genes. *ICN-UCLA Symp. Mol. Cell. Biol.* **18:** 177–185.

Drohan, W., R. Kettmann, D. Colcher, and J. Schlom. 1977. Isolation of the mouse mammary tumor virus sequences not transmitted as germinal provirus in the C3H and RIII mouse strains. *J. Virol.* **21:** 986–995.

Eisenman, R., R. Shaikh, and W.S. Mason. 1978. Identification of an avian oncovirus polyprotein in uninfected chick cells. *Cell* **14:** 89–104.

Elder, J.H., J.W. Gautsch, F.C. Jensen, R.A. Lerner, J.W. Hartley, and W.P. Rowe. 1977. Biochemical evidence that MCF murine leukemia viruses are envelope (*env*) gene recombinants. *Proc. Natl. Acad. Sci.* **74:** 4676–4680.

Ellis, R.W., E. Stockert, and E. Fleissner. 1980. Association of endogenous retroviruses with radiation-induced leukemias of BALB/c mice. *J. Virol.* **33:** 652–660.

Faller, D. and N. Hopkins. 1978a. T_1 oligonucleotide maps of N-, B-, and B→NB tropic murine leukemia viruses derived from BALB/c. *J. Virol.* **26:** 143–152.

———. 1978b. T_1 oligonucleotide maps of Moloney and HIX murine leukemia viruses. *Virology* **90:** 265–273.

Fanning, T.G., J.P. Puma, and R.D. Cardiff. 1980a. Selective amplification of mouse mammary tumor virus in mammary tumors of GR mice. *J. Virol.* **36:** 109–114.

———. 1980b. Identification and partial characterization of an endogenous form of mouse mammary tumor virus that is transcribed into the virion-associated RNA genome. *Nucleic Acids Res.* **8:** 5715–5723.

Fischinger, P.J., P.T. Peebles, S. Nomura, and D.K. Haapala. 1973. Isolation of an RD-114-like oncornavirus from a cat cell line. *J. Virol.* **11:** 978–985.

Frisby, D.P., MacCormick, and R.A. Weiss. 1980. Origin of RAV-0, the endogenous retrovirus of chickens. *Cold Spring Harbor Conf. Cell Proliferation* **7:** 509–517.

Frisby, D.P., R.A. Weiss, M. Roussel, and D. Stehelin. 1979. The distribution of endogenous retrovirus sequences in the DNA of galliform birds does not coincide with avian phylogenetic relationships. *Cell* **17:** 623–634.

Fujita, D.J., Y.C. Chen, R.R. Friis, and P.K. Vogt. 1974. RNA tumor viruses of pheasants: Characterization of avian leukosis subgroups F and G. *Virology* **60:** 558–571.

Furth, J. 1978. The creation of the AKR strain, whose DNA contains the genome of a leukemia virus. In *origins of inbred mice* (ed. H.C. Morse, III.), p. 69–97. Academic Press, New York.

Furth, J., H.R. Seibold, and R.R. Rathobone. 1933. Experimental studies on lymphomatosis of mice. *Am. J. Cancer.* **19:** 521–604.

Gallo, R.C. and F. Wong-Staal. 1980. Molecular biology of primate retroviruses. In *Viral oncology* (ed. G. Klein), pp. 399–431. Raven Press, New York.

Gautsch, J.W., J.H. Elder, F.C. Jensen, and R.A. Lerner. 1980. *In vitro* construction of a B-tropic virus by recombination: B-tropism is a cryptic phenotype of xenotropic murine retroviruses. *Proc. Natl. Acad. Aci.* **77:** 2989–2993.

Gautsch, J.W., J.H. Elder, J. Schindler, F.C. Jensen, and R.A. Lerner. 1978. Structural markers on core protein p30 of murine leukemia virus: Functional correlation with *Fv-1* tropism. *Proc. Natl. Acad. Sci.* **75:** 4170–4174.

Gelb, L.D., J.B. Milstien, M.A. Martin, and S.A. Aaronson. 1973. Characterization of murine leukaemia virus-specific DNA present in normal mouse cells. *Nat. New Biol.* **244:** 76–79.

Gillespie, D., S. Gillespie, R.C. Gallo, J.L. East, and L. Dmochowski. 1973. Genetic origin of RD114 and other RNA tumor viruses assayed by molecular hybridization. *Nat. New Biol.* **244:** 51–54.

Goldberg, R.J., E.M. Scolnick, W.P. Parks, L.A. Yakovleva, and B.A. Lapin. 1974. Isolation of a primate type-C virus from a lymphomatous baboon. *Int. J. Cancer.* **14:** 722–730.

Green, N., H. Hiai, J.H. Elder, R.A. Schwartz, R.H. Khiroya, C.Y. Thomas, P.N. Tsichlis, and J.M. Coffin. 1980. Expression of leukemogenic recombinant viruses associated with a recessive gene in HRS/J mice. *J. Exp. Med.* **152:** 249–264.

Groner, B., E. Buetti, H. Diggelmann, and N.E. Hynes. 1980. Characterization of endogenous and exogenous mouse mammary tumor virus proviral DNA with site-specific molecular clones. *J. Virol.* **36:** 734–745.

Gross, L. 1958. Attempt to recover filterable agent from X-ray-induced leukemia. *Acta Haematol.* **19:** 353–361.

———. 1970. *Oncogenic viruses*, 2nd edition. Pergamon Press, Oxford.

Groudine, M., R. Eisenman, and H. Weintraub. 1981. Chromatin structure of endogenous retroviral genomes and activation by an inhibitor of DNA methylation. *Nature* **292:** 311–317.

Haas, M. 1978. Leukemogenic activity of thymotropic, ecotropic, and xenotropic radiation leukemia virus isolates. *J. Virol.* **25:** 705–709.

Halpern, M.S., D.P. Bolognesi, R.R. Friis, and W.S. Mason. 1975. Expression of the major viral glycoprotein of avian tumor virus in cells of chf(+) chicken embryos. *J. Virol.* **15:** 1131–1140.

Hanafusa, H., T. Miyamoto, and T. Hanafusa. 1970. A cell-associated factor essential for the formation of an infectious form of Rous sarcoma virus. *Proc. Natl. Acad. Sci.* **66:** 314–321.

Hanafusa, H., T. Hanafusa, S. Kawai, and R.E. Luginbuhl. 1974. Genetic control of expression of endogenous virus genes in chicken cells. *Virology* **58:** 439–448.

Hanafusa, H., W.S. Hayward, J.H. Chen, and T. Hanafusa. 1975. Control of expression of tumor virus genes in uninfected chicken cells. *Cold Spring Harbor Symp. Quant. Biol.* **39:** 1139–1144.

Hanafusa, H., T. Aoki, S. Kawai, T. Miyamoto, and R.E. Wilsnack. 1973. Presence of antigen common to avian tumor viral envelope antigen in normal chick embryo cells. *Virology* **56:** 22–32.

Hanafusa, T. and H. Hanafusa. 1973. Isolation of leukosis-type virus from pheasant embryo cells: Probable presence of viral genes in cells. *Virology* **51:** 247–251.

Hanafusa, T., H. Hanafusa, and T. Miyamoto. 1970a. Recovery of a new virus from apparently normal cells by infection with avian tumor viruses. *Proc. Natl. Acad. Sci.* **67:** 1797–1803.

Hanafusa, T., T. Miyamoto, and H. Hanafusa. 1970b. A type of chick embryo cell that fails to support formation of infectious RSV. *Virology* **40:** 55–64.

Hanafusa, T., H. Hanafusa, T. Miyamoto, and E. Fleissner. 1972. Existence and expression of tumor virus genes in chick embryo cells. *Virology* **47:** 475–482.

Hanafusa, T., H. Hanafusa, C.E. Metroka, W.S. Hayward, C.W. Rettenmier, R.C. Sawyer, R.M. Dougherty, and H.S. DiStefano. 1976. Pheasant virus: New class of ribodeoxyvirus. *Proc. Natl. Acad. Sci.* **73:** 1333–1337.

Harbers, K., A. Schnike, H. Stuhlmann, D. Jähner, and R. Jaenisch. 1981. DNA methylation and gene expression: Endogenous retroviral genome becomes infectious after molecular cloning. *Proc. Natl. Acad. Sci.* **78:** 7609–7613.

Harel, L., J. Harel, and J. Huppert. 1967. Partial homology between RNA from Rauscher mouse leukemia virus and cellular DNA. *Biochem. Biophys. Res. Commun.* **28:** 44–49.

Harel, L., J. Harel, F. Lacour, and J. Huppert. 1966. Homologie entre genome du virus de la myeloblastose aviare (AMV) et genome cellulaire. *C. R. Acad. Sci.* **263:**616-619.

Hartley, J.W., N.K. Wolford, L.J. Old, and W.P. Rowe. 1977. A new class of murine leukemia virus associated with development of spontaneous lymphomas. *Proc. Natl. Acad. Sci.* **74:**789–792.

Hayward, W.S. and H. Hanafusa. 1975. Recombination between endogenous and exogenous RNA tumor virus genes as analyzed by nucleic acid hybridization. *J. Virol.* **15:**1367–1377.

———. 1976. Independent regulation of endogenous and exogenous avian RNA tumor virus genes. *Proc. Natl. Acad. Sci.* **73:**2259–2263.

Hayward, W.S., S.B. Braverman, and S.M. Astrin. 1980. Transcriptional products and DNA structure of endogenous avian proviruses. *Cold Spring Harbor Symp. Quant. Biol.* **44:**1111–1121.

Heberling, R.L., S.T. Barker, S.S. Kalter, G.C. Smith, and R.J. Helmke. 1977. Oncornavirus: Isolation from a squirrel monkey (Saimiri sciureus) lung culture. *Science* **195:** 289–292.

Heston, W.E. and W.P. Parks. 1977. Mammary tumors and mammary tumor virus expression in hybrid mice of strains C57BL and GR. *J. Exp. Med.* **146:**1206–1220.

Heston, W., B. Smith, and W.P. Parks. 1976. Mouse mammary tumor virus in hybrids from strains C57BL and GR: Breeding test of backcross segregants. *J. Exp. Med.* **144:** 1022–1030.

Hishinuma, F., P.J. DeBona, S. Astrin, and A.M. Skalka. 1981. Nucleotide sequence of the acceptor site and termini of integrated avian endogenous provirus *ev*-1: Integration creates a 6bp repeat of host DNA. *Cell* **23:**155–164.

Holliday, R. and J.E. Pugh. 1975. DNA modification mechanisms and gene activity during development. *Science* **187:**226–232.

Horan-Hand, P., Y.A. Teramoto, R. Callahan, and J. Schlom. 1980. Interspecies radioimmunoassay for the major internal protein of mammary tumor viruses. *Virology* **101:**61–71.

Howk, R.S., D.H. Troxler, D. Lowy, P.H. Duesberg, and E.M. Scolnick. 1978. Identification of a 30S RNA with properties of a defective type C virus in murine cells. *J. Virol.* **25:**115–123.

Huebner, R.J., G.J. Kelloff, P.S. Sarma, W.T. Lane, H.C. Turner, R.V. Gilden, S. Oroszlan, H. Meier, D.D. Myers, and R.L. Peters. 1970. Group-specific antigen expression during embryogenesis of the genome of the C-type RNA tumor virus: Implications for ontogenesis and oncogenesis. *Proc. Natl. Acad. Sci.* **67:**366–376.

Hughes, S.H., K. Toyoshima, J.M. Bishop, and H.E. Varmus. 1981a. Organization of the endogenous proviruses of chickens: Implications for origin and expression. *Virology* **108:**189–207.

Hughes, S.H., P.K. Vogt, J.M. Bishop, and H.E. Varmus. 1981b. Endogenous proviruses of random-bred chickens and ring-necked pheasants: Analysis with restriction endonucleases. *Virology* **108:**222–229.

Hughes, S.H., F. Payvar, D. Spector, R.T. Schimke, H.L. Robinson, G.S. Payne, J.M. Bishop, and H.E. Varmus. 1979. Heterogeneity of genetic loci in chickens: Analysis of endogenous viral and nonviral genes by cleavage of DNA with restriction endonucleases. *Cell* **18:**347–359.

Humphries, E.H., C. Glover, R.A. Weiss, and J.R. Arrand. 1979. Differences between the endogenous and exogenous DNA sequences of Rous-associated virus-0. *Cell* **18:**803–815.

Hynes, N.E., N. Kennedy, U. Rahmsdorf, and B. Groner. 1981. Hormone-responsive expression of an endogenous proviral gene of mouse mammary tumor virus after molecular cloning and gene transfer into cultured cells. *Proc. Natl. Acad. Sci.* **78:**2038– 2042.

Ihle, J.N., D.R. Joseph, and J.J. Domotor, Jr. 1979. Genetic linkage of C3H/HeJ and

BALB/c endogenous ecotropic C-type viruses to phosphoglucomutase-1 on chromosome 5. *Science* **204:**71–73.

Ishizaki, R. and T. Shimizu. 1970. Observations on the envelope properties of RSV(0). *Virology* **40:**415–417.

Jaenisch, R. 1976. Germ line integration and Mendelian transmission of the exogenous Moloney leukemia virus. *Proc. Natl. Acad. Sci.* **73:**1260–1264.

———. 1977. Germ line integration of Moloney leukemia virus: Effect of homozygosity at the M-MuLV locus. *Cell* **12:**691–696.

———. 1979. Moloney leukemia virus gene expression and gene amplification in preleukemic and leukemic BALB/Mo mice. *Virology* **93:**80–90.

———. 1980a. Retroviruses and embryogenesis: Microinjection of Moloney leukemia virus into midgestation mouse embryos. *Cell* **19:**181–188.

———. 1980b. Germ line integration and Mendelian transmission of exogenous type C viruses. In *Molecular biology of RNA tumor viruses* (ed. J. Stephenson), pp. 131–162. Academic Press, New York.

Jaenisch, R., D. Jähner, and D. Grotkopp. 1980. Derivation of three mouse strains carrying Moloney leukemia virus in their germ line at different genetic loci. *ICN-UCLA Symp. Mol. Cell. Biol.* **18:**265–279.

Jaenisch, R., D. Jähner, P. Nobis, I. Simon, J. Lohler, K. Harbers, and G. Grotkopp. 1981. Chromosomal position and activation of retroviral genomes inserted into the germ line of mice. *Cell* **24:**519–529.

Jähner, D. and R. Jaenisch. 1980. Integration of Moloney leukaemia virus into the germ line of mice: Correlation between site of integration and virus activation. *Nature* **287:**456–458.

Jenkins, N.A., N.G. Copeland, B.A. Taylor, and B.K. Lee. 1981. Dilute (*d*) coat colour mutation of DBA/2J mice is associated with the site of integration of an ecotropic MuLV genome. *Nature* **293:**370–374.

Jones, P.A. and S.M. Taylor. 1980. Cellular differentiation, cytidine analogs and DNA methylation. *Cell* **20:**85–93.

Kang, C.-Y. and H.M. Temin. 1974. Reticuloendotheliosis virus nucleic acid sequences in cellular DNA. *J. Virol.* **14:**1179–1188.

Kawai, S. and H. Hanafusa. 1973. Isolation of defective mutant of avian sarcoma virus. *Proc. Natl. Acad. Sci.* **70:**3493–3947.

Kawashima, K., H. Ikeda, J.W. Hartley, E. Stockert, W.P. Rowe, and L.J. Old. 1976. Changes in expression of murine leukemia virus antigens and production of xenotropic virus in the late preleukemic period in AKR mice. *Proc. Natl. Acad. Sci.* **73:**4680–4684.

Keshet, E. and Y. Shaul. 1981. Terminal direct repeats in a retrovirus-like repeated mouse gene family. *Nature* **289:**83–85.

Keshet, E., Y. Shaul, J. Kaminchik, and H. Aviv. 1980. Heterogeneity of "virus-like" genes encoding retrovirus-associated 30S RNA and their organization within the mouse genome. *Cell* **20:**431–439.

Koshy, R., R.C. Gallo, and F. Wong-Staal. 1980. Characterization of the endogenous feline leukemia virus-related DNA sequences in cats and attempts to identify exogenous viral sequences in tissues of virus-negative leukemic animals. *Virology* **103:**434–445.

Kozak, C.A. and W.P. Rowe. 1978. Genetic mapping of xenotropic leukemia virus-inducing loci in two mouse strains. *Science* **199:**1448–1449.

———. 1979. Genetic mapping of the ecotropic murine leukemia virus-inducing locus of BALB/c mouse to chromosome 5. *Science* **204:**69–71.

———. 1980a. Genetic mapping of xenotropic murine leukemia virus-inducing loci in five mouse strains. *J. Exp. Med.* **152:**219–228.

———. 1980b. Chromosomal mapping of ecotropic and xenotropic leukemia virus inducing loci in the mouse. *ICN-UCLA Symp. Mol. Cell. Biol.* **18:**171–175.

Kuff, E.L., K.K. Lueders, and E.M. Scolnick. 1978. Nucleotide sequence relationship between intracisternal A particles of *Mus musculus* and an endogenous retrovirus (M432) of *Mus cervicolor. J. Virol.* **28:**66–74.

Kuff, E.L., N.A. Wivel, and K.K. Lueders. 1968. The extraction of intracisternal A-particles from a mouse plasma-cell tumor. *Cancer Res.* **28:**2137–2148.

Kuff, E.L., K.K. Lueders, H.L. Ozer, and N.A. Wivel. 1972. Some structural and antigenic properties of intracisternal A particles occurring in mouse tumors. *Proc. Natl. Acad. Sci.* **69:**218–222.

Latarjet, R. and J.-F. Duplan. 1962. Experiment and discussion on leukaemogenesis by cell-free extracts of radiation-induced leukaemia in mice. *Int. J. Radiat. Biol.***5:**339–344.

Lerner, R.A., C.B. Wilson, B.C. Del Villano, P.J. McConahey, and F.J. Dixon. 1976. Endogenous oncornaviral gene expression in adult and fetal mice: Quantitative, histologic, and physiologic studies of the major viral glycoprotein, gp70. *J. Exp. Med.* **143:**151–166.

Levy, J.A. 1973. Xenotropic viruses: Murine leukemia viruses associated with NIH Swiss, NZB, and other mouse strains. *Science* **182:**1151–1153.

———. 1978. Xenotropic type C viruses. *Curr. Top. Microbiol. Immunol.* **79:**109–213.

Levy, J.A. and T. Pincus. 1970. Demonstration of biological activity of a murine leukemia virus of New Zealand Black mice. *Science* **170:**326–327.

Levy, J.A., S.K. Datta, and R.S. Schwartz. 1977. Recovery of xenotropic virus but not ecotropic virus during graft versus host reaction in mice. *Clin. Immunol. Immunopathol.* **7:**262–268

Levy, J.A., J.N. Ihle, O. Oleszko, and R.D. Barnes. 1975. Virus-specific neutralization by a soluble non-immunoglobulin factor found naturally in normal mouse sera. *Proc. Natl. Acad. Sci.* **72:**5071–5075.

Lieberman, M. and H.S. Kaplan. 1959. Leukemogenic activity of filtrates from radiation-induced lymphoid tumors of mice. *Science* **130:**387–388.

Lilly, F. 1970. *Fv-2*: Identification and location of a second gene governing the spleen focus response to Friend leukemia virus in mice. *J. Natl. Cancer Inst.* **45:**163–169.

Linial, M. and P.E. Neiman. 1976. Infection of chick cells by subgroup E viruses. *Virology* **73:**508–520.

Livingston, D.M. and G.J. Todaro. 1973. Endogenous type C virus from a cat cell clone with properties distinct from previously described feline type C virus. *Virology* **53:**142– 151.

Long, C.A., U.J. Dumaswala, S.L. Tancin, and A.B. Vaidya. 1980. Organization and expression of endogenous murine mammary tumor virus genes in mice congenic at the H-2 complex. *Virology* **103:**167–177.

Love, D.N. and R.A. Weiss. 1974. Pseudotypes of vesicular stomatitis virus determined by exogenous and endogenous avian RNA tumor viruses. *Virology* **57:**271–279.

Lovinger, G.G., G. Mark, G.J. Todaro, and G. Schochetman. 1981. 5′-Terminal nucleotide noncoding sequences of retroviruses: Relatedness of two old world primate type C viruses and avian spleen necrosis virus. *J. Virol.* **39:**238–245.

Lowy, D.R. 1978. Infectious murine leukemia virus from DNA of virus-negative AKR mouse embryo cells. *Proc. Natl. Acad. Sci.* **75:**5539–5543.

Lowy, D.R., W.P. Rowe, N. Teich, and J.W. Hartley. 1971. Murine leukemia virus: High-frequency activation in vitro by 5-iododeoxyuridine and 5-bromodeoxyuridine. *Science* **174:**155–156.

Lueders, K.K. and E.L. Kuff. 1977. Sequences associated with intracisternal A particles are reiterated in the mouse genome. *Cell* **12:**963–972.

Lueders, K.K., S. Segal, and E.L. Kuff. 1977. RNA sequences specifically associated with mouse intracisternal A particles. *Cell* **11:**83–94.

Lung, M.L., C. Hering, J.W. Hartley, W.P. Rowe, and N. Hopkins. 1980. Analysis of the genomes of mink cell focus-inducing murine type-C viruses: A progress report. *Cold Spring Harbor Symp. Quant. Biol.* **44:**1269–1274.

Lwoff, A. 1960. Tumor viruses and the cancer problem: A summation of the conference. *Cancer Res.* **20:**820–829.

Mandel, J.L. and P. Chambon. 1979. DNA methylation: Organ specific variations in the methylation pattern within and around ovalbumin and other chicken genes. *Nucleic Acids Res.* **7:**2081–2103.

Manteuil-Brutlag, S., S. Lev, and H.S. Kaplan. 1980. Radiation leukemia virus contains two distinct viral RNAs. *Cell* **19:**643–652.

Massey, R.J., L.O. Arthur, R.C. Nowinski, and G. Schochetman. 1980. Monoclonal antibodies identify individual determinants on mouse mammary tumor virus glycoprotein gp52 with group, class, or type specificity. *J. Virol.* **34:**635–643.

McAllister, R.M., M. Nicolson, M.B. Gardner, R.W. Rongey, S. Rasheed, P.S. Sarma, R.J. Huebner, M. Hatanaka, S. Oroszlan, R.V. Gilden, A. Kabigting, and L. Vernon. 1972. C-type virus released from cultured human rhabdomyosarcoma cells. *Nat. New Biol.* **235:**3–6.

Michalides, R. and J. Schlom. 1975. Relationship in nucleic acid sequences between mouse mammary tumor virus variants. *Proc. Natl. Acad. Sci.* **72:**4635–4639.

Michalides, R., G. Vlahakis, and J. Schlom. 1976. A biochemical approach to the study of the transmission of mouse mammary tumor viruses in mouse strain RIII and C3H. *Int. J. Cancer.* **18:**105–115.

Michalides, R., L. van Deemter, R. Nusse, and R. van Nie. 1980. Identification of the *Mtv-2* gene responsible for the early appearance of mammary tumors in the GR mouse by nucleic acid hybridization. *Proc. Natl. Acad. Sci.* **75:**2368–2372.

Michalides, R., R. Van Nie, R. Nusse, N.E. Hynes, and B. Groner. 1981. Mammary tumor induction loci in GR and DBAf mice contain one provirus of the mouse mammary tumor virus. *Cell* **23:**165–173.

Michalides, R., E. Wagenaar, B. Groner, and N.E. Hynes. 1981. Mammary tumor virus proviral DNA in normal murine tissue and non-virally induced mammary tumors. *J. Virol.* **39:**367–376.

Moll, B., J.W. Hartley, and W.P. Rowe. 1979. Induction of B-tropic and N-tropic murine leukemia virus from B10.BR/SGLI mouse embryo cells by 5-iodo-2′-deoxyuridine. *J. Natl. Cancer Inst.* **63:**213–217.

Moroni, C. and G. Schumann. 1975. Lipopolysaccharide induces C-type virus in short term cultures of BALB/c spleen cells. *Nature* **254:**60–61.

Morris, V.L., C. Kozak, J.C. Cohen, P.R. Shank, P. Jolicoeur, F. Ruddel, and H.E. Varmus. 1979. Endogenous mouse mammary tumor virus DNA is distributed among multiple mouse chromosomes. *Virology* **92:**46–55.

Morris, V., E. Medeiros, G.M. Ringold, J.M. Bishop, and H.E. Varmus. 1977. Comparison of mouse mammary tumor-virus specific DNA in inbred, wild, and Asian mice and in tumors and normal organs from inbred mice. *J. Mol. Biol.* **114:**73–92.

Motta, J.V., L.B. Crittenden, H.G. Purchase, H.A. Stone, and R.L. Witter. 1975. Low oncogenic potential of avian endogenous RNA tumor virus infection or expression. *J. Natl. Cancer Inst.* **55:**685–689.

Muhlbock, O. 1955. Note on a new inbred mouse strain GR/A. *Eur. J. Cancer.* **1:**123–124.

Mullins, J.I., J. Casey, M.O. Nicolson, K.B. Burk, and N. Davidson. 1981. Integration and expression of FeLV proviruses. In *Feline leukemia virus meeting* (ed. W.D. Hardy, Jr. et al.), pp. 373–380. Elsevier/North-Holland, New York. (In press.)

Nandi, S. and C. Helmich. 1974. Transmission of the mammary tumor virus by the GR mouse strain. II. Genetic studies. *J. Natl. Cancer Inst.* **52:**1567–1570.

Nandi, S. and C.M. McGrath. 1973. Mammary neoplasia in mice. *Adv. Cancer Res.* **17:**353–414.

Neiman, P.E. 1973a. Measurement of endogenous leukosis virus nucleotide sequences in the

DNA of normal avian embryos by RNA-DNA hybridization. *Virology* **53:** 196–204.
———. 1973b. Measurement of RD114 virus nucleotide sequences in feline cellular DNA. *Nat. New Biol.* **244:** 62–64.
———. 1978. Mapping by competitive hybridization of sequences which differ between endogenous and exogenous chicken leukosis viruses. *Virology* **85:** 9–16.
Neiman, P.E., S. Das, D. Macdonnell, and C. McMillin-Helsel. 1977. Organization of shared and unshared sequences in the genomes of chicken endogenous and sarcoma viruses. *Cell* **11:** 321–329.
Nowinski, R.C. and E.F. Hays. 1978. Oncogenicity of AKR endogenous leukemia viruses. *J. Virol.* **27:** 13–18.
Nusse, R., J. de Moes, J. Hilkens, and R. van Nie. 1980. Localization of a gene for expression of mouse mammary tumor virus antigens in the GR/MTV-2⁻ mouse strain. *J. Exp. Med.* **152:** 712–719.
O'Donnell, P.V., E. Stockert, Y. Obata, A.B. DeLeo, and L.J. Old. 1980. Murine-leukemia-virus-related cell-surface antigens as serological markers of AKR ecotropic, xenotropic, and dualtropic viruses. *Cold Spring Harbor Symp. Quant. Biol.* **44:** 1255.
Ono, M., M.D. Cole, A.T. White, and R.C.C. Huang. 1980. Sequence organization of cloned intracisternal A particle genes. *Cell* **21:** 465–473.
Orgel, L.E. and F.H.C. Crick. 1980. Selfish DNA: The ultimate parasite. *Nature* **284:** 604–607.
Oroszlan, S., M. Barbacid, T.D. Copeland, S.A. Aaronson, and R.V. Gilden. 1981. Chemical and immunological characterization of the major structural protein (p28) of MMC-1, a rhesus monkey endogenous type C virus: Homology with the major stuctural protein of avian reticuloendotheliosis virus. *J. Virol.* **39:** 845–854.
Pani, P.K. and L.N. Payne. 1973. Further evidence for two loci which control susceptibility of fowl to RSV(RAV-0). *J. Gen. Virol.* **19:** 235–244.
Paterson, B.M., S. Segal, K.K. Lueders, and E.L. Kuff. 1978. RNA associated with murine intracisternal type A particles codes for the main particle protein. *J. Virol.* **27:** 118–126.
Payne, L.N. and R.C. Chubb. 1968. Studies on the nature and genetic control of antigen in normal chick embryos which reacts in the COFAL test. *J. Gen. Virol.* **3:** 379–391.
Payne, L.N., P.K. Pani, and R.A. Weiss. 1971. A dominant epistatic gene which inhibits susceptibility to RSV(RAV-0). *J. Gen. Virol.* **13:** 455–462.
Pincus, T. 1980. The endogenous murine type C viruses. In *Molecular biology of RNA tumor viruses* (ed. J. Stephenson), pp. 77–130. Academic Press, New York.
Pincus, T., J.W. Hartley, and W.P. Rowe. 1971a. A major genetic locus affecting resistance to infection with murine leukemia viruses.I. Tissue culture studies of naturally occurring viruses. *J. Exp. Med.* **133:** 1219–1233.
Pincus, T., W.P. Rowe, and F. Lilly. 1971b. A major genetic locus affecting resistance to infection with murine leukemia viruses. II. Apparent identity to a major locus described for resistance to Friend murine leukemia virus. *J. Exp. Med.* **133:** 1234–1241.
Potter, M. 1978. Comments on the relationship of inbred strains to the genus *Mus*. In *Origins of inbred mice* (ed. H.C. Morse, III), pp. 497–509. Academic Press, New York.
Quint, W., W. Quax, H. van der Putten, and A. Berns. 1981. Characterization of AKR murine leukemia sequences in AKR mouse substrains and structure of integrated recombinant genomes in tumor tissues. *J. Virol.* **39:** 1–10.
Quintrell, N., H.E. Varmus, J.M. Bishop, M.O. Nicolson, and R.M. McAllister. 1974. Homologies among the nucleotide sequences of the genomes of C-type viruses. *Virology* **58:** 569–575.
Rascati, R.J. and R.W. Tennant. 1978. Induction of endogenous murine retrovirus by hydroxyurea and related compounds. *Virology* **87:** 208–211.
Razin, A. and A.D. Riggs. 1980. DNA methylation and gene function. *Science* **210:** 604–610.

Reed, C.L. and F. Rapp. 1976. Induction of murine p30 by superinfecting herpesviruses. *J. Virol.* **19:** 1028–1033.

Rettenmier, C.W. and H. Hanafusa. 1977. Structural protein markers in the avian oncoviruses. *J. Virol.* **24:**850–864.

Rice, N.R., T.I. Bonner, and R.V. Gilden. 1981. Nucleic acid homology between avian and mammalian Type C viruses: Relatedness of reticuloendotheliosis virus cDNA to cloned proviral DNA of the endogenous colobus virus CPC-1. *Virology* **114:** 286–290.

Riggs, A.D. 1975. X inactivation, differentiation, and DNA methylation. *Cytogenet. Cell Gen.* **14:**9–25.

Ringold, G.M. 1979. Glucocorticoid regulation of mouse mammary tumor virus gene expression. *Biochim. Biophys. Acta* **560:**487–508.

Ringold, G.M., P.B. Blair, J.M. Bishop, and H.E. Varmus. 1976. Nucleotide sequence homologies among mouse mammary tumor viruses. *Virology* **70:**550–553.

Robinson, H. 1978. Inheritance and expression of chicken genes that are related to avian leukosis sarcoma viruses. *Curr. Top. Microbiol. Immunol.* **83:** 1–36.

Robinson, H.L., R.E. Eisenman, A. Senior, and S. Ripley. 1979. Low frequency production of recombinant subgroup E avian leukosis virus by uninfected V-15_B chicken cells. *Virology* **99:**21–30.

Robinson, H.L., M.N. Pearson, P.N. Tsichlis, and J.M. Coffin. 1980a. Viral envelope antigens and C regions in nonacute disease associated with avian leukosis virus. In *Viruses in naturally occurring cancer* (ed. M. Essex et al.), pp. 543–551.

Robinson, H.L., C.A. Swanson, J.F. Hruska, and L.B. Crittenden. 1976. Production of unique C-type viruses by chicken cells grown in bromodeoxyuridine. *Virology* **69:**63–74.

Robinson, H.L., M.N. Pearson, D.W. DeSimone, P.N. Tsichlis, and J.M. Coffin. 1980b. Subgroup-E avian-leukosis-virus-associated disease in chickens. *Cold Spring Harbor Symp. Quant. Biol.* **44:** 1133–1142.

Rommelaere, J., D.V. Faller, and N. Hopkins. 1977. RNase T_1-resistant oligonucleotides of Akv-1 and Akv-2 type C viruses of AKR mice. *J. Virol.* **24:**690–694.

———. 1978. Characterization and mapping of RNase T_1-resistant oligonucleotides derived from the genomes of Akv and MCF murine leukemia viruses. *Proc. Natl. Acad. Sci.* **75:**495–499.

Rosenthal, P.N., H.L. Robinson, W.S. Robinson, T. Hanafusa, and H. Hanafusa. 1971. DNA in uninfected and virus-infected cells complementary to avian tumor virus RNA. *Proc. Natl. Acad. Sci.* **68:**2336–2340.

Rosner, M.R., J.-S. Tung, H. Hopkins, and P.W. Robbins. 1980. Relationship of G_{IX} antigen expression to glycosylation of murine leukemia virus glycoprotein. *Proc. Natl. Acad. Sci.* **77:**6420–6424.

Rowe, W.P. 1972. Studies of genetic transmission of murine leukemia virus by AKR mice. I. Crosses with FV-1^n strains of mice. *J. Exp. Med.* **136:** 1272–1285.

Rowe, W.P. and J.W. Hartley. 1972. Studies of genetic transmission of murine leukemia virus by AKR mice. II. Crosses with Fv-1^b strains of mice. *J. Exp. Med.* **136:** 1286–1301.

Rowe, W.P. and C.A. Kozak. 1980. Germ-line reinsertions of AKR murine leukemia virus genomes in Akv-1 congenic mice. *Proc. Natl. Acad. Sci.* **77:**4871–4874.

Rowe, W.P., M.W. Cloyd, and J.W. Hartley. 1980. The status of the association of MCF viruses with leukemogenesis. *Cold Spring Harbor Symp. Quant. Biol.* **44:** 1265–1268.

Rowe, W.P., J.W. Hartley, M.R. Lander, W.E. Pugh, and N. Teich. 1971. Noninfectious AKR mouse embryo cell lines in which each cell has the capacity to be activated to produce infectious murine leukemia virus. *Virology* **46:**866–876.

Scherr, C.J., M.M. Lieber, and G.J. Todaro. 1974. Mixed splenocyte cultures and graft versus host reaction selectivity induce an "S-tropic" murine type-C virus. *Cell* **1:**55–58.

Schlom, J., P. Horan-Hand, Y.A. Teramoto, R. Callahan, G. Todaro, and G. Schidlovsky.

1978. Characterization of a new virus from *Mus cervicolor* immunologically related to the mouse mammary tumor virus. *J. Natl. Cancer Inst.* **61:** 1509–1515.

Scolnick, E.M., R.J. Goldberg, and D. Williams. 1976. Characterization of rat genetic sequences of Kirsten sarcoma virus: Distinct class of endogenous rat type C viral sequence. *J. Virol.* **13:** 1211–1219.

Scolnick, E.M., W.C. Vass, R.S. Howk, and P.H. Duesberg. 1979. Defective retrovirus-like 30S RNA species of rat and mouse cells are infectious if packaged by type C helper virus. *J. Virol.* **29:** 964–972.

Shaikh, R., M. Linial, J. Coffin, and R. Eisenman. 1978. Recombinant avian oncoviruses. I. Alterations in the precursor to the internal structural proteins. *Virology* **87:** 326–338.

Shank, P.R., S.H. Hughes, and H.E. Varmus. 1981. Restriction endonuclease mapping of the DNA of Rous-associated virus 0 reveals extensive homology in structure and sequence with avian sarcoma virus DNA. *Virology* **108:** 177–188.

Shank, P.R., J..C. Cohen, H.E. Varmus, K.R. Yamamoto, and G.M. Ringold. 1978. Mapping of linear and circular forms of mouse mammary tumor virus DNA with restriction endonucleases: Evidence for a large specific deletion occurring at high frequency during circularization. *Proc. Natl. Acad. Sci.* **75:** 2112–2116.

Sherr, C.J., M.M. Lieber, R.E. Benveniste, and G.J. Todaro. 1974. Endogenous baboon type C virus (M7): Biochemical and immunologic characterization. *Virology* **58:** 492–503.

Sherwin, S. and G.J. Todaro. 1979. A new endogenous primate type C virus isolated from the Old World monkey *Colobus polykomos. Proc. Natl. Acad. Sci.* **76:** 5041–5045.

Sherwin, S.A., U.R. Rapp, R.E. Benveniste, A. Sen, and G. Todaro. 1978. Rescue of endogenous 30S retroviral sequences from mouse cells by baboon type C virus. *J. Virol.* **26:** 257–264.

Shoyab, M. and M.A. Baluda. 1976. Ribonucleotide sequence homology among avian oncornaviruses. *J. Virol.* **17:** 106–113.

Skalka, A., P. DeBona, F. Hishinuma, and W. McClements. 1980. Avian endogenous proviral DNA: Analysis of integrated *ev* 1 and a related gs^- chf^- provirus purified by molecular cloning. *Cold Spring Harbor Symp. Quant. Biol.* **44:** 1097–1104.

Smith, E.J. and L.B. Crittenden. 1981. Segregation of chicken endogenous viral loci *ev*-7 and *ev*-12 with the expression of infectious subgroup E avian leukosis virus. *Virology* **112:** 370–374.

Southern, E.M. 1975. Detection of specific sequences among DNA fragments separated by gel electrophoresis. *J. Mol. Biol.* **98:** 503–517.

Stallcup, M.R., J.C. Ring, D.S. Ucker, and K.R. Yamamoto. 1979. Mammary tumor virus genes: Probes for mechanisms of transcriptional regulation. *Cold Spring Harbor Conf. Cell Proliferation* **6:** 919–936.

Steeves, R. and F. Lilly. 1977. Interactions between host and viral genomes in mouse leukemia. *Annu. Rev. Genet.* **11:** 277–296.

Steffen, D. and R.A. Weinberg. 1978. The integrated genome of murine leukemia virus. *Cell* **15:** 1003–1010.

Steffen, D.L., S. Bird, and R.A. Weinberg. 1980. Evidence for the Asiatic origin of endogenous AKR-type murine leukemia proviruses. *J. Virol.* **35:** 824–835.

Steffen, D.L., S. Bird, W.P. Rowe, and R.A. Weinberg. 1979. Identification of DNA fragments carrying ecotropic proviruses of AKR mice. *Proc. Natl. Acad. Sci.* **76:** 4554–4558.

Stephenson, J.R. and S.A. Aaronson. 1972. A genetic locus for inducibility of C-type virus in BALB/c cells: The effect of a nonlinked regulatory gene on detection of virus after chemical activation. *Proc. Natl. Acad. Sci.* **69:** 2798–2801.

———. 1974. Demonstration of a genetic factor influencing release of a xenotropic virus of mouse cells. *Proc. Natl. Acad. Sci.* **71:** 4925–4929.

Stephenson, J.R., S.R. Tronick, R.K. Reynolds, and S.A. Aaronson. 1974. Isolation and characterization of C-type viral gene products of virus-negative mouse cells. *J. Exp. Med.* **139:**427–438.

Stockert, E., L.J. Old, and E.A. Boyse. 1971. The G_{IX} system. A cell surface allo-antigen associated with murine leukemia virus; implications regarding chromosomal integration of the viral genome. *J. Exp. Med.* **133:**1334–1355.

Stuhlman, H., D. Jähner, and R. Jaenisch. 1981. Infectivity and methylation of retroviral genomes is correlated with expression in the animal. *Cell* **26:** 221–232.

Taylor, B.A., H. Meier, and D.D. Myers. 1971. Host-gene control of C-type RNA tumor virus: Inheritance of the group-specific antigen of murine leukemia virus. *Proc. Natl. Acad. Sci.* **68:**3190–3194.

Teich, N., D.R. Lowy, J.W. Hartley, and W.P. Rowe. 1973. Studies of the mechanism of induction of infectious murine leukemia virus from AKR mouse embryo cell lines by 5-iododeoxyuridine and 5-bromodeoxyuridine. *Virology* **51:**163–173.

Temin, H.M. 1964. Homology between RNA from Rous sarcoma virus and DNA from Rous sarcoma virus-infected cells. *Proc. Natl. Acad. Sci.* **52:**323–329.

———. 1980. Origin of retroviruses from cellular moveable genetic elements. Cell **21:** 599–600.

Tennant, R.W. and R.J. Rascati. 1980. Mechanisms of cocarcinogenesis involving endogenous retroviruses. In *Modifiers of chemical carcinogenesis* (ed. T.J. Slaga), vol. 5, pp. 185–205. Raven Press, New York.

Teramoto, Y.A., P. Horan-Hand, R. Callahan, and J. Schlom. 1980a. Detection of novel murine mammary tumor viruses by interspecies immunoassays. *J. Natl. Cancer Inst.* **64:**967–975.

Teramoto, Y.A., D. Medina, C. McGrath, and J. Schlom. 1980b. Noncoordinate expression of murine mammary tumor virus gene products. *Virology* **107:**345–353.

Tereba, T.A. and S.M. Astrin. 1980. Chromosomal localization of *ev*-1, a frequently occurring endogenous retrovirus locus in White Leghorn chickens, by in situ hybridization. *J. Virol.* **35:**888–894.

Tereba, A., L. Skoog, and P.K. Vogt. 1975. RNA tumor virus specific sequences in nuclear DNA of several avian species. *Virology* **65:**524–534.

Todaro, G. 1980. Interspecies transmission of mammalian retroviruses. In *Molecular biology of RNA tumor viruses* (ed. J. Stephenson), pp. 46–76. Academic Press, New York.

Todaro, G.J., S.S. Tevethia, and J.L. Melnick. 1973. Isolation of an RD-114 related cat type-C virus from feline sarcoma virus-transformed baboon cells. *Intervirology* **1:** 399–404.

Todaro, G.J., R.E. Benveniste, S.A. Sherwin, and C.J. Sherr. 1978a. MAC-1, a new genetically transmitted type C virus of primates: "Low frequency" activation from stumptail monkey cell cultures. *Cell* **13:**775–782.

Todaro, G.J., R.E. Benveniste, C.J. Sherr, J. Schlom, G. Schidlovsky, and J.R. Stephenson. 1978b. Isolation and characterization of a new type D retrovirus from the Asian primate, *Presbytis obscurus* (spectacled langur). *Virology* **84:**189–194.

Tooze, J., ed. 1973. *The molecular biology of tumor viruses.* Cold Spring Harbor Laboratory, Cold Spring Harbor, New York.

Tsichlis, P.N. and J.M. Coffin. 1979. Recombination between the defective component of an acute leukemia virus and Rous associated virus an endogenous virus of chickens. *Proc. Natl. Acad. Sci.* **76:**3001–3005.

———. 1980a. Recombinants between endogenous and exogenous avian tumor viruses: Role of the C region and other portions of the genome in the control of replication and transformation. *J. Virol.* **33:**238–249.

———. 1980b. Role of the *C* region in relative growth rates of endogenous and exogenous avian oncoviruses. *Cold Spring Harbor Symp. Quant. Biol.* **44:**1123–1132.

van der Ploeg, L.H.T. and R.A. Flavell. 1980. DNA methylation in the human β globin locus in erythroid and nonerythroid tissues. *Cell* **19:** 947–958.

van der Putten, H., W. Quint, J. Van Raaij, E.R. Maandag, I.M. Verma, and A. Berns. 1981. M-MLV-induced leukemogenesis: Integration and structure of recombinant proviruses in tumors. *Cell* **24:** 729–739.

van Nie, R. and J. de Moes. 1977. Development of a congenic line of the GR mouse strain without early mammary tumours. *Int. J. Cancer* **20:** 588–594.

van Nie, R. and J. Hilgers. 1976. Genetic analysis of mammary tumor induction and expression of mammary tumor virus antigen in hormone-treated ovariectomized GR mice. *J. Natl. Cancer Inst.* **56:** 27–32.

van Nie, R. and A.A. Verstraeten. 1975. Studies of genetic transmission of mammary tumor virus by C3Hf mice. *Int. J. Cancer* **16:** 922–931.

van Nie, R., A.A. Verstraeten, and J. de Moes. 1977. Genetic transmission of mammary tumour virus by GR mice. *Int. J. Cancer* **19:** 383–390.

Varmus, H.E., G. Ringold, and K.R. Yamamoto. 1979. Regulation of mouse mammary tumor virus gene expression by glucocorticoid hormones. In *Glucocorticoid hormone action* (ed. J. Baxter and G. Rousseau) p. 253–278. Spring-Verlag, Berlin..

Varmus, H.E., J.M. Bishop, R.C. Nowinski, and N.H. Sarkar. 1972a. Mammary tumour virus specific nucleotide sequences in mouse DNA. *Nat. New Biol.* **238:** 189–191.

Varmus, H.E., R.A. Weiss, R.R. Friis, W. Levinson, and J.M. Bishop. 1972b. Detection of avian tumor virus-specific nucleotide sequences in avian cell DNAs. *Proc. Natl. Acad. Sci.* **69:** 20–24.

Verstraeten, A.A. and R. van Nie. 1978. Genetic transmission of mammary tumour virus in the DBAF mouse strain. *Int. J. Cancer* **21:** 473–475.

Vogt, P.K. 1967. A virus released by "non producing" Rous sarcoma cells. *Proc. Natl. Acad. Sci.* **58:** 801–808.

Vogt, P.K. and R.R. Friis. 1971. An avian leukosis virus related to RSV(0). Properties and evidence for helper activity. *Virology* **43:** 223–234.

Waalwijk, C. and R.A. Flavell. 1978. DNA methylation at a CCGG sequence in the large intron of the rabbit β globin gene: Tissue-specific variations. *Nucleic Acids Res.* **5:** 4631–4641.

Wang, S.Y., W.S. Hayward, and H. Hanafusa. 1977. Genetic variation in the RNA transcripts of endogenous virus genes in uninfected chicken cells. *J. Virol.* **24:** 64–73.

Weinberg, R.A. 1980. Origins and roles of endogenous retroviruses. *Cell* **22:** 643–644.

Weintraub, H. and M. Groudine. 1976. Chromosomal subunits in active genes have an altered conformation. *Science* **193:** 848–856.

Weiss, R.. 1967. Spontaneous virus production from "non-virus producing" Rous sarcoma cells. *Virology* **32:** 719–723.

———. 1969. The host range of Bryan strain Rous sarcoma virus synthesized in the absence of helper virus. *J. Gen. Virol.* **5:** 511–528.

———. 1973. Some interactions between endogenous and exogenous avian RNA tumor viruses. In *Virus research* (eds. C.F. Fox and W.S. Ribonson), pp. 447–454. Academic Press, New York.

Weiss, R.A. and P.M. Biggs. 1972. Leukosis and Marek's disease viruses of feral red jungle fowl and domestic fowl in Malaya. *J. Natl. Cancer Inst.* **49:** 1713–1725.

Weiss, R.A. and L.N. Payne. 1971. The heritable nature of the factor in chicken cells which acts as a helper virus for Rous sarcoma virus. *Virology* **45:** 508–515.

Weiss, R.A., D. Boettiger, and D.N. Love. 1975. Phenotypic mixing between vesicular stomatitis virus and avian RNA tumor viruses. *Cold Spring Harbor Symp. Quant. Biol.* **39:** 913–918.

Weiss, R.A., W.S. Mason, and P.K. Vogt. 1973. Genetic recombinants and heterozygotes derived from endogenous and exogenous avian RNA tumor viruses. *Virology* **52:** 535–552.

Weiss, R.A., R.R. Friis, E. Katz, and P.K. Vogt. 1971. Induction of avian tumor viruses in normal cells by physical and chemical carcinogens. *Virology* **46:**920–938.
Wilson, D.E. and H. Bauer. 1967. Hybridization of avian myeloblastosis virus RNA with DNA from chick embryo cells. *Virology* **33:**754–757.
Wilson, S.H. and E.L. Kuff. 1972. A novel DNA polymerase activity found in association with intracisternal A-type particles. *Proc. Natl. Acad. Sci.* **69:**1531–1536.
Wong-Staal, F., M.S. Reitz, Jr., C.D. Trainor, and R.C. Gallo. 1975. Murine intracisternal type A particles: A biochemical characterization. J. Virol. **16:**887–896.
Young, H.A., M.L. Wenk, D.G. Goodman, and E.M. Scolnick. 1978. Expression of RNA of an endogenous replication defective retrovirus in rat mammary adenocarcinomas induced by 7, 12-dimethylbenz(*a*)anthracene. *J. Natl. Cancer Inst.* **61:**1329–1337.
Young, H.A., M.A. Gonda, D. De Feo, R.W. Ellis, K. Nagashima, and E.M. Scolnick. 1980. Heteroduplex analysis of cloned rat endogenous replication-defective (30 S) retrovirus and Harvey murine sarcoma virus. *Virology* **107:**89–99.

11

The Search for Human RNA Tumor Viruses

I. INTRODUCTION

With the realization that retrovirus infections are widespread among vertebrate hosts, including some primate species, the search for human retroviruses has not been thwarted through lack of effort. Throughout the 1960s and 1970s, numerous claims have been made for evidence of human retrovirus infection; some proved to involve genuine retroviruses but not human, others were not upheld by more detailed investigation, and still others remain enigmatic as to the provenance of the viruses. At this time, however, it would appear that at least two distinct retroviruses occur as natural infections of human populations. One is a foamy virus (see Chapter 2) with no known associated disease. The other is a C-type oncovirus associated with certain forms of adult T-cell leukemia and lymphoma (see Section V).

A. Epidemiology

Epidemiological studies have not been very helpful in allocating an infectious etiology to human tumors. With most infectious diseases, the transmissible nature of the illness had been obvious before the particular agent was discovered. There have been reports of remarkable clusters in the incidence of children's leukemia and of Hodgkin's disease suggestive of infective transmission (Heath and Hasterlik 1963; Vianna et al. 1971; Dworsky and Henderson 1974; Schimpff et al. 1975), but these studies have been criticized methodologically (Smith and Pike 1976; Mack 1980) and have not been upheld by case-control studies (Alderson and Nayak 1971; Kryscio et al. 1973; P.G. Smith et al. 1977; Alderson 1980). Recent epidemiological evidence of an endemic area in Japan (Uchiyama et al. 1977; Tajima et al. 1979; The T- and B-Cell Malignancy Study Group 1981) for adult T-cell leukemia associated with the retrovirus mentioned above is discussed in Section V.B.

Where tumors are clearly contagious, such as benign warts transmitted by papilloma viruses, the virus etiology of the disease is relatively easy to identify. Where the latent period between infection and presentation of the disease is prolonged, perhaps to a major portion of the natural human life span, identification of the etiological agent is more difficult; for example, the sporadic incidence of shingles would not betray its infectious etiology from epidemiological studies alone. There is a possibility, then, that some forms of human malignant disease which are not apparently clustered might nevertheless be a rare consequence of a widespread, ubiquitous infection. If this were the case, identification of the agent as a causative factor would be more difficult. Even where clustering occurs, as in Burkitt's lymphoma and nasopharyngeal carcinoma, it is easier to identify etiological cofactors (malaria and HLA-type, respectively) than it is to establish the associated virus (Epstein-Barr virus [EBV]) as the principal causative agent. EBV was first identified by electron microscopy of cultured Burkitt lymphoma cells (Epstein et al. 1964) before any seroepidemiological studies were feasible (de Thé 1979). For these reasons, virologists and oncologists have tended to seek evidence for latent retrovirus infection in human tumors without necessarily adducing an infectious etiology first.

B. Virology

Much effort has been placed in the search for human retroviruses in leukemias, lymphomas, and breast cancer because of animal retrovirus models and in pediatric tumors generally because the necessarily shorter period between putative infection and disease might favor a virus etiology rather than other environmental agents. Retroviruses have also been sought in human "autoimmune" diseases because of their association with similar diseases in animals (see Chapter 8), but apart from a possible association with systemic lupus erythematosus (SLE), there is no indication so far of retrovirus involvement.

The major naturally occurring retrovirus diseases of animals are caused by exogenous viruses presenting as endemic or epidemic infections. The viruses may be transmitted horizontally or congenitally, and infection is typically more widespread in the affected population than is the incidence of disease. The tumor cells do not always produce progeny virus, e.g., avian and feline lymphoma (Chapter 8), which should warn us that in humans the tumor tissue may not be the most appropriate for virus isolation. Except in specially selected inbred strains of mice, endogenous viruses do not appear to play an etiological role in naturally occurring malignant disease, although they may be more readily expressed in tumor cells than in normal tissues. An inducible, endogenous retroviral genome has yet to be demonstrated in human cells, but that is not to say that *Homo sapiens* does not harbor such a virus.

Since the vast majority of human tumor cells do not release viral particles, even on prolonged culture in vitro, most investigators have looked for evidence of latent infection using biochemical or immunological probes. But much effort has also been made to rescue infectious retroviruses from human cells and tissues.

Many pitfalls have been encountered in the search for human retroviruses, the major ones being undue enthusiasm over preliminary data and misplaced credulity about the human provenance of virus isolates. Some of the spurious leads will be mentioned here as exemplary fables. Unfortunately, many virologists have become so inured to premature claims for the discovery of yet another human tumor virus that one wit has labeled them "human rumor viruses." It is important, therefore, to ensure that genuinely intriguing evidence receives the critical attention it deserves.

In this chapter we survey briefly the methods used for detecting retroviruses in human tissues before citing a few well-known examples of false leads. Some unsolved problems of human retrovirology are then reviewed, followed by an account of the recent evidence for a human T-cell lymphoma virus. Finally, we discuss the potential for harnessing the molecular genetics of experimental retroviruses to the investigation of nonviral human tumors.

II. METHODOLOGICAL APPROACHES TO THE DETECTION OF HUMAN RETROVIRUSES

A. Electron Microscopy

Viruslike particles have been observed by electron microscopy in thin sections of normal or malignant tissues in vivo, in human tumor cells in culture, and in pelleted preparations of plasma, milk, urine, and ascitic or pleural effusion fluids. Several studies in the 1960s suggested the presence of particles resembling C-type viruses in human leukemic cells and plasma (Burger et al. 1964; Dmochowski et al. 1967; Levine et al. 1967; Seman and Seman 1968) and in urine of leukemic patients (Ames et al. 1966). Similar particles have also been observed in sections of prostatic cancer (Dmochowski and Horoszewicz 1976; Ohtsuki et al. 1977), normal embryonic tissue (Chandra et al. 1970), and in cultures of sarcoma (Morton et al. 1969) and melanoma (Parsons et al. 1974). Particles resembling B-type mouse mammary tumor virus (MMTV) were observed by negative staining in human milk extracts (Feller and Chopra 1969, 1971; Moore et al. 1969, 1971; Schlom et al. 1971, 1972a; Sarkar and Moore 1972) and in thin sections of normal mammary cells in culture (Furmanski et al. 1974). It has been difficult to interpret the appearance of these particles accurately, and their viral nature has therefore been questioned (Arnoult and Haguenau 1966; Prince and Adams 1966; Newell et al. 1968; Calafat and Hageman 1973; Dalton 1975). The most distinctive virion forms are budding particles at the plasma membrane, and these are seldom detected except in cells producing large amounts of virus. Although clear sections through budding particles are diagnostic, the technique is not sensitive, and it will not reveal latent infection where there is no virion maturation.

The observation that C-type particles are frequently seen in the baboon placenta (Kalter et al. 1973a) led to a detailed and exhaustive examination of thin sections of human placentas by Kalter and other investigators. This analysis revealed the presence of complete and budding viruslike particles from occasional cells in a significant proportion of full-term placentas (Kalter et al. 1973b; Dalton et al. 1974; Vernon et al. 1974; Dirksen and Levy 1977). Placental viruslike particles appear to be expressed no more frequently in patients with SLE than in women with normal pregnancies (Imamura et al. 1976; Dirksen and Levy 1977). Infectious virus has not been isolated from placentas and the significance of the particles is not clear. Further evidence for placental retrovirus expression and its possible association with SLE is discussed in a later section.

Electron microscopy has been widely used to confirm the morphology of retroviruses of putative human origin identified by other techniques, e.g., the HeLa virus (Gelderblom et al. 1974b) or HL23V (Hall and Schidlovsky 1976), and viruses secondarily propagated in nonhuman cells. Electron microscopy provided convincing evidence that viruses such as RD114, ESP-1 and HeLa particles were retroviruses (see Section III below), but the technique cannot distinguish human viruses from animal viruses.

B. Reverse Transcriptase Activity and Viruslike RNA Complexes

Since the vast majority of human tumor cells do not release viral particles, most investigators have searched for biochemical markers of latent infection. With the discovery of reverse transcriptase as a unique retroviral enzyme that can be sensitively assayed, much effort was placed on detecting this enzyme activity in human tumor cells resembling the kinds induced by retroviruses in animals, especially leukemias, lymphomas, and mammary tumors. Several reports were published of reverse transcriptase activity in extracts of human tumor cells (Gallo et al. 1970, 1971; Kiessling et al. 1971; Axel et al. 1972a; Baxt et al. 1972; Sarngadharan et al. 1972; Sawada et al. 1977; Sadamori et al. 1981) and under the preleukemic conditions, thrombocythemia (Brodsky et al. 1975), polycythemia vera (Weimann et al. 1975), and myelofibrosis (Steel et al. 1977). In the early reports, many laboratories used experimental template-primer complexes that did not adequately distinguish viral enzyme activity from that of cellular-DNA-dependent DNA polymerases and terminal deoxynucleotidyl transferase (Coleman et al. 1974; B.J. Lewis et al. 1974; McCaffrey et al. 1975; Sarin et al. 1976). Todaro and Gallo (1973), however, claimed that the DNA polymerase activity detected in human acute leukemia cells was immunologically related to reverse transcriptase activity of murine and primate retroviruses.

Subsequently, purified or partially purified polymerases have been prepared that appear to possess biochemical and immunological properties akin to those of primate viral reverse transcriptases. Reverse transcriptase activity has been reported in acute leukemia (Gallagher et al. 1974; Mondal et al. 1975; Witkin et al. 1975) chronic leukemia (Van Muyen et al. 1979), myelofibrosis (Steel et al. 1977), breast carcinoma (Axel et al. 1972a; Gerwin et al. 1973; Ohno et al. 1977), and melanoma and other skin tumors (Balda et al. 1975; Chandra et al. 1978, 1980). Nelson et al. (1978) detected reverse transcriptase activity in normal human placentas, which, as mentioned above, produce occasional particles resembling retroviruses as visualized by electron microscopy.

The reverse transcriptase of retroviruses cannot usually be detected in an enzymically active form until it is proteolytically cleaved from an inactive precursor during packaging into virions (see Chapter 6). One might not therefore expect to detect significant levels of enzyme activity in the absence of viral particles, and indeed a majority of the reports of reverse transcriptase activity in human tumor cells or secretions detected the enzyme in a "particulate" fraction. Schlom and Spiegelman (1971) devised an assay called the simultaneous detection test, which was employed to reveal both the enzyme and the product of its activity in human cells associated with a high-molecular-weight RNA template. This RNA apparently resembled the 70S RNA of retroviral genomes. Positive results with the simultaneous detection test were soon reported by Spiegelman's group and others for a wide variety of human neoplastic cells, including leukemia (Baxt et al. 1972; Gallo et al. 1973; Yaniv et al. 1973), lymphoma (Hehlmann et al. 1972; Kufe et al. 1973; Spiegelman et al. 1973; Chezzi et al. 1976), breast carcinoma (Axel et al. 1972a; Schlom et al. 1972b; Spiegelman et al. 1972; Viola 1973; Michalides et al. 1975), melanoma (Parsons et al. 1974), skin carcinoma (Balda et al. 1975), and lung, gastric, and brain tumors (Cuatico et al. 1973, 1974). Despite the great interest aroused by these reports, in most cases the observations have not been confirmed or further characterized in subsequent studies.

C. Viral Antigens

Although viral RNA and reverse transcriptase are minor components of virions, one would expect much larger amounts of p30 and gp70 to be synthesized in human cells infected with retroviruses. Furthermore, p30 and gp70 or their precursors are frequently expressed in animal retrovirus systems that do not produce complete virions. Provided there was immunological cross-reaction with antibodies to animal retroviral proteins, these antibodies should be useful probes for detecting latent retrovirus infection in human cells. Although numerous papers have reported striking findings of cross-reacting materials, particularly in leukemia and mammary carcinoma, the excitement generated over the human "viral" antigens by and large has not survived their extraction, purification, and characterization (Gardner et al. 1977).

Using antibodies to Rauscher murine leukemia virus (Ra-MLV) and feline RD114 virus, Strand and August (1974b) found cross-reacting antigens by radioimmunoassay in a variety of normal and malignant human tissues, especially in SLE patients. Sherr and Todaro (1974) found antigens in various human tumors related to those of baboon endogenous virus (BaEV) p30, Mellors and Mellors (1976) found a similar antigen in the renal glomeruli of SLE patients, and H. S. Smith et al. (1977) detected a related antigen in a human sarcoma cell line. BaEV and RD114 are antigenically related but do not share many interspecies antigens with the murine and gibbon ape leukemia virus–simian sarcoma-associated virus (GALV-SSAV) groups (Strand and August 1974a). Antigens related to SSAV were also reported. Sherr and Todaro (1975) detected by radioimmunoassay high titers of p30-related antigens in leukocytes of five acute leukemia patients, and Derks et al. (1982) detected a similar antigen in leukemic cells of one patient with chronic myeloid leukemia. Zurcher et al. (1975) used immunofluorescence to detect SSAV-related antigens in cells from bone tumors, and Sawyer et al. (1978) observed a cell-surface antigen akin to gp70 in human placental tissue. Metzgar et al. (1976) detected on leukemic cells membrane antigens that cross-reacted with goat antiserum to purified Friend virus gp70. Adsorption studies indicated that the antigen may also be expressed on normal neutrophils and platelets. Lewis et al. (1974) found a membrane antigen cross-reacting with MLV gp70 on SLE lymphocytes.

Although Strand and August (1974b) and Sherr and Todaro (1974) observed that the human competitor antigens in radioimmunoassays appeared to be proteins with molecular weights of approximately 30,000, in none of the reports was the human antigen thoroughly purified and characterized. Considerable doubt remains as to whether the cross-reactivity was caused by antibodies in the antisera which recognized heterophile antigens. In converse studies, where human antibodies reacting with animal retroviral antigens were detected, this proved eventually to be the case (see Section II.F). Snyder and Fox (1978) have shown that C-type viruses propagated in cell cultures bind or incorporate a fetal serum antigen, which may be carried over in virion purification and may act as a contaminating immunogen when antibodies to "purified" viral antigens are prepared.

Some human cells in which SSAV- or BaEV-related antigens were detected produced complete, infectious virions either spontaneously or following treatment with inducing agents (see Section IV.B). Antigens in human breast carcinoma related to MMTV core and gp52 antigens (Mesa-Tejada et al. 1978; Ohno et al. 1979; Dion et al. 1980) and to Mason-Pfizer monkey virus (MPMV) reverse transcriptase (Ohno and Spiegelman 1977) have also been reported and are discussed in Section IV.A.

D. Nucleic Acid Homology

If humans harbor retroviruses related to those of animal hosts, one should expect to detect them by nucleic acid hybridization methods using animal viral probes. Although normal human DNA, in common with other mammalian DNAs, has conserved cellular genes homologous to viral *onc* genes (Wong-Staal et al. 1981a; Chapter 9), human DNA and RNA do not appear to contain sequences that have substantial homology with animal B-type, C-type, or D-type viruses (Bishop et al. 1974; Gardner et al. 1977; Todaro et al. 1978; Moore et al. 1979; Gallo and Wong-Staal 1980). However, sequences very distantly related to BaEV have been detected in human DNA (Benveniste and Todaro 1976; Wong-Staal et al. 1976; Donehower et al. 1977). An interesting recent report describes the identification and molecular cloning of sequences resembling endogenous retroviral genomes in human DNA (Martin et al. 1981). A sequence extending for nearly 5 kb in African green monkey DNA was identified that had homology with both ecotropic AKR MLV and BaEV. A clone of this monkey DNA sequence was, in turn, used to identify and clone the sequences in normal human DNA, which did not themselves show homology with MLV. These sequences are possibly the same as those showing distant relatedness to BaEV.

Since there is no evidence for endogenous human DNA sequences that have significant homology with known animal viral genomes, the presence of such sequences in tumor tissue should be indicative of retrovirus infection. Early reports of viruslike DNA in human leukemia cells (Baxt and Spiegelman 1972) and mammary carcinoma (Axel et al. 1972b; Vaidya et al. 1974) have not been generally upheld. The probes used may have been contaminated with cDNA of ribosomal RNA; however, this cannot explain the claim that such sequences were present in leukocytes from leukemic patients but not from normal case controls (Baxt and Spiegelman 1972; Baxt et al. 1973). Hybridization of human tumor DNA to simian or murine retroviral probes has been reported in sporadic cases, especially leukemias (Wong-Staal et al. 1976; Reitz et al. 1976; Aulakh and Gallo 1977; Prochownik and Kirsten 1977; Nicolson et al. 1978). Where simian sarcoma virus (SSV) sequences were present in a simian sarcoma virus/simian sarcoma-associated virus (SSV/SSAV) probe, one would expect hybridization to normal and neoplastic human DNA, because the *sis* gene of cellular origin (Chapter 9) is widely conserved among mammalian species, including *H. sapiens* (Wong-Staal et al. 1981a,b).

The lack of convincing evidence of proviral sequences in human tumor cell lines purportedly associated with retrovirus infection had led many critics to question all the evidence for other virus components found in human tissues. Recent evidence from animal systems, however, suggests that the cell clone that eventually becomes a malignant tumor following leukemia virus infection might carry defective genomes, as in gibbons (Wong-Staal et al. 1979) and chickens (Payne et al. 1981), or no detectable virus information at all, as in some feline leukemias (Hardy et al. 1980) (Chapter 8). The availability of molecularly cloned probes to animal retroviruses should aid definitive studies as to whether related sequences are found in human tumor DNA.

E. Rescue and Activation of Retroviral Particles

Many laboratories have reported the production of infectious retroviruses from human cells in sufficient titers to permit detailed characterization. Some proved to be animal retroviruses that had contaminated human cell lines, and three examples are described in Section III. Several investigators have isolated viruses related to the GALV-SSAV and BaEV primate virus groups (Gallagher and Gallo 1975; Nooter et al. 1975; Panem et al. 1975; Teich et al. 1975). Similar particles have been observed in leukemic and preleukemic bone marrow (Mak et al. 1974, 1975; Vosika et al. 1975), in a histiocytic lymphoma cell line (Kaplan et al. 1977; Goodenow and Kaplan 1979), and in an adenocarcinoma cell line (Balabanova et al. 1975), but these have not been successfully serially transmitted as infectious particles to experimental cells in culture. Whether these simian-related viruses represent natural human infections remains controversial, and their properties are discussed in more detail in Section IV.B.

Two isolates of C-type viruses from solid tumors transformed normal cells in vitro (Balabanova et al. 1975; Cook et al. 1978), and cell-free extracts of human osteosarcomas were reported to induce osteosarcomas in hamsters (Finkel et al. 1968; Pritchard et al. 1971). Further reports on these potentially exciting agents have not been forthcoming.

Cocultivation of human tumor cells with "indicator" cell lines has been widely used in attempts to rescue retroviruses believed to be latent in human cells. Cocultivation may seem to be an unnecessarily complicated method of rescuing latent viruses from human cells, because it might lead to recombination of putative human viral genomes with viral genes in the indicator cells. However, it should be remembered that long-term cocultivation has proved sensitive for the rescue from animal cells of endogenous viruses that are otherwise very difficult to isolate (Weiss et al. 1971; Todaro et al. 1978). Keydar et al. (1973) reported the production of virus by embryonic cells cocultivated with breast tumor cells or "infected" with milk from breast cancer patients, but this "virus" has not been further characterized. Gabelman et al. (1975) observed C-type particles after cocultivation of human carcinoma cells derived from a patient with concurrent chronic lymphocytic leukemia with rat XC cells (which contain Rous sarcoma virus [RSV]), but this virus too has not been maintained by passage and probably represents an endogenous rat virus activated in the XC cells. Further viruses were isolated by Nooter et al. (1977, 1978) following cocultivation of human leukemic bone marrow with nonproducer cells containing murine sarcoma virus (MSV). Karpas (1978) described particles that may resemble A particles in a human lymphoblastoid culture from a patient with T-cell leukemia and observed (Karpas et al. 1978) that normal bone-marrow cells become transformed by cocultivation with the lymphoblastoid cells. The cells are apparently negative for EBV nuclear antigen, but evidence is lacking that this transformation system is related to a retrovirus. Miyoshi et al. (1981) also claim that the T-cell lymphoma virus (described in Section V) transforms umbilical-cord leukocytes on cocultivation with lymphoma cells.

With the discovery that latent endogenous virus genomes can be rescued in infectious form by inducing agents (Lowy et al. 1971; Weiss et al. 1971) (see Chapter 10), much effort has been placed—with disappointing results overall—in attempts to activate retroviruses from human cells (Klucis et al. 1976; Stephenson and Aaronson 1976; Gardner et al. 1977; G.J. Todaro, pers. comm.). Numerous human tumor cultures, cell lines, and normal fibroblast strains have been treated with the halogenated pyrimidines, iododeoxyuridine (IdU) and bromodeoxyuridine (BrdU), as activating agents. Holder et al. (1974) activated retrovirus production in a human line HBT-3 with IdU and testosterone; the cell is probably a HeLa variant and the virus, a HeLa virus (see section III.C). Prochownik et al. (1979) induced virus production in HEL-12 human embryonic fibroblasts with IdU, but this cell strain spontaneously produces virus at higher passage (Panem et al. 1977) (see Section IV.B). Bronson et al. (1978, 1979) and Kurth et al. (1980) have used IdU to induce C-type viral particles from human teratocarcinoma cell lines Tera-1 and GH; these particles were not infectious for other cell lines. Arginine deprivation has been used as an inducer of virus in human lymphoblastoid cells by Kotler et al. (1973, 1975, 1977, 1979). One of the lymphoma lines, P3HR-1, also produces C-type particles spontaneously (Kotler et al. 1979; Yaniv et al. 1980). With the recent discovery that endogenous viruses can be efficiently activated by inhibitors of DNA methylation (Groudine et al. 1981), we may expect renewed efforts to activate putative latent human retroviruses.

F. Serological Studies of Human Patients and Populations

Virus infections in host populations are customarily monitored by seroepidemiological studies on antiviral antibodies. Infections of primates with exogenous retroviruses are no exception (Kawakami et al. 1973; Fine et al. 1978). One would therefore expect the examination of human sera for antibodies specific to putative human retroviruses to be a sensitive method for detecting evidence of infection. However, human serological studies have been fraught with difficulties and misleading results. Rigorous seroepidemiological evidence linking a retrovirus to the type of human tumor from which it was isolated will be important in establishing its etiological role. To date, this evidence has been wanting, although the recent serological evidence for human T-cell lymphoma virus infection (Hinuma et al. 1981; Kalyanaraman et al. 1981a; Posner et al. 1981) is beginning to look convincing (see Section V).

Several studies have been made to determine whether human sera contain antibodies reacting specifically with antigens of animal retroviruses. Reports of human antibodies reacting with MMTV are cited in Section IV.A. Radioimmunoassays using purified *gag* or *env* antigens of murine, feline, and simian C-type retroviruses were generally negative (Charman et al. 1974, 1977;

Stephenson and Aaronson 1976; Krakower and Aaronson 1978). However, other studies employing immunoelectron microscopy (Aoki et al. 1976), enzyme-linked assays (Mellors and Mellors 1978), or sensitive radioimmunoprecipitation methods for virions (Snyder et al. 1976; Louie et al. 1976; Kurth et al. 1977, 1979a; Kurth and Mikschy 1978; Ebbesen et al. 1979; Herbrink et al. 1980) have demonstrated the presence of low-titer antibodies reacting with envelope antigens of simian C-type retroviruses. The positive radioimmunoprecipitation studies were controversial because they could not be repeated in all laboratories. Some of the activity was accounted for by the presence of natural human antibodies to fetal calf serum antigens present on the surfaces of culture-propagated viruses, but apparently specific antivirus activity, particularly to the GALV-SSAV and BaEV groups, remained (Kurth et al. 1977; Snyder and Fox 1978). Subsequent studies have resolved the controversy (Barbacid et al. 1980a; Snyder and Fleissner 1980; Löwer et al. 1981): There is general agreement that naturally occurring human antibodies do indeed precipitate gp70 of simian retroviruses, but the antigens recognized are hitherto unidentified heterophile carbohydrate moieties incorporated into the glycosylated gp70 molecules. The carbohydrate antigens are not unique to retroviral gp70; their presence depends on the cell type in which the virus was propagated as well as on the strain of retrovirus.

The demonstration that anti-gp70 specificities in human antisera were not unique to retroviruses suggests that a retrovirus was probably not the initiating immunogen, and therefore these antibodies are not an indicator of human infection. This interpretation is consistent with the findings that such antibodies are ubiquitous in human populations (Löwer et al. 1981). However, there are indications that the titer of the antibodies reacting to simian gp70s is positively correlated with Hodgkin's disease (Ebbesen et al. 1979), acute myelogenous leukemia (Tóth et al. 1980), and testicular teratocarcinoma (Kurth et al. 1980), with pregnancy (Hirsch et al. 1978), and with laboratory workers handling primate retroviruses (Kurth and Mikschy 1978).

Human antibodies reacting with virion core antigens and reverse transcriptases of experimental retroviruses have also been described. Kalyanaraman et al. (1981a) propose that the major core protein, p24, of the putative human T-cell lymphoma virus appears to be a major immunogen in those patients harboring the virus (see Section V), as might be expected for a genuine human infection with an exogenous retrovirus. Mellors and Mellors (1978) and Reynolds and Panem (1981) have studied the specificity of immunoglobulins eluted from glomerulonephritic complexes of autopsies of SLE patients. These authors found that the eluates contained antibodies reacting with p30 of RD114 virus, consistent with their earlier report (Mellors and Mellors 1976) that SLE-affected kidneys contained a p30 antigen related to the RD114/BaEV group. Derks et al. (1982) reported the presence of serum antibodies reacting with SSAV p30 in a patient with chronic myeloid leukemia (CML), whose leukemic cells synthesize a p30 and reverse transcriptase closely related to SSAV.

Prochownik and Kirsten (1976) detected IgG antibodies in the plasma of two of five patients with acute myelogenous leukemia which specifically inactivated reverse transcriptase activity of SSAV, BaEV, and the putative human virus, HEL-12 (see Section IV.B). Investigators in Gallo's laboratory, on the other hand, did not detect significant levels of plasma antibodies to reverse transcriptase in leukemic patients, but they were able to elute IgG from leukocytes that inhibited reverse transcriptase activity (Jacquemin et al. 1978). Antibodies eluted from leukocytes of patients with acute myelogenous leukemia predominantly neutralized the SSAV enzyme, whereas antibodies from leukocytes of CML patients in blast-cell crisis predominantly neutralized feline leukemia virus (FeLV) enzyme. Some normal subjects and CML chronic-phase patients yielded eluted IgG that most strongly neutralized $GALV_{SF}$. The specificity of these cell-bound antibodies to different retroviral polymerases of different species is remarkable; the cell-surface antigens to which the antibodies bind have not been characterized.

One of the most specific serological tests for envelope antigens is neutralization of infectivity of retroviruses or of pseudotypes bearing their glycoproteins. However, nonspecific inactivation due to virion lysis (see below) should not be mistaken for neutralization. The slight reduction of the in vivo titer of MMTV by sera from breast cancer patients (Charney and Moore 1971) was not shown to be specific. Whereas a large number of sera from patients with leukemia and other neoplasms have been negative when tested for neutralization of MSV or vesicular stomatitis virus (VSV) pseudotypes of primate retroviruses (T. J. Schnitzer, pers. comm.), specific neutralization has been observed. Neutralization of VSV pseudotypes with envelope glycoproteins of MPMV or "HeLa virus" (see Section III.C) was observed in very occasional breast cancer patients (Zavada et al. 1972, 1974) and in pregnant women and renal transplant patients (Thiry et al. 1978b,c). The glycoproteins of D-type MPMV and C-type BaEV are immunologically related (Stephenson et al. 1976; Devare et al. 1978; Barbacid et al. 1980b; Fine et al. 1980), and therefore the reactivity of human sera with MPMV might possibly relate to BaEV-like elements in human "infection" (see Section IV.B). However, virus neutralization is usually more type-specific than radioimmunoassays and merits further study with pseudotypes of candidate human viruses.

A curious serological finding was the nonspecific inactivation and lysis of murine, feline, and simian C-type viruses (Welsh et al. 1975, 1976). The lysis is due to antibody-independent binding of the human C1q complement component to gp70, leading to the activation of the classic complement pathway (Cooper et al. 1976). It is not understood why C1q recognizes gp70; possibly the gp70 molecules have a domain resembling the C1q recognition site on the Fc fragment of immunoglobulins. It was suggested (Welsh et al. 1975; Cooper et al. 1976) that the nonspecific lysis of retroviruses by human complement is an adaptive defense system that may protect against viremia and cause the lysis of cells expressing gp70 at the surface. In this case it would be interesting to study complement-deficient patients for evidence of retrovirus infection. Preliminary findings suggest that such patients do not exhibit elevated levels of antibodies reacting with primate retroviruses (Kurth et al. 1979b). Gallagher et al. (1978) have shown a similar lytic activity of gibbon ape sera for retroviral envelopes, yet some of the same gibbons were infected with GALV and synthesized anti-GALV antibodies. The protective effect of the complement-dependent lysis of retrovirus therefore remains doubtful.

Fewer studies have been made on cellular responses than on humoral immunity in humans suspected of harboring retrovirus infections (Black et al. 1974, 1981; Ortaldo et al. 1977; Levin et al. 1978; Thiry et al. 1978a). A recent report (Lopez et al. 1981) identifies in breast cancer patients a T-lymphocyte subset that reacts to MMTV but not to MLV. Other examples of cellular immunity in breast cancer patients are cited in Section IV.A.

A most intriguing recent report concerns the nature of inhibitors of monocyte chemotaxis found in effusion fluids of many kinds of human cancer (Cianciolo et al. 1981). Morphological changes and migration of monocytes can be induced and quantified by the chemoattractant *N*-formyl-methionyl-leucyl-phenylalanine (Cianciolo and Snyderman 1981). Malignant effusions inhibit the morphological polarization of monocytes to a motile configuration, whereas effusions due to benign lesions and bacterial infections have no inhibitory effect. Chromatography of cancerous fluids revealed three peaks of heat-stable inhibitory activity, representing proteins of approximately 200,000, 46,000, and 21,000 daltons. Cianciolo et al. (1981) found that the inhibitory factors could be absorbed by three different monoclonal antibodies reacting to p15(E) of MLV, but not by other monoclonal antibodies, including those specific to MLV gp70. Furthermore, addition of disrupted Ra-MLV virions inhibited human monocyte transformation, and this inhibitor too was absorbed by monoclonal anti-p15(E). Monocyte migration has also been inhibited in mice by MLV proteins (Cianciolo et al. 1980), and FeLV p15(E) has a similar effect (Mathes et al. 1979). There is a wide interspecies reactivity of p15(E) between mammalian C-type and D-type viruses (Thiel et al. 1981). Cianciolo et al. (1981) have demonstrated that potent inhibitory agents for monocyte responsiveness are present in cancerous effusions from a wide variety of human malignancies and that the inhibitors are related antigenically to p15(E). The relationship of the inhibitors to virus-coded proteins and their role in subverting immune responses to cancer remain to be determined.

III. CAUTIONARY TALES OF NOT-SO-HUMAN VIRUSES

A. RD114 Virus

RD114 virus is an isolate of an endogenous xenotropic cat C-type virus that was originally hailed as a human virus. McAllister et al. (1969, 1971) established a cell line (RD) derived from a human rhabdomyosarcoma and developed a metastatic xenograft procedure by injecting RD cells into the brain of a fetal kitten. On reestablishment in culture, the RD cells were found to be releasing C-type viral particles (McAllister et al. 1972) that were unrelated in antigenicity or host range to FeLV or MLV (McAllister et al. 1972, 1973; Oroszlan et al. 1972; Rasheed et al. 1973).

Because of the passage history of the cells from which the virus was isolated and because of its unique immunological properties,

McAllister et al. (1972) suggested that "RD114 virus was either a candidate human virus or a representative of a new feline virus family related to, but distinct from FeLV." The former view was clearly favored, and the correctness of the latter interpretation was not elucidated until data from other laboratories were published more than 1 year later. Two lines of evidence clearly indicated that RD114 virus was feline in origin. First, it was shown that sequences homologous to RD114 genomic RNA were present in normal cat DNA (Neiman 1973; Baluda and Roy-Burman 1973; Fujinaga et al. 1973; Gillespie et al. 1973; Okabe et al. 1973; Ruprecht et al. 1973). Second, xenotropic viruses indistinguishable from RD114 virus were observed to be spontaneously produced or inducible in feline cell lines (Fischinger et al. 1973; Livingston and Todaro 1973; Sarma et al. 1973) and in normal feline cells and tissues (Gardner et al. 1974; Sarma et al. 1974).

It should be noted that at the time RD114 virus was discovered, the concept of xenotropism and the definition of xenotropic murine C-type viruses (Levy 1973) were not developed, although it was known that avian endogenous viruses could best be propagated in foreign cells (Vogt and Friis 1971; Weiss et al. 1971). Furthermore, the only endogenous viruses then known (of chickens and mice) were closely related to exogenous viruses infecting the same species. The discovery in cats of a xenotropic endogenous virus that was only very distantly related to FeLV therefore had no precedent. It was a further surprise to discover in baboons endogenous viruses that were closely related to RD114 virus (Todaro et al. 1973a; Beneveniste et al. 1974; Hellman et al. 1974).

The rescue and amplification of xenotropic endogenous viruses as a by-product of tumor xenograft procedures have been observed frequently since the original observations by McAllister and his colleagues. Although the reisolation of RD114 virus was not repeated in the subsequent transplantation of RD cells into fetal or newborn kittens (Gardner et al. 1973), xenotropic mouse viruses have been isolated several times in human tumor xenografts propagated in mice (Todaro et al. 1973b; Achong et al. 1976; Suzuki et al. 1977; Crawford et al. 1979; Wunderli et al. 1979). One might also expect xenograft procedures to promote the rescue of latent or defective human retroviruses. In this regard the occasional induction of host tumors in xenografted rats and mice (Huebner et al. 1979; Goldenberg and Pavia 1981; Tveit and Pihl 1981) would merit virological analysis.

B. ESP-1 Virus

The ESP-1 virus was first seen in the electron microscope as typical budding and mature forms of C-type particles produced by cells purportedly derived from a lymphoma patient (Priori et al. 1971; Dmochowski and Bowen 1978). The patient was a 5-year-old boy with "American" Burkitt's lymphoma. He had developed a pleural effusion following chemotherapy and died shortly afterwards from disseminated herpes varicella-zoster infection. The ESP-1 culture was initiated from cells tapped from the pleural effusion, but the original cells were not cryopreserved. C-type particles were first observed at the tenth passage, by which time the major cell type was epithelioid. The cells grew vigorously as a cell line and continuously produced retroviral particles, but the yield was low and the cultures were also heavily contaminated with mycoplasma. Chromosome analysis indicated a highly aneuploid human karyotype with fragmented chromosomes. The HLA phenotype was not incompatible with the genotypes of the patient's parents (Dmochowski and Bowen 1978); however, a subline examined by Nelson-Rees and Flandermeyer (1975) contained markers characteristic of HeLa cells.

From the start, the nature of the virus was controversial. Gilden et al. (1971) reported that the *gag* antigens of the virus were closely related to those of MLVs in both species and interspecies determinants, whereas Dmochowski's group (Shigematsu et al. 1971), using immunoferritin electron microscopy techniques, detected only interspecies antigens. Subsequently, Dmochowski and Bowen (1978) observed by immunodiffusion that ESP-1 cells strongly expressed MLV antigens but that the species-specific p30 determinant was only weakly expressed in purified virions. ESP-1 virus contained reverse transcriptase typical of C-type particles (Gallo et al. 1971), which was later reported to be immunologically closely related to MLV enzymes (Dmochowski and Bowen 1978). Genomic homology studies have not been reported. Thus, the virus appears to be of murine origin, growing in human cells of doubtful provenance.

A human cell line, HEK-1 (supposedly derived from embryonic kidney, but possibly a HeLa-cell variant), was maintained in Dmochowski's laboratory and had been deliberately infected with Ra-MLV. It is possible that the human-adapted HEK-1 MLV contaminated the ESP-1 cells. However, the biological properties of the HEK-1 MLV and ESP-1 virus differed. HEK-1 MLV still maintained some properties of ecotropic Ra-MLV, such as XC-cell fusion and rescue of MSV from mouse nonproducer cells. ESP-1 virus was negative for XC-cell fusion and MSV rescue, although, curiously, it acted as a helper for Friend spleen focus-forming virus (SFFV) (Eckner et al. 1974). Antisera that neutralized HEK-1 MLV pseudotypes of SFFV did not neutralize ESP-1 pseudotypes (Eckner et al. 1974). Some differences in detailed ultrastructure between ESP-1 and Ra-MLV were also noted (Dalton 1972). With hindsight, ESP-1 virus would appear to be a xenotropic MLV variant selected for growth in the human cells it contaminated.

C. HeLa Virus

In Moscow, Zhdanov and his colleagues observed retroviral particles in cultures of HeLa cells (Zhdanov et al. 1972, 1973; Ilyin et al. 1973; Bukrinskaya et al. 1974). Other human epithelioid cell lines were also found to be productively or latently infected with a similar virus (Todaro et al. 1970; Zavada et al. 1972; Parks et al. 1973; Miller et al. 1974; Holder et al. 1974), but all of these lines probably represent sublines of HeLa cells (Nelson-Rees et al. 1974; Nelson-Rees and Flandermeyer 1975). Parks et al. (1973) observed that the virus released by a human "amniotic" cell line was related to MPMV. A detailed morphological, biochemical, and immunological characterization was undertaken by Bauer and his colleagues; it showed that the HeLa virus was a D-type virus indistinguishable from MPMV (Bauer et al. 1974; Gelderblom et al. 1974a,b; Watson et al. 1974). Similar findings were reported by Irlin et al. (1973/74) and Priori et al. (1976).

Most of the cell lines producing MPMV-HeLa virus were derived from European substrains of HeLa cells. Presumably, these cells had become contaminated at some stage of their passage history with MPMV from rhesus monkey cells maintained in the same laboratory. MPMV is commonly expressed in cells derived from apparently healthy rhesus monkeys (Ahmed et al. 1974) that have been much used for vaccine production of poliovirus and other agents. Two lessons can be learned from the HeLa virus story. First, nonlytic persistent infections such as those caused by retroviruses can spread from one cell type to another in laboratories without being readily detected. Second, many human cell lines believed to be derived from particular tumors established in culture in fact represent contamination by HeLa cells that outgrow nonestablished cell cultures, appearing as emerging clones of immortal cells.

Zavada et al. (1972, 1974, 1975) prepared envelope pseudotypes of VSV (see Chapter 3) with the glycoproteins of a retrovirus expressed in HeLa cells believed at that time to be human mammary tumor cells. The virus donating the glycoproteins to the pseudotype was almost certainly MPMV. In screening the sera of mammary carcinoma patients, however, Zavada et al. (1972) found that 2 patients out of 400 women had antibodies that strongly neutralized the VSV pseudotype. Could these patients have been infected with a virus related to MPMV? More recently, Thiry et al. (1978a,b,c) have detected neutralizing antibodies to VSV(MPMV) and cell-mediated immune responses to MPMV-infected cells in women with healthy or preeclamptic pregnancies and in renal transplant patients (see Section II.F). These observations await confirmation, but the possibility remains of a human virus antigenically related to MPMV.

IV. ELUSIVE RETROVIRUSES DETECTED IN HUMAN TISSUES

A. Evidence for a Human Mammary Tumor Virus

A great deal of effort has been invested in searching for a retrovirus associated with human breast cancer, but the results have not revealed definitive evidence for such an agent. Two animal viruses have been extensively used as probes for related viruses in man: The Mason-Pfizer monkey virus and the mouse mammary tumor virus. Although MPMV was first isolated from a mammary tumor of a rhesus monkey (Chopra and Mason 1970), it has subsequently been shown to be a common virus of rhesus monkeys (Ahmed et al. 1974; Fine et al. 1978) and is present in many normal tissues; it has not induced breast tumors in experimental infection of primates (Deinhardt 1980). MMTV undoubtedly is the major etiological agent of breast cancer in laboratory mice, and related viruses have been isolated from feral mice of more than one species (see

Chapter 2). The histopathological type of breast tumor induced by MMTV in mice is only rarely found in man, and tumor development in mice depends on several cofactors besides virus infection, chiefly high parity with the concomitant endocrine stimulation it entails (see Chapter 8). As a disease, then, the murine mammary tumor incited by MMTV is not a close model for human mammary carcinoma.

Human breast cancer, however, encompasses a large variety of malignant phenotypes and may reflect a group of cancers with different etiologies, including familial and sporadic presentations. In the search for breast cancer viruses, perhaps not enough attention has been paid to the diversity of the disease. If a B-type virus were transmitted in milk (as in C3H mice) or through the germ cells (as in GR mice), investigation of familial breast cancer (Anderson 1974) would be recommended. Tokuhata (1969) studied the daughters of 550 mothers with breast cancer and found no difference in breast cancer incidence in daughters that were breast fed and daughters that were not. Anderson (1975) was unable to find a significant difference in cancer risk between women who were ever breast fed and those who were never breast fed. Thus, there is no epidemiological evidence to suggest that human breast cancer might have an infectious etiology through milk-borne viruses; indeed, the incidence of breast cancer is relatively low in those countries and communities where breast feeding is common (Fraumeni and Miller 1971), and the major influences on incidence appear to be endocrine and dietary (Armstrong et al. 1981; Pike et al. 1981).

Interest in a retrovirus etiology of human breast cancer was aroused by electron microscope studies of particles resembling B-type retroviruses in human milk (Feller and Chopra 1969, 1971; Moore et al. 1969, 1971; Seman et al. 1971; Sarkar and Moore 1972). Milk is a fine emulsion containing many lipid or membrane-bound particles of approximately the diameter expected for viral particles, and interpretation of this evidence has been difficult (Calafat and Hageman 1973; Dalton 1975). Spiegelman's group and others have reported the biochemical detection of retroviral particles in human milk samples by Schlom and Spiegelman's (1971) "simultaneous detection" of 70S RNA and reverse transcriptase activity (Schlom et al. 1971, 1972a,b,c,; Feldman et al. 1973; Gerwin et al. 1973). Das et al. (1972a) have detected retroviruslike particles in the milk of Parsi women in Bombay. The incidence of breast cancer in the Parsi community is relatively high for India, though not in comparison with Western countries.

Roy-Burman et al. (1973) questioned whether the simultaneous detection test was a reliable and specific indicator of retroviral particles in human milk. However, analysis of the polymerase activity in milk and tumor particles revealed cation and primer-template preferences characteristic of MMTV and MPMV reverse transcriptases (Dion et al. 1974; Ohno et al. 1977; Kantor et al. 1979), and antibody to MPMV reverse transcriptase partially inhibited the enzyme activity of human milk particles (Ohno and Spiegelman 1977). Moreover, nonspecific inhibitors of reverse transcriptase (possibly phosphatase or ribonuclease) have been found to copurify with the enzyme in human milk (McCormick et al. 1974; Sarkar et al. 1973; Fieldsteel 1975; Sanner 1976; Kantor et al. 1979). With removal of the inhibitors, positive results for particulate fractions with enzyme activity are more consistently observed.

In addition to reports of viruslike particles in the milk of normal women, particles were described in human breast tumors or cultures derived from them (Axel et al. 1972a; Spiegelman et al. 1972; Viola 1973; McGrath et al. 1974; Michalides et al. 1975) and from normal mammary epithelial cells cultivated from postnursing lactatory fluids (Furmanski et al. 1974). Molecular hybridization studies indicated significant homology of nucleic acid sequences between MMTV and human breast tumor RNA (Axel et al. 1972b; Spiegelman et al. 1972), between MPMV and breast tumor RNA (Colcher et al. 1974), and between the human milk particles and breast tumor RNA (Das et al. 1972b). Using stringent hybridization conditions, Vaidya et al. (1974) measured MMTV-related RNA in certain human breast carcinomas. On the other hand, MMTV-related DNA in human cells has not been detected by liquid hybridization (Bishop et al. 1974) or more recently by Southern blotting using molecularly cloned probes. It is possible that the early probes yielding positive results were contaminated with cDNA of ribosomal RNA. Spiegelman et al. (1980a,b), nevertheless, cite the early molecular hybridization studies as evidence for a human breast cancer virus related to MMTV.

Viruses that have very little genomic homology may share common antigenic determinants in the virion proteins, e.g., MMTV and MPMV or MPMV and BaEV (Colcher et al. 1977; Devare et al. 1978; Barbacid et al. 1980b; Fine et al. 1980). A search for antigenic cross-reactions between human breast tissues or secretions and antibodies to animal virion proteins might therefore reveal the presence of a human virus too distantly related to be detected by molecular hybridization. Yeh et al. (1975) detected an antigen related to MPMV p27 in malignant breast tissue, and the inhibition of milk-particle polymerase activity by antibody specific to MPMV reverse transcriptase (Ohno and Spiegelman 1977) has already been mentioned. Human milk particles were also found to contain a 27,000-dalton protein similar to MMTV p27 (Müller and Grossman 1972; Furmanski et al. 1976; Zotter et al. 1980). Investigators in other laboratories, however, have been unable to detect MPMV or MMTV p27 in human tumors and secretions (Charman et al. 1977; Hendrick et al. 1978).

Recently, Spiegelman's group reported the presence of a glycoprotein in human mammary carcinomas that reacts with antisera to MMTV gp52 (Mesa-Tejada et al. 1978; Ohno et al. 1979; Spiegelman et al. 1980a,b). The antigen has not yet been extracted and purified from human tumors, but the antigenic moiety shared with MMTV gp52 is not apparently a carbohydrate group. Immunoperoxidase staining of human breast tissues with anti-MMTV-gp52 antibody was positive in about 45% of the breast carcinomas of various types, especially invasive and metastatic tumors, and was negative in normal resting or lactating tissue and in benign lesions such as cystic disease and fibroadenoma. The antibody therefore appears to recognize an antigen expressed specifically in malignant tissue.

Spiegelman and his colleagues have not remarked on the paradox that the restriction of MMTV antigen expression to malignant breast tissue is inconsistent with the wealth of evidence previously published by investigators in his laboratory and others on the presence of MMTV-related particles in human milk from normal women. Yang et al. (1977, 1978) also observed an antigen related to MMTV gp52 expressed in the human mammary tumor MCF-7 cell line (see below). Yang et al. (1978) found that the gp52-related antigen in MCF-7 cells was not expressed in cultured normal mammary epithelial cells, although the normal cells release particles resembling retroviruses (Furmanski et al. 1974), an observation that might explain the paradox noted for Spiegelman's studies. In contrast to the findings of Spiegelman and Yang, Dion and colleagues have detected a human glycoprotein related to MMTV gp52 both in breast carcinoma cells (Black et al. 1976) and in the milk of healthy women (Dion et al. 1980). Presumably, Dion and Spiegelman have developed antisera to MMTV gp52 preparations that recognize different antigenic sites on the related proteins in human tissues. Until these experiments are repeated with monoclonal antibodies specific to MMTV gp52, the possibility remains of a mouse mammary tissue antigen contaminating the gp52 preparations used as immunogens for the antisera, although Dion et al. (1980) claim that the human milk protein and MMTV gp52 share common tryptic peptides. In recent DNA transfection studies (see Section VI.B), Lane et al. (1981) identified a transforming gene shared by MMTV-induced mouse mammary tumors and certain human mammary carcinomas. The transfecting sequences were not linked to the MMTV genome, but they could conceivably encode an antigen assembled into MMTV envelopes that may not be easily distinguished from gp52.

Reports of humoral and cell-mediated immunities of human breast patients reacting to MMTV antigens must also be interpreted with caution until the nature of the human antigens has been more rigorously characterized. Immune responses to MMTV antigens in breast cancer patients have been reported by several investigators (Charney and Moore 1971; Black et al. 1974, 1975, 1976; Bowen et al. 1976; Müller et al. 1976; Newgard et al. 1976; Imai et al. 1979; Witkin et al. 1979; Lopez et al. 1981). The specificity of the cell-mediated reactions was questioned by McCoy et al. (1978), but studies of humoral antibodies were apparently specific to MMTV (Witkin et al. 1979, 1980).

Virological research into human breast cancer has been hampered by the paucity of cell lines that genuinely originate from the mammary gland. One human breast carcinoma cell line that is not a HeLa cell is the MCF-7 line derived from a pleural effusion of a patient with metastatic breast carcinoma (Soule et al. 1973). The MCF-7 cell line retains several morphological and endocrinological features of breast epithelial cells, and it has been examined in detail for the presence of a virus related to MMTV. McGrath et al. (1974) observed the production of retroviral particles from MCF-7 cells which appeared to share antigenic markers with MMTV. Unfortunately, the production of particles from MCF-7 cells appears to be sporadic and has not traveled well to other laboratories. However, a gp52-related antigen (see above) is more readily expressed than whole virions in MCF-7 cells (Yang et al. 1977, 1978). A preliminary report by Viola (1973) on retroviral particles produced by another cell line established from a pleural effusion has not been followed up by a thorough characterization of the viral particles or the cell line releasing them; it was possibly a HeLa-cell contaminant. Keydar et al. (1979) described a third breast carcinoma cell line that may produce retroviral particles. Short-term cultures of normal breast epithelial cells derived from postweaning breast fluids of nursing mothers were briefly described by Furmanski et al. (1974). These cells release particles with 70S RNA and reverse transcriptase activity, but apparently not gp52 related to MMTV as discussed above (Yang et al. 1978). In recent years, techniques for culturing normal and malignant human mammary cells have improved considerably, and more cell types are becoming available for study.

Few attempts have been made to show infectivity in vivo or in vitro for "human" breast retroviruses. Keydar et al. (1973) claimed that human embryonic fibroblasts cocultivated with mammary tumor cells or "infected" with milk from lactating cancer patients frequently produced retroviral particles, whereas control cultures remained virus-free. The virions had a buoyant density of 1.17 g/ml and contained 70S RNA and reverse transcriptase activity, but they were not characterized morphologically or immunologically. If human mammary tumor viruses resemble MMTV, one would not expect the virus to infect cells readily, least of all fibroblastic cells. It is difficult to establish in vitro transmission of even the most virulent strains of MMTV, although xenotropic infection with low productivity of epithelial cells has been obtained (Lasfargues 1976a,b; Vaidya et al. 1976; Ringold et al. 1977).A feline kidney cell line appears to be the best for replication, and high-titer MMTV variants have been selected by passage through these cells (Howard and Schlom 1978). This cell line might be useful for testing the infectivity of the human particles resembling MMTV.

In conclusion, much circumstantial evidence for B-type retroviruses associated with normal and malignant human breast tissues was reported during the 1970s. Regrettably, more rigorous data have not been forthcoming, and little effort has been made to resolve inconsistencies between published results.

B. Viruses Related to GALV/SSAV and BaEV

Viral antigens and viral particles in human tissues and cultures have been detected that are related to the gibbon ape leukemia and simian sarcoma-associated viruses, to the endogenous baboon and cat viruses, or to both virus groups. Antigens related to p30 of BaEV and RD114 were reported in a variety of normal and pathological human tissues by Sherr and Todaro (1974) and Strand and August (1974b). Sherr and Todaro (1975) also published data on the expression of an antigen closely related to GALV p30 in acute myelogenous leukemia cells. In an extensive survey of human tissues, however, Stephenson and Aarsonson (1976) were unable to identify antigens related to BaEV or GALV.

Following reports of reverse transcriptase activity in particulate fractions of human tumors or culture supernatants (see Section II.B), RNA-dependent DNA polymerase was purified directly from spleen biopsies of some preleukemic conditions and from patients with acute myelogenous leukemia (Mondal et al. 1975; Witkin et al. 1975; Steel et al. 1977; Chandra et al. 1980). The purified enzymes have the properties of viral reverse transcriptase and were immunologically related to those of both GALV and BaEV. Investigators in several laboratories had also detected the presence of retroviruslike particles in the medium of cultured leukemia cells (Todaro and Gallo 1973; Gallagher et al. 1974; Mak et al. 1974, 1975; Miller et al. 1974; Gallagher and Gallo 1975; Nooter et al. 1975, 1977; Vosika et al. 1975), lymphoma cells (Kaplan et al. 1977), and embryonic fibroblasts (Panem et al. 1975). Where the particles were produced in sufficient quantities for detailed characterization of their structural antigens, reverse transcriptase, or nucleic acid sequences, they were found to be closely related to GALV/SSAV, but with components also related to BaEV. In at least five distinct isolates from leukemic cells, the viral particles were found to be infectious for cell lines in culture (Nooter et al. 1975, 1977; Teich et al. 1975; Panem et al. 1976; Kaplan 1978). The infectious viruses could be titrated in the XC syncytial plaque assay, which works for the GALV/SSAV group of viruses as well as for ecotropic MLV (see Chapter 3).

It is odd that viruslike particles related to GALV have been found sporadically in such a variety of human tissues when it is clear that viruses of this type are not endogenous to man. Mak et al. (1974, 1975) reported the production of noninfectious particles in bone marrow cultures of a majority of patients with acute or chronic myelogenous and lymphocytic leukemias, irrespective of whether the cultures were made from aspirates taken in relapse or remission; normal bone-marrow cultures, with one exception, were negative. Gallagher and Gallo (1975), on the other hand, observed virus production in only 1 of 16 long-term cultures of leukemic cells from patients with acute myelogenous leukemia. Kaplan et al. (1977, 1979) detected virions in cell lines established from patients with diffuse histiocytic lymphomas and an American Burkitt's lymphoma. Nooter et al. (1975, 1977) isolated infectious viruses from bone-marrow cultures of two cases of children's acute lymphoblastic leukemia. Panem et al. (1975) observed the induction of transient virion production after IdU treatment in four of ten apparently normal fibroblastic cell strains from human fetuses; the virus of one strain, HEL-12, has been characterized. Antigens and viral particles related to BaEV or GALV have also been observed in tissues of patients with SLE (Strand and August 1974b; Mellors and Mellors 1976; Panem et al. 1976).

Thus, the human-tissue isolates related to the exogenous gibbon viruses and endogenous baboon virus do not fit a defined pattern of disease. As we shall discuss, evidence for proviral sequences in most cases is poor. Nor do studies of human antibodies reacting to these viruses help to establish whether they represent natural human infections (see Section III.F). The properties of those human isolates that have been characterized in most detail are briefly described below, and the controversy surrounding their true provenance is reviewed.

1. HL23 Virus

Investigators in Gallo's laboratory established differentiating cultures of leukemic cells from patients with acute myelogenous leukemia, using a medium containing a growth factor secreted by human embryonic cells. The leukemic cells from one patient, HL23, released a retrovirus related to primate viruses (Gallagher and Gallo 1975). This virus isolate, HL23V-1, had the typical morphology of C-type particles, and budding forms were observed (Gallagher and Gallo 1975; Hall and Schidlovsky 1976). However, particle production as measured by reverse transcriptase activity was low and sporadic.

Using cell-free medium harvested from HL23 cells, Teich et al.

(1975) attempted to infect a wide variety of human and animal cells. After transient phases of virion release observed as low titers of reverse transcriptase activity, productive secondary infections became established in four cell types: a human embryonic fibroblast strain (WHE-2), a human rhabdomyosarcoma cell line (A204), a canine thymus cell line (A7573), and a rat kidney cell line (NRK). A more rapid infective transmission was obtained in A204 cells and KNRK cells (nonproducer NRK cells transformed by Kirsten MSV [Ki-MSV]) when these cells were treated with inactivated Sendai virus immediately before infection with HL23 fluids, suggesting that the gp70 in virions released from HL23 cells might be deficient. The KNRK cells, in particular, produced high titers of HL23V-1 and also MSV(HL23V-1) pseudotypes. A wider host range of infectivity was obtained by tertiary infections of cell lines with virus produced by the experimentally infected cells. Additional human cell lines were susceptible to HL23V-1 infection, including cells nonproductively transformed by S^+L^- MSV. HL23V-1 infectivity could be titrated quantitatively by the XC syncytial plaque assay, and MSV(HL23V-1) pseudotypes could be titrated by focus assay on NRK cells and human or quail fibroblasts. Cross-interference of MSV pseudotypes was observed among HL23V-1, GALV, and SSAV. The infectivity of MSV(HL23V-1) pseudotypes was neutralized by goat antiserum to SSAV, but not by serum from the patient from whom HL23 cells were derived. Teich et al. (1975) further showed by immunoassays and by nucleic acid hybridization that HL23V-1 closely resembled SSAV. However, inactivation of HL23V-1 reverse transcriptase activity was noted for antisera to either SSAV or RD114 enzymes, and the A204 and A7573 cells infected with HL23V-1 expressed p30 related to BaEV and RD114, as well as to SSAV.

The HL23V-1 stocks grown by Teich et al. (1975) in the secondarily infected cells were distributed to other laboratories for further characterization. Chan et al. (1976) found that HL23V-1 produced by A204 cells behaved as a mixture of viruses indistinguishable immunologically and in nucleotide sequence from BaEV and SSAV. Okabe et al. (1976) obtained essentially similar results for HL23V-1 grown in A7573 cells, whereas HL23V-1 grown in KNRK cells (which are resistant to BaEV infection) showed immunological reactivity to SSAV only. Whiteley and Naso (1982) have noted some differences in the precursor polyproteins and processing of virion proteins between HL23V and BaEV. One HL23V-1 stock induced sarcomas in marmosets (Bergholz et al. 1977) and transformed foci in fibroblast cultures (Markham et al. 1978); as no other stocks were shown to contain transforming viruses, this stock presumably contained MSV(HL23V-1) pseudotypes rescued from either KNRK cells or S^+L^- canine or human cells.

The very close relationship of HL23V-1 to a mixture of SSAV and BaEV raised the question of whether the virus complex represented a laboratory contamination, initially infecting either HL23 cells or the human embryonic cells used to produce conditioned medium for HL23 cells. The embryonic cells did not release virus or cause infection on cocultivation with human acute myelogenous leukemia cells other than HL23 and were therefore excluded as a source of the virus. Two additional cultures were independently established from peripheral blood and bone marrow, respectively, of the same patient, HL23, taken 14 months after the original biopsy. These cultures also released viruses, HL23V-4 and HL23V-5, which, like HL23V-1, proved to be a mixture of BaEV-related and SSAV-related viruses (Gallagher et al. 1975). At autopsy, hematopoietic tissues of patient HL23 were examined for viral nucleic acid sequences; DNA sequences closely related to BaEV RNA were detected in the spleen (Reitz et al. 1976). Curiously, proviral DNA sequences homologous to SSAV RNA were not detectable in HL23 spleen, although SSAV-related RNA was found both in the spleen and in the cytoplasm of the cultured leukemic cells (Reitz et al. 1976). In a study of eight further myelogenous leukemia patients, extensive hybridization of leukocyte DNA to BaEV probes with high melting temperatures was found in five patients, but not in the other three patients or in normal subjects (Wong-Staal et al. 1976); again, SSAV-related DNA sequences were not detected.

2. *Nooter and Bentvelzen's Viruses*

Following the detection by immunofluorescence (Zurcher et al. 1975) of SSAV-related antigens in cultures of human bone tumor cells, Nooter et al. (1975) reported the isolation of an infectious C-type virus from short-term culture of PHA-stimulated bone-marrow cells from a 4-year-old patient with lymphosarcoma that had progressed to lymphoblastic leukemia. The virus induced syncytia in XC cells cocultivated with the bone-marrow cells. Cocultivation of XC cells with bone-marrow cells of five additional leukemia patients and four normal donors did not lead to virus rescue. The virus was propagated in XC cells and could be secondarily transmitted to human embryonic kidney cells and human embryonic fibroblasts. Indirect immunofluorescence tests indicated that the virus was most closely related to the GALV/SSAV group (Nooter et al. 1975). A second isolate was made 1 month later from the same patient while in remission, by cocultivation of buffy-coat leukocytes with human embryonic fibroblasts. Despite the ability to transmit these isolates to experimental cells, this virus has not been further characterized.

Two years later, Nooter et al. (1977) made further isolations of infectious viruses from cells of two children with acute lymphoblastic leukemia. Bone-marrow cells were cocultivated with canine A7573 cells, and these cells, in turn, were cocultivated with human or rat nonproducer cell lines carrying Ki-MSV. This led to the rescue of MSV pseudotypes that transformed human, rabbit, and rat cells, but not mouse cells. Immunofluorescence and neutralization tests showed that these helper viruses were closely related to SSAV. More detailed immunological and biochemical studies (Koch et al. 1977; Nooter et al. 1978; Nooter 1979; Smith et al. 1979) showed that the virus stocks contained p30, p15, p12, reverse transcriptase, and nucleic acid sequences related to SSAV and also, in one stock, to the BaEV/RD114 group. A rat endogenous virus also became activated in some preparations. The mixture of rat virus, Ki-MSV, and SSAV-like and BaEV-like components has made further analysis and interpretation rather difficult (Nooter 1979).

3. HEL-12 Virus

HEL-12 virus, isolated by Panem et al. (1975), is exceptional in that it originates from human embryonic fibroblasts rather than from leukemic or lymphoma cells. The virus was spontaneously released from late-passage cultures of HEL-12 cells, which are apparently normal fibroblasts derived from the lungs of a spontaneously aborted 8-week-old embryo. HEL-12 virions are typical C-type particles with p30 and reverse transcriptase related to the GALV/SSAV group. Like the HL23V isolates, HEL-12 virions appear to contain nucleic acid sequences and antigens related to, but not identical with, both SSAV and BaEV (Panem et al. 1977;

Prochownik and Kirsten 1977; Panem 1976; Bergholz et al. 1980; Hefti et al. 1980). HEL-12V-related DNA sequences were found in one human osteosarcoma and in one of seven leukemic cell preparations, as well as in HEL-12 cells (Prochownik and Kirsten 1977).

Spontaneous production of HEL-12V from HEL-12 cells was first characterized by transient virus production as measured by reverse transcriptase activity in particulate form in the culture medium. Detailed studies showed that HEL-12 cells proceed through four stages of virus expression (Panem et al. 1977): (1) no detectable viral antigen synthesis; (2) p30 and gp70 expression recorded by immunofluorescence, but no virion production; (3) antigen and virion production; and (4) antigen production and release of virions lacking reverse transcriptase while containing viral RNA. The last stage also does not express enough gp70 at the cell surface to render the cells susceptible to complement-mediated immunolysis with anti-SSAV serum (Bergholz et al. 1980), and by inference, the virions produced at the time lack gp70, as well as reverse transcriptase. The duration of the cycle for virus expression and shutdown takes approximately 140 days, and HEL-12V proviral DNA is present throughout the cycle (Prochownik and Kirsten 1977). A study of cloned HEL-12 cells showed a similar pattern of virus expression (Panem 1976). Treatment of HEL-12 cells with IdU activates virus production earlier than would normally occur, but the release of virus is still transient (Prochownik et al. 1979). During stage 3, when virions containing reverse transcriptase and gp70 are released, some of the particles are infectious and have been transmitted to canine thymus cells, marmoset cells, and early-passage HEL-12 cells (Panem et al. 1976; Bergholz et al. 1980). As with the spontaneous expression of virus in HEL-12 cells, canine cells infected with HEL-12V proceed through the same four stages of expression, although the "cycle" time is reduced to 28 days (Black et al. 1981). Stage-4 HEL-12 cells could also be superinfected with HEL-12V, and they exhibited an accelerated cycle. The transient production of infectious particles and the restriction of reverse transcriptase activity are not understood but may relate to interferon activty.

Using immunological and virological reagents prepared from HEL-12 virus, Panem and her colleagues have detected similar viral antigens and antibodies in tissues obtained from patients with SLE. Eleven specimens of lupus nephropathy showed antigens deposited in the glomeruli that reacted in indirect immunofluorescence tests with antibodies to HEL-12 virions (Panem et al. 1978). IgG antibody eluted from four SLE kidneys reacted with HEL-12V-infected canine cells, but not with control, uninfected canine thymus cells (Panem et al. 1976; Reynolds and Panem 1981). The eluted IgG reacted with purified SSAV p30 and, to a lesser extent, with BaEV p30; gp70 of either virus was not precipitated, and IgG eluted from normal kidneys did not react with viral antigens (Reynolds and Panem 1981). HEL-12V antigens were also detected in the skin of SLE patients (Panem et al. 1978). These findings are reminiscent of those involving the antigens related to RD114 (and hence BaEV) in SLE, reported by Strand and August (1974b) and Mellors and Mellors (1976), and antibodies cross-reacting with RD114 p30, reported by Mellors and Mellors (1978).

Sawyer et al. (1978) detected by immunofluorescence an antigen reacting with anti-HEL-12V antibodies in each of the 24 normal human placentas studied. The antigen is expressed on the villous stromal cells, rather than the syncytiotrophoblast in which budding virions are observed (see Section IV.C).

4. *Kaplan's Viruses*

Kaplan et al. (1977) described the production of C-type particles from SU-DHL-1 lymphoma cells. The SU-DHL-1 cell line was established from a pleural effusion of a 10-year-old boy with diffuse histiocytic lymphoma (Epstein and Kaplan 1974). SU-DHL-1 cells have markers characteristic of lymphoma cells, are aneuploid, and lack EBV nuclear antigen. The virus was first detected as reverse transcriptase activity in particulate fractions of cells and culture fluids. Virions were produced in early (40 days), as well as later, cell passages. The enzyme activity was partially inhibited by antibodies to reverse transcriptase of SSAV or RD114 viruses. Cocultivation of SU-DHL-1 cells with XC cells induced XC-cell fusion. Cocultivation with a variety of human and animal cell lines yielded little evidence of infective transmission. Subsequent studies, however, indicate that the SU-DHL-1 virus can infect and "transform" normal human hematopoietic cells in culture (Kaplan 1978; Kaplan et al. 1979).

The reverse transcriptase of SU-DHL-1 virus has been purified and is most closely related immunologically and by tryptic peptide mapping to those of SSAV and GALV and more distantly to those of BaEV, RD114, and FeLV (Goodenow and Kaplan 1979; Goodenow et al. 1980). Monoclonal antibodies were raised using as immunogen virions purified from 4 liters of culture fluid (Goodenow et al. 1980). Two cloned hybridoma lines produced monoclonal antibodies reacting with reverse transcriptase and p28, respectively. Monoclonal antibody to SU-DHL-1 reverse transcriptase inhibited the enzyme activity of SU-DHL-1 virus most strongly; it also inhibited those of SSAV, GALV, BaEV, and Moloney MLV (Mo-MLV). A 75,000-dalton protein precipitated from labeled extracellular extracts of SU-DHL-1 cells was characterized by tryptic peptides as viral reverse transcriptase. The monoclonal antibody to p28 also precipitated SSAV p28; more limited reaction was observed with BaEV and MLV p30. These monoclonal antibodies could be usefully exploited in comparisons between putative human isolates from different laboratories.

In addition to SU-DHL-1, 7 of 14 further lymphoma cell lines produce low levels of C-type virions (Kaplan et al. 1979). Three of these viruses have been partially characterized and have properties similar to those of SU-DHL-1 virus. One virus is produced by another diffuse histiocytic lymphoma (SU-DHL-10), one by an undifferentiated lymphoma (SU-DUL-1), and a third by an American Burkitt's lymphoma (SU-AmB-3). All the viruses infected and transformed human bone-marrow cells, and SU-AmB-3 virus also induced cell fusion in fu-7 myoblasts (Kaplan et al. 1979). The infected bone-marrow cells underwent morphological changes resembling myelomonocytic leukemia, but they could not be sustained for more than 8 weeks and are thought by these authors to represent a kind of abortive transformation.

5. Significance of Human Isolates

Owing to the close relationship of the human isolates cited above to SSAV, on the one hand, and to BaEV, on the other, it is tempting to assume that these isolates from human cells have arisen as laboratory contaminants. Although several of the isolates exhibited variations in antigenicity or nucleic acid homology with SSAV or BaEV, their propagation in different cells might account for variation by selection or genetic drift. However, the possible human provenance of these viruses should not be so lightly dismissed. Nooter, Panem, and Kaplan, and their associates, had never knowingly handled primate retroviruses before the discovery of their human isolates. Moreover, isolates were made repeatedly from particular cell lines or strains and not from other cells equally susceptible to experimental infection with GALV/SSAV. In the case of patient HL23, SSAV and BaEV RNAs and reverse transcriptase activities could be identified in spleen tissue not cultivated in the laboratory (Reitz et al. 1976). It is strange that SSAV-related DNA was not detected in this or other patients' spleens (Wong-Staal et al. 1976). Similar reverse transcriptase activity has been found in the spleens of other leukemic and preleukemic patients (Witkin et al. 1975; Chandra et al. 1980).

The viruses isolated in the four laboratories cited each displayed very low levels of infectivity, and productive infection of experimental cells was not easily established. HEL-12V infection undergoes a cycle from antigen synthesis to productive infection and back to a nonproductive state (Panem et al. 1977; Black et al. 1981). Infection of cells containing Ki-MSV yielded chronically productive infections (Teich et al. 1975; Nooter et al. 1977, 1978). It is not clear in each case whether the human isolates comprised a mixture of viruses resembling SSAV and BaEV or one virus with properties related to both groups. HL23V-1 propagated in rat cells appeared to lose the BaEV-related component, and this indicates that the original virus was a mixture. It is conceivable, therefore, that humans are commonly infected with these types of viruses but that these viruses are productive only in mixed infection.

A model for the maintenance of infection by a mixed virus population has been established by Schnitzer (1979) in cells that are resistant to infection by either component alone. Using VSV pseudotypes with the envelope properties of primate viruses, Schnitzer et al. (1977) demonstrated that mouse cells were resistant to SSAV infection at the receptor level and to BaEV at a postpenetration stage of the replicative cycle. Schnitzer (1979) therefore tested the efficacy of replication in rodent cells of mixed populations of BaEV and the SSAV-related component of HL23V-1. Whereas a mixture of purely grown BaEV and HL23V-1 could not infect mouse cells, a phenotypically mixed population propagated in bat cells (which support replication of both viruses) would initiate and sustain the synthesis of HL23V-1 in mouse cells. Thus, there is a possibility that some human cells will also sustain productive infection only when mixed infection occurs.

Kaplan's and Nooter's viruses exhibited some capacity to transform normal hematopoietic cells. Many of the primate C-type viruses, including GALV, BaEV, and HL23V-1, are able to block the differentiation of the myelomonocytic cell line HL60 (Collins et al. 1977, 1979). Markham et al. (1979) have observed enhanced proliferation of human B lymphocytes cultured from fresh blood by GALV and SSV. There is, then, evidence that primate retroviruses affect human hematopoietic cell growth and differentiation in vitro and therefore might do so in vivo if natural human infection occurs.

There is little seroepidemiological evidence for human infection with GALV/SSV- or BaEV-related viruses. Initial reports of human antibodies specific to the gp70 of these viruses are probably due to heterophile carbohydrate moieties, although there is some evidence for enhanced antibody titers in certain cancer patients and laboratory workers (see Section II.F). A recent report by Tóth et al. (1980) describes the detection of specific membrane immunofluorescence in cells infected with HL23V-1 or BaEV with antibodies from acute myelogenous leukemia and preleukemic patients. If human subjects were infected with exogenous viruses prenatally, there might generally be immunological tolerance (as seen in chickens infected with leukosis viruses), and the possibility remains that the human placental virions (see Section IV.C) are related to the viruses described here. BaEV is clearly endogenous to baboons; the strong resemblance of a component of the human isolates to BaEV remains puzzling, as closely related genomes are not endogenous to man. However, BaEV-related viruses have spread to other host species in the past, as witnessed by the adoption of RD114-type viruses by ancestral cats (Benveniste and Todaro 1974).

The natural transmission of GALV/SSAV is poorly understood. Lieber et al. (1975) found that a related virus is endogenous to Asian mice, *Mus caroli* and *Mus cervicolor* (Chapter 2). It has been assumed that a murine endogenous virus became an exogenous virus of gibbon apes, perhaps quite recently. In fact, it has not been feasible to study feral gibbons with respect to retrovirus infections, and the provenance of GALV in the colonies of captive gibbons in which it has been found remains unknown (Chapter 2). It is noteworthy, however, that in three of the four colonies, gibbons had been inoculated with human tissues, such as malarial blood or Kuru brain tissue. There is just a possibility that GALV might be an exogenous human retrovirus for which gibbons represent a sensitive indicator species following unwitting experimental infection via human tissues.

SSV and SSAV were first isolated from a New World woolly monkey (Theilen et al. 1971; Wolfe et al. 1971). No studies of other monkeys of this species have been reported, so there is no evidence pertaining to natural retrovirus infections of woolly monkeys. The monkey concerned was a Californian pet in close contact with humans and at one time with a gibbon. It would appear that this monkey became infected with GALV but that the sarcoma-specific *sis* sequences of SSV originated in the monkey (Wong-Staal et al. 1981b).

In addition to the human virus isolates, it is difficult to discount the reports that continue to be published on SSAV/GALV-related virion components associated with occasional human leukemias and lymphomas. Recently, Derks et al. (1982) have reported data on a patient with chronic myeloid leukemia in blast-cell crisis, whose serum contained antibodies specific to SSAV p30 and whose leukemic blood cells expressed p30 and reverse transcriptase related to SSAV. In this case, antibodies and antigens related to the BaEV/RD114 group were not detected. The SSAV-related virions in freshly cultured bone-marrow cells of leukemic cultures (Mak et al. 1974, 1975) are also noteworthy. The polymerases purified from leukemic and myeloproliferative spleens (Mondal et al. 1975; Witkin et al. 1975; Chandra et al. 1980) resemble simian retroviral reverse transcriptase in all properties. Reverse transcriptase activity has been associated with polycythemia vera (Weimann et al. 1975), thrombocythemia (Brodsky et al. 1975), myelofibrosis (Steel et al. 1977; Chandra et al. 1980), and other chronic myeloid and lymphoid proliferative diseases (van Muyen et al. 1979). Perhaps more attention should be given to the study of preleukemic conditions, as leukemic cell clones might not express retroviruses as fully as hematopoietic cells in the proliferative disorders that predispose to leukemia.

In conclusion, the isolation of GALV/SSAV- and BaEV-related viruses from some human hematopoietic malignancies and a human embryo fibroblast culture remains a great enigma. Similar viruses may be expressed in SLE patients, in a minority of leukemia and lymphoma patients, and in some preleukemic conditions. Epidemiological evidence of infection is wanting, but the possibility of a ubiquitous, latent, prenatal infection cannot be ruled out. The development of molecularly cloned viral gene probes, and of monoclonal antibodies to primate retroviruses, has not yet helped to elucidate whether these viruses represent natural human infections. However, these new reagents, and new methods of clonal growth for specific cell types that could harbor the viruses, might reward further investigation into this frustrating area of human tumor virology.

C. Human Placental Virions

Particles resembling C-type viruses in human placentas were first detected by electron microscopy (Kalter et al. 1973b). Budding and complete particles were observed at the basal surface of the syncytiotrophoblast layer (Fig. 11.1) The particles were rare, necessitating the scanning of numerous thin sections of placental tissue and employing many hours of examination under the electron microscope. C-type particles were found in seven of nine full-term pla-

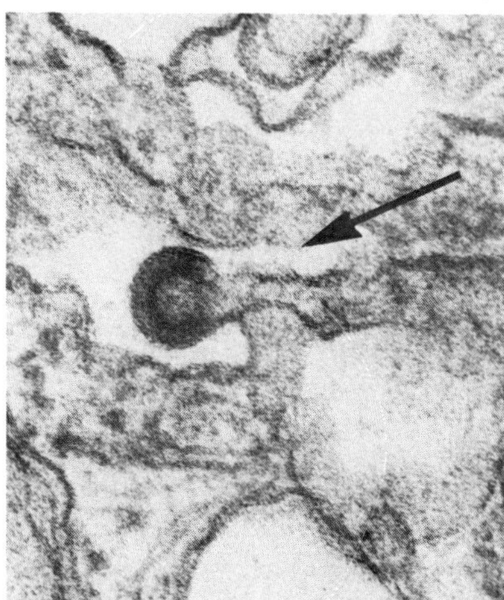

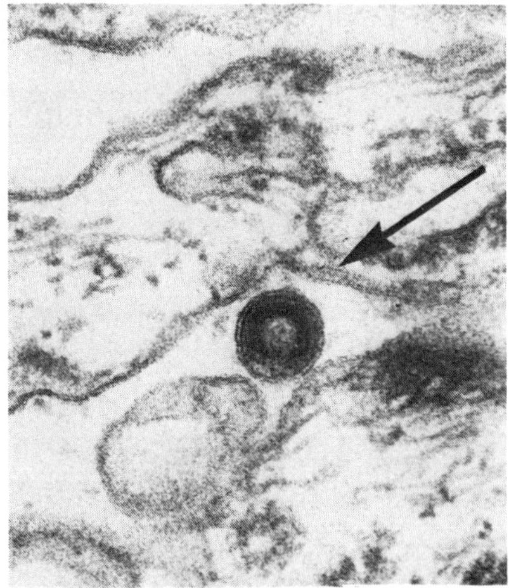

Figure 11.1 C-type viruslike particles in thin sections of syncytiotrophoblast of a normal, full-term human placenta. *(Left)* Budding particle; *(right)* immature particle. Staining was done with uranylacetate and lead citrate. Magnification 100,000×. (Reprinted, with permission, from Dirksen and Levy 1977.)

centas and in the placentas of two pregnancies aborted at 3 months' and 5.5 months' gestation. Dalton et al. (1974) distinguished the human placental particles from typical murine C-type particles by the absence of a distinct space between the nucleocapsid and the envelope. Particles with similar morphologies were observed at high frequency in placentas of baboons (Kalter et al. 1973a; Benveniste et al. 1974) and rhesus monkeys (Schidlovsky and Ahmed 1973; Feldman 1975).

The presence of occasional C-type particles in a majority of full-term human placentas examined was confirmed by Vernon et al. (1974), Imamura et al. (1976), and Dirksen and Levy (1977). In each case, particles with a convincing resemblance to C-type viruses were found mainly in the basal infoldings of the syncytiotrophoblast of the chorionic villi. Because of the possible association of retroviruses with SLE, the placentas from patients with SLE were examined to determine whether they expressed viruslike particles more frequently than do placentas from normal women (Imamura et al. 1976; Dirksen and Levy 1977). In neither study were particles seen with greater frequency in SLE placentas than in normal placental tissue.

Sawyer et al. (1978) detected antigens related to p30 of HEL-12 virus (see Section IV.B) in all normal full-term placentas examined. However, the p30-like antigen was expressed in mesenchymal cells of the fetal villi, and its relationship to the virions expressed in the syncytiotrophoblast layer is not clear. Thiry et al. (1978a,b) have detected both humoral and cell-mediated responses to simian retroviruses in pregnant women. The humoral responses were relatively high in pregnant women with pre-eclamptic toxemia characterized by raised blood pressure, edema, albuminuria, and poor placental function. The antibodies react with MPMV and BaEV. It is not known whether the immune reactions relate specifically to the virions or virus-related antigens expressed in placentas.

The presence of particles resembling C-type virions in human placentas prompted a search for reverse transcriptase activity (Nelson et al. 1978). Extracts from over 100 normal full-term placentas were examined and more than 80% of these placentas contained RNA-dependent DNA polymerase activity. The enzyme activity was specifically stimulated with exogenous rC.dG template primers and was associated with particles banding in sucrose at a density of 1.15–1.17 g/ml, typical of C-type particles. The enzyme activity was not significantly inhibited by antisera specific to GALV/SSAV, BaEV/RD114, or Ra-MLV. However, the absence of enzyme activity in a minority of placentas appeared to be related to the presence of an enzyme inhibitor in the placentas, which also inhibited Ra-MLV reverse transcriptase activity. The inhibitor was studied by Nelson et al. (1981) and was found to copurify with the retroviral particles. Partial characterization of the inhibitor indicated that it is nondialyzable; is insensitive to ether, phospholipase C, and trypsin; and is heat and pH stable. The inhibition of enzyme activity was reversible and could be specifically eliminated by addition of more virus to the reaction. A placenta particularly rich in inhibitor was obtained after normal delivery from a woman who had experienced four previous spontaneous abortions. This prompted Nelson et al. (1981) to speculate that the RNA-dependent DNA polymerase associated with viruslike particles in human placentas may play a role in normal placental development and that its function may be regulated by the inhibitor; excess inhibitor might predispose the fetus to abort.

The human placental virions merit further study. Cocultivation of placental tissue with indicator cell lines susceptible to most primate C-type viruses has not resulted in infectious transmission (J. Kirk and R. A. Weiss, pers. comm.). The particles may represent the expression of a human endogenous C-type virus, and it would be interesting to ascertain whether the syncytiotrophoblast expresses RNA related to the endogenous retroviruslike sequences detected in human DNA by Martin et al. (1981). It would also be interesting to determine whether abnormal trophoblastic tissues, such as those found in some hydatidiform moles and malignant choriocarcinoma, express similar viruslike particles. A preliminary examination of the choriocarcinoma-established cell line, BeWo, has not revealed retroviruses (J. Kirk and R. A. Weiss, pers. comm.). The synthesis of retroviral particles after IdU induction of certain testicular teratocarcinoma cell lines has been described previously (Bronson et al. 1978, 1979; Kurth et al. 1980). It is noteworthy that C-type particles were inducible in Tera-1 cells, but not in Tera-2 cells. Tera-1 cells respond to IdU by differentiating to form, among other tissues, extraembryonic cell types such as yolk-sac and trophoblast, whereas Tera-2 cells are not inducible for cell differentiation. It is conceivable, therefore, that IdU may not directly activate C-type particles in these human tumors but may promote differentiation to a cell type that promotes expression of the placental virion.

V. HUMAN T-CELL LYMPHOMA-LEUKEMIA VIRUSES (HTLV)

In contrast to the viruses discussed in Section IV, the recently discovered C-type virus, HTLV, in mature adult T-cell lymphoma-leukemia has looked convincing from the beginning as an etiological agent of human disease: (1) HTLV is a distinct and unique agent and is associated with a particular kind of malignancy. (2) HTLV is found in each case, and the patients produce specific antiviral antibodies. (3) HTLV appears to infect and transform appropriate target cells in culture. (4) Epidemiological studies indicate that endemic areas of widespread HTLV infection exist in Japan and the West Indies, where the occurrence of the disease has a relatively high incidence. Thus, Koch's postulates have been fulfilled, with the exception that induction of the disease in experimental animals has not yet been reported.

There has been some confusion over the classification of T-cell malignancies with which HTLV is associated. The first isolate (Poiesz et al. 1980b) was obtained from a patient in the United States with cutaneous T-cell lymphoma (CTCL) that appeared as an aggressive form of mycosis fungoides. A second isolate was made from cells of a patient with Sézary T-cell leukemia (Poiesz et al. 1981). Japanese patients are classified as having adult T-cell leukemia (ATL), in which skin lesions are also frequently present (Uchiyama et al. 1977; Kikuchi et al. 1979; Matsumoto et al. 1979; Nakajima et al. 1979; Shimoyama et al. 1979; The T- and B-Cell Malignancy Study Group 1981). Functionally, the Japanese ATL cells appear to behave as "suppressor" cells, whereas their surface phenotype defined by OKT monoclonal antibodies is T4 +, T6 −, T8 − (Takatsuki et al. 1979; Hattori et al. 1981), which is more characteristic of "helper/inducer" cells. A recent study of British patients of West Indian origin by Catovsky et al. (1982) also indicates that the tumor cell-surface phenotype is T4 +, T6 −, T8 −, characteristic of normal helper/inducer cells and Sézary cells. Whereas the adult T-cell lymphoma-leukemia cells have many similarities to those found in typical cases of Sézary syndrome and mycoses fungoides, Catovsky et al. (1982) noted distinctive histopathological features. Moreover, clinical differences were also manifest, the chief ones being hypercalcemia and the rapid progression of the disease. Catovsky et al. (1982) define the disease as T-lymphosarcoma-cell leukemia (T-LCL) but point out that the term adult T-cell lymphoma-leukemia is also appropriate, as the clinical features are those of a malignant lymphoma with leukemic expression. It would appear that clinically and histopathologically, the British and American T-LCL cases are indistinguishable from Japanese ATL and represent a single disease entity with which HTLV is associated.

HTLV was first detected as a C-type viruslike particle in the skin and lymph nodes of patients with mycosis fungoides and Sézary syndrome (van der Loo et al. 1979). As with the discovery of HL23V produced by myeloid leukemia cells (Section IV.B), the development of culture systems for normal and malignant mature T cells was important for virological studies (Poiesz et al. 1980a,b), particularly since HTLV has not yet been propagated in other cell types. The proliferation of mature T cells depends on a specific T-cell growth factor (TCGF), also known as interleukin-2 (Morgan et al. 1976; Mier and Gallo 1980; Ruscetti and Gallo 1981). Normal and malignant T cells can be grown for indefinite periods in culture in the presence of TCGF. Normal T cells in peripheral blood must first be stimulated to divide by inducing agents such as phytohemagglutinin and then can be maintained in a proliferative state by TCGF. Malignant T cells are also usually dependent on TCGF for continued proliferation, but TCGF-independent lines have been isolated which themselves release TCGF constitutively (Gazdar et al. 1980; Poiesz et al. 1980a).

A. Isolation and Characterization of HTLV

The first patient from whom HTLV was isolated was a 28-year-old black American (Poiesz et al. 1980b). A lymphoma cell line, HUT 102, was established in culture from a lymph node biopsy before the patient was treated with whole-body X-irradiation and combination chemotherapy (Gazdar et al. 1980). After 18 months of complete remission and shortly before the disease reappeared systemically, a second cell line, CTCL-3 [cutaneous T-cell lymphoma-3], was established from peripheral blood cells (Poiesz et al.

1980a). The proliferation of HUT 102 cells was initially TCGF-dependent, but after many passages the cells became autonomous; the growth of CTCL-3 has remained TCGF-dependent throughout its passage history (Poiesz et al. 1980a). At first, virus production from HUT 102 cells required IdU induction, but the cell line became a constitutive producer after the 56th passage. CTCL-23 produced virus constitutively after its second passage in culture. Mature and immature forms of C-type particles were seen in electron micrographs of thin sections, with only occasional budding forms. The particles were purified from culture medium and had the buoyant density and 70S RNA typical of retroviruses. RNA-dependent DNA polymerase activity characteristic of viral reverse transcriptase was associated with the particles, showing a preference for Mg^{++} over Mn^{++} under the assay conditions used. The enzyme activity was not inactivated by antisera specific to reverse transcriptases of GALV, SSAV, RD114, Ra-MLV or avian myeloblastosis virus (AMV). SDS-polyacrylamide gel electrophoresis revealed proteins of 52,000, 42,000, 24,000, 19,000, 13,000, and 10,000 daltons associated with virions produced by CTCL-3 cells. The morphological and biochemical characteristics indicate that HTLV most closely resembles bovine leukemia virus (BLV) among the well-known animal retroviruses (Burny et al. 1980) (Chapter 2).

HTLV particles produced by the HUT 102 cell line have been used to characterize the virus in more detail. Reitz et al. (1981) studied the viral genome. A cDNA probe synthesized by the endogenous reverse transcriptase reaction hybridized to completion with HTLV 70S RNA but did not cross-hybridize significantly with 70S RNA prepared from 16 strains of animal B-type, C-type, and D-type viruses, including primate viruses and BLV. Conversely, cDNA probes prepared from SSAV, BaEV, BLV, MPMV, and MMTV did not hybridize with RNA extracted from HUT 102 cells. HTLV therefore does not appear to have sequence homology with previously studied animal retroviruses. Reitz et al. (1981) also probed a variety of normal or malignant human and mammalian DNAs for sequences homologous to HTLV cDNA; no significant homology was found, except in HUT 102 cells. Further studies (Poiesz et al. 1981; R.C. Gallo, pers. comm.) showed that HTLV cDNA hybridized with DNA extracted from T-lymphoma-leukemia cells from a second patient, but not with DNA extracted from an EBV-positive B-lymphoblastoid cell line independently isolated from the same patient. These studies indicate that HTLV gene sequences are not endogenous in humans or in the animal species tested.

HTLV reverse transcriptase purified from HUT 102 particles was characterized in detail by Rho et al. (1981), who confirmed initial studies indicating that HTLV reverse transcriptase is not closely related to enzymes of known B-type, C-type, or D-type retroviruses. In addition to the reverse transcriptase data already reported by Poiesz et al. (1980b), Rho et al. (1981) reported that antisera specific to MPMV, MMTV, BLV, and FeLV did not neutralize HTLV reverse transcriptase activity. The preferred exogenous primer template was poly(C)·oligo(dG), with a relatively high concentration of Mg^{++}. These conditions are favored by B-type and D-type viral reverse transcriptases, and among C-type viruses, by BLV reverse transcriptase (Chapter 2).

Kalyanaraman et al. (1981b) studied the properties of p24, the major core protein of HTLV. A rabbit antiserum to detergent-disrupted HTLV allowed the development of a quantitative radioimmunoassay for p24 and immunologically related proteins, using ^{125}I-labeled p24. The major core proteins of several mammalian B-type, C-type, and D-type viruses, including BLV p24, failed to compete in the HTLV p24 radioimmunoassay. Conversely, HTLV p24 was not precipitated by antisera to major core antigens of other retroviruses. Kalyanaraman et al. (1981b) examined a variety of human lymphoma or lymphoblastoid cells for proteins competing in the p24 radioimmunoassay and found related antigens only in HUT 102 cells and CTCL-2 cells, from which a similar virus was subsequently isolated (Poiesz et al. 1981). Robert-Guroff et al. (1981) prepared a monoclonal antibody to HTLV p19, using disrupted HTLV as the immunogen. As judged by indirect immunofluorescence, the monoclonal antibody recognized antigen in HUT 102, CTCL-2, and CTCL-3 cells, but no related antigen was found in a variety of other human lymphomas and leukemias or in cells infected with nine different strains of mammalian retroviruses. Thus, the major core proteins of HTLV appear to be unique to this virus and to cells infected with the virus.

Gallo and his colleagues have made a further isolate of HTLV from a 64-year-old black female patient originally diagnosed as having Sézary T-cell leukemia (Poiesz et al. 1981). The cell line CTCL-2 (Poiesz et al. 1980a) was established from this patient, and it grew independently of TCGF. The CTCL-2 cells did not release HTLV constitutively, but virus production could be induced by IdU from the second passage onward. HTLV released from induced CTCL-2 cells has nucleic acid sequences, reverse transcriptase, p19, and p24 indistinguishable from those of HUT 102 HTLV. Hybridization studies with cDNA from HUT 102 HTLV show 45% hybridization to HUT 102 DNA and only 21% hybridization to CTCL-2 DNA (Poiesz et el. 1981). These findings suggest either that HTLV proviral sequences are present in only a fraction of the uncloned T-cell cultures or that only a portion of the provirus is preserved in the tumor cells.

The three cell lines, HUT 102, CTCL-2, and CTCL-3, release rather low amounts of HTLV, even after IdU induction (Poiesz et al. 1980b, 1981). The expression of RNA and the presence of proviral DNA do not increase with cell passage, suggesting that long-term culture of these cells does not select for HTLV producer clones. Because only small quantities of virus are synthesized, the cDNA preparations have not been of good quality and the viral genome has not yet been molecularly cloned. Attempts to infect numerous human and animal cell lines have been unsuccessful, but preliminary evidence (R. C. Gallo, pers. comm.) suggests that T lymphocytes from patients' relatives may be susceptible to infection by HTLV. As described below, a Japanese cell line does transmit virus to cord-blood T cells upon cocultivation, leading to the emergence of high-producer cell lines (Miyoshi et al. 1981).

The development of radioimmunoassays for p24 and p19 of HTLV enabled human sera to be studied for the presence of specific antibodies. Posner et al. (1981) used solid-phase radioimmunoassays to screen for antibodies to HTLV antigens in T-cell lymphoma-leukemia patients and in other patients or normal subjects. Sera from a series of 17 patients with CTCL and from 55 normal subjects were tested; sera from two CTCL patients reacted strongly to p24 in the radioimmunoassay. One was serum from the patient from whom the HUT 102 and CTCL-3 cell lines were derived. This serum also reacted with HTLV derived from CTCL-2 cells; unfortunately, serum from that patient was not available. The data are confusing because the CTCL patient serum numbers reported by Posner et al. (1981) do not tally with the CTCL cell culture numbers reported by Poiesz et al. (1980a,b, 1981). It would be interesting to know whether only the two CTCL patients with positive antisera fit the clinicopathological classification of Catovsky et al. (1982) for adult T-cell lymphoma-leukemia thought to be associated with HTLV.

The specificity of the antisera was confirmed by competition radioimmunoassays using lysates of HUT 102 cells and by radioimmunoprecipitation assays of labeled cellular proteins that copurify with HTLV p24 and p19 (Posner et al. 1981). Further tests using a modified radioimmunoprecipitation technique for p24 with the same sera confirmed these results (Kalyanaraman et al. 1981a). In addition, serum from the wife of the first patient contained specific anti-p24 HTLV antibodies. Seven more individuals have subsequently been found to produce anti-p24 serum antibodies (R. C. Gallo, pers. comm.).

The first four virus-positive individuals were blacks born in the Caribbean, except for one white man who spent several years of his youth there (W. A. Blattner and R. C. Gallo, pers. comm.). It is noteworthy that lymphoma among adults has a relatively high incidence in the Caribbean (Hamilton and Persaud 1981). Further studies of p24 antibodies among blacks indicate that the West Indies and southeastern United States are areas of endemic HTLV infection (W. A. Blattner and R. C. Gallo, pers. comm.). The six British cases of adult T-cell lymphoma-leukemia also occurred in blacks from the West Indian Islands and Guyana, and their sera contain high-titer antibodies to HTLV p24 (Catovsky et al. 1982). In summary, a C-type virus first observed serendipitously in a cultured cell line of T-lymphoma cells has encouraged the clinicopathological description of a new disease entity prevalent among people originating from the West Indies or southeastern United States. To what extend the clustering is ethnic as well as environmental remains to be determined.

B. Japanese Adult T-cell Leukemia

In contrast with Western adult T-cell lymphoma-leukemia, the pathological, epidemiological, and serological parameters of the disease in Japan all became apparent before the discovery of a C-type virus released by the malignant cells. ATL is relatively common in Japan. Like the Western cases of T-cell lymphoma-leukemia, Japanese ATL is characterized by rapid progression, poor prognosis, skin lesions, and hypercalcemia (Uchiyama et al.

1977; Kikuchi et al. 1979; Nakajima et al. 1979; Shimoyama et al. 1979; Takatsuki et al. 1979; The T- and B-Cell Malignancy Study Group 1981).

Adult T-cell lymphoma-leukemia was found to occur more commonly than any other leukemia in the Kagoshima (Matsumoto et al. 1979) and Nagasaki (Ichimaru et al. 1979) districts of Kyushu, the most southwestern of the major islands. Indeed, the mortality rate from adult T-cell lymphoma in Kyushu, southern Shikoku, and Okinawa is more than twice that of all Japan (Tajima et al. 1979). Moreover, when the distribution of ATL is mapped according to place of birth and childhood (Fig. 11.2), the clustering of cases in southwestern Japan is even more marked (Uchiyama et al. 1977; Hanaoka et al. 1979; The T- and B-Cell Malignancy Study Group 1981). It appears that an endemic area for ATL exists, which is characterized by high temperatures and much rainfall in summer (Tajima et al. 1979). The clustering of the disease is observed mainly in rural and coastal areas; a relatively high proportion of patients of both sexes worked in agriculture, fisheries, forestry, and primary industries, or grew up in families so engaged

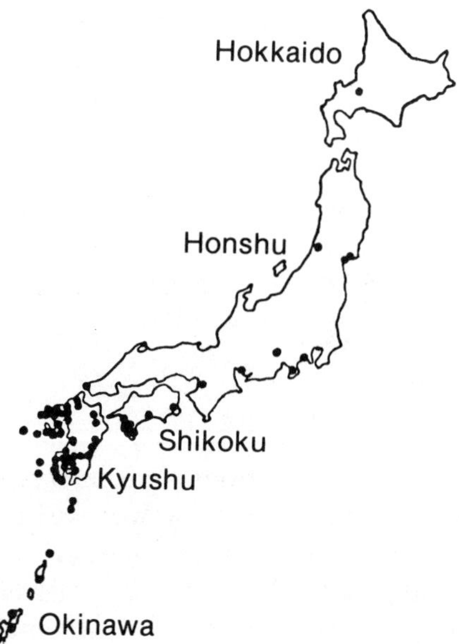

Figure 11.2 Incidence of adult T-cell lymphoma in Japan plotted according to place of patient's birth. (Adapted from Uchiyama et al. 1977 and The T- and B-Cell Malignancy Study Group 1981.)

before migration to industrial centers (The T- and B-Cell Malignancy Study Group 1981). These findings suggest that an environmental etiological agent is endemic in southwestern Japan, possibly transmitted by an insect or helminth vector.

Although the place of birth and childhood showed the greatest geographical clustering, indicating that infection occurred many years before development of the disease, a seasonal peak in the clinical onset of ATL was observed in the summer, in contrast to a small winter peak for the onset of B-cell malignancies (The T- and B-Cell Malignancy Study Group 1981). Several familial cases of ATL were also discovered, suggesting a heritable factor in transmission or susceptibility, but host factors such as HLA-type have not yet been determined.

The discovery of a retrovirus associated with Japanese ATL awaited the reports on American HTLV by Gallo's laboratory. Indeed, an early examination of peripheral blood cultures of two ATL patients failed to detect retroviral particles, although particulate reverse transcriptase activity was found in cultured cells of two myeloma patients examined in the same study (Sawada et al. 1977). The cell line MT-1, established from a Japanese ATL patient, possessed the characteristics of malignant T cells (Miyoshi et al. 1979, 1980). This cell line produced small amounts of C-type viral particles after induction with IdU (Hinuma et al. 1981). MT-1 cells contain viral core proteins and proviral DNA indistinguishable from American HTLV (Gallo et al. 1982). Indirect immunofluorescence with sera from ATL patients demonstrated the presence of a cytoplasmic antigen (ATLA) in 1–5% of the MT-1 cells, and IdU treatment increased the proportion of fluorescing MT-1 cells about fivefold (Hinuma et al. 1981). Anti-ATLA antibodies were found in all 44 patients with ATL and in 32 of 40 patients with nonleukemic lymphoma otherwise resembling ATL. The antibodies were also detected in 26% of the healthy adults living in ATL-endemic areas, but in only 2% of healthy adults living in other areas. Hinuma et al. (1981) therefore proposed that ATLA may be a retroviral antigen associated with ATL. If this is so, it is remarkable that 26% of the normal adults in endemic areas appear to be infected with the virus and produce equivalent titers of antibody to the ATL patients. Preliminary evidence indicates that synthesis of viral antigens can be activated from lymphocytes cultured from healthy, antibody-positive individuals, including blood donors (Miyoshi et al. 1982).

In an independent study, Kalyanaraman et al. (1982) and Robert-Guroff et al. (1982) have assayed sera from Japanese ATL patients and normal subjects for antibodies reacting with HTLV p24 and c19. Sera from six out of six untreated ATL patients contained high-titer anti-p24 antibodies, strongly indicating that Japanese ATL is associated with a virus closely related to the HTLV isolated from American patients. Lower-titer anti-p24 antibodies were found in a small proportion of other types of leukemia. However, sera from all 79 normal Japanese adults, including 39 from the endemic areas for ATL, were negative for p24 antibodies. As this is in contrast with the data obtained by Hinuma et al. (1981) for anti-ATLA antibodies, it raises doubts as to whether ATLA is identical to HTLV p24. There is clearly a need for anti-p24 and anti-ATLA tests to be made on the same set of sera. It is possible that ATLA might be related to HTLV gp55, for which no radioimmunoassays have yet been developed.

Recently, Miyoshi et al. (1981) have developed a second cell line, MT-2, which produces much more C-type virus than MT-1 or the American cell lines. Peripheral blood leukocytes from a 45-year-old female ATL patient were placed in culture and maintained without TCGF. After 2 months, the number of cells decreased considerably, and in the hope of stimulating the growth of the ATL cells, they were cocultivated with the umbilical-cord leukocytes of a male baby. After a further 2 months of coculture, a vigorous, EBV-negative lymphoid cell line with T-cell markers emerged and was designated MT-2. Miyoshi et al. (1981) were surprised to discover that MT-2 cells were male. Almost 100% of the MT-2 cells gave strong fluorescence for ATLA, using reference antisera that did not react with non-ATL T-cell lines. Abundant mature and immature C-type particles were produced by MT-2 cells without IdU activation, although budding particles were rarely seen. A third T-cell line derived from cord-blood cells was developed in a similar way to MT-2 by cocultivation with ATL cells from another patient. This line also produced abundant C-type particles. It would appear, therefore, that some human umbilical-cord T-lymphocytes are susceptible to infection and transformation by ATL virus and support virus replication more efficiently than the original leukemia cells. The virus released from MT-2 cells will be most useful for immunological and molecular genetics studies and for comparison with the American HTLV isolates.

HTLV most closely resembles BLV in biochemical properties. Its pathogenesis and mechanism of spread may also be related to BLV, except that BLV-induced neoplasms are always of the B-cell lineage (Chapter 8). BLV is horizontally transmitted by close contact or, in some regions, possibly by an insect vector, but it probably requires the transfer of infected cells rather than free virus. The tumors, which frequently present cutaneously, take many years to appear, but anti-p24 and anti-gp55 antibodies can be identified long before the disease is manifest. The replication of BLV in lymphocytes in vivo appears to be suppressed not only by antibody, but also by other nonimmunoglobulin inhibitors (Gupta and Ferrer 1982). γ-Interferon is produced in large amounts by human T-lymphoma cells and may inhibit virion maturation. It is therefore exceptional to see release of virus by tumor cells unless they are placed in culture and treated with IdU. It has not been reported whether HTLV is subject to lysis by antibody-independent binding of human complement, as described for simian and murine viruses in Section II.F.

Much remains to be learned about the natural history and epidemiology of HTLV and its relationship to adult T-cell lymphoma-leukemia. It is not known for how long southwestern Japan and the Caribbean have been endemic areas for adult T-cell lymphoma-leukemia. Other endemic areas (possibly southeastern China) may also exist. The incidence of ATL in Japan has risen sharply during the last 30 years (Tajima et al. 1979). As yet, the natural mode of transmission is not known, although HTLV is clearly an exogenous, infectious viral agent. By analogy with BLV, it is possible that HTLV will spread through the human population, owing to modern trends in migration and travel. Bovine leukosis can be controlled by the ruthless elimination of infected cattle from herds, a method unsuitable for the control of human disease! Provided HTLV infection is postnatal, the prospect for developing an effective vaccine using MT-2 or a similar virus isolate, or its cloned genes, should be promising.

VI. HUMAN ONCOGENES

A. Identification and Expression of *c-onc* Genes in Human Tissues and Tumors

As postulated by Weiss (1973), the transforming *(onc)* genes of retroviruses appear to be derived from normal, cellular genes. This was first determined for the *src* gene of RSV with the discovery that sequences homologous to *src* were present in the DNAs of normal chickens (Stehelin et al. 1976) and other vertebrates, including humans (Spector et al. 1978). The oncogenes of three distinct avian acute leukemia viruses were also shown to have homologous cellular genes (Roussel et al. 1979). As described in Chapter 9 (see Tables 9.1 and 9.2), some 15 distinct viral oncogenes *(v-onc)* have now been identified that have cellular homologs *(c-onc)* in host genomes.

Human DNA is no exception in carrying *c-onc* genes, and because *c-onc* sequences are relatively well conserved in evolution, *v-onc* probes derived from animal retroviruses can be exploited to identify homologous human *c-onc* genes and to study their expression in normal and malignant cells. It is not known how many potential *onc* genes exist in vertebrate genomes. Different naturally occurring retroviruses have acted as transducing agents for homologous *c-onc* genes on different occasions (e.g., Fujinami avian sarcoma virus, and Snyder-Theilen and Gardner-Arnstein strains of feline sarcoma virus [Shibuya et al. 1980]), suggesting that a limited number of transducible oncogenes exist in host genomes. Furthermore, as described in Chapter 8, the pathogenesis of nonacute lymphoma viruses involves integration adjacent to, and promotion of genes homologous to, *v-onc* genes found in defective acute leukemia viruses (Hayward et al. 1981). It is therefore reasonable to expect that similar gene activation may operate in some cases of nonviral oncogenesis and that naturally occurring human tumors might be usefully probed for abnormal or ectopic *c-onc* expression.

Human DNA sequences homologous to the following *onc* genes have been detected by molecular hybridization: *src* of RSV (Spector et al. 1978), *myb* of AMV (Bergmann et al. 1981), *abl* of Abelson MLV (Dale and Ozanne 1981), *bas/ras* of BALB and Harvey MSVs, *fes* of Snyder-Theilen feline sarcoma virus (Eva et al. 1982), and *sis* of SSV (Wong-Staal et al. 1981a). Restriction enzyme mapping of human DNA using molecularly cloned probes indicates that most human *c-onc* genes occur at single loci and contain several introns not present in *v-onc* sequences. A detailed analysis of the human *c-sis* gene by Dalla-Favera et al. (1981) following the isolation of a recombinant phage containing the entire human *c-sis* locus shows that it extends over a region of 12 kb, which includes 1.2 kb of *v-sis*-related sequences interrupted by four introns containing *Alu* repeat sequences. There does not appear to be marked polymorphism of *c-onc* genes in human DNA, as judged by restriction mapping within the loci (Wong-Staal et al. 1981a). However, it will be of considerable interest to study possible rearrangements of *c-onc* genes and neighboring sequences in tumor cells.

There is currently much interest in investigating the expression of human *c-onc* genes in normal and neoplastic cells. The presence of RNA transcripts containing homologous sequences has been examined in human cells using molecularly cloned *v-onc* sequences. Eva et al. (1982) probed the expression of *c-myc, c-sis, c-abl,* and *c-bas* (Andersen et al. 1981) in cell lines established from human carcinomas, sarcomas, melanomas, glioblastomas, and a teratocarcinoma. All the cell lines tested by these authors, including normal human fibroblasts, expressed a single 2.7-kb transcript homologous to *myc,* which is presumably the equivalent transcript to those found in avian and rodent cells (see Chapter 9, Table 9.3). However, four cell lines comprising one sarcoma, two carcinomas, and one lymphoblastoid possessed strikingly higher levels of *myc* RNA, as judged semiquantitatively by the intensity of *myc* hybridization to gel-fractionated RNA. Eva et al. (1982) detected a 4.2-kb transcript related to *sis* in 8 of 23 human tumor cell lines examined, including a majority of sarcomas and glioblastomas, but no carcinomas or melanomas. A second, smaller *sis*-related transcript was discernible in a few of the positive cell lines. Transcripts hybridizing to *bas* and *abl* probes were detected in all of the human tumor lines tested and in normal fibroblasts. Both probes hybridized to a complex pattern of transcripts. A curious point not discussed by Eva et al. (1982) is that prominent RNA bands of 7.0, 5.9, and 1.8 kb were evident in Northern blots probed by either *bas* or *abl* clones; it is odd that identical-size transcripts should be detected in human cells when the two oncogenes share no homology.

Cloned *v-onc* probes have also been used to study the expression of *c-onc* homologs in human hematopoietic cells. Westin et al. (1982a) studied the expression of sequences homologous to the *myb* gene of AMV in human hematopoietic cells, including the HL-60 cell line derived from a patient with acute myeloblastic leukemia (Collins et al. 1977). HL-60 cells can be induced to differentiate into granulocytes by dimethylsulfoxide (Collins et al. 1979) or into macrophages by phorbol ester (Rovera et al. 1979). Westin et al. (1982a) found that *myb* expression was high in all proliferating myeloblasts but was suppressed in HL-60 cells after treatment with the inducing agents. Westin et al. (1982b) studied the expression of several *c-onc* sequences in human hematopoietic cells. All proliferating cells, whether derived from normal marrow or from leukemias, expressed multiple-size transcripts of *abl* and *bas* genes and single transcripts of *myc* and *sis* genes. Thus, the expression of these *c-onc* sequences does not appear to be linked specifically with neoplastic cells. Dale and Ozanne (1981) independently cloned the *v-abl* gene and have used it to probe *c-abl* expression in human acute lymphoblastic leukemia cells (B. Ozanne, pers. comm.). Although many leukemic cells expressed low levels of *abl* sequences, two established lines which have properties similar to those of the pre-B cells of murine Abelson leukemias, expressed very high levels.

Studies of the control of expression of *c-onc* homologs in human cells are still in their infancy. Particular attention will be given to cases of expression restricted to specific tumor or normal cell types and to high levels of expression. It will be interesting to see whether ectopic *c-onc* expression might correlate with cytogenetic anomalies in tumors when the chromosomal assignment of human *c-onc* genes is known.

By analogy with the enhanced promotion of *c-onc* genes by retroviruses in avian lymphomagenesis (Hayward et al. 1981) (see Chapter 8), it will be important to ascertain whether the proviral DNA of HTLV is integrated at specific sites in the genome of human T-lymphoma cells. A study of DNA sequences adjacent to the HTLV provirus or of RNA transcribed under the control of HTLV LTR may reveal a human cellular gene that plays a role in the malignant state of mature T cells.

B. Human Transforming Genes Identified by DNA Transfection

The induction of heritable phenotypic transformation by the transfer of DNA has a long history as a genetic tool. The original observations of pneumococcal transformation by Griffith (1928) led to the discovery by Avery et al. (1944) that DNA was the "transforming principle" and hence to the identification of DNA as the chemical repository of genetic information. Ever since Hill and Hillova (1971) first achieved funtional transfection of integrated proviral RSV DNA, there has been interest in the prospect of identifying oncogenes by DNA-transfer techniques. Karpas and Tuckerman (1974) reported the transformation of human fibroblasts by DNA extracted from human rhabdomyosarcoma cells, but this study has not been confirmed and human fibroblasts are notoriously difficult to transform into stable, neoplastic lines even by potent oncogenic viruses. Nicolson et al. (1978) surveyed a number of human sarcomas and leukemias for transforming DNA without success. However, the development of efficient DNA-transfection methods (Graham and van der Eb 1973) and the use of NIH-3T3 recipient cells for neoplastic transformation have more recently led to the development of reliable and consistent transfection assays for nonviral oncogenes in rodent cells transformed by chemical carcinogens (Shih et al. 1979; Cooper et al. 1980).

DNA preparations from a number of human tumor cell lines have recently been shown to transform NIH-3T3 cells in culture. Krontiris and Cooper (1981) and Shih et al. (1981) observed oncogenic transformation following transfection of DNA prepared from the EJ bladder carcinoma line. Murray et al. (1981) found that transfecting DNAs from the colon carcinoma line SW-480, the bladder carcinoma line EJ, and the acute myeloblastic leukemia line HL-60 represented three distinct human transforming genes. Perucho et al. (1981) detected 5 out of 21 human solid tumors with consistent transforming DNA (1 bladder, 1 colon, 2 lung carcinomas, and 1 neuroblastoma). Two lung carcinoma lines and one colon carcinoma line yielded the same transforming DNA, indicating that different kinds of tumors may express similar oncogenes. Oncogenes in soft tissue sarcoma have also been identified by transfection (C. J. Marshall, A. Hall, and R. A. Weiss, pers. comm.). Lane et al. (1981) have studied oncogenes extracted from mammary carcinomas. The transforming activity of DNA extracted from the human mammary carcinoma line MCF-7 was inactivated by the same restriction enzymes as were transforming DNAs of five MMTV-induced mouse mammary carcinomas and one dimethylbenzanthracene-induced mouse mammary carcinoma. These results indicate that the same or closely related transforming genes were activated in the six mouse tumors and the human tumor.

The human oncogenes were passaged by secondary transfection to fresh NIH-3T3 cells, and the secondary transformants contained unique DNA fragments containing only the oncogene and human sequences proximal to it (Murray et al. 1981; Perucho et al. 1981). The highly repetitive *Alu* sequences widely dispersed in human DNA but absent from mouse DNA were found adjacent to the oncogenes; thus the *Alu* sequences can sometimes be used as a tag for the presence, location, and cloning of the transferred human genes.

The transfecting sequences from the mouse mammary tumors studied by Lane et al. (1981) were not linked to exogenous or endogenous MMTV sequences. Similarly, studies with avian bursal lymphoma DNA showed that the oncogenes identified by transfection of NIH-3T3 cells were not linked to retroviral sequences or to the *c-myc* gene that is activated in these tumors (Cooper and Neiman 1981). Attempts to rescue transfected oncogenes with helper retroviruses have been unsuccessful (Shih et al. 1981). From these results it is apparent that the oncogenes revealed by DNA transfection are not part of or linked to retroviruses even when a retrovirus induced the tumor, and their relationship to *c-onc* homologs of *v-onc* genes has yet to be fully evaluated. With the exception of the avian lymphomas and mouse mammary tumors, all of the tumors reported so far as carrying transfectable oncogenes were derived from established cell lines; it will be important to ascertain whether the same genes are expressed in primary tumors.

C. Retroviruses as Vectors for Human Genes

Since retroviruses occasionally serve as transducing agents for cellular oncogenes (Weiss 1973; Stephenson et al. 1979), they might be exploited as vectors for human oncogenes. Avian retroviruses (Stavnezer et al. 1981) and murine retroviruses (Rasheed et al. 1978) incorporate *c-onc* genes from certain cells into their genomes at detectable frequencies. The passage of retroviruses through human cells might therefore give rise to oncogenic transducing viruses, either because the first step in transduction is the incorporation of cellular mRNA into virions (Weiss 1973) or because the provirus integrates near the active oncogene and generates a "hybrid" transcript (Hayward et al. 1981). Furthermore, in vitro genetic manipulation allows genes of extraneous origin to be functionally linked with retroviral genome segments and to come under the control of retroviral LTR sequences, e.g., mouse dihydrofolate reductase (Lee et al. 1981) and herpes simplex virus thymidine kinase (Wei et al. 1981). Cloned *c-onc* genes of normal cells can also be ligated to retroviral LTRs to generate transmissible, oncogenic viruses (Blair et al. 1981). This methodology will be useful for studying the experimental pathogenesis of human cellular oncogenes and other kinds of genes.

VII. EPILOGUE

This volume on retroviruses has encompassed the considerable advances in our understanding of these viruses that have occurred since their discovery 70 years ago. It is to be hoped that the previous chapters have shown what fascinating systems retroviruses provide for studying many aspects of virus-host relationships, molecular genetics of viruses and animal cells, and mechanisms of neoplastic transformation. Retroviruses will no doubt continue to hold the attention of molecular biologists and experimental pathologists for several years to come, independent of their importance in human disease.

Although frustrated in many avenues, the search for human RNA tumor viruses has left some intriguing puzzles to be solved. Yet it has revealed at least one important, if rare, human malignancy that is closely associated with infection by a unique retrovirus. Moreover, the exploitation of retroviruses for probing the organization and expression of human genes active in malignant cells is just beginning.

REFERENCES

Achong, B.G., P.A. Trumper, and B.C. Giovanella. 1976. C-type virus particles in human tumours transplanted into nude mice. *Br. J. Cancer* **34:**203–206.

Ahmed, M., G. Schidlovsky, W. Karol, G. Vidrine, and J.L. Cicmanec. 1974. Occurrence of Mason-Pfizer monkey virus in healthy rhesus monkeys. *Cancer Res.* **34:**3504–3508.

Alderson, M.R. 1980. The epidemiology of leukemia. *Adv. Cancer Res.* **31:**1–76.

Alderson, M.R. and R. Nayak. 1971. A study of space-time clustering in Hodgkin's disease in the Manchester region. *Brit. J. Prev. Soc. Med.* **25:**168–173.

Ames, R.P., J.T. Sobota, R.L. Reagan, and M. Karon. 1966. Virus-like particles and cytopathic activity in urine of patients with leukemia. *Blood* **28:**465–478.

Andersen, P.R., S.G. Devare, S.R. Tronick, R.W. Ellis, S.A. Aaronson, and E.M. Scolnick. 1981. Generation of BALB/-MuSV and Ha-MuSV by type C virus transduction of homologous transforming genes from different species. *Cell* **26:**129–134.

Anderson, D.E. 1974. Genetic study of breast cancer: Identification of a high risk group. *Cancer* **34:**1090–1097.

———. 1975. Genetics and breast cancer. In *Early breast cancer: Detection and treatment* (ed. H.S. Gallager), pp. 41–49. Wiley, New York.

Aoki, T., M.J. Walling, G.S. Bushar, M. Liu, and K.C. Hsu. 1976. Natural antibodies in sera from healthy humans to antigens on surfaces of type C RNA viruses and cells from primates. *Proc. Natl. Acad. Sci.* **73:**2491–2495.

Armstrong, B.K., J.B. Brown, H.T. Clarke, D.K. Crooke, R. Hahnel, J.R. Masarei, and T. Ratajczak. 1981. Diet and reproductive hormones: A study of vegetarian and nonvegetarian postmenopausal women. *J. Natl. Cancer Inst.* **67:**761–767.

Arnoult, J. and F. Haguenau. 1966. Problems raised by the search for virus particles in human leukemia. A study with the electron microscope of blood plasma, cerebrospinal fluid, and megakaryocytes from bone marrow. *J. Natl. Cancer Inst.* **36:**1089–1109.

Aulakh, G.S. and R.C. Gallo. 1977. Rauscher-leukemia-virus-related sequences in human DNA: Presence in some tissues of some patients with hematopoietic neoplasias and absence in DNA from other tissues. *Proc. Natl. Acad. Sci.* **74:**353–357.

Avery, O.T., C.M. MacLeod, and M. McCarty. 1944. Studies on the chemical nature of the substance inducing transformation of pneumococcal types. Induction of transformation by a desoxyribonucleotide acid fraction isolated from Pneumococcus type III. *J. Exp. Med.* **79:** 137–158.

Axel, R., S. Gulati, and S. Spiegelman. 1972a. Particles containing RNA instructed DNA polymerase and virus related RNA in human breast cancers. *Proc. Natl. Acad. Sci.* **69:**3133–3137.

Axel, R., J. Schlom, and S. Spiegelman. 1972b. Presence in human breast cancer of RNA homologous to mouse mammary tumor virus RNA. *Nature* **235:**32–36.

Balabanova, H., M. Kotler, and Y. Becker. 1975. Transformation of cultured human embryonic fibroblasts by oncornavirus-like particles released from a human carcinoma cell line. *Proc. Natl. Acad. Sci.* **72:**2794–2798.

Balda, B.R., R. Hehlmann, J.-R. Cho, and S. Spiegelman. 1975. Oncornavirus-like particles in human skin cancers. *Proc. Natl. Acad. Sci.* **72:**3697–3700.

Baluda, M.A. and P. Roy-Burman. 1973. Partial characterization of RD114 virus by DNA-RNA hybridization studies. *Nat. New Biol.* **244:**59–62.

Barbacid, M., D. Bolognesi, and S.A. Aaronson. 1980a. Humans have antibodies capable of recognizing oncoviral glycoproteins: Demonstration that these antibodies are formed in response to cellular modification of glycoproteins rather than as consequence of exposure to virus. *Proc. Natl. Acad. Sci.* **77:**1617–1621.

Barbacid, M., L.K. Long, and S.A. Aaronson. 1980b. Major structural proteins of type B, type C, and type D oncoviruses share interspecies antigenic determinants. *Proc. Natl. Acad. Sci.* **77:**72–76.

Bauer, H., J.H. Daams, K.F. Watson, K. Mölling, H. Gelderblom, and W. Schäfer. 1974. Oncornavirus-like particles in HeLa cells. II. Immunological characterization of the virus. *Int. J. Cancer* **13:**254–261.

Baxt, W. and S. Spiegelman. 1972. Nuclear DNA sequences present in human leukemic cells and absent in normal leukocytes. *Proc. Natl. Acad. Sci.* **69:**3737–3741.

Baxt, W., R. Hehlmann, and S. Spiegelman. 1972. Human leukaemic cells contain reverse transcriptase associated with a high molecular weight virus-related RNA. *Nat. New Biol.* **240:**72–75.

Baxt, W.G., A.W. Yates, H.J. Wallace, J.F. Holland, and S. Spiegelman. 1973. Leukemia specific DNA sequences in leukocytes of the leukemic member of identical twins. *Proc. Natl. Acad. Sci.* **70:**2629–2632.

Benveniste, R.E. and G.J. Todaro. 1974. Evolution of C-type viral genes: Inheritance of exogenously acquired viral genes. *Nature* **252:**456–459.

———. 1976. Evolution of type C viral genes: Evidence for an Asian origin of man. *Nature* **261:**101–108.

Benveniste, R.E., M.M. Lieber, D.M. Livingston, C.J. Sherr, G.J. Todaro, and S.S. Kalter. 1974. Infectious C-type virus isolated from a baboon placenta. *Nature* **248:**17–20.

Bergholz, C.M., J.T. Reynolds, and S. Panem. 1980. Biological and antigenic characteristics of HEL-12 virus. *J. Gen. Virol.* **50:**247–257.

Bergholz, C.M., L.G. Wolfe, F. Deinhardt, B. Thakkar, and B. Marczynska. 1977. Oncogenicity in marmosets of HL-23V, a type C oncornavirus isolated from human leukemic cells, and comparison with simian sarcoma virus type 1 (SSV-1/SSAV-1). *J. Natl. Cancer Inst.* **58:**1041–1046.

Bergmann, D.G., L.M. Souza, and M.A. Baluda. 1981. Vertebrate DNAs contain nucleotide sequences related to the transforming gene of avian myeloblastosis virus. *J. Virol.* **40:**450–455.

Bishop, J.M., N. Quintrell, E. Medeiros, and H.E. Varmus. 1974. Of birds and mice and men: Comments on the use of animal models and molecular hybridization in the search for human tumor viruses. *Cancer* **34:**1421–1426.

Black, M.M., D.H. Moore, B. Shore, R.E. Zachrau, and H.P. Leis, Jr. 1974. Effect of murine milk samples and human breast tissues on human leukocyte migration indices. *Cancer Res.* **34:**1054–1060.

Black, M.M., R.E. Zachrau, B. Shore, D.H. Moore, and H.P. Leis, Jr. 1975. Prognostically favorable immunogens of human breast cancer tissue: Antigenic similarity to murine mammary tumor virus. *Cancer* **35:**121–128.

Black, M.M., R.E. Zachrau, A.S. Dion, B. Shore, D.L. Fine, H.P. Leis, and C.J. Williams. 1976. Cellular hypersensitivity to gp55 of RIII-murine mammary tumor virus and gp55-like protein of human breast cancer. *Cancer Res.* **36:**4137–4142.

Black, R.J., J.W.-T. Yang, and S. Panem. 1981. Restricted HEL-12 virus infection in *de novo* infected human and canine cells. *J. Gen. Virol.* **57:**343–355.

Blair, D.G., M. Oskarsson, T.G. Wood, W.L. McClements, P.J. Fischinger, and G.G. Vande Woude. 1981. Activation of the transforming potential of a normal cell sequence: A molecular model for oncogenesis. *Science* **212:**941–943.

Bowen, J.M., L. Dmochowski, M.F. Miller, E.S. Priori, G. Seman, M.L. Dodson, and K. Maryama. 1976. Implication of humoral antibody in mice and humans to breast tumor and mouse mammary tumor virus-associated antigens. *Cancer Res.* **36:**759–764.

Brodsky, I., A.A. Fuscaldo, B.J. Erlick, E.W. Kingsbury, G.M. Schultz, and K.E. Fuscaldo. 1975. Analysis of platelets from patients with thrombocythemia for reverse transcriptase and virus-like particles. *J. Natl. Cancer Inst.* **55:**1069–1974.

Bronson, D.L., E.E. Fraley, J. Fogh, and S.S. Kalter. 1979. Induction of retrovirus particles in human testicular tumor (Tera-1) cell cultures: An electron microscope study. *J. Natl. Cancer Inst.* **63:**337–339.

Bronson, D.L., D.M. Ritzi, E.E. Fraley, and A.J. Dalton. 1978. Morphologic evidence for retrovirus production by epithelial cells derived from a human testicular tumor metastasis. *J. Natl. Cancer Inst.* **60:**1305–1308.

Bukrinskaya, A.G., G.G. Miller, E.N. Lebedeva, and V.M. Zhdanov. 1974. Intracellular virus-specific structures and RNAs in oncornavirus-producing human cells. *J. Virol.* **13:**478–487.

Burger, C.L., W.W. Harris, N.G. Anderson, T.W. Bartlett, and R.M. Kniseley. 1964. Virus-like particles in human leukemic plasma. *Proc. Soc. Exp. Biol. Med.* **115:**151–156.

Burny, A., C. Bruck, H. Chantrenne, Y. Cleuter, D. Dekegel, J. Ghysdael, R. Kettman, M. Leclercq, J. Leunen, M. Mammerickx, and D. Portelle. 1980. Bovine leukemia virus: Molecular biology and epidemiology. In *Viral oncology* (ed. G. Klein), pp. 231–289. Raven Press, New York.

Calafat, J. and P.C. Hageman. 1973. Remarks on virus-like particles in human milk. *Nature* **242:**260–262.

Catovsky, D., M.F. Greaves, M. Rose, D.A.G. Galton, A.W.G. Goolden, D.R. McCluskey, J.M. White, I. Lampert, G. Bourikas, R. Ireland, J.M. Bridges, W.A. Blattner, and R.C. Gallo. 1982. Adult T-cell lymphoma-leukemia in blacks from the West Indies. *Lancet* (in press).

Chan, E., W.T. Peters, R.W. Sweet, T. Ohno, D.W. Kuse, S. Spieglman, R.C. Gallo, and R.E. Gallagher. 1976. Characterization of a virus (HL23V) isolated from cultured acute myelogenous leukemia cells. *Nature* **260:**266–268.

Chandra, P., S. Balikcioglu, and B. Mildner. 1978. Biochemical and immunological characterization of a reverse transcriptase from human melanoma tissue. *Cancer Lett.* **5:**299–310.

Chandra, P., L.K. Steel, H. Laube, S. Balikcioglu, B. Mildner, U. Ebener, K. Weite, and A. Vogel. 1980. Immunological characterization of reverse transcriptases from human tumors: Evidence for subgroup-specific interspecies antigenic determinants on the reverse transcriptase molecule. *Cold Spring Harbor Conf. Cell Proliferation* **7:**775–791.

Chandra, S., T. Liszczak, W. Korol, and E.M. Jensen. 1970. Type-C particles in human tissues. I. Electron microscopic study of embryonic tissues *in vivo* and *in vitro*. *Int. J. Cancer* **6:**40–45.

Charman, H.P., N. Kim, M. White, and R.V. Gilden. 1974. Failure to detect in human sera antibodies cross-reactive with group-specific antigens of murine leukemia virus. *J. Natl. Cancer Inst.* **52:**1409–1413.

Charman, H.P., R. Rahman, M.H. White, N. Kim, and R.V. Gilden. 1977. Radioimmunoassay for the major structural protein of Mason-Pfizer monkey virus: Attempts to detect the presence of antigen or antibody in humans. *Int. J. Cancer* **19:**498–504.

Charney, J. and D.H. Moore. 1971. Neutralization of murine mammary tumour virus by sera of women with breast cancer. *Nature* **229:**627–628.

Chezzi, C., G. Dettori, V. Manzari, A.M. Agliano, and A. Sanna. 1976. Simultaneous detection of reverse transcriptase and high molecular weight RNA in tissue of patients with Hodgkin's disease and patients with leukemia. *Proc. Natl. Acad. Sci.* **73:**4649–4652.

Chopra, H.C. and M.M. Mason. 1970. A new virus in a spontaneous mammary tumor of a rhesus monkey. *Cancer Res.* **30:**2081–2086.

Cianciolo, G.J. and R. Snyderman. 1981. Monocyte responsiveness to chemotactic stimuli in vitro is a property of a subpopulation of human mononuclear cells which can respond to multiple chemoattractants. *J. Clin. Invest.* **67:**60–68.

Cianciolo, G.J., T.J. Matthews, D.P. Bolognesi, and R. Snyderman. 1980. Macrophage accumulation in mice is inhibited by low molecular weight products from murine leukemia viruses. *J. Immunol.* **124:**2900–2905.

Cianciolo, G., J. Hunter, J. Silva, J.S. Haskill, and R. Snyderman. 1981. Inhibitors of monocyte responses to chemotaxins are present in human cancerous effusions and react with monoclonal antibodies to the p15(E) structural protein of retroviruses. *J. Clin. Invest.* **68:**831–844.

Colcher, D., Y.A. Teramoto, and J. Schlom. 1977. Inter-species radioimmunoassay for the major structural proteins of primate type-D retroviruses. *Proc. Natl. Acad. Sci.* **74:**5739–5743.

Colcher, D., S. Spiegelman, and J. Schlom. 1974. Sequence homology between the RNA of Mason-Pfizer monkey virus and the RNA of human malignant breast tumors. *Proc. Natl. Acad. Sci.* **71:**4975–4979.

Coleman, M.S., J.J. Hutton, P. DeSimone, and F.J. Bollum. 1974. Terminal deoxyribonucleotidyl transferase in human leukemia. *Proc. Natl. Acad. Sci.* **71:**4404–4408.

Collins, S.J., R.C. Gallo, and R.E. Gallagher. 1977. Continuous growth and differentiation of human myeloid leukaemic cells in suspension culture. *Nature* **270:**347–349.

Collins, S.J., F.W. Ruscetti, R.E. Gallagher, and R.C. Gallo. 1979. Normal functional characteristics of cultured human promyelocytic leukemia cells (HL-60) after induction of differentiation by dimethysulfoxide. *J. Exp. Med.* **149:**969–974.

Cook, B., F. O'Sullivan, J. Leung, P. Morse, B. Graham, and A.L. Chapman. 1978. Transformation of human embryo cells with the use of cell-free extracts of a human rhabdomyosarcoma cell line (HUS-2). *J. Natl. Cancer Inst.* **60:**979–984.

Cooper, G.M. and P.E. Neiman. 1981. Two distinct candidate transforming genes of lymphoid leukosis virus-induced neoplasms. *Nature* **292:**857–858.

Cooper, G.M., S. Okenquist, and L. Silverman. 1980. Transforming activity of DNA of chemically transformed and normal cells. *Nature* **284:**418–421.

Cooper, N.R., F.C. Jensen, R.M. Welsh, Jr., and M.B.A. Oldstone. 1976. Lysis of RNA tumor viruses by human serum: Direct antibody-independent triggering of the classical complement pathway. *J. Exp. Med.* **144:**970–984.

Crawford, D.H., B.G. Achong, N.M. Teich, S. Finerty, J.L. Thompson, M.A. Epstein, and B.C. Giovanella. 1979. Identification of murine endogenous xenotropic retrovirus in cultured multicellular tumour spheroids from nude-mouse-passaged nasopharyngeal carcinoma. *Int. J. Cancer* **23:**1–7.

Cuatico, W., J.-R. Cho, and S. Spiegelman. 1973. Particles with RNA of high molecular weight and RNA-directed DNA polymerase in human brain tumors. *Proc. Natl. Acad. Sci.* **70:**2789–2793.

———. 1974. Evidence of particle-associated RNA-directed DNA polymerase and high molecular weight RNA in human gastrointestinal and lung malignancies. *Proc. Natl. Acad. Sci.* **71:**3304–3308.

Dale, B. and B. Ozanne. 1981. Characterization of mouse cellular deoxyribonucleic acid homologous to Abelson murine leukemia virus-specific sequences. *Mol. Cell. Biol.* **1:**731–742.

Dalla-Favera, R., E.P. Gelman, R.C. Gallo, and F. Wong-Staal. 1981. A human *onc* gene homologous to the transforming gene *(v-sis)* of simian sarcoma virus. *Nature* **293:**31–35.

Dalton, A.J. 1972. Observations on the details of ultrastructure of a series of type C viruses. *Cancer Res.* **32:**1351–1353.

———. 1975. Microvesicles and vesicles of multivesicular bodies versus "virus-like" particles. *J. Natl. Cancer Inst.* **54:**1137–1145.

Dalton, A.J., A. Hellman, S.S. Kalter, and R.J. Helmke. 1974. Ultrastructural comparison of placental virus with several type-C oncogenic viruses. *J. Natl. Cancer Inst.* **52:**1379–1381.

Das, M.R., A.B. Vaidya, S.M. Sirsat, and D.H. Moore. 1972a. Polymerase and RNA studies on milk virions from women of the Parsi community. *J. Natl. Cancer Inst.* **48:**1191–1196.

Das, M.R., E. Sadavisan, R. Koshy, A.B. Vaidya, and S.M. Sirsat. 1972b. Homology between RNA from human malignant breast tissue and DNA synthesized by milk particles. *Nature* **239:**92–95.

Deinhardt, F. 1980. Biology of primate retroviruses. In *viral oncology* (ed. G. Klein), pp. 357–398. Raven Press, New York.

Derks, J.P.A., L. Hofmans, H.W. Bruning, and J.J. Rood. 1982. Synthesis of a viral protein with a molecular weight of 30,000 (p30) by leukemic cells and antibodies cross-reacting with simian sarcoma virus p30 in serum of a chronic myeloid leukemia patient. *Cancer Res.* **42:**681–686.

de Thé, G. 1979. The epidemiology of Burkitt's lymphoma: Evidence for a causal association with Epstein-Barr virus. *Epidemiol. Rev.* **1:**32–54.

Devare, S.G., R.E. Hanson, Jr., and J.R. Stephenson. 1978. Primate retroviruses: Envelope glycoproteins of endogenous type C and type D viruses possess common interspecies antigenic determinants. *J. Virol.* **26:**316–324.

Dion, A.S., A.B. Vaidya, and G.S. Fout. 1974. Cation preferences for poly(rC) · oligo(dG)-directed DNA synthesis by RNA tumor viruses and human milk particulates. *Cancer Res.* **34:**3509–3515.

Dion, A.S., D.C Farwell, A.A. Pomenti, and A.J. Girardi. 1980. A human protein related to the major envelope protein of murine mammary tumor virus: Identification and characterization. *Proc. Natl. Acad. Sci.* **77:**1301–1305.

Dirksen, E.R. and J.A. Levy. 1977. Virus-like particles in placentas from normal individuals and patients with systemic lupus erythematosus. *J. Natl. Cancer Inst.* **59:**1187–1192.

Dmochowski, L. and J.M. Bowen. 1978. Viruses and human cancer: The history and current status of ESP-1. *Prog. Exp. Tumor Res.* **21:**160–195.

Dmochowski, L. and J.S. Horoszewicz. 1976. Viral oncology of prostatic cancer. *Semin. Oncol.* **3:**141–150.

Dmochowski, L., T. Yumoto, C.E. Grey, R.L. Hales, P.L. Langford, H.G. Taylor, E.J. Freireich, C.C. Schullenberger, J.A. Shively, and C.D. Howe. 1967. Electron microscopic studies of human leukemia and lymphoma. *Cancer* **20:**760–777.

Donehower, L., F. Wong-Staal, and D. Gillespie. 1977. Divergence of baboon endogenous type C virogenes in primates: Genomic viral RNA in molecular hybridization experiments. *J. Virol.* **21:**932–941.

Dworsky, R.L. and B.E. Henderson. 1974. Hodgkin's disease clustering in families and communities. *Cancer Res.* **34:**1161–1163.

Ebbesen, P., C. Due, J. Hesse, R. Kurth, G.R. Noble, R. Gallagher, A. Voller, and G. Jensen. 1979. Elevated titer of antibodies to simian sarcoma virus envelope antigen (gp70) and normal response to influenza virus in untreated Danish Hodgkin's patients. *Int. J. Cancer* **24:**1–5.

Eckner, R.J., E.S. Priori, W.A. Mirand, and L. Dmochowski. 1974. Studies on the biological and antigenic properties of ESP-1 type C virus particles. *Cancer Res.* **34:**2521–2529.

Epstein, A.L. and H.S. Kaplan. 1974. Biology of the human malignant lymphomas. I. Establishment in continuous cell culture and heterotransplantation of diffuse histiocytic lymphomas. *Cancer* **34:**1851–1972.

Epstein, M.A., B.G. Achong, and Y.M. Barr. 1964. Virus particles in cultured lymphoblasts from Burkitt's lymphoma. *Lancet* **1:**702–703.

Eva, A., K.C. Robbins, P.R. Andersen, A. Srinivasan, S.R. Tronick, E.P. Reddy, N.W. Ellmore, A.T. Galen, J.A. Lautenberger, T.S. Papas, E.H. Westin, F. Wong-Staal, R.C. Gallo, and S.A. Aaronson. 1982. Cellular genes analogous to retroviral *onc* genes are transcribed in human tumour cells. *Nature* **295:**116–119.

Feldman, D. 1975. An electron microscope study of virus particles in rhesus monkey placenta. *Proc. Natl. Acad. Sci.* **71:**118–121

Feldman, S.P., J. Schlom, and S. Spiegelman. 1973. Further evidence for oncornaviruses in human milk: The production of cores. *Proc. Natl. Acad. Sci.* **70:**1976–1980.

Feller, W.F. and H.C. Chopra. 1969. Studies of human milk in relation to the possible viral etiology of breast cancer. *Cancer* **24:**1250–1254.

———. 1971. Virus-like particles in human milk. *Cancer* **28:**1425–1430.

Fieldsteel, A.H. 1974. Nonspecific antiviral substances in human milk active against arbovirus and murine leukemia virus. *Cancer Res.* **34:**712–715.

Fine, D.L., L.O. Arthur, and G. Schochetman. 1980. Functionally conserved determinants on gp70s of endogenous primate retroviruses. *Virology* **101:**176–184.

Fine, D.L., S.G. Devare, L.O. Arthur, H.P. Charman, and J.R. Stephenson. 1978. Type D retroviruses: Occurrence of natural antibodies to Mason-Pfizer monkey virus in rhesus monkeys. *Virology* **86:**567–571.

Finkel, M.P., B.O. Biskis, and C. Farrell. 1968. Osteosarcomas appearing in Syrian hamsters after treatment with extracts of human osteosarcomas. *Proc. Natl. Acad. Sci.* **60:**1223–1230.

Fischinger, P.J., P.T. Peebles, S. Nomura, and D.K. Haapala. 1973. Isolation of an RD-114-like oncornavirus from a cat cell line. *J. Virol.* **11:**978–985.

Fraumeni, J.F. and R.W. Miller. 1971. Breast cancer from breast feeding. *Lancet* **2:**1196–1197.

Fujinaga, K., A. Rankin, H. Yamazaki, K. Sekikawa, J. Bragdon, and M. Green. 1973. RD-114 virus: Analysis of viral gene sequences in feline and human cells by DNA-DNA reassociation kinetics and RNA-DNA hybridization. *Virology* **56:**484–495.

Furmanski, P., C.P. Loeckner, C. Longley, L.J. Larson, and M.A. Rich. 1976. Identification and isolation of the major core protein from the oncornavirus-like particle in human milk. *Cancer Res.* **36:**4001–4007.

Furmanski, P., C. Longley, D. Fouchey, R. Rich, and M.A. Rich. 1974. Normal human mammary cells in culture: Evidence for oncornavirus-like particles. *J. Natl. Cancer Inst.* **52:**975–977.

Gabelman, N., S. Waxman, W. Smith, and S.D. Douglas. 1975. Appearance of C-type virus-like particles after co-cultivation of a human tumor cell line with rat (XC) cells. *Int. J. Cancer* **16:**355–369.

Gallagher, R.E. and R.C. Gallo. 1975. Type C RNA tumor virus isolated from cultured human acute myelogenous leukemia cells. *Science* **187:**350–353.

Gallagher, R.E., A.W. Schrecker, C.A. Walter, and R.C. Gallo. 1978. Oncornavirus lytic activity in the serum of gibbon apes. *J. Natl. Cancer Inst.* **60:**677–682.

Gallagher, R.E., S.Z. Salahuddin, W.T. Hall, K.B. McCredie, and R.C. Gallo. 1975. Growth and differentiation in culture of leukemic leukocytes from a patient with acute myelogenous leukemia and reidentification of type C virus. *Proc. Natl. Acad. Sci.* **72:**4137–4141.

Gallagher, R.E., G.J. Todaro, R.G. Smith, D.M. Livingston, and R.C. Gallo. 1974. Relationship between RNA-directed DNA polymerase (reverse transcriptase) from human acute leukemic blood cells and primate type-C viruses. *Proc. Natl. Acad. Sci.* **71:**1309–1313.

Gallo, R.C. and F. Wong-Staal. 1980. Molecular biology of primate retroviruses. In *Viral oncology* (ed. G. Klein), pp. 399–431. Raven Press, New York.

Gallo, R.C., S.S. Yang, and R.C. Ting. 1970. RNA dependent polymerase in human acute leukemic cells. *Nature* **228:**927–929.

Gallo, R.C., W.A. Blattner, M.S. Reitz, Jr., and Y. Ito. 1982. HTLV: The virus of adult T-cell leukaemia in Japan and elsewhere. *Lancet* **1:**683.

Gallo, R.C., N.R. Miller, W.C. Saxinger, and D. Gillespie. 1973. Primate RNA tumor virus-like DNA synthesized endogenously by RNA-dependent DNA polymerase in virus-like particles from fresh human acute leukemic blood cells. *Proc. Natl. Acad. Sci.* **70:**3219–3224.

Gallo, R.C., P.S. Sarin, P.T. Allen, W.A. Newton, E.S. Priori, J.M. Bowen, and L. Dmochowski. 1971. Reverse transcriptase in type C virus particles of human origin. *Nat. New Biol.* **232:**140–142.

Gardner, M.B., E.Y. Johnson, S. Rasheed, and R.M. McAllister. 1973. Intracerebral transplantation of human rhabdomyosarcoma cells into fetal and newborn kittens. *Int. J. Cancer.* **12:**563–567.

Gardner, M.B., S. Rasheed, R.W. Rongey, H.P. Charman, B. Alena, R.V. Gilden, and R.J. Huebner. 1974. Natural expression of feline type-C virus genomes. Prevalence of detectable FeLV and RD-114 gs antigen, type-C virus particles and infectious virus in postnatal and fetal cats. *Int. J. Cancer.* **14:**97–105.

Gardner, M.B., S. Rasheed, S. Shimizu, R.W. Rongey, B.E. Henderson, R.M. McAllister, V. Klement, H.P. Charman, R.V. Gilden, R.L. Heberling, and R.J. Huebner. 1977. Search for RNA tumor virus in humans. *Cold Spring Harbor Conf. Cell Proliferation* **4:**1235–1251.

Gazdar, A.F., D.N. Carney, P.A. Bunn, E.K. Russell, E.S. Jaffe, G.P. Schechter, and J.G. Guccion. 1980. Mitogen requirements for the in vitro propagation of cutaneous T-cell lymphomas. *Blood* **55:**409–417.

Gelderblom, H., H. Ogura, and H. Bauer. 1974a. On the occurrence of oncornavirus-like particles in HeLa cells. *Cytobiologie* **8:**339–344.

Gelderblom, H., H. Bauer, H. Ogura, R. Wigand, and A.B. Fischer. 1974b. Detection of oncornavirus-like particles in HeLa cells. I. Fine structure and comparative morphological classification. *Int. J. Cancer* **13:**246–253.

Gerwin, B.I., P.S. Ebert, H.C. Chopra, S.G. Smith, J.P. Kvedar, S. Albert, and M.J. Brennan. 1973. DNA polymerase activities of human milk. *Science* **180:**198–201.

Gilden, R.V., W.P. Parks, R.J. Huebner, and G.J. Todaro. 1971. Murine leukaemia virus group-specific antigen in the C-type virus-containing human cell line, ESP-1. *Nature* **233:**102–103.

Gillespie, D., S. Gillespie, R.C. Gallo, J.L. East, and L. Dmochowski. 1973. Genetic origin of RD114 and other RNA tumor viruses assayed by molecular hybridization. *Nat. New Biol.* **244:**51–54.

Goldenberg, D.M. and R.A. Pavia. 1981. Malignant potential of murine stromal cells after transplantation of human tumors into nude mice. *Science* **212:**65–67.

Goodenow, R.S. and H.S. Kaplan. 1979. Characterization of the reverse transcriptase of a type C RNA virus produced by a human lymphoma cell line. *Proc. Natl. Acad. Sci.* **76:**4971–4975.

Goodenow, R.S., S. Brown, R. Levy, and H.S. Kaplan. 1980. Partial characterization of the virion proteins of a type-C RNA virus produced by a human histiocytic lymphoma cell line. *Cold Spring Harbor Conf. Cell Proliferation* **7:**737–752.

Graham, F.L. and A.J. van der Eb. 1973. A new technique for the assay of infectivity of human adenovirus 5 DNA. *Virology* **52:**456–467.

Griffith, S. 1928. The significance of pneumococcal types. *J. Hyg.* **27:**113–159.

Groudine, M., R. Eisenman, and H. Weintraub. 1981. Chromatin structure of endogenous retrovirus genes and activation by an inhibitor of DNA methylation. *Nature* **292:**311–317.

Gupta, P. and J.F. Ferrer. 1982. Expression of bovine leukemia virus genome is blocked by a nonimmunoglobulin protein in plasma from infected cattle. *Science* **215:**405–407.

Hall, W.T. and G. Schidlovsky. 1976. Typical type C virus in human leukemia. *J. Natl. Cancer Inst.* **56:**639–642.

Hamilton, P.J.S. and V. Persaud. 1981. Cancer among blacks in the West Indies. In *Cancer among black populations* (ed. C. Mettlin and G.P. Murphy), pp. 1–15. A.R. Liss, New York.

Hanaoka, M., M. Sakaki, H. Matsumoto, H. Tanakawa, H. Yamabe, K. Tomimoto, C. Tasaka, H. Fujiwara, T. Uchiyama, and K. Takatsuki. 1979. Adult T-cell leukemia: Histological classification and characteristics. *Acta Pathol. Jpn.* **29:**723–738.

Hardy, W.D., A.J. McClelland, E.E. Zuckerman, H.W. Snyder, E.G. MacEwen, D.P. Francis, and M. Essex. 1980. Immunology and epidemiology of feline leukemia virus nonproducer lymphosarcomas. *Cold Spring Harbor Conf. Cell Proliferation* **7:**677–698.

Hattori, T., T. Uchiyama, T. Toibana, K. Takatsuki, and H. Uchino. 1981. Surface phenotype of Japanese adult T-cell leukemia cells characterized by monoclonal antibodies. *Blood* **58:**645–647.

Hayward, W.S., B.G. Neel, and S.M. Astrin. 1981. Activation of a cellular *onc* gene by promoter insertion in ALV-induced lymphoid leukosis. *Nature* **290:**475–480.

Heath, C.W., Jr. and R.S. Hasterlik. 1963. Leukemia among children in a suburban community. *Am. J. Med.* **34:**796–812.

Hefti, E., J.T. Reynolds, S. Panem, and W.H. Kirsten. 1980. Characterization of unique nucleotide sequences and antigenic determinants of a type-C virus isolated from normal human cells (HEL-12 virus). *Cold Spring Harbor Conf. Cell Proliferation* **7:**729–736.

Hehlmann, R., D. Kufe, and S. Spiegelmann. 1972. Viral-related RNA in Hodgkin's disease and other human lymphomas. *Proc. Natl. Acad. Sci.* **69:**1727–1731.

Hellman, A., P.T. Peebles, J.E. Strickland, A.K. Fowler, S.S. Kalter, S. Oroszlan, and R.V. Gilden. 1974. Baboon virus isolate M-7 with properties similar to feline virus RD-114. *J. Virol.* **14:**133–138.

Hendrick, J.-C., C. Francois, C.-M. Calberg-Bacq, C. Colin, P. Franchimont, L. Gosselin, S. Kozma, and P.M. Osterrieth. 1978. Radioimmunoassay for protein p28 of murine mammary tumor virus in organs and serum of mice and search for related antigens in human sera and breast cancer extracts. *Cancer Res.* **38:**1826–1831.

Herbrink, P., J.E.T. Moen, J. Brouwer, and S.O. Warnaar. 1980. Detection of antibodies cross-reactive with type C RNA tumor viral p30 protein in human sera and exudate fluids. *Cancer Res.* **40:**166–173.

Hill, M. and J. Hillova. 1971. Production virale dans les fibroblastes de poule traites par l'acide desoxyribonucleique de cellules XC de rat transformees par le virus de Rous. *C.R. Acad. Sci.* **272:**3094–3097.

Hinuma, Y., K. Nagata, M. Hanaoka, M. Nakai, T. Matsumoto, K.-I. Kinoshita, S. Shirakawa, and I. Miyoshi. 1981. Adult T-cell leukemia: Antigen in an ATL cell line and detection of antibodies to the antigen in human sera. *Proc. Natl. Acad. Sci.* **78:**6476–6480.

Hirsch, M.S., A.P. Kelly, D.S. Chapin, T.C. Fuller, P.H. Black, and R. Kurth. 1978. Immunity to antigens associated with primate C-type oncoviruses in pregnant women. *Science* **199:**1337–1340.

Holder, W.D., W.G. Robey, and G.F. Vande Woude. 1974. Activation of a C-type virus from the human carcinoma cell line HBT-3 by iododeoxyuridine and testosterone. *Nature* **249:**759–762.

Howard, D.K. and J. Schlom. 1978. Isolation of host-range variants of mouse mammary tumor viruses that efficiently infect cells *in vitro*. *Proc. Natl. Acad. Sci.* **75:**5718–5722.

Huebner, R.J., D.C. Fish, D. Djurickovic, R.W. Trimmer, A.L. Bare, R.M. Bare, and G.T. Smith. 1979. Induction of rat sarcomas in rats treated with antithymocyte sera after transplantation of human cancer cells. *Proc. Natl. Acad. Sci.* **76:**1793–1794.

Ichimaru, M., K. Kinoshita, S. Kamihira, S. Ikeda, Y. Yamada, and T. Amagasaki. 1979. T-cell malignant lymphoma in Nagasaki district and its problems. *Jpn. J. Clin. Oncol.* **9:**337–346.

Ilyin, K.V., A.F. Bykovsky, and V.M. Zhdanov. 1973. An oncornavirus isolated from human cancer cell line. *Cancer* **32:**89–96.

Imai, M., C. Yamada, S. Saga, S. Nagayoshi, and M. Hoshino. 1979. Immunological cross reaction between sera from patients with breast cancer and mouse mammary tumor virus. *Gann* **70:**63–74.

Imamura, M., P.E. Phillips, and R.C. Mellors. 1976. The occurrence and frequency of type C virus-like particles in placentas from patients with systemic lupus erythematosus and from normal subjects. *Am. J. Pathol.* **83:**383–394.

Irlin, I.S., K.V. Ilyin, A.F. Bykovsky, G.G. Miller, M.Y. Volkova, T.F. Lozinsky, and V.M. Zhdanov. 1973/74. Common antigens in oncornaviruses from continuous human cell lines and Mason-Pfizer virus. *Intervirology* **2:**95–99.

Jacquemin, P.C., C. Saxinger, and R.C. Gallo. 1978. Surface antibodies of human myelogenous leukaemia leukocytes reactive with specific typc-C viral reverse transcriptases. *Nature* **276:**230–236.

Kalter, S.S., R.J. Helmke, R.L. Heberling, M. Panigel, P.J. Felsburg, and L.R. Axelrod. 1973a. Observations of apparent C-type particles in baboon (*Papio cynocephalus*) placentas. *Science* **179:**1332–1333.

Kalter, S.S., R.J. Helmke, R.L. Heberling, M. Panigel, A.K. Fowler, J.E. Strickland, and A. Hellman. 1973b. C-type particles in normal human placentas. *J. Natl. Cancer Inst.* **50:**1081–1084.

Kalyanaraman, V.S., M.G. Sarngadharan, P.A. Bunn, J.D. Minna, and R.C. Gallo. 1981a. Antibodies in human sera reactive against an internal structural protein of human T-cell lymphoma virus. *Nature* **294:**271–273.

Kalyanaraman, V.S., M.G. Sarngadharan, Y. Nakao, Y. Ito, and R.C. Gallo. 1982. Natural antibodies to the structural core protein (p24) of the human T-cell leukemia (lymphoma) retrovirus (HTLV) found in sera of leukemia patients in Japan. *Proc. Natl. Acad. Sci.* **79:**(in press).

Kalyanaraman, V.S., M.G. Sarngadharan, B. Poiesz, F.W. Ruscetti, and R.C. Gallo. 1981b. Immunological properties of a type C retrovirus isolated from cultured human T-lymphoma cells and comparison to other mammalian retroviruses. *J. Virol.* **38:**906–915.

Kantor, J.A., Y.-H. Lee, J.G. Chirikjian, and W.F. Feller. 1979. DNA polymerase with characteristics of reverse transcriptase purified from human milk. *Science* **204:**511–513.

Kaplan, H.S. 1978. Studies of an RNA virus isolated from a human histiocytic lymphoma cell line. *Cold Spring Harbor Conf. Cell Proliferation* **5:**695–706.

Kaplan, H.S., R.S. Goodenow, S. Gartner, and M.M. Bieber. 1979. Biology and virology of the human malignant lymphomas. *Cancer* **43:**1–24.

Kaplan, H.S., R.S. Goodenow, A.L. Epstein, S. Gartner, A. Declève, and P.N. Rosenthal. 1977. Isolation of a type of C RNA virus from an established human histiocytic lymphoma cell line. *Proc. Natl. Acad. Sci.* **74:**2564–2568.

Karpas, A. 1978. New virus expressed in cultured human leukaemic myeloblasts. *Lancet* **2:**110.

Karpas, A. and E. Tuckerman. 1974. Transformation of human fibroblasts with DNA of cultured human rhabdomyosarcoma cells. *Lancet* **1:**1138–1141.

Karpas, A., T.G. Wreghitt, and J. Nagington. 1978. Transformation of normal bone-marrow cells by a leukaemic cell line associated with a presumptive new human virus. *Lancet* **2:**1016–1019.

Kawakami, T.G., P.M. Buckley, T.S. McDowell, and A. DePaoli. 1973. Antibodies to simian C-type virus antigen in sera of gibbons (*Hylobates* sp.). *Nat. New Biol.* **246:**105–107.

Keydar, I., L. Chen, S. Karby, F.R. Weiss, J. Delarea, M. Radu, S. Chaitcik, and H.J. Brenner. 1979. Establishment and characterization of a cell line of human breast carcinoma origin. *Eur. J. Cancer* **15:**659–670.

Keydar, J., Z. Gilead, S. Karby, and E. Harel. 1973. Production of virus by embryonic cultures co-cultivated with breast tumor cells or infected with milk from breast cancer patients. *Nat. New Biol.* **241:**49–52.

Kiessling, A.A., G.H. Weber, A.O. Deeney, E.A. Possehl, and G.S. Beaudreau. 1971. Deoxyribonucleic acid polymerase activity associated with a plasma particulate fraction from patients with chronic lymphocytic leukemia. *J. Virol.* **7:**221–226.

Kikuchi, M., T. Matsui, N. Matsui, E. Sato, M. Tokunaga, K. Hasui, M. Ichimaru, K. Kinoshita, and S. Kamihira. 1979. T-cell malignancies in adults: Histopathological studies of lymph nodes in 110 patients. *Jpn. J. Clin. Oncol.* **9:**407–422.

Klucis, E., L. Jackson, and P.G. Parsons. 1976. Survey of human lymphoblastoid cell lines and primary cultures of normal and leukaemic leukocytes for oncornavirus production. *Int. J. Cancer* **18:**413–420.

Koch, G., K. Nooter, P. Bentvelzen, and J.J. Haaijman. 1977. Serological characterization of a putative human C-type oncornavirus by means of the Sepharose bead immunofluorescence assay. *Eur. J. Cancer* **13:**1397–1403.

Kotler, M., H. Balabanova, A. Friedman, and Y. Becker. 1979. Retrovirus-like particles in EBV negative Burkitt's lymphoma cell line but not in EBV DNA positive lines from patients with ataxia telangiectasia and Down's syndrome. *Br. J. Cancer* **39:**414–421.

Kotler, M., H. Balabanova, Z. Ben-Moyal, A. Friedman, and Y. Becker. 1977. Properties of the oncornavirus particles isolated from P3HR-1 and Raji human lymphoblastoid cell lines. *Isr. J. Med. Sci.* **13:**740–746.

Kotler, M., H. Balabanova, E. Weinberg, A. Friedman, and Y. Becker. 1975. Oncornavirus-like particles released from arginine-deprived human lymphoblastoid cell lines. *Proc. Natl. Acad. Sci.* **72:**4592–4596.

Kotler, M., E. Weinberg, O. Haspel, U. Olshevsky, and Y. Becker. 1973. Particles released from arginine deprived human leukemic cells. *Nat. New Biol.* **244:**197–200.

Krakower, J.M. and S.A. Aaronson. 1978. Seroepidemiologic assessment of feline leukaemia virus infection risk for man. *Nature* **273:**463–464.

Krontiris, T.G. and G.M. Cooper. 1981. Transforming activity of human tumor DNAs. *Proc. Natl. Acad. Sci.* **78:**1181–1184.

Kryscio, R.J., M.H. Myers, S.T. Prusiner, H.W. Heise, and B.W. Christine. 1973. The space-time distribution of Hodgkin's disease in Connecticut, 1940–1969. *J. Natl. Cancer Inst.* **50:**1107–1110.

Kufe, D., I.T. Magrath, J.L. Ziegler, and S. Spiegelman. 1973. Burkitt's tumors contain particles encapsulating RNA-instructed DNA polymerase and high molecular weight virus-related RNA. *Proc. Natl. Acad. Sci.* **70:**737–741.

Kurth, R. and U. Mikschy. 1978. Human antibodies reactive with purified envelope antigens of primate type C tumor viruses. *Proc. Natl. Acad. Sci.* **75:**5692–5696.

Kurth, R., A. Huesgen, F. Katz, and J. Löwer. 1979a. Comparison of radioimmunoprecipitation assays for the detection of human anti-tumor virus antibodies. *J. Immunol. Methods* **30:**355–366.

Kurth, R., N.M. Teich, R. Weiss, and R.T.D. Oliver. 1977. Natural human antibodies reactive with primate type-C viral antigens. *Proc. Natl. Acad. Sci.* **74:**1237–1241.

Kurth, R., H. Gelderblom, A. Huesgen, F. Katz, F.R. Sailer, M.W. Steward, and W. Vetterman. 1979b. Recognition of simian sarcoma virus antigen by human sera. In *Modern trends in human leukemia* (ed. R. Neth et al.), vol. 3, pp. 385–394. Springer, Heidelberg.

Kurth, R., R. Löwer, R. Harzmann, R. Pfeiffer, C.G. Schmidt, J. Fogh, and H. Frank. 1980. Oncornavirus synthesis in human teratocarcinoma cultures and an increased antiviral immune reactivity in corresponding patients. *Cold Spring Harbor Conf. Cell Proliferation* **7:**835–846.

Lane, M.A., A. Sainten, and G.M. Cooper. 1981. Activation of related transforming genes in mouse and human mammary carcinomas. *Proc. Natl. Acad. Sci.* **78:**5185–5189.

Lasfargues, E.Y., A.B. Vaidya, J.C. Lasfargues, and D.H. Moore. 1976a. In vitro susceptibility of mink lung cells to the mouse mammary tumor virus. *J. Natl. Cancer Inst.* **57:**447–449.

Lasfargues, E.Y., J.C. Lasfargues, A.S. Dion, A.E. Greene, and D.H. Moore. 1976b. Experimental infection of a cat kidney cell line with mouse mammary tumor virus. *Cancer Res.* **36:**67–72.

Lee, F., R. Mulligan, P. Berg, and G. Ringold. 1981. Glucocorticoids regulate expression of dihydrofolate reductase cDNA in mouse mammary tumour virus chimaeric plasmids. *Nature* **294:**228–232.

Levin, A.C., R.J. Massey, and F. Deinhardt. 1978. Spontaneous human mononuclear cell cytotoxicity to cultured tumor cells: Reproducibility of serial measurements with the use of a chromium-51-release microcytotoxicity assay. *J. Natl. Cancer Inst.* **60:**1283–1294.

Levine, P.H., J.S. Horoszewicz, J.T. Grace, Jr., L.S. Chai, R.R. Ellison, and J.F. Holland. 1967. Relationship between clinical status of leukemic patients and virus-like particles in their plasma. *Cancer* **20:**1563–1577.

Levy, J.A. 1973. Xenotropic viruses: Murine leukemia viruses associated with NIH Swiss, NZB, and other mouse strains. *Science* **182:**1151–1153.

Lewis, B.J., J.W. Abrell, R.G. Smith, and R.C. Gallo. 1974. Human DNA polymerase III (R-DNA polymerase): Distinction from DNA polymerase I and reverse transcriptase. *Science* **183:**867–869.

Lewis, R.M., W. Tannenberg, C. Smith, and R.S. Schwartz. 1974. C-type viruses in systemic lupus erythematosus. *Nature* **252:**78–79.

Lieber, M.M., C.J. Sherr, G.J. Todaro, R.E. Benveniste, R. Callahan, and H.G. Coon. 1975. Isolation from the Asian mouse *Mus caroli* of an endogenous type C virus related to infectious primate type C viruses. *Proc. Natl. Acad. Sci.* **72:**2315–2319.

Livingston, D.M.. and G.J. Todaro. 1973. Endogenous type C virus from a cat cell clone with properties distinct from previously described feline type C virus. *Virology* **53:**142–151.

Lopez, D.M., W.P. Parks, M.A. Silverman, and J.A. Distasio. 1981. Lymphoproliferative responses to mouse mammary tumor virus in lymphocyte subsets of breast cancer patients. *J. Natl. Cancer Inst.* **67:**353–358.

Louie, S., J.E. Curtis, J.E. Till, and E.A. McCulloch. 1976. Antibodies in human sera to oncornavirus-like proteins from normal or leukemic marrow cell cultures. *J. Exp. Med.* **144:**1243–1253.

Löwer, J., E.A. Davidson, N.M. Teich, R.A. Weiss, A.P. Joseph, and R. Kurth. 1981. Heterophil human antibodies recognize oncovirus envelope antigens: Epidemiological parameters and immunological specificity of the reaction. *Virology* **109:**409–417.

Lowy, D.R., W.P. Rowe, N. Teich, and J.W. Hartley. 1971. Murine leukemia virus: High frequency activation in vitro by 5′-iododeoxyuridine and 5-bromodeoxyuridine. *Science* **174:**155–156.

Mack, T.M. 1980. Epidemiology of Hodgkin's disease in young adults: Compatability with various infectious-disease models. *Cold Spring Harbor Conf. Cell Proliferation* **7:**1221–1230.

Mak, T.W., S. Kurtz, J. Manaster, and D. Housman. 1975. Viral-related information in oncornavirus-like particles isolated from cultures of marrow cells from leukemic patients in relapse and remission. *Proc. Natl. Acad. Sci.* **72:**623–627.

Mak, T.W., J. Manaster, A.F. Howatson, E.A. McCulloch, and J.E. Till. 1974. Particles with characteristics of leukoviruses in cultures of marrow cells from leukemic patients in remission and relapse. *Proc. Natl. Acad. Sci.* **71:**4336–4340.

Markham, P.D., W. Dodge, S.Z. Salahuddin, and R.E. Gallagher. 1978. An *in vitro* transformation assay for SiSV-1 and HL23V using feline embryonic fibroblasts. *Proc. Soc. Exp. Biol. Med.* **157:**312–318.

Markham, P.D., F. Ruscetti, S.Z. Salahuddin, R.E. Gallagher, and R.C. Gallo. 1979. Enhanced induction of growth of B lymphoblasts from fresh human blood by primate type-C retroviruses (gibbon ape leukemia virus and simian sarcoma virus). *Int. J. Cancer* **23:**148–156.

Martin, M.A., T. Bryan, S. Rasheed, and A.S. Khan. 1981. Identification and cloning of endogenous retroviral sequences present in human DNA. *Proc. Natl. Acad. Sci.* **78:**4892–4896.

Mathes, L.E., R.G. Olsen, L.C. Hebebrand, E.A. Hoover, J.P. Schaller, P.W. Adams, and W.S. Nichols. 1979. Immunosuppressive properties of a virion polypeptide, a 15,000-dalton protein, from feline leukemia virus. *Cancer Res.* **39:**950–955.

Matsumoto, M., K. Nomura, T. Matsumoto, K. Nishioka, S. Hanada, H. Furusho, H. Kikuchi, Y. Yato, A. Utsunomiya, T. Uematsu, M. Iwahashi, S. Hashimoto, and K. Yunoki. 1979. Adult T-cell leukemia-lymphoma in Kagoshima district, southwestern Japan: Clinical and hematological characteristics. *Jpn. J. Clin. Oncol.* **9:**325–336.

McAllister, R.M., J. Melnyk, J.Z. Finklestein, E.C. Adams, Jr., and M.B. Gardner. 1969. Cultivation in vitro of cells derived from a human rhabdomyosarcoma. *Cancer* **24:**520–526.

McAllister, R.M., W.A. Nelson-Rees, E.Y. Johnson, R.W. Rongey, and M.B. Gardner. 1971. Disseminated rhabdomyosarcomas formed in kittens by cultured human rhabdomyosarcoma cells. *J. Natl. Cancer Inst.* **47:**603–611.

McAllister, R.M., M. Nicolson, M.B. Gardner, S. Rasheed, R.W. Rongey, W.D. Hardy, Jr., and R.V. Gilden. 1973. RD-114 virus compared with feline and murine type-C viruses released from RD cells. *Nat. New Biol.* **242:**75–78.

McAllister, R.M., M.O. Nicolson, M.B. Gardner, R.W. Rongey, S. Rasheed, P.S. Sarma, R.J. Huebner, M. Hatanaka, S. Oroszlan, R.V. Gilden, A. Kabigting, and L. Vernon. 1972. C-type virus released from cultured human rhabdomyosarcoma cells. *Nat. New Biol.* **235:**3–6.

McCaffrey, R., T.A. Harrison, R. Parkman, and D. Baltimore. 1975. Terminal deoxynucleotidyl transferase activity in human leukemic cells and in normal human thymocytes. *N. Engl. J. Med.* **292:**775–780.

McCormick, J.J., L.J. Larson, and M.A. Rich. 1974. RNase inhibition of reverse transcriptase activity in human milk. *Nature* **251:**737–740.

McCoy, J.L., J.H. Dean, G.B. Cannon, L.J. Jerome, T.C. Alford, W.P. Parks, R.V. Gilden, S.T. Oroszlan, and R.B. Herberman. 1978. Leukocyte migration inhibition and lymphocyte blastogenesis responses in breast carcinoma patients to mouse mammary tumor virus and to virion gp52 antigen and Rauscher murine leukemia virus-Kirsten sarcoma virus gp69/71 antigen. *J. Natl. Cancer Inst.* **60:**1259–1267.

McGrath, C.M., P.M. Grant, H.D. Soule, T. Glancy, and M.A. Rich. 1974. Replication of oncornavirus-like particle in human breast carcinoma cell line, MCF-7. *Nature* **252:**247–250.

Mellors, R.C. and J.W. Mellors. 1976. Antigen related to mammalian type-C RNA viral p30 proteins is located in renal glomeruli in human systemic lupus erythematosus. *Proc. Natl. Acad. Sci.* **73:**233–237.

———. 1978. Type C RNA virus-specific antibody in human systemic lupus erythematosus demonstrated by enzymoimmunoassay. *Proc. Natl. Acad. Sci.* **75:**2463–2467.

Mesa-Tejada, R., I. Keydar, M. Ramanarayanan, T. Ohno, C. Fenoglio, and S. Spiegelman. 1978. Detection in human breast carcinomas of an antigen immunologically related to a group specific antigen of mouse mammary tumor virus. *Proc. Natl. Acad. Sci.* **75:**1529–1533.

Metzgar, R.S., T. Mohanakumar, and D.P. Bolognesi. 1976. Relationships between membrane antigens of human leukemic cells and oncogenic RNA virus structural components. *J. Exp. Med.* **143:**47–63.

Michalides, R., S. Spiegelman, and J. Schlom. 1975. Biochemical characterization of putative subviral particulates from human malignant breast tumors. *Cancer Res.* **35:**1003–1008.

Mier, J.W. and R.C. Gallo. 1980. Purification and some characteristics of human T-cell growth factor from phytohemagglutinin-stimulated lymphocyte conditioned media. *Proc. Natl. Acad. Sci.* **77:**6134–6138.

Miller, G.G., V.M. Zhdanov, T.F. Lozinsky, M.Y. Volkova, K.V. Ilyin, D.B. Golubev, I.S. Irlin, and A.F. Bykovsky. 1974. Production of an oncornavirus by the continuous human cell line, Detroit-6. *J. Natl. Cancer Inst.* **52:**357–361.

Miyoshi, I., M. Fujishita, H. Taguchi, Y. Ohtsuki, T. Akogi, Y.M. Morimoto, and A.

Nagasaki. 1982. Caution against blood transfusions from donors seropositive to adenovirus T-cell leukaemia-associated antigens. *Lancet* **1:** 683–684.
Miyoshi, I., I. Kubonishi, M. Sumida, S. Hiraki, T. Tsubota, I. Kimura, K. Miyamoto, and J. Sato. 1980. A novel T-cell line derived from adult T-cell leukemia. *Gann* **71:** 155–156.
Miyoshi, I., I. Kubonishi, S. Yoshimoto, T. Akagi, Y. Ohtsuki, Y. Shiraishi, K. Nagata, and Y. Hinuma. 1981. Type C virus particles in a cord T-cell line derived by cocultivating normal human cord leukocytes and human leukaemic T cells. *Nature* **294:**770–771.
Miyoshi, I., I. Kubonishi, M. Sumida, S. Yoshimoto, S. Hiraki, T. Tsubota, H. Kobashi, M. Lai, T. Tanaka, I. Kimura, K. Miyamoto, and J. Sato. 1979. Characteristics of a leukemic T-cell line derived from adult T-cell leukemia. *Jpn. J. Clin. Oncol.* **9:**485–494.
Mondal, H., R.E. Gallagher, and R.C. Gallo. 1975. RNA directed DNA polymerase from human leukemic blood cells and from primate type-C virus producing cells; high and low molecular weight forms with variant biochemical and immunological properties. *Proc. Natl. Acad. Sci.* **72:** 1194–1198.
Moore, D.H., N.H. Sarkar, C.E. Kelly, N. Pillsbury, and J. Charney. 1969. Type B particles in human milk. *Texas Rep. Biol. Med.* **27:** 1027–1039.
Moore, D.H., C.A. Long, A.B. Vaidya, J.B. Sheffield, A.S. Dion, and E.Y. Lasfargues. 1979. Mammary tumor viruses. *Adv. Cancer Res.* **29:**347–418.
Moore, D.H., J. Charney, B. Kramarsky, E.Y. Lasfargues, N.H. Sarkar, M.J. Brennan, J.H. Burrows, S.M. Sirsat, J.C. Paymaster, and A.B. Vaida. 1971. Search for a human breast cancer virus. *Nature* **229:**611–615.
Morgan, D.A., F.W. Ruscetti, and R. Gallo. 1976. Selective growth of T-lymphocytes from normal human bone marrow. *Science* **193:** 1007–1008,
Morton, D., W.T. Hall, and R.A. Malmgren. 1969. Human liposarcomas: Tissue cultures containing foci of transformed cells with viral particles. *Science* **165:**813–816.
Müller, M. and H. Grossman. 1972. An antigen in human breast cancer sera related to the murine mammary tumour virus. *Nature* **237:** 116–117.
Müller, M., S. Zotter, and C. Kemmer. 1976. Specificity of human antibodies to intracytoplasmic type-A particles in the murine mammary tumor virus. *J. Natl. Cancer Inst.* **56:**295–303.
Murray, M.J., B.-Z. Shilo, C. Shih, D. Cowing, H.W. Hsu, and R.A. Weinberg. 1981. Three different human tumor cell lines contain different oncogenes. *Cell* **25:**355–362.
Nakajima, H., T. Nagatani, and R. Nagai. 1979. Histopathological and immunological studies of malignant lymphoma of the skin. *Jpn. J. Clin. Oncol.* **9:**373–386.
Neiman, P.E. 1973. Measurement of RD114 virus nucleotide sequences in feline cellular DNA. *Nat. New Biol.* **244:**62–64.
Nelson, J., J.-A. Leong, and J.A. Levy. 1978. Normal human placentas contain RNA-directed DNA polymerase activity like that in viruses. *Proc. Natl. Acad. Sci.* **75:**6263–6267.
Nelson, J.A., J.A. Levy, and J.C. Leong. 1981. Human placentas contain a specific inhibitor of RNA-directed DNA polymerase. *Proc. Natl. Acad. Sci.* **78:** 1670–1674.
Nelson-Rees, W.A. and R.R. Flandermeyer. 1975. HeLa cultures defined. *Science* **191:**96–98.
Nelson-Rees, W.A., R.R. Flandermeyer, and P.K. Hawthorne. 1974. Banded marker chromosomes as indicators of intraspecies cellular contamination. *Science* **184:** 1093–1096.
Newell, G.R., W.W. Harris, K.O. Bowman, C.W. Boone, and N.G. Anderson. 1968. Evaluation of "viruslike" particles in the plasmas of 255 patients with leukemia and related diseases. *N. Engl. J. Med.* **278:** 1185–1191.
Newgard, K.W., R.D. Cardiff, and P.B. Blair. 1976. Human antibodies binding to the mouse mammary tumor virus: A nonspecific reaction? *Cancer Res.* **36:**765–768.

Nicolson, M.O., R.V. Gilden, H. Charman, N. Rice, R. Heberling, and R.M. McAllister. 1978. Search for infective mammalian type-C virus-related genes in the DNA of human sarcomas and leukemias. *Int. J. Cancer* **21:**700–706.

Nooter, K. 1979. *Studies on the role of RNA tumor viruses in human leukemia.* Radiobiological Institute of the Organization for Health Research TNO. Rijswijk, The Netherlands.

Nooter, K., P. Bentvelzen, C. Zurcher, and J. Rhim. 1977. Detection of human C-type "helper" viruses in human leukemic bone marrow with murine sarcoma virus-transformed human and rat non-producer cells. *Int. J. Cancer* **19:**59–65.

Nooter, K., A.M. Aarssen, P. Bentvelzen, F.G. de Groot, and F.G. van Pelt. 1975. Isolation of infectious C-type oncornavirus from human leukaemic bone marrow cells. *Nature* **256:**595–597.

Nooter, K., J. Overdevest, R. Dubbes, G. Koch, P. Bentvelzen, C. Zurcher, J. Coolen, and J. Calafat. 1978. Type-C oncovirus isolate from human leukemic bone marrow: Further in vitro and in vivo characterization. *Int. J. Cancer* **21:**27–34.

Ohno, T. and S. Spiegelman. 1977. Antigenic relatedness of the DNA polymerase of human breast cancer particles to the enzyme of the Mason-Pfizer monkey virus. *Proc. Natl. Acad. Sci.* **74:**2144–2148.

Ohno, T., R.W. Sweet, R. Hu, D. Dejak, and S. Spiegelman. 1977. Purification and characterization of the DNA polymerase of human breast cancer particles. *Proc. Natl. Acad. Sci.* **74:**764–768.

Ohno, T., R. Mesa-Tejada, I. Keydar, M. Ramanarayanan, J. Bausch, and S. Spiegelman. 1979. Human breast carcinoma antigen is immunologically related to the polypeptide of the group-specific glycoprotein of mouse mammary tumor virus. *Proc. Natl. Acad. Sci.* **76:**2460–2464.

Ohtsuki, Y., G. Seman, L. Dmochowski, J.M. Bowen, and D.E. Johnson. 1977. Virus-like particles in a case of human prostate carcinoma. *J. Natl. Cancer Inst.* **58:**1493–1496.

Okabe, H., R.V. Gilden, and M. Hatanaka. 1973. Extensive homology of RD114 virus DNA with RNA of feline origin. *Nat. New Biol.* **244:**54–56.

Okabe, H., R.V. Gilden, M. Hatanaka, J.R. Stephenson, R.E. Gallagher, R.C. Gallo, S.R. Tronick, and S.A. Aaronson. 1976. Immunological and biochemical characterisation of type C viruses isolated from cultured human AML cells. *Nature* **260:**264–266.

Oroszlan, S., D. Bova, M.H.M. White, R. Toni, C. Foreman, and R.V. Gilden. 1972. Purification and immunological characterization of the major internal protein of the RD-114 virus. *Proc. Natl. Acad. Sci.* **69:**1211–1215.

Ortaldo, J.R., R.K. Oldham, G.C. Cannon, and R.B. Herberman. 1977. Specificity of natural cytotoxic reactivity of normal human lymphocytes against a myeloid leukemia cell line. *J. Natl. Cancer Inst.* **59:**77–82.

Panem, S. 1976. Spontaneous type C virus expression in human embryonic lung cells (HEL-12): Comparison of cloned and mixed cell populations. *ICN-UCLA Symp. Mol. Cell Biol.* 409–417.

Panem, S., N.G. Ordonez, H. Dalton, and K. Soltani. 1978. Viral immune complexes in systemic lupus erythematosus: C-type viral complex deposition in skin. *J. Invest. Dermatol.* **71:**260–262.

Panem, S., E.V. Prochownik, W.H. Knish, and W.H. Kirsten. 1977. Cell generation and type C virus expression in the human embryonic cell strain HEL-12. *J. Gen. Virol.* **35:**487–495.

Panem, S., E.V. Prochownik, F.R. Reale, and W.H. Kirsten. 1975. Isolation of type-C virions from a normal human fibroblast strain. *Science* **189:**297–299.

Panem, S., N.G. Ordonez, W.H. Kirsten, A.I. Katz, and B.H. Spargo. 1976. C-type virus expression in systemic lupus erythematosus. *N. Engl. J. Med.* **295:**470–475.

Parks, W.P., R.V. Gilden, A.F. Bykovsky, G.G. Miller, V.M. Zdhanov, V.D. Soloviev, and

E.M. Scolnick. 1973. Mason-Pfizer virus characterization: A similar virus in a human amniotic cell line. *J. Virol.* **12:**1540–1547.

Parsons, P.G., P. Goss, and J.H. Pope. 1974. Detection in human melanoma cell lines of particles with some properties in common with RNA tumour viruses. *Int. J. Cancer* **13:**606–618.

Payne, G.S., S.A. Courtneidge, L.B. Crittenden, A.M. Fadly, J.M. Bishop, and H.E. Varmus. 1981. Analysis of avian leukosis virus DNA and RNA in bursal tumors: Viral gene expression is not required for maintenance of the tumor state. *Cell* **23:**311–322.

Perucho, M., M. Goldfarb, K. Shimizu, C. Lama, J. Fogh, and M. Wigler. 1981. Human-tumor-derived cell lines contain common and different transforming genes. *Cell* **27:**467–476.

Pike, M.C., P.K. Siiteri, and C.W. Welsch, eds. 1981. Hormones and breast cancer. *Banbury Rep.* **8:**1–491.

Poiesz, B.J., F.W. Ruscetti, J.W. Mier, A.M. Woods, and R.C. Gallo. 1980a. T-cell lines established from human T-lymphocytic neoplasias by direct response to T-cell growth factor. *Proc. Natl. Acad. Sci.* **77:**6815–6819.

Poiesz, B.J., F.W. Ruscetti, M.S. Reitz, V.S. Kalyanaraman, and R.C. Gallo. 1981. Isolation of a new type of C retrovirus (HTLV) in primary uncultured cells of a patient with Sézary T-cell leukaemia. *Nature* **294:**268–271.

Poiesz, B.J., F.W. Ruscetti, A.F. Gazdar, P.A. Bunn, J.D. Minna, and R.C. Gallo. 1980b. Detection and isolation of type C retrovirus particles from fresh and cultured lymphocytes of a patient with cutaneous T-cell lymphoma. *Proc. Natl. Acad. Sci.* **77:**7415–7419.

Posner, L.E., M. Robert-Guroff, V.S. Kalyanaraman, B.J. Poiesz, F.W. Ruscetti, B. Fossieck, P.A. Bunn, J.D. Minna, and R.C. Gallo. 1981. Natural antibodies to the human T cell lymphoma virus in patients with cutaneous T cell lymphomas. *J. Exp. Med.* **154:**333–346.

Prince, A.M. and W.R. Adams. 1966. Virus-like particles in human plasma and serum: Role of platelet lysosomes. *J. Natl. Cancer Inst.* **37:**153–166.

Priori, E.S., L. Dmochowski, B. Myers, and J.R. Wilbur. 1971. Constant production of type C virus particles in a continuous tissue culture derived from pleural effusion cells of a lymphoma patient. *Nat. New Biol.* **232:**61–62.

Priori, E., K.V. Ilyin, L. Dmochowski, and D.L. Fine. 1976. Immunological relationship between an oncornavirus isolate from HEp-2 cells, Mason-Pfizer monkey virus, and human tumor cells. In *Comparative leukemia research 1975* (ed. J. Clemmesen and D.S. Yohn), pp. 488–490. Karger, Basel.

Pritchard, D.J., C.A. Reilly, and M.P. Finkel. 1971. Evidence for a human osteosarcoma virus. *Nat. New Biol.* **234:**126–127.

Prochownik, E.V. and W.H. Kirsten. 1976. Inhibition of reverse transcriptases of primate type C viruses by 7S immunoglobulin from patients with leukaemia. *Nature* **260:**64–67.

———. 1977. Nucleic acid sequences of primate type C viruses in normal and neoplastic human tissues. *Nature* **267:**175–177.

Prochownik, E.V., S. Panem, and W.H. Kirsten. 1979. Type C virus induced by iododeoxyuridine in the human embryonic cell strain HEL-12. *J. Gen. Virol.* **42:**399–403.

Rasheed, S., M.G. Gardner, and R.J. Huebner. 1978. In vitro isolation of stable rat sarcoma virus. *Proc. Natl. Acad. Sci.* **75:**2972–2976.

Rasheed, S., R.M. McAllister, B.E. Henderson, and M.B. Gardner. 1973. In vitro host range and serological studies on RD-114 virus. *J. Natl. Cancer Inst.* **51:**1383–1385.

Reitz, M.S., Jr., B.J. Poiesz, F.W. Ruscetti, and R.C. Gallo. 1981. Characterization and distribution of nucleic acid sequences of a novel type C retrovirus isolated from neoplastic human T lymphocytes. *Proc. Natl. Acad. Sci.* **78:**1887–1891.

Reitz, M.S., N.R. Miller, F. Wong-Staal, R.E. Gallagher, R.C. Gallo, and D.H. Gillespie. 1976. Primate type-C virus nucleic acid sequences (woolly monkey and baboon types) in tissues from a patient with acute myelogenous leukemia and in viruses isolated from cultured cells of the same patient. *Proc. Natl. Acad. Sci.* **78:**2113–2117.

Reynolds, J.T. and S. Panem. 1981. Characterization of antibody to C-type virus antigens isolated from immune complexes in kidneys of patients with systemic lupus erythematosus. *Lab. Invest.* **44:**410–419.

Rho, H.M., B. Poiesz, F.W. Ruscetti, and R.C. Gallo. 1981. Characterization of the reverse transcriptase from a new retrovirus (HTLV) produced by a human cutaneous T-cell lymphoma cell line. *Virology* **112:**355–360.

Ringold, G.M., R.D. Cardiff, H.E. Varmus, and K.R. Yamamoto. 1977. Infection of cultured rat hepatoma cells by mouse mammary tumor viruses. *Cell* **10:**11–18.

Robert-Guroff, M., F.W. Ruscetti, L.E. Posner, B.J. Poiesz, and R.C. Gallo. 1981. Detection of the human T-cell lymphoma virus p19 in cells of some patients with cutaneous T-cell lymphoma and leukemia using a monoclonal antibody. *J. Exp. Med.* **154:**1957–1964.

Robert-Guroff, M., Y. Nakao, K. Notake, Y. Ito, A. Sliski, and R.C. Gallo. 1982. Natural antibodies to human retrovirus HTLV in a cluster of Japanese patients with adenovirus T-cell leukemia. *Science* **295:**975–978.

Roussel, M., S. Saule, C. Lagrou, C. Rommens, H. Beug, T. Graf, and D. Stehelin. 1979. Three new types of viral oncogenes of cellular origin specific for haematopoietic cell transformation. *Nature* **281:**452–455.

Rovera, G., D. Santoli, and C. Dansky. 1979. Human promyelocytic leukemia cells in culture differentiate into macrophage-like cells when treated with a phorbol diester. *Proc. Natl. Acad. Sci.* **76:**1279–1283.

Roy-Burman, R., R.W. Rongey, B.E. Henderson, and M.B. Gardner. 1973. Attempts to detect RNA tumour virus in human milk. *Nat. New Biol.* **244:**146.

Ruprecht, R.M., N.C. Goodman, and S. Spiegelman. 1973. Determination of natural host taxonomy of RNA tumor viruses by molecular hybridization: Application to RD114, a candidate human virus. *Proc. Natl. Acad. Sci.* **70:**1437–1441.

Ruscetti, F.W. and R.C. Gallo. 1981. Human T-lymphocyte growth factor: Regulation of growth and function of T lymphocytes. *Blood* **57:**379–394.

Sadamori, N., H. Nonaka, M. Ichimaru, H. Igarashi, M. Hirota, and H. Sawada. 1981. Familial acute myelogenous leukemia associated with RNA virus and polymorphism of 1qh+. *Cancer Genet. Cytogenet.* **4:**23–30.

Sanner, T. 1976. Removal of inhibitors against RNA-directed DNA polymerase activity in human milk. *Cancer Res.* **36:**405–408.

Sarin, P.S., P.N. Anderson, and R.C. Gallo. 1976. Terminal deoxynucleotidyl transferase activities in human blood leukocytes and lymphoblast cell lines: High levels in lymphoblast cell lines and in blast cells of some patients with chronic myelogenous leukemia in acute phase. *Blood* **47:**11–20.

Sarkar, N.H. and D.H. Moore. 1972. On the possibility of a human breast cancer virus. *Nature* **236:**103–106.

Sarkar, N.H., J. Charney, A.S. Dion, and D.H. Moore. 1973. Effect of human milk on the mouse mammary tumor virus. *Cancer Res.* **33:**626–629.

Sarma, P.S., J. Tseng, Y.K. Lee, and R.V. Gilden. 1973. Virus similar to RD114 virus in cat cells. *Nat. New Biol.* **244:**56–59.

Sarma, P.S., A. Sharar, J. Tseng, P.J. Price, and M. Gardner, 1974. Studies on the prevalence of endogenous type C virus RD 114 in cats. *Proc. Soc. Exp. Biol. Med.* **145:**757–762.

Sarngadharan, M.G., P.S. Sarin, M.S. Reitz, and R.C. Gallo. 1972. Reverse transcriptase activity of human acute leukemic cells. Purification of the enzyme response to AMV 70S RNA, and characterization of the DNA product. *Nat. New Biol.* **240:**67–72.

Sawada, H., M. Tashima, T. Nakamura, T. Uchiyama, K. Sagawa, K. Takatsuki, H.

Uchino, and Y. Ito. 1977. RNA-reverse transcriptase complex from cultured human myeloma-leukemia cells. *Int. J. Cancer* **20:**15–20.

Sawyer, M.H., N.E. Nachlas, Jr., and S. Panem. 1978. C-type viral antigen expression in human placenta. *Nature* **275:**62–64.

Schidlovsky, G. and M. Ahmed. 1973. C-type virus particles in placentas and fetal tissues of rhesus monkeys. *J. Natl. Cancer Inst.* **51:**225–233.

Schimpff, S.C., C.R. Schimpff, D.M. Brager, and P.H. Wiernik. 1975. Leukemia and lymphoma patients linked by prior social contact. *Lancet* **1:**124–129.

Schlom, J. and S. Spiegelman. 1971. Simultaneous detection of reverse transcriptase and high molecular weight RNA unique to oncogenic RNA viruses. *Science* **174:**840–843.

Schlom, J., S. Spiegelman, and D.H. Moore. 1971. RNA-dependent DNA polymerase activity in virus-like particles isolated from human milk. *Nature* **231:**97–100.

———. 1972b. Detection of high-molecular-weight RNA in particles from human milk. *Science* **175:**542–544.

———. 1972c. Reverse transcriptase and high molecular weight RNA in particles from mouse and human milk. *J. Natl. Cancer Inst.* **48:**1197–1203.

Schlom, J., D. Colcher, and S. Spiegelman, S. Gillespie, and D. Gillespie. 1972a. Quantitation of RNA tumor viruses and virus-like particles in human milk by hybridization to polyadenylic acid sequences. *Science* **179:**696–698.

Schnitzer, T.J. 1979. Phenotypic mixing between two primate oncoviruses. *J. Gen. Virol.* **42:**199–206.

Schnitzer, T.J., R.A. Weiss, and J. Zavada. 1977. Pseudotypes of vesicular stomatitis virus with the envelope properties of mammalian and primate retroviruses. *J. Virol.* **23:**449–454.

Seman, G. and C. Seman. 1968. Electron microscopic search for virus particles in patients with leukemia and lymphoma. *Cancer* **22:**1033–1045.

Seman, G., H.S. Gallager, J.M. Lukeman, and L. Dmochowski. 1971. Studies on the presence of particles resembling RNA virus particles in human breast tumors, pleural effusions, their tissue cultures and milk. *Cancer* **28:**1431–1442.

Sherr, C.J. and G.J. Todaro. 1974. Type-C virus antigens in man. Antigens related to endogenous primate virus in human tumors. *Proc. Natl. Acad. Sci.* **71:**4703–4707.

———. 1975. Primate type C virus p30 antigen in cells from human with acute leukemia. *Science* **187:**855–857.

Shibuya, M., T. Hanafusa, H. Hanafusa, and J.R. Stephenson. 1980. Homology exists among the transforming sequences of avian and feline sarcoma virus. *Proc. Natl. Acad. Sci.* **77:**6536–6540.

Shigematsu, T., E.S. Priori, L. Dmochowski, and J.R. Wilbur. 1971. Immunelectron microscopic studies of type C virus particles in ESP-1 and HEK-1-HRLV cell lines. *Nature* **234:**412–414.

Shih, C., L.C. Padhy, M. Murray, and R.A. Weinberg. 1981. Transforming genes of carcinomas and neuroblastomas introduced into mouse fibroblasts. *Nature* **290:**261–264.

Shih, C., B.-Z. Shilo. M.P. Goldfarb, A. Dannenberg, and R.A. Weinberg. 1979. Passage of phenotypes of chemically transformed cells via transformation of DNA and chromatin. *Proc. Natl. Acad. Sci.* **76:**5714–5718.

Shimoyama, M., K. Minato, H. Saito, T. Kitahara, C. Konda, M. Nakazawa, S. Watanabe, N. Inada, T. Nagatani, K. Deura, and A. Mikata. 1979. Comparisons of clinical, morphologic, and immunologic characteristics of adult T-cell leukemia-lymphoma and cutaneous T-cell lymphoma. *Jpn. J. Clin. Oncol.* **9:**357–372.

Smith, H.S., J.L. Riggs, and E.L. Springer. 1977. Expression of antigenic crossreactivity to RD 114 p30 protein in a human fibrosarcoma cell line. *Proc. Natl. Acad. Sci.* **74:**744–748.

Smith, P.G., and M.C. Pike. 1976. Current epidemiological evidence for transmission of Hodgkin's disease. *Cancer Res.* **36:**660–662.

Smith, P.G., M.C. Pike, L.J. Kinlen, A. Jones, and R. Harris. 1977. Contacts between young people with Hodgkin's disease. A case-control study. *Lancet* **2:**59–62.

Smith, R.G., K. Nooter, P. Bentvelzen, M. Robert-Guroff, K. Harewood, M.S. Reitz, S.A. Lee, and R.C. Gallo. 1979. Characterization of a type-C virus produced by co-cultures of human leukemic bone-marrow and fetal canine thymus cells. *Int. J. Cancer* **24:**210–217.

Snyder, H.W., Jr., and E. Fleissner. 1980. Specificity of human antibodies to oncovirus glycoproteins: Recognition of antigen by natural antibodies directed against carbohydrate structures. *Proc. Natl. Acad. Sci.* **77:**1622–1626.

Snyder, H.W., Jr., and M. Fox. 1978. Characterization of a fetal calf serum derived molecule reactive with human natural antibodies: Its occurrence in tissue-culture grown, type C RNA viruses. *J. Immunol.* **120:**646–651.

Snyder, H.W., Jr., T. Pincus, and E. Fleissner. 1976. Specificities of human immunoglobulins reactive with antigens in preparations of several mammalian type-C viruses. *Virology* **75:**60–73.

Soule, H.D., J. Vazquez, A. Long, S. Albert, and M. Brennan. 1973. A human cell line from a pleural effusion derived from a breast carcinoma. *J. Natl. Cancer Inst.* **51:**1409–1416.

Spector, D.H., H.E. Varmus, and J.M. Bishop. 1978. Nucleotide sequences related to the transforming gene of avian sarcoma virus are present in the DNA of uninfected vertebrates. *Proc. Natl. Acad. Sci.* **75:**4102–4106.

Spiegelman, S., R. Axel, and J. Schlom. 1972. Virus-related RNA in human and mouse mammary tumors. *J. Natl. Cancer Inst.* **48:**1205–1211.

Spiegelman, S., D. Kufe, R. Hehlmann, and W.P. Peters. 1973. Evidence for RNA tumor viruses in human lymphomas including Burkitt's disease. *Cancer Res.* **33:**1515–1526.

Speigelman, S., I. Keydar, R. Mesa-Tejada, T. Ohno, M. Ramanarayanan, R. Nayak, J. Bausch, and C. Fenoglio. 1980a. Possible diagnostic implications of a mammary tumor virus related protein in human breast cancer. *Cancer* **46:**879–892.

Spiegelman, S., R. Mesa-Tejada, T. Ohno, M. Ramanarayanan, R. Nayak, J. Bausch, C. Fenoglio, and I. Keydar. 1980b. The presence and clinical implications of a virus-related protein in human breast cancer. *Cold Spring Harbor Conf. Cell Proliferation* **7:**1149–1167.

Stavnezer, E., D.S. Gerhard R.C. Binari, and I. Balazs. 1981. Generation of transforming viruses in cultures of chicken fibroblasts infected with an avian leukosis virus. *J. Virol.* **39:** 920–934.

Steel, L.K., H. Laube, and P. Chandra. 1977. Biochemical and serological characteristics of reverse transcriptase from human spleen in a case of childhood myelofibrotic syndrome. *Cancer Lett.* **2:**291–298.

Stehelin, D., H.E. Varmus, J.M. Bishop, and P.K. Vogt. 1976. DNA related to the transforming gene(s) of avian sarcoma virus is present in normal avian DNA. *Nature* **260:**170–173.

Stephenson, J.R. and S.A. Aaronson. 1976. Search for antigens and antibodies crossreactive with type C viruses of the woolly monkey and gibbon ape in animal models and in human. *Proc. Natl. Acad. Sci.* **73:**1725–1729.

———. 1977. Endogenous C-type viral expression in primates. *Nature* **266:**469–472.

Stephenson, J.R., A.S. Khan, W.J.M. van de Ven, and F.H. Reynolds, Jr. 1979. Type C retroviruses as vectors for cloning cellular genes with probable transforming function. *J. Natl. Cancer Inst.* **63:**1111–1119.

Strand, M. and J.T. August. 1974a. Structural proteins of mammalian oncogenic RNA viruses: Multiple antigenic determinants of the major internal protein and envelope glycoprotein. *J. Virol.* **13:**171–180.

———. 1974b. Type-C RNA virus gene expression in human tissue. *J. Virol.* **14:** 1584–1596.

Suzuki, T., K. Yanagihara, K. Yoshida, T. Seido, N. Kuga, Y. Shimosato, and S. Oboshi. 1977. Infectious murine type-C viruses released from human cancer cells transplanted into nude mice. *Gann* **68:**99–106.

Tajima, K., S. Tominaga, T. Kuroishi, H. Shimizu, and T. Suchi. 1979. Geographical features and epidemiological approach to endemic T-cell leukemia/lymphoma in Japan. *Jpn. J. Clin. Oncol.* **9:**495–504.

Takatsuki, K., T. Uchiyama, T. Ueshima, and T. Hattori. 1979. Adult T-cell leukemia: Further clinical observations and cytogenic and functional studies of leukemic cells. *Jpn. J. Clin. Oncol.* **9:**317–324.

Teich, N.M., R.A. Weiss, S.Z. Salahuddin, R.E. Gallagher, D.H. Gillespie, and R.C. Gallo. 1975. Infective transmission and characterisation of a C-type virus released by cultured human myeloid leukaemia cells. *Nature* **256:**551–555.

The T- and B-Cell Malignancy Study Group. 1981. Statistical analysis of immunologic, clinical and histopathologic data on lymphoid malignancies in Japan. *Jpn. J. Clin. Oncol.* **11:**15–38.

Theilen, G.H., D. Gould, M. Fowler, and D.L. Dungworth. 1971. C-type virus in tumor tissue of a woolly monkey (Lagothrix spp.) with fibrosarcoma. *J. Natl. Cancer Inst.* **47:**881–889.

Thiel, H.J., E.M. Broughton, T.J. Matthews, W. Schäfer, and D.P. Bolognesi. 1981. Interspecies reactivity of type C and and D retrovirus p15(E) and p15(C) proteins. *Virology* **111:**270–274.

Thiry, L., S. Sprecher-Goldberger, M. Bossens, and F. Neuray. 1978a. Cell-mediated immune response to simian oncornavirus antigens in pregnant women. *J. Natl. Cancer Inst.* **60:**527–532.

———. 1978b. Immune response to primate oncornaviruses in pre-eclampsia. *Lancet* **1:**1268.

Thiry, L., S. Sprecher-Goldberger, M. Bossens, J. Cogniaux-Le Clerc, and P. Vereerstraeten. 1978c. Neutralization of Mason-Pfizer virus by sera from patients treated for renal disease. *J. Gen. Virol.* **41:**587–597.

Todaro, G.J. and R.C. Gallo. 1973. Immunological relationship of DNA polymerase from human acute leukemia cells and primate and mouse leukemia virus reverse transcriptase. *Nature* **244:**206–209.

Todaro, G.J., V. Zeve, and S.A. Aaronson. 1970. Virus in cell culture derived from human tumour patients. *Nature* **226:**1047–1049.

Todaro, G.J., S.S. Tevethia, and J.L. Melnick. 1973a. Isolation of an RD-114 related type-C virus from feline sarcoma virus-transformed baboon cells. *Intervirology* **1:**399–404.

Todaro, G.J., R.E. Benveniste, S.A. Sherwin, and C.J. Sherr. 1978. MAC-1, a new genetically transmitted type C virus of primates: "Low frequency" activation from stumptail monkey cell cultures. *Cell* **13:**775–782.

Todaro, G.J., P. Arnstein, W.P. Parks, E.H. Lennette, and R.J. Huebner. 1973b. A type C virus in human rhabdomyosarcoma cells after inoculation into NIH Swiss mice treated with anti-thymocyte serum. *Proc. Natl. Acad. Sci.* **70:**859–862.

Tokuhata, G.K. 1969. Morbidity and mortality among offspring of breast cancer mothers. *Am. J. Epidemiol.* **89:**139–153.

Tóth, D., J. Kiss, L. Váczi, Z. Madár, J. Jakó, and K. Rák. 1980. Specific antibodies to viruses HL-23 and BILN in the blood plasma of patients with acute myelogenous leukaemia and with potential preleukaemia. *Acta Microbiol. Acad. Sci. Hung.* **27:**147–153.

Tveit, K.M. and A. Pihl. 1981. Do cell lines in vitro reflect the properties of the tumours of origin? A study of lines derived from human melanoma xenografts. *Br. J. Cancer* **44:**775–786.

Uchiyama, T., J. Yodoi, K. Sagawa, K. Takatsuki, and H. Uchino. 1977. Adult T-cell leukemia: Clinical and hematologic features of 16 cases. *Blood* **50:**481–492.

Vaidya, A.B., M.M. Black, A.S. Dion, and D.H. Moore. 1974. Homology between human breast tumour RNA and mouse mammary virus genome. *Nature* **249:**565–567.

Vaidya, A.B., E.Y. Lasfargues, G. Heubel, J.C. Lasfargues, and D.H. Moore. 1976. Murine mammary tumor viruses: Characterization of infection of nonmurine cells. *J. Virol.* **18:**911–917.

van der Loo, E.M., G.N. van Muijen, W.A. van Vloten, W. Beens, E. Scheffer, and C.J. Meijer. 1979. C-type virus-like particles specifically localized in Langerhans cells and related cells of skin and lymph nodes of patients with mycosis fungoides and Sezary's syndrome. A morphological and biochemical study. *Virchows Arch. B Cell Pathol.* **31:**193–203.

van Muijen, G.N.P., J. te Velde, G.J. den Ottolander, A. Brand, N. Koopman-Broekhuyzen, A. Schaberg, and S.O. Warnaar. 1979. On the presence of reverse transcriptase in myelo- and lymphoproliferative disorders. *Cancer* **43:**1682–1688.

Vernon, M.L., J.M. McMahon, and J.J. Hackett. 1974. Additional evidence of type-C particles in human placentas. *J. Natl. Cancer Inst.* **52:**987–989.

Vianna, N.J., P. Greenwald, and J.N.P. Davies. 1971. Extended epidemic of Hodgkin's disease in high school students. *Lancet* **1:**1209–1210.

Viola, M.C. 1973. Reverse transcriptase and 70S RNA in supernatant from a human cell line. *J. Natl. Cancer Inst.* **50:**1175–1178.

Vogt, P.K. and R.R. Friis. 1971. An avian leukosis virus related to RSV(O): Properties and evidence for helper activity. *Virology* **43:**223–234.

Vosika, G.J., W. Krivit, J.M. Gerrard, P.F. Coccia, M.E. Nesbit, J.J. Coalson, and B.J. Kennedy. 1975. Oncornavirus-like particles from cultured bone marrow cells preceding leukemia and malignant histiocytosis. *Proc. Natl. Acad. Sci.* **72:**2804–2808.

Watson, K.F., K. Mölling, H. Gelderblom, and H. Bauer. 1974. Oncornavirus-like particles in HeLa cells. III. Biochemical characterization of the virus. *Int. J. Cancer* **13:**262–267.

Wei, C.-M., M. Gibson, P.G. Spear, and E.M. Scolnick. 1981. Construction and isolation of a transmissible retrovirus containing the *src* gene of Harvey murine sarcoma virus and the thymidine kinase gene of herpes simplex virus type 1. *J. Virol.* **39:**935–944.

Weimann, B.J., J. Schmidt, N. Kluge, W. Ostertag, and D.I. Wolfrum. 1975. RNA-dependent DNA polymerase from a cell line derived from the bone marrow of a patient with polycythemia vera. *Eur. J. Biochem.* **59:**581–588.

Weiss, R.A. 1973. Transmission of cellular genetic elements by RNA tumour viruses. In *Possible episomes in eukaryotes* (ed. L.G. Silvestri), pp 130–141. North-Holland, Amsterdam.

Weiss, R.A., R.R. Friis, E. Katz, and P.K. Vogt. 1971. Induction of avian tumor viruses in normal cells by physical and chemical carcinogens. *Virology* **46:**920–938.

Welsh, R.M., N.R. Cooper, F.C. Jensen, and M.B.A. Oldstone. 1975. Human serum lyses RNA tumor viruses. *Nature* **257:**612–614.

Welsh, R.M., Jr., A.F.C. Jensen, N.R. Cooper, and M.B. Oldstone. 1976. Inactivation and lysis of oncornaviruses by human serum. *Virology* **74:**432–440.

Westin, E.H., R.C. Gallo, S.K. Ariya, A. Eva, L.M. Souza, M. Baluda, S.A. Aaronson, and F. Wong-Staal. 1982a. Differential expression of the AMV gene in human hematopoietic cells. *Proc. Natl. Acad. Sci.* **79:**(in press).

Westin, E.H., F. Wong-Staal, E.P. Gelmann, R. Dalla-Favera, T. Papas, J.A. Lautenberger, A. Eva. P. Reddy, S. Tronick, S.A. Aaronson, and R.C. Gallo. 1982b. Expression of cellular homologues of retroviral *onc* genes in human hematopoietic cells. *Proc. Natl. Acad. Sci.* **79:**(in press).

Whiteley, S.A. and R.B. Naso. 1981. A comparative analysis: The intracellular precursor polyproteins of baboon endogenous retroviruses and the human viral isolate HL23V. *J. Virol.* (in press).

Witkin, S.S., T. Ohno, and S. Spiegelman. 1975. Purificaton of RNA-instructed DNA polymerase from human leukemic spleens. *Proc. Natl. Acad. Sci.* **72:**4133–4136.

Witkin, S.S., R.A. Egeli, N.H. Sarkar, R.A. Good, and N.K. Day. 1979. Virolysis of mouse mammary tumor virus by sera from breast cancer patients. *Proc. Natl. Acad. Sci.* **76:**2984–2987.

Witkin, S.S., N.H. Sarkar, D.W. Kinne, R.A. Good, and N.K. Day. 1980. Antibodies reactive with the mouse mammary tumor virus in sera of breast cancer patients. *Int. J. Cancer* **25:**721–725.

Wolfe, L.G., F. Deinhardt, G.H. Theilen, H. Rabin, T. Kawakami, and L.K. Bustad. 1971. Induction of tumors in marmoset monkeys by simian sarcoma virus, type 1 *(Lagothrix)*: A preliminary report. *J. Natl. Cancer Inst.* **47:**1115–1120.

Wong-Staal, F., D. Gillespie, and R.C. Gallo. 1976. Proviral sequences of baboon endogenous type C RNA virus in DNA of human leukaemic tissues. *Nature* **262:**190–195.

Wong-Staal, F., M.S. Reitz, Jr., and R.C. Gallo. 1979. Retrovirus sequences in a leukemic gibbon and its contact: Evidence for partial provirus in the nonleukemic gibbon. *Proc. Natl. Acad. Sci.* **76:**2032–2036.

Wong-Staal, F., G. Dalla Favera, R. Franchini, E.P. Gellman, and R.C. Gallo. 1981a. Three distinct genes in human DNA related to the transforming genes of mammalian sarcoma retroviruses. *Science* **213:**226–228.

Wong-Staal, F., G. Dalla Favera, E.P. Gellman, V. Manzari, S. Szala, S.F. Josephs, and R.C. Gallo. 1981b. The *v-sis* transforming gene of simian sarcoma virus is a new onc gene of primate origin. *Nature* **294:**273–275.

Wunderli, H., D.D. Mickey, and D.F. Paulson. 1979. C-type virus particles in urogenital tumours after heterotransplantation into nude mice. *Br. J. Cancer* **39:**35–42.

Yang, N.-S., C.M. McGrath, and P. Furmanski. 1978. Presence of a mouse mammary tumor virus-related antigen in human breast carcinoma cells and its absence from normal mammary epithelial cells. *J. Natl. Cancer Inst.* **61:**1205–1208.

Yang, N.-S., H.D. Soule, and C.M. McGrath. 1977. Expression of murine mammary tumor virus-related antigens in human breast carcinoma (MCF-7) cells. *J. Natl. Cancer Inst.* **59:**1357–1367.

Yaniv, A., T. Gotlieb-Stematsky, A. Vonsover, and K. Perk. 1980. Evidence for type-C retrovirus production by Burkitt's lymphoma-derived cell line. *Int. J. Cancer* **25:**205–211.

Yaniv, A., S.C. Gulati, A. Burny, and S. Spiegelman. 1973. Detection of complexes containing 70S RNA and reverse transcriptase in human leukemic plasma. *Intervirology* **1:**317–328.

Yeh, J., M. Ahmed, S.A. Mayyasi, and A.A. Alessi. 1975. Detection of an antigen related to Mason-Pfizer virus in malignant human breast tumors. *Science* **190:**583–584.

Zavada, J., J. Bubenik, R. Widmaier, and Z. Zavadova. 1975. Phenotypically mixed vesicular stomatitis virus particles produced in human tumor cell lines. *Cold Spring Harbor Symp. Quant. Biol.* **39:**907–912.

Zavada, J., Z. Zavadova, A. Malir, and A. Kocent. 1972. VSV pseudotype produced in cell line derived from human mammary carcinoma. *Nat. New Biol.* **240:**124–125.

Zavada, J., Z. Zavadova, R. Widmaier, J. Bubenik, M. Indrova, and C. Altaner. 1974. A transmissible antigen detected in two cell lines derived from human tumours. *J. Gen. Virol.* **24:**327–337.

Zhdanov, V.M., V.D. Soloviev, T.A. Bektemirov, F.P. Filatov, and A.V. Bykovsky. 1972. Isolation of a leukovirus from a continuous human cell line. *Arch. Gesamte Virusforsch.* **39:**309–316.

Zhdanov, V.M., V.O. Soloviev, T.A. Bektemirov, K.V. Ilyin, A.F. Bykovsky, N.P. Mazurenko, I.S. Irlin, and F.I. Yershov. 1973. Isolation of oncornaviruses from continuous human cell cultures. *Intervirology* **1:** 19–26.

Zotter, S., C. Kemmer, A. Lossnitzer, H. Grossmann, and B.A. Johannsen. 1980. Mouse mammary tumour virus-related antigen in core-like density fractions from large samples of women's milk. *Eur. J. Cancer* **16:**455–467.

Zurcher, C., J. Brinkhof, P. Bentvelzen, and J.C.H. de Man. 1975. C-type virus antigens detected by immunofluorescence in human bone tumour cultures. *Nature* **254:**457–459.

Appendixes

APPENDIX A
Nomenclature

Communication among retrovirologists has been greatly simplified over the past decade by the general acceptance of conventional names for structural and genetic features of viral genomes, for viral mutants, and for virus-coded proteins. As a convenient summary to assist reading of the text and use of the ensuing Appendixes, we provide here the major definitions and rules that now govern the appellation of retroviral genes, noncoding regions of genomes, mutants, and proteins; in some cases, references are provided for more detailed explanations of these terms and symbols.

1. Structural and Genetic Features of Retroviral Genomes

A full account of the properties of retroviral genomes is provided in Chapter 4. Here, we simply reiterate the definitions of regions of the genome important for interpretation of the maps and sequences presented in Appendixes B through F.

a. The Regions of Replication-competent Retroviral RNA

Cap site: The penultimate nucleotide at the 5′ end of the viral RNA subunit, presumably the initiating nucleotide in an RNA transcript of proviral DNA; linked to a methylated "cap" ribonucleotide by a 5′-5′ linkage.

R: A short sequence (13–60 nucleotides) repeated at both ends of the RNA subunit, exclusive of the cap nucleotide at the 5′ terminus and the poly(A) tract at the 3′ terminus; also present twice in viral DNA as part of the LTR.

U_5: A sequence of about 80–120 nucleotides, positioned between R and PB(–), present once in viral RNA and twice in the viral

DNA product of reverse transcription; it forms part of the LTR.

PB(−): A region (usually 18 nucleotides) adjacent to U_5 and complementary to the 3′ terminus of the host tRNA species, which functions as primer for synthesis of the minus (−) strand of viral DNA.

L: The untranslated region of a few hundred nucleotides between PB(−) and the initiation codon for the first coding region of the viral genome (*gag*).

gag: The first of three coding domains of a replication-competent genome (Baltimore 1975); encodes a polyprotein whose products form the major structural proteins of the virus core and contribute the principal *g*roup-specific *a*nti*g*enic determinants.

pol: The second coding domain, encoding part of a polyprotein also containing *gag* peptides, whose cleavage products include virion-associated, RNA-directed DNA *pol*ymerase (reverse transcriptase).

env: The third coding domain, encoding a polyprotein whose products are the major structural proteins of the viral *enve*lope and induce the major neutralizing and type-specific antibodies.

S_d (donor splice site): A site (or sites) at which a 5′ portion of the genome is joined to a portion of the 3′ end of viral RNA to form a spliced, subgenomic messenger RNA; the major S_d is positioned near the 5′ terminus, probably within L or *gag;* depending on the virus strain.

S_a (acceptor splice site): A site (or sites) at which portions of the 3′ end of viral RNA are joined to S_d to form subgenomic mRNAs.

PB(+): The purine-rich sequence of 7–18 nucleotides on the 5′ side of U_3 believed to be the sequence of an as yet unidentified primer for synthesis of the plus (+) strand of viral DNA.

U_3: A sequence of several hundred (~170–1200) nucleotides positioned between PB(+) and R near the 3′ end of viral RNA, present once in viral RNA and twice in the viral DNA product of reverse transcription; it forms part of the LTR.

Poly(A) tract: A homopolymer of 50–200 adenylic acid residues added posttranscriptionally next to the R sequence at the 3′ end of the viral RNA; the poly(A) tract and cap nucleotide are not encoded in the viral genome, although a signal for polyadenylation (AAUAAA) is generally present about 15–20 nucleotides from the 3′ end of the heteropolymeric sequence.

b. Region of Retroviral Genomes Peculiar to Their DNA Forms

LTR (long terminal repeat): A domain of several hundred (~270–1300) base pairs composed of U_3-R-U_5 (5′ → 3′) and found at both ends of the unintegrated linear DNA product of reverse transcription; the LTR unit is also found in closed circular retroviral DNA (in one copy or two) and at both ends of integrated (proviral) DNA; in proviral DNA, the 5′ LTR lacks 2 nucleotides from the 5′ end of U_3 and the 3′ LTR lacks 2 bp from the 3′ end of U_5.

IR (inverted repeat): Short sequences (~5–23 bp) that form a perfect (or slightly imperfect) inverted repeat at the ends of the LTR unit; the IRs form a palindromic sequence when two complete LTRs are joined in circular DNA; 2 bp are missing from the IRs in proviral DNA.

Circular junction: The point at which LTRs are joined in circular DNA containing two LTRs.

Provirus: The integrated form of viral DNA.

2. A Nomenclature for *onc* Sequences

All structural proteins of retroviruses identified to date can be assigned to the coding domains encompassed by the terms *gag, pol,* and *env* (see above and Chapters 4 and 6). Although the individual domains may exhibit no structural homology when different virus isolates are compared, the functional homology has proved sufficiently strong (see Chapter 7) to vindicate the decision to use these three terms when referring to the genetic composition of a diverse collection of retroviruses. However, many retroviruses contain and use a set of coding sequences in addition to *gag, pol,* and *env,* and these sequences appear to share some important features: They encode a protein (or proteins) unnecessary for virus replication but probably required for the induction and maintenance of the transformed phenotype, and they are closely related to sequences that occur in the uninfected host cell but are distinct from the genome of any identified endogenous proviruses. These sequences are generically termed *onc* sequences or genes. Because of the importance of distinguishing among the relatively large number of different *onc* genes (at least 13 *onc* genes have been identified in over 20 transforming retrovirus isolates), a system for naming individual viral *onc* genes and for distinguishing them from their cellular homologs has recently been proposed (Coffin et al. 1981) and is used throughout this volume (see Chapter 9). According to the proposed system:

> *onc* genes will be given trivial three letter designations. These names are not meant to imply specific diseases, target cells, or functions, rather they are to be simply names of sequences which are not derived from viral replicative information and which encode a protein (or a portion of a polyprotein) likely to be involved in transformation of the infected cell. The system also distinguishes the viral from the related cellular sequences and, where necessary, the sequences in related viral strains from one another.

Names proposed and in general use as of mid-1981 are tabulated in Chapter 9 (Tables 9.1 and 9.2); others will no doubt be added in the near future.

> The names of these sequences are to be generated according to the following guidelines.
>
> 1. The names should be 3 letters, lowercase italics.
> 2. The names should be *trivial;* that is, no target cell specificity or functional significance is implied, and they are to be considered as names of coding sequences only.
> 3. They are to be derived in some mnemonic way from the name of the prototype virus or viruses or some other memorable feature of the viruses.
> 4. Related sequences in different viruses from the same species are to be called by the same name, in a way that should point to the same cell sequence and the same or a closely related protein product, although it should not be necessary to have identified all of these to assign a name.
> 5. When necessary for clarity, the differences between inserts in related viruses can be indicated by prefixing the name with the abbreviation or name for the virus or virus strain.
> 6. The related sequence found in the cell of origin will be designated with a lower case *c*- preceding the sequence names, e.g., *c-src*. The animal species of the cellular homologue should be indicated in parenthesis following the name of the sequence (e.g., *c-src* (chicken)). The unadorned name will indicate the viral sequence only; however, where helpful for emphasis it may be prefixed with *v*- (e.g., *v-src*).
> 7. Protein products will be designated according to current convention using the approximate molecular weight ($\times 10^{-3}$) preceded by p (for protein), pp (for phosphoprotein), or P (for polyprotein), and followed by

name of the gene in superscript. Thus $pp60^{src}$, $p150^{c\text{-}abl}$, $P120^{gag\text{-}abl}$ stand for the product of *src*, the product of the cell sequences related to *abl*, and the polyprotein containing both *gag* and *abl* specific information, respectively.

8. Should the same virus be found to have two *independently expressed* inserts (i.e., coding for different proteins through distinct mRNAs), then they can be distinguished by affixing -A, -B, etc. to the name (e.g., avian erythroblastosis virus *erb*-A and *erb*-B).
9. Names along the same lines can also be given to nontransforming inserts if found in retroviruses or deliberately put there, but should be limited to genetically significant regions, i.e., those with a protein (or functional RNA) product.
10. In the case where somewhat different yet related inserts are found in viruses of different species, different names may be used (Shibuya et al. 1980).
11. Strict genetic evidence is not required to assign a name, but it should be shown a) that the region is not-viral, and b) that is has either a protein or functional RNA product or a genetically identifiable function.

3. Nomenclature for Viral Mutants

Thus far, a formal nomenclature for viral mutants has been devised only for mutants of avian retroviruses, in view of the large numbers of such mutants (see Chapter 7 and accompanying tables). We present below an abbreviated version of the rules proposed by Vogt et al. (1974) and widely used by students of avian viruses.

Laboratory code letter. Each laboratory isolating conditional or nonconditonal mutants of avian leukosis and sarcoma viruses selects two capital letters which will be listed, preferably in italic type, before the mutant number. The current laboratory code is BE = Bethesda, John P. Bader; BK = Berkeley, G.S. Martin; BO = Boston, John Coffin; CU = Champagne-Urbana, Illinois, Michael Weber; FL = Gainesville, Florida, Carlo Moscovici; GI = Giessen, Robert R. Friis; LA = Los Angeles, Peter K. Vogt; LO = London, Robin A. Weiss and John A. Wyke; MA = Madison, Howard M. Temin; MI = Miami, M.M. Siegel; NE = New York, Alan Goldberg; NY = New York, Hidesaburo Hanafusa and Teruko Hanafusa; OS = Osaka, Kumao Toyoshima; PA = Paris, Philippe Vigier, Jean-Michel Biquard, and George Calothy; PH = Philadelphia, D. Boettiger and William S. Mason; RO = Rochester, New York, Piero Balduzzi; SE = Seattle, Maxine Linial; SF = San Francisco, Harold Varmus; ST = Stanford, William Robinson; TK = Tokyo, Sadaaki Kawai; TU = Tubingen, Thomas Graf. New laboratory code letters should be registered with Peter K. Vogt to avoid duplication.

Mutant number. Investigators may assign any number to a new mutant isolated in their laboratory. However, a given mutant number or number-letter combination may be issued only once by the same laboratory. This restriction should apply to all avian RNA tumor viruses encompassing conditional and nonconditional mutants and sarcoma, as well as leukosis, virus mutants.

Mutant category. Several categories of mutants have been recognized. These include temperature-sensitive (*ts*) conditional mutants, and nonconditional mutants such as transformation-defective (*td*) derivatives of avian sarcoma viruses, replication defectives (*rd*), coordinately defective (*cd*) viruses, which neither transform nor replicate, and mutants in focus morphology (fusiform, *morph*^{f}, or *ff*). In general, a suitable abbreviation of the mutant category should be incorporated in the designation of each mutant. This abbreviation should consist of lowercase italic letters (preferably two) to be placed without a hyphen before the laboratory code letter (e.g., *ts*LA335 = temperature-sensitive mutant 335 isolated in laboratory LA).

Wild-type strain. If mutants of several wild-type strains are described, it may be desirable to include an abbreviation of the strain in the mutant designation. This abbreviation should follow the mutant number. [See Chapter 7.]

Mutant subgroup. The envelope subgroup of a mutant may be included in the designation of individual mutants. It should then be appended, by using a hyphen, as a capital letter (Roman type) to mutant number of wild-type strain designation, (e.g., LA335-C or LA335PR-C).

Double mutants. If a second mutation is introduced in a mutant virus, a supplementary number should be attached to the first mutant number by using a hyphen. This supplementary number is subject to the same restrictions stipulated for the mutant number (see above); i.e., it cannot be a mutant number already used by the same laboratory. Thus, ambiguity is avoided if the two mutations are separated by recombination. The second number may also include information on the category of the new mutant (e.g., LA335-*td*121 = a transformation defective derivative of LA335 isolated in laboratory LA). If the secondary mutation is isolated in a different laboratory, the appropriate laboratory code letter should precede the secondary mutant number (e.g., LA335-NY4 = a transformation-defective derivative isolated from LA335 in laboratory NY). Mutant viruses which are isolated as bona fide single mutations but later found to carry multiple mutations should be marked by a lowercase Roman "m" (for multiple) after the mutant number (e.g., LA334m). If the two mutations of a double mutant are separated, e.g., by recombination, they should each be assigned a separate number. This could be done simply by adding a digit to the old mutant number, bearing in mind that the newly created number must not coincide with one previously used by the same laboratory (e.g., LA334m yields LA3341 and 3342).

4. Nomenclature for Retroviral Proteins

Soon after the introduction of high-resolution techniques for separation of viral proteins, it became apparent that confusion about the identities of viral proteins could only be avoided by a standardized nomenclature. The proposal made by August et al. (1974) after a meeting of interested parties has been generally accepted and supplies the basic rules governing usage throughout this book (see, especially, Chapters 6 and 9).

> It was suggested that the viral proteins be designated according to their apparent molecular weights in thousands. Proteins should be designated by a lowercase 'p' and glycoprotein by a 'gp' placed before the number indicating the molecular weight. Where the content leaves any ambiguity about the virus of origin, the name of the virus from which the proteins are derived can be prefixed to the protein designation. For example, the MLV protein of molecular weight 30,000 would be referred to as MLV p30. [The current nomenclature agreed upon for the major proteins of avian and murine viruses is shown in the tables in Chapter 6.] For designation of proteins by either the gel filtration or gel electrophoresis techniques it was suggested that the molecular weights be assigned according to the currently accepted figures for the avian and murine viral proteins.
>
> The antigenic determinants of the viral proteins have been characterized as type-specific, group-specific, and interspecies. We propose that when the antigenic determinants of a given protein are under consideration they be referred to in relation to this common nomenclature, e.g., p30 type, or p30 group, or p30 interspecies. The advantage of this usage is that it clearly identifies an antigen as a property of a given protein. Moreover, it can accommodate without ambiguity the presence of multiple antigenic determinants in a single protein that now appears to be a general property of virion proteins.
>
> Additional information concerning the structural role of a protein or its properties can be added in parentheses at the investigator's discretion. This could be either a phrase, e.g., MLV p30 (major core protein) or, if desired, an abbreviated symbol. For example, it was agreed that a constituent of intact viral cores may be indicated by the capital letter C, e.g, MLV p30(C). The letter E may designate a protein of the viral envelope and the letter N the major constituent of the viral ribonucleoprotein, e.g., MLV p10(N). This latter is by analogy to the nomenclature that has been adapted the ribonucleoproteins of influenza and rhabdoviruses.
>
> There are two advantages in this system: (1) It is flexible, i.e., a newly identified polypeptide can be added easily without disturbing the designations already in use, and (2) some physicochemical information about the protein is conveyed by its name. However, it is not the intent of this scheme to give precise values to molecular weights but to provide a generally applicable nomenclature to facilitate scientific exchange. In this regard there are certain specific problems. One is the choice between results obtained from gel filtration in guanidine hydrochloride as compared to those from polyacrylamide gel electrophoresis in the presence of sodium dodecyl sulfate. It was agreed that the molecular weights of the smaller components (10,000–30,000) should be designated by the results of guanidine hydrochloride gel filtration,

as the resolution of proteins by this method may be superior in this range. However, in a higher molecular-weight range (30,000–100,000) the resolution of the guanidine hydrochloride procedure is inferior, and gel electrophoresis is the method of choice. A second problem is that it is known that the molecular-weight estimates of glycoproteins by sodium dodecyl sulfate-polyacrylamide gel electrophoresis are often incorrect, presumably because of reduced binding of detergent to the carbohydrate component, leading to falsely high apparent molecular weights. Nevertheless, because the electrophoretic method offers good resolution of higher molecular-weight proteins, it was agreed that apparent molecular weights by this method should be used to designate viral glycoproteins. It is recognized that, because of the use of the gel filtration procedure as a reference, the molecular-weight values of smaller viral proteins may not correlate precisely with globular protein standards when measured by the polyacrylamide gel electrophoresis procedure.

Within this framework, additional, generally accepted conventions have arisen. Superscripts are used to indicate the coding region from which proteins were derived (as in $pp60^{src}$ or $p30^{gag}$). Proteins likely or proven to be precursors to more mature forms are designated by Pr, rather than p (as in $Pr76^{gag}$ or $Pr180^{gag\text{-}pol}$); other polyproteins not shown to be further processed are designated by a capital P (as in $P140^{gag\text{-}fps}$). A p is prefixed to a name to indicate that the protein is phosphorylated (as in $pp19^{gag}$) and a g is prefixed to indicate that it is glycosylated (as in $gp85^{env}$ or $gPr92^{env}$).

REFERENCES

August, J.T., D.P. Bolognesi, E. Fleissner, R.V. Gilden, and R.C. Nowinski. 1974. A proposed nomenclature for the virion proteins of oncogenic RNA viruses. *Virology* **60:**595–601.

Baltimore, D. 1975. Tumor viruses: 1974. *Cold Spring Harbor Symp. Quant. Biol.* **39:**1187–1200.

Coffin, J.M., H.E. Varmus, J.M. Bishop, M. Essex, W.D. Hardy, G.S. Martin, N.E. Rosenberg, E.M. Scolnick, R.A. Weinberg, and P.K. Vogt. 1981. A proposal for naming host cell-derived inserts in retrovirus genomes. *J. Virol.* **40:**953–957.

Shibuya, H., T. Hanafusa, H. Hanafusa, and J.R. Stephenson. 1980. Homology exists among the transformants of avian and feline sarcoma viruses. *Proc. Natl. Acad. Sci.* **77:**6536–6570.

Vogt, P.K., R.A. Weiss, and H. Hanafusa. 1974. A proposal for numbering mutants of avian leukosis and sarcoma viruses. *J. Virol.* **13:**551–554.

APPENDIX B

Restriction Maps of Representative Retroviral Proviruses and Cellular Oncogenes

1. Rous-associated Viruses
2. Acute Transforming Avian Retroviruses
3. Avian Viruses Not from the ASV-ALV Group
4. Murine Viruses I
5. Murine Viruses II
6. Murine Viruses III
7. Feline Viruses
8. Other Mammalian Retroviruses
9. Cellular Oncogenes I
10. Cellular Oncogenes II
11. Endogenous Proviruses Present in White Leghorn Chickens

The restriction maps presented here provide reasonable guides to some of the best-studied retroviral genomes. However, caution must be exercised in using these maps. In most cases, the maps are derived from a single virus isolate or from a single cloned viral DNA molecule. Since retroviruses exhibit considerable restriction site polymorphism, even within strains, the presence or absence of a particular restriction site should be confirmed experimentally in each instance. Furthermore, the maps shown here are necessarily incomplete; when no site for a particular enzyme is shown, it should not be assumed that no sites for that enzyme occur in the viral DNA.

In all cases, LTRs are depicted as compound boxes, with U_3 as an open box and R + U_5 as a closed box. (The nucleotide sequences of several of these LTRs are presented in Appendix D; inspection of these sequences provides additional information about the number and position of restriction sites.) The drawings have been made according to the accompanying scales. With the exception of *Eco*RI (sometimes shown as RI), the conventional names for restriction enzymes are employed throughout. Discussion of the methods by which the maps are derived can be found in Chapter 5 and in the cited references. The references listed here are by no means complete; they are meant to guide the reader to the source of the map presented. In many instances, the illustrated map was chosen arbitrarily since similar maps were available from multiple sources.

1. Restriction Maps of Rous-associated Viruses

The maps of RAV-1 and RAV-2 were provided by G. Payne (Payne et al., *Cell* **23,** 311, 1981, and unpubl.) and the map of RAV-0 was that derived by Shank et al. (*Virol.* **108,** 177, 1980). (See also Ju et al., *J. Virol.* **33,** 1026, 1980; Humphries et al., *Cell* **18,** 803, 1979.)

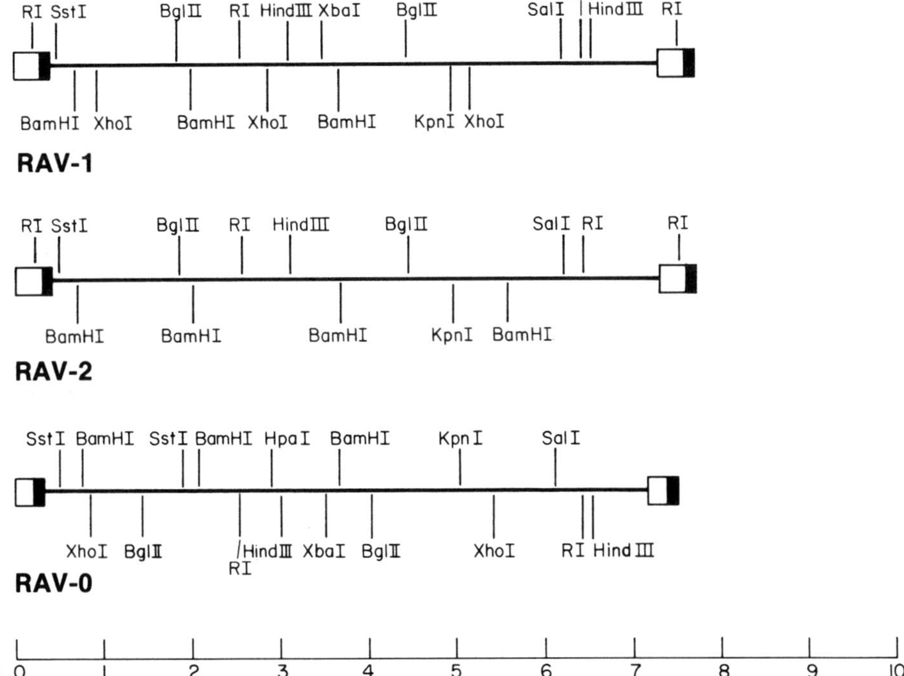

2. Restriction Maps of Acute Transforming Avian Retroviruses

The AMV map is derived principally from Souza et al. (*Proc. Natl. Acad. Sci.* **77,** 5177, 1980) with slight modifications suggested by T. Gonda (pers. comm.). The AEV map is from Vennstrom et al. (*J. Virol.* **36,** 575, 1980); the MC29 map is from Vennstrom et al. (*J. Virol.* **39,** 635, 1981). The map of RSV is a compilation of the data of Taylor et al. (*J. Virol.* **26,** 479, 1978), Shank et al. (*Cell* **15,** 1383, 1978), and DeLorbe et al.(*J. Virol.* **36,** 50, 1980) and is most applicable to the SR-A strain of RSV. Extensive polymorphism has been documented for the several studied strains of RSV, particularly in regions outside *gag* and *pol* (cf. Shank et al., *Cell* **15,** 1383, 1978; Lerner et al., *J. Virol.* **42,** 346, 1982; Katz et al., *J. Virol.* **42,** 346, 1982; and the sequence of PrC-RSV in Appendix E). The viral oncogenes are shown as a solid bar. The oncogenes are: for AMV, *myb*; for AEV, *erb*-A and *erb*-B; for MC-29, *myc*; and for RSV, *src*.

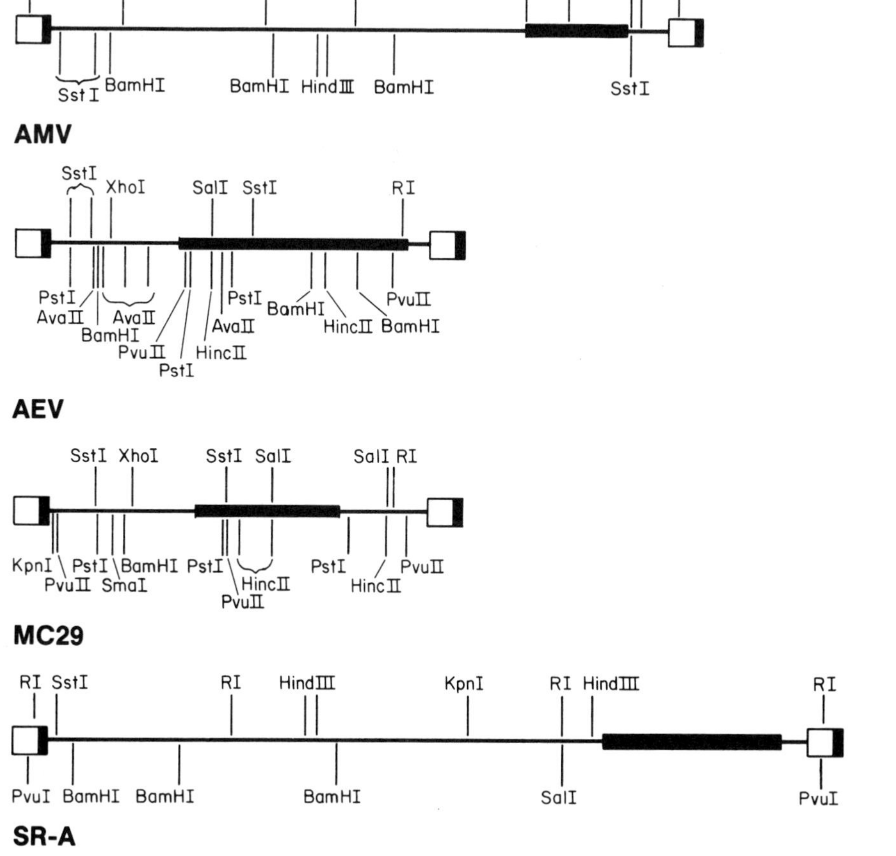
HindIII
XhoI
RI
XbaI
KpnI
RI
XbaI
XhoI
HindIII
SstI
BamHI
BamHI
HindIII
BamHI
SstI
AMV
SstI
XhoI
SalI
SstI
RI
PstI
AvaII
AvaII
BamHI
PvuII
PstI
HincII
AvaII
PstI
BamHI
HincII
BamHI
PvuII
AEV
SstI
XhoI
SstI
SalI
SalI
RI
KpnI
PvuII
PstI
SmaI
BamHI
PstI
PvuII
HincII
PstI
HincII
PvuII
MC29
RI
SstI
RI
HindIII
KpnI
RI
HindIII
RI
PvuI
BamHI
BamHI
BamHI
SalI
PvuI
SR-A
kb 0 1 2 3 4 5 6 7 8 9 10

3. Avian Viruses Not from the ASV-ALV Group

The oncogene, *v-rel,* present in REV-T, is shown as a thick bar. The SNV map is from O'Rear et al. (*Cell* **20,** 423, 1980); the REV-A and REV-T maps are from Chen et al. (*J. Virol.* **40,** 800, 1981); for more detailed maps, see Rice et al. (*J. Virol.* **42,** 237, 1982).

SstI
SalI
BglII
AvrII
Bst(E)II
HindIII
/Bst(E)II
BglII
SstI
BamHI
KpnI
XbaI
BamHI
XbaI
PstI
BamHI
PstI
KpnI
XhoI
BamHI
PstI
BamHI
AvrII
BamHI

SNV

SstI
SalI
XhoI
HindIII
HindIII
SstI
KpnI
KpnI
KpnI

REV-A

SstI
SalI
HindIII
SstI
KpnI
KpnI
RI
ClaI
RI

REV-T

kb 0 1 2 3 4 5 6 7 8 9 10

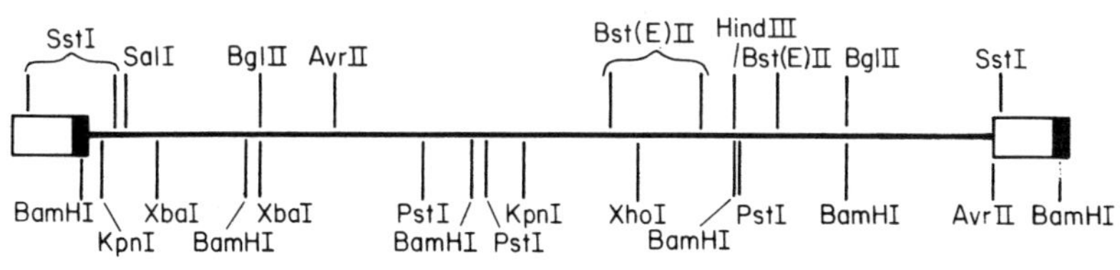

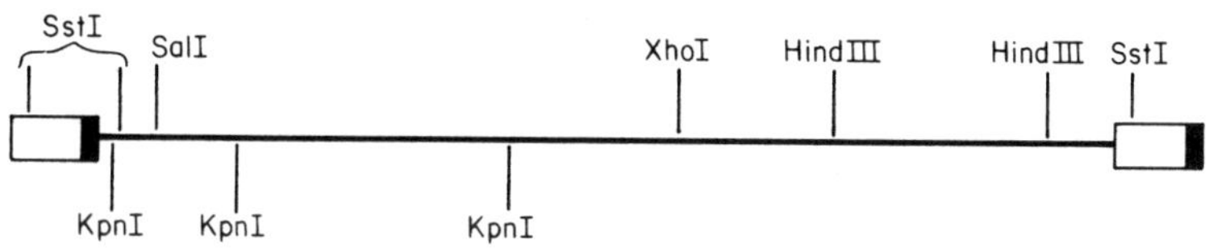

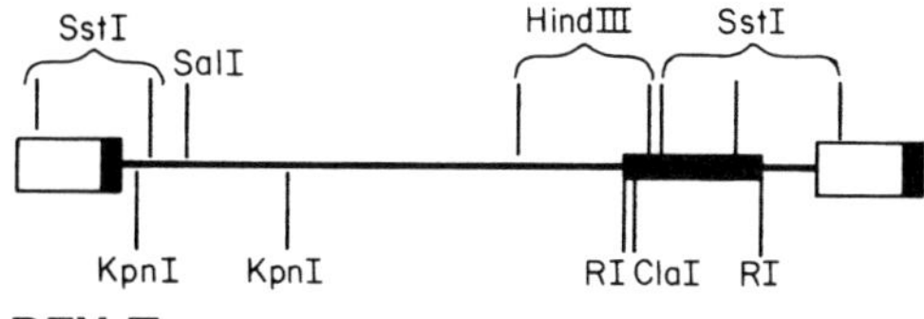

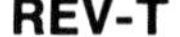

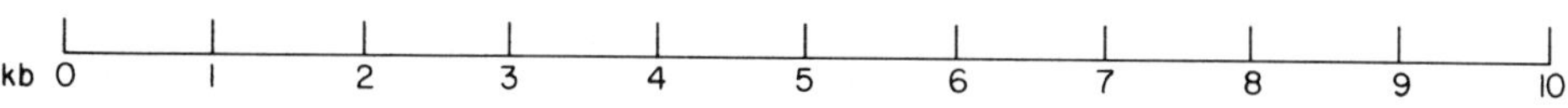

4. Murine Viruses (I)

The MMTV map is derived from studies of MMTV(C3H) and MMTV(GR) by Shank et al. (*Proc. Natl. Acad. Sci.* **75,** 2112, 1978) and J.C. Cohen et al. (*Cell* **16,** 333, 1979); the map is representative of MMTV(C3H). Additional mapping of horizontally transmitted and endogenous genomes can be found in J.C. Cohen et al. (*J. Virol.* **32,** 483, 1979); Groner and Hynes (*J. Virol.* **33,** 1013, 1980); Groner et al. (*J. Virol.* **36,** 734, 1980); Donehower et al. (*Cold Spring Harbor Symp. Quant. Biol.* **44,** 1153, 1980); Majors and Varmus (*Nature* **289,** 253, 1981); Hynes et al. (*Proc. Natl. Acad. Sci.* **78,** 2038, 1981); and Etkind et al. (*J. Virol* **41,** 855, 1982).

The maps of an ecotropic endogenous viral genome and of the Friend strain of MLV genome are from Chattopadhyay et al. (*J. Virol.* **39,** 777, 1981). The map of Mo-MLV DNA is derived from Verma and McKennet (*J. Virol.* **26,** 630, 1978), Gilboa et al. (*Cell* **16,** 863, 1979), and Yoshimura and Weinberg (*Cell* **16,** 323, 1979); more detailed information and maps of additional MLV genomes can be found in the cited references and in Chattopadhyay et al. (*Virology* **113,** 465, 1981; *Nature* **295,** 25, 1982).

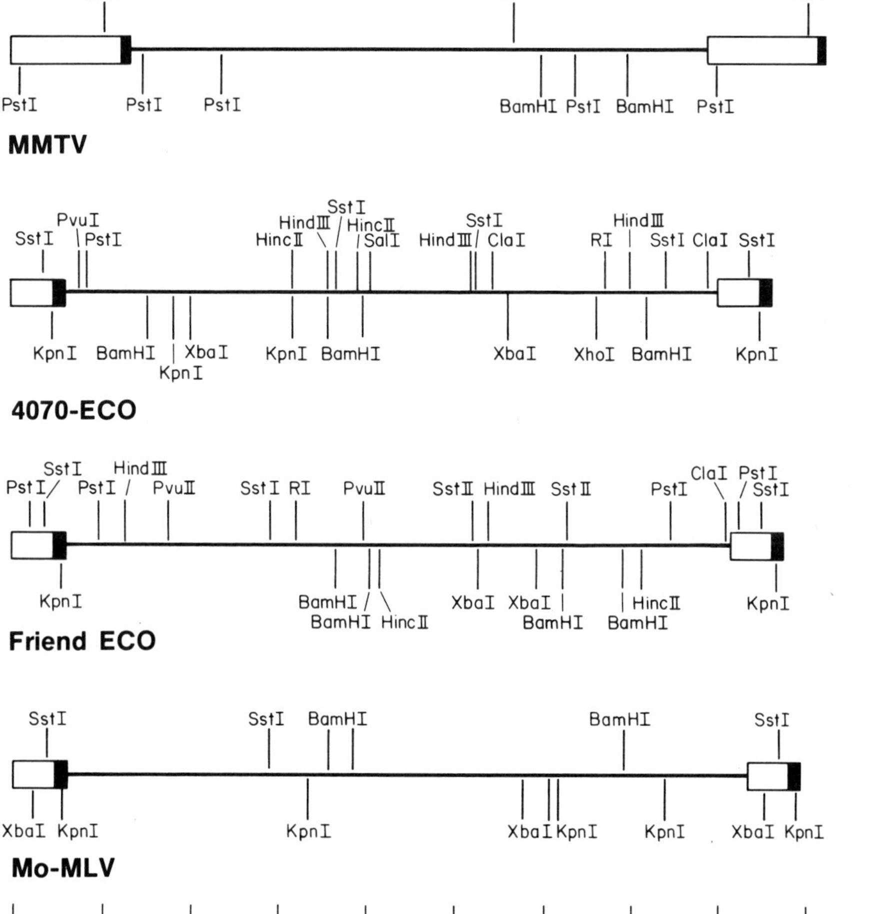
SstI
RI
SstI
PstI
PstI
PstI
BamHI PstI BamHI PstI
MMTV
SstI
PvuI
PstI
HindIII
SstI
HincII
HincII
SalI
HindIII
SstI
ClaI
RI
HindIII
SstI ClaI SstI
KpnI BamHI XbaI
KpnI
KpnI BamHI
XbaI
XhoI BamHI
KpnI
4070-ECO
PstI SstI
PstI HindIII
PvuII
SstI RI
PvuII
SstII HindIII SstII
PstI
ClaI PstI SstI
KpnI
BamHI
BamHI HincII
XbaI XbaI
BamHI
HincII
BamHI
KpnI
Friend ECO
SstI
SstI BamHI
BamHI
SstI
XbaI KpnI
KpnI
XbaI KpnI
KpnI
XbaI KpnI
Mo-MLV
kb 0 1 2 3 4 5 6 7 8 9 10

5. Murine Viruses II

The regions of mink-cell focus-forming virus (MCF) derived from the xenotropic parent are shown as an open bar, and the regions derived from the ecotropic parent are shown by a solid line. The data are taken from Chattopadhyay et al. (*Virology* **113,** 465, 1981).

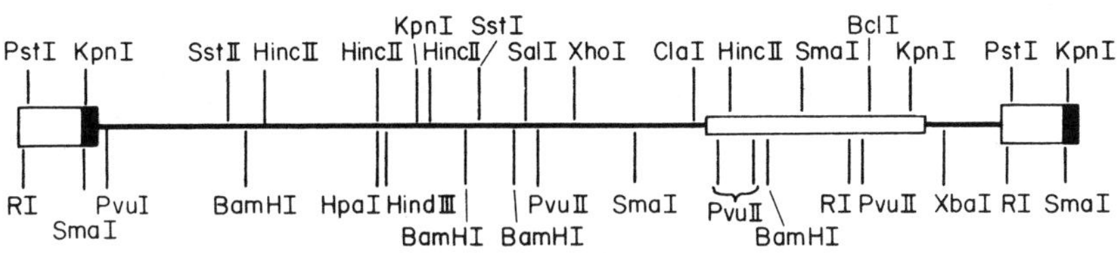

MCF M116

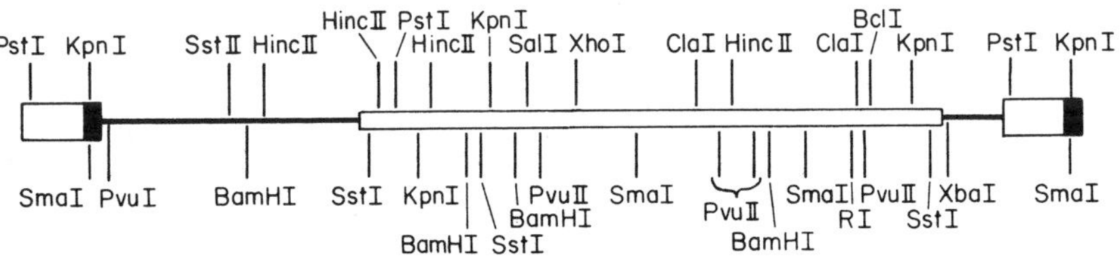

MCF 247

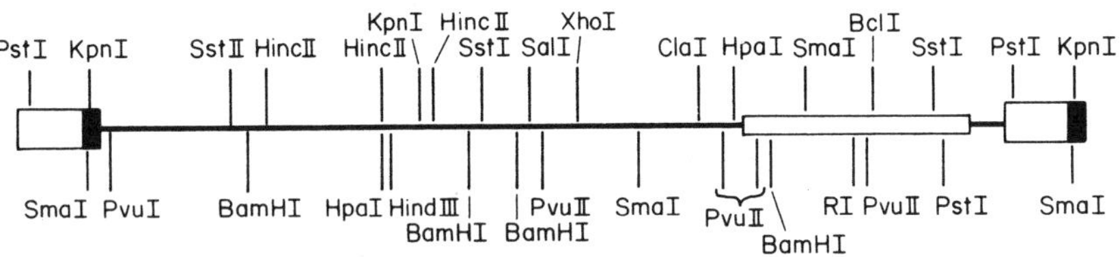

MCF 13

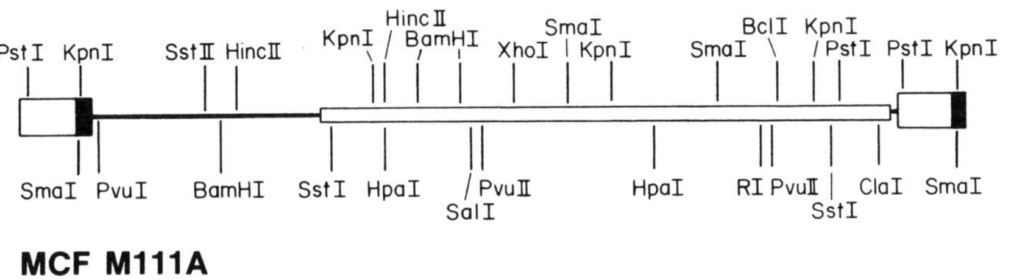

MCF M111A

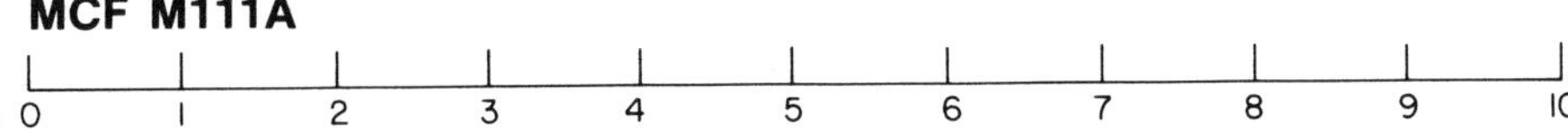

6. Murine Viruses III

The viral oncogenes are shown as thick bars. The oncogenes are: for Mo-MSV, *mos*; for BALB MSV, *bas*; and for Ha-MSV, *v-Ha-ras*. The Mo-MSV 124 map is from Verma et al. (*Proc. Natl. Acad. Sci.* **77,** 1773, 1980); the BALB MSV map is from P.R. Andersen et al. (*J. Virol.* **40,** 431, 1981). The Ha-MSV map is from Goldfarb and Weinberg (*J. Virol.* **32,** 30, 1979), Hager et al. (*J. Virol.* **31,** 795, 1979), and Ellis et al. (*J. Virol.* **36,** 408, 1980). The Ki-MSV map is from N. Tsuchida (pers. comm.). The precise extent of the oncogene in Ki-MSV was not available, and the barred region denoting *v-Ki-ras* was therefore omitted. The SFFV map is from A. Bernstein (pers. comm.).

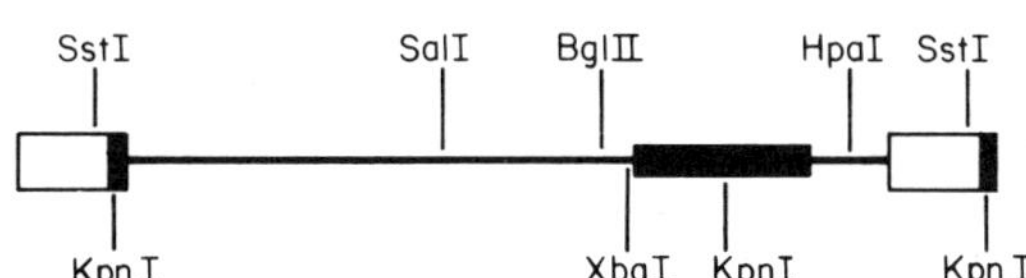

Mo-MSV-124

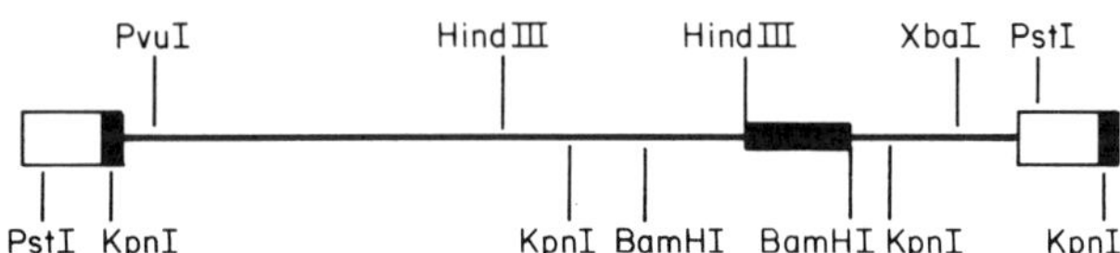

BALB MSV

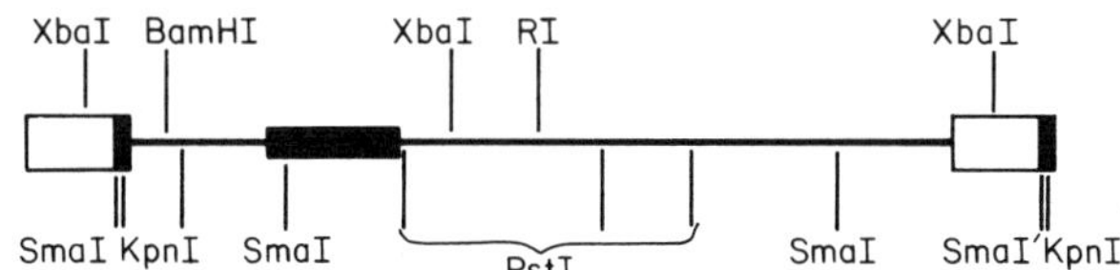

Ha-MSV

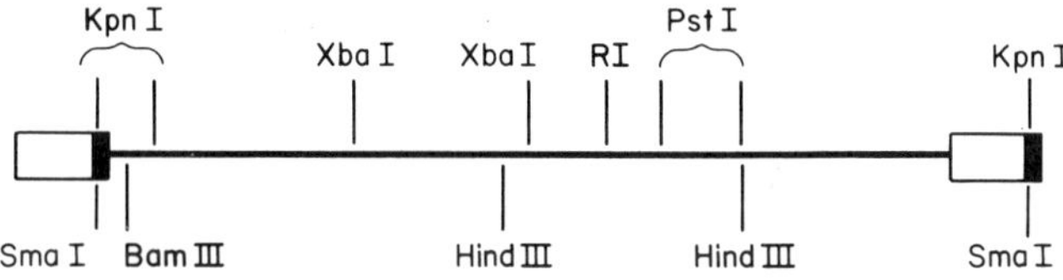

Ki-MSV

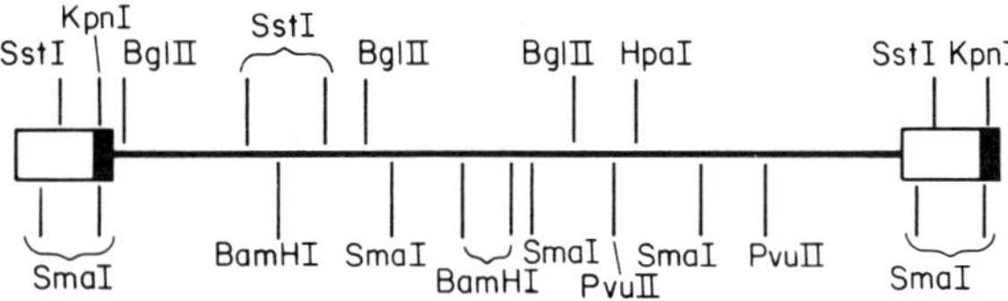

SFFV

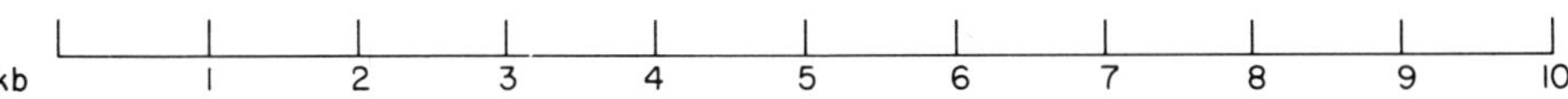

7. Feline Viruses

The viral oncogenes are shown as thick bars. The oncogenes are: for ST-FeSV, *ST-fes*; for GA-FeSV, *GA-fes*; and for SM-FeSV, *SM-fms*. The RD114 map is from J. Mullins (pers. comm.). The ST-FeLV and ST-FeSV maps are from Sherr et al. (*J. Virol.* **32,** 200, 1980). The GA-FeLV map is from Mullins et al. (*Nucleic Acids Research* **8,** 3287, 1980; see also Mullins et al., *J. Virol.* **36,** 688, 1981); the GA-FeSV map from Fedele et al. (*Proc. Natl. Acad. Sci.* **78,** 4036, 1981). The SM-FeSV map is from Donner et al. (*J. Virol.* **41,** 489, 1982).

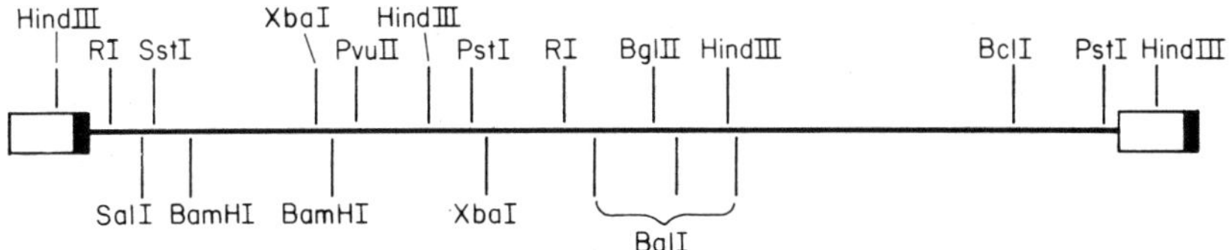

RD114

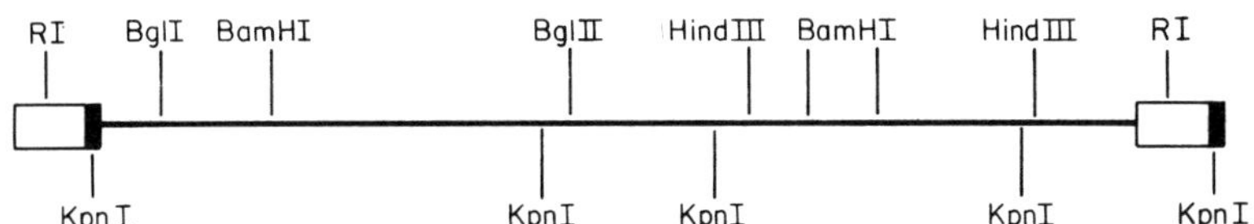

ST-FeLV

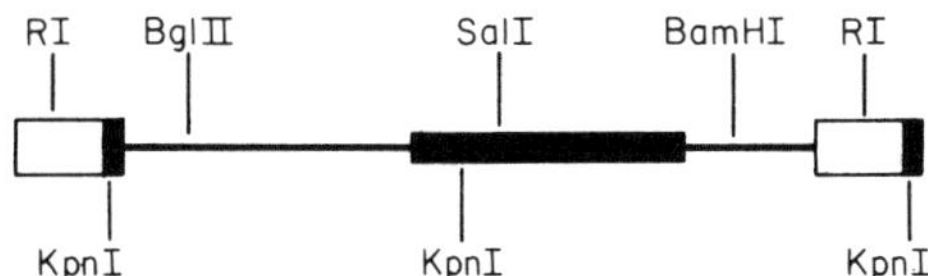

ST-FeSV

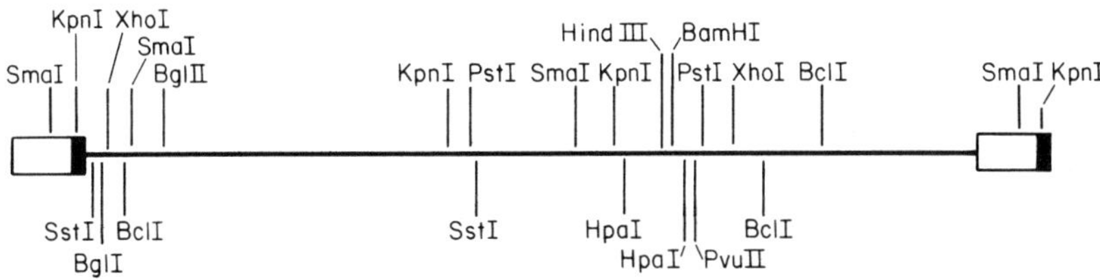

GA-FeLV

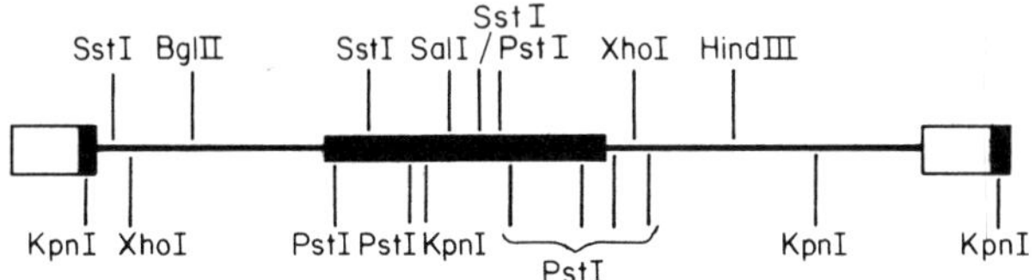

GA-FeSV

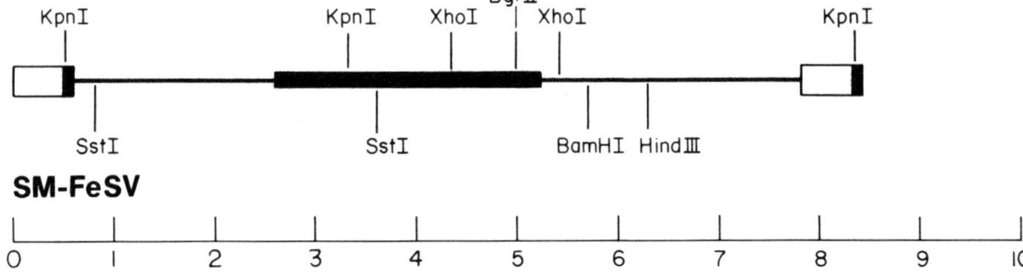

8. Other Mammalian Retroviruses

The map of BaEV is from M. Cohen et al. (*Proc. Natl. Acad. Sci.* **78,** 5207, 1981). The maps of GaLV and of the helper virus (SSAV) are from Trainor et al. (*J. Virol.* **41,** 298, 1982). The visna virus map is from Harris et al. (*Virology* **113,** 573, 1981). Unintegrated linear visna virus DNA has a single-stranded gap near the middle of the genome; the position of the single-stranded region is marked.

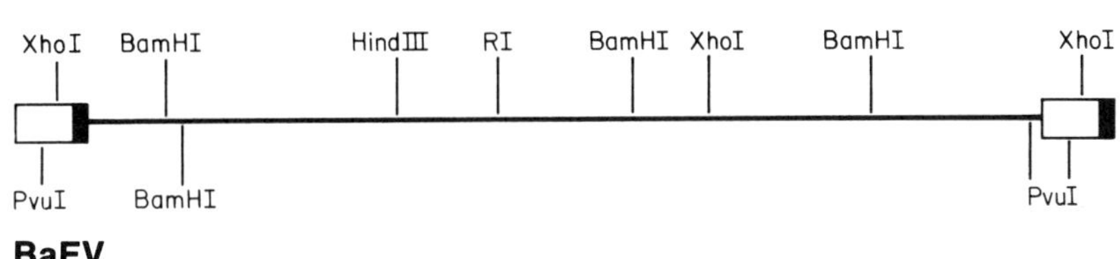

BaEV

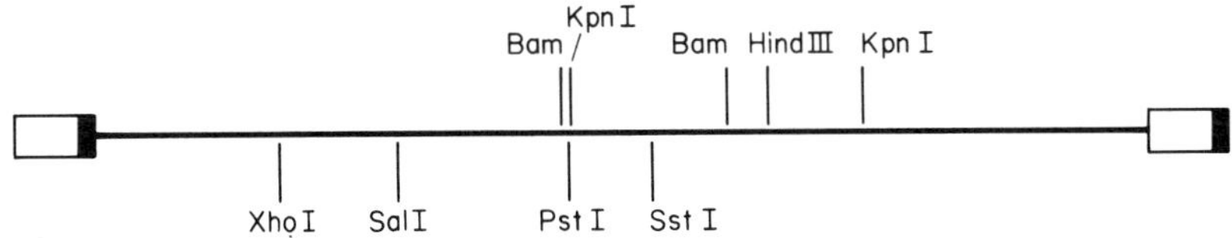

GaLV-Seato

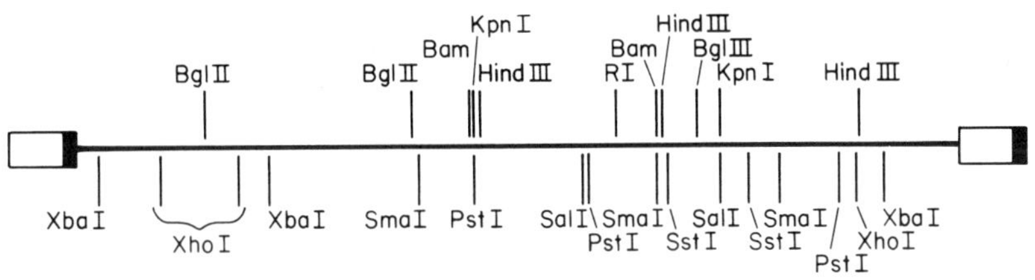

SSAV

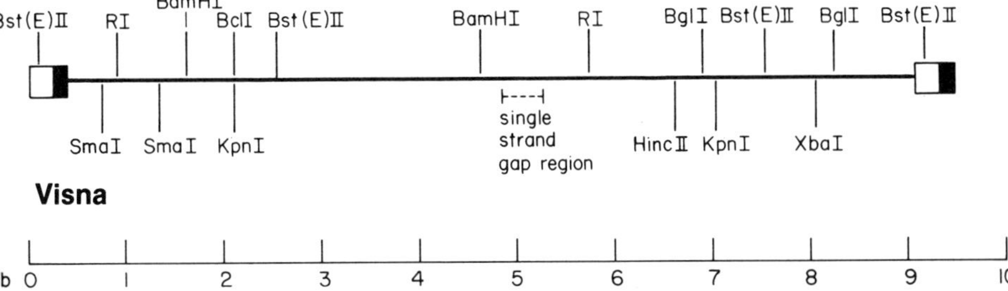

Visna

9. Cellular Oncogenes I

Exons are shown as thick bars on these maps, and intervening sequences and flanking sequences are shown as thin lines. The maps are for the form of these oncogenes present in chickens. The *c-src* map is from Shalloway et al. (*Cell* **24,** 531, 1981; see also Parker et al., *Proc. Natl. Acad. Sci.* **75,** 5842, 1981; Takeya et al., *Mol. Cell. Biol.* **1,** 1024, 1981). The *c-myb* map is from T. Gonda (pers. comm.) and the *c-rel* map is from I. Chen and H. Temin (pers. comm.).

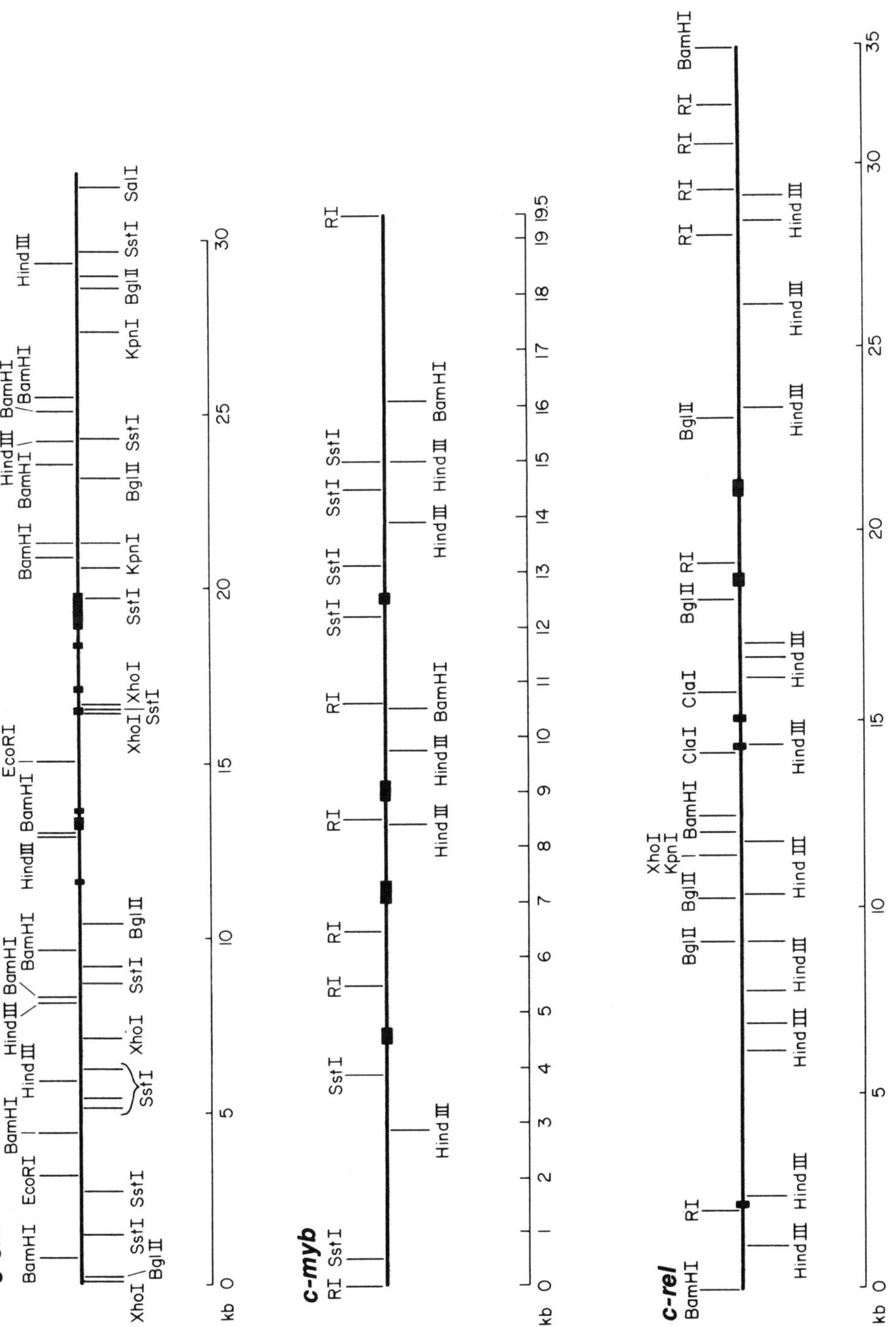
c-myb
c-rel
kb

10. Cellular Oncogenes II

In these drawings each of the *c-onc* genes is paired with the homologous *v-onc.* Again exons are shown as thick bars, and introns and flanking regions as a thin line. The *v-myc*/*c-myc* (chicken) comparison is from B. Neel (pers. comm.) (see also Robins et al., *J. Virol.* **41,** 635, 1982; Payne et al., *Nature* **295,** 209, 1982). The *v*-Harvey-*ras* and the two highly homologous *c-ras* (rat) genes are from DeFeo et al. (*Proc. Natl. Acad. Sci.* **78,** 3328, 1981) and the *v-mos*/*c-mos* (mouse) comparison was drawn from the sequence data of van Beveren et al. (*Nature* **289,** 258, 1981, and pers. comm. and Appendix E).

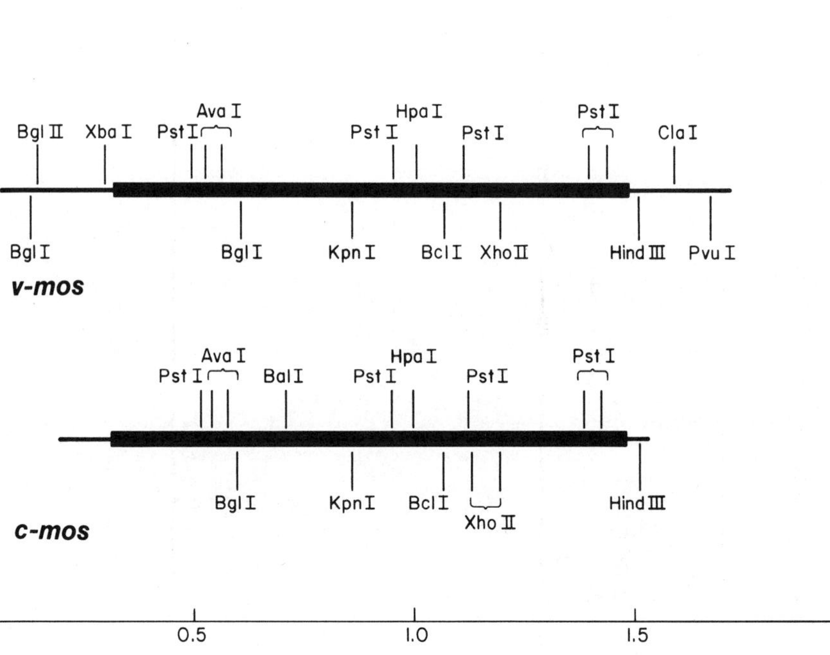

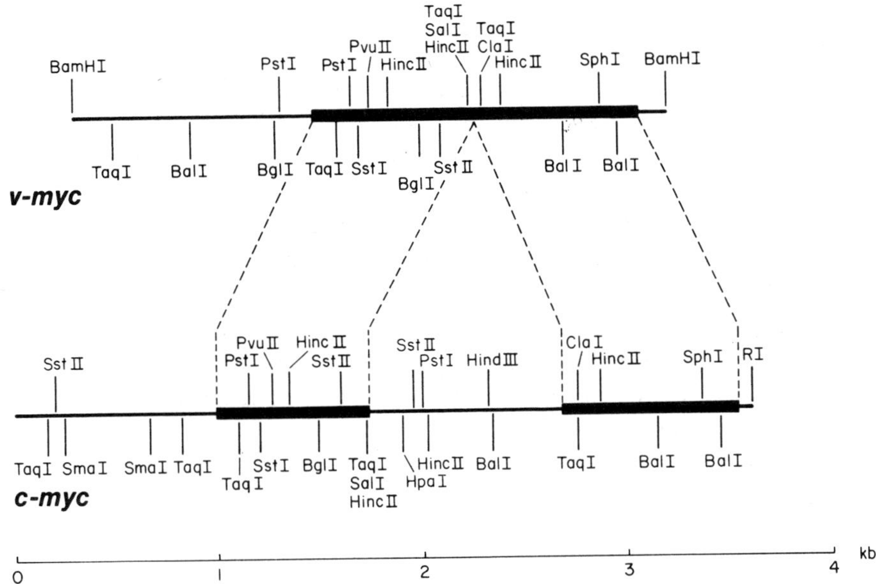

v-myc
c-myc
kb
0
1
2
3
4

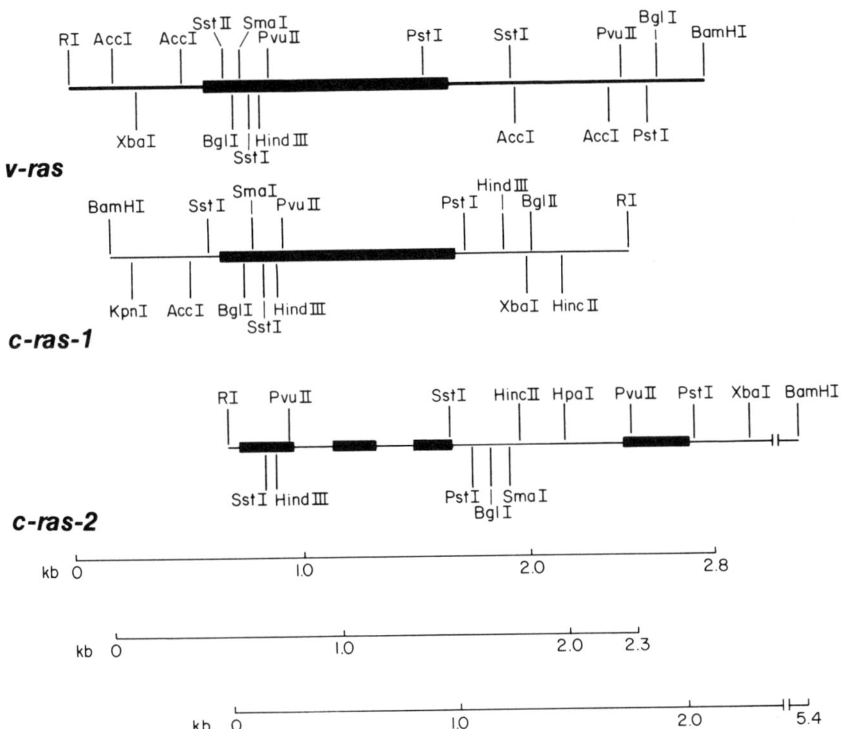

v-ras
c-ras-1
c-ras-2
kb 0 1.0 2.0 2.8
kb 0 1.0 2.0 2.3
kb 0 1.0 2.0 5.4

11. Endogenous Proviruses Present in White Leghorn Chickens

The drawings are to scale. Proviral DNA is shown as thick lines, and the LTRs as thin vertical boxes; U_3 is an open box, and U_5 a filled box. Cell DNA is shown as thin lines. For proviruses which have sustained deletions (*ev*-3, *ev*-4, *ev*-5, and *ev*-6), the approximate size of the deleted viral sequences is shown as an open box. In some cases restriction sites could not be placed unambiguously on the map; in these cases the size of the hybridizing fragment is listed in kb at the left of the drawing (i.e., *ev*-1 *Sst*I, 11). If a particular provirus is associated with a known phenotype, this is also listed (i.e., *ev*-1, gs^-chf^-). One of the proviruses has not been given an *ev* number designation, and this provirus has been labeled "3" in the drawing. The two elements at the bottom of the drawing, *ev*-15 and *ev*-16 hybridize only with probes specific for the endogenous virus LTR, and may consist of an LTR not associated with any other viral DNA sequence. The data presented here are from Hughes et al. (*Virology* **108,** 189, 1981) (for further discussion and additional references see Chapter 10).

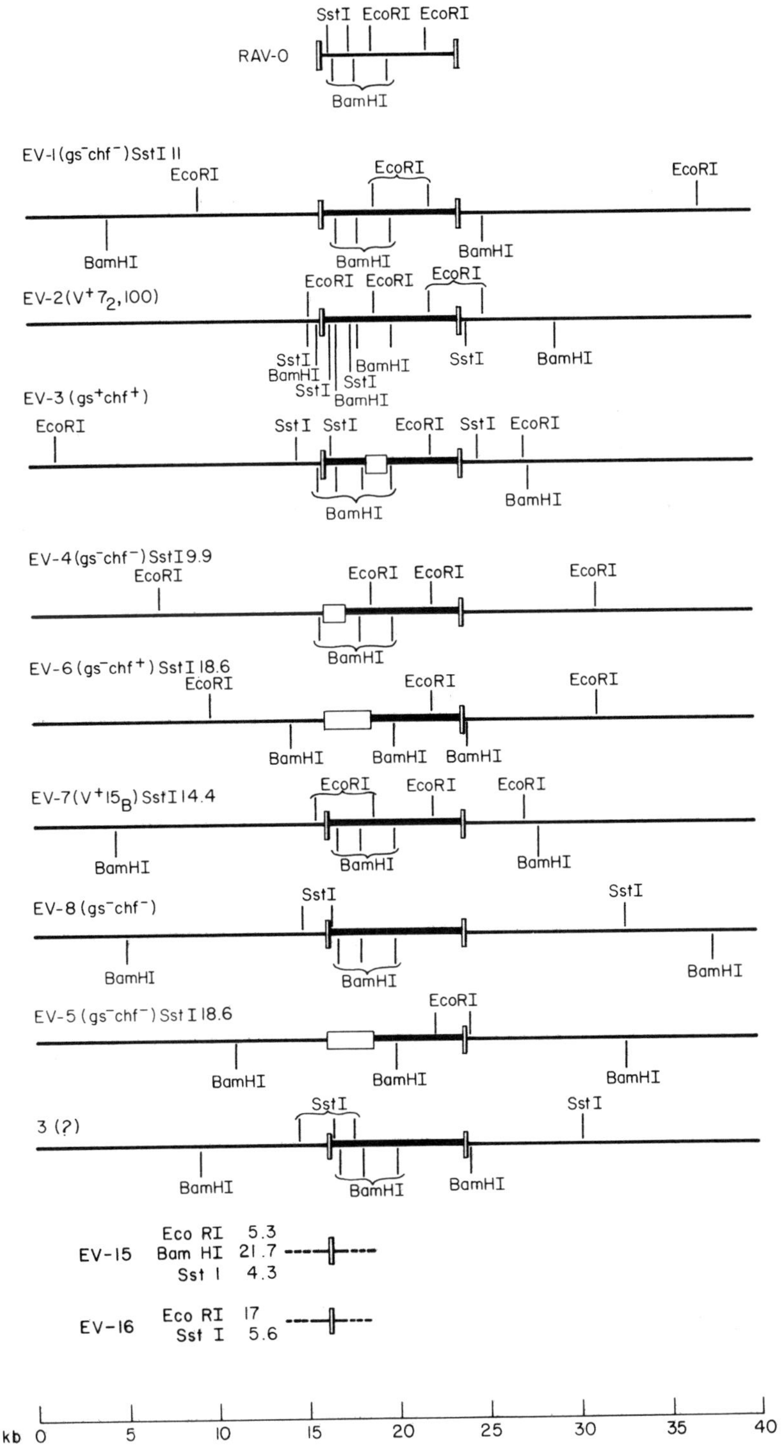

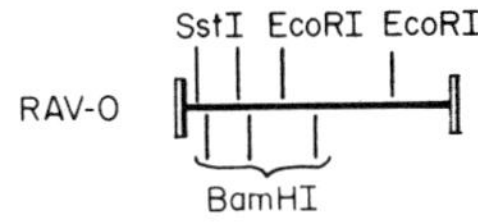

SstI EcoRI EcoRI
RAV-0
BamHI
EV-1(gs⁻chf⁻)SstI 11
EcoRI
EcoRI
EcoRI
BamHI
BamHI
BamHI
EV-2(V⁺7₂,100)
EcoRI EcoRI
EcoRI
SstI
BamHI
SstI
BamHI
SstI
BamHI
SstI
BamHI
EV-3 (gs⁺chf⁺)
EcoRI
SstI SstI
EcoRI SstI EcoRI
BamHI
BamHI
EV-4(gs⁻chf⁻)SstI 9.9
EcoRI
EcoRI EcoRI
EcoRI
BamHI
EV-6 (gs⁻chf⁺) SstI 18.6
EcoRI
EcoRI
EcoRI
BamHI BamHI BamHI
EV-7(V⁺15B) SstI 14.4
EcoRI
EcoRI
EcoRI
BamHI
BamHI
BamHI
EV-8 (gs⁻chf⁻)
SstI
SstI
BamHI
BamHI
BamHI
EV-5 (gs⁻chf⁻) Sst I 18.6
EcoRI
BamHI
BamHI
BamHI
3 (?)
SstI
SstI
BamHI
BamHI
BamHI
EV-15
Eco RI 5.3
Bam HI 21.7
Sst I 4.3
EV-16
Eco RI 17
Sst I 5.6
kb 0 5 10 15 20 25 30 35 40

APPENDIX C
tRNA Primers

1. General tRNA Structure
2. $tRNA^{Pro}_{1,2}$
3. $tRNA^{Lys}_{3}$
4. $tRNA^{Trp}_{1}$

A general model of a tRNA molecule is shown in the conventional cloverleaf form. Each of the four arms is labeled and conserved bases are shown. When the tRNA is bound to retrovirus viral RNA as a primer, the 3′ end of the tRNA, including the first half of the TΨC arm, up to the m_1A, is hydrogen-bonded to the complementary region (the primer binding site) on viral RNAs. The RSV virus primer is $tRNA^{Trp}$ (Harada et al., *J. Biol. Chem.* **250,** 3487, 1975). The MLV and REV primers are both $tRNA^{Pro}_{1,2}$(Peters et al., *J. Virol.* **21,** 1031, 1977; Harada et al., *J. Biol. Chem.* **24,** 10979, 1979; Peters and Dahlberg, *J. Virol.* **31,** 398, 1979; Peters and Glover, *J. Virol.* **33,** 708, 1980) and the MTV primer is $tRNA^{Lys}_{3}$ (Peters and Glover, *J. Virol.* **35,** 31, 1980).

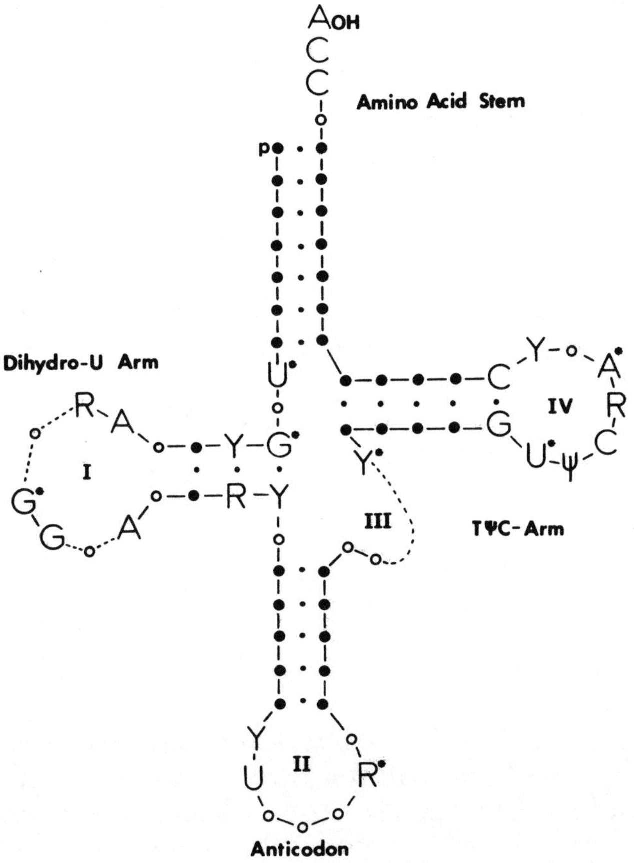

Amino Acid Stem

Dihydro-U Arm

TΨC-Arm

Anticodon

GENERAL tRNA STRUCTURE

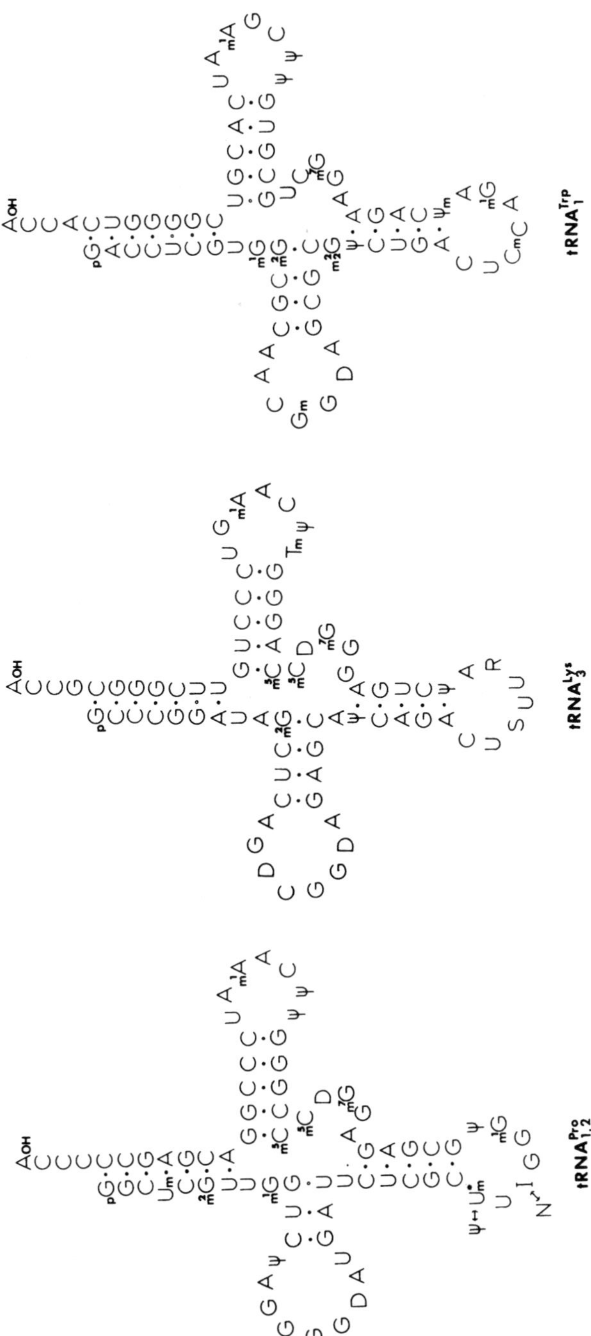
tRNA$^{Trp}_{1}$
tRNA$^{Lys}_{3}$
tRNA$^{Pro}_{1,2}$

APPENDIX D
Sequences of Retroviral LTRs

1. Sequence of the Rous Sarcoma Virus LTR
2. Sequence of the LTR of Chicken Endogenous Provirus *ev*-1
3. Sequence of Spleen Necrosis Virus LTR
4. Sequences of Ecotropic MLV and MSV LTRs
5. Sequence of the Mouse Mammary Tumor Virus LTR

The sequences of retroviral LTRs are given for the coding strands of proviruses and are presented as though each LTR were present in circular DNA bearing one copy of the LTR (see Chapter 5, Fig. 5.4). Structural features are indicated as described below. There is considerable variation in the length and sequence of the LTRs from different isolates of the same retrovirus, with most of the differences occurring in the U_3 region; hence deviation from the sequences presented here should be anticipated in new isolates.

For several of the LTRs presented, alternative sequences were available; the sequences employed were chosen arbitrarily. The nature of sequence variation in the LTRs can be better appreciated by consulting the alternative references listed for each LTR sequence.

The numbering of nucleotides in the format used here is arbitrary and does not begin with the first residue of the LTR in most cases. Definition of most of the symbols can be found in Chapter 4 and Appendix A. Sequences shown here generally include the polypurine tract (PPT) adjacent to the 5′ boundary of the LTR and the tRNA primer binding site (PBS) at the 3′ boundary. (The 5′ and 3′ boundaries are indicated by vertical arrows.) The PPT is an A-G-rich sequence of up to 20 nucleotides; the PBS is an 18-nucleotide sequence that is perfectly complementary to the 18 nucleotides at the 3′ terminus of the appropriate tRNA primer (see Appendix C). These sites are important in the initiation of synthesis of plus and minus strands of viral DNA, thereby determining the LTR boundaries (see Chapter 5). Whenever the data permit, vertical arrows denote the boundaries of U_3 and R and of R and U_5. The former boundary is the site at which RNA synthesis begins, and its definition requires examination of the capped 5′ terminus of viral RNA or the 3′ end of "strong stop," minus-strand DNA. The latter boundary is determined by the site of polyadenylation at the 3′ end of viral RNA; the position of this site appears to be heterogeneous in some virus strains. Inverted repeats are invariably found at the ends of LTRs and are indicated here by horizontal arrows, with closed boxes identifying mismatched bases within the repeats.

1. Sequence of the Rous Sarcoma Virus LTR

The LTR sequence shown here is derived from a circular molecule bearing two LTRs in tandem, cloned from quail cells infected by the SR-A strain of RSV (Swanstrom et al., *Proc. Natl. Acad. Sci.* **78,** 124, 1981). Similar data have been reported by Ju and Skalka (*Cell* **22,** 379, 1980), Yamamoto et al. (*Proc. Natl. Acad. Sci.* **77,** 176, 1980), Highfield et al. (*J. Virol.* **36,** 271, 1980), and Katz et al. (*J. Virol.* **42,** 346, 1982). The site of polyadenylation is heterogeneous in RSV (Schwartz et al., *Proc. Natl. Acad. Sci.* **74,** 998, 1977); R can be 16, 19, or 21 bases long. In this figure, the boundary between R and U_5 has been placed 21 bases from the end of U_3. The corresponding sequences of the PR-C strain of RSV are presented in Appendix E as part of the complete sequence of the genome.

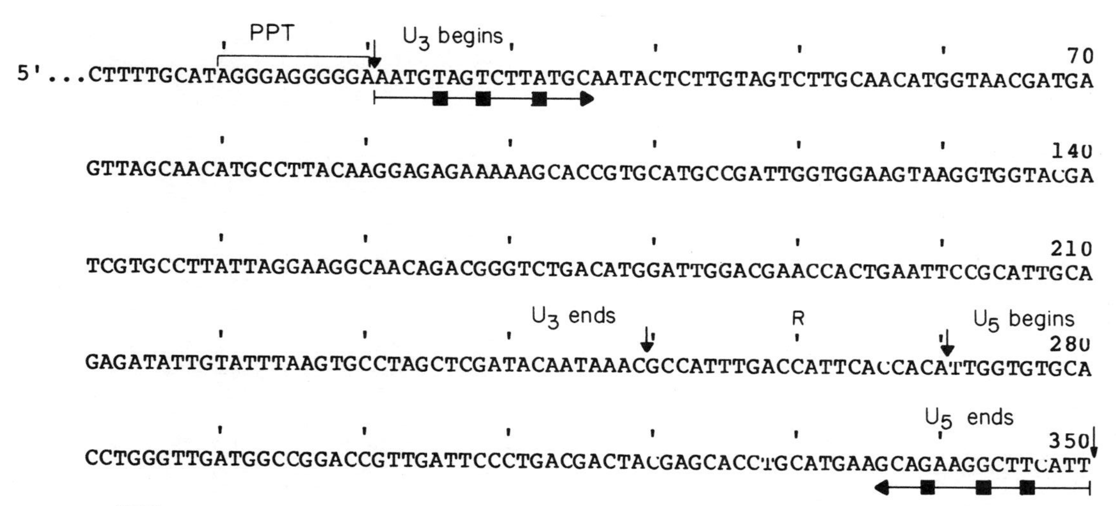

Figure D.1. RSV

2. Sequence of the LTR of the Chicken Endogenous Provirus *ev*-1

The sequence of the endogenous provirus, *ev*-1, was determined by Hishinuma et al. (*Cell* **23,** 155, 1981) and has been oriented to conform with the format described in the introduction to this section. The boundaries of R were positioned by comparison with the features of the RSV LTR. The sequence of the LTR of the closely related virus RAV-0, the product of the endogenous locus *ev*-2, is also available (Hughes, *J. Virol.,* in press, 1982). The only differences in the RAV-0 sequence are an additional A (after position 50 in the *ev*-1 sequence) and five substitutions (C for T at position 7, A for G at position 16, T for A at position 57, A for G at position 187, and T for C at position 214). A schematic diagram comparing this sequence with that of an endogenous virus LTR can be found in Figure 10.1.

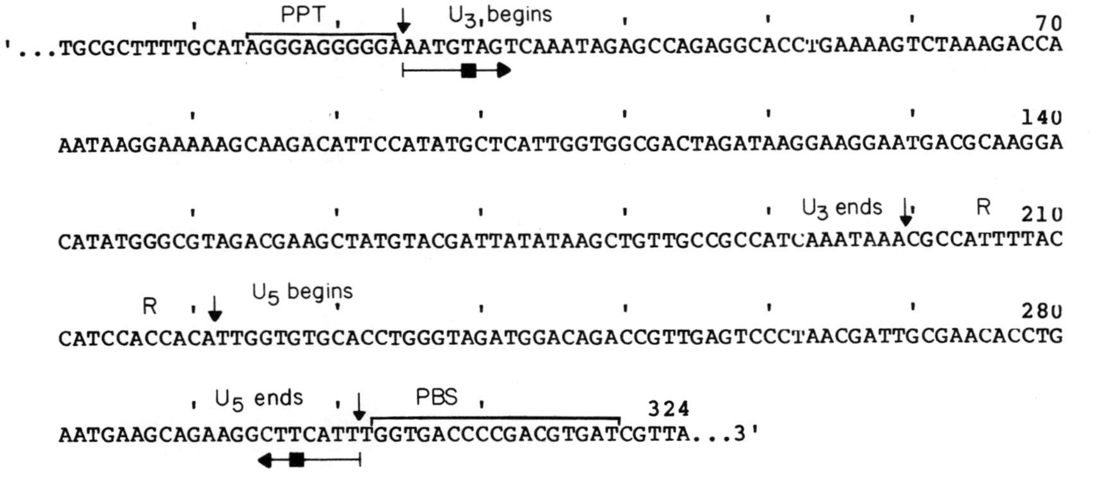

Figure D.2. ev-1 LTR

3. Sequence of the Spleen Necrosis Virus LTR

The data of Shimotohno et al. (*Nature* **285,** 550, 1980), obtained by sequencing both LTRs of a provirus cloned from SNV-infected chicken cells, have been oriented to conform to the format used for other sequences (see introduction to this section). The polypurine tract (PPT) is relatively short in the SNV genome, and the boundaries of R are approximate.

```
PPT          U3 begins                                                    70
5'...CAGTGGGGAATGTGGAGGGAGCTCTGGGGGAAATAGCGCTGGCTCGCAACTGCTATATTAGCTTCTGTA

                                                                         140
CTCATGCTTGCTTGCCTGGCCACTAACCGCCATATTAGCTTCTGTACACATGCTTGCTTGCCGTAGCCGC

                                                                         210
CATTGTACTTGATATGCCATTTCTCGGAATCGGCATCAAGTTTCGCTTCTCGAGAGCAAGCCCACAAACC

                                                                         280
ACAAAAGGAAACGCGCACCGAAGGCAAGCATCAGACCACTTGCGCCATCCAATCATGAACGGACAAGAGA

                                                                         350
TCGGACTATCATACTGGAGCCAATGGTTGTAAAGGGCAGATGCTACTCTCCAATGAGGGAAAATGTCATG

                                        U3 ends         R begins
                                                                         420
TAACACCCTGTAAGCTGTAAGAGGCTATATAAGCCGGGTACATCTCTTGCTCGGGGTCGCCGTCCTGCAC

                                                R ends          U5 begins
                                                                         490
ATTGTTGTTGTGACGTGCGGCCCAGATTCGAATCTGTAATAAAACTTTTTCTTCTGAATCCTCAGATTGG

                                                                         560
CAGTGAGAGGAGATTTTGTTCGTGGTGTTGGCTGGCCTACTGGGTGGGCGCAGGGATCCGGACTGAATCC

U5 ends                  PBS
                                           603
GTAGTACTTCGGTACAACATTTGGGGGCTCGTCCGGGATACCC...3'
```

Figure D.3. SNV

4. Sequences of Ecotropic MLV and MSV LTRs

LTRs of ecotropic MLV DNAs (from AKR and Moloney strains) and of Moloney strain of MSV have been sequenced by several investigators. (See Dhar et al., *Proc. Natl. Acad. Sci.* **77,** 3937, 1980; Reddy et al., *Proc. Natl. Acad. Sci.* **77,** 5234, 1980 and *Science* **214,** 445, 1981; and van Beveren et al., *Proc. Natl. Acad. Sci.* **77,** 3307, 1980 and *J. Virol.* **41,** 542, 1982, and Appendix E for sequences in addition to those presented here.) The LTR sequences are provided here without the primer binding site or polypurine tract; these are shown as part of the complete sequences of Mo-MSV and Mo-MLV DNA in Appendix E. The beginning of R (the cap site for viral RNA) is approximate; alternative GC dinucleotides are nearby and could represent the true 5′ boundary of R. The 3′ boundary of R is also not known precisely and has been estimated from the position of a CA dinucleotide about 20 nucleotides downstream from the presumptive polyadenylation signal, AATAAA and from Coffin et al. (*Cell* **13,** 761, 1978). The MLV/MSV LTRs often contain direct repeats of about 50 to 100 nucleotides in length within the U_3 region; these repeat units are indicated by boxed sequences labeled "DR." The following pages show the sequences of three LTRs of this class. (A) pMLV 201 contains Mo-MLV DNA cloned from the products of reverse transcription in vitro; the LTR sequence was originally determined by Sutcliffe et al. (*Proc. Natl. Acad. Sci.* **77,** 3302, 1980) and later modified by van Beveren et al. (*J. Virol.* **41,** 542, 1982). The cloned DNA lacks the 2 bp expected at the 3′ end of the LTR; these have been supplied to simplify comparison with other LTRs. No extensive direct repeat is present in this LTR. (B) pMSV-12 contains DNA derived from circular molecules present in cells acutely infected with Mo-MSV strain 124 (Verma et al., *Proc. Natl. Acad. Sci.* **77,** 1773, 1980). This clone was found to have two separated LTRs in opposite orientations, indicative of an autointegration event of the type first described by Shoemaker et al. (*Proc. Natl. Acad. Sci.* **77,** 3932, 1980). The LTR sequence shown here was determined by Van Beveren et al. (*J. Virol.* **41,** 542, 1982) and the 2 bp missing from the 3′ end of the LTR as a result of the autointegration event have been added. This LTR shows a 57-bp direct repeat. (C) AKR 614 is a provirus from mouse cells recently infected with the AKR strain of MLV, cloned in phage λ by Lowy et al. (*Proc. Natl. Acad. Sci.* **77,** 614, 1980). The sequence of the LTR was determined by Van Beveren et al. (*J. Virol.* **41,** 542, 1982) and reveals a 99-bp direct repeat with two mismatches.

```
   U3 begins                                                        70
5'...AATGAAAGACCCCACCTGTAGGTTTGGCAAGCTAGCTTAAGTAACGCCATTTTGCAAGGCATGGAAAAAT

                                                                   140
ACATAACTGAGAATAGAAAAGTTCAGATCAAGGTCAGGAACAGATGGAACAGCTGAATATGGGCCAAACA

                                                                   210
GGATATCTGTGGTAAGCAGTTCCTGCCCCGGCTCAGGGCCAAGAACAGATGGTCCCCAGATGCGGTCCAG

                                                                   280
CCCTCAGCAGTTTCTAGAGAACCATCAGATGTTTCCAGGGTGCCCCAAGGACCTGAAATGACCCTGTGCC

                                                                   350
TTATTTGAACTAACCAATCAGTTGCCTTCTCGCTTCTGTTCGCGCGCTTCTGCTCCCCGAGCTCAATAAA

            U3 ends    ↓ R                                         420
AGAGCCCACAACCCCTCACTCGGGGCGCCAGTCCTCCGATTGACTGAGTCGCCCGGGTACCCGTGTATCC
           R ends        U5 begins
                                                                   490
AATAAACCCTCTTGCAGTTGCATCCGACTTGTGGTCTCGCTGTTCCTTGGGAGGGTCTCCTCTGAGTGAT

          U5 ends           519
TGACTACCCGTCAGCGGGGGTCTTTCATT...3'
```

Figure D.4.A. MLV

```
   U3 begins                                                         70
5'..AATGAAAGACCCCACCCGTAGGTGGCAAGCTAGCTTAAGTAACGCCACTTTGCAAGGCATGGAAAAATAC

                                                                    140
ATAACTGAGAATAGAAAAGTTCAGATCAAGGTCAGGAACAAAGAAACAGCTGAATACCAAACAGGATATC

                        DR                                          210
TGTGGTAAGCGGTTCCTGCCCCGGCTCAGGGCCAAGAACAGATGAGACAGCTGAGTGATGGGCCAAACAG

                        DR                                          280
GATATCTGTGGTAAGCAGTTCCTGCCCCGGCTCGGGGCCAAGAACAGATGGTCCCCAGATGAGGTCCAGC

                                                                    350
CCTCAGCAGTTTCTAGTGAATCATCAGATGTTTCCAGGGTGCCCCAAGGACCTGAAAATGACCCTGTACC

                                                                    420
TTATTTGAACTAACCAATCAGTTCGCTTCTCGCTTCTGTTCGCGCGCTTCCGCTCTCCGAGCTCAATAAA

           U3 ends          R begins                                490
AGAGCCCACAACCCCTCACTCGGCGCGCCAGTCTTCCGATAGACTGCGTCGCCCGGGTACCCGTATTCCC

          R ends          U5 begins                                 560
AATAAAGCCTCTTGCTGTTTGCATCCGAATCGTGGTCTCGCTGTTCCTTGGGAGGGTCTCCTCTGAGTGA

                     U5 ends   589
TTGACTACCCACGACGGGGGTCTTTCATT..3'
```

Figure D.4.B. MSV

```
   U3 begins                                                          70
5'...AATGAAAGACCCCTTCATAAGGCTTAGCCAGCTAACTGCAGTAACGCCATTTTGCAAGGCATGGAAAAT

                                                                     140
ACCAGAGCTGATGTTCTCAGAAAAACAAGAACAAGGAAGTACAGAGAGGCTGGAATGTACCGGGACTAGG

                               DR                                    210
GCCAAACAGGATATCTGTGGTCAAGCACTAGGGCCCCGGCCCAGGGCCAAGAACAGATGGTCCCCAGAAA

                                           DR                        280
CAGAGAGGCTGGAAAGTACCGGGACTAGGGCCAAACAGGATATCTGTGGTCAAGCACTAGGGCCCCGGCC

                                                                     350
CAGGGCCAAGAACAGATGGTCCCCAGAAATAGCTAAAACAACAACAGTTTCAAGAGACCCAGAAACTGTC

                                                                     420
TCAAGGTTCCCCAGATGACCGGGGATCAACCCCAAGCCTCATTTAAACTAACCAATCAGCTCGCTTCTCG

                                                 U3 ends        R begins
                                                                     490
CTTCTGTACCCGCGCTTATTGCTGCCCAGCTCTATAAAAAGGTAAGAACCCCACACTCGGCGCGCCAGT

                                          R ends         U5 begins
                                                                     560
CCTCCGATAGACTGAGTCGCCCGGGTACCCGTGTATCCAATAAAGCCTTTTGCTGTTGCATCCGAATCGT

                                                     U5 ends   626
GGTCTCGCTGATCCTTGGGAGGGTCTCCTAAGAGTGATTGACTGCCCAGCCTGGGGGTCTTTCATT...3'
```

Figure D.4.C. AKR

5. Sequence of the Mouse Mammary Tumor Virus LTR

The sequence illustrated here is based principally upon the published results of Donehower et al. (*J. Virol.* **37,** 226, 1981), obtained with circular DNA bearing two LTRs cloned from cells infected with MMTV(C3H); the sequence has been modified slightly, according to unpublished results of J. Majors and L. Donehower (pers. comm.). The sequence has several unusual features: a relatively large U_3 domain (ca. 1195 bp), inverted repeats in which the two terminal nucleotides are not matched; and a long open reading frame (978 bp), beginning with the ATG at position 28 and concluding with the TAG at position 985. The boundary between R and U_5 is not known precisely; it is based upon the position of a CA dinucleotide following the putative polyadenylation signal (AGTAAA) and is in approximate accord with the published results of Klemenz et al. (*Mol. Biol. Rep.* **7,** 123, 1981). The cardinal features of the LTR of this virus strain (including the open reading frame) are preserved in the other MMTV LTRs that have been sequenced: MMTV(GR) (H. Diggelmann, pers. comm.) and endogenous MMTV proviruses known as GR-40, or unit II, and as unit V (Kennedy et al., *Nature* **295,** 622, 1982; L. Donehower and G. Hager, pers. comm.).

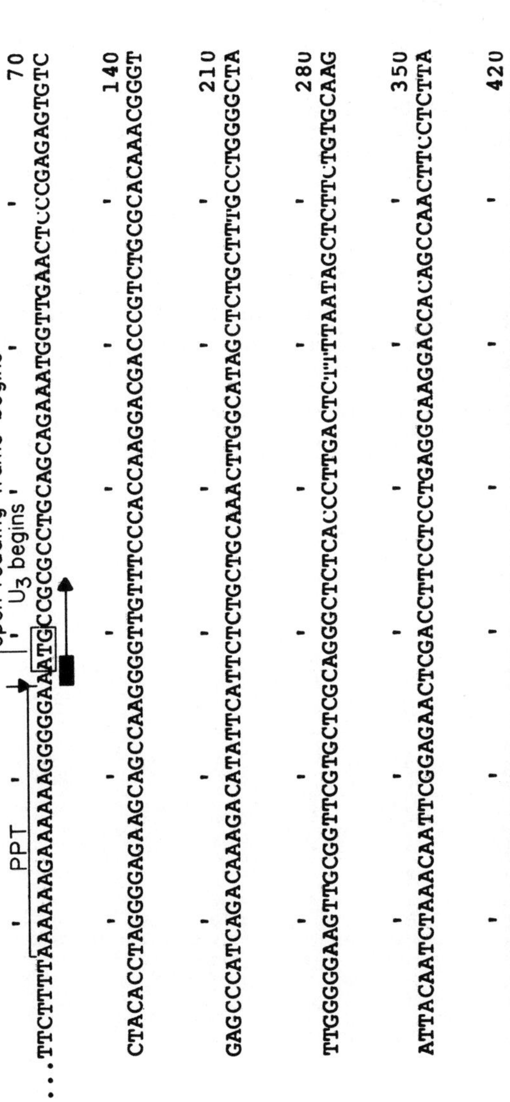
open reading frame begins
PPT
U3 begins
70
5'...TTCTTTTAAAAAAGAAAAAAGGGGAAATGCCGCGCCTGCAGCAGAAATGGTTGAACTCCCGAGAGTGTC
140
CTACACCTAGGGGAGAAGCAGCCAAGGGGTTGTTTCCCACCAAGGACGACCCGTCTGCGCACAAACGGGT
210
GAGCCCATCAGACAAAGACATATTCATTCTCTGCTGCAAACTTGGCATAGCTCTGCTTTGCCTGGGGCTA
280
TTGGGGGAAGTTGCGGTTCGTGCTCGCAGGGCTCTCACCCTTGACTCTTTTAATAGCTCTTCTGTGCAAG
350
ATTACAATCTAAACAATTCGGAGAACTCGACCTTCCTCCTGAGGCAAGGACCACAGCCAACTTCCTCTTA
420
CAAGCCGCATCGATTTTGTCCTTCAGAAATAGAAATAAGAATGCTTGCTAAAAATTATATTTTTACCAAT
490
AAGACCAATCCAATAGGTAGATTATTAGTTACTATGTTAAGAAATGAATCATTATCTTTTAGTACTATTT

```
                                                                     560
TTACTCAAATTCAGAAGTTAGAAATGGGAATAGAAAATAGAAAGAGACGCTCAACCTCAATTGAAGAACA

                                                                     630
GGTGCAAGGACTATTGACCACAGGCCTAGAAGTAAAAAAGGAAAAAAGAGTGTTTTTGTCAAAATAGGA

                                                                     700
GACAGGTGGTGGCAACTAGGGACTTATAGGGGACCTTACATCTACAGACCAACAGATGCCCCCTTACCAT

                                                                     770
ATACAGGAAGATATGACTTAAATTGGGATAGGTGGGTTACAGTCAATGGCTATAAAGTGTTATATAGATC

                                                                     840
CCTCCCTTTTCGTGAAAGACTCGCCAGAGCTAGACCTCCTTGGTGTATGTTGTCTCAAGAAGAAAAAGAC

                                                                     910
GACATGAAACAACAGGTACATGATTATATTTATCTAGGAACAGGAATGCACTTTTGGGGAAAGATTTTCC
```

```
                                                                    980
ATACCAAGGAGGGGACAGTGGCTGGACTAATAGAACATTATTCTCCAAAAACTTATGGCATGAGTTATTA

open reading frame ends
                                                                   1050
TGAATAGCCTTTATTGGCCCAACCTTGCGGTTCCCAGGGCTTAAGTAAGTTTTTGGTTACAAACTGTTCT

                                                                   1120
TAAAACGAGGATGTGAGACAAGTGGTTTCCTGACTTGGTTTGGTATCAAAGGTTCTGATCTGAGCTCTGA

                                                                   1190
GTGTTCTATTTTCCTATGTTCTTTTGGAATTTATCCAAATCTTATGTAAATGCTTATGTAAACCAAGATA

            U3 ends                R           U5 begins
                                                                   1260
TAAAAGAGTGCTGATTTTTTGAGTAAACTTGCAACAGTCCTAACATTCACCTCTTGTGTGTTTGTGTCTG

                                                                   1330
TTCGCCATCCCGTCTCCGCTCGTCACTTATCCTTCACTTTCCAGAGGGTCCCCCCGCAGACCCCGGCGAC

           U5 ends  13|56        PBS
CTCAGGTCGGCCGACTGCGGCAGCTGGCGCCCGAACAGGGACCT...3'
```

Figure D.5. MMTV

APPENDIX E

Complete Nucleotide Sequences of Three Retroviral Genomes and a Cellular *onc* Gene

1. The Complete Nucleotide Sequence of the Pr-C Strain of Rous Sarcoma Virus
2. The Complete Sequence of Moloney Murine Leukemia Virus
3. The Complete Nucleotide Sequence of Moloney Murine Sarcoma Virus, Clone 124, Unintegrated Circular DNA Containing Two LTRs
4. Nucleotide Sequence of *c-mos*

Three retroviral genomes have been entirely sequenced: Rous sarcoma virus (RSV), Moloney murine leukemia virus (Mo-MLV), and Moloney murine sarcoma virus (Mo-MSV). In addition, the complete nucleotide sequence of the cellular homolog of the oncogene carried by Mo-MSV, *c-mos,* has been determined. In all cases, the sequence of only one strand, the coding strand, is provided here. The sequences are written for a DNA copy—that is, Ts are used instead of Us. The proposed amino acid sequences for known genes are given; also, correlations with protein sequence will be discussed briefly in the legends for the individual sequences and in the section devoted to amino acid sequence (Appendix F).

1. The Complete Nucleotide Sequence of the Pr-C Strain of Rous Sarcoma Virus

The sequence is presented as a DNA version of the entire viral RNA genome. The sequence begins with the R sequence "R" at the 5′ end of the genome. The precise boundary between R and U_5 (here marked with an arrow) is dependent on the extent of the R sequence at the 3′ end of viral RNA (see Appendix D). The 3′ end of U_5 forms an imperfect inverted repeat with U_3 (12 of 15 bases); inverted repeats of this sort are present in the LTRs of all retroviruses (see Appendix D). A horizontal arrow marks the inverted repeat; the mismatched bases are indicated by boxes. Just beyond U_5 is the primer binding site (PBS). Approximately 280 bases beyond U_5 is the beginning of the *gag* coding region, at position 379. Just past the initiation site for *gag* is the upstream splice site for the *env* and *pol* messages at position 397; it is marked by a vertical arrow and "SD." The proteolytic cleavage sites that produce the various *gag* polypeptides are marked by vertical arrows. p19^{gag} is encoded from 379 to 904 and p27^{gag} from 1097 to 1816; the coding region for p10^{gag} lies between these domains. The p12^{gag} sequence commences at position 1843 and the p15^{gag} sequence begins at 2111. The *gag* gene terminates with a TAG codon at position 2483. The start of the *pol* gene is 20 bases from the last sense codon in *gag*, implying that the mechanism which generates the *gag-pol* fusion protein (Pr180$^{gag\text{-}pol}$) also changes the translational frame. The *pol* gene ends with a TAA codon at position 5188.

The sequence coding for the major mature viral glycoprotein, gp85^{env}, begins at position 5245 with the Asp codon, GAT (marked "gp85"). However, the aminoterminal portion of the primary translation product of *env* is removed by proteolytic cleavage. Preceding the GAT codon at position 5246 is an in-phase open reading frame that begins after the TGA termination codon at position 5042 and contains an ATG codon at position 5054. This open reading frame overlaps the carboxy terminus of the *pol* gene but is in a different reading frame. The candidate splice acceptor site (SA) for the *env* message is at position 5078, which would join position 5078 to position 397 near the 5′ end of viral RNA (see Hackett et al., *J. Virol.* **41**, 527, 1982). This joining would remove the candidate ATG at position 5054. However, the first 6 amino acids of *gag* are encoded before position 397; thus, the primary translation product of the *env* gene seems to have an amino terminus encoded by *gag* (D. Schwartz and E. Hunter, pers. comm.). The amino acid sequence of the signal peptide of the *env* gene product is not displayed in the figure. The sequence of $gp37^{env}$ begins at position 6269 (marked "gp37").

The *src* gene begins at position 7129 and terminates with a TAA codon at position 8707. Unlike the product of *env*, the product of *src*, $pp60^{src}$, appears to be encoded in the genome by contiguous sequence; the splice acceptor site (SA) for *src* in RNA has been located about 75 nucleotides upstream from the initiation site (at position 7053; D. Schwartz; J. Sorge; R. Swanstrom; all pers. comm.), so that the *gag* ATG from the leader sequence is followed in the same reading frame by the TGA at position 7063.

Between the end of *src* and the beginning of U_3 is a noncoding region about 350 bases long. Adjacent to U_3, there is a polypurine tract (PPT); polypurine tracts are found at this position in all known retroviral genomes (see Appendix D). The first 15 bases of U_3 form an imperfect inverted repeat with U_5; 12 of the 15 are matched. The 3′ end of RSV RNA is heterogeneous (see Appendix D.1 for discussion and references).

This sequence, which is not yet published, was determined mainly by analysis of cDNA made in vitro from PrC-RSV RNA and was generously provided by D. Schwartz, R. Tizard, and W. Gilbert. Czernilofsky et al. (*Nature* **287**, 198, 1980) have published a sequence for *src* and the 3′ terminus of *env* from the SRA strain of RSV; Swanstrom et al. (*J. Virol.* **41**, 535, 1982) have reported the DNA sequences of 1010 nucleotides corresponding to the 5′ end of SR-A RSV RNA.

```
          R                U5 begins                                                     U5 ends
GCCATTTTACCATTCACCACATTGGTGTGCACCTGGCTTGATGGCCGGACCGTCGATTCCCTAACGATTGCGAACACCTGAATGAAGCAG    90

           PBS
AAGGCTTCATTTGGTGACCCCGACGTGATAGTTAGGGAATAGTGGTCGGCCACAGACGGCGTGGCGATCCTGCCCTCATCCGTCTCGCTT   180

ATTCGGGGAGCGGACGATGACCCTAGTAGAGGGGGCTGCGGCTTAGGAGGGCAGAAGCTGAGTGGCGTCGGAGGGAGCTCTACTGCAGGG   270

AGCCCAGATACCCTACCGAGAACTCAGAGAGTCGTTGGAAGACGGGAAGGAAGCCCGACGACTGAGCAGTCCACCCCAGGCGTGATTCTG   360
                   P19          SD
                  MetGluAlaValIleLysValIleSerSerAlaCysLysThrTyrCysGlyLysThrSerProSerLysLys
GTCGCCCGGTGGATCAAGCATGGAAGCCGTCATAAAGGTGATTTCGTCCGCGTGTAAAACCTATTGCGGGAAAACCTCTCCTTCTAAGAA   450

GluIleGlyAlaMetLeuSerLeuLeuGlnLysGluGlyLeuLeuMetSerProSerAspLeuTyrSerProGlySerTrpAspProIle
GGAAATAGGGGCCATGTTGTCCCTCTTACAAAAGGAAGGGTTGCTTATGTCTCCCTCAGACTTATATTCCCCGGGGTCCTGGGATCCCAT   540

ThrAlaAlaLeuSerGlnArgAlaMetIleLeuGlyLysSerGlyGluLeuLysThrTrpGlyLeuValLeuGlyAlaLeuLysAlaAla
TACCGCGGCGCTATCCCAGCGGGCTATGATACTTGGGAAATCGGGAGAGTTAAAAACCTGGGGATTGGTTTTGGGGGCATTGAAGGCGGC   630

ArgGluGluGlnValThrSerGluGlnAlaLysPheTrpLeuGlyLeuGlyGlyGlyArgValSerProProGlyProGluCysIleGlu
TCGAGAGGAACAGGTTACATCTGAGCAAGCAAAGTTTTGGTTGGGATTAGGGGGAGGGAGGGTCTCTCCCCCAGGTCCGGAGTGCATCGA   720

LysProAlaThrGluArgArgIleAspLysGlyGluGluValGlyGluThrThrValGlnArgAspAlaLysMetAlaProGluGluThr
GAAACCAGCAACGGAGCGGCGAATCGACAAAGGGGAGGAAGTGGGAGAAACAACTGTGCAGCGAGATGCGAAGATGGCGCCGGAGGAAAC   810

AlaThrProLysThrValGlyThrSerCysTyrHisCysGlyThrAlaIleGlyCysAsnCysAlaThrAlaSerAlaProProProPro
GGCCACACCTAAAACCGTTGGCACATCCTGCTATCATTGCGGAACAGCTATTGGCTGTAATTGCGCCACAGCCTCGGCTCCTCCTCCTCC   900
P19      P10
TyrValGlySerGlyLeuTyrProSerLeuAlaGlyValGlyGluGlnGlnGlyGlnGlyGlyAspThrProProGlyAlaGluGlnSer
TTATGTGGGGAGTGGTTTGTATCCTTCCCTGGCGGGGGTGGGAGAGCAGCAGGGCCAGGGGGGTGACACACCTCCGGGGGCGGAACAGTC   990

ArgAlaGluProGlyHisAlaGlyGlnAlaProGlyProAlaLeuThrAspTrpAlaArgValArgGluGluLeuAlaSerThrGlyPro
AAGGGCGGAGCCAGGGCATGCGGGTCAGGCTCCTGGGCCGGCCCTGACTGACTGGGCAAGGGTCAGGGAGGAGCTTGCGAGTACTGGTCC   1080
      P10         P27
ProValValAlaMetProValValIleLysThrGluGlyProAlaTrpThrProLeuGluProLysLeuIleThrArgLeuAlaAspThr
GCCCGTGGTGGCCATGCCTGTAGTGATTAAGACAGAGGGACCCGCTTGGACCCCTCTGGAGCCAAAATTGATCACAAGACTGGCTGATAC   1170
```

```
 ValArgThrLysGlyLeuArgSerProIleThrMetAlaGluValGluAlaLeuMetSerSerProLeuLeuProHisAspValThrAsn
GGTCAGGACCAAGGGCTTACGATCCCCGATTACTATGGCAGAAGTGGAAGCGCTTATGTCCTCCCCGCTGCTGCCGCATGACGTCACGAA   1260

 LeuMetArgValIleLeuGlyProAlaProTyrAlaLeuTrpMetAspAlaTrpGlyValGlnLeuGlnThrValIleAlaAlaAlaThr
TCTAATGAGAGTTATTTAGGGCCTGCCCCATATGCCTTATGGATGGACGCTTGGGGAGTCCAACTCCAGACAGTTATAGCGGCAGCCAC   1350

 ArgAspProArgHisProAlaAsnGlyGlnGlyArgGlyGluArgThrAsnLeuAsnArgLeuLysGlyLeuAlaAspGlyMetValGly
TCGCGACCCCCGACACCCAGCGAACGGTCAAGGGCGGGGGAACGGACTAATTTGAATCGCTTAAAGGGCTTAGCTGATGGGATGGTGGG   1440

 AsnProGlnGlyGlnAlaAlaLeuLeuArgProGlyGluLeuValAlaIleThrAlaSerAlaLeuGlnAlaPheArgGluValAlaArg
CAACCCACAGGGTCAGGCCGCATTATTAAGACCGGGGGAATTGGTTGCTATTACGGCGTCGGCTCTCCAGGCGTTTAGAGAGGTTGCCCG   1530

 LeuAlaGluProAlaGlyProTrpAlaAspIleMetGlnGlyProSerGluSerPheValAspPheAlaAsnArgLeuIleLysAlaVal
GCTGGCGGAACCTGCAGGTCCATGGGCGGACATCATGCAGGGACCATCTGAGTCCTTTGTTGATTTTGCCAATCGGCTTATAAAGGCGGT   1620

 GluGlySerAspLeuProProSerAlaArgAlaProValIleIleAspCysPheArgGlnLysSerGlnProAspIleGlnGlnLeuIle
TGAGGGGTCAGATCTCCCGCCTTCCGCGCGGGCTCCGGTGATCATTGACTGCTTTAGGCAGAAGTCACAGCCAGATATTCAGCAGCTTAT   1710

 ArgThrAlaProSerThrLeuThrThrProGlyGluIleIleLysTyrValLeuAspArgGlnLysThrAlaProLeuThrAspGlnGly
ACGGACAGCACCCTCCACGCTGACCACCCCAGGAGAGATAATTAAATATGTGCTAGACAGGCAGAAGACTGCCCCTCTTACGGATCAAGG   1800
      P27     ↓                          ↓ P12
 IleAlaAlaAlaMetSerSerAlaIleGlnProLeuIleMetAlaValValAsnArgGluArgAspGlyGlnThrGlySerGlyGlyArg
CATAGCCGCGGCCATGTCGTCTGCTATCCAGCCCTTAATTATGGCAGTAGTCAATAGAGAGAGGGATGGACAAACTGGGTCGGGTGGTCG   1890

 AlaArgGlyLeuCysTyrThrCysGlySerProGlyHisTyrGlnAlaGlnCysProLysLysArgLysSerGlyAsnSerArgGluArg
TGCCCGAGGGCTCTGCTACACTTGTGGATCCCCGGGACATTATCAGGCGCAGTGCCCGAAAAAACGGAAGTCAGGAAACAGCCGTGAGCG   1980

 CysGlnLeuCysAsnGlyMetGlyHisAsnAlaLysGlnCysArgLysArgAspGlyAsnGlnGlyGlnArgProGlyLysGlyLeuSer
ATGTCAGTTGTGTAACGGGATGGGACACAACGCTAAACAGTGTAGGAAGCGGATGGCAACCAGGGCCAACGCCCAGGAAAAGGTCTCTC   2070
                                   P12   ↓    P15
 SerGlyProTrpProGlyProGluProProAlaValSerLeuAlaMetThrMetGluHisLysAspArgProLeuValArgValIleLeu
TTCGGGGCCGTGGCCCGGCCCTGAGCCACCTGCCGTCTCGTTAGCGATGACAATGGAACATAAAGATCGCCCCTTGGTTAGGGTCATTCT   2160

 ThrAsnThrGlySerHisProValLysGlnArgSerValTyrIleThrAlaLeuLeuAspSerGlyAlaAspIleThrIleIleSerGlu
GACTAACACTGGGAGTCATCCGGTCAAACAGCGTTCGGTGTATATCACCGCGCTGTTGGACTCTGGAGCGGACATCACTATTATTTCAGA   2250
```

```
 GluAspTrpProThrAspTrpProValMetGluAlaAlaAsnProGlnIleHisGlyIleGlyGlyGlyIleProMetArgLysSerArg
GGAGGATTGGCCCACCGATTGGCCAGTGATGGAGGCCGCGAACCCGCAGATCCATGGGATAGGAGGGGAATTCCCATGCGAAAATCTCG   2340

 AspMetIleGluLeuGlyValIleAsnArgAspGlySerLeuGluArgProLeuLeuLeuPheProAlaValAlaMetValArgGlySer
TGACATGATAGAGTTGGGGGTTATTAACCGAGACGGGTCTTTGGAGCGACCCCTGCTCCTCTTCCCCGCAGTAGCTATGGTTAGAGGGAG   2430
                                          P15
 IleLeuGlyArgAspCysLeuGlnGlyLeuGlyLeuArgLeuThrAsnLeu***
                                                                ThrValAlaLeuHisLeu
TATCCTAGGAAGAGATTGTCTGCAGGGCCTAGGGCTCCGCTTGACAAATTTATAGGGAGGGCCACTGTTCTCACTGTTGCGCTACATCTG   2520

AlaIleProLeuLysTrpLysProAspHisThrProValTrpIleAspGlnTrpProLeuProGluGlyLysLeuValAlaLeuThrGln
GCTATTCCGCTCAAATGGAAGCCAGACCACACGCCTGTGTGGATTGACCAGTGGCCCCTCCCTGAAGGTAAACTTGTAGCGCTAACGCAA   2610

LeuValGluLysGluLeuGlnLeuGlyHisIleGluProSerLeuSerCysTrpAsnThrProValPheValIleArgLysAlaSerGly
TTAGTGGAAAAAGAATTACAGTTAGGACATATAGAACCTTCACTTAGTTGTTGGAACACACCTGTCTTCGTGATCCGGAAGGCTTCCGGG   2700

SerTyrArgLeuLeuHisAspLeuArgAlaValAsnAlaLysLeuValProPheGlyAlaValGlnGlnGlyAlaProValLeuSerAla
TCTTACCGCTTACTGCATGATTTGCGCGCTGTTAACGCCAAGCTTGTTCCTTTTGGGGCCGTCCAACAGGGGGCGCCAGTTCTCTCCGCG   2790

LeuProArgGlyTrpProLeuMetValLeuAspLeuLysAspCysPhePheSerIleProLeuAlaGluGlnAspArgGluAlaPheAla
CTCCCGCGTGGCTGGCCCCTGATGGTCTTAGACCTCAAGGATTGCTTCTTTTCTATCCCTCTTGCGGAACAAGATCGCGAAGCTTTTGCA   2880

PheThrLeuProSerValAsnAsnGlnAlaProAlaArgArgPheGlnTrpLysValLeuProGlnGlyMetThrCysSerProThrIle
TTTACGCTCCCCTCTGTGAATAACCAGGCCCCCGCTCGAAGATTCCAATGGAAGGTCTTGCCCCAAGGGATGACCTGTTCTCCCACTATC   2970

CysGlnLeuValValGlyGlnValLeuGluProLeuArgLeuLysHisProSerLeuCysMetLeuHisTyrMetAspAspLeuLeuLeu
TGTCAGTTGGTAGTGGGTCAGGTACTTGAGCCCTTGCGACTCAAGCACCCATCTCTGTGCATGTTGCATTATATGGATGATCTTTTGCTA   3060

AlaAlaSerSerHisAspGlyLeuGluAlaAlaGlyGluGluValIleSerThrLeuGluArgAlaGlyPheThrIleSerProAspLys
GCCGCCTCAAGTCACGATGGGTTGGAAGCGGCAGGGGAGGAGGTTATCAGTACATTGGAAAGAGCCGGGTTCACTATTTCGCCTGATAAG   3150

ValGlnArgGluProGlyValGlnTyrLeuGlyTyrLysLeuGlySerThrTyrValAlaProValGlyLeuValAlaGluProArgIle
GTCCAGAGGGAGCCCGGAGTACAATATCTTGGGTACAAGTTAGGCAGTACGTATGTAGCACCCGTAGGCCTGGTAGCAGAACCCAGGATA   3240
```

AlaThrLeuTrpAspValGlnLysLeuValGlySerLeuGlnTrpLeuArgProAlaLeuGlyIleProProArgLeuMetGlyProPhe
GCCACCTTGTGGGATGTTCAAAAGCTGGTGGGGTCACTTCAGTGGCTTCGCCCAGCGTTAGGAATCCCGCCACGACTGATGGGCCCCTTC 3330

TyrGluGlnLeuArgGlySerAspProAsnGluAlaArgGluTrpAsnLeuAspMetLysMetAlaTrpArgGluIleValArgLeuSer
TATGAGCAGTTACGAGGGTCAGATCCTAACGAGGCGAGGGAATGGAATCTAGACATGAAAATGGCCTGGAGAGAGATCGTACGGCTTAGC 3420

ThrThrAlaAlaLeuGluArgTrpAspProAlaLeuProLeuGluGlyAlaValAlaArgCysGluGlnGlyAlaIleGlyValLeuGly
ACCACTGCTGCCT GGAACGATGGGACCCTGCCCTGCCTCTGGAAGGAGCGGTCGCTAGATGTGAACAGGGGGCAATAGGGGTTTTGGGA 3510

GlnGlyLeuSerThrHisProArgProCysLeuTrpLeuPheSerThrGlnProThrLysAlaPheThrAlaTrpLeuGluValLeuThr
CAGGGACTGTCCACACACCCAAGGCCATGCTTGTGGTTATTCTCCACCCAACCCACCAAGGCGTTTACTGCTTGGTTAGAAGTGCTCACC 3600

LeuLeuIleThrLysLeuArgAlaSerAlaValArgThrPheGlyLysGluValAspIleLeuLeuLeuProAlaCysPheArgGluAsp
CTTTTGATTACTAAGCTACGTGCTTCGGCAGTGCGAACCTTTGGCAAGGAGGTCGATATCCTCCTGTTGCCTGCATGCTTTCGGGAGGAC 3690

LeuProLeuProGluGlyIleLeuLeuAlaLeuLysGlyPheAlaGlyLysIleArgSerSerAspThrProSerIlePheAspIleAla
CTTCCGCTCCCAGAGGGGATCCTGTTAGCCCTTAAGGGGTTTGCAGGAAAAATCAGGAGTAGTGACACGCCATCTATTTTTGACATTGCG 3780

ArgProLeuHisValSerLeuLysValArgValThrAspHisProValProGlyProThrValPheThrAspAlaSerSerSerThrHis
CGTCCACTGCATGTTTCTCTGAAAGTGAGGGTTACCGACCACCCTGTGCCGGGACCCACTGTCTTTACTGACGCCTCCTCAAGCACCCAT 3870

LysGlyValValValTrpArgGluGlyProArgTrpGluIleLysGluIleAlaAspLeuGlyAlaSerValGlnGlnLeuGluAlaArg
AAGGGGGTGGTAGTCTGGAGGGAGGGCCCAAGGTGGGAGATAAAAGAAATAGCTGATTTGGGGGCAAGTGTACAACAACTGGAAGCACGC 3960

AlaValAlaMetAlaLeuLeuLeuTrpProThrThrProThrAsnValValThrAspSerAlaPheValAlaLysMetLeuLeuLysMet
GCTGTGGCCATGGCACTTCTGCTGTGGCCGACAACGCCCACTAATGTAGTGACTGACTCCGCGTTTGTTGCGAAAATGTTACTCAAGATG 4050

GlyGlnGluGlyValProSerThrAlaAlaAlaPheIleLeuGluAspAlaLeuSerGlnArgSerAlaMetAlaAlaValLeuHisVal
GGACAGGAGGGAGTCCCGTCTACAGCGGCGGCTTTTATTTTAGAGGATGCGTTAAGCCAAAGGTCAGCCATGGCCGCCGTTCTCCACGTG 4140

ArgSerHisSerGluValProGlyPhePheThrGluGlyAsnAspValAlaAspSerGlnAlaThrPheGlnAlaTyrProLeuArgGlu
CGGAGTCATTCTGAAGTGCCAGGGTTTTTCACAGAAGGAAATGACGTGGCAGATAGCCAAGCCACCTTCCAAGCGTATCCCTTGAGAGAG 4230

AlaLysAspLeuHisThrAlaLeuHisIleGlyProArgAlaLeuSerLysAlaCysAsnIleSerMetGlnGlnAlaArgGluValVal
GCTAAAGATCTTCATACCGCTCTCCATATTGGACCCCGCGCGCTATCCAAAGCGTGTAATATATCTATGCAGCAGGCTAGGGAGGTTGTT 4320

```
GlnThrCysProHisCysAsnSerAlaProAlaLeuGluAlaGlyValAsnProArgGlyLeuGlyProLeuGlnIleTrpGlnThrAsp
CAGACCTGCCCGCATTGTAATTCAGCCCCTGCGTTGGAGGCCGGAGTAAACCCTAGGGGTTTGGGACCCCTACAGATATGGCAGACAGAC   4410

PheThrLeuGluProArgMetAlaProArgSerTrpLeuAlaValThrValAspThrAlaSerSerAlaIleValValThrGlnHisGly
TTTACGCTTGAGCCTAGAATGGCCCCCCGTTCCTGGCTCGCTGTTACTGTGGATACCGCCTCATCAGCGATAGTCGTAACTCAGCATGGC   4500

ArgValThrSerValAlaValGlnHisHisTrpAlaThrAlaIleAlaValLeuGlyArgProLysAlaIleLysThrAspAsnGlySer
CGTGTCACATCGGTTGCTGTACAACATCATTGGGCCACGGCTATCGCCGTTTTGGGAAGACCAAAGGCCATAAAAACAGATAATGGGTCC   4590

CysPheThrSerLysSerThrArgGluTrpLeuAlaArgTrpGlyIleAlaHisThrThrGlyIleProGlyAsnSerGlnGlyGlnAla
TGCTTCACGTCTAAATCCACGCGAGAGTGGCTCGCGAGATGGGGGATAGCACACACCACCGGGATTCCGGGTAATTCCCAGGGTCAAGCT   4680

MetValGluArgAlaAsnArgLeuLeuLysAspArgIleArgValLeuAlaGluGlyAspGlyPheMetLysArgIleProThrSerLys
ATGGTAGAGCGGGCCAACCGGCTCCTGAAAGATAGGATCCGTGTGCTTGCGGAGGGGGACGGCTTTATGAAAAGAATCCCCACCAGCAAA   4770

GlnGlyGluLeuLeuAlaLysAlaMetTyrAlaLeuAsnHisPheGluArgGlyGluAsnThrLysThrProIleGlnLysHisTrpArg
CAGGGGGAACTATTAGCCAAGGCAATGTATGCCCTCAATCACTTTGAGCGTGGTGAAAACACGAAAACACCGATACAAAAACACTGGAGA   4860

ProThrValLeuThrGluGlyProProValLysIleArgIleGluThrGlyGluTrpGluLysGlyTrpAsnValLeuValTrpGlyArg
CCTACCGTTCTTACAGAAGGACCCCCGGTTAAAATACGAATAGAGACAGGGGAGTGGAAAAAGGATGGAACGTGCTGGTCTGGGGACGA   4950

GlyTyrAlaAlaValLysAsnArgAspThrAspLysValIleTrpValProSerArgLysValLysProAspIleThrGlnLysAspGlu
GGTTATGCCGCTGTGAAAAACAGGGACACTGATAAGGTTATTTGGGTACCCTCTCGAAAAGTTAAACCGGACATCACCCAAAAGGATGAG   5040
                                                  ↓SA
ValThrLysLysAspGluAlaSerProLeuPheAlaGlyIleSerAspTrpIleProTrpGluAspGluGlnGluGlyLeuGlnGlyGlu
GTGACTAAGAAAGATGAGGCGAGCCCTCTTTTTGCAGGCATTTCTGACTGGATACCCTGGGAAGACGAGCAAGAAGGACTCCAAGGAGAA   5130

ThrAlaSerAsnLysGlnGluArgProGlyGluAspThrLeuAlaAlaAsnGluSer***
ACCGCTAGCAACAAGCAAGAAAGACCCGGAGAAGACACCCTTGCTGCCAACGAGAGTTAATTATATTCTCATTATTGGTGTCCTGGTCTT   5220
                  gp 85
                          AspValHisLeuLeuGluGlnProGlyAsnLeuTrpIleThrTrpAlaAsnArgThrGlyGlnThr
GTGTGAGGTTACGGGGGTAAGAGCTGATGTTCACTTACTCGAGCAGCCAGGGAACCTTTGGATTACATGGGCCAACCGTACAGGCCAAAC   5310

AspPheCysLeuSerThrGlnSerAlaThrSerProPheGlnThrCysLeuIleGlyIleProSerProIleSerGluGlyAspPheLys
GGATTTCTGCCTCTCTACACAGTCAGCCACCTCCCCTTTTCAAACATGTTTGATAGGTATCCCGTCTCCTATTTCCGAAGGTGATTTTAA   5400
```

```
 GlyTyrValSerAspThrAsnCysSerThrValGlyThrAspArgLeuValLeuSerAlaSerIleThrGlyGlyProAspAsnSerThr
GGGATATGTTTCTGATACAAATTGCTCCACTGTGGGAACTGACCGGTTAGTCTTGTCAGCCAGCATTACCGGCGGCCCTGACAACAGCAC     5490

 ThrLeuThrTyrArgLysValSerCysLeuLeuLeuLysLeuAsnValSerMetTrpAspGluProProGluLeuGlnLeuLeuGlySer
CACCCTCACTTATCGAAAGGTTTCATGCCTGCTGTTAAAGCTGAACGTCTCCATGTGGGATGAGCCACCTGAACTGCAGCTGCTAGGTTC     5580

 GlnSerLeuProAsnValThrAsnIleThrGlnValSerGlyValAlaGlyGlyCysValTyrPheAlaProArgAlaThrGlyLeuPhe
CCAGTCTCTCCCTAACGTTACTAACATTACTCAGGTCTCTGGCGTGGCCGGGGGATGTGTATATTTCGCCCCAAGGGCCACTGGCCTGTT     5670

 LeuGlyTrpSerLysGlnGlyLeuSerArgPheLeuLeuArgHisProPheThrSerThrSerAsnSerThrGluProPheThrValVal
TTTAGGTTGGTCTAAACAAGGTCTCTCGCGGTTCCTCCTCCGTCACCCCTTTACCTCCACCTCTAACTCCACGGAACCGTTCACGGTGGT     5760

 ThrAlaAspArgHisAsnLeuPheMetGlySerGluTyrCysGlyAlaTyrGlyTyrArgPheTrpGluIleTyrAsnCysSerGlnThr
GACAGCGGATAGACACAATCTTTTTATGGGGAGTGAGTACTGTGGTGCATATGGCTACAGATTTTGGGAAATATATAACTGCTCACAGAC     5850

 ArgAsnThrTyrArgCysGlyAspValGlyGlyThrGlyLeuProGluThrTrpCysArgGlyLysGlyGlyIleTrpValAsnGlnSer
TAGGAATACTTACCGCTGTGGAGACGTGGGAGGTACTGGCCTCCCTGAAACCTGGTGCAGAGGAAAAGGAGGTATATGGGTTAATCAATC     5940

 LysGluIleAsnGluThrGluProPheSerPheThrAlaAsnCysThrGlySerAsnLeuGlyAsnValSerGlyCysCysGlyGluPro
AAAGGAAATTAATGAGACAGAGCCGTTCAGTTTTACTGCGAACTGTACTGGCAGTAATTTGGGTAATGTCAGCGGATGTTGCGGAGAACC     6030

 IleThrIleLeuProLeuGlyAlaTrpIleAspSerThrGlnGlySerPheThrLysProLysAlaLeuProProAlaIlePheLeuIle
AATCACGATTCTCCCACTAGGGGCATGGATCGACAGTACGCAAGGTAGTTTCACTAAACCAAAAGCGCTACCACCCGCAATTTTCCTCAT     6120

 CysGlyAspArgAlaTrpGlnGlyIleProSerArgProValGlyGlyProCysTyrLeuGlyLysLeuThrMetLeuAlaProAsnHis
TTGTGGGGATCGCGCATGGCAAGGAATTCCCAGTCGTCCGGTAGGGGGCCCCTGCTATTTAGGCAAGCTTACCATGTTAGCACCCAACCA     6210

                                                               ↓ Gp37
 ThrAspIleLeuLysIleLeuAlaAsnSerSerArgThrGlyIleArgArgLysArgSerValSerHisLeuAspAspThrCysSerAsp
TACAGATATTCTCAAAATACTTGCTAATTCGTCGCGGACAGGTATAAGACGTAAACGAAGCGTCTCACACCTGGATGATACATGCTCAGA     6300

 GluValGlnLeuTrpGlyProThrAlaArgIlePheAlaSerIleLeuAlaProGlyValAlaAlaAlaGlnAlaLeuArgGluIleGlu
TGAAGTACAGCTTTGGGGTCCTACAGCAAGAATCTTTGCATCTATCTTAGCCCCGGGGGTAGCAGCTGCGCAAGCCTTAAGAGAAATTGA     6390

 ArgLeuAlaCysTrpSerValLysGlnAlaAsnLeuThrThrSerLeuLeuGlyAspLeuLeuAspAspValThrSerIleArgHisAla
GAGACTAGCCTGTTGGTCCGTTAAACAGGCTAACTTGACAACATCACTCCTCGGGGACTTATTGGATGATGTCACGAGTATTCGACACGC     6480
```

ValLeuGlnAsnArgAlaAlaIleAspPheLeuLeuLeuAlaHisGlyHisGlyCysGluAspValAlaGlyMetCysCysPheAsnLeu
GGTCCTGCAGAACCGAGCGGCTATTGACTTCTTGCTTCTAGCTCACGGCCATGGCTGTGAGGACGTTGCCGGAATGTGTTGTTTCAATCT 6570

SerAspHisSerGluSerIleGlnLysLysPheGlnLeuMetLysLysHisValAsnLysIleGlyValAspSerAspProIleGlySer
GAGTGATCACAGTGAATCTATACAGAAGAAGTTCCAGCTAATGAAGAAACATGTCAATAAGATCGGCGTGGACAGCGACCCAATCGGAAG 6660

TrpLeuArgGlyIlePheGlyGlyIleGlyGluTrpAlaValHisLeuLeuLysGlyLeuLeuLeuGlyLeuValValIleLeuLeuLeu
TTGGCTGCGAGGGATATTCGGGGGAATAGGGGAATGGGCCGTTCATCTGCTAAAAGGACTGCTTTTGGGGCTTGTAGTTATTTTATTGCT 6750

LeuValCysLeuProCysLeuLeuGlnPheValSerSerSerIleArgLysMetIleAsnSerSerIleAsnTyrHisThrGluTyrArg
ACTGGTGTGCCTGCCTTGCCTTTTACAATTTGTGTCTAGTAGTATTCGAAAGATGATTAATAGTTCAATCAACTATCATACTGAATACAG 6840

LysMetGlnGlyGlyAlaVal***
GAAGATGCAGGGCGGAGCAGTCTAGAGCTCAGTTATAATAATCCTGCGAATCGGGCTGTAACGGGGCAAGGCTTGACCGAGGGGACTATA 6930

ACATGTATAGGCGAAAAGCGGGGTCTCGGTTGTAACGCGCTTAGGAAGTCCCCTCGAGGTATGGCAGATATGCTCTTGCATAGGGGGAAA 7020

↓SA
AAATGTAGTCTTAATATTGTCTGTGTGCTGCAGGAGCTAAGCTGACTCTGCTGGTGGCCTCGCGTACCACTGTGGCCAGGCGGTAGCTGG 7110

MetGlySerSerLysSerLysProLysAspProSerGlnArgArgHisSerLeuGluProProAspSerThr
GACGTGCAGCCGACCACCATGGGGAGCAGCAAGAGCAAGCCTAAGGACCCCAGCCAGCGCCGGCACAGCCTGGAGCCACCCGACAGCACC 7200

HisHisGlyGlyPheProAlaSerGlnThrProAspGluThrAlaAlaProAspAlaHisArgAsnProSerArgSerPheGlyThrVal
CACCACGGGGGATTCCCAGCCTCGCAGACCCCCGACGAGACAGCAGCCCCCGACGCACACCGCAACCCCAGCCGCTCCTTCGGGACCGTG 7290

AlaThrGluProLysLeuPheTrpGlyPheAsnThrSerAspThrValThrSerProGlnArgAlaGlyAlaLeuAlaGlyGlyValThr
GCCACCGAGCCCAAGCTCTTCTGGGGCTTCAACACTTCTGACACCGTCACGTCGCCGCAGCGTGCCGGGGCACTGGCTGGCGGCGTCACC 7380

ThrPheValAlaLeuTyrAspTyrGluSerTrpThrGluThrAspLeuSerPheLysLysGlyGluArgLeuGlnIleValAsnAsnThr
ACTTTCGTGGCTCTCTACGACTACGAGTCCTGGACTGAAACGGACTTGTCCTTCAAGAAAGGAGAACGCCTGCAGATTGTCAACAACACG 7470

GluGlyAspTrpTrpLeuAlaHisSerLeuThrThrGlyGlnThrGlyTyrIleProSerAsnTyrValAlaProSerAspSerIleGln
GAAGGTGACTGGTGGCTGGCTCATTCCCTCACTACAGGACAGACGGGCTACATCCCCAGTAACTATGTCGCGCCCTCAGACTCCATCCAG 7560

AlaGluGluTrpTyrPheGlyLysIleThrArgArgGluSerGluArgLeuLeuLeuAsnProGluAsnProArgGlyThrPheLeuVal
GCTGAAGAGTGGTACTTTGGGAAGATCACTCGTCGGGAGTCCGAGCGGCTGCTGCTTAACCCCGAAAACCCCCGGGGAACCTTCTTGGTC 7650

```
ArgLysSerGluThrAlaLysGlyAlaTyrCysLeuSerValSerAspPheAspAsnAlaLysGlyProAsnValLysHisTyrLysIle
CGGAAGAGCGAGACGGCAAAGGGTGCCTATTGCCTCTCCGTTTCTGACTTTGACAACGCCAAGGGGCCCAATGTGAAGCACTACAAGATC    7740

TyrLysLeuTyrSerGlyGlyPheTyrIleThrSerArgThrGlnPheGlySerLeuGlnGlnLeuValAlaTyrTyrSerLysHisAla
TACAAGCTGTACAGCGGCGGCTTCTACATCACCTCACGCACACAGTTCGGCAGCCTACAGCAGCTGGTGGCCTACTACTCCAAACATGCT    7830

AspGlyLeuCysHisArgLeuAlaAsnValCysProThrSerLysProGlnThrGlnGlyLeuAlaLysAspAlaTrpGluIleProArg
GATGGCTTGTGCCACCGCCTGGCCAACGTCTGCCCCACGTCCAAGCCCCAGACCCAGGGACTCGCCAAGGACGCGTGGGAAATCCCCCGG    7920

GluSerLeuArgLeuGluAlaLysLeuGlyGlnGlyCysPheGlyGluValTrpMetGlyThrTrpAsnAspThrThrArgValAlaIle
GAGTCGCTACGGCTGGAGGCGAAGCTGGGGCAGGGCTGCTTTGGAGAGGTCTGGATGGGGACCTGGAACGACACCACCAGAGTGGCCATA    8010

LysThrLeuLysProGlyThrMetSerProGluAlaPheLeuGlnGluAlaGlnValMetLysLysLeuArgHisGluLysLeuValGln
AAGACTCTGAAGCCCGGCACCATGTCCCCGGAGGCCTTCCTGCAGGAAGCCCAAGTGATGAAGAAGCTCCGGCATGAGAAGCTGGTTCAG    8100

LeuTyrAlaValValSerGluGluProIleTyrIleValIleGluTyrMetSerLysGlySerLeuLeuAspPheLeuLysGlyGluMet
CTGTACGCAGTGGTGTCGGAAGAGCCCATCTACATCGTCATTGAGTACATGAGCAAGGGGAGCCTCCTGGATTTCCTGAAGGGAGAGATG    8190

GlyLysTyrLeuArgLeuProGlnLeuValAspMetAlaAlaGlnIleAlaSerGlyMetAlaTyrValGluArgMetAsnTyrValHis
GGCAAGTACCTGCGGCTGCCACAGCTCGTCGATATGGCTGCTCAGATTGCATCCGGCATGGCCTATGTGGAGAGAATGAACTACGTGCAC    8280

ArgAspLeuArgAlaAlaAsnIleLeuValGlyGluAsnLeuValCysLysValAlaAspPheGlyLeuAlaArgLeuIleGluAspAsn
CGAGACCTGCGGGCGGCCAACATCCTGGTGGGGGAGAACCTGGTGTGCAAGGTGGCTGACTTCGGGCTGGCACGCCTCATCGAGGACAAC    8370

GluTyrThrAlaArgGlnGlyAlaLysPheProIleLysTrpThrAlaProGluAlaAlaLeuTyrGlyArgPheThrIleLysSerAsp
GAGTACACAGCACGGCAAGGTGCCAAGTTCCCCATCAAGTGGACAGCCCCCGAGGCAGCCCTCTATGGCCGGTTCACCATCAAGTCGGAT    8460

ValTrpSerPheGlyIleLeuLeuThrGluLeuThrThrLysGlyArgValProTyrProGlyMetValAsnArgGluValLeuAspGln
GTCTGGTCCTTCGGCATCCTGCTGACTGAGCTGACCACCAAGGGCCGGGTGCCATACCCAGGGATGGTCAACAGGGAGGTGCTGGACCAG    8550

ValGluArgGlyTyrArgMetProCysProProGluCysProGluSerLeuHisAspLeuMetCysGlnCysTrpArgLysAspProGlu
GTGGAGAGGGGCTACCGCATGCCCTGCCCGCCCGAGTGCCCCGAGTCGCTGCATGACCTCATGTGCCAGTGCTGGCGGAAGGACCCTGAG    8640
```

```
GluArgProThrPheLysTyrLeuGlnAlaGlnLeuLeuProAlaCysValLeuGluValAlaGlu***
GAGCGGCCCACCTTTAAGTACCTGCAGGCCCAGCTGCTCCCTGCTTGTGTGTTGGAGGTCGCTGAGTAAGTACGAGGCGTGACCTACAAT   8730

TGCTCAAATAATGCTTCTGTAGAAATTGTTTAGCATTAGGCGTCCTGCGTTGCTCCGCGATGTACGGGTCAGGTATAATGTGCAGTTTGA   8820

CTGAGGGGACCATGATGTGTATAGGCGTCAAGCGGGGCTTCGGTTGTACGCGGATAGGAATCCCCTCAGGACAATTCTGCTTGGAATATG   8910

ATGGCGTCTTCCCTGTTTTGCCCTTAGACTATTCGAGTTGCCTCTGTGGATTAGGGCTGGAGGCAGCACGGATAGTCTGATGGCCAAATA   9000
                                                    PPT   |--■--■--■-->  U3 begins
AGGCAGGCAAGACAGCTATTTGTAACTGCGAAATACGCTTTTGCATAGGGAGGGGAAATGTAGTCTTATGCAATACTCCTGTAGTCTTG   9090

CAACATGCTTATGTAACGATGAGTTAGCAATATGCCTTACAAGGAAAGAAAAGGCACCGTGCATGCCGATTGGTGGTAGTAAGGTGGTAC   9180

GATCGTGCCTTATTAGGAAGGTATCAGACGGGTCTAACATGGATTGGACGAACCACTGAATTCCGCATCGCAGAGATATTGTATTTAAGT   9270
     U3 ends         ↓  R
GCCTAGCTCGATACAATAAACGCCATTTTACCATT
```

Figure E.1. RSV nucleotide sequence.

2. The Complete Sequence of Moloney Murine Leukemia Virus

The sequence has been arranged to correspond with a genomic copy of viral RNA. The sequence begins with R, which is marked "R" on the sequence. On the 3′ side of R is U_5, and the 3′ end of U_5 forms an imperfect inverted repeat with the 5′ end of U_3. The inverted repeats (marked "IR") lie next to the primer binding site (marked "primer") and the unmarked polypurine tract adjacent to U_3. The major product of *gag*, $Pr65^{gag}$, begins with the sequence of $p15^{gag}$ at position 624; translation presumably initiates at the preceding ATG codon. The positions of the known amino termini of p12, p30, and p10, and the carboxy terminus of p10 are denoted by arrows. Direct sequencing of $Pr65^{gag}$ (Appendix F) has confirmed the nucleotide sequence shown here. An additional, glycosylated product of *gag*, $gP85^{gag}$, has been identified on the plasma membrane of MLV-infected cells and shown to be longer than $Pr65^{gag}$ at the amino terminus (see Chapter 6 for discussion and references). It is not known how this protein is made; however, the predicted translational product of the available open reading frame continuous with and preceding p15 is provided in the figure. *gag* terminates with a TAG codon at position 2235 and is followed by a long open reading frame (*pol*) beginning at the next available codon position, 2238. The 5′ boundary of *pol* cannot be precisely specified since the amino terminus of reverse transcriptase has not been determined and the mechanism for bypassing the *gag* termination codon to make $Pr180^{gag\text{-}pol}$ is not known (for further discussion, see Chapters 5 and 6). The *pol* domain terminates with a TAA codon at position 5835. The *env* gene commences at 5777, so that the amino terminus of the primary translation product, $gPr80^{env}$, is encoded in a reading frame that overlaps a different frame used for the carboxy terminus of the *pol* product. Arrows indicate the cleavage sites used to generate the amino termini of the mature *env* proteins, $gp70^{env}$ and p15(E), as well as the R peptide. A possible splice acceptor site for generation of *env* mRNA is marked "acceptor" at position 5500. *env* is followed by a short untranslated region, including the polypurine tract, then U_3.

The sequence given here was derived from a cloned circular species of Mo-MLV DNA with a single LTR by Shinnick et al. (*Nature* **293,** 543, 1981); the cloning and characterization of the DNA was reported by Berns et al. (*J. Virol.* **36,** 254, 1980) and by Van Beveren et al. (*Nature* **289,** 258, 1981). The sequenced clone is not infectious, indicating an unidentified lesion, which has been located within the 5′ two-thirds of the genome, as discussed by Shinnick et al. (*Nature* **293,** 543, 1981).

(cap)GCGCCAGTCCTCCGATTGACTGAGTCGCCCGGGTACCCGTGTATCCAATAAACCCTCTTGCAGTTGCATCCGACTTGTGGTCTCGCTGTTCCTTGGGAGGGTCTCCTCTGAGTGATTGAC
R U5 120

IR
TACCCGTCAGCGGGGGTCTTTCATTTGGGGGCTCGTCCGGGATCGGGAGACCCCTGCCCAGGGACCACCGACCCACCACCGGGAGGTAAGCTGGCCAGCAACTTATCTGTGTCTGTCCGA
primer 240

LeuThrSerSerValSerGlyGlyProValValGluLeuThrSerSerGluHisProAlaAlaThrLeu
TTGTCTAGTGTCTATGACTGATTTTATGCGCCTGCGTCGGTACTAGTTAGCTAACTAGCTCTGTATCTGGCGGACCCGTGGTGGAACTGACGAGTTCGGAACACCCGGCCGCAACCCTGG
360

GlyAspValProGlyThrSerGlyAlaValPheValAlaArgProGluSerLysAsnProAspArgPheGlyLeuPheGlyAlaProProLeuGluGluGlyTyrValValLeuValGly
GAGACGTCCCAGGGACTTCGGGGGCCGTTTTTGTGGCCCGACCTGAGTCCAAAAATCCCGATCGTTTTGGACTCTTTGGTGCACCCCCCTTAGAGGAGGGATATGTGGTTCTGGTAGGAG
480

AspGluAsnLeuLysGlnPheProProProSerGluPheLeuLeuSerValTrpAspArgSerArgAlaAlaArgLeuValCysCysSerIleValLeuCysCysLeuCysLeuThrVal
ACGAGAACCTAAAACAGTTCCCGCCTCCGTCTGAATTTTTGCTTTCGGTTTGGGACCGAAGCCGCGCCGCGCGTCTTGTCTGCTGCAGCATCGTTCTGTGTTGTCTCTGTCTGACTGTGT
600

p15
PheLeuTyrLeuSerGluAsnMetGlyGlnThrValThrThrProLeuSerLeuThrLeuGlyHisTrpLysAspValGluArgIleAlaHisAsnGlnSerValAspValLysLysArg
TTCTGTATTTGTCTGAGAATATGGGCCAGACTGTTACCACTCCCTTAAGTTTGACCTTAGGTCACTGGAAAGATGTCGAGCGGATCGCTCACAACCAGTCGGTAGATGTCAAGAAGAGAC
720

ArgTrpValThrPheCysSerAlaGluTrpProThrPheAsnValGlyTrpProArgAspGlyThrPheAsnArgAspLeuIleThrGlnValLysIleLysValPheSerProGlyPro
GTTGGGTTACCTTCTGCTCTGCAGAATGGCCAACCTTTAACGTCGGATGGCCGCGAGACGGCACCTTTAACCGAGACCTCATCACCCAGGTTAAGATCAAGGTCTTTTCACCTGGCCCGC
840

HisGlyHisProAspGlnValProTyrIleValThrTrpGluAlaLeuAlaPheAspProProProTrpValLysProPheValHisProLysProProProProLeuProProSerAla
ATGGACACCCAGACCAGGTCCCCTACATCGTGACCTGGGAAGCCTTGGCTTTTGACCCCCCTCCCTGGGTCAAGCCCTTTGTACACCCTAAGCCTCCGCCTCCTCTTCCTCCATCCGCCC
960

p12
ProSerLeuProLeuGluProProArgSerThrProProArgSerSerLeuTyrProAlaLeuThrProSerLeuGlyAlaLysProLysProGlnValLeuSerAspSerGlyGlyPro
CGTCTCTCCCCCTTGAACCTCCTCGTTCGACCCCGCCTCGATCCTCCCTTTATCCAGCCCTCACTCCTTCTCTAGGCGCCAAACCTAAACCTCAAGTTCTTTCTGACAGTGGGGGGCCGC
1080

LeuIleAspLeuLeuThrGluAspProProProTyrArgAspProArgProProProSerAspArgAspGlyAsnGlyGlyGluAlaThrProAlaGlyGluAlaProAspProSerPro
TCATCGACCTACTTACAGAAGACCCCCCGCCTTATAGGGACCCAAGACCACCCCCTTCCGACAGGGACGGAAATGGTGGAGAAGCGACCCCTGCGGGAGAGGCACCGGACCCCTCCCCAA
1200

```
                                                                   p30
MetAlaSerArgLeuArgGlyArgArgGluProProValAlaAspSerThrThrSerGlnAlaPheProLeuArgAlaGlyGlyAsnGlyGlnLeuGlnTyrTrpProPheSerSerSer
TGGCATCTCGCCTACGTGGGAGACGGGAGCCCCCTGTGGCCGACTCCACTACCTCGCAGGCATTCCCCCTCCGCGCAGGAGGAAACGGACAGCTTCAATACTGGCCGTTCTCCTCTTCTG
                                                                                                                     1320

AspLeuTyrAsnTrpLysAsnAsnAsnProSerPheSerGluAspProGlyLysLeuThrAlaLeuIleGluSerValLeuIleThrHisGlnProThrTrpAspAspCysGlnGlnLeu
ACCTTTACAACTGGAAAAATAATAACCCTTCTTTTTCTGAAGATCCAGGTAAACTGACAGCTCTGATCGAGTCTGTTCTCATCACCCATCAGCCCACCTGGGACGACTGTCAGCAGCTGT
                                                                                                                     1440

LeuGlyThrLeuLeuThrGlyGluGluLysGlnArgValLeuLeuGluAlaArgLysAlaValArgGlyAspAspGlyArgProThrGlnLeuProAsnGluValAspAlaAlaPhePro
TGGGGACTCTGCTGACCGGAGAAGAAAAACAACGGGTGCTCTTAGAGGCTAGAAAGGCGGTGCGGGGCGATGATGGGCGCCCCACTCAACTGCCCAATGAAGTCGATGCCGCTTTTCCCC
                                                                                                                     1560

LeuGluArgProAspTrpAspTyrThrThrGlnAlaGlyArgAsnHisLeuValHisTyrArgGlnLeuLeuLeuAlaGlyLeuGlnAsnAlaGlyArgSerProThrAsnLeuAlaLys
TCGAGCGCCCAGACTGGGATTACACCACCCAGGCAGGTAGGAACCACCTAGTCCACTATCGCCAGTTGCTCCTAGCGGGTCTCCAAAACGCGGGCAGAAGCCCCACCAATTTGGCCAAGG
                                                                                                                     1680

ValLysGlyIleThrGlnGlyProAsnGluSerProSerAlaPheLeuGluArgLeuLysGluAlaTyrArgArgTyrThrProTyrAspProGluAspProGlyGlnGluThrAsnVal
TAAAAGGAATAACACAAGGGCCCAATGAGTCTCCCTCGGCCTTCCTAGAGAGACTTAAGGAAGCCTATCGCAGGTACACTCCTTATGACCCTGAGGACCCAGGGCAAGAAACTAATGTGT
                                                                                                                     1800

SerMetSerPheIleTrpGlnSerAlaProAspIleGlyArgLysLeuGlyArgLeuGluAspLeuLysAsnLysThrLeuGlyAspLeuValArgGluAlaGluLysIlePheAsnLys
CTATGTCTTTCATTTGGCAGTCTGCCCCAGACATTGGGAGAAAGTTAGGGAGGTTAGAAGATTTAAAAAACAAGACGCTTGGAGATTTGGTTAGAGAGGCAGAAAAGATCTTTAATAAAC
                                                                                                                     1920

ArgGluThrProGluGluArgGluGluArgIleArgArgGluThrGluGluLysGluGluArgArgArgThrGluAspGluGlnLysGluLysGluArgAspArgArgArgHisArgGlu
GAGAAACCCCGGAAGAAAGAGAGGAACGTATCAGGAGAGAAACAGAGGAAAAAGAAGAACGCCGTAGGACAGAGGATGAGCAGAAAGAGAAAGAAAGAGATCGTAGGAGACATAGAGAGA
                                                                                                                     2040
              p10
MetSerLysLeuLeuAlaThrValValSerGlyGlnLysGlnAspArgGlnGlyGlyGluArgArgArgSerGlnLeuAspArgAspGlnCysAlaTyrCysLysGluLysGlyHisTrp
TGAGCAAGCTATTGGCCACTGTCGTTAGTGGACAGAAACAGGATAGACAGGGAGGAGAACGAAGGAGGTCCCAACTCGATCGCGACCAGTGTGCCTACTGCAAAGAAAAGGGGCACTGGG
                                                                                                                     2160
                                                                           pol
AlaLysAspCysProLysLysProArgGlyProArgGlyProArgProGlnThrSerLeuLeuThrLeuAspAsp***GlyGlyGlnGlyGlnAspProProProGluProArgIleThr
CTAAAGATTGTCCCAAGAAACCACGAGGACCTCGGGGACCAAGACCCCAGACCTCCCTCCTGACCCTAGATGACTAGGGAGGTCAGGGTCAGGACCCCCCCCTGAACCCAGGATAACCC
                                                                                                                     2280

LeuLysValGlyGlyGlnProValThrPheLeuValAspThrGlyAlaGlnHisSerValLeuThrGlnAsnProGlyProLeuSerAspLysSerAlaTrpValGlnGlyAlaThrGly
TCAAAGTCGGGGGGCAACCCGTCACCTTCCTGGTAGATACTGGGGCCCAACACTCCGTGCTGACCCAAAATCCTGGACCCCTAAGTGATAAGTCTGCCTGGGTCCAAGGGGCTACTGGAG
                                                                                                                     2400
```

```
GlyLysArgTyrArgTrpThrThrAspArgLysValHisLeuAlaThrGlyLysValThrHisSerPheLeuHisValProAspCysProTyrProLeuLeuGlyArgAspLeuLeuThr
GAAAGCGGTATCGCTGGACCACGGATCGCAAAGTACATCTAGCTACCGGTAAGGTCACCCACTCTTTCCTCCATGTACCAGACTGTCCCTATCCTCTGTTAGGAAGAGATTTGCTGACTA
                                                                                                                     2520

LysLeuLysAlaGlnIleHisPheGluGlySerGlyAlaGlnValMetGlyProMetGlyGlnProLeuGlnValLeuThrLeuAsnIleGluAspGluHisArgLeuHisGluThrSer
AACTAAAAGCCCAAATCCACTTTGAGGGATCAGGAGCTCAGGTTATGGGACCAATGGGGCAGCCCCTGCAAGTGTTGACCCTAAATATAGAAGATGAGCATCGGCTACATGAGACCTCAA
                                                                                                                     2640

LysGluProAspValSerLeuGlySerThrTrpLeuSerAspPheProGlnAlaTrpAlaGluThrGlyGlyMetGlyLeuAlaValArgGlnAlaProLeuIleIleProLeuLysAla
AAGAGCCAGATGTTTCTCTAGGGTCCACATGGCTGTCTGATTTTCCTCAGGCCTGGGCGGAAACCGGGGGCATGGGACTGGCAGTTCGCCAAGCTCCTCTGATCATACCTCTGAAAGCAA
                                                                                                                     2760

ThrSerThrProValSerIleLysGlnTyrProMetSerGlnGluAlaArgLeuGlyIleLysProHisIleGlnArgLeuLeuAspGlnGlyIleLeuValProCysGlnSerProTrp
CCTCTACCCCCGTGTCCATAAAACAATACCCCATGTCACAAGAAGCCAGACTGGGGATCAAGCCCCACATACAGAGACTGTTGGACCAGGGAATACTGGTACCCTGCCAGTCCCCCTGGA
                                                                                                                     2880

AsnThrProLeuLeuProValLysLysProGlyThrAsnAspTyrArgProValGlnAspLeuArgGluValAsnLysArgValGluAspIleHisProThrValProAsnProTyrAsn
ACACGCCCCTGCTACCCGTTAAGAAACCAGGGACTAATGATTATAGGCCTGTCCAGGATCTGAGAGAAGTCAACAAGCGGGTGGAAGACATCCACCCCACCGTGCCCAACCCTTACAACC
                                                                                                                     3000

LeuLeuSerGlyLeuProProSerHisGlnTrpTyrThrValLeuAspLeuLysAspAlaPhePheCysLeuArgLeuHisProThrSerGlnProLeuPheAlaPheGluTrpArgAsp
TCTTGAGCGGGCTCCCACCGTCCCACCAGTGGTACACTGTGCTTGATTTAAAGGATGCCTTTTTCTGCCTGAGACTCCACCCCACCAGTCAGCCTCTCTTCGCCTTTGAGTGGAGAGATC
                                                                                                                     3120

ProGluMetGlyIleSerGlyGlnLeuThrTrpThrArgLeuProGlnGlyPheLysAsnSerProThrLeuPheAspGluAlaLeuHisArgAspLeuAlaAspPheArgIleGlnHis
CAGAGATGGGAATCTCAGGACAATTGACCTGGACCAGACTCCCACAGGGTTTCAAAAACAGTCCCACCCTGTTTGATGAGGCACTGCACAGAGACCTAGCAGACTTCCGGATCCAGCACC
                                                                                                                     3240

ProAspLeuIleLeuLeuGlnTyrValAspAspLeuLeuLeuAlaAlaThrSerGluLeuAspCysGlnGlnGlyThrArgAlaLeuLeuGlnThrLeuGlyAsnLeuGlyTyrArgAla
CAGACTTGATCCTGCTACAGTACGTGGATGACTTACTGCTGGCCGCCACTTCTGAGCTAGACTGCCAACAAGGTACTCGGGCCCTGTTACAAACCCTAGGGAACCTCGGGTATCGGGCCT
                                                                                                                     3360

SerAlaLysLysAlaGlnIleCysGlnLysGlnValLysTyrLeuGlyTyrLeuLeuLysGluGlyGlnArgTrpLeuThrGluAlaArgLysGluThrValMetGlyGlnProThrPro
CGGCCAAGAAAGCCCAAATTTGCCAGAAACAGGTCAAGTATCTGGGGTATCTTCTAAAAGAGGGTCAGAGATGGCTGACTGAGGCCAGAAAAGAGACTGTGATGGGGCAGCCTACTCCGA
                                                                                                                     3480

LysThrProArgGlnLeuArgGluPheLeuGlyThrAlaGlyPheCysArgLeuTrpIleProGlyPheAlaGluMetAlaAlaProLysTyrProLeuThrLysThrGlyThrLeuPhe
AGACCCCTCGACAACTAAGGGAGTTCCTAGGGACGGCAGGCTTCTGTCGCCTCTGGATCCCTGGGTTTGCAGAAATGGCAGCCCCCTTGTACCCTCTCACCAAAACGGGGACTCTGTTTA
                                                                                                                     3600
```

AsnTrpGlyProAspGlnGlnLysAlaTyrGlnGluIleLysGlnAlaLeuLeuThrAlaProAlaLeuGlyLeuProAspLeuThrLysProPheGluLeuPheValAspGluLysGln
ATTGGGGCCCAGACCAACAAAAGGCCTATCAAGAAATCAAGCAAGCTCTTCTAACTGCCCCAGCCCTGGGGTTGCCAGATTTGACTAAGCCCTTTGAACTCTTTGTCGACGAGAAGCAGG
3720

GlyTyrAlaLysGlyValLeuThrGlnLysLeuGlyProTrpArgArgProValAlaTyrLeuSerLysLysLeuAspProValAlaAlaGlyTrpProProCysLeuArgMetValAla
GCTACGCCAAAGGTGTCCTAACGCAAAAACTGGGACCTTGGCGTCGGCCGGTGGCCTACCTGTCCAAAAAGCTAGACCCAGTAGCAGCTGGGTGGCCCCCTTGCCTACGGATGGTAGCAG
3840

AlaIleAlaValLeuThrLysAspAlaGlyLysLeuThrMetGlyGlnProLeuValIleLeuAlaProHisAlaValGluAlaLeuValLysGlnProProAspArgTrpLeuSerAsn
CCATTGCCGTACTGACAAAGGATGCAGGCAAGCTAACCATGGGACAGCCACTAGTCATTCTGGCCCCCCATGCAGTAGAGGCACTAGTCAAACAACCCCCCGACCGCTGGCTTTCCAACG
3960

AlaArgMetThrHisTyrGlnAlaLeuLeuLeuAspThrAspArgValGlnPheGlyProValValAlaLeuAsnProAlaThrLeuLeuProLeuProGluGluGlyLeuGlnHisAsn
CCCGGATGACTCACTATCAGGCCTTGCTTTTGGACACGGACCGGGTCCAGTTCGGACCGGTGGTAGCCCTGAACCCGGCTACGCTGCTCCCACTGCCTGAGGAAGGGCTGCAACACAACT
4080

CysLeuAspIleLeuAlaGluAlaHisGlyThrArgProAspLeuThrAspGlnProLeuProAspAlaAspHisThrTrpTyrThrAspGlySerSerLeuLeuGlnGluGlyGlnArg
GCCTTGATATCCTGGCCGAAGCCCACGGAACCCGACCCGACCTAACGGACCAGCCGCTCCCAGACGCCGACCACACCTGGTACACGGATGGAAGCAGTCTCTTACAAGAGGGACAGCGTA
4200

LysAlaGlyAlaAlaValThrThrGluThrGluValIleTrpAlaLysAlaLeuProAlaGlyThrSerAlaGlnArgAlaGluLeuIleAlaLeuThrGlnAlaLeuLysMetAlaGlu
AGGCGGGAGCTGCGGTGACCACCGAGACCGAGGTAATCTGGGCTAAAGCCCTGCCAGCCGGGACATCCGCTCAGCGGGCTGAACTGATAGCACTCACCCAGGCCCTAAAGATGGCAGAAG
4320

GlyLysLysLeuAsnValTyrThrAspSerArgTyrAlaPheAlaThrAlaHisIleHisGlyGluIleTyrArgArgArgGlyLeuLeuThrSerGluGlyLysGluIleLysAsnLys
GTAAGAAGCTAAATGTTTATACTGATAGCCGTTATGCTTTTGCTACTGCCCATATCCATGGAGAAATATACAGAAGGCGTGGGTTGCTCACATCAGAAGGCAAAGAGATCAAAAATAAAG
4440

AspGluIleLeuAlaLeuLeuLysAlaLeuPheLeuProLysArgLeuSerIleIleHisCysProGlyHisGlnLysGlyHisSerAlaGluAlaArgGlyAsnArgMetAlaAspGln
ACGAGATCTTGGCCCTACTAAAAGCCCTCTTTCTGCCCAAAAGACTTAGCATAATCCATTGTCCAGGACATCAAAAGGGACACAGCGCCGAGGCTAGAGGCAACCGGATGGCTGACCAAG
4560

AlaAlaArgLysAlaAlaIleThrGluThrProAspThrSerThrLeuLeuIleGluAsnSerSerProTyrThrSerGluHisPheHisTyrThrValThrAspIleLysAspLeuThr
CGGCCCGAAAGGCAGCCATCACAGAGACTCCAGACACCTCTACCCTCCTCATAGAAAATTCATCACCCTACACCTCAGAACATTTTCATTACACAGTGACTGATATAAAGGACCTAACCA
4680

LysLeuGlyAlaIleTyrAspLysThrLysLysTyrTrpValTyrGlnGlyLysProValMetProAspGlnPheThrPheGluLeuLeuAspPheLeuHisGlnLeuThrHisLeuSer
AGTTGGGGGCCATTTATGATAAAACAAAGAAGTATTGGGTCTACCAAGGAAAACCTGTGATGCCTGACCAGTTTACTTTTGAATTATTAGACTTTCTTCATCAGCTGACTCACCTCAGCT
4800

PheSerLysMetLysAlaLeuLeuGluArgSerHisSerProTyrTyrMetLeuAsnArgAspArgThrLeuLysAsnIleThrGluThrCysLysAlaCysAlaGlnValAsnAlaSer
TCTCAAAAATGAAGGCTCTCCTAGAGAGAAGCCACAGTCCCTACTACATGCTGAACCGGGATCGAACACTCAAAAATATCACTGAGACCTGCAAAGCTTGTGCACAAGTCAACGCCAGCA
4920

LysSerAlaValLysGlnGlyThrArgValArgGlyHisArgProGlyThrHisTrpGluIleAspPheThrGluIleLysProGlyLeuTyrGlyTyrLysTyrLeuLeuValPheIle
AGTCTGCCGTTAAACAGGGAACTAGGGTCCGCGGGCATCGGCCCGGCACTCATTGGGAGATCGATTTCACCGAGATAAAGCCCGGATTGTATGGCTATAAATATCTTCTAGTTTTTATAG
5040

AspThrPheSerGlyTrpIleGluAlaPheProThrLysLysGluThrAlaLysValValThrLysLysLeuLeuGluGluIlePheProArgPheGlyMetProGlnValLeuGlyThr
ATACCTTTTCTGGCTGGATAGAAGCCTTCCCAACCAAGAAAGAAACCGCCAAGGTCGTAACCAAGAAGCTACTAGAGGAGATCTTCCCCAGGTTCGGCATGCCTCAGGTATTGGGAACTG
5160

AspAsnGlyProAlaPheValSerLysValSerGlnThrValAlaAspLeuLeuGlyIleAspTrpLysLeuHisCysAlaTyrArgProGlnSerSerGlyGlnValGluArgMetAsn
ACAATGGGCCTGCCTTCGTCTCCAAGGTGAGTCAGACAGTGGCCGATCTGTTGGGGATTGATTGGAAATTACATTGTGCATACAGACCCCAAAGCTCAGGCCAGGTAGAAAGAATGAATA
5280

ArgThrIleLysGluThrLeuThrLysLeuThrLeuAlaThrGlySerArgAspTrpValLeuLeuLeuProLeuAlaLeuTyrArgAlaArgAsnThrProGlyProHisGlyLeuThr
GAACCATCAAGGAGACTTTAACTAAATTAACGCTTGCAACTGGCTCTAGAGACTGGGTGCTCCTACTCCCCTTAGCCCTGTACCGAGCCCGCAACACGCCGGGCCCCCATGGCCTCACCC
5400

ProTyrGluIleLeuTyrGlyAlaProProProLeuValAsnPheProAspProAspMetThrArgValThrAsnSerProSerLeuGlnAlaHisLeuGlnAlaLeuTyrLeuValGln
CATATGAGATCTTATATGGGGCACCCCCGCCCCTTGTAAACTTCCCTGACCCTGACATGACAAGAGTTACTAACAGCCCCTCTCTCCAAGCTCACTTACAGGCTCTCTACTTAGTCCAGC
acceptor
5520

HisGluValTrpArgProLeuAlaAlaAlaTyrGlnGluGlnLeuAspArgProValValProHisProTyrArgValGlyAspThrValTrpValArgArgHisGlnThrLysAsnLeu
ACGAAGTCTGGAGACCTCTGGCGGCAGCCTACCAAGAACAACTGGACCGACCGGTGGTACCTCACCCTTACCGAGTCGGCGACACAGTGTGGGTCCGCCGACACCAGACTAAGAACCTAG
5640

GluProArgTrpLysGlyProTyrThrValLeuLeuThrThrProThrAlaLeuLysValAspGlyIleAlaAlaTrpIleHisAlaAlaHisValLysAlaAlaAspProGlyGlyGly
AACCTCGCTGGAAAGGACCTTACACAGTCCTGCTGACCACCCCCACCGCCCTCAAAGTAGACGGCATCGCAGCTTGGATACACGCCGCCCACGTGAAGGCTGCCGACCCCGGGGGTGGAC
5760
env
MetAlaArgSerThrLeuSerLysProLeuLysAsnLysValAsnProArgGlyProLeuIleProLeuIleLeuLeuMetLeuArgGlyValSerThrAlaSer
gp70
*ProSerSerArgLeuThrTrpArgValGlnArgSerGlnAsnProLeuLysIleArgLeuThrArgGluAlaPro****
CATCCTCTAGACTGACATGGCGCGTTCAACGCTCTCAAAACCCCTTAAAAATAAGGTTAACCCGCGAGGCCCCCTAATCCCCTTAATTCTTCTGATGCTCAGAGGGGTCAGTACTGCTTC
5880

ProGlySerSerProHisGlnValTyrAsnIleThrTrpGluValThrAsnGlyAspArgGluThrValTrpAlaThrSerGlyAsnHisProLeuTrpThrTrpTrpProAspLeuThr
GCCCGGCTCCAGTCCTCATCAAGTCTATAATATCACCTGGGAGGTAACCAATGGAGATCGGGAGACGGTATGGGCAACTTCTGGCAACCACCCTCTGTGGACCTGGTGGCCTGACCTTAC
6000

ProAspLeuCysMetLeuAlaHisHisGlyProSerTyrTrpGlyLeuGluTyrGlnSerProPheSerSerProProGlyProProCysCysSerGlyGlySerSerProGlyCysSer
CCCAGATTTATGTATGTTAGCCCACCATGGACCATCTTATTGGGGCTAGAATATCAATCCCCTTTTTCTTCTCCCCCGGGCCCCCTTGTTGCTCAGGGGGCAGCAGCCCAGGCTGTTC
6120

ArgAspCysGluGluProLeuThrSerLeuThrProArgCysAsnThrAlaTrpAsnArgLeuLysLeuAspGlnThrThrHisLysSerAsnGluGlyPheTyrValCysProGlyPro
CAGAGACTGCGAAGAACCTTTAACCTCCCTCACCCCTCGGTGCAACACTGCCTGGAACAGACTCAAGCTAGACCAGACAACTCATAAATCAAATGAGGGATTTTATGTTTGCCCCGGGCC
6240

HisArgProArgGluSerLysSerCysGlyGlyProAspSerPheTyrCysAlaTyrTrpGlyCysGluThrThrGlyArgAlaTyrTrpLysProSerSerSerTrpAspPheIleThr
CCACCGCCCCCGAGAATCCAAGTCATGTGGGGGTCCAGACTCCTTCTACTGTGCCTATTGGGGCTGTGAGACAACCGGTAGAGCTTACTGGAAGCCCTCCTCATCATGGGATTTCATCAC
6360

ValAsnAsnAsnLeuThrSerAspGlnAlaValGlnValCysLysAspAsnLysTrpCysAsnProLeuValIleArgPheThrAspAlaGlyArgArgValThrSerTrpThrThrGly
AGTAAACAACAATCTCACCTCTGACCAGGCTGTCCAGGTATGCAAAGATAATAAGTGGTGCAACCCCTTAGTTATTCGGTTTACAGACGCCGGGAGACGGGTTACTTCCTGGACCACAGG
6480

HisTyrTrpGlyLeuArgLeuTyrValSerGlyGlnAspProGlyLeuThrPheGlyIleArgLeuArgTyrGlnAsnLeuGlyProArgValProIleGlyProAsnProValLeuAla
ACATTACTGGGGCTTACGTTTGTATGTCTCCGGACAAGATCCAGGGCTTACATTTGGGATCCGACTCAGATACCAAAATCTAGGACCCCGCGTCCCAATAGGGCCAAACCCCGTTCTGGC
6600

AspGlnGlnProLeuSerLysProLysProValLysSerProSerValThrLysProProSerGlyThrProLeuSerProThrGlnLeuProProAlaGlyThrGluAsnArgLeuLeu
AGACCAACAGCCACTCTCCAAGCCCAAACCTGTTAAGTCGCCTTCAGTCACCAAACCACCCAGTGGGACTCCTCTCTCCCCTACCCAACTTCCACCGGCGGGAACGGAAAATAGGCTGCT
6720

AsnLeuValAspGlyAlaTyrGlnAlaLeuAsnLeuThrSerProAspLysThrGlnGluCysTrpLeuCysLeuValAlaGlyProProTyrTyrGluGlyValAlaValLeuGlyThr
AAACTTAGTAGACGGAGCCTACCAAGCCCTCAACCTCACCAGTCCTGACAAAACCCAAGAGTGCTGGTTGTGTCTAGTAGCGGGACCCCCCTACTACGAAGGGGTTGCCGTCCTGGGTAC
6840

TyrSerAsnHisThrSerAlaProAlaAsnCysSerValAlaSerGlnHisLysLeuThrLeuSerGluValThrGlyGlnGlyLeuCysIleGlyAlaValProLysThrHisGlnAla
CTACTCCAACCATACCTCTGCTCCAGCCAACTGCTCCGTGGCCTCCCAACACAAGTTGACCCTGTCCGAAGTGACCGGACAGGGACTCTGCATAGGAGCAGTTCCCAAAACACATCAGGC
6960

LeuCysAsnThrThrGlnThrSerSerArgGlySerTyrTyrLeuValAlaProThrGlyThrMetTrpAlaCysSerThrGlyLeuThrProCysIleSerThrThrIleLeuAsnLeu
CCTATGTAATACCACCCAGACAAGCAGTCGAGGGTCCTATTATCTAGTTGCCCCTACAGGTACCATGTGGGCTTGTAGTACCGGGCTTACTCCATGCATCTCCACCACCATACTGAACCT
7080

p15E

ThrThrAspTyrCysValLeuValGluLeuTrpProArgValThrTyrHisSerProSerTyrValTyrGlyLeuPheGluArgSerAsnArgHisLysArgGluProValSerLeuThr
TACCACTGATTATTGTGTTCTTGTCGAACTCTGGCCAAGAGTCACCTATCATTCCCCCAGCTATGTTTACGGCCTGTTTGAGAGATCCAACCGACACAAAAGAGAACCGGTGTCGTTAAC
7200

```
 LeuAlaLeuLeuLeuGlyGlyLeuThrMetGlyGlyIleAlaAlaGlyIleGlyThrGlyThrThrAlaLeuMetAlaThrGlnGlnPheGlnGlnLeuGlnAlaAlaValGlnAspAsp
CCTGGCCCTATTATTGGGTGGACTAACCATGGGGGGAATTGCCGCTGGAATAGGAACAGGGACTACTGCTCTAATGGCCACTCAGCAATTCCAGCAGCTCCAAGCCGCAGTACAGGATGA
                                                                                                                       7320

 LeuArgGluValGluLysSerIleSerAsnLeuGluLysSerLeuThrSerLeuSerGluValValLeuGlnAsnArgArgGlyLeuAspLeuLeuPheLeuLysGluGlyGlyLeuCys
TCTCAGGGAGGTTGAAAAATCAATCTCTAACCTAGAAAAGTCTCTCACTTCCCTGTCTGAAGTTGTCCTACAGAATCGAAGGGGCCTAGACTTGTTATTTCTAAAAGAAGGAGGGCTGTG
                                                                                                                       7440

 AlaAlaLeuLysGluGluCysCysPheTyrAlaAspHisThrGlyLeuValArgAspSerMetAlaLysLeuArgGluArgLeuAsnGlnArgGlnLysLeuPheGluSerThrGlnGly
TGCTGCTCTAAAAGAAGAATGTTGCTTCTATGCGGACCACACAGGACTAGTGAGAGACAGCATGGCCAAATTGAGAGAGAGGCTTAATCAGAGACAGAAACTGTTTGAGTCAACTCAAGG
                                                                                                                       7560

 TrpPheGluGlyLeuPheAsnArgSerProTrpPheThrThrLeuIleSerThrIleMetGlyProLeuIleValLeuLeuMetIleLeuLeuPheGlyProCysIleLeuAsnArgLeu
ATGGTTTGAGGGACTGTTTAACAGATCCCCTTGGTTTACCACCTTGATATCTACCATTATGGGACCCCTCATTGTACTCCTAATGATTTTGCTCTTCGGACCCTGCATTCTTAATCGATT
                                                                                                                       7680
                                                                               R
 ValGlnPheValLysAspArgIleSerValValGlnAlaLeuValLeuThrGlnGlnTyrHisGlnLeuLysProIleGluTyrGluPro***
AGTCCAATTTGTTAAAGACAGGATATCAGTGGTCCAGGCTCTAGTTTTGACTCAACAATATCACCAGCTGAAGCCTATAGAGTACGAGCCATAGATAAAATAAAAGATTTTATTTAGTCT
                                                                                                                       7800
                    IR
CCAGAAAAAGGGGGGAATGAAAGACCCCACCTGTAGGTTTGGCAAGCTAGCTTAAGTAACGCCATTTTGCAAGGCATGGAAAAATACATAACTGAGAATAGAGAAGTTCAGATCAAGGTC
                                      U3                                                                               7920

AGGAACAGATGGAACAGCTGAATATGGGCCAAACAGGATATCTGTGGTAAGCAGTTCCTGCCCCGGCTCAGGGCCAAGAACAGATGGAACAGCTGAATATGGGCCAAACAGGATATCTGT
                                                                                                                       8040

GGTAAGCAGTTCCTGCCCCGGCTCAGGGCCAAGAACAGATGGTCCCCAGATGCGGTCCAGCCCTCAGCAGTTTCTAGAGAACCATCAGATGTTTCCAGGGTGCCCCAAGGACCTGAAATG
                                                                                                                       8160

ACCCTGTGCCTTATTTGAACTAACCAATCAGTTCGCTTCTCGCTTCTGTTCGCGCGCTTCTGCTCCCCGAGCTCAATAAAAGAGCCCACAACCCCTCACTCGGGGCGCCAGTCCTCCGAT
                                                                                                   U3                  8280

TGACTGAGTCGCCCGGGTACCCGTGTATCCAATAAACCCTCTTGCAGTTGCA(PolyA)
                      R                     8332
```

3. The Complete Nucleotide Sequence of Moloney Murine Sarcoma Virus, Clone 124, Unintegrated Circular DNA Containing Two LTRs

The viral DNA sequence was determined by Van Beveren et al. (*Cell* **27,** 97, 1981) from a cloned circular DNA species of Mo-MSV, strain 124; a similar sequence has been published by Reddy et al. (*Science* **214,** 445, 1981). The results are presented as if the sequence were from a provirus. The sequence starts with an unexpected "A" residue found at the junction of the two LTRs in the molecular clone. Only the coding strand is shown in the figure. Several features of the LTRs (residues 2–590 and 5245–5833) are indicated. The site of initiation of viral RNA synthesis, marked CAP, defines the boundary between U_3 and R; the boundary between U_5 and R is known only approximately (ca. positions 515 and 5757). The ends of U_3 and U_5 form a perfect inverted repeat of 13 bases; these sequences have been overlined. Two sequences that form a direct repeat in the U_3 region (56 out of 58 residues match) are marked by arrows and "d.r." Closely related murine retroviral LTRs may have only one copy of this sequence or a repeat of a different size (see Appendix D). The CAT box and the TATA box, thought to be important in the initiation of transcription, are marked, as are the signal for polyadenylation (poly[A]), the primer binding site (PBS), a potential linkage site for the formation of dimeric virion RNA (DLS), and the polypurine tract implicated in the priming of plus-strand DNA (origin [+] strand). Substantial differences (deletions and substitutions) between this sequence and that of Mo-MLV clone-1 DNA are indicated; when the deleted sequences include one copy of a sequence repeated in Mo-MLV, the residual repeat sequence is boxed. (Further comparison can be made with the Mo-MLV sequence on the preceding pages; full explanations are presented in *Cell* **27,** 97, 1981.) Regions capable of encoding large polypeptides are shown. The *gag* gene, which encodes a polypeptide of 61,100 daltons, begins at nucleotide 1042 and ends with a TAG codon at 2656. Cleavage sites for the *gag* polypeptides are shown (see Appendix F). Also marked are coordinates for an open reading frame that might encode a 17,300-dalton protein, called X, a hypothetical remnant of the *pol* gene product. The coding region begins at 2970 and terminates with a TGA codon at position 3450.

The *v-mos* gene begins at position 3875 and terminates with a TAG codon at position 4997; the gene product is 40,900 daltons. The sites of recombination between the parental virus, Mo-MLV, and the *c-mos* oncogene are marked by arrows labeled "substitution II" (see also the *c-mos* sequence in this section of the appendix). The first 14 bases of the *v-mos* coding domain are derived from the 5′ end of the Mo-MLV *env* gene.

The nucleotide sequence in the region of the *gag* gene was confirmed in many areas using protein sequence data (Oroszlan et al., *Proc. Natl. Acad. Sci.* **75,** 1404, 1978; Henderson et al., *J. Biol. Chem.* **256,** 8400, 1981; Versteegen et al., *J. Biol. Chem.* 1982, in press; S. Oroszlan, pers. comm.). The nucleotide sequence at the 3′ terminus of the *v-mos* gene has been confirmed by immunoprecipitation of polypeptides synthesized in vitro, using antibodies raised against a synthetic peptide whose sequence was specified by the nucleotide sequence (Papkoff et al., *Cell* **27,** 109, 1981).

```
   →5' LTR          U3 begins
A|A A T G A A A G A C C C C A C C C G T A G G T G G C A A G C T A G C T T A A G T A A C G C C A C T T T G C A A G G C A
                 10                  20                  30                  40                  50                  60

T G G A A A A A T A C A T A A C T G A G A A T A G A A A A G T T C A G A T C A A G G T C A G G A A C A A A G A A A C A G
                 70                  80                  90                 100                 110                 120

            →d.r.
C T G A A T A|C C A A A C A G G A T A T C T G T G G T A A G C G G T T C C T G C C C C G G C T C A G G G C C A A G A A C
                130                 140                 150                 160                 170                 180

d.r.←                             →d.r.
A G A T G|A G A C A G C T G A G T G A T G G G|C C A A A C A G G A T A T C T G T G G T A A G C A G T T C C T G C C C C G
                190                 200                 210                 220                 230                 240

                              d.r.←
G C T C G G G G C C A A G A A C A G A T G|G T C C C C A G A T G C G G T C C A G C C C T C A G C A G T T T C T A G T G A
                250                 260                 270                 280                 290                 300

A T C A T C A G A T G T T T C C A G G G T G C C C C A A G G A C C T G A A A A T G A C C C T G T A C C T T A T T T G A A
                310                 320                 330                 340                 350                 360

     "CAT-box"                                                                                         "TATA-box"
C T A A[C C A A T]C A G T T C G C T T C T C G C T T C T G T T C G C G C G C T T C C G C T C T C C G A G C T[C A A T A A]
                370                 380                 390                 400                 410                 420

                  U3 ends              CAP      R begins
                                        ↓
[A]A G A G C C C A C A A C C C C T C A C T C G G C G C G C C A G T C T T C C G A T A G A C T G C G T C G C C C G G G T A
                430                 440                 450                 460                 470                 480

                  poly (A)      R ends                      U5 begins
C C C G T A T T C C C[A A T A A A]G C C T C T T G C T G T T T G C A T C C G A A T C G T G G T C T C G C T G T T C C T T
                490                 500                 510                 520                 530                 540
```

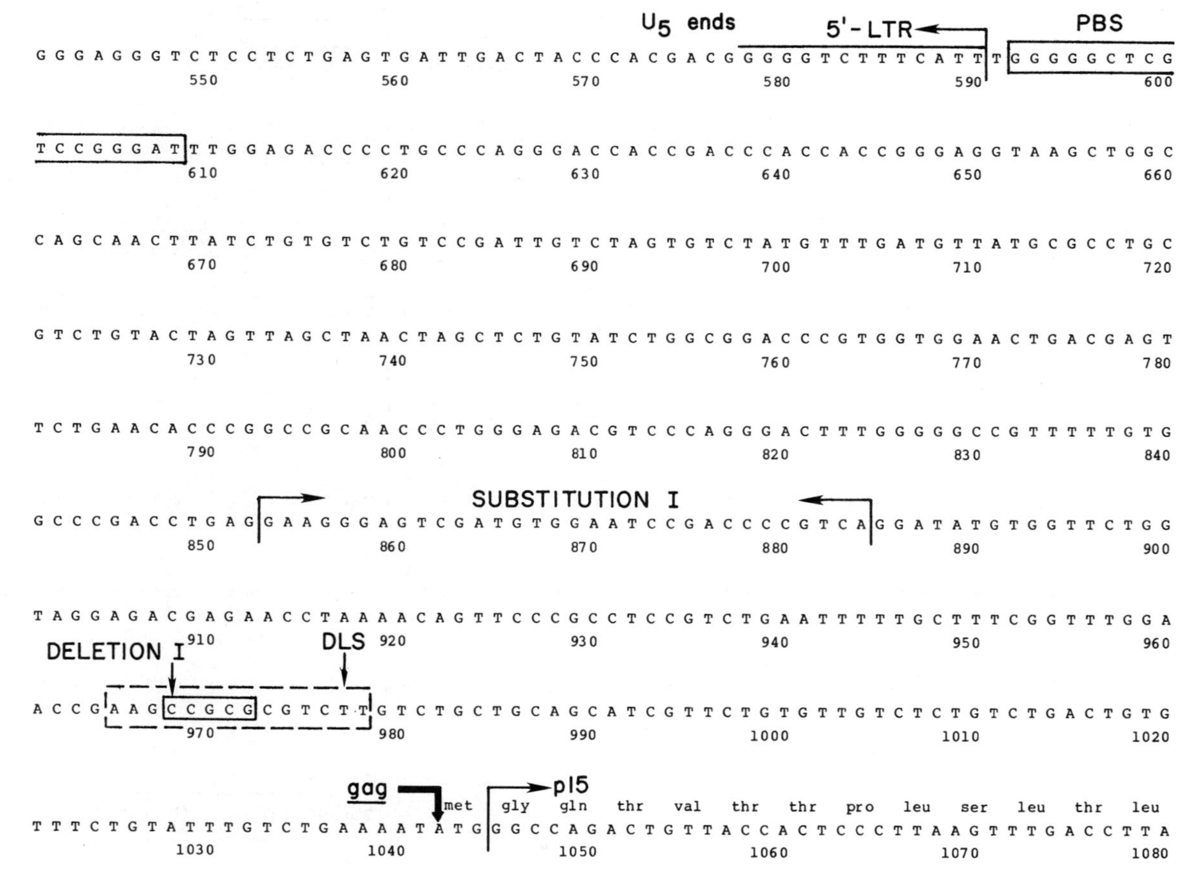
U5 ends
5'-LTR
PBS
GGAGGGTCTCCTCTGAGTGATTGACTACCCACGACGGGGGTCTTTCATTTGGGGGCTCG
550 560 570 580 590 600
TCCGGGATTTGGAGACCCCTGCCCAGGGACCACCGACCCACCACCGGGAGGTAAGCTGGC
610 620 630 640 650 660
CAGCAACTTATCTGTGTCTGTCCGATTGTCTAGTGTCTATGTTTGATGTTATGCGCCTGC
670 680 690 700 710 720
GTCTGTACTAGTTAGCTAACTAGCTCTGTATCTGGCGGACCCGTGGTGGAACTGACGAGT
730 740 750 760 770 780
TCTGAACACCCGGCCGCAACCCTGGGAGACGTCCCAGGGACTTTGGGGGCCGTTTTTGTG
790 800 810 820 830 840
SUBSTITUTION I
GCCCGACCTGAGGAAGGGAGTCGATGTGGAATCCGACCCCGTCAGGATATGTGGTTCTGG
850 860 870 880 890 900
TAGGAGACGAGAACCTAAAACAGTTCCCGCCTCCGTCTGAATTTTTGCTTTCGGTTTGGA
910 920 930 940 950 960
DELETION I
DLS
ACCGAAGCCGCGCGTCTTGTCTGCTGCAGCATCGTTCTGTGTTGTCTCTGTCTGACTGTG
970 980 990 1000 1010 1020
gag
p15
met gly gln thr val thr thr pro leu ser leu thr leu
TTTCTGTATTTGTCTGAAAATATGGGCCAGACTGTTACCACTCCCTTAAGTTTGACCTTA
1030 1040 1050 1060 1070 1080

```
asp   his   trp   lys   asp   val   glu   arg   leu   ala   his   asn   gln   ser   val   asp   val   lys   lys   arg
G A T C A C T G G A A A G A T G T C G A G C G G C T C G C T C A C A A C C A G T C G G T A G A T G T C A A G A A G A G A
                1090                1100                1110                1120                1130                1140

arg   trp   val   thr   phe   cys   ser   ala   glu   trp   pro   thr   phe   asn   val   gly   trp   pro   arg   asp
C G T T G G G T T A C C T T C T G C T C T G C A G A A T G G C C A A C C T T T A A C G T C G G A T G G C C G C G A G A C
                1150                1160                1170                1180                1190                1200

gly   thr   phe   asn   arg   asp   leu   ile   thr   gln   val   lys   ile   lys   val   phe   ser   pro   gly   pro
G G C A C C T T T A A C C G A G A C C T C A T C A C C C A G G T T A A G A T C A A G G T C T T T T C A C C T G G C C C G
                1210                1220                1230                1240                1250                1260

his   gly   his   pro   asp   gln   val   pro   tyr   ile   val   thr   trp   glu   ala   leu   ala   phe   asp   pro
C A T G G A C A C C C A G A C C A G G T C C C C T A C A T C G T G A C C T G G G A A G C C T T G G C T T T T G A C C C C
                1270                1280                1290                1300                1310                1320

pro   pro   trp   val   lys   pro   phe   val   his   pro   lys   pro   pro   pro   pro   leu   leu   pro   ser   ala
C C T C C C T G G G T C A A G C C C T T T G T A C A C C C T A A G C C T C C G C C T C C T C T T C T T C C A T C C G C G
                1330                1340                1350                1360                1370                1380

                                                                                                  p15 <--+--> p12
pro   ser   leu   pro   leu   glu   pro   pro   leu   ser   thr   pro   pro   gln   ser   ser   leu   tyr | pro   ala
C C G T C T C T C C C C C T T G A A C C T C C T C T T T C G A C C C C G C C T C A A T C C T C C C T T T A T|C C A G C C
                1390                1400                1410                1420                1430                1440

leu   thr   pro   ser   leu   gly   ala   lys   pro   lys   pro   gln   val   leu   ser   asp   ser   gly   gly   pro
C T C A C T C C T T C T T T G G G C G C C A A A C C T A A A C C T C A A G T T C T T T C T G A C A G T G G G G G C C C G
                1450                1460                1470                1480                1490                1500
```

```
leu ile asp leu leu thr glu asp pro pro pro tyr arg asp pro arg pro pro pro ser
C T C A T C G A C C T A C T T A C A G A A G A C C C C C C G C C T T A T A G G G A C C C A A G A C C A C C C C C T T C C
                1510                1520                1530                1540                1550                1560

asp arg asp gly asp ser gly glu ala thr pro ala gly glu ala pro asp pro ser pro
G A C A G G G A C G G A G A T A G T G G A G A A G C G A C C C C T G C G G G A G A G G C A C C G G A C C C C T C C C C A
                1570                1580                1590                1600                1610                1620

met ala ser arg leu arg gly arg arg glu pro pro val ala asp ser thr thr ser gln
A T G G C A T C T C G C C T G C G T G G G A G A C G G G A G C C C C C T G T G G C C G A C T C C A C T A C C T C G C A G
                1630                1640                1650                1660                1670                1680

p12 <----|----> p30
ala phe | pro leu arg thr gly gly asn gly gln leu gln tyr trp pro phe ser ser ser
G C A T T C | C C C C T C C G C A C A G G A G G A A A C G G A C A G C T T C A A T A C T G G C C G T T C T C C T C T T C T
                1690                1700                1710                1720                1730                1740

asp leu tyr asn trp lys asn asn asn pro ser phe ser glu asp pro gly lys leu thr
G A C C T T T A C A A C T G G A A A A A T A A T A A C C C T T C T T T T T C T G A A G A T C C A G G T A A A C T G A C A
                1750                1760                1770                1780                1790                1800

ala leu ile glu ser val leu ile thr his gln pro thr trp asp asp cys gln gln leu
G C T C T G A T C G A G T C T G T C C T C A T C A C C C A T C A G C C C A C C T G G G A C G A C T G T C A G C A G C T G
                1810                1820                1830                1840                1850                1860

leu gly thr leu leu thr gly glu glu lys gln arg val leu leu glu ala arg lys ala
T T G G G G A C T C T G C T G A C C G G G G A A G A A A A A C A A C G G G T G C T C T T A G A G G C T A G A A A G G C G
                1870                1880                1890                1900                1910                1920
```

```
val   arg   gly   asp   asp   gly   arg   pro   thr   gln   leu   pro   asn   glu   val   asp   ala   ala   phe   pro
G T G C G G G G C G A T G A T G G G C G C C C C A C T C A A C T G C C C A A T G A A G T C G A T G C C G C T T T T C C C
                  1930                          1940                          1950                          1960                          1970                          1980

leu   glu   arg   pro   asp   trp   glu   tyr   thr   thr   gln   ala   gly   arg   asn   his   leu   val   his   tyr
C T C G A G C G C C C A G A C T G G G A G T A C A C C A C C C A G G C A G G T A G G A A C C A C C T A G T C C A C T A T
                  1990                          2000                          2010                          2020                          2030                          2040

arg   gln   leu   leu   ile   ala   gly   leu   gln   asn   ala   gly   arg   ser   pro   thr   asn   leu   ala   lys
C G C C A G T T G C T C A T A G C G G G T C T C C A A A A C G C G G G C A G A A G C C C C A C C A A T T T G G C C A A G
                  2050                          2060                          2070                          2080                          2090                          2100

val   lys   gly   ile   thr   gln   gly   pro   asn   glu   ser   pro   ser   ala   phe   leu   glu   arg   leu   lys
G T A A A A G G A A T A A C A C A A G G G C C C A A T G A G T C T C C C T C G G C C T T C C T A G A G A G A C T T A A G
                  2110                          2120                          2130                          2140                          2150                          2160

glu   ala   tyr   arg   arg   tyr   thr   pro   tyr   asp   pro   glu   asp   pro   gly   gln   glu   thr   asn   val
G A A G C C T A T C G C A G G T A C A C T C C T T A T G A C C C T G A G G A C C C A G G G C A A G A A A C T A A T G T G
                  2170                          2180                          2190                          2200                          2210                          2220

ser   met   ser   phe   ile   trp   gln   ser   ala   pro   asp   ile   gly   arg   lys   leu   glu   arg   leu   glu
T C T A T G T C T T T C A T T T G G C A G T C T G C C C C A G A C A T T G G G A G A A A G T T A G A G A G G T T A G A A
                  2230                          2240                          2250                          2260                          2270                          2280

asp   leu   arg   asn   lys   thr   leu   gly   asp   leu   val   arg   glu   ala   glu   arg   ile   phe   asn   lys
G A T T T G A G A A A C A A G A C G C T T G G A G A T T T G G T T A G A G A G G C A G A A A G G A T C T T T A A T A A A
                  2290                          2300                          2310                          2320                          2330                          2340
```

```
arg   glu   thr   pro   glu   glu   arg   glu   glu   arg   ile   arg   arg   glu   arg   glu   glu   lys   glu   glu
C G A G A A A C C C C G G A A G A A A G A G A G G A A C G T A T C A G G A G A G A A A G A G A G G A A A A G G A A G A A
               2350                2360                2370                2380                2390                2400

arg   arg   arg   thr   glu   asp   glu   gln   lys   glu   lys   glu   arg   asp   arg   arg   arg   his   arg   glu
C G C C G T A G G A C A G A G G A T G A G C A G A A A G A G A A A G A A A G A G A T C G T A G G A G A C A T A G A G A G
               2410                2420                2430                2440                2450                2460

                p30 <------|------> p10
met   ser   arg   leu   leu | ala   thr   val   val   ser   gly   gln   arg   gln   asp   arg   gln   glu   gly   glu
A T G A G C A G G C T A T T G|G C C A C T G T C G T T A G T G G A C A G A G A C A G G A T A G A C A G G A A G G A G A A
               2470                2480                2490                2500                2510                2520

arg   arg   arg   ser   gln   leu   asp   cys   asp   gln   cys   thr   tyr   cys   glu   glu   gln   gly   his   trp
C G A A G G A G G T C C C A A C T C G A C T G C G A C C A G T G T A C C T A C T G C G A A G A A C A A G G G C A C T G G
               2530                2540                2550                2560                2570                2580

ala   lys   asp   cys   pro   lys   arg   pro   arg   gly   pro   arg   gly   pro   arg   pro   gln   thr   ser   leu
G C T A A A G A T T G T C C C A A G A G A C C A C G A G G A C C T C G G G G A C C A A G A C C C C A G A C C T C C C T C
               2590                2600                2610                2620                2630                2640

p10 <--|
leu   | thr   leu   asp   asp   ***
C T G|A C C C T A G A T G A C T A G G G A G G T C A G G G T C A G G A G C C C C C C C T G A A C C C A G G A T A A C C
               2650                2660                2670                2680                2690                2700

                                                                                         DELETION II
C T C A A A G T C G G G G G G C A A C C C G T C A C C T T C C T G G T A G A T A C[T G G G G C C C A]G A C C A A C A A A
               2710                2720                2730                2740                2750                2760

A G G C C T A T C A A G A A A T C A A G C A A G T T C T T C T A A C T G C C C C A G C C C T G G G G T T G C C A G A T T
               2770                2780                2790                2800                2810                2820
```

```
T G A C T A A G C C C T T T G A A C T C T T T G T C G A C G A G A A G C A G G G C T A C G C C A A A G G T G T C C T A A
                  2830                2840                2850                2860                2870                2880

C G C A A A A A C T G G G A C C T T G G C G T C G G C C G G T G G C C T A C C T G T C C A A A C A G C T A G A C C C A G
                  2890                2900                2910                2920                2930                2940

                                                    "Protein X"
                                                           met   val   ala   ala   ile   ala   val   leu   thr   lys   asp
T A G C A G C T G G G T G A C C C C C T T G C C T A C G G A T G G T A G C A G C C A T T G C C G T A C T G A C A A A G G
                  2950                2960                2970                2980                2990                3000

   ala   gly   lys   leu   thr   met   gly   gln   pro   leu   val   ile   leu   ala   pro   his   ala   val   glu   ala
A T G C A G G C A A G C T A A C C A T G G G A C A G C C A C T A G T C A T T C T G G C C C C C C A T G C A G T A G A G G
                  3010                3020                3030                3040                3050                3060

   leu   val   lys   gln   pro   pro   asp   arg   trp   leu   ser   asn   ala   arg   met   thr   his   tyr   gln   ala
C A C T A G T C A A A C A A C C C C C C G A C C G C T G G C T T T C C A A C G C C C G G A T G A C T C A C T A T C A G G
                  3070                3080                3090                3100                3110                3120

   leu   leu   leu   asp   thr   asp   arg   val   gln   phe   arg   pro   val   val   ala   leu   asn   pro   ala   thr
C C T T G C T T T T G G A C A C G G A C C G G G T C C A G T T C A G A C C G G T G G T A G C C C T G A A C C C G G C T A
                  3130                3140                3150                3160                3170                3180

   leu   leu   pro   leu   pro   glu   lys   gly   leu   gln   his   asn   cys   leu   asp   ile   leu   ala   glu   ala
C G C T G C T C C C A C T G C C T G A G A A A G G G C T G C A A C A C A A C T G C C T T G A T A T C C T G G C C G A A G
                  3190                3200                3210                3220                3230                3240

   his   gly   thr   arg   pro   asp   leu   thr   asp   gln   pro   leu   pro   asp   ala   asp   his   thr   trp   tyr
C T C A T G G A A C C C G A C C C G A C C T A A C G G A C C A G C C G C T C C C A G A C G C C G A C C A C A C C T G G T
                  3250                3260                3270                3280                3290                3300
```

```
      thr   asp   gly   ser   ser   leu   leu   gln   glu   gly   gln   arg   lys   ala   gly   ala   ala   val   thr   thr
A C A C G G A T G G A A G C A G T C T T T T A C A A G A G G G A C A G C G T A A G G C G G G A G C T G C G G T G A C C A
                3310                3320                3330                3340                3350                3360

           DELETION III                                                                                  DELETION IV
                                                                                                              |
      glu   thr   glu   lys   pro   ser   gln   pro   arg   lys   lys   thr   ala   lys   val   val   asn   leu   pro   gln
C C G A G A C C G[A G]A A G C C T T C C C A A C C A A G A A A A A A A A C C G C C A A G G T C G T A A▼A T C T T C C C C
                3370                3380                3390                3400                3410                3420

      val   arg   his   ala   ser   gly   ile   gly   asn   ***
A G G T T C G G C A T G C T T C A G G T A T T G G A A C T G A C A A T G G G C C T G C C T T C G T C T C C A A G G T G
                3430                3440                3450                3460                3470                3480

A G T C A G A C A G T G G C C G A T C T G T T G G G G A T T G A T T G G A A A T T A C A T T G T G C A T A C A G A C C C
                3490                3500                3510                3520                3530                3540

C A A A G C T C A G G C C A G G T A G A A A G A A T A A A T A G A A C C A T C A A G G A G A C T T T A A C T A A A T T A
                3550                3560                3570                3580                3590                3600

A C G C T T G C A A C T G G C T C T A G G G A C T G G G T G C T C C T A C T C C C C T T A G C C C T G T A T C G A G C C
                3610                3620                3630                3640                3650                3660

C G C A A C A C G C C G G G C C C C C A T G G C C T C A C C C C A T A T G A G A T C T T A T G T G G G C A C C C C C G
                3670                3680                3690                3700                3710                3720

C C C C T T G T A A A C T T C C C T G A C C C T G A C A T G A C A A G A G T T A C T A A C A G C C C C T C T C T C C A A
                3730                3740                3750                3760                3770                3780
```

```
G C T C A C A T A C A G G C T C T C T A C T T A G T C C A G C A C G A A G T C T G G A G A C C T C T G G C G G C A G C C
                  3790                3800                3810                3820                3830                3840

                  DELETION V                         v-mos^Mo                    → SUBSTITUTION II
                                                      met   ala   his   ser   thr | pro   cys   ser   gln
T A C C A A G A A C A A C[T G G A C C]A T C C T C T A G A C T G A C A T G G C G C A T T C A A C|G C C A T G C T C C C A
                  3850                3860                3870                3880                3890                3900

 thr   ser   leu   ala   val   pro   asn   his   phe   ser   leu   val   ser   his   val   thr   val   pro   ser   glu
A A C T T C C C T G G C T G T T C C T A A T C A T T T C T C C C T A G T G T C T C A T G T G A C T G T C C C A T C T G A
                  3910                3920                3930                3940                3950                3960

 gly   val   met   pro.  ser   pro   leu   ser   leu   cys   arg   tyr   leu   pro   arg   glu   leu   ser   pro   ser
G G G T G T A A T G C C T T C G C C T C T A A G C C T G T G T C G C T A C C T C C C T C G T G A G C T G T C G C C A T C
                  3970                3980                3990                4000                4010                4020

 val   asp   ser   arg   ser   cys   ser   ile   pro   leu   val   ala   pro   arg   lys   ala   gly   lys   leu   phe
G G T A G A C T C G C G G T C C T G C A G C A T T C C T T T G G T G G C C C C G A G G A A G G C A G G G A A G C T C T T
                  4030                4040                4050                4060                4070                4080

 leu   gly   thr   thr   pro   pro   arg   ala   pro   gly   leu   pro   arg   arg   leu   ala   trp   phe   ser   ile
C C T G G G G A C C A C T C C T C C T C G G G C T C C C G G A C T G C C A C G C C G G C T G G C C T G G T T C T C C A T
                  4090                4100                4110                4120                4130                4140

 asp   trp   glu   gln   val   cys   leu   met   his   arg   leu   gly   ser   gly   gly   phe   gly   ser   val   tyr
A G A C T G G G A A C A G G T A T G T C T G A T G C A T A G G C T G G G C T C T G G A G G G T T T G G C T C G G T G T A
                  4150                4160                4170                4180                4190                4200

 lys   ala   thr   tyr   his   gly   val   pro   val   ala   ile   lys   gln   val   asn   lys   cys   thr   glu   asp
C A A A G C C A C T T A C C A C G G T G T T C C T G T G G C C A T C A A G C A A G T A A A C A A G T G C A C C G A G G A
                  4210                4220                4230                4240                4250                4260
```

```
leu   arg   ala   ser   gln   arg   ser   phe   trp   ala   glu   leu   asn   ile   ala   gly   leu   arg   his   asp
C C T A C G T G C A T C C C A G C G G A G T T T C T G G G C T G A A C T G A A C A T T G C A G G A C T A C G C C A C G A
                  4270                4280                4290                4300                4310                4320

asn   ile   val   arg   val   val   ala   ala   ser   thr   arg   thr   pro   glu   asp   ser   asn   ser   leu   gly
C A A C A T A G T T C G G G T T G T G G C T G C C A G C A C G C G C A C G C C C G A A G A C T C C A A C A G C C T A G G
                  4330                4340                4350                4360                4370                4380

thr   ile   ile   met   glu   phe   gly   gly   asn   val   thr   leu   his   gln   val   ile   tyr   asp   ala   thr
T A C C A T A A T C A T G G A G T T T G G G G G C A A C G T G A C T C T A C A C C A A G T C A T C T A C G A T G C C A C
                  4390                4400                4410                4420                4430                4440

arg   ser   pro   glu   pro   leu   ser   cys   arg   lys   gln   leu   ser   leu   gly   lys   cys   leu   lys   tyr
C C G C T C A C C G G A G C C T C T C A G C T G C A G A A A A C A A C T A A G T T T G G G G A A G T G C C T C A A G T A
                  4450                4460                4470                4480                4490                4500

ser   leu   asp   val   val   asn   gly   leu   leu   phe   leu   his   ser   gln   ser   ile   leu   his   leu   asp
T T C C C T A G A T G T T G T T A A C G G C C T G C T T T T T C T C C A C T C A C A A A G C A T T T T G C A C T T G G A
                  4510                4520                4530                4540                4550                4560

leu   lys   pro   ala   asn   ile   leu   ile   ser   glu   gln   asp   val   cys   lys   ile   ser   asp   phe   gly
C C T G A A G C C A G C G A A C A T T T T G A T T A G T G A G C A G G A C G T T T G T A A G A T C A G T G A C T T C G G
                  4570                4580                4590                4600                4610                4620

cys   ser   gln   lys   leu   gln   asp   leu   arg   gly   arg   gln   ala   ser   pro   pro   his   ile   gly   gly
C T G C T C C C A G A A G C T G C A G G A T C T G C G G G G C C G G C A G G C G T C C C C T C C C C A C A T A G G G G G
                  4630                4640                4650                4660                4670                4680
```

```
 thr tyr thr his gln ala pro glu ile leu lys gly glu ile ala thr pro lys ala asp
C A C G T A C A C G C A C C A A G C T C C G G A G A T C C T A A A A G G A G A G A T T G C C A C G C C C A A A G C T G A
4690 4700 4710 4720 4730 4740

 ile tyr ser phe gly ile thr leu trp gln met thr thr arg glu val pro tyr ser gly
C A T C T A C T C T T T T G G A A T C A C C C T G T G G C A G A T G A C T A C C A G A G A G G T G C C T T A C T C C G G
4750 4760 4770 4780 4790 4800

 glu pro gln tyr val gln tyr ala val val ala tyr asn leu arg pro ser leu ala gly
C G A A C C T C A G T A C G T G C A G T A T G C A G T G G T A G C C T A C A A T C T G C G T C C C T C A C T G G C A G G
4810 4820 4830 4840 4850 4860

 ala val phe thr ala ser leu thr gly lys ala leu gln asn ile ile gln ser cys trp
A G C G G T G T T C A C C G C C T C C C T G A C T G G A A A G G C A C T G C A G A A C A T C A T C C A G A G C T G C T G
4870 4880 4890 4900 4910 4920

 glu ala arg gly leu gln arg pro ser ala glu leu leu gln arg asp leu lys ala phe
G G A G G C C C G C G G C C T G C A G A G G C C G A G T G C A G A A C T G C T C C A A A G G A C C T C A A G G C T T T
4930 4940 4950 4960 4970 4980

 arg gly thr leu gly ***
C C G A G G G A C A C T A G G C T G A C T C C A T C G A G C C A G T G T A G A G A T A A G C T T T T G T T T C T G T T T
4990 5000 5010 5020 5030 5040
```

SUBSTITUTION II

```
A T T T T T T A T G G G A C C C C T T A T T G T A C T C C T A A T G A T T T T G C T C T T C G G A C C C T G C A T T C T
5050 5060 5070 5080 5090 5100

T A A T C G A T T A G T C C A A T T T G T T A A A G A C A G G A T A T C A G T G G T C C A G G C T C T A G C T T T G A C
5110 5120 5130 5140 5150 5160
```

```
                                                                    poly (A)
TCAACAATAT CACCAGCTGA AGCCTATAGA GTACGAGCCA TAGTTAA[AAT AAA]AGATTTT
      5170       5180       5190       5200       5210       5220

ORIGIN (+) STRAND         → 3'-LTR                  U3 begins
ATTTAGTCTC CAGAAAAAGG GGGG|AATGAA AGACCCCACC CGTAGGTGGC AAGCTAGCTT
      5230       5240       5250       5260       5270       5280

AAGTAACGCC ACTTTGCAAG GCATGGAAAA ATACATAACT GAGAATAGAA AAGTTCAGAT
      5290       5300       5310       5320       5330       5340

                               → d.r.
CAAGGTCAGG AACAAAGAAA CAGCTGAATA|CCAAACAGGA TATCTGTGGT AAGCGGTTCC
      5350       5360       5370       5380       5390       5400

                        d.r. ←                        → d.r.
TGCCCCGGCT CAGGGCCAAG AACAGATG|AG ACAGCTGAGT GATGGG|CCAA ACAGGATATC
      5410       5420       5430       5440       5450       5460

                                             d.r. ←
TGTGGTAAGC AGTTCCTGCC CCGGCTCGGG GCCAAGAACA GATG|GTCCCC AGATGCGGTC
      5470       5480       5490       5500       5510       5520

CAGCCCTCAG CAGTTTCTAG TGAATCATCA GATGTTTCCA GGGTGCCCCA AGGACCTGAA
      5530       5540       5550       5560       5570       5580

                              "CAT-box"
AATGACCCTG TACCTTATTT GAACTAA[CCA AT]CAGTTCGC TTCTCGCTTC TGTTCGCGCG
      5590       5600       5610       5620       5630       5640

                 "TATA-box"         U3 ends             CAP   R begins
                                                          ↓
CTTCCGCTCT CCGAGCT[CAA TAAA]AGAGCC CACAACCCCT CACTCGGCGC GCCAGTCTTC
      5650       5660       5670       5680       5690       5700
```

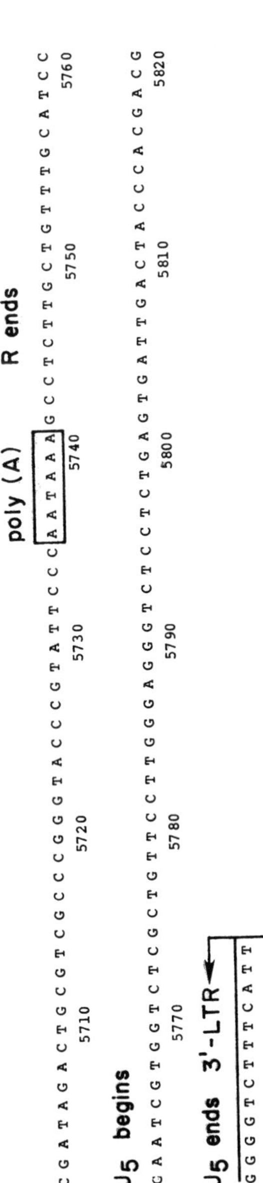
poly (A)
R ends
C G A T A G A C T G C G T C G C C C G G G T A C C C G T A T T C C C A A T A A A G C C T C T T G C T G T T T G C A T C C
5710 5720 5730 5740 5750 5760
U5 begins
C A A T C G T G G T C T C G C T G T T C C T T G G G A G G G T C T C C T C T G A G T G A T T G A C T A C C C A C G A C G
5770 5780 5790 5800 5810 5820
U5 ends 3'-LTR
G G G G T C T T T C A T T
5830

4. Nucleotide Sequence of *c-mos*

Nucleotide number 1 is 174 nucleotides upstream from the region of homology with *v-mos* in the genome of Mo-MSV-124. The region of overlap with *v-mos* is marked by arrows. Underlinings indicate the in-frame stop codons upstream and downsteam from the first available initiator codon (which is boxed).

A potential polyadenylation signal (residues 1389–1394) is shown by a bracket. These data were derived from a cloned *Eco*RI fragment containing the mouse *c-mos* gene by Van Beveren et al. (*Nature* **289,** 258, 1981). An additional 85 nucleotides included in this figure were provided by C. Van Beveren (pers. comm.). See Chapter 9 for discussion of the expression and oncogenic potential of *c-mos.*

```
A G C T G T G A G C A A T C G T T T C A T C T G A G A C T G C C A G G C T T C A T C T G C A C C C C C A A C C C C A C C
                 10                  20                  30                  40                  50                  60

                                                                                                met  trp  leu  val
T G A C T T A T T T T T T A A A A A A G A A A C A C C T T G T G G A G T A G T G A T A G C A C A G [A T G] T G G C T G G T
                 70                  80                  90                  100                 110                 120

 leu  arg  ile  lys  glu  glu  gly  lys  gly  thr  gly  ile  glu  gly  ser  asn  leu  gln  pro  cys
T T T G A G A A T C A A G G A A G A A G G A A A G G A A C T G G G A T T G A A G G C A G C A A T C T T C A G C C A T G
                 130                 140                 150                 160                 170                 180

 ser  gln  thr  ser  leu  ala  val  pro  thr  his  phe  ser  leu  val  ser  his  val  thr  val  pro
C T C C C A A A C T T C C C T G G C T G T T C C T A C T C A T T T C T C C C T A G T G T C T C A T G T G A C T G T C C C
                 190                 200                 210                 220                 230                 240

 ser  glu  gly  val  met  pro  ser  pro  leu  ser  leu  cys  arg  tyr  leu  pro  arg  glu  leu  ser
A T C T G A G G G T G T A A T G C C T T C G C C T C T A A G C C T G T G T C G C T A C C T C C C T C G T G A G C T G T C
                 250                 260                 270                 280                 290                 300

 pro  ser  val  asp  ser  arg  ser  cys  ser  ile  pro  leu  val  ala  pro  arg  lys  ala  gly  lys
G C C A T C G G T G G A C T C G C G G T C C T G C A G C A T T C C T T T G G T G G C C C C G A G G A A G G C A G G A A
                 310                 320                 330                 340                 350                 360

 leu  phe  leu  gly  thr  thr  pro  pro  arg  ala  pro  gly  leu  pro  arg  arg  leu  ala  trp  phe
G C T C T T C C T G G G G A C C A C T C C T C C T C G G G C T C C C G G A C T G C C A C G C C G G C T G G C C T G G T T
                 370                 380                 390                 400                 410                 420

 ser  ile  asp  trp  glu  gln  val  cys  leu  met  his  arg  leu  gly  ser  gly  gly  phe  gly  ser
C T C C A T A G A C T G G G A A C A G G T A T G T C T G A T G C A T A G G C T G G G C T C T G G A G G G T T T G G C T C
                 430                 440                 450                 460                 470                 480

 val  tyr  lys  ala  thr  tyr  his  gly  val  pro  val  ala  ile  lys  gln  val  asn  lys  cys  thr
G G T G T A T A A A G C C A C T T A C C A C G G T G T T C C T G T G G C C A T C A A G C A A G T A A A C A A G T G C A C
                 490                 500                 510                 520                 530                 540

 lys  asp  leu  arg  ala  ser  gln  arg  ser  phe  trp  ala  glu  leu  asn  ile  ala  arg  leu  arg
C A A G G A C C T A C G T G C A T C C C A G C G G A G T T T C T G G G C T G A A C T G A A C A T T G C A A G A C T A C G
                 550                 560                 570                 580                 590                 600

 his  asp  asn  ile  val  arg  val  val  ala  ala  ser  thr  arg  thr  pro  glu  asp  ser  asn  ser
C C A C G A C A A C A T A G T T C G G G T T G T G G C T G C C A G C A C G C G C A C G C C C G A A G A C T C C A A C A G
                 610                 620                 630                 640                 650                 660
```

```
   leu   gly   thr   ile   ile   met   glu   phe   gly   gly   asn   val   thr   leu   his   gln   val   ile   tyr   gly
C C T A G G T A C C A T A A T C A T G G A G T T T G G G G G C A A C G T G A C T C T A C A C C A A G T C A T C T A C G G
                 670                 680                 690                 700                 710                 720

   ala   thr   arg   ser   pro   glu   pro   leu   ser   cys   arg   glu   gln   leu   ser   leu   gly   lys   cys   leu
T G C C A C C C G C T C A C C G G A G C C T C T C A G C T G C A G A G A A C A A C T G A G T T T G G G G A A G T G C C T
                 730                 740                 750                 760                 770                 780

   lys   tyr   ser   leu   asp   val   val   asn   gly   leu   leu   phe   leu   his   ser   gln   ser   ile   leu   his
C A A G T A T T C C C T A G A T G T T G T T A A C G G C C T G C T T T T T C T C C A C T C A C A A A G C A T T T T G C A
                 790                 800                 810                 820                 830                 840

   leu   asp   leu   lys   pro   ala   asn   ile   leu   ile   ser   glu   gln   asp   val   cys   lys   ile   ser   asp
C T T G G A C C T G A A G C C A G C G A A C A T T T T G A T C A G T G A G C A A G A C G T T T G T A A G A T C A G T G A
                 850                 860                 870                 880                 890                 900

   phe   gly   cys   ser   gln   lys   leu   gln   asp   leu   arg   cys   arg   gln   ala   ser   pro   his   his   ile
C T T C G G C T G C T C C C A G A A G C T G C A G G A T C T G C G G T G C C G G C A G G C G T C C C C T C A C C A C A T
                 910                 920                 930                 940                 950                 960

   gly   gly   thr   tyr   thr   his   gln   ala   pro   glu   ile   leu   lys   gly   glu   ile   ala   thr   pro   lys
A G G G G G C A C G T A C A C G C A C C A A G C T C C G G A G A T C C T G A A A G G A G A G A T T G C C A C G C C C A A
                 970                 980                 990                1000                1010                1020

   ala   asp   ile   tyr   ser   phe   gly   ile   thr   leu   trp   gln   met   thr   thr   arg   glu   val   pro   tyr
A G C T G A C A T C T A C T C T T T T G G A A T C A C C C T G T G G C A G A T G A C C A C C A G G G A G G T G C C T T A
                1030                1040                1050                1060                1070                1080

   ser   gly   glu   pro   gln   tyr   val   gln   tyr   ala   val   val   ala   tyr   asn   leu   arg   pro   ser   leu
C T C C G G C G A A C C T C A G T A C G T G C A G T A T G C A G T G G T T G C C T A C A A T C T G C G C C C C T C A C T
                1090                1100                1110                1120                1130                1140

   ala   gly   ala   val   phe   thr   ala   ser   leu   thr   gly   lys   ala   leu   gln   asn   ile   ile   gln   ser
G G C A G G A G C G G T G T T C A C C G C C T C C C T G A C T G G A A A G G C A C T G C A G A A C A T C A T C C A G A G
                1150                1160                1170                1180                1190                1200

   cys   trp   glu   ala   arg   ala   leu   gln   arg   pro   gly   ala   glu   leu   leu   gln   arg   asp   leu   lys
C T G C T G G G A G G C C C G C G C C C T G C A G A G G C C G G G T G C A G A A C T G C T C C A A A G G G A C C T C A A
                1210                1220                1230                1240                1250                1260

   ala   phe   arg   gly   ala   leu   gly   ***
G G C T T T C C G A G G G G C A C T A G G C T G A C T C C A T C G A G C C G A T G T A G A G A T A A G C T T T T T G T C
                1270                1280                1290                1300                1310                1320
```

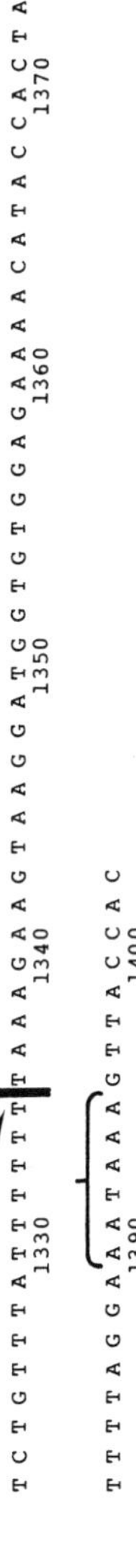
T C T G T T T T A T T T T T T T A A A G A A G T A A G G A T G G T G T G G A G A A A A C A T A C C A C T A G G C A T A T
1330
1340
1350
1360
1370
1380
T T T T A G G A A A T A A A G T T A C C A C
1390
1400

APPENDIX F

Amino Acid Sequences of Retroviral Structural Proteins

All the amino acid sequences presented in this section were derived directly (rather than inferred from nucleic acid sequence; see Appendix E). Protein sequence, when available, is a valuable guide for nucleic acid sequencing; conversely nucleic acid sequence can aid protein sequence determination. The protein and nucleic sequences presented here and in Appendix E are in complete agreement.

1. The Complete Amino Acid Sequence of Ra-MLV and Mo-MLV Pr65^{gag}

The Mo-MLV Pr65^{gag} sequence differs from that of Ra-MLV at those positions where the altered amino acid is shown under the Ra-MLV Pr65^{gag} sequence. The complete structure of Ra-MLV Pr65^{gag} was determined by sequencing the internal structural proteins p15, p12, p30, and p10, and analyzing a variant of p10 having a four-amino-acid extension at its carboxy terminus. The structural proteins of Mo-MLV have also been completely (p12) or partially (p15, p30, p10) sequenced. Arrows indicate the cleavage sites that have been defined from the amino- and carboxyterminal sequences of the structural proteins (Oroszlan et al., *Proc. Natl. Acad. Sci.* **75,** 1404, 1978) and from the DNA sequence of Mo-MSV (Van Beveren et al., *Cell* **27,** 97, 1981), which is in full agreement with the amino acid sequence. In the p15 region and at a few points in the p30 sequence, the Mo-MSV DNA sequence was used to align the peptides. The DNA sequence for Mo-MLV (Shinnick et al., *Nature* **293,** 543, 1981) is also in full agreement with the protein sequence data. The Pr65^{gag} polyproteins of Ra-MLV and Mo-MLV show approximately 91% identity; the most variable region is p12. The amino acid sequence differences between the fully processed structural proteins are as follows: in p15, 14 out of 130, or 10.8%; in p12, 20 out of 84, or 23.8%; in p30, 12 out of 263, or 4.6%; and in p10, 3 out of 56, or 5.4%. The amino terminus of p15 is blocked.

The data shown here are from L.E. Henderson, T.D. Copeland, G.W. Smythers, R.C. Sowder, and S. Oroszlan, (unpubl.); Versteegen et al. (*J. Biol. Chem.,* 1982 [in press]); and Henderson et al. (*J. Biol. Chem.* **256,** 8400, 1981).

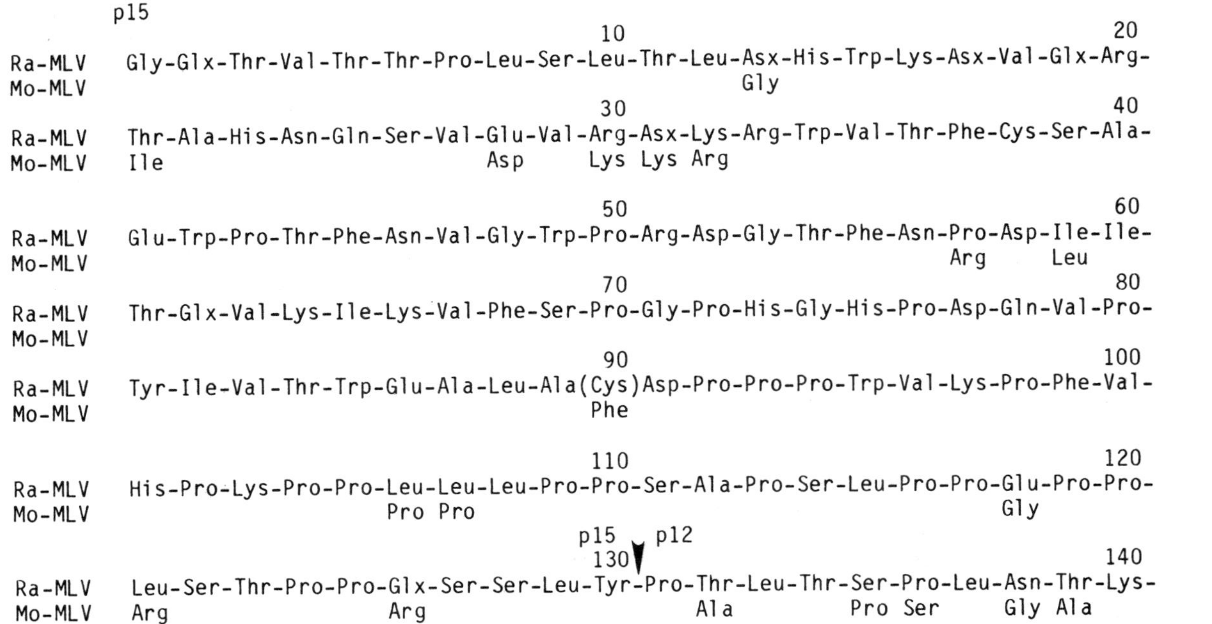
p15
10 20
Ra-MLV Gly-Glx-Thr-Val-Thr-Thr-Pro-Leu-Ser-Leu-Thr-Leu-Asx-His-Trp-Lys-Asx-Val-Glx-Arg-
Mo-MLV Gly
30 40
Ra-MLV Thr-Ala-His-Asn-Gln-Ser-Val-Glu-Val-Arg-Asx-Lys-Arg-Trp-Val-Thr-Phe-Cys-Ser-Ala-
Mo-MLV Ile Asp Lys Lys Arg
50 60
Ra-MLV Glu-Trp-Pro-Thr-Phe-Asn-Val-Gly-Trp-Pro-Arg-Asp-Gly-Thr-Phe-Asn-Pro-Asp-Ile-Ile-
Mo-MLV Arg Leu
70 80
Ra-MLV Thr-Glx-Val-Lys-Ile-Lys-Val-Phe-Ser-Pro-Gly-Pro-His-Gly-His-Pro-Asp-Gln-Val-Pro-
Mo-MLV
90 100
Ra-MLV Tyr-Ile-Val-Thr-Trp-Glu-Ala-Leu-Ala(Cys)Asp-Pro-Pro-Pro-Trp-Val-Lys-Pro-Phe-Val-
Mo-MLV Phe
110 120
Ra-MLV His-Pro-Lys-Pro-Pro-Leu-Leu-Leu-Pro-Pro-Ser-Ala-Pro-Ser-Leu-Pro-Pro-Glu-Pro-Pro-
Mo-MLV Pro Pro Gly
p15 p12
130 140
Ra-MLV Leu-Ser-Thr-Pro-Pro-Glx-Ser-Ser-Leu-Tyr-Pro-Thr-Leu-Thr-Ser-Pro-Leu-Asn-Thr-Lys-
Mo-MLV Arg Arg Ala Pro Ser Gly Ala

```
                                                150                                     160
Ra-MLV      Pro-Arg-Pro-Gln-Val-Leu-Pro-Asp-Ser-Gly-Gly-Pro-Leu-Val-Asp-Leu-Leu-Thr-Glu-Asp-
Mo-MLV          Lys                 Ser                         Ile

                                                170                                     180
Ra-MLV      Pro-Pro-Pro-Tyr-Arg-Asp-Pro-Gly-Pro-Pro-Ser-Ser-Asp-Gly-Asn-Gly-Asn-Ser-Gly-Glu-
Mo-MLV                                  Arg         Pro         Arg Asp         Gly

                                                190                                     200
Ra-MLV      Val-Ala-Pro-Thr-Glu-Gly-Ala-Pro-Asp-Ser-Ser-Pro-Met-Val-Ser-Arg-Leu-Arg-Gly-Arg-
Mo-MLV      Ala Thr     Ala Gly Glu             Pro             Ala

                                                            p12  v  p30
                                                210                                     220
Ra-MLV      Arg-Glu-Pro-Pro-Val-Ala-Asp-Ser-Thr-Thr-Ser-Gln-Ala-Phe-Pro-Leu-Arg-Leu-Gly-Gly-
Mo-MLV                                                                      Ala
                                                230                                     240
Ra-MLV      Asn-Gly-Gln-Leu-Gln-Tyr-Trp-Pro-Phe-Ser-Ser-Ser-Asp-Leu-Tyr-Asn-Trp-Lys-Asn-Asn-
Mo-MLV
                                                250                                     260
Ra-MLV      Asn-Pro-Ser-Phe-Ser-Glu-Asp-Pro-Gly-Lys-Leu-Thr-Ala-Leu-Ile-Glu-Ser-Val-Leu-Leu-
Mo-MLV                                                                              Ile

                                                270                                     280
Ra-MLV      Thr-His-Gln-Pro-Thr-Trp-Asp-Asp-Cys-Gln-Gln-Leu-Leu-Gly-Thr-Leu-Leu-Thr-Gly-Glu-
Mo-MLV
```

```
                                            290                                    300
Ra-MLV   Glu-Lys-Gln-Arg-Val-Leu-Leu-Glu-Ala-Arg-Lys-Ala-Val-Arg-Gly-Glu-Asp-Gly-Arg-Pro-
Mo-MLV
                                            310                                    320
Ra-MLV   Thr-Gln-Leu-Pro-Asn-Asp-Ile-Asn-Asp-Ala-Phe-Pro-Leu-Glu-Arg-Pro-Asp-Trp-Asp-Tyr-
Mo-MLV                       Glu Val Asp Ala

                                            330                                    340
Ra-MLV   Asn-Thr-Gln-Arg-Gly-Arg-Asn-His-Leu-Val-His-Tyr-Arg-Gln-Leu-Leu Leu-Ala-Gly-Leu-
Mo-MLV   Thr         Ala
                                            350                                    360
Ra-MLV   Gln-Asn-Ala-Gly-Arg-Ser-Pro-Thr-Asn-Leu-Ala-Lys-Val-Lys-Gly-Ile-Thr-Gln-Gly-Pro-
Mo-MLV
                                            370                                    380
Ra-MLV   Asn-Glu-Ser-Pro-Ser-Ala-Phe-Leu-Glu-Arg-Leu-Lys-Glu-Ala-Tyr-Arg-Arg-Tyr-Thr-Pro-
Mo-MLV
                                            390 CHO                                400
Ra-MLV   Tyr-Asp-Pro-Glu-Asp-Pro-Gly-Gln-Glu-Thr-Asn-Val-Ser-Met-Ser-Phe-Ile-Trp-Gln-Ser-
Mo-MLV
                                            410                                    420
Ra-MLV   Ala-Pro-Asp-Ile-Gly-Arg-Lys-Leu-Glu-Arg-Leu-Glu-Asp-Leu-Lys-Ser-Lys-Thr-Leu-Gly-
Mo-MLV                                                              Asn
                                            430                                    440
Ra-MLV   Asp-Leu-Val-Arg-Glu-Ala-Glu-Lys-Ile-Phe-Asn-Lys-Arg-Glu-Thr-Pro-Glu-Glu-Arg-Glu-
Mo-MLV
```

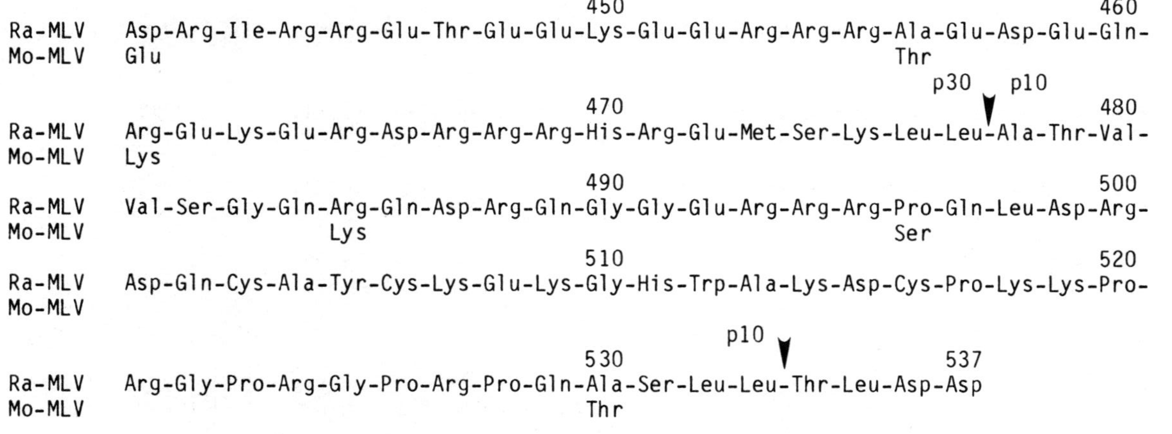

Figure F.1. Amino acid sequence of Ra-MLV and Mo-MLV $Pr65^{gag}$.

2. Classification of Mammalian C-type Retroviruses Based on the Alignment of the Aminoterminal Sequences of the Internal Structural Protein p30 (Oroszlan et al., *Virology* 115, 262, 1981)

In this classification scheme, the p30 sequences within a single subgroup are aligned without deletions or insertions. In the alignment of the subgroups, gaps have been introduced as indicated by hyphen (-). The number of amino acids deleted are as follows: seven in subgroup I, eight in subgroup II, none in subgroup III, and one in subgroup IV. Abbreviations: Ra, Rauscher; Mo, Moloney; MLV, mouse leukemia virus; FeLV, feline leukemia virus (Theilen strain); BaEV, baboon endogenous virus; RD-114, feline endogenous virus; GaLV, gibbon ape leukemia virus; SSAV, simian sarcoma-associated virus; MMC-1, endogenous type-C virus of *Macaca mulatta;* MAC-1, endogenous C-type virus of *Macaca arcotoides;* CPC-1, endogenous C-type virus of *Colobus polykomos.* In subgroup I, all mouse p30s have identical sequences except at position 4 where the p30s of AKR-MLV, Gross-MLV, and Ra-MLV contain Leu; Ra-MLV, NZB-MLV, and Mo-MLV contain Ala; and wild mouse LMV has Ser. FeLV p30 differs from Mo-MLV in the six positions indicated. The rat C-type virus also belongs to subgroup I (Oroszlan et al., *J. Biol. Chem.* **250,** 6232, 1975). In subgroup II, BaEV and RD-114 p30s differ from each other only in position 17 (Copeland et al., *Virology* **109,** 13, 1981). In subgroup III, GaLV and SSAV p30s are identical (Oroszlan et al., *Virology* **77,** 413, 1977). In subgroup IV, MMC-1 p30 differs from MAC-1 in position 15 and both differ from CPC-1 in positions 13–15 (Oroszlan et al., *J. Virol.* **115,** 262, 1981). The avian reticuloendotheliosis (REV-A) p30 more closely resembles mammalian p30s than the avian C-type virus protein homolog p27 (Hunter et al., *Proc. Natl. Acad. Sci.* **75,** 2708, 1978); the REV-A p30 is more closely related to the p30s of the *Macaca colobus* virus subgroup (63% homology) than to the other mammalian viruses (Oroszlan et al., *J. Virol.* **39,** 845, 1981). REV-A is therefore best classified as a C-type virus belonging to subgroup IV. The amino acids that are identical in P30s of REV-A and subgroup IV are underlined in the REV-A p30 sequence.

```
Subgroup I      1         5             10            15             20            25            30

    Ra-MLV              Leu
    Mo-MLV    ProLeuArgAlaGlyGly - - - - - AsnGly - - GlnLeuGlnTyrTrpProPheSerSerSerAspLeuTyrAsnTrpLys
    FeLV                Glu   Pro                Asn      ArgPro                      Ala

Subgroup II

    BaEV                                                  Ile
              ProLeuArgThrVal - - - - - - AsnArg - - Thr    GlnTyrTrpProPheSerAlaSerAspLeuTyrAsnTrpLys
    RD-114                                                  Val

Subgroup III

    GaLV
              ProLeuArgAlaIleGlyProProAlaGluProAsnGlyLeuValProLeuGlnTyrTrpProPheSer X AlaAspLeuTyr
    SSAV

Subgroup IV

    MMC-1                                              His
    MAC-1     ProLeuArgGluIleGlySerLeuAspAspThr - GlyLeuSerArgLeuMetTyrTrpProPheSerThrSerAspLeuTyrAsnTrpLys
    CPC-1                                         AlaProPro

Common        ProLeuArg                                             TyrTrpProPheSer     AspLeuTyrAsnTrpLys
______________

    REV-A     ProLeuArgGluThrGlyGluArgAspMetGly - GlyArgProMetArgThrTyrValProPheThrThrSerAspLeuTyrAsnTrpLys
```

Figure F.2. Alignment of aminoterminal sequences of p30.

3. Alignment of the Aminoterminal Sequences of Mammalian C-type Virus Glycoproteins

Common amino acids are enclosed in the box. Amino acids marked "X" were undefined; the asterisk (*) indicates a deletion. The amino terminus of the MMTV gp52^{env} (not shown) can be found in Arthur et al. (*J. Virol.* **41,** 414, 1982).

The data shown in the figure are from Oroszlan et al. (In *Biosynthesis, modifications, and processing of cellular and viral polyproteins* [eds. G. Koch and D. Richter], Academic Press, Inc., New York, 1980, pp. 219–232; Henderson et al., *Virology* **85,** 319, 1978; and Linder et al., *J. Virol.* **42,** 1982 [in press.]).

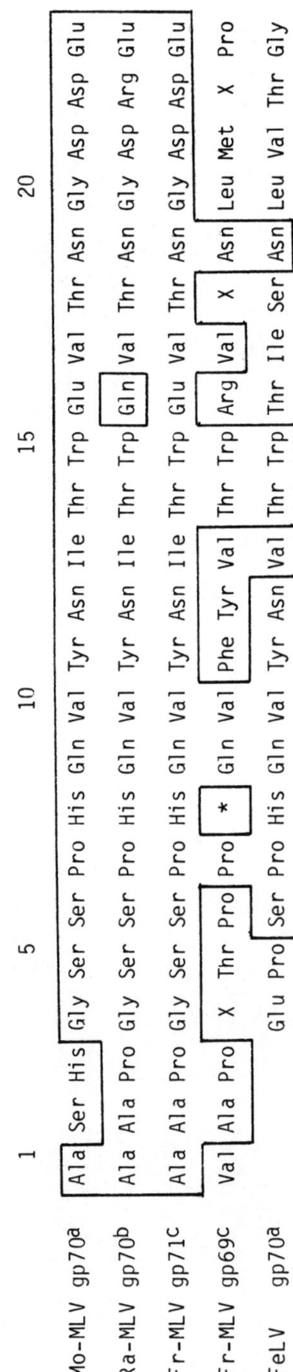

Figure F.3. Aminoterminal sequences of mammalian C-type viral glycoproteins.

Index